Neuro Quick Reference*

12 Pairs of Cranial Nerves/Functions

I	Olfactory	Sense of smell
II	Optic	Vision
III	Oculomotor	Eye movements, regulation of size of pupil, accommodation
IV	Trochlear	Eye movements
V	Trigeminal	Chewing movements
VI	Abducens	Abduction of eye
VII	Facial	Facial expression, secretion of saliva and tears
VIII	Vestibulocochlear	Vestibular branch: Balance/equilibrium Cochlear/auditory branch: Hearing
IX	Glossopharyngeal	Swallowing, secretion of saliva
X	Vagus	Slows heart, increases peristalsis, and contracts muscles for voice production
XI	Accessory	Shoulder movements, turning movements of head
XII	Hypoglossal	Tongue movements

31 Pairs of Spinal Nerves

Cervical:	1–8
Thoracic:	1–12
Lumbar:	1–5
Sacral:	1–5
Coccygeal:	1
Total:	**31**

Ascending Tracts of the Spinal Cord

Lateral spinothalamic
Ventral spinothalamic
Fasciculi gracilis and cuneatus
Spinocerebellar

Descending Tracts of the Spinal Cord

Lateral corticospinal (or crossed pyramidal)
Ventral corticospinal (direct pyramidal)
Lateral reticulospinal
Medial reticulospinal
Rubrospinal

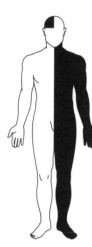

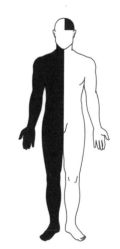

Right Brain Damage

(Stroke on right side of the brain)
- Paralyzed left side: Hemiplegia
- Left-sided neglect
- Spatial-perceptual deficits
- Tends to deny or minimize problems
- Rapid performance, short attention span
- Impulsive, safety problems
- Impaired judgment
- Impaired time concepts

Left Brain Damage

(Stroke on left side of the brain)
- Paralyzed right side: Hemiplegia
- Impaired speech/language/aphasias
- Impaired right/left discrimination
- Slow performance, cautious
- Aware of deficits: Depression, anxiety
- Impaired comprehension related to language, math

NEUROSCIENCE NURSING

A SPECTRUM OF CARE

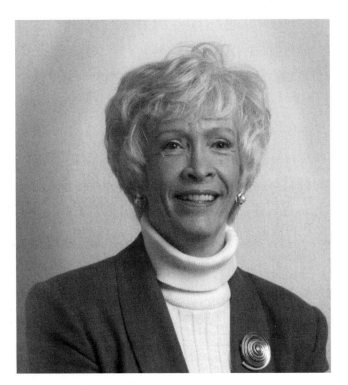

Ellen Barker, MSN, RN, is an Advanced Practice Nurse (APN) with prescriptive authority in private practice. She is the founder and president of Neuroscience Nursing Consultants in Greenville, Delaware. In addition to her practice, Ellen is a certified Life Care Planner (CLCP), a Legal Nurse Consultant (LNC), and a Certified Neuroscience Nurse (CNRN), and she is certified by the American Board of Disability Analysts (ABDA). The services she provides include providing office or home appointments for patients/families with neurologic disorders, teaching, conducting workshops, consulting for hospital and health care facilities, case management for neuroscience patients, legal nurse consulting, and life care planning. Ellen is recognized nationally as an expert in neuroscience nursing and neurorehabilitation and lectures across the United States, including Hawaii, bringing her enthusiasm and passion to promote the practice of neuroscience nursing.

Ellen graduated from the College of Nursing at the University of Delaware and completed her graduate studies at Widener University with a clinical specialty in Neuroscience Nursing and Neurorehabilitation, to include Burn, Emergency, and Trauma Management.

In addition to her professional activities, Ellen volunteers for many statewide health organizations. She is the founder of the Delaware Stroke Initiative (DSI). In addition, she serves on the professional board of the Delaware chapter of the Multiple Sclerosis Society and other state nonprofit organizations.

Ellen's publications include more than 70 articles and chapters that appear regularly in journals and textbooks. She is past editor of the *Journal of Neuroscience Nursing* and currently serves on the editorial board for the nursing journal *RN*. With her dynamic classroom presentations and extensive background, Ellen is frequently sought by hospitals and health care facilities as a speaker to promote advanced knowledge and excellence in neuroscience nursing and neurorehabilitation. She has been a long-term advocate for certification in neuroscience nursing and has presented her "Neuroscience Nursing Review Course" to hundreds of audiences all across the country.

Ellen is a member of numerous professional organizations, contributing her leadership and her inspiration to share her extensive knowledge and expertise. She has received numerous awards and recognitions for her leadership role as a nurse.

Third Edition

NEUROSCIENCE NURSING

A SPECTRUM OF CARE

Ellen Barker, MSN, APN, CNRN, CLCP, ABDA
President
Neuroscience Nursing Consultants
Greenville, Delaware

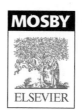

MOSBY

ELSEVIER

11830 Westline Industrial Drive
St. Louis, Missouri 63146

NEUROSCIENCE NURSING: A SPECTRUM OF CARE, THIRD EDITION   ISBN: 978-0-323-04401-1

Previous editions copyrighted 2002 and 1994.

Library of Congress Control Number: 2007924220

ISBN: 978-0-323-04401-1

Executive Publisher: Barbara Nelson Cullen
Senior Developmental Editor: Jennifer Ehlers
Publishing Services Manager: Jeff Patterson
Senior Project Manager: Clay S. Broeker
Design Direction: Margaret Reid
Cover Designer: Margaret Reid

Printed in the United States of America

Last digit is the print number: 9 8 7 6 5 4 3 2

The third edition of *Neuroscience Nursing: A Spectrum of Care* is dedicated to *You,* the reader. The enthusiastic response from thousands of readers year after year has been the inspiration, motivation, and spirit that have guided me to accept the awesome responsibility of writing, editing, and seeking the contributions of outstanding authors to complete this latest volume. I trust that you will locate important information throughout the 25 chapters, which translate the latest scientific principles and technological advances to your clinical practice to help improve the lives of those individuals with neurologic disorders entrusted to your expert care. Thank you!

Contributors

Ellen Barker, MSN, APN, CNRN, CLCP, ABDA
President
Neuroscience Nursing Consultants
Greenville, Delaware
Neuroanatomy and Physiology of the Nervous System; The Adult Neurologic Assessment; Neurodiagnostic Studies; Central Nervous System Metabolic Disorders: Syndrome of Inappropriate Antidiuretic Hormone and Diabetes Insipidus; Altered States of Consciousness and Sleep; Cranial Surgery; Intracranial Pressure and Monitoring; Neurorehabilitation; Cranial Nerve Deficits; Stroke Management; Management of Aneurysms, Subarachnoid Hemorrhage, and Arteriovenous Malformation; Management of the Neuroscience Patient With Pain; Management of Seizures and Epilepsy; Legal Issues and Life Care Planning for the Neuroscience Patient

Aliza Bitton Ben-Zacharia, NP
The Mount Sinai Medical Center
Department of Neurology
New York, New York
Inflammatory Demyelinating Diseases

Michele J. Bergman, RN
Craig Hospital
Englewood, Colorado
Neurotrauma: Spinal Injury

Cynthia Blank-Reid, MSN, RN, CEN
Temple University Hospital
Philadelphia, Pennsylvania
Neuroscience Critical Care Management; Neurotrauma: Traumatic Brain Injury

Eileen M. Bohan, BSN, RN
Department of Neurosurgery
Johns Hopkins University School of Medicine
Baltimore, Maryland
Brain Tumors

Henry Brem, MD
Director of Neurosurgery
The Johns Hopkins Hospital
Baltimore, Maryland
Brain Tumors

Janet S. Cellar, RN, MSN
Wesley Woods Health Center
Department of Neurology
Atlanta, Georgia
Management of Dementia and Motor Neuron Disease

Maura L. Del Bene, MS, RN, NP-P
Clinical Research Nurse
MDA/ALS Research Center
Columbia-Presbyterian Medical Center
Neurological Institute of New York
New York, New York
Inflammatory Demyelinating Diseases

Allyson Delaune, BSN
Department of Neurosurgery
Louisiana State University
Shreveport, Louisiana
Cranial Surgery; Management of Aneurysms, Subarachnoid Hemorrhage, and Arteriovenous Malformation

Gary L. Gallia, MD
Department of Neurosurgery
Johns Hopkins Medicine
Baltimore, Maryland
Brain Tumors

Alberto Iaia, MD
Neuroscience Institute of Delaware
Greenville, Delaware
Neurodiagnostic Studies

Kelly Johnson, MSN, RN, CFNP, CRRN, CNAA
Craig Hospital
Englewood, Colorado
Neurotrauma: Spinal Injury

Jean M. Jones, JD, RN
Janet, Jenner, & Suggs, LLC
Baltimore, Maryland
Legal Issues and Life Care Planning for the Neuroscience Patient

Lewis J. Kaplan, MD
Associate Professor and Director
Emergency General Surgery
Yale University School of Medicine
New Haven, Connecticut
Neuroscience Critical Care Management

Jaffar Khan, MD
The ALS Center at Emory University
Atlanta, Georgia
Management of Dementia and Motor Neuron Disease

Diana Abson Kraemer, MD
Harborview Medical Center
University of Washington
Seattle, Washington
Management of Seizures and Epilepsy

James J. Lah, MD, PhD
The ALS Center at Emory University
Atlanta, Georgia
Management of Dementia and Motor Neuron Disease

Marcia S. Lorimer, RN, MSN
School of Nursing
Duke University Medical Center
Durham, North Carolina
Neuromuscular Junction and Muscle Disease

Brian N. Maddux, MD, PhD
Movement Disorders Center
The Neurological Institute
University Hospitals Case Medical Center
Cleveland, Ohio
*Management of Parkinson's Disease and
    Movement Disorders*

Robin N. McClelland, RN, MSN
Temple University Hospital
Philadelphia, Pennsylvania
Neurotrauma: Traumatic Brain Injury

Anne G. Miers, MSN, RN, CNRN, APRN
St. Mary's Hospital–Mayo Clinic
Rochester, Minnesota
*Nontraumatic Disorders of the Spine;
    Peripheral Nerve Disorders*

Kelly Mowrey, RN, MS, ANP-C, CNRN
Craig Hospital
Englewood, Colorado
Neurotrauma: Spinal Injury

Anil Nanda, MD, FACS
Professor and Chairman
Department of Neurosurgery
Louisiana State University
Shreveport, Louisiana
*Cranial Surgery; Management of Aneurysms,
    Subarachnoid Hemorrhage, and Arteriovenous
    Malformation*

Margaret Pass, RN, MS, CIC
Infection Control Epidemiologist
Johns Hopkins Medical Institutions
Baltimore, Maryland
Central Nervous System Infections

Promod Pillai, MD
Department of Neurosurgery
Louisiana State University
Shreveport, Louisiana
*Management of Aneurysms, Subarachnoid Hemorrhage,
    and Arteriovenous Malformation*

Meraida Polak, RN, BSN
Research Nurse
The ALS Center at Emory University
Atlanta, Georgia
Management of Dementia and Motor Neuron Disease

David E. Riley, MD
Director
Movement Disorders Center
The Neurological Institute
University Hospitals Case Medical Center
Cleveland, Ohio
*Management of Parkinson's Disease and
    Movement Disorders*

Donald B. Sanders, MD
Professor
Department of Neurology
Duke University Medical Center
Durham, North Carolina
Neuromuscular Junction and Muscle Disease

Thomas A. Santora, MD
Temple University Hospital
Philadelphia, Pennsylvania
*Neuroscience Critical Care Management;
    Neurotrauma: Traumatic Brain Injury*

Bernadette Tucker-Lipscomb, RN, MSN
Duke University Medical Center and Health Center
Durham, North Carolina
Neuromuscular Junction and Muscle Disease

Christina M. Whitney, RN, DNSc
Movement Disorders Center
The Neurological Institute
University Hospitals Case Medical Center
Cleveland, Ohio
*Management of Parkinson's Disease and
    Movement Disorders*

Joyce S. Willens, PhD, RN
College of Nursing
Villanova University
Villanova, Pennsylvania
Management of the Neuroscience Patient With Pain

Consultants

Lee Dresser, MD
Neurologist
Wilmington Neurology Consultants
Newark, Delaware

Mary Johnson, MN, RN, CS, CNRN
Senior Care Specialist
University of Iowa
Iowa City, Iowa

Darcy Reisman, PhD, PT
Assistant Research Professor
Department of Physical Therapy
University of Delaware
Newark, Delaware

Peter Rossi, MD
Neurologist, Neurorehabilitation
Medical Director, Neurorehabilitation Services
Rehabilitation of the Pacific
Honolulu, Hawaii

Karen Stolka, RD, LDN
Clinical Dietitian Specialist
Johns Hopkins University Hospital
Baltimore, Maryland

James Wooten, PharmD
Assistant Professor
University of Missouri School of Medicine
Kansas City, Missouri

Reviewers

Kathleen Martin Adamski, RN, MN, CNRN
Lead Nursing Instructor
Nursing Department
Walla Walla Community College
Walla Walla, Washington

Mary Kay Bader, MSN, RN, CCRN, CNRN
Neuroscience Clinical Nurse Specialist
Mission Hospital Regional Medical Center
Mission Viejo, California

Janice M. Buelow
Assistant Professor
Department of Adult Health
Indiana University School of Nursing
Indianapolis, Indiana

Barbara Fitzsimmons, RN, MS, CNRN
Nurse Educator
The Johns Hopkins Hospital
Baltimore, Maryland

Ellie Franges, RN, MSN, CRNP
Nurse Practitioner, Neurosurgery
St. Luke's Hospital and Health Network
Bethlehem, Pennsylvania

Paula Gisler, RN
Administrative Director
The Neuroscience Center at Central Baptist Hospital
Lexington, Kentucky

Ginny Wacker Guido, JD, MSN, RN, FAAN
Associate Dean
University of North Dakota College of Nursing
Grand Forks, North Dakota

W. Andrew Kofke, MD, MBA, FCCM
Professor
Department of Anesthesiology and Critical Care
University of Pennsylvania
Philadelphia, Pennsylvania

Judi Kuric, PhD, MSN, RN, APRN, BC,
    CRRN-A, CNRN
Assistant Professor
University of Southern Indiana School of Nursing and
    Health Professions
Acute Care Nurse Practitioner
NeuroRehab Solutions
Evansville, Indiana

Kathy Lupica, RN, MSN
Nurse Practitioner/Clinical Nurse Specialist
Cleveland Clinic Cancer Center
Brain Tumor Institute
Cleveland, Ohio

Karen March, RN, MN, CNRN, CCRN
Integra Lifesciences
Clinical Faculty, Biobehavioral Nursing
University of Washington
Seattle, Washington

Barbara Martindale, RN, BHSA, CCRN,
    CNRN, CWCN
Assistant Nurse Manager
North Broward Medical Center
Pompano Beach, Florida

Meraida Polak, RN, BSN
Research Nurse
The ALS Center at Emory University
Atlanta, Georgia

Amy Perrin Ross, APRN, MSN, CNRN, MSCN
Neuroscience Program Coordinator
Loyola University Medical Center
Maywood, Illinois

Marianne Shaughnessy, PhD, RN, CRNP
Assistant Professor
University of Maryland
Baltimore, Maryland

Paula Sherwood, PhD, RN, CNRN
Research Assistant Professor
School of Nursing
University of Pittsburgh
Pittsburgh, Pennsylvania

Angela Starkweather, PhD, ACNP, CCRN, CNRN
Assistant Professor
Intercollegiate College of Nursing
Washington State University
Spokane, Washington

Chris Stewart-Amidei, RN, APN, MSN, CNRN,
    CCRN, CS
Clinical Nurse Specialist
Department of Neurosurgery
University of Chicago
Chicago, Illinois

Andrea Strayer, MS, CNRN
Nurse Practitioner
University of Wisconsin Hospitals and Clinics
Department of Neurological Surgery
Madison, Wisconsin

Michelle VanDenmark, MSN, RN, CNRN
Sioux Valley Hospital
University of South Dakota Medical Center
Sioux Falls, South Dakota

Readers of the third edition of *Neuroscience Nursing* will benefit from the contribution and expertise of 32 authors who have shared their extensive knowledge and experience to promote the comprehensive management of disorders that affect the nervous system. A new feature in this addition is the review of each chapter by four highly specialized health care providers to insert additions where appropriate in order to advance the reader's knowledge of nutrition, neuropharmacology, neurorehabilitation, and special considerations for the older adult with neurologic disorders.

Obesity, or less-than adequate-diet, and poor nutrition have become a national health crisis. Neurologic patients are at higher risk, making diet a major component of nursing management, health education, and follow-up for disease prevention and recovery after a neurologic illness. Through education, more patient responsibility can be emphasized. Readers will find nutritional considerations throughout the book.

The media and medical community have focused increasing attention on the safety and efficacy of current and new drugs, with reports of civil and criminal actions resulting from medication errors. Nurses have become acutely aware of medication errors that increase morbidity and mortality, making it essential to have extensive knowledge of drugs for safe administration and the need for close monitoring and follow-up. Increasing numbers of individuals are turning to complementary and alternative medicine, making the Alerts and Tips on drugs included in this volume essential reading.

Until we find a cure for some of the catastrophic neurologic disorders (stroke, spinal injury, multiple sclerosis, and other disabling conditions), new and exciting therapies in neurorehabilitation give hope for restoring function. Introducing the new concepts for neurorehabilitation can be initiated in the critical care phase and reinforced throughout each stage of recovery. Discussion of neurorehabilitation, an important nursing component, is included throughout the book.

Beginning in January of 2006, 6000 individuals turn 60 each day, creating a stronger need than ever before to understand the special needs of older Americans with neurologic disorders. In 5 years, the first wave of baby boomers will reach 65. With advanced age will come a rising tide of hypertension and complex chronic medical problems that have the potential to overwhelm the health care system unless we take steps now to prepare.

While each chapter in the third edition of *Neuroscience Nursing* has retained the basic format of the previous edition, this edition presents the latest evidence-based neuroscience medicine and technological advances that impact and influence the delivery of the best patient care. Neuroscience nurses have worked tirelessly to advance this specialty and are recognized as the preeminent providers of this very specialized care. Neuroscience nursing continues to evolve as the most exciting, challenging, and rewarding area of practice. Nurses have shown their dedication to advancing the specialty in hospitals across the country by taking leadership roles in designing and planning neuroscience centers of excellence and establishing neuroscience institutes.

The demand for new and experienced neuroscience nurses has never been higher and reinforces the need to promote our specialty and to encourage nursing students to pursue careers as neuroscience nurses. The number of nurses practicing in this specialty is growing, with more nurses obtaining the CNRN certification, conducting research, pursuing advanced degrees to qualify as an advanced practice nurse (APN) or nurse practitioner (NP), and obtaining academic appointments (PhD) to teach neuroscience nursing topics and offer students innovative neuroscience opportunities.

Up-to-date information on the latest research, technologies, and resources is needed to meet the many challenges facing nurses committed to serving this patient population. The third edition brings all these elements together in each chapter for a quick reference or for detailed content with tables, algorithms, boxes, clinical pathways, and special features. Regardless of the area of practice, every nurse can easily locate the section of their interest, whether acute, nonacute, rehabilitation, home care, or case management, to review chapters from leading expert authors who have researched and compiled data from the latest literature and their personal knowledge from years of practice.

The highest level of knowledge and skills to successfully manage patients from admission to neurorehabilitation and back to their community are included with emphasis on special considerations for nutrition, older adults, case management, rehabilitation, and health teaching.

Part One is considered the foundation of the practice and will familiarize the clinician with basic and fundamental neuroanatomy and physiology, neurologic assessment, and neurodiagnostic studies. The new addition of eight pages of color plates in this section are designed to dramatize the incredible structures of the nervous system along with other important illustrations of interest. The ability to understand and to complete a thorough neurologic assessment described in Chapter 2 is absolutely essential to the practice.

Universal electronic medical records are beginning to replace the outdated paper charting and will improve accuracy, provide an extensive health database, prevent many medical errors, decrease problems with illegible handwriting, and provide rapid communication among health care providers that can revolutionize the health care system. Patients may soon arrive at their health care provider's facility with a computer stick that contains their entire medical record.

Practical tips and techniques are included in most chapters. The incredible advances in the ability to accurately and rapidly diagnose patient problems are detailed in Chapter 3. Rapid and accurate diagnosis has contributed to saving lives, decreasing the time from symptom onset to aggressive intervention to give the patient the best chance for decreased suffering, increased survival, and highest quality of life.

Part Two, the body of the text, compiles the latest information from research, best practice, and literature as a guide to help provide clinicians with the knowledge base for management of the neuroscience patient's complex, complicated care. Patients need our expertise and support to navigate the often-fragmented and difficult health care system and to recover or to learn how to live as near normal a life as possible, with full knowledge of their neurologic disorder and treatments. Each individual with a neurologic disease or condition, and his or her family, requires a special, individualized plan of care from the day of symptom onset and diagnosis to recovery. If the neurologic disease is terminal and shortens life expectancy, special considerations for patient care and our sensitivity and compassion are needed for the patient and family through the terminal phase or impending death. The authors have compiled chapters that cover the neurologic disorders to assist the nurse in confidently and competently delivering care and experiencing the satisfaction that comes from personal pride when the majority of patient's improve and recover.

In Part Three, the reader has access to common conditions with the latest information on pain, headache, seizures, and epilepsy. These conditions have the potential to completely alter an individual's life. The more we know about these conditions, the better we can assist patients in undergoing early diagnostic studies, seeking the most appropriate treatment, and learning to cope and successfully manage their lives, in spite of pain or seizures. Not every community offers all the latest interventions and treatments for these conditions. It is important for every nurse to know about the nearest facility in the region for referral and follow-up. It is not uncommon for patients who have recovered from a catastrophic illness to later discover that they may never be totally pain free or seizure free and require close monitoring and lifetime treatments.

Part Four, covering legal considerations and life care planning, contains important content that is more relevant than ever in today's climate and deals with issues of consent, life support, living wills, power of attorney, plan of care, and identification of individuals who can benefit from a life care plan following a catastrophic illness or chronic neurologic illness. End-of-life issues and death with dignity are topics covered in our professional literature and also in the media. Our practice today need not be overshadowed by fear of litigation when we follow standards of care and with full awareness of state practice acts and patients' legal rights.

As the editor, it is with great pride and excitement that I join with all the authors in sharing everything that compels us to practice in this specialty and hopefully to motivate and inspire each reader to realize how important they are as members of the team who each day work tirelessly to advocate for preserving what is best in our practice while embracing new and innovative ways to deliver the best care to our patients and their families.

Sincerely,
Ellen Barker
Editor

Acknowledgments

I would like to express my sincere thanks to each of the contributing authors, who are impressive practitioners with individual areas of specialized expertise in the neurosciences. They have shared their knowledge and years of experience to provide readers in-depth information presented in the most current evidence-based format to promote the best patient care for the complicated needs of neuroscience patients.

Book and chapter reviewers were the other group of experts to contribute to the writing of this edition, with blind reviews of content offering excellent comments for the authors. A unique aspect of the text is the careful scrutiny and review by the four consultants who reviewed each chapter to edit or contribute to special patient considerations or needs of the elderly, rehabilitation, nutrition, and neuropharmacology. Several chapters were also reviewed for content and recommendations by experts in neurology and neurorehabilitation with their names acknowledged at the end of the respective chapters.

Special thanks go to Barbara Nelson Cullen, Executive Publisher for Nursing at Elsevier, Philadelphia, Pennsylvania. After a lengthy luncheon discussion, Barbara offered me the opportunity to serve as editor of the third edition of *Neuroscience Nursing: A Spectrum of Care.* Her support and extensive background with nursing textbooks, combined with years of experience as an executive publisher, have been the guiding light for the overall project from the first day. Jennifer Ehlers, Senior Developmental Editor in Philadelphia, also played an important role in helping me to complete this work. She always had a solution for each daunting task or problem.

There are many behind the scenes staff at Elsevier to whom I am so grateful and who have contributed in many ways to finalize the work. The overall design and beautiful cover were created by Designer Margaret Reid. Hours of editing and proofreading have been completed under the able direction of Clay Broeker, Senior Project Manager in St. Louis, Missouri.

I have learned a great deal with each edition, and as with earlier editions, I am still in awe at the huge leap from the typed pages generated on the authors' computers to the final edition of a polished hardcover textbook that will have a history of its own for many years to come.

Contents

Part Two

Neurologic Disorders

Neuroanatomy and Assessment

ELLEN BARKER

CHAPTER 1

Neuroanatomy and Physiology of the Nervous System

At the heart of neuroscience nursing is the study of the science of the brain and nervous system. Knowledge of the neuroanatomy and physiology of the nervous system is central to clinicians who encounter patients with dysfunction of the brain and the spinal cord. The neuroanatomic basis for each of the diseases and conditions reviewed in this book will provide the foundation essential for the specialty practice of neuroscience nursing and how diseases of the nervous system interfere with normal function.

The **nervous system** receives stimuli from the environment, processes and interprets these stimuli, and organizes the appropriate responses. The activity of the nervous system is manifested by what is called "behavior." Any behavior requires the activity of all brain regions. The human brain is capable of making complex decisions, thinking logically, feeling deep emotions, and carrying out multiple and demanding tasks. The brain largely remains a mystery that continues to challenge us to study and learn its secrets.

The brain can be described both **phylogenetically** in terms of evolution in animals and **embryologically** as it develops in humans. The brain is thought to grow and change or reorganize throughout life, a feature called **plasticity.** The more a brain is stretched to do mental activities, the more it stays vital and healthy.

Neuroscience is a relatively new science and is concerned with the development, chemistry, structure, function, and pathology of the nervous system. An increased understanding of the anatomy and the intricacies of the nervous system and the application of this knowledge will help health care professionals further improve the care of the neuroscience patient. The intent of this chapter is to assist the reader in acquiring a thorough foundation of basic principles and a core of fundamental knowledge that is relevant to understanding the structure and function of the nervous system. The reader is encouraged to refer to this chapter to correlate neuroanatomy and neurophysiology with the clinical presentation of the neuroscience patient.

Knowledge of normal neuroanatomic structures and functions helps the nurse clinician to better appreciate and quickly recognize the characteristic signs and symptoms of neurologic dysfunctions. The nurse clinician will also be able to understand the neurodiagnostic studies that create clear images of the living spinal cord and the brain to compare and contrast normal versus abnormal images. Recognition of a patient's changing condition or a neurologic emergency that correlates with neuroanatomic changes enhances the clinician's ability to respond appropriately and communicate effectively with the clinical health care team. In some situations, this could mean the difference between life and death.

BONES OF THE CRANIUM

The human skull consists of 28 bones. The skull is divided into two major sections: the *supratentorial space* above the tentorium and the *infratentorial space* below the tentorium. The supratentorial space contains the cerebral hemispheres and the diencephalon. The infratentorial space contains the cerebellum and the brainstem.[2]

The skull is divided into two major divisions: the bony structure of the **cranium** and the **facial skull** to protect the brain (Fig. 1-1). The oval skull is supported below by the vertebral column. The bone of the cranium consists of three layers: the **outer table,** which is made up of hard cortical bone; the **diploë** middle layer, which is made up of soft cancellous bone; and the **inner table,** which is made up of hard cortical or compact bone (Fig. 1-2).

The facial part of the skull is made up of 14 bones, including the anterior part of the frontal bone, the nasal bone, the zygomatic bone, the maxilla bone, the mandible bone, and two orbital openings. Eight cranial bones encase the brain: **frontal bone,** two **parietal bones,** two **temporal bones, occipital bone, sphenoid bone,** and **ethmoid bone** (see Fig. 1-1). The **frontal bone** is a single cranial bone that protects the frontal lobe. The frontal portion forms the forehead above the orbits of the eyes and then curves inferiorly and posteriorly to become the roof of the orbit on each side of the nasal bone. The **supraorbital notch** in the roof of the orbits carries the supraorbital artery and vein. Within the anterior part of the skull is a cavity, the **frontal sinus,** which drains into the nasal cavity. The frontal bone is joined posteriorly with the parietal bones at the **coronal suture** (see Fig. 1-1).

The **sphenoid bone** occupies a central portion of the skull and resembles the shape of a winged bat (Fig. 1-3). The

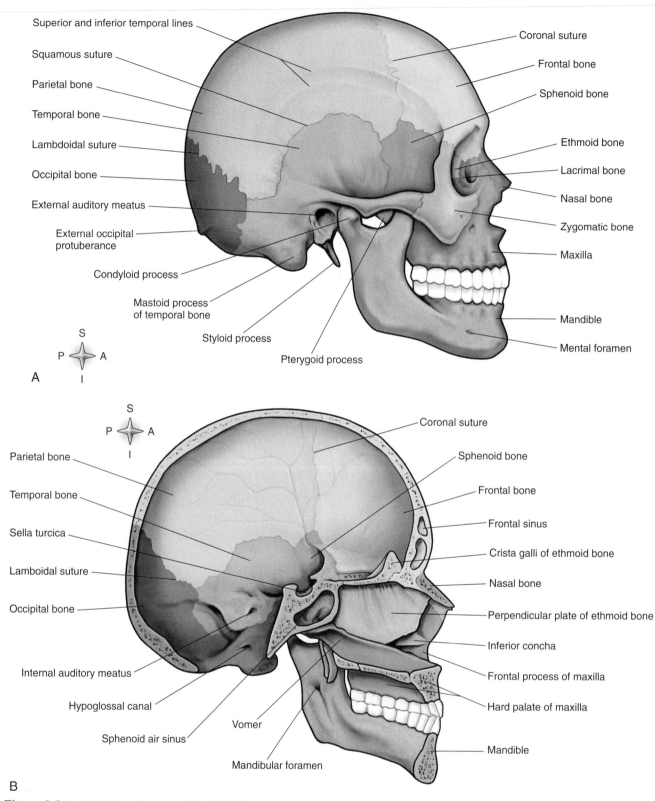

Superior and inferior temporal lines

Squamous suture

Parietal bone

Temporal bone

Lambdoidal suture

Occipital bone

External auditory meatus

External occipital
protuberance

Condyloid process

Mastoid process
of temporal bone

Styloid process

Pterygoid process

Coronal suture

Frontal bone

Sphenoid bone

Ethmoid bone

Lacrimal bone

Nasal bone

Zygomatic bone

Maxilla

Mandible

Mental foramen

S
P ✛ A
I

A

S
P ✛ A
I

Parietal bone

Temporal bone

Sella turcica

Lamboidal suture

Occipital bone

Internal auditory meatus

Hypoglossal canal

Sphenoid air sinus

Vomer

Mandibular foramen

Coronal suture

Sphenoid bone

Frontal bone

Frontal sinus

Crista galli of ethmoid bone

Nasal bone

Perpendicular plate of ethmoid bone

Inferior concha

Frontal process of maxilla

Hard palate of maxilla

Mandible

B

Figure 1-1 A, Skull view from the right side. **B,** Left half of the skull viewed from within.
(From Thibodeau GA, Patton K: Anatomy and physiology, *ed 5, St Louis, 2003, Mosby.)*

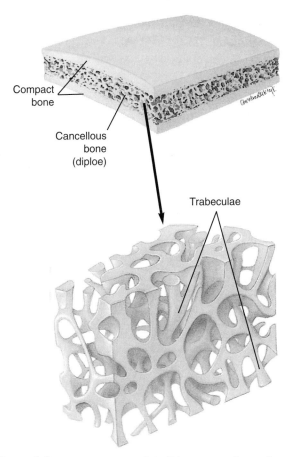

Figure 1-2 The three layers of skull bone: outer layer of compact bone surrounding cancellous bone. Note the fine structure of compact and cancellous bone.
(From Thibodeau GA, Patton K: Anatomy and physiology, *ed 5, St Louis, 2003, Mosby.)*

part that is hollow is called the **sphenoid sinus.** The sphenoid bone has a greater and lesser wing on each side, with a space between known as the **superior orbital fissure** that carries vessels and nerves to the orbit. The so-called "legs" of the sphenoid bone are known as the medial and lateral **pterygoid plates,** to which are attached a muscle of the pharynx and a pair of masticating muscles.

The paired **parietal bones** form the sides of the cranium and fuse at the top (see Fig. 1-1). These two bones make up the major portions of the calvaria, or skullcap, that protects the parietal lobe and parts of the frontal lobes. The parietal bones articulate with the occipital, frontal, temporal, and sphenoid bones.

The two **temporal bones** are large bones that form a major part of the lateral walls and base of the skull (see Fig. 1-3). The temporal bone contains cavities and recesses associated with the ear. Each temporal bone consists of four portions: mastoid, squamous, petrous, and tympanic. Behind the flap of the ear is the **mastoid process** of the temporal bone (see Fig. 1-1). A hollow section of this process contains air cells. The **zygomatic process** projects anteriorly from the **squamous** portion of the temporal bone. In addition, branches

of the middle meningeal arteries create grooves internally over time in the squamous portion. If a fracture occurs across one of these grooves, an epidural hemorrhage may result. The **petrous** portion houses the internal ear that contains the vestibular organs of equilibrium, the organs of hearing, and structures of the middle ear. Canals for cranial nerves VII and VIII and the internal carotid arteries also are located in the petrous portion. The **tympanic** portion of the temporal bone houses the tympanic membrane (eardrum).

The **ethmoid bone** is a delicate structure with thin plates and many air cells. It contains the **crista galli** for olfaction sensations, the **cribriform plate** through which olfactory nerves pass, **air cells,** and the midline **perpendicular plate,** which forms part of the nasal septum.

The **occipital bone** is the posterior aspect of the skull (see Fig. 1-3). A projection of bone called the **external occipital protuberance** is prominent at the upper border of the neck. In the base of the skull is the great foramen, or **foramen magnum,** which marks the boundary between the brain and the spinal cord (see Fig. 1-3). On either side of the foramen are processes that make up the **condyles;** these condyles allow the skull to articulate with the atlas (the first cervical vertebra that articulates with the occipital bone).

Sutures

The fontanelles of the newborn close at approximately 2 years of age; they fill with fibrous tissue that is eventually replaced by bone. These four joints are called **sutures** (Fig. 1-4; see also Fig. 1-1). The **coronal suture** is the ossification that extends ear-to-ear between the frontal bone and the parietal bones.

The **sagittal suture** runs midline from anterior to posterior at the top of the skull and is formed from ossification of the parietal bones. The **lambdoidal suture** is formed at the ossification juncture between the two parietal bones and the triangular occipital bone. The **squamosal suture** runs anterior to posterior from the ossification between the parietal and temporal bones and the temporal and occipital bones.

Cranial Fossa

The interior of the skull is compartmentalized into three cranial fossae. At the basilar skull, the bony structures are divided into fossae as part of the interior of the skull.[2] The three **cranial fossae** are the **anterior, middle,** and **posterior** (see Fig. 1-2). The **anterior** or **frontal fossa** is the smallest and primarily supports the frontal lobe. It is composed of the frontal bone and portions of the sphenoid and ethmoid bones, cribiform plates that contain the olfactory bulbs, and orifices for the olfactory nerves. The deeper **middle fossa** supports the temporal lobes, occipital lobe, and parietal lobes. The **posterior fossa,** the deepest and largest, supports the brainstem (midbrain, pons, and medulla) and cerebellum. Only 2 of 12 cranial nerves are located entirely outside the posterior fossa. The foramen magnum lies in the center of the posterior fossa.

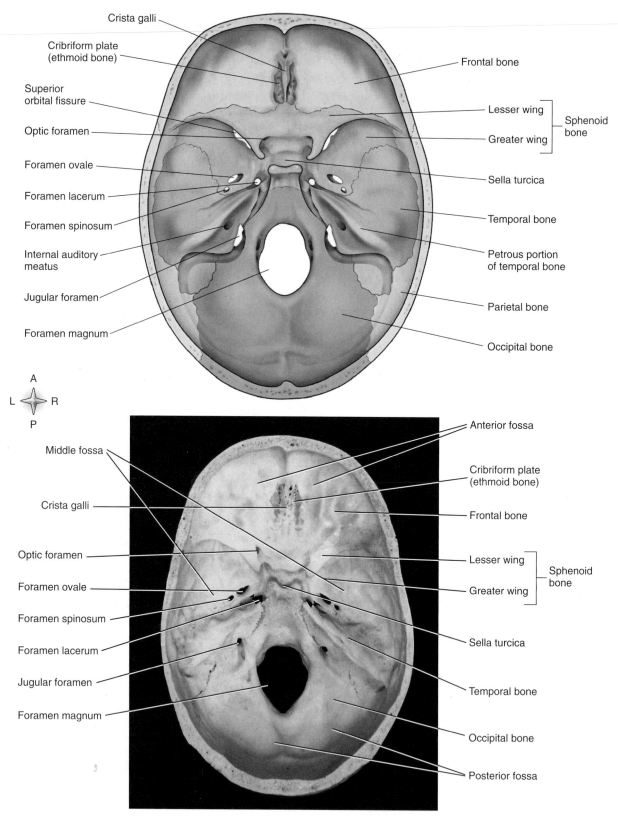

Figure 1-3 Floor of the cranial cavity.
(From Thibodeau GA, Patton K: Anatomy and physiology, ed 5, St Louis, 2003, Mosby.)

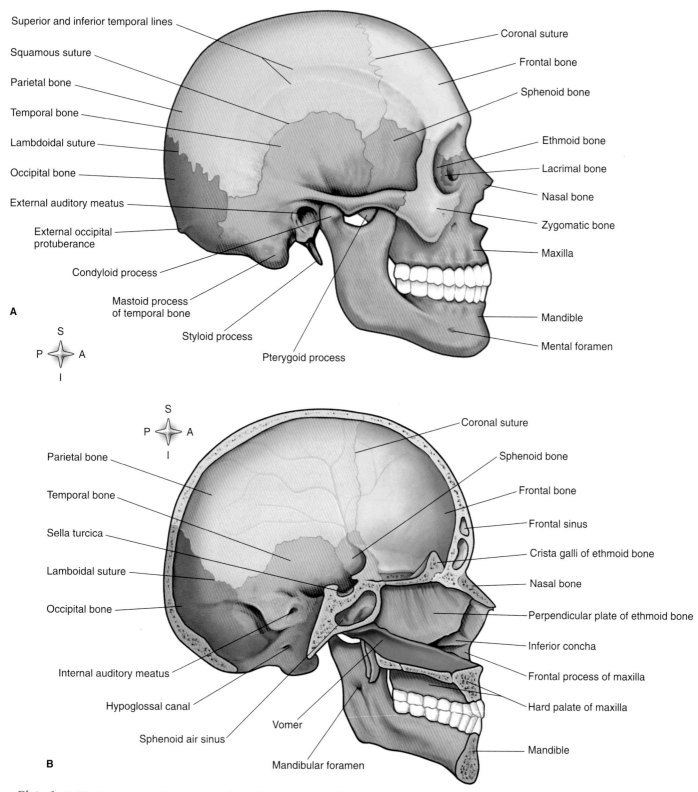

Superior and inferior temporal lines

Squamous suture

Parietal bone

Temporal bone

Lambdoidal suture

Occipital bone

External auditory meatus

External occipital protuberance

Condyloid process

Mastoid process of temporal bone

Styloid process

Pterygoid process

Coronal suture

Frontal bone

Sphenoid bone

Ethmoid bone

Lacrimal bone

Nasal bone

Zygomatic bone

Maxilla

Mandible

Mental foramen

A

S
P ← → A
I

S
P ← → A
I

Parietal bone

Temporal bone

Sella turcica

Lamboidal suture

Occipital bone

Internal auditory meatus

Hypoglossal canal

Sphenoid air sinus

Vomer

Mandibular foramen

Coronal suture

Sphenoid bone

Frontal bone

Frontal sinus

Crista galli of ethmoid bone

Nasal bone

Perpendicular plate of ethmoid bone

Inferior concha

Frontal process of maxilla

Hard palate of maxilla

Mandible

B

Plate 1 A, Skull view from the right side. **B,** Left half of the skull viewed from within.
(From Thibodeau GA, Patton K: Anatomy and physiology, ed 5, St Louis, 2003, Mosby.)

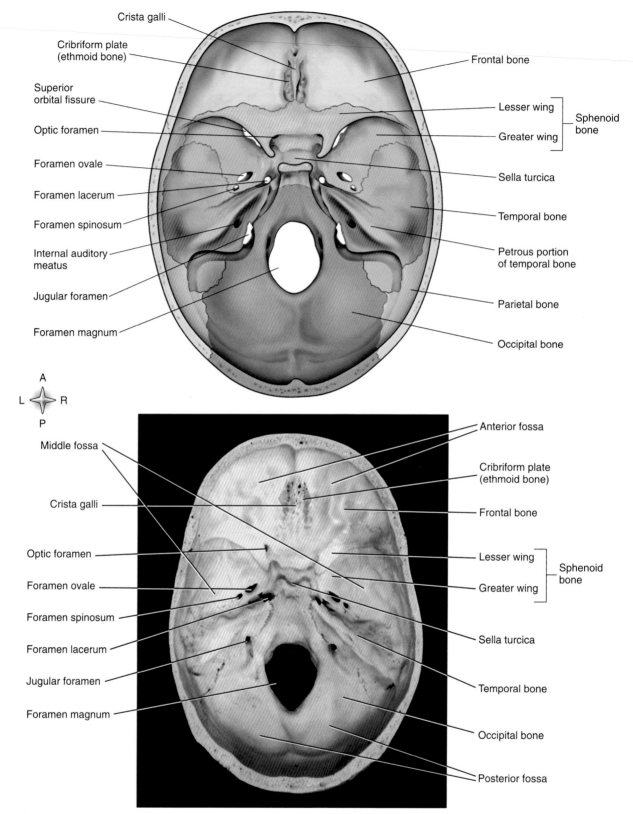

Plate 2 Floor of the cranial cavity.
(From Thibodeau GA, Patton K: Anatomy and physiology, *ed 5, St Louis, 2003, Mosby.)*

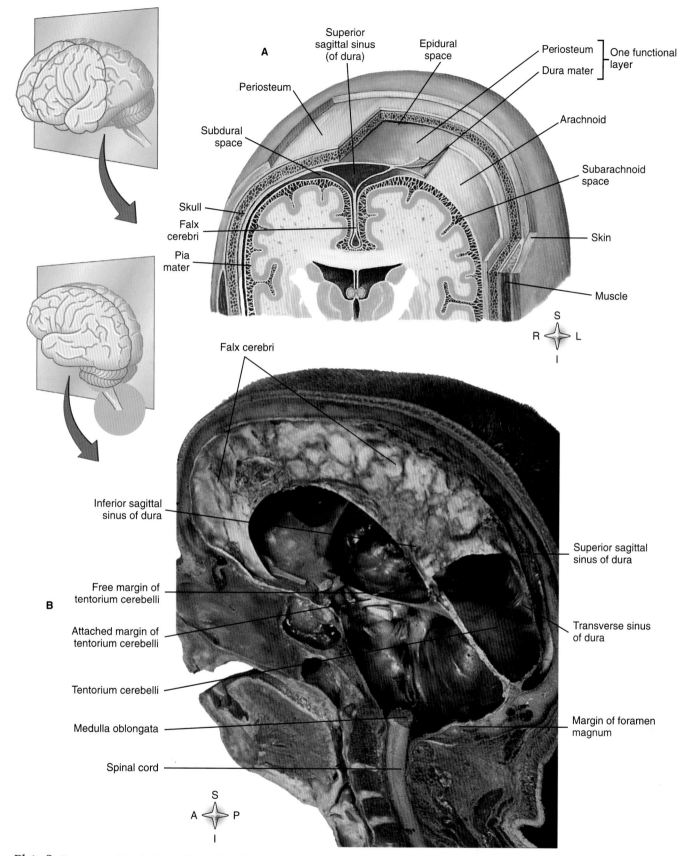

Plate 3 Coverings of the brain. **A,** Frontal section of the superior portion of the head, as viewed from the front. Both the bony and the membranous coverings of the brain can be seen. **B,** Tranverse section of the skull, viewed from below. The dura has been retained in this specimen to show how it lines the inner roof of the cranium and the falx cerebri extending inward.
(From Thibodeau GA, Patton K: Anatomy and physiology, *ed 5, St Louis, 2003, Mosby.)*

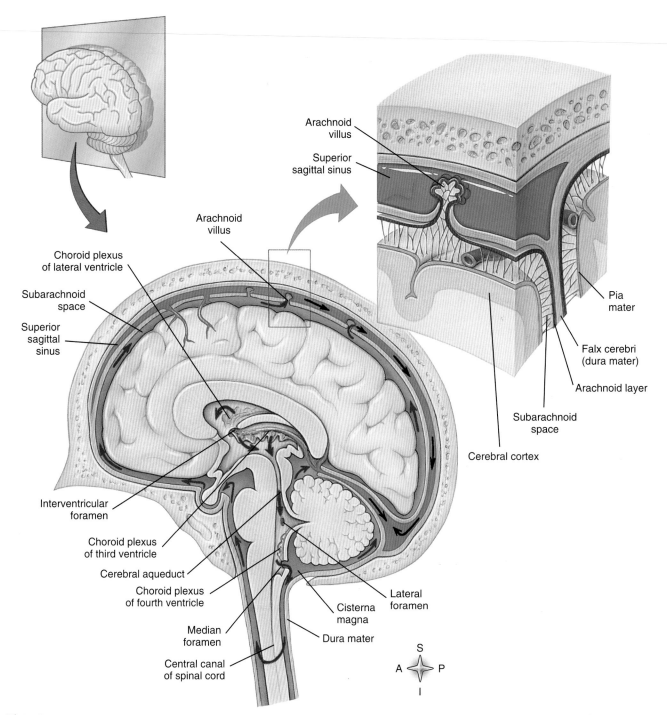

Arachnoid villus

Superior sagittal sinus

Arachnoid villus

Choroid plexus of lateral ventricle

Subarachnoid space

Superior sagittal sinus

Pia mater

Falx cerebri (dura mater)

Arachnoid layer

Subarachnoid space

Cerebral cortex

Interventricular foramen

Choroid plexus of third ventricle

Cerebral aqueduct

Choroid plexus of fourth ventricle

Median foramen

Lateral foramen

Cisterna magna

Dura mater

Central canal of spinal cord

S
A — P
I

Plate 4 Flow of cerebrospinal fluid (CSF). The fluid produced by filtration of blood by the choroid plexus of each ventricle flows inferiorly through the lateral ventricles, interventricular foramen, third ventricle, cerebral aqueduct, fourth ventricle, and subarachnoid space and to the blood.
(From Thibodeau GA, Patton K: Anatomy and physiology, *ed 5, St Louis, 2003, Mosby.)*

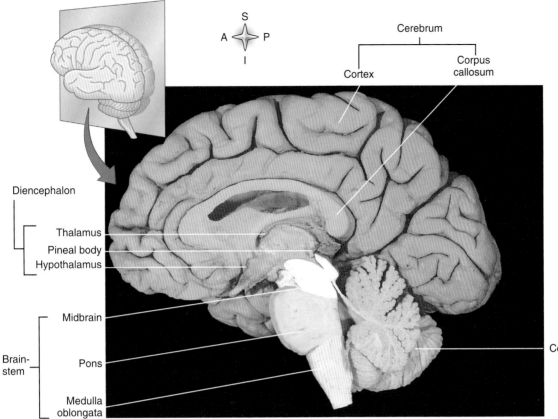

Plate 5 Divisions of the brain. A midsagittal section of the brain reveals features of its major divisions. *(From Thibodeau GA, Patton K:* Anatomy and physiology, *ed 5, St Louis, 2003, Mosby.)*

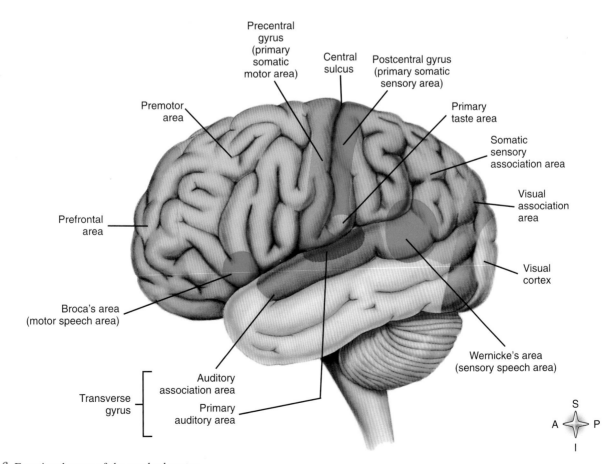

Plate 6 Functional areas of the cerebral cortex. *(From Thibodeau GA, Patton K:* Anatomy and physiology, *ed 5, St Louis, 2003, Mosby.)*

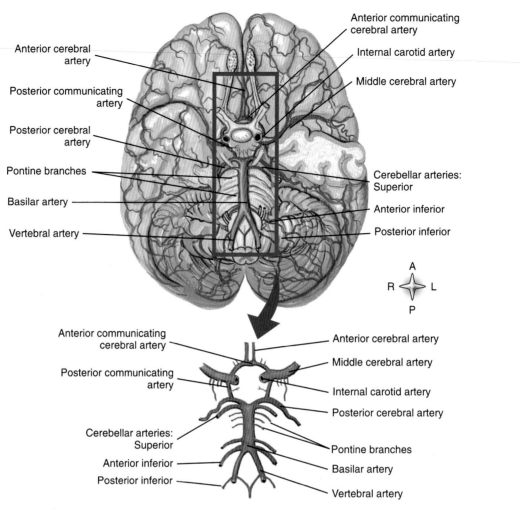

Plate 7 Arteries at the base of the brain. The arteries that compose the circle of Willis are the two anterior cerebral arteries joined to each other by the anterior communicating cerebral artery and to the posterior cerebral arteries by the posterior communicating arteries. *(From Thibodeau GA, Patton K:* Anatomy and physiology, *ed 5, St Louis, 2003, Mosby.)*

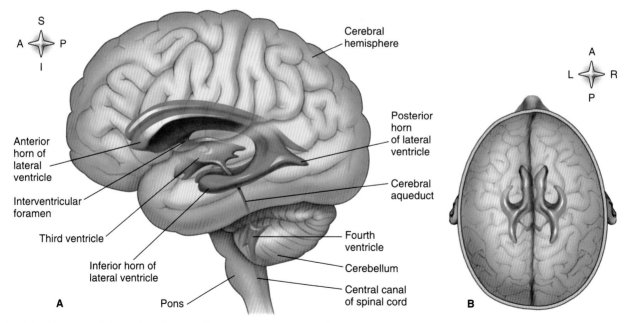

Plate 8 Fluid spaces of the brain. The large figure **(A)** shows the ventricles highlighted within the brain in a left lateral view. The small figure **(B)** shows the ventricles from above. *(From Thibodeau GA, Patton K:* Anatomy and physiology, *ed 5, St Louis, 2003, Mosby.)*

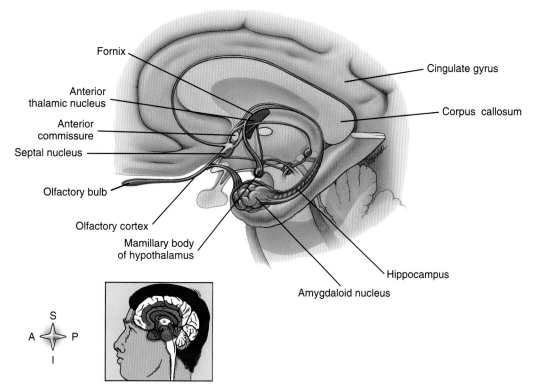

Fornix

Cingulate gyrus

Anterior thalamic nucleus

Corpus callosum

Anterior commissure

Septal nucleus

Olfactory bulb

Olfactory cortex

Mamillary body of hypothalamus

Hippocampus

Amygdaloid nucleus

S

A ← → P

I

Plate 9 Structures of the limbic system.
(From Thibodeau GA, Patton K: Anatomy and physiology, *ed 5, St Louis, 2003, Mosby.)*

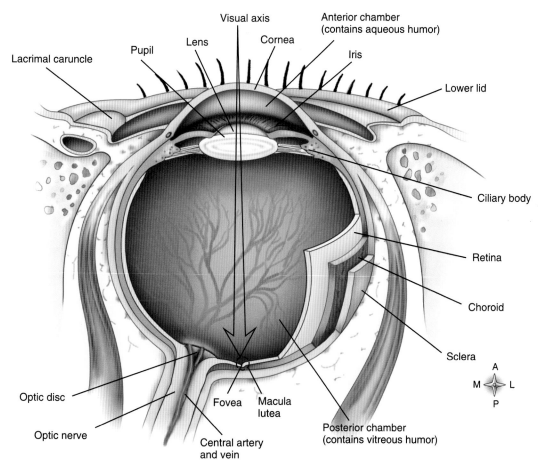

Visual axis

Anterior chamber (contains aqueous humor)

Lens

Cornea

Pupil

Iris

Lacrimal caruncle

Lower lid

Ciliary body

Retina

Choroid

Sclera

Optic disc

Fovea

Macula lutea

Posterior chamber (contains vitreous humor)

Optic nerve

Central artery and vein

A

M ← → L

P

Plate 10 Horizontal section through the right eyeball. The eye is viewed from above.
(From Thibodeau GA, Patton K: Anatomy and physiology, *ed 5, St Louis, 2003, Mosby.)*

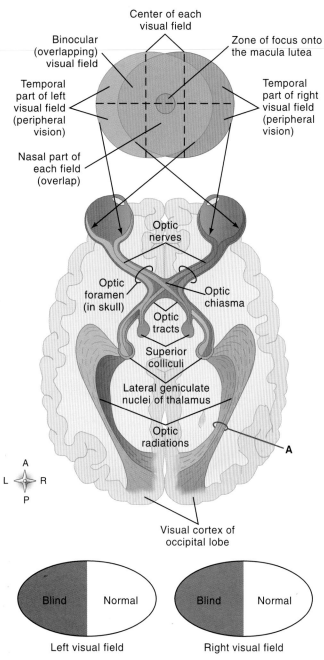

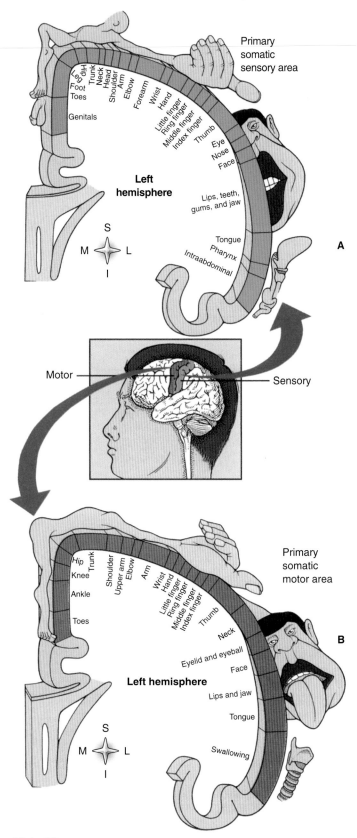

Plate 11 Visual fields and neuronal pathways of the eye. Note the structures that make up each pathway: optic nerve, optic chiasma, lateral geniculate body of thalamus, optic radiations, and visual cortex of occipital lobe. Fibers from the nasal portion of each retina cross over to the opposite side at the optic chiasma and terminate in the lateral geniculate nuclei. Location of a lesion in the visual pathway determines the resulting visual defect. Damage at point *A*, for example, would cause blindness in the right nasal and left temporal visual fields, as the ovals beneath indicate. (Trace the visual pathway from point A back to the visual field map to see why this is so. What would be the effect of pressure on the optic chiasma—by a pituitary tumor, for instance? Answer: It would produce blindness in both temporal fields. Why? Because it destroys fibers from the nasal side of both retinas.)

(From Thibodeau GA, Patton K: Anatomy and physiology, *ed 5, St Louis, 2003, Mosby.)*

Plate 12 Primary somatic sensory **(A)** and motor **(B)** areas of the cortex. The body parts illustrated here show which parts of the body are "mapped" to specific areas of each cortical area. The exaggerated face indicates that more cortical area is devoted to processing information to/from the many receptors and motor units of the face than the leg or arm, for example.

(From Thibodeau GA, Patton K: Anatomy and physiology, *ed 5, St Louis, 2003, Mosby.)*

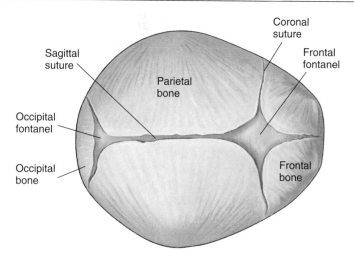

Figure 1-4 Infant skull with sutures viewed from above. *(From Thibodeau GA, Patton K:* Anatomy and physiology, *ed 5, St Louis, 2003, Mosby.)*

STRUCTURES OF THE SPINE

The spine, also called the **vertebral column,** is a flexible, S-shaped column approximately 2 feet in length. The spine consists of 33 bones called **vertebrae** that are separated by **intervertebral disks** (Fig. 1-5). It articulates with the skull above and terminates with the wedge-shaped coccygeal bones, which are fused in the adult.

The vertebral column is similar to a hollow tube and creates a passageway (spinal canal) to encase and protect the spinal cord. Intervertebral foramina along the sides allow the spinal nerves to exit the spinal cord. The vertebral column is made up of 33 bones during early development. In adults, the upper 24 vertebrae articulate and the lower are formed by fusion of the bones. Vertebrae are stacked on top of one another and consist of five regions: **cervical (C1–C7), thoracic or dorsal (T1–T12), lumbar (L1–L5), sacral (S1–S5, fused),** and one **coccygeal (fused from four).** With the exception of C1 and C2, all vertebrae are very similar. A typical vertebra consists of a **vertebral body, vertebral arch, spinous process, pair of lamina, articulating facet joints, transverse process,** and **pair of pedicle** (see Chapter 12).

The seven cervical vertebrae are small and increase in mass from C1 to C7 (Fig. 1-6). The first cervical vertebra (C1) is called the **atlas.** It supports the head, is ringlike in structure, has no vertebral body or spinous process, and allows flexion and extension of the head. The second cervical vertebra (C2) is called the **axis.** It has a toothlike upward projection called a dens (odontoid), which unites with C1 to form a pivot and allow rotation of the head. These first two vertebra are linked together and to the skull by ligaments. The lower cervical vertebrae (C3 to C7) allow flexion, extension, and rotation of the head. Foramina in the transverse processes allow passage of the vertebral arteries to supply blood to the brain.

Each of the 12 thoracic vertebrae are attached to a rib. The thoracic vertebrae increase in size as they progress down the spinal column. They allow flexion and rotation of the trunk, but the ribs limit lateral bending. The thoracic curvature is concave. The five lumbar vertebrae are large, support the thorax, rest on the sacrum, and allow flexion and extension but limit rotation. The five sacral vertebrae fuse to form the sacrum with attachments to the hips. These vertebrae accommodate a division of the fifth sacral nerve and bear the weight of the torso. The coccyx vertebrae are fused and have no pedicles, laminae, or spinous processes.

Spinal Disks

The **intervertebral disks** serve to cushion and separate the bony vertebrae and absorb stress. These fibrocartilaginous, mostly avascular disks have an inner, spongy **nucleus pulposus** surrounded by tough concentric fibrous tissue called the **annulus fibrosus,** which conforms to the size of the disks (Fig. 1-7). The annulus tissue forms strong bands to contain the nucleus. As an individual ages, however, the disks narrow as they dry out and calcium is laid down at the margins of the vertebral bodies, causing osteophytes that compress the nerve roots. With age, the disks lose the ability to imbibe water, leading to less viscosity. The annulus tissue may start to break down and allow portions of the disk to herniate. The disks add height to the spinal column but shrink with age as the result of a loss of water content; this causes a loss of height for the individual.

Spinal Ligaments

Without the **spinal ligaments,** the vertebral column would not be able to adequately support the torso (Fig. 1-8). The **anterior longitudinal ligament** extends along the anterior surface of the vertebra from the axis to the sacrum. The **posterior longitudinal ligament** is situated within the spinal canal and extends along the posterior surface of the vertebra from the axis to the sacrum. Other important ligaments are the **ligamentum flava;** these yellow elastic tissues are interposed between the lamina and attached to their anterior surface to support upright posture.

DEVELOPMENT OF THE NERVOUS SYSTEM

The basic function of the nervous system is to rapidly regulate, and thereby integrate, the activities of the different parts of the body. Functionally, rapid communication is possible because nervous tissue has much more developed excitability and conductivity characteristics than any other type of tissue.[4] Cell division of the fertilized ovum begins before it reaches the uterus. After becoming implanted in the uterus, a layer of cells develops and forms the **embryonic disk.** The embryonic disk becomes trilaminar during the third week of development, and at this stage the three primary tissues of the embryo (**ectoderm, endoderm,** and **mesoderm**) can be distinguished.[4]

The nervous system (brain and spinal cord) develops from the ectoderm, the outermost of the three germ layers

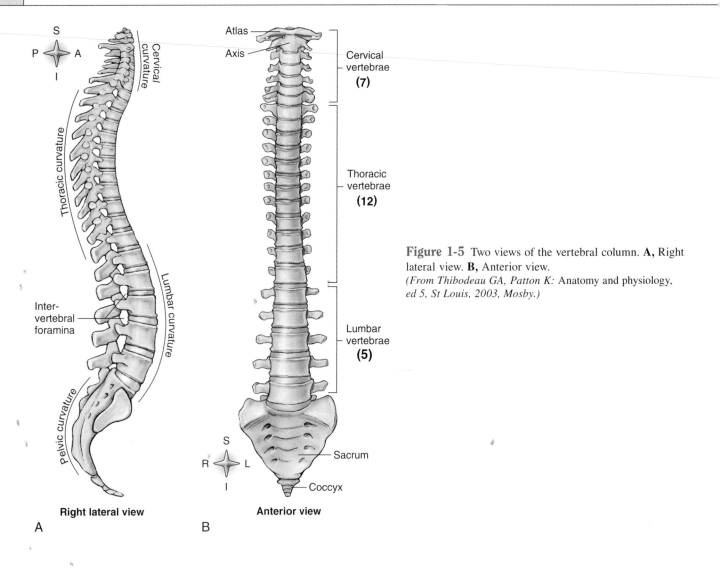

Atlas
Axis
Cervical vertebrae (7)
Cervical curvature
Thoracic vertebrae (12)
Thoracic curvature
Inter-vertebral foramina
Lumbar vertebrae (5)
Lumbar curvature
Pelvic curvature
Sacrum
Coccyx

Right lateral view

Anterior view

A

B

Figure 1-5 Two views of the vertebral column. **A,** Right lateral view. **B,** Anterior view.
(From Thibodeau GA, Patton K: Anatomy and physiology, *ed 5, St Louis, 2003, Mosby.)*

of the embryo. Actual nerve tissue is ectodermal in origin and consists of two basic kinds of cells: nerve cells, or neurons, which are the conducting units of the system, and neuroglia, which are the connecting and supporting cells.[3] It is one of the earliest systems to develop, beginning in the fourth week of gestation. The neural plate forms during the third week of embryonic development.[4] The neural ectoderm is initially a flat layer of cells, but through growth and fusion it becomes a hollow tube that sinks below the surface ectoderm to develop into the brain and spinal cord (Fig. 1-9).

The **neural tube** is hollow throughout its development and develops into virtually the entire central nervous system (CNS). The spaces within the neural tube are called **vesicles.** These persist in the adult brain as the **ventricular spaces.** Around the end of the first gestational month, a series of bulges anterior to the first cervical somites appear. **Somites** are any of the paired segmented masses of mesodermal tissue that form along the length of the neural tube during the early stage of embryonic development.[1] Prenatal events such as the mother's exposure to drugs or toxins can lead to developmental abnormalities.

As the neural folds fuse to form the neural tube, laterally located cells are pinched off the neural tube and migrate throughout the embryo. These **neural crest** cells contribute to the formation of the sensory and autonomic ganglia, peripheral nerves, adrenal medulla, pigment cells, and skeletal and muscular structures of the head and neck.

Primary Brain Vesicles

As the rostral, or head end, of the neural tube develops into the brain, it expands to form **three primary brain vesicles.** The most rostral vesicle is the **prosencephalon** (forebrain), followed by the **mesencephalon** (midbrain) and the **rhombencephalon** (hindbrain). The cavities of these vesicles become the ventricles.

Secondary Brain Vesicles

As development continues into the fifth week, the three primary brain vesicles differentiate into **five secondary brain vesicles.** The prosencephalon subdivides into three secondary vesicles: a pair of **telencephalic vesicles** and the

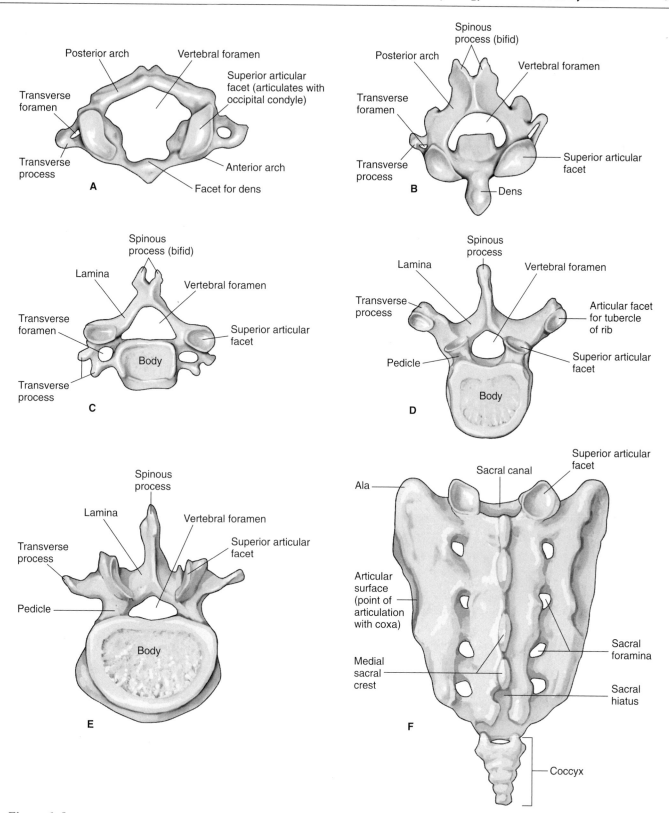

Figure 1-6 Vertebrae. **A,** Atlas (first cervical vertebra), superior view. **B,** Axis (second cervical vertebra), slightly posterior and superior view. **C,** Fifth cervical vertebra, superior view. **D,** Thoracic vertebra, superior view. **E,** Lumbar vertebra, superior view. **F,** Sacrum and coccyx, posterior view.
(From Thibodeau GA, Patton K: Anatomy and physiology, *ed 5, St Louis, 2003, Mosby.)*

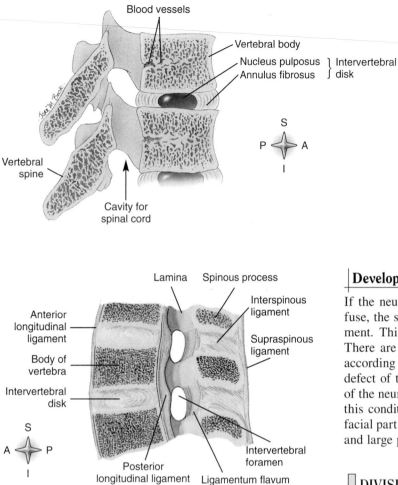

Figure 1-7 Saggital section of vertebra. *(From Thibodeau GA, Patton K:* Anatomy and physiology, *ed 5, St Louis, 2003, Mosby.)*

Figure 1-8 Vertebrae and their ligaments. *(From Thibodeau GA, Patton K:* Anatomy and physiology, *ed 5, St Louis, 2003, Mosby.)*

unpaired **diencephalon.** Each telencephalic vesicle subsequently develops into a **cerebral hemisphere** and **basal ganglia,** and the diencephalon develops into the **dorsal thalamus, hypothalamus, subthalamus,** and **epithalamus.** The rhombencephalon becomes subdivided into the metencephalon (which gives rise to the **pons** and **cerebellum**) and the **myelencephalon** (which differentiates into the **medulla**) (Fig. 1-10). The mesencephalon remains undivided and gives rise to the adult **midbrain.**

Flexures

Because space within the cranial vault is limited, the developing brain must fold in on itself to fit into the space provided. Therefore several flexures develop in the neural tube. The **cervical flexure** occurs between the medulla and spinal cord in the myelencephalon. The **cephalic flexure** occurs between the midbrain and diencephalon, and the **rhombencephalic flexure** occurs between the metencephalon and myelencephalon. These flexures allow the brain to fold more compactly to fit into the intracranial space (Fig. 1-11).

Developmental Anomalies

If the neural folds at the caudal end of the embryo fail to fuse, the spinal cord does not complete its normal development. This results in a condition known as **spina bifida.** There are several levels of spina bifida, which are graded according to the severity of the spinal cord defect and the defect of the overlying vertebral column. If the rostral end of the neural tube fails to close, **anencephaly** may occur. In this condition, which is usually incompatible with life, the facial part of the skull forms but the roof of the cranial vault and large portions of the brain remain defective or absent.

DIVISIONS OF THE NERVOUS SYSTEM

The nervous system is organized to detect changes (stimuli) in the internal and external environment, evaluate that information, and possibly respond by initiating changes in muscles or glands.[3] The nervous system consists of two main divisions: the central nervous system and the peripheral nervous system (Fig. 1-12).

Central Nervous System

The **central nervous system (CNS)** includes the brain and spinal cord. The **brain** is one of the largest organs in adults and allows us to interact with the outside world. The brain is contained in the skull, and the spinal cord is located within the vertebral canal. The brain can be subdivided into several parts, each with specific functions. The largest portion of the brain consists of the cerebrum made up of paired **cerebral hemispheres, cortex,** and **corpus callosum.** Inferior and medial to the cerebral hemispheres is the **diencephalon,** which consists of the dorsal **thalamus, hypothalamus, subthalamus,** and **pineal gland** or **epithalamus.** Inferior to the diencephalon is the brainstem comprising **midbrain, pons,** and **medulla oblongata.** Posterior to the pons and medulla is the **cerebellum**[2] (Fig. 1-13).

The medulla continues through the foramen magnum of the skull and is continuous with the spinal cord. The **spinal**

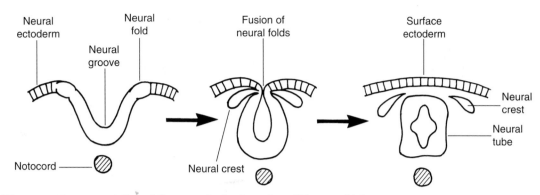

Figure 1-9 Diagrammatic representation of the stages in the formation of the neural tube.

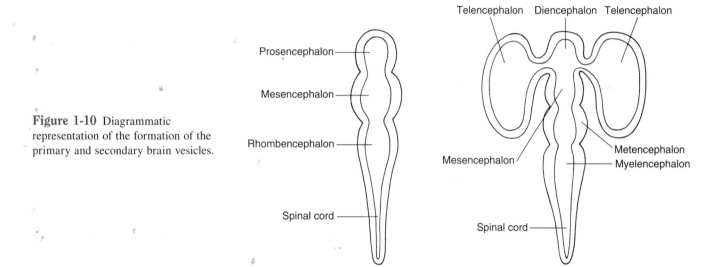

Figure 1-10 Diagrammatic representation of the formation of the primary and secondary brain vesicles.

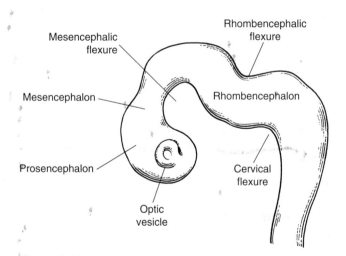

Figure 1-11 Lateral view of the neural tube showing the development of flexures at 36 days of gestation. The mesencephalic and cervical flexures are concave ventrally, whereas the rhombencephalic flexure is concave dorsally.

cord is roughly 18 inches (42 to 45 cm) long and extends from the foramen magnum of the skull to the intervertebral disk between vertebrae L1 and L2 (Fig. 1-14). Like the brain, the spinal cord is surrounded by three meningeal layers. The subarachnoid space contains approximately 75 ml of cerebrospinal fluid to protect the cord.

Peripheral Nervous System

The **peripheral nervous system (PNS)** consists of the nerves located outside the cranial cavity and vertebral column that includes the cranial and spinal nerves, peripheral nerves, neuromuscular junctions, muscles, autonomic nervous system, and enteric nervous system. It is through the peripheral nerves that information is conducted toward (afferent) and away from (efferent) the CNS from communication with the skin, muscles, and other structures in the body. The peripheral nerves are composed of many axons and either originate or terminate within the CNS. The peripheral nerves are divided into two groups: **cranial nerves** and **spinal nerves** (see Fig. 1-12). Twelve pairs of cranial nerves that

Central Nervous System   **Peripheral Nervous System**

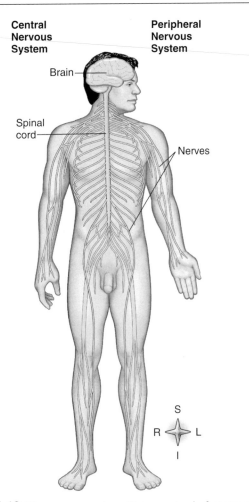

Brain

Spinal cord

Nerves

S

R ⊕ L

I

Figure 1-12 The nervous system. Major anatomic features of the human nervous system include the brain, the spinal cord, and each of the individual nerves. The brain and spinal cord make up the central nervous system (CNS) and all the nerves and their branches make up the peripheral nervous system (PNS). Nerves originating from the brain are classified as *cranial nerves,* and nerves originating from the spinal cord are called *spinal nerves.* *(From Thibodeau GA, Patton K:* Anatomy and physiology, *ed 5, St Louis, 2003, Mosby.)*

originate from the brain emerge from the brain and travel through the various foramina of the skull before traveling in the periphery. The cranial nerves are primarily involved with the innervation of structures in the head and neck (with the exception of the vagus nerve) and the transmission of both sensory and motor information to and from the brain (Fig. 1-15).

Innervation of the body below the neck is handled primarily by 31 pairs of spinal nerves connected by their roots. These nerves emerge from the spinal cord at each vertebral level and leave the vertebral canal by passing through the intervertebral foramina. The spinal nerves are responsible for the formation of the various nerve plexuses that innervate the skin and muscles throughout the body. Each spinal nerve consists of both ventral (motor) and dorsal root (sensory) components.

Autonomic Nervous System

The **autonomic nervous system (ANS)** is a specialized part of the nervous system that consists of afferent and efferent pathways. The ANS regulates involuntary body functions, for example, the activity of the cardiac muscles, smooth muscles, and glands. It controls the activities of the viscera at an unconscious level (Fig. 1-16). The major **effector organs** of the ANS are **smooth muscle, cardiac muscle,** and **glands.** The ANS is made up of two neuron chains that carry messages from the CNS to the peripheral effector organs. The two efferent divisions of the ANS are the **sympathetic** and **parasympathetic.** These parallel systems regulate visceral organs by acting in cooperative opposing manners.[2] The ANS can also be considered to include afferent pathways for visceral receptors.

Sympathetic Division

The **sympathetic division** of the ANS prepares the body to meet crisis situations. It is sometimes called the "flight or fight" system because it prepares the body physiologically to either fight or run away from danger. It receives input from the thoracic and lumbar spinal cord. Both of these reactions require the same physiologic adjustments. The sympathetic division of the ANS elevates the heart rate and blood pressure, increases respirations, dilates the pupil of the eye, shunts blood to the muscles and skin, and inhibits the digestion of food.

Parasympathetic Division

The **parasympathetic division** of the ANS is for nonemergencies—the "rest and digest" response. It receives input from the cervical and sacral spinal cord and operates during moments of calm. It tends to promote activities that restore the body's energy sources. Activities controlled by the parasympathetic division of the ANS include slowing the heart rate, lowering the blood pressure, decreasing respirations, shunting blood from the periphery to the internal organs, constricting the pupil, and increasing the activity of the gastrointestinal tract.

In both divisions of the ANS there is a two-neuron chain that carries information from the CNS to the periphery. The first neuron in the chain is called the **preganglionic neuron** and has cell bodies located in the CNS. The cell bodies of the sympathetic division of the ANS are located in the spinal cord in spinal segments T1 to L2 (the **thoracolumbar** division). The cell bodies of the parasympathetic division of the ANS are located in the nuclei of cranial nerves III, VII, IX, and X or in spinal cord segments S2, S3, and S4 (the **craniosacral** division).

The preganglionic axons of both divisions of the ANS course out to the periphery in the cranial nerves and spinal nerves to terminate on the cell bodies of the second neuron in the chain—the postganglionic neuron. The **postganglionic cell bodies** are distributed throughout the body in the various autonomic ganglia. The axons that arise from these postganglionic cell bodies innervate the specific effector organs of the ANS (e.g., smooth muscles, cardiac muscles, and glands). In the parasympathetic division of

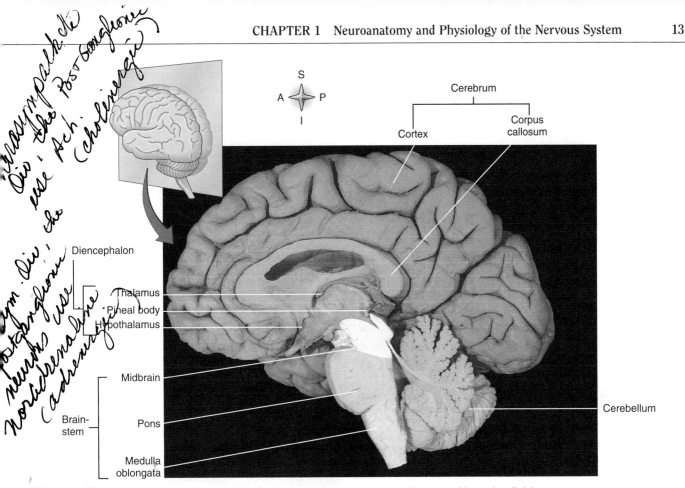

Figure 1-13 Divisions of the brain. A midsagittal section of the brain reveals features of its major divisions. *(From Thibodeau GA, Patton K: Anatomy and physiology, ed 5, St Louis, 2003, Mosby.)*

the ANS the postganglionic neurons use acetylcholine as their transmitter. Hence this division of the ANS (in addition to being called *craniosacral*) is called the **cholinergic** division. The sympathetic division of the ANS is called not only *thoracolumbar* but also **adrenergic** because its postganglionic neurons use noradrenaline as their neurotransmitter (see Fig. 1-16).

ANATOMY OF THE NERVOUS SYSTEM

Meninges

The brain and spinal cord are protected by the skull and vertebral column and enclosed in connective tissue membranes called **meninges.** This series of connective tissue that covers the brain includes the **dura mater, arachnoid,** and **pia mater** (Fig. 1-17). The meninges are important because they are often the source of tumors known as **meningiomas.** Meningiomas are not usually malignant or invasive but may cause considerable problems by exerting pressure on certain areas of the nervous system.

Dura Mater

The dura mater is the outermost meningeal covering and is arranged in two layers. This tough, inelastic, white fibrous coat lines the cranial cavity and vertebral canal and is

regarded as bilaminar, or composed of two layers. It forms a continuous membranous sac and delineates the CNS from the PNS. The outer periosteal layer adheres to the skull and forms its periosteum, whereas the inner meningeal layer is in contact with the arachnoid. The two layers of dura adhere to each other except at the sites of formation of the **dural venous sinuses.** The dura has been described as being like a thin leathery bag around the brain. The **epidural space** is located between the dura mater and the skull.

The meningeal layer of the dura mater produces a number of prominent folds that subdivide the interior of the cranial cavity. Four such folds can be identified. The largest and most prominent of these is the **falx cerebri** (see Fig. 1-17). This fold is located along the sagittal suture of the skull, where it separates the right and left cerebral hemispheres in the longitudinal fissure of the brain. The next largest meningeal fold is the **tentorium cerebelli,** a small triangular process that is a double, horizontally oriented fold that divides the posterior cranial fossa into its superior and inferior compartments, or **supratentorial** and **infratentorial** structures. The cerebellum occupies the compartment inferior to the tentorium cerebelli, and the occipital lobes of the cerebrum are located superior to the tentorium cerebelli. The two remaining and less prominent folds are the **diaphragma sellae,** which forms a partial covering or roof over the sella turcica covering the pituitary body, and the **falx cerebelli,** which is attached posteriorly to the internal occipital

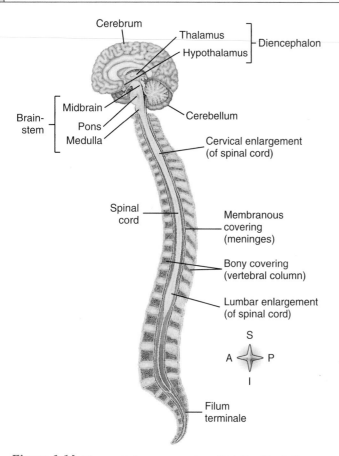

Figure 1-14 The central nervous system. Details of both the brain and the spinal cord are easily seen in this figure. *(From Thibodeau GA, Patton K:* Anatomy and physiology, *ed 5, St Louis, 2003, Mosby.)*

protuberance and incompletely separates the cerebellum into right and left halves (see Fig. 1-17).

Arachnoid

The arachnoid is a thin, avascular, transparent connective tissue membrane that encloses the brain and is interposed between the pia mater and the dura mater. It bridges sulci and other surface irregularities. The arachnoid is separated from the dura mater by only a thin film of fluid. Thus the **subdural space** is only a "potential space" of fluid collection. The arachnoid is attached to the underlying pia mater by a series of thin trabeculae. The space between the arachnoid and the underlying pia mater is considerable and is called the **subarachnoid space.** It is normally filled with **cerebrospinal fluid (CSF).** Cerebral vessels or aneurysms can rupture here, causing subarachnoid hemorrhage.

The subarachnoid space and its CSF form a hydrostatic cushion around the brain, which serves to protect the brain from blows to the skull. The subarachnoid space underlying the superior sagittal sinus contains arachnoid villi, which are sites for CSF absorption into the superior sagittal sinus (see Fig. 1-19). The arachnoid villi move CSF from the subarachnoid space to the venous system in a "one-way" valve to allow the CSF to enter the sinus and mix with venous blood.

The subarachnoid space extends into the vertebral canal and also surrounds the spinal cord.

The **basilar cisterns** are pools of CSF at the base of the brain and around the brainstem where the pia and arachnoid are widely separated. The largest dilation of the subarachnoid space is located posteroinferior to the cerebellum and is known as the **cisterna magna** or **cerebellomedullary cistern** (see Fig. 1-19). The remaining cisterns are known as the **interpeduncular, pontine,** and **superior cistern.** This dilation of the subarachnoid space, which is filled with the cauda equina, is called the **lumbar cistern.** Samples of the CSF may be safely removed from the lumbar cistern below the L3 vertebral level.

Pia Mater

The **pia mater** is the meningeal layer that is closely adherent to the surface of the brain and follows the gyri and sulci patterns—the hills and valleys of the brain. It contains a fine network of blood vessels and intervenes into the sulci of the brain (see Fig. 1-17). The foot processes of astrocytes abut against the pia mater on the surface of the brain and spinal cord, forming the **pia-glial membrane.**

Ventricular System and Cerebrospinal Fluid

The hollow tube in the developing brain develops to form the ventricular system. The **ventricles** of the adult brain are fluid-filled cavities or hollow spaces lined by ependyma and contain specialized epithelium called the **choroid plexus** that produces about 80% of the CSF (Figs. 1-18 and 1-19). The arachnoid villi (which can be seen in the small box in Fig. 1-19) allow absorption of CSF into the superior sagittal sinus where it continues its pathway, if uninterrupted, back to the heart.

Choroid Plexus

The **choroid plexus** is a pink, cauliflower- or seaweed-like tissue found within the ventricles of the brain. It consists of sheets of cuboidal epithelium that project into the lumen of the ventricular spaces and are responsible for the production of CSF in the CNS (see Fig. 1-19).

Cerebrospinal Fluid

CSF is a clear fluid similar to an ultrafiltrate of blood plasma but contains lower concentrations of potassium, bicarbonate, calcium, and glucose and higher concentrations of magnesium and chloride. CSF functions to preserve homeostasis in the nervous system, provide buoyancy for the brain, cushion the brain from impact with bones of the skull, and drain unwanted substances away from the brain. It is a transudate of the blood plasma and is secreted into the ventricles at a rate of approximately 0.3 to 0.4 ml/min, or more than 400 ml/day. Approximately 150 ml of CSF circulates within the ventricles of the brain and the subarachnoid space surrounding the brain, with about 30 ml within the intraventricular space. The total volume of CSF is renewed more than three times per day. Pulsation of the choroid plexus may contribute to the movement of CSF within the ventricles.

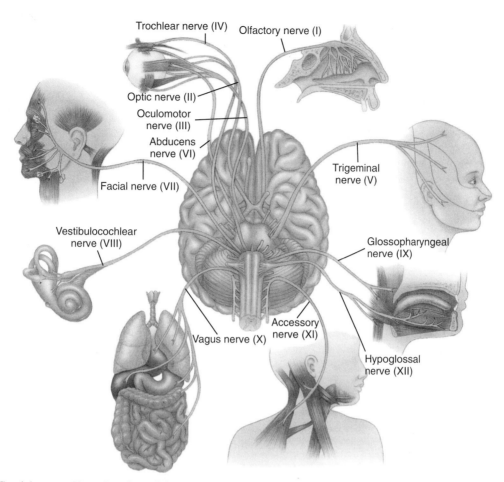

Figure 1-15 Cranial nerves. Ventral surface of the brain showing attachment of the cranial nerves. *(From Thibodeau GA, Patton K: Anatomy and physiology, ed 5, St Louis, 2003, Mosby.)*

Approximately 20% of the CSF may be derived from the capillary bed of the brain and metabolic water production, ependymal cells lining the ventricles or blood vessels of the brain and spinal cord. CSF fluid volume produced within the capillary beds of the brain may in fact contribute to the overall bulk weight of the brain itself.

Lateral Ventricles

The two **lateral ventricles** are the largest and are located in the cerebral hemispheres. They are roughly C shaped and follow the contours of the cerebral hemisphere (see Figs. 1-18 and 1-19). Each lateral ventricle has an **anterior horn** that projects into the frontal lobe and a **posterior horn** that projects into the occipital lobe. The **inferior horn** of the lateral ventricles extends into the temporal lobe. All three horns of the ventricular system unite in the **body** of the lateral ventricle, which is located in the parietal lobe. They are lined by ependymal cells. The lateral ventricles produce CSF by the choroid plexus that flows into the third ventricle through the interventricular foramina or **foramina of Monro.**

Third Ventricle

The **third ventricle,** located in the midline of the diencephalon, is surrounded by the thalamus and hypothalamus (see Figs. 1-18 and 1-19). The **pineal gland** is attached to the roof of the third ventricle. The third ventricle is a narrow cleft that collects CSF from the two lateral ventricles that flows from the caudal regions of the third ventricle through the cerebral aqueduct.

The **cerebral aqueduct** is surrounded by the midbrain. The cerebral aqueduct is a narrow part of the ventricular system that interconnects the third and fourth ventricles (see Fig. 1-19).

Fourth Ventricle

The **fourth ventricle** is a pyramid-shaped space surrounded by the cerebellum, pons, and medulla (see Figs. 1-18 and 1-19). CSF that flows into the fourth ventricle can enter the subarachnoid space by flowing through one of three foramina that open into it from the fourth ventricle. There is a single midline or median foramen, the **foramen of Magendie,** and a pair of lateral foramina, the **foramina of Luschka,** that allow the CSF to continue its pathway. Tufts of choroid plexus from the fourth ventricle occasionally project through the foramina into the subarachnoid space.

Flow of Cerebrospinal Fluid

CSF flows from the lateral ventricles through the interventricular foramina and into the third ventricle. The choroid

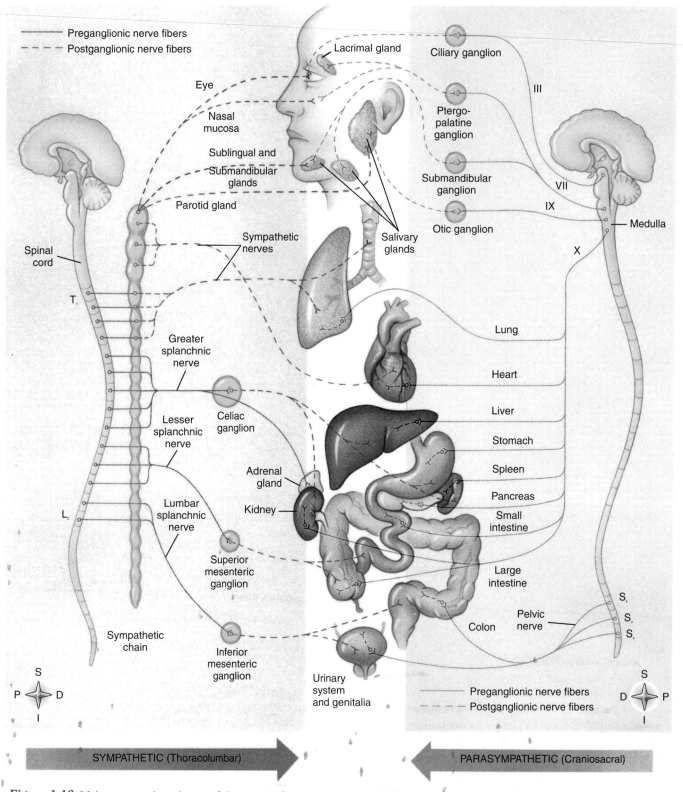

Figure 1-16 Major autonomic pathways of the autonomic nervous system (ANS). *(From Thibodeau GA, Patton K: Anatomy and physiology, ed 5, St Louis, 2003, Mosby.)*

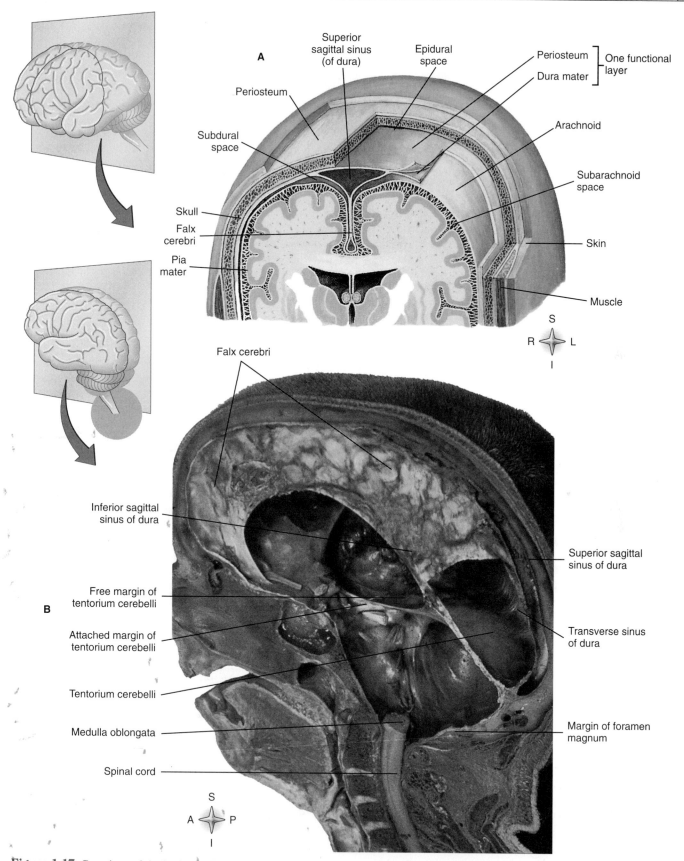

Figure 1-17 Coverings of the brain. **A,** Frontal section of the superior portion of the head, as viewed from the front. Both the bony and the membranous coverings of the brain can be seen. **B,** Tranverse section of the skull, viewed from below. The dura has been retained in this specimen to show how it lines the inner roof of the cranium and the falx cerebri extending inward.
(From Thibodeau GA, Patton K: Anatomy and physiology, *ed 5, St Louis, 2003, Mosby.)*

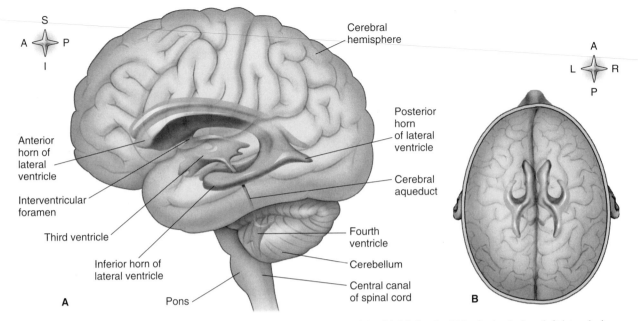

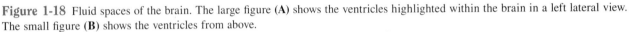

Figure 1-18 Fluid spaces of the brain. The large figure **(A)** shows the ventricles highlighted within the brain in a left lateral view. The small figure **(B)** shows the ventricles from above. *(From Thibodeau GA, Patton K:* Anatomy and physiology, *ed 5, St Louis, 2003, Mosby.)*

plexus of the third ventricle also adds CSF to the volume; the CSF flows from the third ventricle into the fourth ventricle via the cerebral aqueduct. CSF may escape into the subarachnoid space through one of the three openings in the roof of the fourth ventricle. If the flow of CSF into the fourth ventricle is blocked (e.g., a tumor of the pineal gland obstructs the cerebral aqueduct), it builds up in the more rostral ventricles, which results in **hydrocephalus.**

The CSF is absorbed from the subarachnoid space by specialized epithelial structures called **arachnoid granulations,** which project into the dural venous sinuses. The CSF that is absorbed by the arachnoid granulations is secreted back into the venous blood of the dural venous sinuses. This produces a turnover of CSF, with production in the ventricles and secretions into the dural sinuses (see Fig. 1-19).

Neurons

Neurons are highly specialized cells in the brain, spinal cord, and spinal ganglia. It has been estimated that the brain produces approximately 100 billion cells during its development, including neurons. The brain changes with aging as the volume of brain tissue decreases and neurons die. **Neurons** are the functional cells of the nervous system and are specialized for the reception of stimuli, integration, and transmission or conduction of information. Unmyelinated neurons are darker in color than myelinated neurons with their glistening white color, and appear gray, as in the neocortex or gray matter. There is a great variety of neuron types, depending on the size, shape, and number of processes and function.

A neuron consists of a **cell body,** or **perikaryon,** and elongated processes that emanate from the perikaryon (Fig. 1-20). Neurons have receptive neurites or processes called **dendrites,** which radiate from a central portion of the cell and conduct impulses toward the perikaryon. Neurons also have a single process called the **axon,** which conveys impulses away from the perikaryon. Axons extend for variable distances and break into axon terminals that form junctions called synapses. Every neuron possesses at least one dendrite and one axon. Neurons may have more than one dendrite, but they have only one axon. The most common type of neuron in the cerebral cortex is the pyramidal cell, which is a neuron with a pyramid-shaped cell body in the gray matter of the cerebral cortex.

Neurons can be classified according to the direction in which they conduct impulses or according to their number of processes. In general, three types of neurons are identified in the nervous system on the basis of their shape and number of processes (Fig. 1-21).

Pseudounipolar, or **unipolar, neurons** are those that appear to have only one process originating from the perikaryon. This single process, which morphologically resembles an axon, divides into two. One branch goes to the skin in the periphery, where it is associated with sensory endings. The other branch enters the nervous system, where it synapses on other neurons in the CNS. Pseudounipolar neurons are typically found in the sensory ganglia of the peripheral nerves. All primary sensory afferent neurons and some autonomic neurons are unipolar.

Bipolar neurons have two processes emanating from the cell body. One process is functionally the dendrite and is associated with sensory endings, whereas the other process is functionally an axon. Bipolar neurons have a limited distribution in the nervous system and are largely associated with the retina of the eye and the primary sensory neurons of the auditory and olfactory systems.

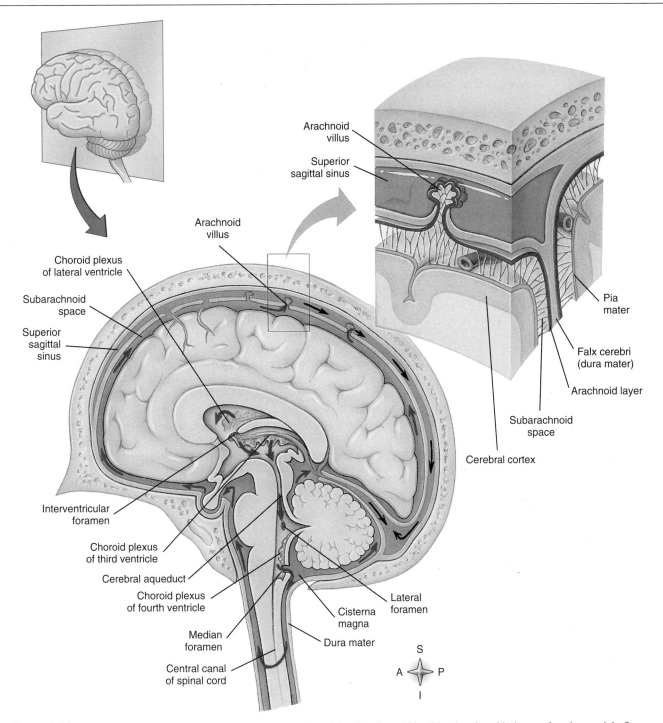

Figure 1-19 Flow of cerebrospinal fluid (CSF). The fluid produced by filtration of blood by the choroid plexus of each ventricle flows inferiorly through the lateral ventricles, interventricular foramen, third ventricle, cerebral aqueduct, fourth ventricle, and subarachnoid space and to the blood.
(From Thibodeau GA, Patton K: Anatomy and physiology, *ed 5, St Louis, 2003, Mosby.)*

Multipolar neurons are the most numerous neurons in the nervous system. These neurons possess many dendrites but only a single axon. They are found throughout the CNS and PNS.

Perikaryon
The perikaryon of a typical neuron contains the same organelles as any other cell in the body. Each cell has a **cell membrane** that consists of lipoproteins. The most prominent feature of the cell is a large, round, distinctive **nucleus** and a prominent, darkly staining **nucleolus. Chromatin** is the material within the cell nucleus from which the chromosomes are formed. It consists of strands of **deoxyribonucleic acid (DNA),** which is the carrier of genetic information. **Ribonucleic acid (RNA)** is found in both the nucleus and the cytoplasm of cells; it transmits genetic instructions from

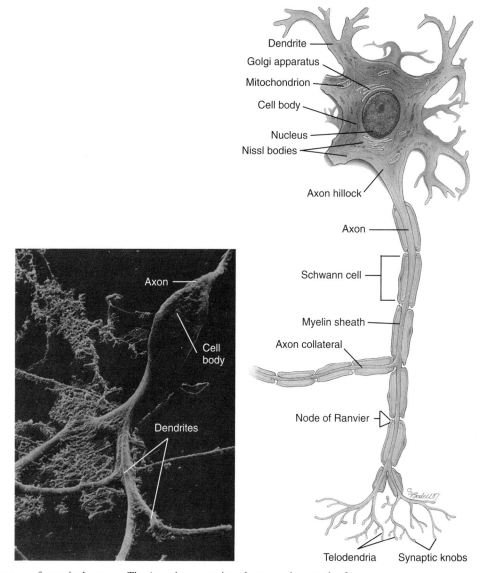

Figure 1-20 Structure of a typical neuron. The *inset* is a scanning electron micrograph of a neuron. *(From Thibodeau GA, Patton K:* Anatomy and physiology, *ed 5, St Louis, 2003, Mosby.)*

the nucleus to the cytoplasm. In the cytoplasm, RNA functions in the assembly of proteins.

The cytoplasm of the perikaryon contains the usual complement of organelles. The most prominent of these is the **chromophilic** substance, also known as Nissl substance. Chromophilic substance is **rough endoplasmic reticulum (RER),** an important organelle in protein synthesis. Numerous mitochondria produce energy to drive the many activities of the neuron, and a **Golgi complex** is present for "packaging" the proteins produced in the RER.

Neurofilaments are solid, rodlike structures that form the so-called **cytoskeleton** and give shape to the neuron and its processes. **Neurotubules** are hollow, tubelike structures that

give shape to the neuron and also function in the transport of material within the neuron.

Dendrites

Dendrites are short, multiple branching (treelike) processes that are receptive neurons, which radiate from a central portion of the cell. They conduct impulses toward the cell body. The axons and dendrites of the neuron contain many of the same organelles found in the cytoplasm of the perikaryon (see Figs. 1-20 and 1-21). Dendrites, the processes that carry impulses to the perikaryon, contain **mitochondria, RER, neurotubules,** and **neurofilaments.** Near the synapses, the dendrite may demonstrate modification of its

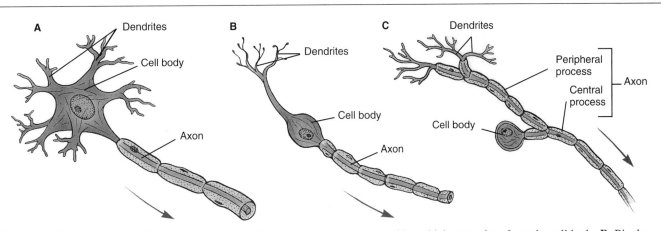

Figure 1-21 Structural classification of neurons. **A,** Multipolar neuron: neuron with multiple extensions from the cell body. **B,** Bipolar neuron: neuron with exactly two extensions from the cell body. **C,** Unipolar neuron: neuron with only one extension from the cell body. The central process is an axon; the peripheral process is a modified axon with branched dendrites at its extremity. (The *arrow* shows the direction of impulse travel.)
(From Thibodeau GA, Patton K: Anatomy and physiology, ed 5, St Louis, 2003, Mosby.)

cell membrane in the form of **dendritic spines,** which provide abundant surface area for contacts with other neurons.

Action Potential

An **action potential** is an electric impulse that consists of a self-propagating series of **polarizations** and **depolarizations** that are transmitted across the cell membranes of a nerve fiber. The outer surface of the cell membrane bears a positive charge, whereas the inner surface of the membrane is negatively charged. Inside the cell, the concentration of potassium is about 50 times higher and the sodium concentration is about 10 times lower than on the outside. The interior of a cell at rest is −60 to −70 mV and is negative with respect to the extracellular fluid. This steady-state transmembrane voltage is called a **resting membrane potential.**

When a neuron becomes active (i.e., during the transmission of a nerve impulse), the permeability of the membrane to sodium changes. When the membrane potential is reduced to approximately −50 mV, a process called depolarization, voltage-sensitive channels open and allow sodium and calcium ions to flow in. Potassium channels open to increase the outflow of potassium. The process continues until the cell repolarizes to its resting state. If the cell becomes more negative (through the influx of chloride ions and the outflow of potassium ions), it is hyperpolarized.

Axons

An axon is a single long process that conveys impulses away from the cell body. Axons range from a few micrometers to several feet in length (see Figs. 1-20 and 1-21). They tend to be very long processes. The length of an axon is maintained by the presence of neurofilaments and neurotubules. The axon attaches to the perikaryon at the **axon hillock.** This region is largely devoid of organelles and is the region of the axon where action potentials are generated. The distal end of the axon is a specialized region that contributes to the formation of the **synapse.** The synapse is the point through which impulses are transmitted from one neuron to another.

In the region of the synapse, the axonal membrane is thickened and the cytoplasm contains many mitochondria and small, membrane-bound structures called **synaptic vesicles.** The synaptic vesicles contain vesicles filled with minute amounts of chemical substances called **neurotransmitters.** When released from the synapse, these chemicals excite the next neuron in the chain and generate an action potential, thus continuing the flow of neural impulses. Some neurotransmitters (e.g., acetylcholine) are complex proteins, whereas other neurotransmitters are modified amino acids (Table 1-1). When the action potential arrives at the foot of a cell, it attaches to special receptors on the surface of a dendrite, cell body, axon, or another **synaptic terminal.**

Many axons in both the CNS and PNS are ensheathed by a coating known as **myelin.** Speed of conduction depends on the size of the axon and myelin thickness. Myelin is the white matter formed by special supporting cells called **neurolemmocytes (Schwann cells)** in the PNS and **oligodendrocytes** in the CNS. These cells approach axons and wrap them with successive layers of cell membrane to cover and insulate the axons (Fig. 1-22). Myelin is not continuous from the beginning to the end of the axon but instead is interrupted at regular intervals. These interruptions in the myelin sheath are called the **nodes of Ranvier.** Impulses that travel along myelinated axons jump from one node of Ranvier to another. This is known as **saltatory conduction** and is very rapid.

Supportive Cells: Neuroglia

The supporting cells of the nervous system are the **neuroglia,** which literally means "nerve glue." These specialized cells form the background for the activity of neurons. The number of glial cells is up to 10 times greater than the number of neurons in the nervous system. The various morphologic types of glia have specific functions. There are five major types of glial cells in the CNS: astrocytes, oligodendrocytes, phagocytic microglial cells, ciliated ependymal cells, and Schwann cells (see Fig. 1-22). Glial cells are important by virtue of the fact that they are capable of division and replacing themselves

TABLE 1-1	Examples of Neurotransmitters	
Neurotransmitter	Location*	Function*
Small-Molecule Transmitters		
Acetylcholine	Junctions with motor effectors (muscles, glands); many parts of brain	Excitatory or inhibitory; involved in memory
Amines		
Serotonin	Several regions of the CNS	Mostly inhibitory; involved in moods and emotions, sleep
Histamine	Brain	Mostly excitatory; involved in emotions and regulation of body temperature and water balance
Dopamine	Brain; autonomic system	Mostly inhibitory; involved in emotions/moods and in regulating motor control
Epinephrine	Several areas of the CNS and in the sympathetic division of the ANS	Excitatory or inhibitory; acts as a hormone when secreted by sympathetic neurosecretory cells of the adrenal gland
Norepinephrine	Several areas of the CNS and in the sympathetic division of the ANS	Excitatory or inhibitory; regulates sympathetic effectors; in brain, involved in emotional responses
Amino Acids		
Glutamate (glutamic acid)	CNS	Excitatory; most common excitatory neurotransmitter in CNS
Gamma-aminobutyric acid (GABA)	Brain	Inhibitory; most common inhibitory neurotransmitter in brain
Glycine	Spinal cord	Inhibitory; most common inhibitory neurotransmitter in spinal cord
Other Small Molecules		
Nitric oxide (NO)	Uncertain	May be a signal from postsynaptic to presynaptic neuron
Large-Molecule Transmitters		
Neuropeptides		
Vasoactive intestinal peptide (VIP)	Brain; some ANS and sensory fibers; retina; gastrointestinal tract	Function in nervous system uncertain
Cholecystokinin (CCK)	Brain; retina	Function in nervous system uncertain
Substance P	Brain, spinal cord, sensory pain pathways; gastrointestinal tract	Mostly excitatory; transmits pain information
Enkephalins	Several regions of CNS; retina; intestinal tract	Mostly inhibitory; act like opiates to block pain
Endorphins	Several regions of CNS; retina; intestinal tract	Mostly inhibitory; act like opiates to block pain

From Thibodeau GA, Patton K: *Anatomy and physiology,* ed 5, St Louis, 2003, Mosby, p 365.
*These are examples only; most of these neurotransmitters are also found in other locations, and many have additional functions.

throughout adulthood. Hence the majority of CNS tumors are of glial origin. The number of glial cells has been estimated to be over 900 billion. The ability to divide also makes glial cells susceptible to abnormal cell division for cancer.

Astrocytes

Astrocytes are 10 times more prevalent than neurons and are widespread, performing many roles throughout the CNS. The cells are the largest and most numerous of the glial cells. They derive their name from the Greek word *astron*, which means stellate or star shaped. Astrocytes contain many processes that radiate from the center of the cell into brain tissue (see Fig. 1-22, *A*). They are thought to nourish the neurons by taking glucose from the blood, converting it to lactic acid, and delivering it to connecting neurons. Astrocytes have numerous microfilaments in their cytoplasm, which is thought to give them some rigidity and contribute to the physical support of neural elements in the CNS. Astrocytes form tight sheaths around the brain's blood capillaries interposed between neurons and blood vessels in the CNS. This functions as one of the morphologic elements to form the blood-brain barrier. The **blood-brain barrier (BBB)** is a restrictive barrier that prevents toxic substances from readily entering the extracellular space of the nervous system. Tight junctions of the brain capillaries and foot processes of the astrocytes are major structural elements of the blood-brain barrier.

Because of their proximity to the blood vessels, astrocytes are also thought to contribute to the nutritional needs of neurons. In injured regions of the CNS, astrocytes have been observed to develop phagocytic properties and contribute to reactive gliosis and scar formation that forms after a surgical incision or healing from a CNS injury.

Oligodendrocytes

Oligodendrocytes are very small cells found throughout the CNS. They have a small, rounded nucleus, and very few

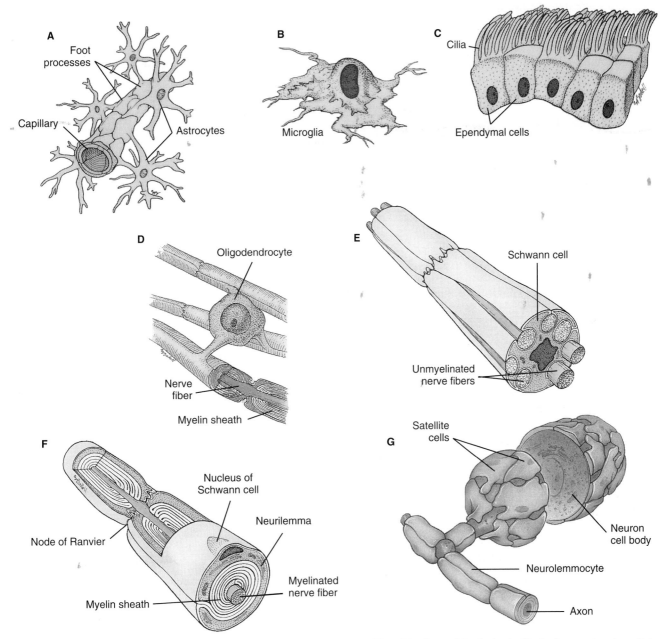

Figure 1-22 Types of glia. **A,** Astrocytes attached to the outside of a capillary blood vessel in the brain. **B,** A phagocytic microglial cell. **C,** Ciliated ependymal cells forming a sheet that usually lines fluid cavities in the brain. **D,** Oligodendrocyte with processes that wrap around nerve fibers in the CNS to form myelin sheaths. **E,** Schwann cell supporting a bundle of nerve fibers in the PNS. **F,** Another type of Schwann cell wrapping around a peripheral nerve fiber to form a thick myelin sheath. **G,** Satellite cells, another type of Schwann cell, surround and support cell bodies of neurons in the PNS.
(From Thibodeau GA, Patton K: Anatomy and physiology, ed 5, St Louis, 2003, Mosby.)

cytoplasmic processes emanate from the cell. In fact, the name *oligodendrocyte* means "few treelike processes." These cells are common in the white matter of the brain and spinal cord (see Fig. 1-22, *D*). Their main function is to produce the fatty myelin sheath in the CNS. Within the CNS, oligodendrocyte processes enwrap axons and lay down several layers of cell membrane to myelinate the axons. In contrast to the neurolemmocyte or Schwann cell, which produces myelin in the PNS and can myelinate only one axon, an oligodendrocyte can myelinate multiple axons. Oligodendrocytes do not produce a basement membrane around the outside of the myelin sheath, unlike neurolemmocytes or Schwann cells, which do produce a basement membrane in the PNS. The regeneration of transected axons is therefore more successful in the PNS, because the basement membrane forms a tunnel through which the regenerating axon can grow outward to reach its effector organ. In the CNS, where the oligodendrocytes do not produce a basement membrane around the outside of the myelin sheath, regenerating axons do not have a tunnel to guide their regeneration.

Microglia

Microglia are small, circulating, and quiescent until needed for their "phagocytic" activity as scavengers. Both astrocytes and oligodendrocytes develop from ectoderm. **Microglia** are mesodermally derived glial cells found mostly in the gray matter that enter the nervous system along with the blood vessels (see Fig. 1-22, *B*). These stationary cells are small and macrophage-like and are difficult to view in brain sections. When called to action from inflamed or degenerating brain tissue, however, they enlarge and become phagocytic. They are the scavengers of the nervous system, phagocytosing debris, microorganisms, and dead cells.

Ependyma

The **ependyma** cells are columnar-shaped to cuboidal-shaped cells that line the ventricles and fluid-filled cavities of the brain and spinal cord. These cells have **microvilli** and **cilia** that probably function in aiding the circulation of CSF within these cavities (see Fig. 1-22, *B*).

Schwann Cells

The Schwann cells are found only in the PNS. They form the myelin sheath around the axons of myelinated peripheral neurons and are the source of myelin. Schwann cells support bundles of nerve fibers in the PNS (see Fig. 1-22, *E*). Other types of Schwann cells called satellite cells surround the cell body of a neuron in regions called ganglia (see Fig. 1-22, *G*).

Spinal Cord

Location and Shape

The **spinal cord** is a long oval-shaped cylinder approximately 1 cm in diameter lodged in the vertebral canal. The average length is 42 to 45 cm, with a weight of approximately 30 g. The cord is an extension superiorly of the medulla oblongata of the brain and tapers as it descends through the foramen magnum at the base of the skull and terminated inferiorly at the level of L1. There are two prominent enlargements along its length in the cervical and the lumbar regions (Fig. 1-23; see also Fig. 1-14). It does not completely fill the spinal cavity, occupying only two thirds of the spinal canal. The spinal cavity also contains the meninges, CSF, a cushion of adipose tissue, and blood vessels.[3] The spinal cord is wrapped in meninges that protect and support it within the bony covering. The dura mater covering the spinal cord consists of only one layer and terminates caudally as a sac at the S2 vertebral level. The dura mater extends along each nerve root and becomes continuous with the tissue surrounding each spinal nerve.

The arachnoid covers the spinal cord; it is continuous from the brain above through the foramen magnum and ends at the S2 vertebral level. The arachnoid also continues along the spinal nerve roots. The pia mater is a vascular membrane close to the spinal cord and becomes thickened on each side between nerve roots to form the **ligamentum denticulatum.** This support allows the spinal cord to be suspended in the middle of the dural sheath. The pia mater extends along each nerve root.

The spinal cord is a relay system that conducts sensory and motor impulses to and from the brain and controls many

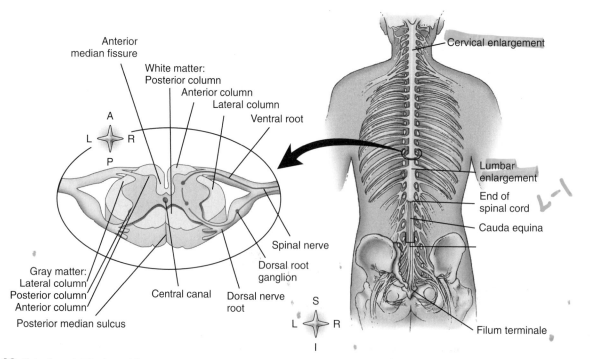

Figure 1-23 Spinal cord. The inset illustrates a transverse section of the spinal cord shown in the broader view. (*From Thibodeau GA, Patton K:* Anatomy and physiology, *ed 5, St Louis, 2003, Mosby.*)

reflexes. Thirty-one pairs of spinal nerves originate and exit from the cord. Unlike the brain, the inner core consists of an H-shaped gray matter consisting of nerve cell bodies, neuroglia, and blood vessels surrounded by an outer covering of white matter (Fig. 1-24).

Cerebrospinal Fluid

Protection of the spinal cord is provided by the CSF, which surrounds the spinal cord in the subarachnoid space. The CSF escapes from the ventricles via the foramina in the fourth ventricle and enters the subarachnoid space to circulate around the spinal cord (see Fig. 1-19).

Extent

The spinal cord is the most inferior part of the CNS and is located within and protected by the vertebral column. Phylogenetically, it is the oldest part of the CNS. The spinal cord is the structure through which information is channeled from the brain to the muscles in the periphery of the body and through which sensation from the body tissues are sent to the brain. The upper end of the spinal cord is located at the **foramen magnum** of the skull. Its lower, tapered end is known as the **conus medullaris** and is located opposite the intervertebral disk between vertebrae L1 and L2. Inferior or caudal to the spinal cord, the dura mater forms the **dural sac,** which extends to the lower border of S2. The dural sac contains the **filum terminale,** a large number of lumbosacral nerve roots which extends from the lower end of the spinal cord surrounding the filum terminale, which is known as the **cauda equina.** It is so named because it resembles a horse's tail. The sac contains CSF. A spinal needle inserted into the lumbar cistern, or subarachnoid space within the dural sac, may create a slight sensation as the needle passes among the nerve roots to allow safe sampling of CSF.

The spinal cord can be divided into 31 segments (Fig. 1-25). Spinal segments are designated by a letter and a number (e.g., C5 is the fifth cervical cord segment, T11 is the eleventh thoracic spinal cord segment). Each segment of the spinal cord gives off a pair of spinal nerves. There are 8 cervical spinal nerves beginning with a nerve that is above C1 and a nerve below C1 (C1–C8), 12 thoracic spinal nerves (T1–T12), 5 lumbar nerves (L1–L5), 5 sacral nerves (S1–S5), and 1 coccygeal pair of spinal nerves. The spinal nerves course outward from the spinal cord to innervate the muscles and skin of the body below the neck. Each spinal nerve and spinal cord segment is responsible for the innervation of muscles and skin in a corresponding body segment.

Enlargements

Although the overall shape of the spinal cord is cylindric, two local swellings are to be noted. The cervical region of the spinal cord demonstrates a **cervical enlargement** between C5 and T1. This enlargement is due to the presence of additional neurons for the innervation of the upper limbs. Likewise, the **lumbar enlargement,** located between L3 and S3, is produced by the presence of additional neurons for the innervation of the lower limbs.

Cross-Sectional Anatomy

A typical cross section through the spinal cord is round or oval and reveals a central, butterfly-shaped area of gray matter that is composed largely of cell bodies, dendrites, synapses, and unmyelinated axons (see Fig. 1-24). The **gray matter** of the spinal cord is divided into **dorsal, ventral,** and lateral horns. Ten distinct cellular laminae within the spinal gray

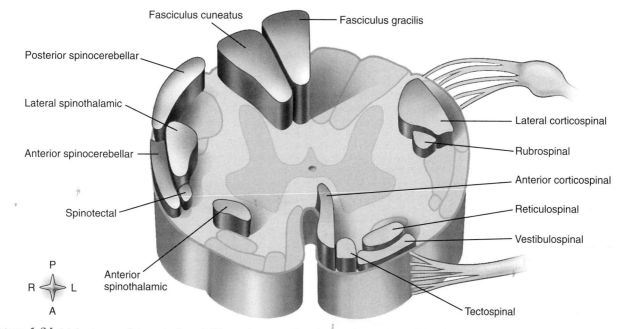

Figure 1-24 Major tracts of the spinal cord. The major ascending (sensory) tracts are highlighted in blue. The major descending (motor) tracts are highlighted in red.
(From Thibodeau GA, Patton K: Anatomy and physiology, ed 5, St Louis, 2003, Mosby.)

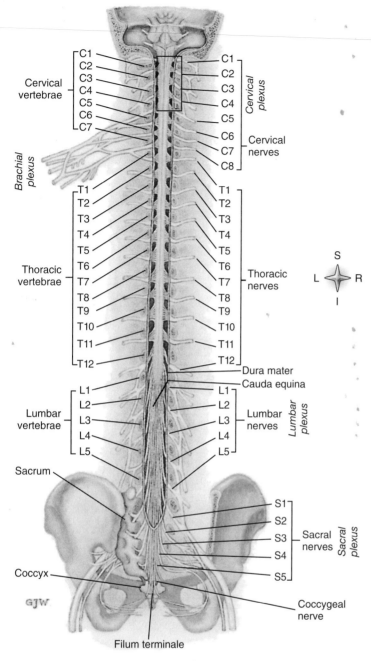

C1
C2
C3
C4
C5
C6
C7

Cervical
vertebrae

C1
C2
C3
C4
C5

Cervical plexus

C6
C7
C8

Cervical
nerves

Brachial plexus

T1
T2
T3
T4
T5
T6
T7
T8
T9
T10
T11
T12

Thoracic
vertebrae

T1
T2
T3
T4
T5
T6
T7
T8
T9
T10
T11
T12

Thoracic
nerves

Dura mater
Cauda equina

L1
L2
L3
L4
L5

Lumbar
vertebrae

L1
L2
L3
L4
L5

Lumbar
nerves

Lumbar plexus

Sacrum

S1
S2
S3
S4
S5

Sacral
nerves

Sacral plexus

Coccyx

Coccygeal
nerve

GJW

Filum terminale

S
L ✦ R
I

Figure 1-25 Spinal nerves. Each of 31 pairs of spinal nerves exits the spinal cavity from the intervertebral foramina. The names of the vertebrae are given on the left and the names of the corresponding spinal nerves on the right. Note that after leaving the spinal cavity, many of the spinal nerves interconnect to form networks called *plexuses*.

matter have been used to describe cell groups and are referred to as **Rexed's laminae I to X.** There are differences in each laminar cell group throughout the spinal cord segments.

Neurotransmitters

Neurotransmitters are chemicals that modify or result in the transmission of nerve impulses between synapses that allow cells to talk to each other. They are released from synaptic knobs into synaptic clefts to bridge the gap between neurons. Excitatory neurotransmitters decrease the negativity of postsynaptic membrane potential, and inhibitory transmitters increase such potentials. Two major excitatory amino acids, **glutamate** and **aspartate,** play an important role as neurotransmitters in the spinal cord (see Table 1-1).

Gray and White Matter

Within each of the horns of the gray matter, functional clusters of neurons are localized to form **nuclei,** aggregates of cell bodies within the CNS that serve specific functions. For example, within the ventral horn of gray matter are distinct nuclei that are responsible for the innervation of specific skeletal muscles.

White matter consists of longitudinally oriented axons that convey messages up and down the spinal cord. It is through these pathways that the spinal cord communicates with the brain. The white matter of the spinal cord is divided into three gross regions called **funiculi.** The dorsal funiculus, which expands on either side of the midline, is located between the dorsal horns of the gray matter. The dorsal and lateral funiculi are clearly separated from one another by the dorsal horns of the gray matter, but separation of the lateral and ventral funiculi is less distinct. Within each of the three funiculi, axons are organized into functionally related bundles called **fasciculi,** or tracts (see Fig. 1-24).

Fasciculi

Fasciculi are composed of axons that have similar cell bodies of origin and cell bodies of termination and serve specific sensory or motor functions. An example of a spinal cord fasciculus is the **lateral spinothalamic tract.** This tract arises from cell bodies in the dorsal horn of the gray matter in the spinal cord. It travels upward through the spinal cord in the lateral funiculus, continues uninterrupted through the brainstem, and terminates in the dorsal thalamus. This tract is the main pathway for conveying pain information from the spinal cord. The various fasciculi that travel in the spinal cord are discussed in later sections of this chapter.

Typical Spinal Nerve

There are **31 pairs of spinal nerves** attached to the spinal cord along its entire length, and they are numbered according to the level of the vertebral area where they emerge: 8 cervical, 12 thoracic, 5 lumbar, 5 sacral, and 1 coccygeal. These nerves carry information from the periphery to the spinal cord and from the spinal cord to the periphery. The spinal nerves innervate the skin and musculature of the entire body below the neck.

Communication takes place between nerves when a **plexus** or network of nerves interjoin. A plexus can be formed by a primary branch of the trunks of nerves (e.g., the cervical, brachial, lumbar, and sacral plexuses). The nerves divide, join, and divide again in a braided effect (Figs. 1-26, 1-27, and 1-28). The anatomy of the plexuses is very complex, and a plexopathy involves more than one spinal or peripheral nerve. Therefore plexopathies are more difficult to recognize and localize than are lesions of the spinal roots or peripheral nerves.

Each spinal nerve consists of a dorsal root and a ventral root. The **dorsal root** enters the dorsal surface of its spinal cord segment. The dorsal root of the spinal nerve carries sensory information into the spinal cord. Cell bodies that have their axons in the dorsal root of the spinal nerve are pseudounipolar neurons located in the **dorsal root ganglia.** The **ventral root** of the spinal nerve is attached to the spinal cord at the junction between the lateral and ventral funiculi. The ventral root consists largely of axons that arise from the cells in the lateral and anterior horn of the gray matter. These are the axons of multipolar neurons that are destined to innervate skeletal muscle and structures of the ANS. The union of the dorsal and ventral roots is the formation of the **spinal nerve.**

After emerging from the intervertebral foramen, the spinal nerve divides into its two terminal branches. The smaller of the two is the **dorsal primary ramus,** which is responsible for innervating a narrow strip of skin and muscle along the dorsal aspect of the vertebral column. The larger branch is the **ventral primary ramus** and is responsible for

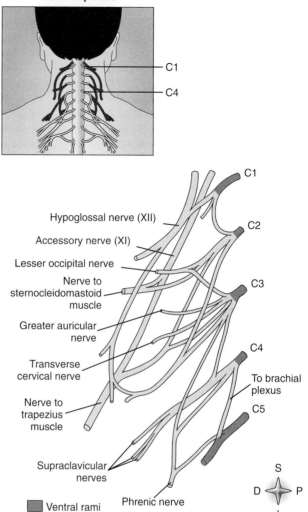

Cervical plexus

Figure 1-26 Cervical plexus. Ventral rami of the first four cervical spinal nerves (C1–C4) exchange fibers in this plexus found deep within the neck. Notice that some of the fibers from C5 enter this plexus to form a portion of the phrenic nerve. *(From Thibodeau GA, Patton K:* Anatomy and physiology, *ed 5, St Louis, 2003, Mosby.)*

innervating muscle and skin along the anterior and lateral body wall and the upper and lower extremities. Each of the spinal nerves has one or more **communicating rami** through which axons of the autonomic preganglionic neurons travel to the ganglia of the ANS.

Typical Spinal Reflex Arc

The **spinal reflex arc** is a protective mechanism to help the body avoid serious tissue damage. If an individual's hand touches a hot stove, the hand is immediately withdrawn without any thought on the part of the individual. The spinal reflex arc, like other reflex arcs, consists of several components (Fig. 1-29).

Sensory endings in the skin detect painful stimuli and generate impulses in afferent neurons, which conduct the painful stimuli toward the spinal cord. These impulses enter the dorsal horn of gray matter of the spinal cord through the

Brachial plexus

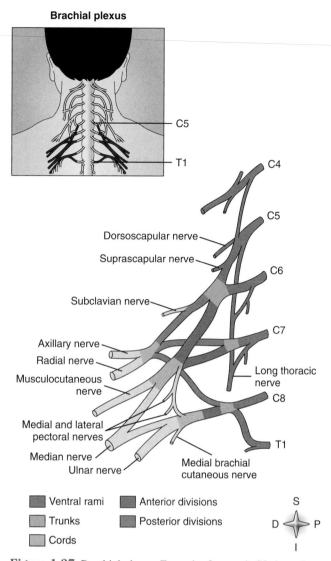

Figure 1-27 Brachial plexus. From the five rami, C3 through T1, the plexus forms three "trunks," each of which, in turn, subdivides into an anterior and a posterior "division." The divisional branches then reorganize into three "cords." The cords give rise to the individual nerves that exit this plexus.
(*From Thibodeau GA, Patton K:* Anatomy and physiology, *ed 5, St Louis, 2003, Mosby.*)

dorsal root of the spinal nerve. Very often, but not always, the incoming afferent neuron synapses on an **interneuron.**

The **interneuron** modifies the signal of the afferent neuron before passing it on to the neurons in the ventral horn of gray matter, where it activates motor neurons to skeletal muscles to complete the reflex arc. These motor/efferent neurons send their axons into the **ventral roots** of the spinal nerves to reach the appropriate skeletal muscles, resulting in the withdrawal of the hand from the hot stove.

Brainstem

The **brainstem** is the central core of the brain and consists of the **medulla, pons,** and **midbrain** (see Fig. 1-13). Although

Lumbosacral plexus

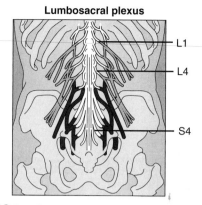

Figure 1-28 Lumbosacral plexus. This plexus is formed by the combination of the lumbar plexus with the sacral plexus. Notice that the ventral rami split into anterior and posterior "divisions" before reorganizing into the various individual nerves that exit this plexus.
(*From Thibodeau GA, Patton K:* Anatomy and physiology, *ed 5, St Louis, 2003, Mosby.*)

each of these regions has intrinsic structures that are related to specific functions of the region, each region also contains the various ascending and descending pathways that carry information between the spinal cord and the brain. The brainstem contains essential brain functions of wakefulness and breathing, conduction of all body motor and sensory tracts, and the origin of all cranial nerves except for cranial nerve I (smell) and II (vision). For example, the systems that control the sleep-wake cycle are believed to be located in the brainstem. Lack of brainstem reflexes (e.g., pupils, corneal, gag, and lack of spontaneous breathing in a comatose patient) are signs of brain death.

Limbic Lobe Versus Limbic System
Limbus is Latin for "border." The **limbic lobe** is a complex, ill-defined area or ring of cortical tissue that is mostly composed of the cingulate gyrus and the parahippocampal gyri of the temporal lobe; it is partially hidden by the brainstem (Fig. 1-30). The limbic lobe and many of the structures with which it is interconnected (e.g., hippocampus, thalamus, olfactory) make up the **limbic system.** This system is thought to play a major role in the primitive emotional response to either hypothalamic activity or to higher thought processes, memory, emotions of feeding behavior, sense of smell, fear, rage, aggression, and fundamental behaviors that ensure the survival of the species (e.g., feeding, mating, and motivation). Limbic lobe seizure activity occurs in this area.

Reticular Formation Versus Reticular Activating System
The **reticular formation** is a phylogenetically primitive network of small neurons that extend throughout the brainstem and into the spinal cord. Impulses from this diffuse network of neurons ascend and descend through a myriad of synapses with facilitatory or inhibitory influences. The reticular formation controls breathing, the heartbeat, blood

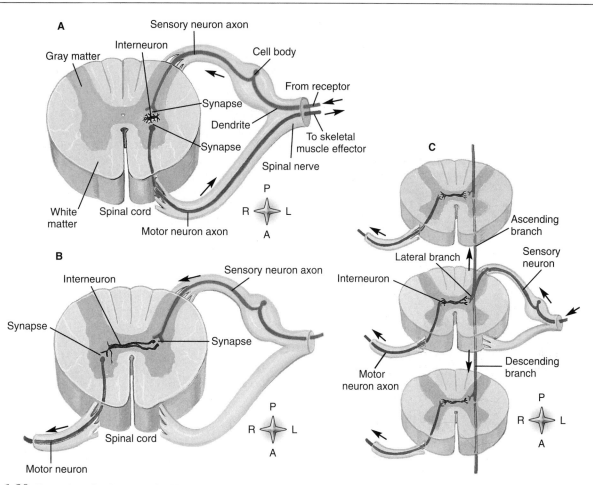

Figure 1-29 Examples of reflex arcs. **A,** Three-neuron ipsilateral reflex arc. Sensory information enters on the same side of the CNS as the motor information leaves the CNS. **B,** Three-neuron contralateral reflex arc. Sensory information enters the opposite side of the CNS from the side that motor information exits the CNS. **C,** Intersegmental reflex arc. Divergent branches of a sensory neuron bring information to several segments of the CNS at the same time. Motor information leaves each segment on the opposite side of the CNS. *(From Thibodeau GA, Patton K: Anatomy and physiology, ed 5, St Louis, 2003, Mosby.)*

pressure, level of consciousness (LOC), and other functions. The **reticular activating system (RAS)** is a functional rather than a morphologic system in the brain. It is thought to ascend and project through thalamic nuclei to the cerebral cortex with a network of nerve fibers in the thalamus, hypothalamus, and brainstem (Fig. 1-31). An intact RAS is essential for wakefulness, attention, concentration, and introspection.

Medulla

The **medulla,** the most inferior part of the brainstem, is located at the foramen magnum of the skull and is continuous with the spinal cord inferiorly. Sections of the caudal end of the medulla resemble those of the upper end of the spinal cord, but the morphology changes greatly as one progresses in a rostral direction along the medulla. The aggregates of neurons that make up the horns of gray matter in the spinal cord become more distinctive as they give rise to the numerous cranial nerve nuclei. The individual fasciculi that

course within the white matter of the spinal cord become separated from one another and are more easily identified (Fig. 1-32).

General Features

The surface features of the medulla are distinctively different from those of the spinal cord. Whereas the spinal cord is round and cylindric in shape, the medulla is more irregular. The central canal of the spinal cord opens into the **fourth ventricle,** which is located on the dorsal aspect of the medulla. The majority of nuclei within the medulla are the nuclei of the origin and termination of the cranial nerves. The remainder of the nuclei in the medulla mediate specific sensory, motor, and integrative functions of the medulla.

The white matter on the ventral aspect of the medulla aggregate into two stout bundles of fibers called the **pyramids.** The axons that make up the pyramids continue into the spinal cord as the **corticospinal tracts.** Lateral to each pyramid is a small oval swelling, the **inferior olive.** The

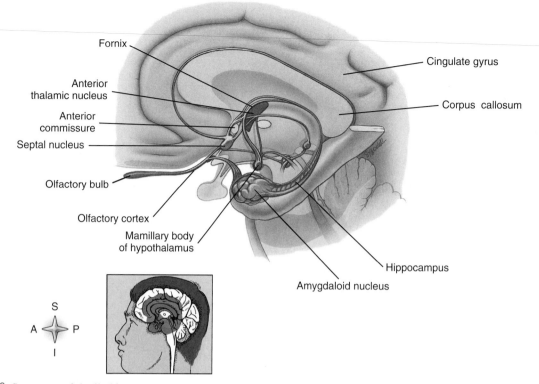

Figure 1-30 Structures of the limbic system.
(From Thibodeau GA, Patton K: Anatomy and physiology, ed 5, St Louis, 2003, Mosby.)

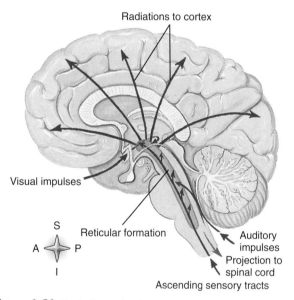

Figure 1-31 Reticular activating system (RAS). Consists of centers in the brainstem reticular formation plus fibers that conduct to the centers from below and fibers that conduct from the centers to widespread areas of the cerebral cortex. Functioning of the RAS is essential for consciousness.
(From Thibodeau GA, Patton K: Anatomy and physiology, ed 5, St Louis, 2003, Mosby.)

neurons that make up the inferior olive send their axons to the cerebellum in the **inferior cerebellar peduncles.** The groove between the inferior olive and the pyramid is called the **preolivary sulcus.** The fibers of the **hypoglossal nerve (cranial nerve [CN] XII)** emerge from the medulla in the preolivary sulcus (see Fig. 1-15). The groove posterior to the olive is the **postolivary sulcus,** through which the **spinal accessory (CN XI), vagus (CN X),** and **glossopharyngeal (CN IX) nerves** emerge from the brainstem. The roof of the fourth ventricle in the rostral end of the medulla is very thin and attenuated and is known as the **inferior medullary vellum.**

Functions

The medulla contains centers for the regulation of the basic rhythm of respiration, rate and strength of the heartbeat (cardiac center), and diameter of the blood vessels (vasomotor area). In addition, neurons of the medulla regulate the reflexes of vomiting, sneezing, swallowing, and coughing. Four of the 12 pairs of cranial nerves have their origin in the medulla: the hypoglossal nerve (CN XII), spinal accessory nerve (CN XI), vagus nerve (CN X), and glossopharyngeal nerve (CN IX) (see Fig. 1-15).

Associated Cranial Nerves

Hypoglossal Nerve (CN XII). The **hypoglossal nerve** (CN XII) is a motor nerve that originates from the cells of the hypoglossal nucleus in the floor of the fourth ventricle. Axons of the hypoglossal nerve course through the medulla to emerge

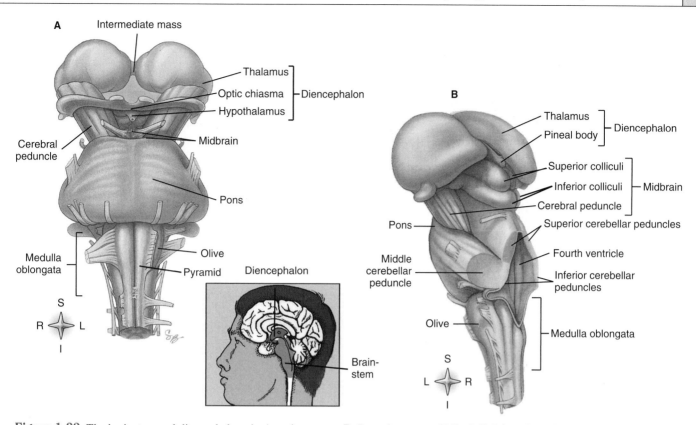

Figure 1-32 The brainstem and diencephalon. **A,** Anterior aspect. **B,** Posterior aspect (shifted slightly to lateral). *(From Thibodeau GA, Patton K:* Anatomy and physiology, *ed 5, St Louis, 2003, Mosby.)*

in the preolivary sulcus. Each hypoglossal nerve leaves the skull by passing through the **hypoglossal canal** to provide motor innervation to the intrinsic and extrinsic muscles of the corresponding half of the tongue. Injury to one hypoglossal nucleus or nerve results in paralysis of the ipsilateral half of the tongue. If a patient with a hypoglossal nerve is asked to protrude his or her tongue, the tongue will deviate toward the side of the injury because of the unopposed action of the contralateral genioglossus muscle (see Fig. 1-15).

Spinal Accessory Nerve (CN XI). The **spinal accessory nerve** (CN XI) is a pure motor nerve consisting of two parts. It emerges onto the surface of the medulla in the postolivary sulcus and leaves the skull through the jugular foramen along with the vagus and glossopharyngeal nerves. Each spinal accessory nerve innervates the ipsilateral **trapezius** and **sternocleidomastoid** muscles. Injury to one spinal accessory nerve results in paralysis of these muscles ipsilaterally, and the patient becomes unable to shrug his or her shoulder or turn his or her head to the opposite side (see Fig. 1-15).

Vagus Nerve (CN X). The **vagus nerve** (CN X), one of the most complex of the cranial nerves, has both sensory and motor functions. Some of the motor fibers of the vagus arise from the **nucleus ambiguus** and innervate many of the muscles of the **pharynx** as well as the **intrinsic muscles of the larynx.** The remainder of the motor fibers of the vagus nerve arise from the **dorsal motor nucleus of the vagus.** The remainder of the motor fibers of the vagus nerve arise from the **dorsal motor nucleus of the vagus** and are preganglionic, parasympathetic axons that terminate in the

ganglia located within the walls of the thoracic and abdominal viscera innervated by the vagus.

The sensory neurons of the vagus nerve carry sensations of touch and pain from the skin around the ear. In addition, the vagus nerve carries sensory information from all of the viscera it innervates to provide sensory input for visceral reflexes. Taste sensations from the root of the tongue and epiglottic region are also carried in the vagus nerve.

Each vagus nerve leaves the skull through one of the jugular foramina to course through the neck in a carotid sheath. The nerves are widely distributed throughout the thorax and abdomen. Unilateral destruction of one vagus nerve as it emerges from the brainstem results in paralysis of all of the muscles innervated by it. Most significant is the paralysis of the ipsilateral vocal cord, which then remains adducted. Bilateral destruction of both vagus nerves can result in asphyxiation, because both vocal cords will be adducted, resulting in blockage of the glottis and obstruction of the airway (Fig. 1-33).

Glossopharyngeal Nerve (CN IX). The **glossopharyngeal nerve** (CN IX) is similar in its composition to the vagus nerve. Motor fibers of the glossopharyngeal nerve originate from the rostral end of the nucleus ambiguus to innervate one muscle of the pharynx, the stylopharyngeus. In addition, preganglionic parasympathetic axons arising from the inferior salivatory nucleus travel in the glossopharyngeal nerve for innervation of the parotid gland.

Somatic sensory neurons are located in the superior ganglion of the glossopharyngeal nerve. Like those of the vagus,

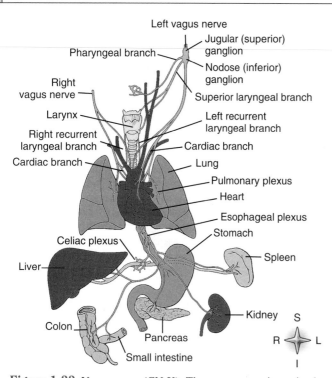

Figure 1-33 Vagus nerve (CN X). The vagus nerve is a mixed cranial nerve with many widely distributed branches—hence the name *vagus,* which is the Latin word for "wanderer." *(From Thibodeau GA, Patton K:* Anatomy and physiology, *ed 5, St Louis, 2003, Mosby.)*

these neurons carry general information from the skin around the ear. Other sensory fibers are distributed to sensory endings in the carotid sinus and constitute an important afferent component of the **carotid sinus reflex.** The glossopharyngeal nerve contains a special afferent branch, the carotid sinus nerve. This branch innervates the carotid body and carotid sinus, which are **chemoreceptor** and **baroreceptor centers**. Elevation of carotid arterial pressure stimulates the carotid sinus nerve; these impulses go to the medulla and to the vagus and its distribution to the ganglion cells in the wall of the heart to slow the heart rate and reduce blood pressure.

The **carotid body** contains special chemoreceptors that respond to changes in the carbon dioxide and oxygen content of the blood. Activation of these chemoreceptors sends impulses through the glossopharyngeal nerve to the nucleus of the solitary tract; these impulses go to the "respiratory center" of the medulla, where they influence the rate of respiration.

Taste sensations from the taste buds of the posterior one third of the tongue (see Fig. 1-15) are also carried in the glossopharyngeal nerve. The fibers of the glossopharyngeal nerve enter and leave the medulla in the postolivary sulcus. Each nerve leaves the skull through one of the jugular foramina of the skull. Unilateral destruction of a glossopharyngeal nerve as it emerges from the brainstem results in loss of the **gag reflex** and the carotid sinus reflex unilaterally.

Pons

General Features

The **pons** is located rostral to the medulla and is separated from it by the **inferior pontine sulcus** ventrally and the **stria medullaris** of the fourth ventricle dorsally. The word *pons* is Latin for "bridge." This designation is derived from the fact that the majority of nerve fibers on the ventral aspect of the pons connect the pons to the cerebellum. These fibers form a "bridge" between the brainstem and the cerebellum known as the **middle cerebellar peduncle.** The **tegmentum** of the pons is located dorsally and contributes to the floor of the fourth ventricle. It also contains a number of pathways that continue into the pons from the medulla. Like the medulla, the pons has a number of nuclei associated with specific cranial nerves. At the rostral end of the pons, the fourth ventricle narrows to become the **cerebral aqueduct.** This region of the pons is known as the **isthmus** region and is separated from the midbrain by the **superior pontine sulcus** (see Figs. 1-13 and 1-32).

Functions

In conjunction with the rhythmicity area of the medulla, the **pneumotaxic area** (controls the rate of respiration) and **apneustic area** (controls the length of respiration) of the pons contribute to the control of respirations through pathways that traverse the pontine reticular formation. CNs VIII, VII, VI, and V are associated with this region and are discussed in the following sections.

Associated Cranial Nerves

Vestibulocochlear Nerve (CN VIII). The **vestibulocochlear nerve** (CN VIII) enters the brainstem in the region of the **pontomedullary junction.** As its name implies, this cranial nerve is associated with the special senses of equilibrium, balance, and hearing. It is frequently injured together with the facial nerve in fractures of the middle fossa of the base of the skull or blows to the head. The **vestibular ganglion** of CN VIII contains bipolar neurons that send their peripheral processes into the **semicircular canals, sacculus,** and **utricle,** where they terminate in special sensory endings that detect changes in head position relative to gravity and changes in the angular acceleration of the body. The central processes terminate in the vestibular nuclei located in the pons and upper medulla. Information received from the vestibular portion of CN VIII by the vestibular nuclei is relayed to the cerebellum for reflex adjustment of muscle tone and posture, thus keeping the body in balance.

The bipolar neurons of the vestibulocochlear nerve that are related to hearing have their cell bodies located in the **spiral ganglion.** The spiral ganglion is embedded in the bone of the inner ear that is part of the **cochlea.** The peripheral processes of these neurons are associated with the specialized receptors in the cochlea. They respond to vibration of the **tympanic membrane,** which in turn stimulates wave motion in the **endolymph.** The central processes of these neurons enter the brainstem in the auditory nerve, where they synapse in the dorsal and ventral cochlear nuclei (see Fig. 1-15).

Facial Nerve (CN VII). The **facial nerve** (CN VII) has both sensory and motor functions. The motor fibers of the facial nerve that arise from the **superior salivatory nucleus** of the pons are preganglionic, parasympathetic neurons that control the **lacrimal glands** and the submandibular and sublingual **salivary glands.** The remaining motor fibers of the facial nerve arise from the **facial nucleus** in the tegmentum of the pons. These neurons course rostrally and dorsally in the pontine tegmentum, where they loop over the **abducens nucleus** before leaving the pons in the cerebellopontine (CP) angle. They innervate the muscles of facial expression, as well as a number of other muscles in the face.

The sensory fibers in the facial nerve originate in the **geniculate ganglion,** which is located within the temporal bone of the skull. Some of these sensory neurons innervate the skin lining the external auditory meatus, from which they carry general sensory information. The remaining sensory neurons of the facial nerve carry taste sensations from the anterior two thirds of the tongue.

Each facial nerve leaves the pons in the pontomedullary junction to enter the **internal acoustic meatus** along with the vestibulocochlear nerve. The facial nerve gives off a number of branches within the temporal bone. The main stem of the facial nerve, containing axons from the nucleus of the facial nerve, leaves the skull through the **stylomastoid foramen** and branches on the surface of the face to provide motor innervation to the muscles of facial expression.

Destruction of the facial nerve in the posterior cranial fossa as it enters the internal acoustic meatus results in the loss of all sensory and motor functions of the nerve. Destruction of individual branches results in the loss of specific functions. The main trunk of the facial nerve is often compressed or injured as it emerges from the stylomastoid foramen of the skull, which results in paralysis of the muscles of facial expression ipsilaterally in a condition known as **Bell's palsy.** It is more frequently paralyzed than any other cranial nerve (see Fig. 1-15).

Abducens Nerve (CN VI). The **abducens nerve** (CN VI) has a pure motor function. Arising from the abducens nucleus in the pons, the fibers emerge from the brainstem ventrally at the pontomedullary junction. The nerve courses forward from the pons to enter the orbit of the skull through the superior orbital fissure. In the orbit, the abducens nerve provides innervation to the ipsilateral **lateral rectus muscle.** This muscle abducts the pupil of the eye from the midline. Injury or destruction of the abducens nerve in either the brainstem or the orbit results in paralysis of the lateral rectus muscle. A CN VI palsy results from a fracture at the base of the skull. The unopposed action of the medial rectus muscle results in the pupil of the eye being adducted (internal strabismus) when at rest (see Fig. 1-15).

Trigeminal Nerve (CN V). The **trigeminal nerve** (CN V) is the largest of the cranial nerves. It is called the "great sensory nerve of the face" because its major function is to carry sensory information from the skin and mucous membranes of the head and neck. In addition to its sensory function, the trigeminal nerve is responsible for the innervation of eight pairs of muscles in the head, including the four pairs of muscles of **mastication.**

The cell bodies of most of the sensory fibers of the trigeminal nerve are located in the **trigeminal ganglion.** The peripheral processes of these neurons are organized into three divisions. From superior to inferior, these divisions are the **ophthalmic, maxillary,** and **mandibular** divisions. The ophthalmic division carries sensory innervation from the skin of the upper face and forehead, bridge of the nose, cornea, and eyelid. The maxillary division carries sensory innervation from the upper jaw, cheek, and upper teeth, as well as the mucous membranes of the palate, nasal cavity, and nasal sinuses. The mandibular division carries sensory innervation from the lower jaw and associated skin of the face, lower teeth, and mucous membranes of the oral cavity.

The central processes of the sensory neurons of the trigeminal nerve constitute the **portio major** of the nerve. The portio minor, or motor part of the trigeminal nerve, accompanies the mandibular division of the nerve in the periphery (see Fig. 1-15).

Trigeminal neuralgia (tic douloureux) is a condition in which spontaneous pain impulses arise in one or more divisions of the trigeminal facial nerve. Pain radiates along the course of the branch of the nerve from the angle of the jaw (see Chapter 16).

Midbrain

The midbrain, located immediately rostral to the pons, is a short, constricted part of the brainstem (see Figs. 1-13 and 1-32).

General Features

The dorsal surface of the midbrain or tectum consists of four rounded masses. The caudal pair of eminences is the **inferior colliculi,** and the rostral pair is the **superior colliculi.** The superior colliculi are divided into a superficial area for the processing of visual stimuli and a deeper portion for the integration of visual and auditory motor reflexes. The inferior colliculi are auditory relay nuclei. They receive fibers from the optic nerve and serve as reflex centers for eye movements and blinking. The **cerebral aqueduct,** a portion of the ventricular system of the brain, runs through the center of the midbrain (see Figs. 1-18 and 1-19).

In the tegmentum of the midbrain are a number of nuclei, including the red nuclei (which give rise to the rubrospinal tracts) and those nuclei related to specific cranial nerves.

The **substantia nigra** is located on the dorsal aspect of the **cerebral peduncles.** The cerebral peduncles are thick columns of tissue on the ventral aspect of the midbrain. The neurons of the substantia nigra contain melanin and are therefore black. Degeneration of the neurons in the substantia nigra is the basis of parkinsonism.

Large fiber bundles occupy the ventral surface of each cerebral peduncle. Many of the axons in these bundles synapse in the pontine nuclei. Some of the fibers of the cerebral peduncles become the pyramids in the medulla and continue into the spinal cord as the corticospinal tracts.

Associated Cranial Nerves

Two pairs of cranial nerves (CN IV and CN III) are associated with the midbrain.

Trochlear Nerve (CN IV). The more caudal of the cranial nerves is the **trochlear nerve** (CN IV), which is the longest of the cranial nerves. Each trochlear nerve arises from one of the **trochlear nuclei.** They course dorsally and cross one another in the roof of the midbrain at the **pontomesencephalic junction.** The trochlear nerves are the only cranial nerves that exit from the dorsal surface of the brainstem. Dysfunction may cause giddiness when descending steps due to double vision when looking downward. They leave the cranial cavity by passing through the superior orbital fissure.

On entering the orbit, each trochlear nerve innervates one of the extraocular eye muscles, the superior oblique. The action of the superior oblique muscle is to direct the pupil of the eye down and out. Because of their emergence from the dorsal aspect of the brainstem and their long intracranial course, the trochlear nerves are particularly vulnerable to injury. Injuries to these nerves are difficult to detect because other extraocular eye muscles can compensate for the movement produced by the superior oblique (see Fig. 1-15).

Oculomotor Nerve (CN III). The **oculomotor nerve** (CN III) is a motor nerve that provides innervation to some of the muscles that move the eye. Each oculomotor nerve arises from the oculomotor nucleus to emerge on the ventral surface of the midbrain in the **interpeduncular fossa.** The nerves leave the cranial cavity by passing into the orbit through the superior orbital fissure. Within the orbit, each oculomotor nerve innervates four of the extraocular eye muscles: superior rectus, medial rectus, inferior rectus, and inferior oblique. In addition, the oculomotor nerve innervates the levator palpebrae superior muscle, which lifts the upper eyelid.

Some fibers of the oculomotor nerve arise from the **Edinger-Westphal nuclei,** which are located in the tegmentum of the midbrain. These parasympathetic preganglionic neurons control both the constrictor pupillae muscles of the eye, which decrease the diameter of the pupil, and the ciliary muscles, which control the thickness of the lens.

Lesions of the oculomotor nerve that result in paralysis of the medial rectus will result in unopposed activity of the lateral rectus; the pupil is then abducted at rest (external strabismus). In addition, destruction of the oculomotor nerve results in the loss of parasympathetic innervation of the constrictor pupillae muscles, resulting in dilation of the pupils by the sympathetic division of the ANS (see Fig. 1-15).

Diencephalon

The region immediately rostral to the midbrain is the **diencephalon.** The major divisions of the diencephalon are the **thalamus, hypothalamus, epithalamus,** and **subthalamus.** These structures surround the third ventricle (Fig. 1-34).

General Features and Subdivisions
Dorsal Thalamus. The right and left **thalami** surround the third ventricle. In about 20% of the population, they are connected to one another via the **interthalamic adhesion,** a mass of gray matter that occupies the third ventricle. The dorsal thalamus is a relay center for the sensory and motor pathways. All sensory information coming into the brain

from the spinal cord or the cranial nerves is processed in the dorsal thalamus before being sent to the cerebrum. The only exception to this is the sense of smell (olfaction), which enters the cerebral cortex directly. In addition, the motor areas of the cerebrum and cerebellum send information to the dorsal thalamus. In this way, the dorsal thalamus also serves as a motor relay center. Feelings of well-being or malaise are thought to originate in the dorsal thalamus. The appreciation of **temperature, pain,** and **light touch** is also thought to be an important function of the dorsal thalamus.

Hypothalamus. The **hypothalamus** is located ventral to the dorsal thalamus. The hypothalamus is the CNS regulatory center for the ANS. Consequently, a number of visceral activities are associated with the hypothalamus. Control of **water balance, temperature regulation, sexual activity, cardiovascular regulation,** and **activity of the gastrointestinal tract** have been identified as functions of the hypothalamus. The hypothalamus exerts its control through descending pathways that influence the activity of neurons of the ANS.

The identification of feeding and satiety centers in the hypothalamus suggests possible CNS causes of certain eating disorders such as anorexia and bulimia. In addition, the hypothalamus is known to control the release of certain hormones from the pituitary gland, which makes it difficult to separate certain glandular disorders from neural disorders (see Fig. 1-34).

Epithalamus. The **pineal gland** and its associated structures constitute the **epithalamus.** The pineal gland is thought to respond to the cycle of light in the environment through input from the visual system. It is also thought to regulate the onset of puberty in humans. Deposits of an amorphous substance in the pineal gland, called "brain sand," result in calcification of the gland and are easily identifiable on x-ray examination. Shifts of the pineal gland from its midline position usually indicate intracranial disease (see Fig. 1-34).

Subthalamus. The **subthalamus** is a small nuclear group of neurons that is considered part of the basal ganglia. It has motor functions and is discussed later in this chapter with the motor systems.

Associated Cranial Nerves
Optic Nerve (CN II). The **optic nerve** (CN II) is associated with the diencephalon and is the special sensory nerve for vision (see Fig. 1-15). The optic nerve and the visual pathway are discussed in greater detail later in this chapter.

Cerebrum

General Features and Subdivisions
The **cerebrum** is the most highly evolved part of the brain in humans. The cerebral cortex is the organ of thought and consists of two cerebral hemispheres. These two hemispheres appear the same but are functionally different. The **left hemisphere** is thought to be involved in language, recognition of printed words and numbers, prosody, memory related to language, and complex movement sequences and gestures such as writing. The left hemisphere is the dominant hemisphere for language for almost all right-handed adults and for many left-handed adults.

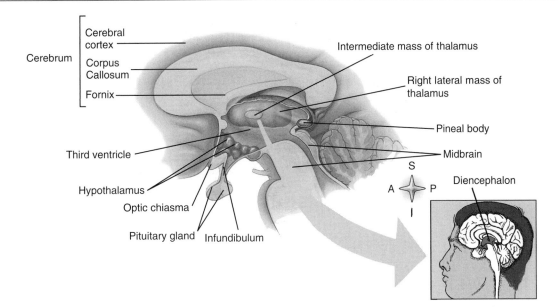

Figure 1-34 Diencephalon and surrounding structures. This midsagittal section highlights the largest regions of the diencephalon, the thalamus and hypothalamus, but also shows the smaller optic chiasm and pineal body. Note the position of the diencephalon between the midbrain and the cerebrum. Compare this view of the diencephalon with that in Figure 1-32. *(From Thibodeau GA, Patton K: Anatomy and physiology, ed 5, St Louis, 2003, Mosby.)*

The **right hemisphere** controls spatial abilities and drawing and is specialized to process figures and faces and memory of places. The clinician should be alert to these differences following injury (e.g., stroke or acquired brain injury).

The cerebral cortex is the thin layer or mantle of gray substance covering the surface of each hemisphere, folded into gyri that are separated by sulci. The cerebral cortex is an aggregation of neuron cell bodies that form the surface of the two cerebral hemispheres. The surface of each cerebral hemisphere is highly convoluted. These convolutions, or **gyri,** are separated by shallow grooves called **sulci.** Deeper sulci are called **fissures.** In histologic section, the surface of the cerebrum can be seen as covered with a thick layer of gray matter known as the **cerebral cortex** that covers the surface of each cerebral hemisphere. Like gray matter elsewhere in the brain, the cerebral cortex consists of cell bodies, dendrites, unmyelinated axons, and synapses. The cerebral cortex is responsible for thinking and the higher mental functions; for general movement; for visceral functions, perception, and behavioral reactions; and for the association and integration of these functions. Beneath the cortex is a layer of **medullary white matter** consisting of axons that are largely myelinated and that arise from various parts of the nervous system. The connection between the cortical areas is as important as or more important than an individual cortical area because it allows many different areas to communicate. This connection is carried out by the white matter, which consists of bundles of axons that are extensions of neurons. White matter tracts can be very short, connecting adjacent cortical areas, or very long, connecting distant cortical or subcortical regions. The degree of white matter disruption can be directly correlated with the degree of neurologic impairment following brain injury. The primary somatic

motor area has been mapped according to the specific areas of the body it controls (Fig. 1-35).

The cerebral hemispheres are divided into lobes that are named for the bones of the skull with which they are associated—**frontal, parietal, occipital,** and **temporal lobes.** In general, the right cerebral hemisphere receives sensory information from and controls motor activity for the left side of the body, whereas the left cerebral hemisphere receives sensory information from and controls motor activity for the right side of the body.

Frontal Lobe

The **frontal lobe** of each cerebral hemisphere is located beneath the frontal bone of the skull and rests on the orbit of the eye in the anterior cranial fossa of the skull. The rostral boundary of the frontal lobe is the **frontal pole.** Caudally, the frontal lobe ends in a sulcus **(central sulcus),** which courses along the lateral surface of the cerebral hemisphere (see Fig. 1-35).

The major functions ascribed to the frontal lobe are the initiation of motor activity and voluntary movement, personality and mood, initiative, "executive function," planning, concentration, insight, social behavior, speech, conscious thought, abstract thinking, and judgment. The gyrus immediately in front of the central sulcus, the **precentral gyrus,** has been identified as the primary motor area of the cerebrum. This primary voluntary motor area has a somatotopic organization that is often referred to as *Homunculus,* or little man (Fig. 1-36). This is based largely on the observation that stimulation of this region elicits motor responses in muscles on the opposite side of the body. Secondary and supplementary motor areas also have been identified in the frontal lobe. These regions are believed to largely direct the primary motor cortex in the execution of various motor programs.

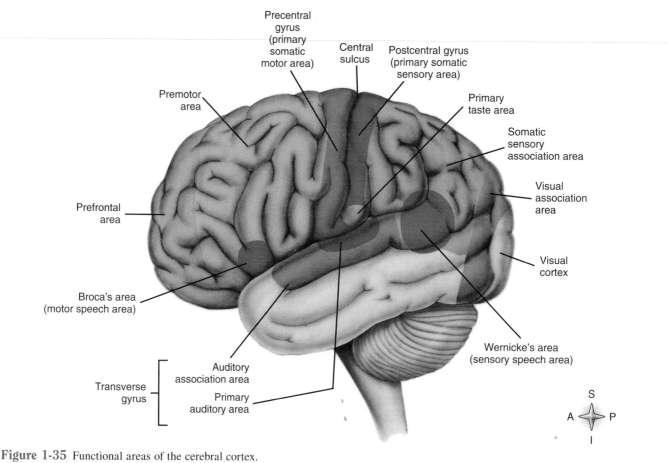

Figure 1-35 Functional areas of the cerebral cortex.
(From Thibodeau GA, Patton K: Anatomy and physiology, ed 5, St Louis, 2003, Mosby.)

The **frontal eye fields,** which are located in the caudal part of the middle frontal gyrus, have been identified for the initiation of conjugate, voluntary deviation of the eyes to the opposite side. The **prefrontal area** of the frontal lobe is believed to be concerned with affective reactions to the present based on experience.

Parietal Lobe. The **parietal lobes** are located beneath the parietal bones of the skull within the middle cranial fossa. The rostral boundary of each parietal lobe is the **central sulcus** (see Fig. 1-35). The caudal boundary of the parietal lobe is not sharply demarcated on the lateral surface of the cerebral hemisphere, but on the medial aspect of the cerebral hemisphere the parietal and occipital lobes are clearly separated by the **parieto-occipital fissure.**

The parietal lobes include the **primary somatosensory area** of the brain, which is located in the **postcentral gyrus.** The primary somatosensory area is the region in which general sensory information from the opposite side of the body is processed. It also functions in the localization of sensory information to the body surface.

In addition to the primary somatosensory area, a **secondary somatosensory area** has been identified in each parietal lobe. The exact role of this region in sensory perception is not known, but it is thought to be involved in the less discriminative aspects of sensation. Much of the parietal cortex constitutes the **somesthetic association cortex.** The

somesthetic association cortex allows familiar objects to be recognized by holding or touching them, largely based on experience. Lesions of the parietal association cortex result in an inability to understand the significance of sensory inputs. Such a deficit is called an **agnosia.**

The parietal lobes are the areas most commonly involved in strokes, which often result in bizarre behaviors by the patient. Patients with parietal strokes often are unable to distinguish between the right and left sides of their bodies, tell time, or recognize familiar objects held in their hands.

Occipital Lobe. The **occipital lobe** of each cerebral hemisphere is wedge shaped and extends from the parieto-occipital fissure rostrally to the **occipital pole** caudally. The **calcarine sulcus** divides the medial surface of each occipital lobe into superior and inferior portions (see Fig. 1-35).

The occipital lobe contains the **primary visual cortex** for the perception and interpretation of visual input from the eyes. This area is on the medial surface of each occipital lobe and borders the calcarine fissure. Projections from the visual pathway must reach this area of the occipital lobe for vision to occur. The lateral surface of the occipital lobe is the visual association cortex, which stores information from previous visual experiences. The **occipital eye center,** located within the occipital lobe, receives inputs from the superior colliculus of the midbrain and causes reflex movement of the eyes to track moving objects in the visual field.

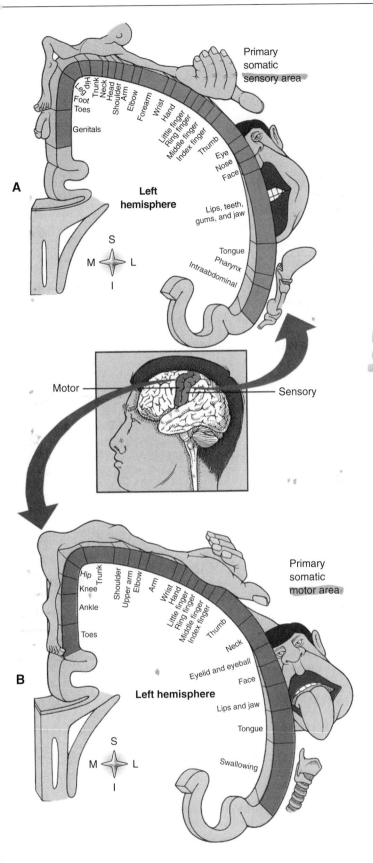

Temporal Lobe. The **temporal lobe** is located in the middle cranial fossa beneath the temporal bone. It is separated from the rest of the cerebral hemisphere by the **lateral fissure (of Sylvius).** If the cerebral hemisphere is likened to a boxing glove or mitten, the hand part of the glove or mitten would include the frontal, parietal, and occipital lobes, and the temporal lobe would be the thumb (see Fig. 1-35).

The major function of the temporal lobe is localized in the **primary auditory area,** which is located in the **transverse temporal gyri (of Heschl)** in the floor of the lateral fissure. This region of cortex receives inputs from the auditory pathway and is involved in the processing of auditory information. The **auditory association cortex** of the temporal lobe is important in language function.

The **hippocampus** is located medially in the temporal lobe. Phylogenetically, it is an older part of the cerebrum and is involved in emotion and sexual behavior. The hippocampus coordinates these responses through its connections with the hypothalamus via the **fornix.** Long-term memory is thought to be functionally related to the association cortex within all areas of the cerebrum, but recent memory processing is thought to be largely the role of the hippocampus and its related structures. Bilateral damage to the temporal lobe may result in memory loss, particularly long-term memory loss (see Chapter 11).

Insular Gyri. Deep within the medial wall of the lateral fissure of the cerebral hemisphere is a collection of gyri that are not considered to be part of any of the four lobes. These are the **insular gyri,** three or four parallel gyri that course along the side of the cerebral hemisphere deep within the lateral fissure. The exact function of the insular gyri is not known.

Associated Cranial Nerves

Olfactory Nerve (CN I). The **olfactory nerve** (CN I) is the only cranial nerve to have direct connections with the cerebrum. It is concerned with the special sensation of smell. It is not actually a nerve at all but instead consists of numerous nerve cells located in the mucosa of the roof of the nasal cavity. These cells pierce the cribriform plate of the ethmoid bone to enter the olfactory bulb in the anterior cranial fossa. Olfactory impulses are transmitted from the olfactory bulbs into the temporal lobe of the cerebrum via the **olfactory tracts.** Olfaction is the only sensation that does not pass through the thalamus before reaching the cerebrum.

Cerebral White Matter

The **cerebral white matter** is made up of the fibers that allow the cerebrum to communicate with the rest of the CNS.

Figure 1-36 Primary somatic sensory (**A**) and motor (**B**) areas of the cortex. The body parts illustrated here show which parts of the body are "mapped" to specific areas of each cortical area. The exaggerated face indicates that more cortical area is devoted to processing information to/from the many receptors and motor units of the face than the leg or arm, for example.
(From Thibodeau GA, Patton K: Anatomy and physiology, ed 5, St Louis, 2003, Mosby.)

The fibers that make up the cerebral white matter can be classified into three major groups according to their origins and terminations.

Association Fibers

The association bundles allow for the exchange of information between lobes within each hemisphere. **Association fibers** connect the adjacent gyri and lobes of the same cerebral hemisphere. Short association fibers interconnect adjacent gyri, and the long association fibers interconnect the lobes within a cerebral hemisphere. The major association bundle in the cerebrum is the **superior longitudinal fasciculus (SLF),** which interconnects the parietal, temporal, occipital, and frontal lobes. Other, less prominent association bundles are also present.

Commissural Fibers

Commissural fibers, which cross the midline, interconnect equivalent regions of the right and left cerebral hemispheres. The largest of these bundles of fibers is the massive **corpus callosum,** which can best be observed on the medial surface of a brain cut in the sagittal plane (see Fig. 1-30). The corpus callosum is a transverse band of nerve fibers that join the cerebral hemispheres. It is located at the bottom of the longitudinal fissure between the two hemispheres and is covered by the cingulate gyrus. The corpus callosum is divided into the **genu** (which interconnects the frontal lobes anteriorly), the **body** (which interconnects the parietal lobes), and the **splenium** (which interconnects the occipital lobes posteriorly). The two temporal lobes are connected by a separate commissure **(anterior commissure),** which is located inferior to the genu of the corpus callosum.

Projection Fibers

Projection fibers connect the cerebral cortex with lower brain centers in the brainstem and spinal cord. Some of these fibers arise from cells of the cerebral cortex and project downward to lower brain levels, where they influence the activities of various nuclei in the brainstem and spinal cord. Other projection fibers arise from cells in the nuclei of lower brain levels and convey information upward to the cerebral cortex. Within the cerebral hemisphere, most projection fibers are organized into a wide band of white matter called the **internal capsule.**

The **internal capsule** is L shaped in horizontal sections of the brain. It is divided into the **anterior limb, genu,** and **posterior limb.** The internal capsule is bounded medially by the dorsal thalamus, anteriorly by the caudate nucleus, and laterally by the lentiform nucleus. The latter two nuclei are part of the basal ganglia, which are discussed in the next section. The majority of fibers in the anterior limb of the internal capsule are **frontopontine fibers,** which arise in the frontal cortex and terminate in the pontine nuclei of the ventral pons. The **pontine nuclei** send input into the cerebellum; thus the frontopontine fibers provide a pathway for the motor cortex to influence the activity of the cerebellum. **Corticobulbar** and **corticospinal** fibers leave the motor cortex of the cerebrum and then project through the genu and posterior limb of the internal capsule to influence the activity

of the motor nuclei of the cranial nerves (corticobulbar fibers) and the cells in the anterior horns of the gray matter in the spinal cord (corticospinal fibers). The posterior limb of the internal capsule carries fibers from the dorsal thalamus to the general sensory areas of the parietal lobe; the **retrolenticular** part carries fibers for the visual pathway from the dorsal thalamus to the occipital lobe, and the **sublenticular** part carries projection fibers from the auditory nuclei of the dorsal thalamus to the temporal lobe of the brain.

Basal Ganglia

Islands of gray matter located deep within the white matter of the hemispheres are called cerebral nuclei or **basal ganglia.** Collectively, the basal ganglia constitute the **corpus striatum,** the **amygdaloid nucleus,** and the **claustrum** (Fig. 1-37). These structures are thought to represent a phylogenetically old motor system in the brain in which "programs" for stereotypic and repetitive movements originate. The basal ganglia controls and is programmed for automatic movement. The basal ganglia exert their influence on the motor cortex of the cerebrum through their connections with the motor nuclei of the dorsal thalamus. The amygdaloid nucleus is buried medially in the temporal lobe. The claustrum is a thin layer of gray matter located just beneath the **insular gyri.** Its function is poorly understood. The largest portion of the basal ganglia is the corpus striatum, which is made up of the **lentiform nucleus** and the **caudate nucleus.** The caudate nucleus is located rostral to the anterior limb of the internal capsule; the lentiform nucleus, consisting of the **globus pallidus** and **putamen,** is located lateral to the internal capsule. The most important are the caudate nucleus, the putamen, and the pallidum. The basal ganglia is surrounded by the rings of the limbic system and lie between the thalamus of the diencephalons and the white matter of the hemisphere.

Like the cerebellum, the basal ganglia influence activity indirectly by their connections with the dorsal thalamus and the cerebral cortex, particularly the motor cortex. Lesions of the basal ganglia result in a variety of **dyskinesias** of movement disorders that are characterized by the presence of "tremors at rest." The patient displays a number of brisk, jerky movements **(choreiform movements);** slow, sinuous movements **(athetoid movements);** or other inappropriate and purposeless movements.

BLOOD SUPPLY OF THE CENTRAL NERVOUS SYSTEM

The **blood supply** of the CNS is derived from two major sets of arteries. The brain receives about 20% of the total resting cardiac output. For the blood supply of the posterior system, two vertebral arteries join at the lower brainstem to form the basilar artery. The **vertebrobasilar system** of vessels supplies blood posteriorly to the caudal parts of the brain (e.g., to perfuse the occipital lobe) and the spinal cord. The blood supply of the anterior system arises from the bifurcation of the common carotid artery that divides into the anterior and middle cerebral arteries. Anteriorly, the **internal carotid**

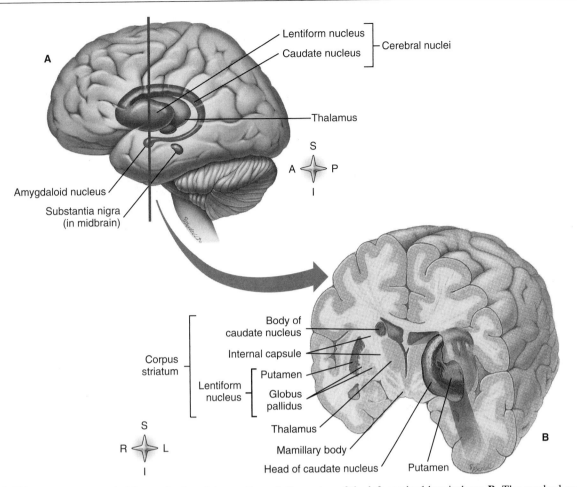

Figure 1-37 Cerebral nuclei. **A,** The cerebral nuclei seen through the cortex of the left cerebral hemisphere. **B,** The cerebral nuclei seen in frontal (coronal) section of the brain.
(From Thibodeau GA, Patton K: Anatomy and physiology, *ed 5, St Louis, 2003, Mosby.)*

system of vessels supplies blood to the rostral parts of the brain. These two systems interconnect with one another at the base of the brain to form the **cerebral arterial circle (circle of Willis)** (Fig. 1-38). The circle of Willis is formed by interconnections of the internal carotid, anterior cerebral, posterior cerebral, basilar, anterior communicating, and posterior communicating arteries. The circle of Willis allows for distribution of blood across the brain.

Vertebral Arteries

The paired **vertebral arteries** arise from the subclavian arteries and course upward in the transverse cervical foramina. After piercing the posterior atlanto-occipital membrane, they ascend through the foramen magnum of the skull on the anterior surface of the spinal cord and medulla and supply approximately 50 to 100 ml/min of blood to the brain.

Each vertebral artery gives off **anterior** and **posterior** spinal arteries. The right and left anterior spinal arteries unite with one another to form a single anterior spinal artery that courses inferiorly in the anterior median sulcus of the spinal cord to supply the anterior two thirds of the spinal

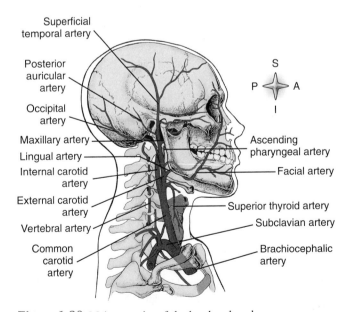

Figure 1-38 Major arteries of the head and neck.
(From Thibodeau GA, Patton K: Anatomy and physiology, *ed 5, St Louis, 2003, Mosby.)*

cord. The branches of the vertebral arteries provide the principal blood supply for virtually the entire cervical spinal cord.

The posterior spinal arteries retain their individuality, and each courses inferiorly on the posterior surface of the spinal cord medial to the dorsal roots of the spinal nerves. The spinal arteries, at the point at which they arise from the vertebral arteries, supply only the upper cervical spinal cord. As they course inferiorly, they are reinforced at periodic intervals by the **radicular arteries,** which are branches of the segmental arteries of the aorta.

The **posteroinferior cerebellar arteries (PICA),** which also arise from the vertebral arteries, supply blood to the posterior parts of the cerebellum and the lateral region of the medulla. The vertebral arteries fuse with one another on the basilar surface of the pons to form the unpaired or single **basilar artery.** Branches of the basilar artery include the **anterior-inferior cerebellar artery (AICA),** which supplies the inferior surface of the cerebellum, the upper medulla, and the caudal pons. The **internal auditory** or **labyrinthine artery,** which enters the internal acoustic meatus, supplies the auditory nerve. Its occlusion can lead to vertigo and ipsilateral deafness. **Pontine branches** of the basilar artery supply the pons, and the **superior cerebellar artery (SCA)** supplies the superior surface of the cerebellum. The basilar artery terminates by dividing into a pair of **posterior** cerebral arteries, which supply blood to the occipital lobes of the cerebrum and to the inferior surface of the temporal lobes (Fig. 1-39).

Internal Carotid Arteries

The **internal** and **external carotid arteries** arise from the bifurcation of the **common carotids.** The external carotid arteries supply blood to the face and neck, and the internal carotids ascend in the neck without providing any branches. The brain receives approximately 750 to 800 ml/min of blood, or about 15% to 25% of the resting cardiac output. Each internal carotid artery supplies approximately 250 ml/min of blood to the brain.

The first branches to arise from the internal carotid arteries are the **hypophyseal arteries,** which supply the hypophysis. The **ophthalmic arteries** arise from the internal carotids immediately after they enter the middle cranial fossa. The ophthalmic arteries enter the orbit by passing through the optic canals and supply structures within the orbit. At the base of the brain, each internal carotid gives off a **posterior communicating** branch that anastomoses with a posterior cerebral branch of the **basilar artery.**

Each internal carotid artery terminates by dividing into **anterior** and **middle cerebral arteries (MCAs).** The MCAs are the largest of the terminal branches. They course within the lateral fissure of the cerebral hemisphere, giving off frontal, parietal, and occipital branches that ramify on the lateral surface of the cerebral hemisphere. They are the principal blood supply of the parietal lobe. It has been recognized that nearly 90% of all strokes involve the MCA of the brain.

The two anterior cerebral arteries run along the base of the brain to meet in the midline, where they are connected to one another by the small **anterior communicating artery (ACA).** Each anterior cerebral artery courses upward along the genu of the corpus callosum, supplying cortical branches to the medial face of the cerebral hemisphere. An important branch of the anterior cerebral artery is the **recurrent artery (of Heubner),** a branch that supplies blood to the caudate nucleus, putamen, and portions of the internal capsule. The anterior cerebral artery and its branches are the major blood supply for the medial aspects of the frontal lobes and motor cortex.

Blood-Brain Barrier

For the most part, the capillaries of the brain are impermeable and have a continuous endothelium, tight junctional complexes, and a complete basement membrane. Immediately surrounding the capillaries are the processes of astrocytes. All of these elements contribute to the formation of a restrictive barrier that prevents the free movement of material (e.g., oxygen and glucose) from the bloodstream into the brain. The **blood-brain barrier (BBB)** protects the brain from toxic elements entering the brain that may be circulating in the blood. Although the BBB protects the nervous system, it also hinders the effective use of certain drug therapies in the treatment of nervous system problems, such as malignant brain tumors. The BBB must be altered for some drugs to be able to reach the brain in therapeutic doses. Breakdown of the BBB can occur with brain injury.

Collateral Circulation in the Brain

The arteries of the brain and spinal cord are called **end arteries.** The individual branches of each artery do not anastomose with one another in the formation of a collateral circulation. Therefore when one of the major branches of an end artery becomes blocked, the brain tissue served by that artery becomes infarcted and dies. There are, however, connections between the vertebrobasilar and internal carotid systems of each side of the base of the brain. These vessels constitute the cerebral arterial circle.

The **arterial circle (of Willis)** consists of a circle of vessels that surround the stalk of the hypophysis. It is formed by anastomoses between the right and left posterior cerebral, posterior communicating and internal carotid, anterior cerebral and anterior communicating, anterior cerebral and internal carotid, and posterior communicating and posterior cerebral arteries (see Fig. 1-39).

Venous Drainage From the Brain

Numerous unnamed veins drain venous blood from the CNS. The majority of them drain into a system of **dural venous sinuses,** large venous channels that are formed within the folds of the dura mater. These sinuses provide a low-pressure channel for the movement of large volumes of blood from the cranial cavity back to the general circulation.

The largest and most prominent of the dural sinuses is the **superior sagittal sinus (SSS),** which is located in the superior margin of the falx cerebri. This sinus runs from the crista

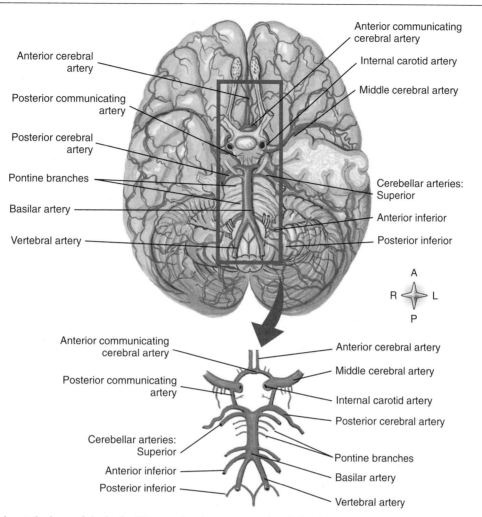

Figure 1-39 Arteries at the base of the brain. The arteries that compose the circle of Willis are the two anterior cerebral arteries joined to each other by the anterior communicating cerebral artery and to the posterior cerebral arteries by the posterior communicating arteries.
(From Thibodeau GA, Patton K: Anatomy and physiology, *ed 5, St Louis, 2003, Mosby.)*

galli of the ethmoid bone anteriorly to the tentorium cerebelli. The **inferior sagittal sinus** courses in the inferior edge of the falx cerebri and ends in the **straight sinus** at the anterior edge of the tentorium cerebelli (Fig. 1-40). Most of the large **cerebral veins** that drain blood from the cerebral hemispheres flow into the **great cerebral vein (of Galen),** which in turn drains into the straight sinus. The straight sinus courses posteriorly through the tentorium cerebelli and unites with the superior sagittal sinus adjacent to the internal occipital protuberance in the formation of the **confluence of the sinuses.** The two **transverse sinuses** course laterally from the confluence along the posterior edge of the tentorium cerebelli.

As they near the temporal bone, the transverse sinuses take on an S-shaped configuration to become the **sigmoid sinuses.** The sigmoid sinuses leave the skull through the **jugular foramina** as the **internal jugular veins.** A pair of **cavernous sinuses,** one located on each side of the sella turcica, communicate with the **ophthalmic veins** in the orbit and with the transverse sinuses via the **petrosal sinuses. Emissary veins** also carry blood from the deep layers of the scalp into the dural venous sinuses. Because venous blood flows relatively freely through the dural sinuses and because they and the veins that drain from the face and scalp have no valves, infections on the surface of the scalp and face have the potential to spread into the dural venous sinuses. Because of the communication between these vessels, an open scalp wound following traumatic head injury has the potential to cause a serious CNS infection. Such a situation is relatively serious and can result in dire consequences, such as meningitis.

SOMATIC SENSORY PATHWAYS IN THE CENTRAL NERVOUS SYSTEM

The transmission of sensory information from the skin of the body involves complex neural pathways that originate in the sensory receptors of the skin, muscles, and joints and that involve chains of several neurons before reaching the cerebral cortex. The sensory information is refined and modified as it is transmitted upward through the ascending pathways of the spinal cord and brainstem.

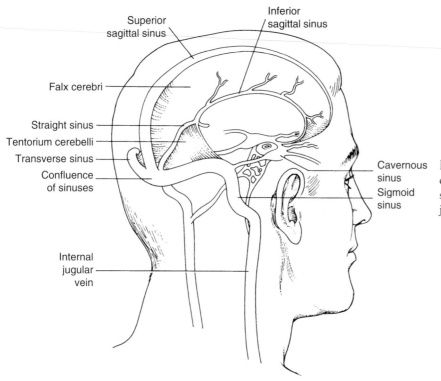

Superior sagittal sinus

Inferior sagittal sinus

Falx cerebri

Straight sinus

Tentorium cerebelli

Transverse sinus

Confluence of sinuses

Internal jugular vein

Cavernous sinus

Sigmoid sinus

Figure 1-40 Diagram showing the pattern of distribution of the major dural venous sinuses and their connection to the internal jugular veins.

In general, there are two major somatic sensory systems to consider. The older, **spinothalamic system** is for the transmission of **protopathic sensibility. Protopathic sensations** include such modalities as **pain, temperature,** and **crude (nondiscriminative) touch.** The phylogenetically newer system is for the transmission of **epicritic sensibility. Epicritic sensations** include **position sense (proprioception), movement sense (kinesthesia),** and **discriminative touch (two-point discrimination).**

In general, the skin over the entire surface of the body is endowed with several different types of sensory endings. **Free naked nerve endings** are largely thought to respond to painful stimuli and to act as pain receptors, but they may also be involved in touch. In addition, other specialized epithelial endings carry touch sensations. These include **tactile corpuscles (of Meissner), lamellated corpuscles (of Pacini),** and **peritrichal endings** surrounding the base of all hairs on the body. The tactile corpuscles are thought to be the most involved in discriminative touch because they are densely distributed over areas of the body that are very sensitive, such as the fingers, hands, toes, lips, and face.

Neuromuscular spindles, neurotendinous spindles (Golgi tendon organs), and endings in the capsules of the joints and tendons are thought to be responsible for the transmission of proprioceptive and kinesthetic information.

In general, epicritic and protopathic sensations use different pathways in the spinal cord. In addition, the pathways for these sensibilities from the skin and mucous membranes of the head differ from those that carry these same sensations from the skin and muscles of the body below the neck.

Epicritic Sensibility

As discussed earlier, epicritic sensibility includes the modalities of proprioception, kinesthesia, and discriminative touch. **Proprioception** is the ability to perceive the position of a body part in space. **Kinesthesia** is the ability to sense the location and rate of movement of a body part in space. **Discriminative touch** is the ability to detect two points applied to the skin simultaneously as two separate points. This is the basis of the ability to distinguish textures and differences in surfaces simply by feel.

Epicritic sensibility from the body arises in the many receptors located in the skin, in the tactile corpuscles for discriminative touch, and in the various endings associated with the muscles, tendons, and joints for proprioception and kinesthesia. The first-order neurons that have this pathway are the pseudounipolar neurons. Their cell bodies are located in the dorsal root ganglia or spinal nerves; their peripheral processes terminate in the tactile corpuscles, lamellated corpuscles, and neurotendinous organs; and their central processes travel in the dorsal root of the spinal nerve.

In general, these neurons are the largest of the dorsal root ganglia, and they have large **group-A fibers** that are heavily myelinated. The central processes of these primary sensory neurons tend to be localized in the medial aspect of the dorsal root. After entering the spinal cord, each process bifurcates into (1) a short ascending branch that enters the spinal cord gray matter and is involved in reflex arcs, and (2) a long ascending branch that enters the ipsilateral white matter of the dorsal funiculus of the spinal cord. The long ascending fiber is involved in the transmission of epicritic sensory information up through the spinal cord. In the upper thoracic and cervical regions of the spinal cord, the dorsal funiculus of white matter can be subdivided into two distinct bundles: a medially placed **fasciculus gracilis** that consists of fibers from the lower body, and a laterally placed **fasciculus cuneatus** that consists of fibers from the upper body.

The fasciculus gracilis and fasciculus cuneatus ascend through the spinal cord to reach the lower medulla. In the medulla, the axons of these two fasciculi synapse in the **nucleus gracilis** and **nucleus cuneatus,** respectively. The nucleus gracilis and nucleus cuneatus are the locations of the cell bodies of the second-order neurons for the pathway of epicritic sensation. The axons that arise from the cells of these nuclei course ventrally in the medulla and cross the midline as the **internal arcuate** fibers to form the **medial lemniscus** on the opposite side of the medulla. The medial lemniscus ascends through the brainstem uninterrupted until it reaches the dorsal thalamus. The axons of the medial lemniscus synapse in the **ventral posterolateral nucleus (VPL)** of the dorsal thalamus. The cells of the VPL give rise to axons that enter the **posterior limb of the internal capsule** and that terminate in the body area of the **primary somatosensory cortex** of the parietal lobe.

In summary, epicritic sensibility below the neck is carried by a three-neuron chain from the periphery to the cerebral cortex. The primary or first-order neuron has its cell body in the dorsal root ganglia, the second-order neuron has its cell body in the nucleus gracilis or cuneatus, and the third-order neuron has its cell body in the ventral posterolateral nucleus of the dorsal thalamus. The transmission of information remains ipsilateral until it reaches the second-order neuron, which crosses in the medulla.

Epicritic sensibility from the skin and mucous membranes of the head originates from the activation of sensory endings that are primarily associated with the trigeminal nerve but also include minor contributions from the facial, glossopharyngeal, and vagus nerves. The cell bodies of the first-order neurons are located in the ganglia of the respective nerves. The axons that carry information for discriminative touch terminate in the **chief sensory nucleus** of the trigeminal nerve, which is located in the pons. Axons arising from the cells of the chief sensory nucleus of the trigeminal nerve cross the midline to form the **ventral trigeminothalamic tract.** The ventral trigeminothalamic tract ascends through the brainstem medial to the medial lemniscus. Like the medial lemniscus, it terminates in the dorsal thalamus, specifically in the **ventral posteromedial nucleus of the dorsal thalamus (VPM).** The VPM gives off axons that enter the **genu of the internal capsule** to course upward to the face area of the primary somatosensory cortex of the **parietal lobe.**

Protopathic Sensibility

Protopathic sensibility involves the transmission of pain, thermal sensation, and crude (nondiscriminative) touch. Specific endings have not been proven for the reception of thermal sensation. **Crude touch** is probably mediated by naked nerve endings and by the peritrichal endings on hairs and other touch receptors in the skin.

Pain is thought to be mediated largely by free, naked nerve endings in the skin. These receptors are associated with two types of fibers: lightly myelinated fibers of the **group-A type** and thin unmyelinated fibers of the **group-C type** (see Chapter 23). The distinction of two types of pain fibers may explain the difference in the affective qualities of pain. **A fibers** are concerned with the experience of acute pain, which is often sharp and well localized, whereas **C fibers** are used in the transmission of chronic pain, which is described as diffuse, dull, aching, and poorly localized.

The cell bodies of the first-order neurons that are associated with pain receptors are located in the dorsal root ganglia of the spinal nerves. These cell bodies are small or intermediate in size. The central processes of these neurons tend to be localized in the lateral portion of the dorsal root of the spinal nerve. After entering the spinal cord, these fibers bifurcate into two short divisions that travel up and down the spinal cord in a tract located just dorsal to the dorsal horn of the gray matter, the **dorsolateral fasciculus.** The majority of these fibers terminate in the dorsal horn of the gray matter, particularly in the region known as the **substantia gelatinosa.** The various connections made in the dorsal horn of gray matter are important in the formation of reflexes and in the modulation of pain information as it comes into the spinal cord.

Eventually, the pain impulses reach cell bodies located deep within the gray matter of the dorsal horn. These cell bodies give off axons that cross the spinal cord in the **ventral white commissure** and ascend in the lateral funiculus of the spinal cord as the **spinothalamic tract.** The spinothalamic tract ascends through the entire length of the spinal cord and brainstem. In the brainstem, the spinothalamic tract becomes located dorsal to the medial lemniscus. It finally terminates in the VPL—the same thalamic nucleus in which the medial lemniscus terminates. The axons that arise in the VPL and project to the primary somatosensory cortex are important in the ability to localize pain on the body surface. In addition to the VPL, pain impulses reach other thalamic nuclei and are projected to wide areas of the cerebral cortex.

Pain from the head regions is carried largely by fibers of the **trigeminal nerve.** The cell bodies of the first-order neurons of the pain pathway are located in the ganglion of the trigeminal nerve. The central processes of pain fibers enter the pons in the trigeminal nerve. These axons form the **spinal trigeminal tract,** which descends into the medulla. The axons of the spinal trigeminal tract terminate in the **nucleus of the spinal trigeminal tract.** In many ways, this nucleus resembles the dorsal horn of the gray matter in the spinal cord. Axons arise from the cells of the nucleus of the spinal trigeminal tract and cross the midline to enter the **ventral trigeminothalamic tract,** which ascends on the opposite side of the brainstem to terminate in the VPM of the dorsal thalamus. The VPM projects third-order axons to the head area of the primary somatosensory area of the parietal lobe.

Modulation of Pain Pathways

The activity of the pain pathway is modified at many points along the way. The brain possesses a system of intrinsic structures that inhibit the transmission of pain through the CNS. Many axons that arise from the neurons of the sensory cortex project downward to the sensory nuclei of the brainstem and spinal cord, particularly the chief sensory nucleus of the trigeminal nerve, the spinal nucleus of the trigeminal nerve, the nucleus gracilis and nucleus cuneatus, and the dorsal horn of the gray matter in the spinal cord. These projection fibers are thought to modulate and refine the transmission of sensory information. Pathways arising from the **raphe nuclei** and **periaqueductal gray** of the midbrain have a powerful influence in inhibiting the upward transmission of pain impulses.

The neurons in these regions possess **opiate receptors** and respond to morphine and morphine-like substances by releasing intrinsic substances known as **enkephalins** and **endorphins.** Enkephalins and endorphins are able to inhibit the transmission of pain through the pain pathways.

The sensation of crude touch, or light touch, is difficult to evaluate. It is probably mediated by touch receptors in the skin and by the peritrichal endings around the bases of hairs. Crude touch is related to the feeling of itching or tickling in the skin. The pathway for crude touch follows the same neurons used for pain and temperature and travels over the same pathways. Loss of touch sensation is difficult to demonstrate in persons with lesions in the nervous system, because touch is carried by both the spinothalamic system and the medial lemniscus.

MOTOR PATHWAYS IN THE CENTRAL NERVOUS SYSTEM

Lower Motor Neurons

Cell bodies of neurons located in the various motor nuclei of cranial nerves and the anterior horns of the spinal cord directly innervate skeletal muscle. These neurons are called **lower motor neurons (LMNs),** and they are the last neurons to carry information from the nervous system out to the muscles.

There are two types of LMNs. **Alpha motor neurons,** which are large and heavily myelinated, innervate most fibers in any given muscle. The **gamma motor neurons** are smaller in diameter and innervate small muscle cells within the **muscle spindles.** Muscles that are involved in gross movements, such as the gluteus maximus, have motor units. Muscles that are involved in fine motor control, such as the intrinsic muscles in the hand, have small motor units. Stimulation of the alpha motor neurons results in contraction of the skeletal muscles that they innervate.

For the spinal nerves, the cell bodies of the alpha and gamma motor neurons are located in the **anterior horn of the gray matter** in the spinal cord. Individual clusters of neurons constitute the nuclei that innervate specific skeletal muscles. In general, the neurons that innervate proximal musculature are located medially in the anterior horn, and those that innervate the more distal muscles are located laterally in the anterior horn. The neurons that innervate the extensor muscles are located dorsal to those that innervate the flexor muscles. This organization of the anterior horn of gray matter in the spinal cord is called **somatotopic organization** (see Fig. 1-36).

All skeletal muscle must be innervated to survive. If the nerve that innervates a particular skeletal muscle is severed or crushed, a **lower motor lesion** will occur. Such denervated muscles demonstrate flaccid paralysis, a loss of muscle tone **(atonia),** a loss of muscle tendon reflexes **(areflexia),** and progressive degeneration of the muscles **(atrophy).** LMN lesions are often associated with spinal cord injury or tumors, polio, and surgery to the aorta in which the blood supply of the spinal cord is interrupted. In lower motor neuron paralysis the reflex arcs are permanently damaged, causing decreased muscle tone and flaccidity and diminished or absent reflexes.

Upper Motor Neurons

Because the LMNs send instructions for muscles to contract, it follows that certain pathways in the CNS influence the activity of the LMNs to facilitate and inhibit muscle contractions. Several known pathways that arise from higher brain centers influence the activity of the LMNs. These pathways constitute the **upper motor neurons (UMNs),** which are axons of neurons in the cerebrum that travel in the corticospinal tract in the motor region of cranial nuclei or the spinal cord. UMN paralysis is an injury to or lesion in the brain and spinal cord that causes damage to the cell bodies, axons, or both of the UMNs, which extend from the cerebral cortex to the cells in the spinal column that cause weakness or paralysis.

The **corticospinal tract** is an important pathway that originates from cells in the cerebral cortex of the primary motor area and the premotor area of the frontal lobe. **Corticobulbar fibers** also arise from this region. Corticobulbar fibers terminate in the motor nuclei of the cranial nerves, whereas corticospinal fibers terminate in the anterior horns of the gray matter of the spinal cord.

Corticobulbar and corticospinal fibers course downward to the brainstem through the internal capsule. In the midbrain they are located on the ventral aspect of the cerebral peduncle and continue downward through the ventral pons. In the medulla, the corticospinal fibers become aggregated into a stout bundle located on the ventral aspect of the medulla. This bundle is called the **pyramid.** Most fibers in the pyramids of the lower medulla are corticospinal because the corticobulbar fibers have synapsed in the cranial nerve motor nuclei along the way.

The two pyramids partially cross one another in the **decussation of the pyramids** found in the caudal medulla. Most fibers (90%) cross in the decussation and enter the lateral funiculus of the spinal cord to form the **lateral corticospinal tract.** These fibers continue through the spinal cord and terminate in the anterior horn of the gray matter. The uncrossed fibers (10%) constitute the **ventral corticospinal tract,** whose fibers eventually cross at the level of the spinal cord, where they terminate. Most corticospinal fibers terminate in the gray matter of the upper levels of the spinal cord. They have a profound influence on the muscles that are involved in fine, discrete movement of the hand.

Tracts and Pathways

The **rubrospinal tracts** originate in the red nuclei of the midbrain, cross the midline in the ventral tegmental decussation, and descend through the brainstem to reach the spinal cord. The exact location and course of these tracts in humans is unknown, although studies in animals suggest that the rubrospinal tracts have a profound effect on the activity of the LMNs that innervate the flexor muscles.

The **vestibulospinal tracts** arise from neurons of the vestibular nuclei in the medulla. These uncrossed pathways descend through the brainstem to terminate in the gray matter of the ipsilateral spinal cord. Vestibulospinal neurons influence the LMNs that innervate extensor muscles. The vestibulospinal tract is largely responsible for helping maintain balance and resist the effects of gravity.

The **tectospinal tract** arises from neurons located in the roof of the midbrain (tectum). The axons of this pathway terminate largely in the motor cranial nerve nuclei of the brainstem and the gray matter of the upper cervical spinal cord. This tract produces motor responses to auditory and visual stimuli that help to fix the gaze on moving objects in the visual field or to turn the head in the direction of a sound.

The **reticulospinal pathways** arise from the central core of the brainstem, the reticular formation. The reticular formation is phylogenetically the oldest part of the nervous system. It consists of polyneuronal, polysynaptic pathways that run up and down the brainstem parallel to the long ascending and descending pathways. Anatomically, the pathways of the reticular formation are difficult to demonstrate. Physiologic data are usually given as proof of their existence. The reticulospinal pathways include two pathways that originate in the reticular formation of the pons and cerebellum, respectively. These two pathways are thought to modify tendon reflex activity and therefore adjust muscle tone. See Table 1-2 for major ascending tracts of the spinal cord.

TABLE 1-2	Major Ascending Tracts of the Spinal Cord			
Name	**Function**	**Location**	**Origin**	**Termination**
Lateral spinothalamic	Pain, temperature, and crude touch opposite side	Lateral white columns	Posterior gray column opposite side	Thalamus
Anterior spinothalamic	Crude touch and pressure	Anterior white columns	Posterior gray column opposite side	Thalamus
Fasciculi gracilis and cuneatus	Discriminating touch and pressure sensations, including vibration, stereognosis, and two-point discrimination; also conscious kinesthesia	Posterior white columns	Spinal ganglia same side	Medulla
Anterior and posterior spinocerebellar	Unconscious kinesthesia	Lateral white columns	Anterior or posterior gray column	Cerebellum
Spinotectal	Touch related to visual reflexes	Lateral white columns	Posterior gray columns	Superior colliculus (midbrain)
Lateral corticospinal (or crossed pyramidal)	Voluntary movement, contraction of individual or small groups of muscles, particularly those moving hands, fingers, feet, and toes of opposite side	Lateral white columns	Motor areas or cerebral cortex opposite side from tract location in cord	Lateral or anterior gray columns
Anterior corticospinal (direct pyramidal)	Same as lateral corticospinal except mainly muscles of same side	Anterior white columns	Motor cortex but on same side as location in cord	Lateral or anterior gray columns
Reticulospinal	Maintain posture during movement	Anterior white columns	Reticular formation (midbrain, pons, and medulla)	Anterior gray columns
Rubrospinal	Coordination of body movement and posture	Lateral white columns	Red nucleus (of midbrain)	Anterior gray columns
Tectospinal	Head and neck movement during visual reflexes	Anterior white columns	Superior colliculus (midbrain)	Medulla and anterior gray columns
Vestibulospinal	Coordination of posture/balance	Anterior white columns	Vestibular nucleus (pons, medulla)	Anterior gray columns

From Thibodeau GA, Patton K: *Anatomy and physiology,* ed 5, St Louis, 2003, Mosby, pp 382–383.

Role of the Cerebellum

The **cerebellum,** the second largest part of the brain, indirectly influences the activity of skeletal muscles for an essential role in movement (see Figs. 1-13 and 1-18). The cerebellum is not part of the brainstem but is attached to the brainstem via a large number of nerve fibers called *peduncles.* The cerebellum indirectly influences the activity of skeletal muscles. The fibers do not cross; the right hemisphere controls the skeletal muscles on the right side, and the left hemisphere controls the skeletal muscles on the left side. It is generally divided into a right and left lobe that is connected by a narrow midline portion called the **vermis.** Gray matter makes up the covering and white matter the interior. Cerebellar influence is not exerted at the level of the LMNs but rather by influencing the activity of the motor cortex. The primary functions of the cerebellum are to coordinate somatic muscle activity, regulate muscle tone, and maintain balance and equilibrium.

The oldest part of the cerebellum is the **flocculonodular lobe.** This portion of the cerebellum receives most of its information from the **semicircular canals, saccule,** and **utricle** via the vestibular nuclei. It functions to maintain equilibrium or balance. The **anterior lobe** of the cerebellum is mainly involved with the regulation of muscle tone. The **posterior lobe** of the cerebellum functions in the coordination of skilled movements.

The cerebellum receives sensory information from muscle spindle organs and other sensory receptors in the muscles and tendons. This information is sent either directly into the cerebellum or into other brainstem nuclei that have connections with the cerebellum. The main nuclei that send information into the cerebellum are the **inferior olivary nuclei,** the **pontine nuclei,** and the **vestibular nuclei.**

The fibers that enter the cerebellum from the vestibular nuclei and the inferior olivary nuclei course in the inferior cerebellar **peduncle.** Those arising in the pontine nuclei course in the middle cerebellar peduncle. Information about the degree of contraction of individual skeletal muscles is processed and modified in the cerebellar cortex. Axons arising from the cells of the cerebellar cortex are projected to the deep cerebellar nuclei. Axons arising from the deep cerebellar nuclei travel in the superior cerebellar peduncle to course upward in the brainstem and terminate in the ventral lateral and ventral posterior nuclei of the dorsal thalamus. Axons that arise from these nuclei project upward to the motor areas of the cerebral cortex. Thus the cerebellum receives information about the degree of contraction and tension in skeletal muscles. It uses this information not to influence the LMNs directly but rather to influence the activity of the motor complex. Lesions of the cerebellum may be characterized by a loss of equilibrium, a loss of muscle tone, and the onset of "intention tremors."

SPECIAL SENSES

Vision

Vision depends on the ability of the eye to collect light rays and focus them on the retina. The **retina** is the special sensory epithelium that lines the inside of the eyeball and generates the visual impulses that are sent to the occipital lobe over the visual pathway.

Eye and Retina

The posterior four fifths of the outer coat of the globe of the eye is white and opaque and is called the **sclera** (Fig. 1-41). The **sclera** is the tough inelastic white opaque membrane covering the posterior five sixths of the eye bulb. The **retina** is the 10-layered delicate nervous tissue membrane of the eye that is continuous with the optic nerve. The retina receives images and transmits them through the optic nerve to the brain. The anterior one fifth of the globe is transparent and is called the **cornea.** Light rays that enter the eye are refracted by the cornea, lens, iris, and internal transport material (humors). Focusing is accomplished by means of refraction, and the image is focused onto the retina by the **biconcave lens.** This lens is located posterior to the **iris,** which is the colored part of the eye. In the center of the iris is the **pupil,** an opening through which the light rays must pass to reach the lens. The iris contains circular and radially arranged smooth muscle cells that control the diameter of the pupil. Stray or aberrant light rays are absorbed by the **choroid,** a heavily pigmented layer that is located between the sclera and the retina.

The image that is focused on the retina is inverted and reversed from left to right. The retina is a complex sensory receptor containing five different types of neural cells. The outer layer of the retina is the layer of **rod** cells and **cone** cells. These specialized neural cells are the actual sensory receptors of the eye. Rod cells, which number about 130 million per eye, function best in dim light and are important in night vision. Cone cells, which number about 7 million per eye, function best in bright light and are necessary for sharp, color vision. In the posterior wall of the eyeball and in direct line with the visual axis is a disc-shaped region that is somewhat yellowish in color. This region is called the **macula lutea.** A depression in the center of the macula, the **fovea centralis,** is the area of greatest visual acuity because it contains only cone receptors. If a hole develops in the macula, loss of vision will occur.

Within the retina, rod and cone cells synapse on bipolar neurons, which in turn synapse with ganglion cells. The axons of the ganglion cells make up the **optic nerve.** The point on the retina where all of the axons of the ganglion cells converge to form the optic nerve is called the **optic papilla.** This region is devoid of rod and cone cells and is therefore the **"blind spot."** As the axons of the ganglion cells leave the eyeball to enter the optic nerve, they acquire a coating of myelin. Horizontal and amacrine cells contribute to the processing of visual stimuli in the retina.

Visual Pathway

The optic nerve emerges from the posterior aspect of the eyeball and courses through the orbit (Fig. 1-42). The retina of the eye develops from the CNS, and therefore the optic nerve is different from other peripheral nerves in that it does not possess an **epineurium** but rather is enclosed in a sheath of dura mater. In addition, the axons of the optic nerve are

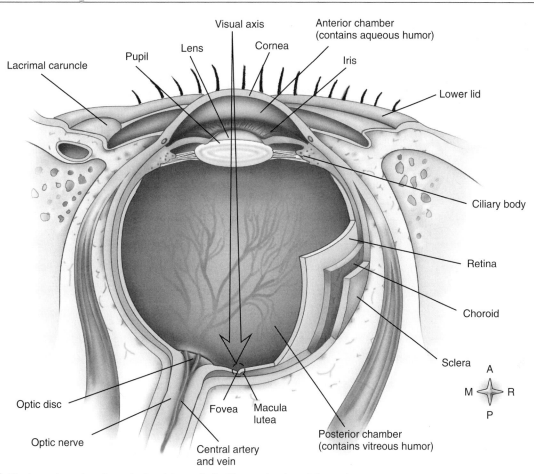

Figure 1-41 Horizontal section through the right eyeball. The eye is viewed from above. (*From Thibodeau GA, Patton K:* Anatomy and physiology, *ed 5, St Louis, 2003, Mosby.*)

not myelinated by neurolemmocytes as are regular peripheral nerves but instead are myelinated by oligodendrocytes as are other axons in the CNS. In this regard, the optic nerve is more like a brain tract than a true peripheral nerve.

Each optic nerve leaves the orbit through the **optic canal.** Just anterior to the infundibulum of the pituitary gland, the two optic nerves partially decussate to form the **optic chiasm.** The optic chiasm consists of axons from ganglion cells of the nasal retina of each eye. These axons cross the midline to join uncrossed axons in the optic nerve of the contralateral eye in the formation of the **optic tract.**

The optic tract consists of crossed axons from the **nasal retina** of each eye and uncrossed axons from the temporal retina of each eye. Because of the crossing of fibers in the optic chiasm, all visual information from the right side of the **visual field** is localized in the left optic tract, and all images from the left side of the visual field are localized in the right optic tract. This crossing over of axons in the optic chiasm is the basis of binocular vision and allows for good depth perception.

Most of the axons of the optic tract terminate in the **lateral geniculate body,** one of the nuclei of the dorsal thalamus. A small bundle of axons from each optic tract, known as the **brachium of the superior colliculus,** bypass the lateral geniculate body to enter the **superior colliculus**

of the midbrain. These axons are important in providing input to the superior colliculus to coordinate reflex movement of the eyes and head in response to moving objects in the visual field. Any moving object in the visual field will cause the head and eyes to be directed toward it until the brain can assess the object and decide whether to continue looking at it.

The axons that arise from the lateral geniculate carry the visual information to the **primary visual cortex** in the occipital lobe. Because these axons terminate in the occipital lobe cortex that borders the **calcarine fissure,** the pathway is called the **geniculocalcarine tract.**

Visual Cortex
The upper and lower borders of the calcarine fissure constitute the primary visual cortex. This area is located largely on the medial face of the occipital lobe. The largest area of the calcarine cortex is devoted to macular vision. As stated earlier, the macula is the area of greatest visual acuity even though it is the smallest part of the retina.

Retinotopic Organization of the Visual System
If the eye were bisected in its midsagittal plane, the half of the eye adjacent to the nose would be the nasal half of the eye, and the lateral half would be the temporal half of the

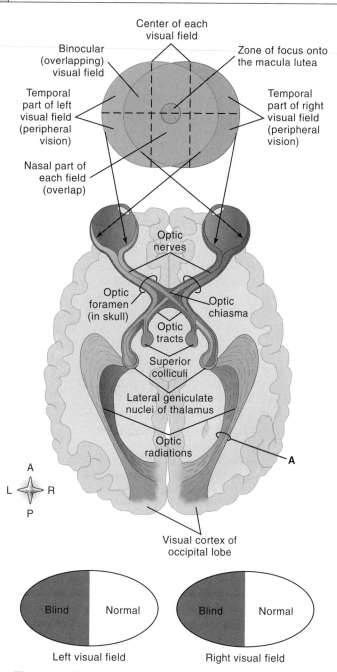

Center of each
visual field

Binocular
(overlapping)
visual field

Zone of focus onto
the macula lutea

Temporal part of left
visual field (peripheral vision)

Temporal part of right
visual field (peripheral vision)

Nasal part of
each field
(overlap)

Optic
nerves

Optic
foramen
(in skull)

Optic
chiasma

Optic
tracts

Superior
colliculi

Lateral geniculate
nuclei of thalamus

Optic
radiations

A

A
L ✦ R
P

Visual cortex of
occipital lobe

Blind   Normal

Left visual field

Blind   Normal

Right visual field

Figure 1-42 Visual fields and neuronal pathways of the eye. Note the structures that make up each pathway: optic nerve, optic chiasma, lateral geniculate body of thalamus, optic radiations, and visual cortex of occipital lobe. Fibers from the nasal portion of each retina cross over to the opposite side at the optic chiasma and terminate in the lateral geniculate nuclei. Location of a lesion in the visual pathway determines the resulting visual defect. Damage at point *A*, for example, would cause blindness in the right nasal and left temporal visual fields, as the ovals beneath indicate. (Trace the visual pathway from point A back to the visual field map to see why this is so. What would be the effect of pressure on the optic chiasma—by a pituitary tumor, for instance? Answer: It would produce blindness in both temporal fields. Why? Because it destroys fibers from the nasal side of both retinas.)
(From Thibodeau GA, Patton K: Anatomy and physiology, *ed 5, St Louis, 2003, Mosby.)*

eye. Because the lens inverts the images and reverses them from left to right, the **nasal half of the retina sees the temporal visual field,** and the **temporal half of the retina sees the nasal field.** Each eye has its own visual field; if each eye is alternately opened and closed, it is noted that, for the most part, the visual fields of the two eyes overlap. When both eyes are open and looking straight ahead, the brain processes the information from each individual eye and forms a single visual image. Because of the decussation of nasal retinal fibers in the optic chiasm, everything on the left side of the visual field is being "seen" by the right occipital lobe, and vice versa. If either optic nerve is destroyed, the patient loses vision in that eye. The nasal retina of each eye looks at the edges of the visual field, and these axons are contained in the optic chiasm. Therefore if the optic chiasm is destroyed, the patient loses vision in the periphery of the visual field and experiences "tunnel vision," or **heteronymous hemianopsia.** Lesions of the optic tract, lateral geniculate nucleus, geniculocalcarine tract, or visual cortex result in the loss of vision in the contralateral visual field (**homonymous hemianopsia).**

In addition, the loss of certain visual reflexes is evident with lesions of the visual system. Visual reflexes are discussed later in this chapter (see Fig. 1-42).

Hearing

Hearing, or **audition,** is another of the important sensations. The auditory system includes the **external ear, middle ear,** and **inner ear,** as well as the **auditory nerve** and **auditory pathway** in the CNS. The external ear is concerned mainly with the collection and conduction of sound waves, which cause vibration of the **tympanic membrane** at the lateral end of the **auditory canal.** The three bones of the middle ear cavity form a chain that connects the tympanic membrane with the **oval window of the cochlea.** The **malleus** is connected to the tympanic membrane. The **incus** is connected to both the malleus and **stapes,** and the **footplate of the stapes** is connected to the oval window of the cochlea. This arrangement of ossicles transmits sound waves to the cochlea, where the sensory end organ of the auditory system is located (Fig. 1-43).

Cochlea

The **cochlea** consists of a bony spiral that resembles a snail's shell with two and a half turns from base to apex. The central bony core of the cochlea is the **modiolus,** through which the nerves and blood vessels reach the sensory epithelium within the cochlea. The **membranous labyrinth,** which is divided into three compartments, lines the interior of the cochlea. The uppermost compartment is the **scala vestibuli,** and the lowermost compartment is the **scala tympani.** The **cochlear duct** is located between these two vestibuli. The scala vestibuli and scala tympani are continuous at the apex of the spiral of the cochlea. They contain a fluid called **perilymph.**

The cochlear duct is closed off from the scala vestibuli and tympani, but it also contains fluid called **endolymph.** The sensory epithelium (**organ of Corti**) is located in the

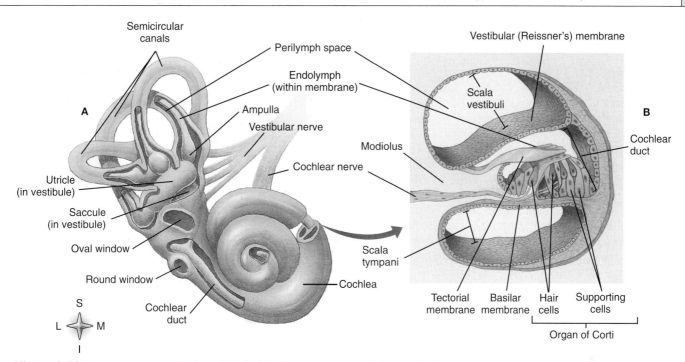

Figure 1-43   The inner ear. **A,** The bony labyrinth is the hard outer wall of the entire inner ear and includes semicircular canals, vestibule, and cochlea. Within the bony labyrinth is the membranous labyrinth, which is surrounded by perilymph and filled with endolymph. Each ampulla in the vestibule contains a crista ampullaris that detects changes in head position and sends sensory impulses through the vestibular nerve to the brain. **B,** The inset shows a section of the membranous cochlea. Hair cells in the organ of Corti detect sound and send the information through the cochlear nerve. The vestibular and cochlear nerves join to form the eighth cranial nerve (CN VIII).
(From Thibodeau GA, Patton K: Anatomy and physiology, *ed 5, St Louis, 2003, Mosby.)*

cochlear duct. This epithelium rests on a **basement membrane,** a gelatinous sheet that is attached to the inner edge of the cochlear duct.

In addition to the hair cells, a number of supportive cells are found in the organ of Corti. Dendritic terminals of primary sensory neurons are associated with the base of each hair cell. Vibrations of the tympanic membrane are transferred to the oval window by the three ear ossicles. Vibration of the stapes in the oval window sets up a wave motion in the perilymph of the cochlea. This wave motion is similar to that observed when a stone is thrown into a body of water and concentric waves spread outward. The wave in the perilymph displaces the basilar membrane and its attached hair cells. This movement causes the hairs of the hair cells to bend, thus generating impulses in the dendritic terminals of the primary auditory neurons (see Fig. 1-43).

Auditory Pathway

The cell bodies of the primary auditory neurons are located in the **spiral ganglion** of the cochlea. These are bipolar neurons whose peripheral processes are located at the base of the hair cells and whose central processes are located in the **auditory** or **cochlear nerve.** The cochlear nerves enter the brainstem at the **pontomedullary junction,** where the axons of the primary sensory neurons terminate in either the dorsal or **ventral cochlear nucleus.**

Axons arising from both the dorsal and ventral cochlear nuclei carry auditory impulses upward through the brainstem in the **lateral lemniscus.** Auditory information is both crossed and uncrossed in the lateral lemniscus. For this reason, destruction of one lateral lemniscus causes diminished hearing in both ears but more pronounced loss on the side of the lesion. Along the lateral lemniscus are a number of relays in which the auditory impulses are refined. All fibers of each lateral lemniscus eventually reach the **inferior colliculi.** Axons arising from the cells of the inferior colliculi form the **brachium of the inferior colliculus** and continue to carry the auditory impulses upward to the **medial geniculate nuclei** of the dorsal thalamus. Cells of the medial geniculate nuclei send their axons into the **sublenticular portion of the internal capsule** to continue the auditory pathway to the **primary auditory cortex** located in the **transverse temporal gyri** of the cerebrum.

Auditory Reflexes

Some of the fibers from the inferior colliculus synapse in the superior colliculus to activate the **tectospinal pathway.** This pathway causes reflex turning of the head and eyes in the direction of sudden or loud noises.

Equilibrium

Equilibrium is the special somatic sense of balance. This system helps the body to remain properly oriented with respect to gravity through reflex adjustments of muscle tone. In addition to the sensory input received from the muscles and the visual system, the vestibular system has its own specialized receptors in the inner ear.

Receptors

The specific receptors for the vestibular system include the **saccule, utricle,** and **semicircular canals.** The saccule and utricle consist of localized swellings of the membranous labyrinth, each of which contains a patch of sensory epithelium called the **macula.** The cells of the macula of the saccule and utricle are **hair cells** similar to those found in the cochlea. The hairs of the macular cells are embedded in a gel-like membrane; this membrane contains small calcium concretions resembling sand that are called **otoliths.** Gravity pulls on the otoliths when the head is bent forward, backward, or from side-to-side, thus bending the hair cells and initiating impulses in the primary sensory receptors located at the bases of the hair cells. In this way, the vestibular apparatus detects changes in head position.

While the saccule and utricle detect changes in head position, the three semicircular canals detect alterations in the angular momentum of the body in space. These canals are continuous with the membranous labyrinth and are roughly perpendicular to each other to correspond to the three planes of space. A localized expansion in each of the semicircular canals (the **ampulla**) contains a raised patch of sensory epithelium. Like the saccule and utricle, this sensory epithelium consists of hair cells with apical hairs embedded in a gelatinous membrane called the **cupola.** The cupola projects into the lumen of the semicircular canal and is bathed by the endolymph. As the body is accelerated through space, the endolymph in the semicircular canals begins to move, thereby displacing the cupola and activating the hair cells to generate impulses in the primary sensory endings.

Vestibular Pathway

The primary sensory neurons of the vestibular system are located in the **vestibular ganglion,** which is embedded in the temporal bone near the **internal auditory meatus.** The peripheral processes of these neurons are associated with the bases of the hair cells of the saccule and utricle and the ampullae of the semicircular canals. The central processes of these neurons form the vestibular part of the **vestibulocochlear nerve.** This nerve enters the brainstem at the pontomedullary junction. The majority of vestibular fibers terminate in the floor of the medulla. A small portion of the fibers course into the cerebellum to terminate in the vestibular part of the cerebellum (the flocculonodular lobe). Axons arising in the flocculonodular lobe course back to the vestibular nuclei.

The vestibular nuclei maintain connections with the cerebellum and the motor neurons of the spinal cord. Two major pathways that originate in the vestibular nuclei are the **medial longitudinal fasciculus (MLF)** and the **lateral vestibulospinal tract.**

The MLF interconnects the vestibular nuclei with the motor nuclei that innervate the extraocular eye muscles. Specifically, these nuclei are the oculomotor, trochlear, and abducens nuclei. The purpose of the MLF is to coordinate conjugate movements of the eye in accordance with head movements, thereby maintaining the ability to visually fix on an object while the head moves. When spinning in a circle, a person usually focuses on one point on the horizon until the head reaches its maximum point of lateral excursion. The head and eyes then snap to a new point, and so on.

The fibers of the MLF continue into the spinal cord as the medial vestibulospinal tract. Stimulation of the vestibular apparatus or nerve can lead to rapid oscillations of the eye. This phenomenon is known as **nystagmus.**

The **lateral vestibulospinal tract** arises from the cells of the vestibular nuclei, particularly the **lateral vestibular nucleus.** This pathway, which descends uncrossed through the brainstem and spinal cord, has a profound influence on the anterior horn cells that innervate extensor muscles in the limbs. Extension of the muscles on one side of the body assists the individual in resisting the effects of centrifugal force and angular momentum.

Cortical Connections

The exact way in which vestibular information reaches the cerebrum is not clearly understood. It is believed that information from the vestibular system reaches the parietal lobe; the **superior temporal gyrus** also receives vestibular input because stimulation of this area results in reports of dizziness, or *vertigo.*

NEUROANATOMY OF SOME COMMON REFLEXES

In general, reflexes generally occur at the unconscious level and require at least two neurons to be operational. The sensory neuron of a reflex arc is called the **afferent limb** of the reflex, and the motor neuron is called the **efferent limb** of the reflex. Sensory impulses arise in the afferent limb of the reflex. This neuron synapses on the cell body of the efferent neuron, either directly or through the intermediary of an association neuron. The impulses are then carried over the afferent limb of the reflex, resulting in a motor response.

Blink Reflex

The **blink reflex** protects the cornea from irritation and drying. Irritation of the cornea results in a brisk closing of the upper eyelid. This action places a thin layer of tears over the cornea, thus relieving the irritation. The afferent limb of the blink reflex is carried by axons of the ophthalmic division of the trigeminal nerve. Within the pons, impulses are transferred to the neurons that make up the motor nucleus of the facial nerve, specifically to those neurons that innervate the orbicularis oculi muscle. Activation of these neurons results in contraction of the orbicularis oculi muscle, which closes the eye. The blink reflex, or **corneal reflex** as it is called, can be tested by drawing a wisp of sterile cotton across the cornea. Loss of the blink reflex indicates a lesion of the trigeminal nerve, the facial nerve, or their central connections. (See Chapter 2 for more information on the neuroassessment of the blink reflex.)

Pupillary Light Reflex

Shining a light into one pupil of the eye causes the pupils of both eyes to rapidly and briskly constrict. This is known as the **pupillary light reflex.** Constriction of the pupil into which the light is shining is called the **direct response;** constriction of the opposite pupil is called the **consensual response.** This reflex produces adjustments to the diameter of the pupil to regulate the amount of light entering the eye.

The afferent limb of the reflex arises in the ganglion cells of the retina that send their axons into the optic nerve, optic chiasm, and optic tract. Some axons in the optic tract continue into the brachium of the superior colliculus to enter the midbrain. Here the impulses are passed into an area of the midbrain called the **pretectal region.** Neurons in the pretectal region process the incoming sensory impulses and send them to the **Edinger-Westphal nuclei** of both eyes. Impulses arising from these nuclei travel in the oculomotor nerves (CN III) to reach the ciliary ganglia. From the ciliary ganglia, the impulses travel into the eye, where they cause the pupils to constrict by activation of the constrictor pupillae muscle. Loss of the pupillary light reflex may result from lesions of the optic nerve, brachium of the superior colliculus, pretectal region, or oculomotor nerve. (See Chapter 2 for more information on the neuroassessment of the blink reflex.)

Accommodation Convergence

The pupils of the eye also constrict when the gaze is directed from far to near. This is known as the **accommodation convergence response.** It can be tested by asking the patient to direct his or her gaze from a distant point (e.g., the wall of the room) to a finger held up in front of his or her nose. In this response, the lens thickens and the pupils converge and constrict. The neuroanatomic pathway is essentially the same as for the pupillary light reflex. One difference, however, is that this pathway seems to bypass the pretectal region. This is based on the observation that lesions of the pretectal region, such as may occur in syphilis, interrupt the pathway for the light reflex but not the pathway for accommodation-convergence. Such a condition is called an **Argyll-Robertson pupil,** a pupil that does not constrict to light but does constrict for accommodation.

Emetic Reflex

The **emetic reflex** is the expulsion of gastric contents, or vomiting. It originates in many places but most often from afferents in the lining of the upper gastrointestinal (GI) tract. The afferent impulses are carried over the vagus nerve (CN X) to the medulla, where the vomiting or emetic center is located. This center organizes the motor response by sending impulses to the motor nuclei that control the contraction of the diaphragm and the anterolateral muscles of the abdominal wall. In addition, motor impulses are sent to the smooth muscles of the GI tract to initiate reverse peristalsis, which results in the ejection of gastric contents. The medullary emetic center also receives input from the vestibular system, olfactory system, and visual system.

Sneezing and Coughing Reflexes

The reflexes of **sneezing** and **coughing** are similar in that they both involve the forcible expulsion of air from the respiratory tract as the result of irritation. Sneezing is initiated by irritation of the sensory endings of the trigeminal nerve, which are located in the mucosa of the nasal cavity. Coughing is initiated by irritation of the sensory endings in the mucosa of the pharynx or larynx. In both instances, there is a momentary closing of the glottic opening by the vocal folds and a simultaneous contraction of the diaphragm and abdominal musculature. This results in a buildup of pressure in the abdominal cavity and is followed by an immediate opening of the glottis caused by abduction of the vocal folds and a brisk and violent rush of air through the respiratory tree. The purpose of this reflex is to expel the irritant from the respiratory passage.

Carotid Sinus Reflex

Control of blood pressure is regulated by a number of neural and hormonal factors. One major neural reflex is the **carotid sinus reflex.** Stretch receptors in the wall of the carotid sinus, located at the bifurcation of the common carotid artery, are innervated by afferent fibers of the glossopharyngeal nerve (CN IX). Additional pressure receptors are also localized in the wall of the aorta and the walls of the great vessels of the right side of the heart. These receive afferent innervation by the vagus nerve (CN X). These **baroreceptors** respond to increases in blood pressure in the great vessels by sending impulses over their respective cranial nerves into the medulla. Within the medulla, the motor response of the reflex is organized in the cardiac inhibitory center. This center sends impulses to the motor nucleus of the vagus nerve, which in turn conducts the efferent impulses to the heart to slow its contraction and reduce blood pressure. In addition, the afferent impulses from the carotid sinus and the other baroreceptors cause depression of the vasomotor center in the medulla, resulting in decreased sympathetic activity and dilation of the peripheral vessels. This phenomenon also contributes to a decrease in blood pressure.

Tendon Reflexes

All skeletal muscles in the body are composed of two types of muscle fibers: **intrafusal** and **extrafusal.** The bulk of a muscle consists of extrafusal muscle fibers. Extrafusal muscle fibers are innervated by the large alpha motor neurons of the anterior horn of the spinal cord, and they provide the powerful contracting force of the muscle.

Intrafusal muscle fibers are located within muscle spindles, small sensory receptors embedded within the mass of the muscle. Intrafusal muscle fibers are innervated by the gamma motor neurons and are arranged parallel to special sensory endings in the muscle spindle. Tension in the intrafusal muscle fibers stretches the sensory endings, causing them to send impulses into the spinal cord. These sensory impulses are carried to the spinal cord by large myelinated afferent nerve fibers that synapse on the alpha motor neurons that innervate the extrafusal muscle fibers. This causes the muscle to contract, thereby relieving the tension in the muscle spindle. This arrangement is the basis of most muscle tendon reflexes in the body.

When the tendon of a specific muscle is tapped, the muscle usually responds with a brisk and strong contraction. This is known as a **tendon reflex,** of which the patellar tendon reflex is the best example. The afferent limb of this reflex is in the **muscle spindle,** which contains a stretch receptor. Stretching the tendon of the muscle with the tap of the percussion hammer elicits a barrage of impulses in the afferent fibers that are connected to the annulospiral endings in the muscle spindle. The afferent impulses course over the spinal nerves that make up the peripheral nerve (L2, L3, L4) and synapse in the anterior horn of the gray matter in the appropriate spinal segments. Here the alpha motor neurons that innervate the quadriceps femoris muscle are activated. Impulses travel from those neurons into the ventral roots of the spinal nerves (L2, L3, and L4) and into the peripheral nerve innervating the quadriceps femoris muscle (femoral muscle). The entire muscle contracts, resulting in the relief of tension in the receptor.

CONCLUSION

Neuroanatomy is the foundation of neuroscience nursing. The ability to correctly correlate the anatomic site of injury or pathologic lesion is essential to effective patient management. Neuroanatomy is less overwhelming and more fascinating when the clinician and reader begin to appreciate the intricate organization of the brain and spinal cord. This review can be used as a quick reference for the experienced clinician or basic learning for the novice to better understand the anatomy and function of the brain and spinal cord. As we continue to put together all the pieces that form the mosaic of the brain and spinal cord, this process demonstrates how little we know and how much more we need to learn as scientists continue to try to unravel the mystery of the nervous system.

Neuroanatomy is fascinating and exciting. As the clinician applies knowledge and understanding of neuroanatomy to individual patients with neurologic disorders, patient man-

agement and treatment become harmonious with the clinical presentation and patient's response.

Health teaching is an important component of neuroscience patient management. The clinician who demonstrates a thorough understanding of neuroanatomy and the neurologic disease process will possess valuable tools for teaching and clinical practice.

REFERENCES

1. Athni SS, Churches IM, Loftus B: Neuroanatomy. In Rolak LA, editor: *Neurology secrets,* ed 3, Philadelphia, 2001, Hanley & Belfus.
2. Slazinski T, Littlejohns LR: Anatomy of the nervous system. In Bader MK, Littlejohn LR, editors: *AANN core curriculum for neuroscience nurses,* ed 4, St Louis, 2004, Saunders.
3. Thibodeau G, Patton K: Tissues. In Thibodeau G, Patton K: *Anatomy and physiology,* St Louis, 2003, Mosby.
4. Zuccarelli L: Cellular physiology of the nervous system. In Bader MK, Littlejohn LR, editors: *AANN core curriculum for neuroscience nursing,* ed 4, St Louis, 2004, Elsevier.

SUGGESTED READINGS

Frackowiak RSJ, Friston KJ, Frith CD, Dolan RJ, Price CJ, Zeki S, Asburner J, Perry W (editors): *Human brain function,* ed 2, Boston, 2004, Elsevier.

Gilman S, Newman SW: *Manter and Gatz's essential of clinical neuroanatomy and neurophysiology,* ed 10, Philadelphia, 2003, FA Davis.

Johnson MH, Yuko M, Gilmore RO: *Brain development and cognition,* ed 2, Malden, MA, 2002, Blackwell Publishers.

Kiernan JA: *The human nervous system, an anatomical viewpoint,* ed 8, Philadelphia, 2004, Harper & Row.

Nolte J: *The human brain,* ed 5, St Louis, 2002, Mosby.

Paxinos G, Mai J (editors): *The human nervous system,* ed 2, Boston, 2004, Elsevier.

Rolak LA: *Neurology secrets,* ed 3, Philadelphia, 2001, Hanley & Belfus.

Snell RS: *Clinical neuroanatomy for medical students,* ed 5, Philadelphia, 2001, Lippincott Williams & Wilkins.

Waxman SG: *Clinical neuroanatomy,* ed 25, New York, 2003, McGraw-Hill.

CHAPTER 2

The Adult Neurologic Assessment

The goal of a neurologic assessment is to thoroughly evaluate a patient so that a comprehensive picture of the individual's neurologic condition, disease, symptoms, and state of health can be used by the health care team. The hallmark for optimal care begins with the neurologic assessment followed by the documentation of findings. The initial assessment serves as the baseline to screen for abnormal findings. These data (information) are collected and analyzed for further investigation of the nature and extent of any neurologic abnormalities. Critical thinking skills are needed to interpret and integrate the assessment finding and provide a scientific basis for completing an individualized plan of care to help the patient reach outcome goals.

Patient management is guided by the use of evidence-based medicine, standardized clinical pathways, hospital policies and procedure, or predetermined protocols. This includes physician and health care provider orders initiated after the initial assessment of presenting complaints and diagnoses and follow-up assessments based on the patient's condition and response to treatment. For example, assessments could be a "standard" for a general assessment conducted every 4 hours, or a flexible "problem-focused" system for nursing staff to individualize care delivery designed to increase clinicians' efficiency and effectiveness.[5] The neurologic assessment of an individual with a known or suspected neurologic disorder begins the moment the clinician meets the patient and begins a conversation or observation. Special skills are required by the clinician to collect a thorough history; listen carefully to the patient's responses and follow up with appropriate questions. Taking time to collect a comprehensive history and developing extensive knowledge of the neurologic disease helps the interdisciplinary team to make an accurate statement of the correct diagnosis and to treat the patient with effective therapies.

Once the history is recorded, the assessment of the patient then becomes more focused and reassessments identify complications that may impede progress and recovery. The patient's assessment proceeds in a systematic manner using the necessary components of the neurologic assessment described in this chapter (Box 2-1).

The steps of the nursing process are applied as an organizational framework to (1) generate a database from the patient's history; (2) develop a list of actual and/or potential problems using nursing diagnoses with expected outcomes; (3) design a plan of care; (4) initiate appropriate treatments; (5) determine rehabilitation potential; and (6) evaluate the clinical management to achieve expected patient outcomes or address variances.

Patient assessment helps determine the kind of care that is required to meet a patient's initial needs, as well as serial assessments in response to care and any changes in the patient's status. The assessment is completed as soon as possible (i.e., following a hospital admission) for effective and efficient patient care while the initial and continuously occurring data are analyzed for decision making about the best course of treatment. Each patient's physical status, psychologic status, and social status are assessed, with reassessments made at regular intervals in the course of care or if there is a significant change in a patient's condition or diagnosis. A concern for the patient's comfort and privacy must be maintained, with modifications made to adapt to the patient's limitations, pain, and discomfort.

There are situations where a **"neuro check"** may be ordered for a brief neurologic assessment. It may only include the level of consciousness (LOC), movement of the extremities (voluntary versus involuntary), and pupil check for equality, reactivity to light, and ability to accommodate.

This chapter offers guidelines for the assessment of an adult patient in a variety of clinical settings. It is important for the clinician to correlate knowledge of normal neuroanatomy and physiology with clinical findings to locate clinically significant abnormalities of the nervous system. It is also important for the clinician to know how to use the appropriate neurologic examination instruments. Concise, accurate, and thorough documentation of the findings is necessary to communicate the patient's neurologic status to other members of the professional team.

PURPOSE OF THE NEUROLOGIC ASSESSMENT

The basic purpose of the neurologic assessment is to identify normal versus abnormal neurologic functions. It is important to know the location, nature, and effect of the lesion or area of the nervous system that is affected and to analyze results of neurodiagnostic studies. After completion of a detailed assessment, the clinician should identify abnormal signs and symptoms, interpret the findings for further investigation, and discuss with the treating team to develop an individualized plan of care for successful management. It is important to recognize how the neurologic disorder has affected the

BOX 2-1	The Neurologic Assessment

Begins on Admission
- Present with symptom(s)
- Chief patient complaint

Elicit Neurologic History
- Basic background history
- Allergies
- Recreational substances
- Medications
- Onset, location, duration
- Pattern of disease progression
- Characteristics
- Mental status
- Interventions

Complaint or Symptoms Related to
- Traumatic
- Vascular
- Epileptic
- Inflammatory
- Infective
- Neoplastic
- Degenerative
- Genetic/congenital pain

Components of the Neurologic Assessment
- Consciousness
- Cranial nerves
- Pupillary
- Sensory status
- Motor status
- Reflexes
- Autonomic responses
- Pain
- Vital signs

Determine Location(s) or Region Affected
- Level of peripheral nervous system affected
- Level of central nervous system affected

Document Findings and Problem List
- Expected outcomes
- Plan of care
- Outcomes in response to treatment and therapeutic interventions
- Improvement
- Resolution of problems
- Neurologic rehabilitation
- Recovery
- Chronic state or unavoidable death

Discharge

BOX 2-2	Tools for the Neurologic Assessment

- Penlight or small flashlight
- Equipment to test sharp and dull sensation (e.g., broken wooden tongue depressor or cotton-tipped applicator)
- Tuning fork (e.g., 128 or 256 Hz tuning fork)
- Ophthalmoscope
- Stethoscope
- Odoriferous but nonirritating substances (e.g., crushed cloves, coffee, or wintergreen)
- Otoscope
- Eye chart (e.g., Snellen or handheld Rosenbaum; sterile cotton swabs) or printed material
- Reflex hammer
- Measuring tape
- Tongue depressors
- Miscellaneous: cotton balls, pen or pencil and paper or chart to record date (optional), test tubes for cold and warm water

BOX 2-3	Goals of the Neurologic Assessment

- Determine the diagnosis and appropriate triage
- Utilize rapid assessment for emergency lifesaving treatment of critically ill
- Identify abnormal versus normal neurologic functions
- Identify any abnormal signs and symptoms
- Develop a problem list of actual or potential problems
- Interpret findings for further investigation
- Establish and document the baseline for follow-up and focused serial assessments
- Coordinate appropriate management decisions to improve outcome
- Recognize early complications promptly
- Monitor trends of improvement or deterioration to help predict recovery and outcomes
- Identify functional restoration, rehabilitation potential, or life care planning (LCP) needs
- Identify response to treatments, medications, and therapies
- Define knowledge deficits for future health teaching

individual's level of functional ability and impaired his or her capacity for self-care. Age, culture, the absence or presence of pain, the medications the individual is taking, the rapport between the patient and practitioner, and the health care setting should all be considered when performing the assessment.

For patients with a serious or life-threatening injury or illness, the assessment is performed quickly and is accompanied by diagnostic studies for the purpose of rapid diagnosis and emergent treatment. The bedside clinician's assessment identifies response to treatments, medications, therapies, and early trends of deterioration or improvement. In the home setting, the clinician may perform a neurologic assessment to closely monitor the patient's long-term recovery and responses. The office or outpatient clinician, as well as the case manager or disease management clinician, may need to assess for early signs of complications that could result in rehospitalization unless the patient is treated promptly. The life care planner (LCP) performs a neurologic assessment to develop long-term needs based on the life expectancy of a patient with a catastrophic neurologic disease or injury (see Chapter 25). The clinician may modify the assessment in each particular setting, but the purpose remains the same.

The tools listed in Box 2-2 are used in examination of the nervous system; the clinician selects the tool based on the patient's clinical condition, the physical environment or setting, and the purpose of the assessment. Each of the goals listed in Box 2-3 serves an important role in the overall care of the patient.

PERFORMANCE OF THE ADULT NEUROLOGIC ASSESSMENT

The neurologic assessment begins when the clinician first interacts with the patient. Observation of the patient's general appearance, skin color, facial expression, attention span, eye contact, response to verbal stimuli, cognition, behavior, emotional status, coordination, balance and symmetry of movement, demeanor, dress, personal hygiene or cleanliness, speech patterns, and ability to follow commands should be noted.

Components of a neurologic assessment include the patient's neurologic history, basic background history, mental status, motor function and gait of extremities, sensory function, cranial nerves (including pupils and brainstem function), deep tendon reflexes (based on clinician's skill level), autonomic responses, vital signs, cerebellar function and coordination, spinal cord function, and pain. Each of these components is discussed in detail later in this chapter. After the clinician is familiar with all of these components, the assessment can be individualized by choosing the components necessary for the patient being examined. Any component of the assessment that the patient is unable to complete should be deferred until a later time.

There are also situations where a **screening** is performed (e.g., blood pressure screening) as a preliminary step for the purpose of early detection that may require further investigation of a large sample of the population to detect a specific disease or problem such as stroke. A simple **neurologic screening** can be part of a health checkup or wellness check, or it may be done in the case of a minor complaint to determine the need for a comprehensive neurologic assessment.

Screenings vary from setting to setting and may include an overall observation of the individual's appearance; cognition along with the level of consciousness, memory, attention, and judgment; emotional status; speech and language; motor status for tone and strength; sensory status for superficial pain and touch; and cranial nerve (CN) evaluation of CN II (vision); CNs III, IV, and VI (eye movements); CN V (sensation to face); CN VII (facial weakness); and CN VIII (hearing).

History

The history is the most important part of the evaluation.[2] No examination can be complete without a history, and no history can be too complete. The importance of the history is emphasized by the fact that in the great majority of cases many neuroscience health care professionals rely primarily on the history to form the diagnosis.

The neurologic, personal, and social history includes questions on environmental or occupational exposure. The patient's hand, eye, and foot dominance should be noted. The clinician should ask about a family history of problems with dexterity and dominance, as well as check the patient's history concerning past ability for self-care, home and financial management ability, and shopping and communication skills.

An essential component of the neurologic assessment is the history of the neurologic illness. The history can be obtained from the patient, if possible, or from family or significant others, particularly if the patient's condition makes him or her a poor historian (Box 2-4). When using

---

BOX 2-4	Neurologic History

- History of present complaint
- Time course and progression (e.g., appeared suddenly or over a period of time)
- Signs and symptoms: include date of onset, severity, localization, extension, duration, and frequency
- Associated complaints, especially pain, headache, seizures, or changes in eating or sleeping patterns
- Screen for other neurologic complaints because patient may have more than one neurologic disorder
- Current neurologic state
- Loss of feeling, numbness, or tingling of the arms and legs
- Difficulty with walking, gait, balance, or coordination
- Weakness on one or both sides of the body
- Changes in vision, decrease in vision, or double vision (diplopia) in one or both eyes
- Difficulty with memory or ability to communicate or understand
- Change in personality
- Change in hearing, decrease in hearing, or ringing (tinnitus) in one or both ears
- Changes in or loss of smell or taste
- Changes in speech, decrease in swallowing, or aspiration
- Loss of bladder/bowel control or sexual function

- Loss of consciousness or feelings of light-headedness, dizziness, or vertigo
- Smoking history, use of alcohol, alcoholism, or use of illicit and mood-altering drugs
- Medical or metabolic disorders (e.g., excessive weight loss or gain, excessive thirst, thyroid disease, hypertension, or diabetes mellitus)
- Precipitating, aggravating, or alleviating factors
- Past and current treatment with prescription, over-the-counter, herbal, or alternative therapies
- Remissions or exacerbations
- Family history, with familial or hereditary occurrence of similar problems (e.g., stroke, ruptured aneurysm, neurofibromatosis, Huntington's chorea, muscular dystrophy, or Tay-Sachs disease)
- Absenteeism and interference with work, school, and recreational activities or activities of daily living (ADLs)
- Learning disorders, being held back in school, special education
- Education, vocation, highest level of education received
- Exposure to chemicals, toxins, fertilizers, lead, asbestos, high-energy electrical fields, pollutants
- Sexual history and risk factors for sexually transmitted diseases, including human immunodeficiency virus (HIV) infection

- Focus on patterns of past injuries (e.g., slips, trips, or falls), age-related senile gait, arthritis, muscle wasting or weakness, footdrop, ataxia, incoordination, tremors, increased lower extremity muscle tone, spastic paresis or paraparesis, difficulty sitting down or arising from a chair, difficulty navigating stairs, or parkinsonian gait
- Inquire about clumsiness; decreased performance in activities of daily living (ADLs); meal preparation; driving a car; use of public transportation; social withdrawal; decreased ability to see, smell, hear, or think; memory loss; confusion; and inability to make decisions
- Ask about any increase in social or home use of alcohol and wine, or cigarette, cigar, or pipe smoking
- Inquire about "accidents" (e.g., bowel and bladder incontinence) and use of protective undergarments
- Describe a transient ischemic attack (TIA) and ask if patient has experienced any TIA episodes or recent onset of dizziness or vertigo, tremors, or weakness
- Ask direct questions about poor appetite; restricted dietary intake; problems with eating, chewing, or swallowing; malabsorption or diarrhea; weight loss or gain; and feelings of low energy, loneliness, hopelessness, and helplessness; such questions may lead to admissions of depression and even thoughts of suicide, or use of medications to enhance sexuality
- Observe closely for behavior and response to questions
- Validate answers with others who are familiar with patient

the patient as the source of the history, validation of the information from family members or significant others may be necessary.

If other individuals are needed for the patient's history, the clinician should select the individual who is in the most immediate contact with the patient on a daily basis. Information about behavioral or personality changes, memory, hearing loss, changes in speech and language, mood swings, and seizures are best elicited from family members. These questions may be most applicable with older adult patients (Box 2-5).

Remembering the mnemonic OLD CARTS helps to prompt historical questions about the patient's complaint in terms of the following:

Onset
Location
Duration
Characteristics
Aggravating/Associated factors
Relieving factors
Temporal factors
Severity of symptoms

Assessment of Mental Status

The **mental status** is related to the mood and thoughts of an individual. Abnormalities may reflect a neurologic disease, psychiatric illness, or psychiatric illness secondary to a neurologic disease (e.g., depression following a stroke).[2] The **mental status examination (MSE)** assesses the higher cortical functions of thinking and reasoning. The goal is to determine deviations from normal, taking into consideration the patient's age, culture, education, and occupation. Conditions to observe for are signs of confusion, dementia, attention, perseveration, and resistance to interference. The MSE attempts to distinguish focal neurologic deficits, diffuse neurologic deficits, and primary or secondary psychiatric illness.[2]

Level of Consciousness

The **level of consciousness (LOC)** is the most important component of the neurologic assessment. **Consciousness** is the state of awareness of self, the environment, and responses to the environment; **coma** is the opposite of consciousness, or the total absence of awareness of self and the environment, even when the patient is externally stimulated. **Attention** refers to the ability to focus on a specific object, issue, or activity. There are two components of attention: alertness and directed attention (DA).[1] **Alertness** refers to a patient's overall ability to attend to environmental stimuli. **Directed attention** is thought to be the mechanism that inhibits irrelevant stimuli.

Between the extreme states of consciousness and coma are a variety of altered states of consciousness. Consciousness is a sensitive indicator of cortical function and is easily disrupted by neurologic damage or disease. When neurologic damage such as a structural lesion has occurred, a coma may result. This lesion can be either **supratentorial** (above the tentorium) or **infratentorial** (below the tentorium). Other causes of coma may be metabolic or psychiatric (Table 2-1). Important clues from the assessment of consciousness are used for all aspects of the neurologic examination.

Changes in the LOC during serial assessment, although often subtle, are essential indicators of improvement or deterioration in the patient's condition. Management decision making is guided by the degree of impairment of consciousness. The lower the LOC, the more intensive the clinical workup and nursing care will be. Finally, the LOC, in conjunction with pupillary reactivity and other brainstem signs, is a key component in the prediction of outcome.

Whatever the choice of LOC assessment tools, the goal of assessment of this parameter is to identify subtle changes in consciousness responses.

Components of Consciousness. There are two major components of consciousness: (1) arousal and (2) awareness of self and the environment with the ability to respond, or the content of consciousness. Consciousness is a function of the reticular formation, which has its origin in the brainstem. Fibers of the reticular formation in the upper brainstem, thalamus, and hypothalamus, called the **reticular activating system (RAS),** provide for the first component, arousal. Awareness comes with the integration of the reticular formation and RAS and higher cortical function.

Arousal, which includes the ability to respond to stimuli, is a state of responsiveness to sensory stimulation. Arousal requires both hemispheres and upper brainstem to be intact.[9] Observation is focused on the patient's ability to respond to

TABLE 2-1	Differential Characteristics of States Causing Sustained Unconsciousness
Mechanism	**Manifestations**
Supratentorial mass lesions compressing or displacing the diencephalon or brainstem	Initiating signs usually of focal cerebral dysfunction
	Signs of dysfunction progress rostrally to caudally
	Neurologic signs at any given time point to one anatomic area (e.g., diencephalon, mesencephalon, medulla)
	Motor signs often asymmetric
Infratentorial mass of destruction causing coma	History of preceding brainstem dysfunction or sudden onset of coma
	Localizing brainstem signs precede or accompany onset of coma and always include oculovestibular abnormality
	Cranial nerve palsies, usually presenting "bizarre" respiratory patterns that appear at onset
Metabolic coma	Confusion and stupor commonly precede motor signs
	Motor signs are usually symmetric
	Pupillary reactions are usually preserved
	Asterixis, myoclonus, tremor, and seizures are common
	Acid-base imbalance with hyperventilation or hypoventilation is common
Psychiatric unresponsiveness	Lids close actively
	Pupils reactive or dilated (cycloplegics)
	Oculocephalic reflexes are unpredictable; oculovestibular reflexes are physiologic (nystagmus is present)
	Motor tone is inconsistent or normal
	Eupnea or hyperventilation is usual
	No pathologic reflexes are present
	Electroencephalogram is normal

Modified from Plum F, Posner J: *The diagnosis of stupor and coma*, ed 3, Philadelphia, 1980, Oxford University Press.

noxious stimuli in an appropriate manner.[8] Arousal is best seen in the examination of patients in a persistent vegetative state (PVS). Patients in a vegetative state have brainstem function that allows for relatively normal life-sustaining functions, such as respiration and circulation. An apparent wake-sleep cycle is noted in these patients by observing periods of increased activity and periods of decreased activity. Reflex-type reaction to noise, lights, or noxious stimuli is also noted, but no meaningful interaction with the observer or these stimuli occurs.

Awareness is the orientation to person, place, and time and implies interaction with and reaction to environmental stimuli. After awareness is determined, the LOC is evaluated further. Conscious behavior depends on the presence in the cerebral hemispheres of relatively intact functional areas that interact extensively with each other, as well as with the deeper activating systems of the upper brainstem.[8]

Categories of Consciousness. A variety of tools and scales have been devised to describe the patient's LOC. Table 2-2 lists terms commonly used to describe LOCs. Patients are often difficult to categorize under these descriptions, and the descriptions alone may not be detailed enough to adequately communicate the patient's true state of consciousness. The key to communication of an LOC assessment is for the clinician to specifically describe the patient's response to a specific stimulus. For example, to record "The patient moans and withdraws from noxious stimuli" gives the next clinician a more complete picture of the patient than saying, "The patient is obtunded." It is essential to include both the

TABLE 2-2	Terms Describing Levels of Consciousness
Term	**Description**
Alert	Patient responds immediately to minimal external stimuli and is keenly aware of the environment.
Confused	Patient is disoriented to time or place but usually oriented to person, with impaired judgment and decision making and decreased attention span.
Delirious	Patient is disoriented to time, place, and person with loss of contact with reality and often has auditory or visual hallucinations.
Lethargic	Patient displays a state of severe drowsiness or inaction in which the patient needs an increased stimulus to be awakened.
Obtunded	Patient displays dull indifference to external stimuli, and response is minimally maintained. Able to arouse with stimulation and questions are answered with a minimal response.
Stuporous	Deep sleep, patient can be aroused only by vigorous and continuous external stimuli. Motor response is often withdrawal or localizing to stimulus.
Comatose	Vigorous stimulation fails to produce any verbal or voluntary neural response and patient cannot be aroused; eyes closed.

TABLE 2-3	Glasgow Coma Scale Categories	
Category	**Response**	**Score**
Eye opening	Spontaneous—eyes open spontaneously without verbal or noxious stimulation	4
	To speech—eyes open with verbal stimuli but not necessarily to command	3
	To pain—eyes open with various forms of noxious stimuli	2
	None—no eye opening with any type of stimulation	1
Verbal response	Oriented—aware of person, place, time, reason for hospitalization, and personal data	5
	Confused—answers not appropriate to question but correct use of language	4
	Inappropriate words—disorganized, random speech, no sustained conversation	3
	Incomprehensible sounds—moans, groans, and mumbles incomprehensibly	2
	None—no verbalization, even to noxious stimulation	1
Best motor response	Obeys commands—performs simple tasks on command and able to repeat task on command	6
	Localizes to pain—organized attempt to localize and remove painful stimuli	5
	Withdraws from pain—withdraws extremity from source of painful stimuli	4
	Abnormal flexion—decorticate posturing that occurs spontaneously or in response to noxious stimuli	3
	Extension—decerebrate posturing that occurs spontaneously or in response to noxious stimuli	2
	None—no response to noxious stimuli; flaccid	1

Modified from Teasdale G, Jennett B: Assessment of coma and impaired consciousness—a practical scale, *Lancet* 2:81, 1974.

response and the stimulus that was required to produce the response.

Glasgow Coma Scale. The **Glasgow Coma Scale (GCS)** is a practical standarized system for assessing the degree of consciousness and is the most widely recognized LOC assessment tool.[10] This scored scale is based on evaluation of three categories: eye opening, verbal response, and best motor response (Table 2-3). The highest possible score on the GCS is 15, and the lowest score is 3. Generally, a GCS score of 8 or less indicates a coma. Originally the scoring system was developed to assist with general communication of the severity of neurologic injury in patients with traumatic brain injury (TBI). Adapted and modified, this scale has become the basis of many neurologic assessment flow sheets (Fig. 2-1).

When using the GCS for serial assessment, the clinician should remember several points. The GCS is an LOC assessment tool only and should never be considered a complete neurologic examination. It is not a sensitive tool for evaluation of altered sensorium. The GCS does not account for possible aphasia and is not a good indicator of lateralization of neurologic deterioration, since the GCS records only the "best" motor response. Lateralization involves decreasing motor response on one side or changes in pupillary reaction. (Also see Chapter 6 to review the new FOUR Score coma scale.)

For example, a patient with a GCS score of 10 (e.g., eye opening—2; verbal response—3; motor response—5), localizing to pain on both sides at the last examination, may now be localizing to pain on the right but demonstrating abnormal flexion (decorticate posturing) on the left. Examination of the pupils may also show a change and reveal a right pupil that is 2 mm larger than the left and sluggishly reactive. Because the GCS records only the best motor response, this patient could have a GCS score of 10, just as in the previous assessment. The patient's deteriorating condition points to an expanding mass lesion on the right side of the brain, but the GCS score alone would never indicate this.

The GCS is often used incorrectly in the evaluation of patients with spinal cord injuries. A patient with a complete C5 or C6 vertebral injury but no head injury should have a GCS score of 15. Confusion arises with the motor portion of the GCS. A score of 6 on the motor examination implies that the patient is able to respond to verbal commands accurately. Although the patient with this level of spinal cord injury is not able to wiggle the fingers or toes, he or she is able to perform such functions as sticking out the tongue and raising the eyebrows. Often clinicians will score the motor portion as 1—no response to noxious stimuli; flaccid. This results in a GCS score of 9, which falsely implies a significant alteration in consciousness. The clinician needs to remember that the GCS is assessing the LOC, not motor function of the extremities. It should be kept in mind, however, that a patient may have a dual diagnosis of head injury and spinal cord injury and would be appropriately assessed using the GCS and a complete spine assessment (see Chapter 14).

Approach to the Patient. Evaluation of the LOC is most accurate when the patient is stimulated to a maximal state of arousal. To identify subtle changes in consciousness, the clinician should never begin a serial assessment with the assumption that the patient will perform at the same level as during the last assessment. Each assessment should be started as if the patient were intact neurologically.

The **first level of response** is when the clinician approaches the patient, positioned in a comfortable manner, and observes for a response by the patient to the clinician's physical presence using a normal speaking voice. If the patient does not respond, the clinician should call out the patient's name. For the **second level,** if there is no response, a louder verbal stimulus or shouting is used. The **third level** requires tactile stimulation with a gentle shaking of the patient to elicit a

THE JOHNS HOPKINS HOSPITAL
DEPARTMENT OF NEUROSCIENCE NURSING

MULTIPLE DAY FLOWSHEET

ASSESSMENT   *for addressograph plate*

If assessment meets normal criteria place a check (✔) next to the assessment parameter. Total assessment needs to be completed every 24 hours. If abnormal assessment, place an asterisk (*) next to parameter and record findings in progress note. If abnormal assessment remains unchanged from shift to shift, draw an arrow (→) beside the assessment parameter. For Neurological section, chart actual findings where appropriate.

	Assessment — DATE / TIME								
Neurological/Sensory									
MENTAL STATUS	Alert, oriented to person, place and time								
	Answers questions appropriately for age								
COMA SCALE	Best Motor								
	Best Verbal								
	Eye Opening								
	GCS Total								
	Stimulation								
MOTOR STRENGTH	Right Arm	5/5 5/5 5/5	5/5 5/5 5/5	5/5 5/5	5/5 5/5	5/5 5/5	5/5	5/5 5/5	5/5 5/5
	Left Arm	5/5 5/5 5/5	5/5 5/5 5/5	5/5 5/5	5/5 5/5	5/5 5/5	5/5	5/5 5/5	5/5 5/5
	Right Leg	5/5 5/5 5/5	5/5 5/5 5/5	5/5 5/5	5/5 5/5	5/5 5/5	5/5	5/5 5/5	5/5 5/5
	Left Leg	5/5 5/5 5/5	5/5 5/5 5/5	5/5 5/5	5/5 5/5	5/5 5/5	5/5	5/5 5/5	5/5 5/5
	Absence of Drift								
	Fall Risk Assessment Score								
Pupillary Reaction, CN III	Right Size/Reaction								
	Left Size/Reaction								
CRANIAL NERVES (CN)	CN II (Vision, visual fields)								
	CN III, IV, VI (Extraocular movements)								
	CN V (Facial sensation)								
	CN VII (Facial symmetry)								
	CN VIII (Hearing, balance)								
	CN IX, X (Gag)								
	(Cough)								
	CN XI (Shoulder shrug)								
	CN XII (Tongue midline)								
CEREBELLAR	Rapid Alternating Movements; Finger-to-nose; Heel/shin								
SENSORY	Pain goal (as appropriate)								
	Pain rating score								
	Pain free or pain goal achieved								
	Absence of paresthesias								
RESPIRATORY	Unlabored respirations								
	Absence of cough								
	Tracheostomy/Stoma (Size: _____)								
	Oxygen: _____								
	Breath sounds clear								
	Registered Nurse Initials / Licensed Practical Nurse Initials								

Glasgow Coma Scale (GCS)		**Stimulation**	**Motor Strength**	**Pupils**		**Phlebitis Scale**	
Motor	**Verbal**		5 - Normal	Reaction / Equality / Size		**Grade**	**Clinical Criteria**
6 - Obeys Command	5 - Oriented		4 - Movement against resistance, less than normal	B - Brisk	P - Pinpoint	0	No symptoms
5 - Localizes Pain	4 - Confused	V - Voice		S - Sluggish	S - Small	1	Erythema at access site with or without pain
4 - Withdrawal	3 - Inappropriate Words	ST - Shout	3 - Movement against gravity, but not resistance	F - Fixed	M - Moderate	2	Pain at access site with erythema and/or edema
3 - Flexion to Pain	2 - Incomprehensible Sounds	SK - Shake	2 - Movement, but not against gravity	= - Equal	L - Large	3	Pain at access site with erythema and/or edema Streak formation Palpable venous cord
2 - Extension to Pain	1 - None	P - Pain	1 - Flicker of muscle	≠ - Unequal			
1 - None			0 - No movement	**Pain Scale**		4	Pain at access site with erythema and/or edema Streak formation Palpable venous cord greater than 1 inch in length Purulent drainage
Eyes				0 - No Pain			
4 - Spontaneously	2 - To Pain			10 - Worst Pain			
3 - To Speech	1 - None						

FORM #JHH-05-996-0002 (1/05)   JH1889T - 996

Figure 2-1 Neuroscience nursing flow sheet.
(Used with permission from Johns Hopkins Hospital, Department of Neuroscience Nursing, Baltimore, MD.)   *Continued*

PATIENT NAME:

_____

HISTORY NUMBER:

_____

ASSESSMENT

Braden Risk Assessment Score: Assess the following factors daily. Patients with a total of 16 or less are considered to be at risk of developing pressure ulcers. Place on Pressure Ulcer Prevention Standard.

		1	2	3	4
SENSORY PERCEPTION	Ability to respond meaningfully to pressure-related discomfort.	Completely Limited	Very limited	Slightly Limited	No Impairment
MOISTURE	Degree to which skin is exposed to moisture	Constantly Moist	Very Moist	Occasionally Moist	Rarely Moist
ACTIVITY	Degree to physical activity	Bedrest	Chairfast	Walks Occasionally	Walks Frequently
MOBILITY	Ability to change and control body position	Completely Immobile	Very Limited	Slightly Limited	No Limitations
NUTRITION	Usual food intake pattern	Very Poor	Probably Inadequate	Adequate	Excellent
FRICTION and SHEAR		Problem	Potential Problem	No Apparent Problem	**Total Score**

If assessment meets normal criteria place a check (✔) next to assessment parameter. If abnormal assessment, place an asterisk (*) next to parameter and record findings in progress note. If abnormal assessment remains unchanged from shift to shift, draw an arrow (→) beside the assessment parameter and record findings in progress note.

ASSESSMENT	DATE / TIME													
Cardiovascular														
Absence of edema														
Skin warm and dry														
Radial pulses regular and palpable														
Gastrointestinal														
Appetite appropriate														
Nutritional intake sufficient														
Swallows without difficulty														
Absence of nausea and vomiting														
Abdomen non-distended														
Elimination within own normal pattern, consistency and color														
Last bowel movement: _____														
Nasogastric tube/Gastric tube/Jejunostomy tube														
Bowel sounds present times 4 quadrants														
Genitourinary														
Urinary output quantity sufficient, clear yellow to amber, without burning, urgency or frequency														
Intermittent catheterization:_____														
Indwelling catheter (Size: _____)														
Musculoskeletal														
Absence of skeletal deformity														
Moves all extremities														
Integumentary														
Skin intact														
Procedure site clean: _____														
Absence of pallor, cyanosis, jaundice, erythema or edema														
Braden Risk Assessment Score														
Vascular Access Device(s): _____														
Phlebitis Score (as appropriate)														
Drains: _____														
Psychosocial														
Appearance, behavior and verbalization are appropriate to the situation and age of patient														
Family/significant others interactions are appropriate to the situation														
Ready, willing and able to learn														
Registered Nurse Initials / **Licensed Practical Nurse Initials**														

FORM #JHH-05-996-0002 (1/05)   JH1943T - 996

Figure 2-1, cont'd

PATIENT NAME: _____   **HISTORY NUMBER:** _____

DATE														
TIME														
Plans of Care (POC)														
Enteral Tube Feed Standard														
Fall Prevention Intervention - Low														
Fall Prevention Intervention - Moderate														
Fall Prevention Intervention - High														
Isolation (Specify: _____)														
Oxygen Therapy Standard														
Patient Controlled Analgesia Standard (Specify: _____)														
Post-Operative Standard														
Pressure Ulcer Prevention Standard														
Pulse Oximeter Standard														
Respiratory Standard - Low														
Respiratory Standard - Moderate														
Respiratory Standard - High														
Restraint Standard														
Seizure Standard														
Tracheostomy Standard														
Vascular Access Device Standard														
Additional POC:														
Registered Nurse Initials														

Date	Time	Assessment / Problem	Admission, Transfer, Transport, Discharge Note/Plans/ Interventions/Response to Interventions/ Progress Towards Expected Outcomes

Figure 2-1, cont'd

response. Finally, if none of these levels has aroused the patient, the clinician should use the **fourth level,** or noxious stimuli (e.g., a "central" painful stimulation with supraorbital pressure, sternal rub, squeezing the trapezius, or pinching the inner aspect of the arm), unless contraindicated, to obtain a maximal patient response to stimuli. Observe for bilateral responses. If an asymmetric or only a unilateral response is noted, it is appropriate to apply peripheral stimuli (e.g., nailbed compression). This approach will better detect subtle improvements, as well as deterioration in neurologic functioning.

Orientation. A patient is assessed for orientation to time (either the day of the week or the day of the month, the month, or the year), place (hospital or home address, city, and state), and person (full name). Orientation to time is often lost first and may be impaired early, even in mild organic brain syndromes. Orientation to time may also be lost in hospitalized patients, particularly those in a critical care environment. This type of disorientation is less often a result of cerebral dysfunction than of sleep deprivation or sensory overload. Loss of orientation to place may occur with a moderate disturbance of cerebral function. Disorientation to person is the last orientation parameter lost and occurs with severe cerebral dysfunction, such as obtundation, delirium, or dementia. An isolated loss of orientation to person should be highly suspect.

Confusion is a mental state characterized by disorientation to time, place or person, or situation. Confusion may cause bewilderment, perplexity, lack of orderly thought, and the inability to choose or act decisively. Confusion may result from an organic mental disorder or accompany severe emotional stress or psychologic disorders. As a nursing diagnosis, *confusion* has been defined as the abrupt onset of a cluster of global, transient changes and disturbances in attention, cognition, psychomotor activity, and level of consciousness, or it may result from disturbances in the sleep/wake cycle. Confusion may be acute or chronic. Disorientation is a state of mental confusion that may occur in organic mental disorders, drug or alcohol intoxication, or severe stress.

Speech and Language. Communication is one of the highest cortical functions of the human being. Communication, also known as language, is made up of four major functions: listening, reading, speaking, and writing. These four functions are integrated with each other and conscious experiences to form a central language process. A change in language can be the first and only neurologic deficit. Dysarthria is poorly articulated speech, resulting from interference in the control and execution over the muscles of speech, usually caused by damage to the central or peripheral motor nerve. The individual may exhibit loss of clear articulation, phonation, or breath control. Types of dysarthrias range from flaccid with a hypernasal characteristic, to spastic with slurred speech, to ataxic with prolonged speech patterns, to hypokinetic dysarthria that is flat speech often with a rush of words. Hyperkinetic dysarthria is an abnormal speech rhythm that can be fast or slow. Some individuals may have combinations of dysarthrias with mixed characteristics.

Disturbances of the dominant hemisphere, which is responsible for the complex process of interpretation and formulation of language symbols, lead to aphasia, or the inability to communicate (Table 2-4). Difficulty in communication is known as *dysphasia*. Writing is usually the most impaired modality in aphasia. **Apraxia of speech** is motor speech characterized by substitutions, additions, repetitions, and prolongations of sounds resulting from impairment in the organization or programming of previously learned patterns of movement. Profanity and the ability to carry a tune are often well preserved.

As indicated in the preceding paragraph, language function resides predominantly in the dominant hemisphere. The left hemisphere contains language in almost all right-handed

TABLE 2-4	Classification of Common Aphasias					
Aphasia	Speech Production	Repetition	Verbal Comprehension	Naming	Reading	Writing
Expressive, Broca's, motor	Impaired	Impaired	Normal	May be impaired	Variable, may be impaired	Impaired
Receptive, Wernicke's, sensory	Normal	Impaired	Impaired	Impaired	Impaired	Impaired
Conduction	Normal	Impaired	Normal	May be impaired	Normal or variable	Impaired
Transcortical motor	Impaired	Normal	Normal	May be impaired	May be impaired	Impaired
Transcortical sensory	Normal	Normal	Impaired	Impaired	Impaired	Impaired
Transcortical mixed	Impaired	Normal	Impaired	Impaired	Impaired	Impaired
Anomic	Normal	Normal	May be impaired	May be impaired	Impaired	May be impaired
Global	Impaired	Impaired	Impaired	Impaired	Impaired	Impaired

From Weiderholt WC: *Neurology for the non-neurologist,* Philadelphia, 1988, WB Saunders.

individuals and in 70% of patients who are left-handed or ambidextrous.[2]

Specifically, these functions lie at the junction of the frontal, temporal, and parietal lobes, with deep connections between these regions. There are a variety of types of aphasias, but all disturbances in speech and language processing are due either to the inability to correctly receive and incorporate information (receptive aphasia) or to the inability to correctly communicate information (expressive aphasia).

Receptive Aphasia. **Receptive aphasia,** also known as **Wernicke's aphasia, sensory aphasia,** or **fluent aphasia,** results from damage in the parietal and/or posterior temporal lobes. In receptive aphasia the ability to comprehend written language (alexia) or verbal language is impaired. The patient converses fluently but without clear meaning. Although the patient may be able to participate in reflexive conversational exchanges, such as "Hello, how are you? Fine, thank you," more difficult conversation is often meaningless. The words are pronounced correctly, but the string of words does not make a concrete thought or a clear sentence. In receptive aphasia the patient often does not recognize the deficit and may appear unconcerned about errors or lapses in speech. Give a simple command or ask the patient simple questions or questions with yes/no answers. If the patient does not understand, repeat louder. Ask the patient if he or she is having difficulty finding the right words. To assess word-finding or naming ability, ask the patient to name as many animals as he or she can think of in 1 minute. Normally a patient should name 18 to 22 animals.[2]

Expressive Aphasia. **Expressive aphasia** or **motor aphasia,** also known as **Broca's aphasia** or **nonfluent aphasia,** results from damage to Broca's area, which is the inferior and posterior portions of the dominant frontal lobe. Broca's aphasia may be associated with hemiplegia. In expressive aphasia the patient's comprehension and ability to conceptualize are relatively preserved, but the ability to form language and express thoughts is impaired. The speech pattern is slow, produced with great effort, and poorly articulated. The patient is not able to produce 50 words per minute. Disturbed coordination (**dyspraxia**) of speaking and breathing alter the rhythm of speech. Writing is also usually impaired in expressive aphasia and is called **dysgraphia.**

Expressive aphasia is often accompanied by a right hemiparesis that is worse in the arm than in the leg. Frustration, anger, and depression are frequently seen with expressive aphasia, since the patient is acutely aware of the deficit.

Other Aphasias. Other types of aphasias occur because of damage in the conduction pathways or nearby cortical fiber tracts.

Conduction aphasia is caused by a lesion between Broca's and Wernicke's areas. Speech is fluent, but abnormalities appear in repetition and writing.

Transcortical aphasias are aphasias occurring because of damage adjacent to either Broca's or Wernicke's area. These sensory or motor aphasias are rare and similar to aphasias of the adjacent area except that repetition, or the repeating of words, is normal.

Global aphasia results from a very large lesion involving the frontal, parietal, and temporal lobes. In global aphasia, all language functions are impaired. Global aphasia is a severe disorder of both expression and comprehension and is associated generally with destruction of both Broca's and Wernicke's areas.

Amnesic, or **anomic, aphasia** may be expressive or receptive and results in the inability to name objects. The patient may have fluent speech devoid of meaningful words and extreme word-finding difficulty.[9] The area involved in anomic aphasia has not been localized, but the lesion may be posterior. Anomic aphasia occurs with preservation of the ability to understand and repeat words; the difficulty is in the use of nouns (nominal or substantive words).

Assessment Parameters

The assessment of the patient's ability to verbally comprehend and communicate is an essential element in a complete neurologic examination but also has far-reaching implications in the planning, intervention, and evaluation of clinical management. Listen and evaluate speech in context to the clinical setting. Expressive aphasia is generally easier to recognize, since the patient is often hemiparetic and struggling to speak. Receptive aphasia can occur without obvious focal motor or sensory abnormalities because the lesion is usually in the temporal or parietal lobe, away from the motor and sensory pathways. Frequently, speech deficits or disorders are initially misinterpreted as confusion.

Assessment of speech and language occurs during the entire neurologic examination. When evaluating the appropriateness of the patient's memory, LOC, ability to relate a history, or ability to follow commands, the clinician is also evaluating the patient's speech and language. In each communication with the patient, the clinician includes the parameters listed in Box 2-6.

Other items that could affect the patient's ability to communicate include a deteriorating LOC, loss of hearing or vision, and unfamiliarity with the chosen language. Asking the patient to write or read a paragraph is an excellent screening test because a patient who is aphasic in spoken language is unable to read and write normally. If speech abnormalities are suspected, the patient should be referred to a speech therapist for a complete evaluation. To test reading, ask the patient to read a sentence. Dyslexia is impairment in the ability to read as a result of a variety of pathologic conditions, some of which are associated with the CNS. Individu-

BOX 2-6	Key Areas of Assessment: Speech and Language
Comprehension	Reading/writing
Content	Repetition
Effort	Speech volume
Flow	Speed/rate
Fluency	Spontaneity
Grammar	Syntax
Naming	Timing (latencies)
Paraphasias	Vocabulary
Phonation (breathiness, resonance, nasality)	Word choice
	Word output
Prosody (inflection)	

als with dyslexia often reverse letters and words and cannot adequately distinguish the letter sequences in written words and have difficulty determining left from right.

Memory. **Memory** is a complex, integrated function involving the limbic system, the temporal lobe, the prefrontal area, and cortical association areas. It is the primary cognitive process associated with learning. Poor performance may indicate organic brain disease. Memory and learning are closely related insofar as memory is the process whereby learned information is stored in the central nervous system (CNS) for future retrieval. Memory is thought to involve the encoding, storage, and retrieval of information. Memory is evaluated in three areas: retention, recent memory, and remote memory. Inform the patient that you will be asking questions that might range from very simple, current events to events that occurred many years ago.

Retention. Retention (immediate recall) is assessed by asking the patient to repeat a given sequence of digits (e.g., "seven, two, six, four, nine") both forward and in reverse. This type of immediate recall addresses issues of attention span, as well as intellectual functioning. Retention may also be tested by asking the patient to repeat a sentence or to carry out a three-part command, such as "Stand up, touch your forehead, and turn to the left." The retention function is impaired when a primary sensory receiving area of the cortex is affected. Impairment is manifested as inattentiveness, distractibility, or failure to focus on the stimulus and how many errors are made and how many times you have to repeat instructions.[2]

Recent Memory. Recent, or short-term, memory may be assessed by asking the patient to describe what he or she ate for breakfast or news events from the past few days. The patient is asked to remember three things, such as bell, book, and candle, and is then asked to recall them after 5 minutes. You might ask the patient to remember the location of a fictitious address and to repeat it back to you. Recent memory is also assessed by having the patient describe the course of the current illness. Impairment of recent memory usually implies bilateral medial temporal lobe dysfunction.[1] Patients with a receptive speech deficit will have difficulty with this task.

Remote Memory. Of the three types of memory assessed, remote, or long-term, memory is the one requiring the most validation by someone close to the patient. With remote memory testing, the patient is asked such things as the names and ages of children, siblings, or parents, or the date of graduation from high school. Impairment of remote memory implies widespread and severe brain dysfunction and is often seen with advanced dementia.

General Knowledge. Assessment of the patient's **general fund of knowledge** should be individualized to the patient's intellectual level, social and cultural background, and general interests. The main purpose of assessing general information is to determine whether the patient has an adequate fund of knowledge commensurate with his or her intellectual level and experiences. General information, once accumulated, is not lost until there is a severe loss of brain substance or severe impairment of function. The patient can be asked to name the current president of the United States, the number of days in a week, the number of weeks in a year, or local

current events. Patients may be clever in concealing memory loss with expressions such as "You know what I mean."

Calculation. The patient's intellectual level and educational background also should be considered when assessing calculation. The most common way of testing calculation is by serial subtraction of 7s from 100. Other examples are to ask the patient to multiply 5 times 13, to divide 38 by 2, or to add 33 and 49. These calculations may be too difficult for some patients and they can be assessed by simple multiplication questions. A patient's ability to calculate may be disturbed in diffuse brain disease and in focal lesions of the dominant hemisphere in the region of the angular gyrus.[7]

Abstraction and Judgment. **Abstraction** and **judgment** describe the ability to project into the future and draw on experience in response to a described situation. Abstract thoughts test for frontal lobe function and are useful with frontal lobe lesions and dementia.[2] Interpretation of similarities in word pairs can be used as a test for abstraction. For example, the patient might be presented with word pairs such as orange/banana or horse/dog, where the answers should be "Both an orange and a banana are fruits" and "A horse and a dog are both animals."

Tell the patient that you would like him or her to explain some proverbs, such as "A rolling stone gathers no moss" or "A stitch in time saves nine." Abstraction and judgment require an intact frontal lobe. Judgment is often poor in organic brain disease, mental retardation, and psychotic states. A patient with impaired brain function will have difficulty performing on an abstract level and will be vague or will respond concretely.[7]

Assessment of Motor Function

The patient's motor status is assessed to determine movement and strength of extremities and the ability to move spontaneously or as a result of stimulation. The examiner evaluates involuntary movements, muscle symmetry, atrophy, and gait. The clinician must consider the age, physical build, gender, occupation, activity level, and nutrition of the patient. The successful performance of any motor function involves interaction of the muscles, neuromuscular junction, peripheral nerves, central nerve pathways (both pyramidal and extrapyramidal), cerebellum, and motor cortex of the frontal lobe. Because these systems are all integrated, the clinician must understand what each contributes to the final motor response. The level of the nervous system affected can be determined by the distribution and pattern of weakness. There are five patterns of muscular weakness: upper motor neuron (UMN), lower motor neuron (LMN), muscle disease, neuromuscular junction, and functional weakness that is not in a distribution that can be understood on an anatomic basis.[2] The basic methods of inspection, palpation, and percussion are used for the examination of muscles.[1] **Handedness** should be noted at the beginning of the assessment. Explain or demonstrate to the patient that you will be assessing simple movements, performing range of motion (ROM), and comparing the patient's strength from the right side to the left side and upper extremities versus lower extremities as you observe and feel the patient's muscles.

Motor System Components

Voluntary motor movements originate in the motor cortex of the frontal lobe of the brain. Certain parts of the nervous system are primarily responsible for muscle activity. These are the upper motor neurons, both the pyramidal and the extrapyramidal systems, the lower motor neurons, and the cerebellum. The components of the motor assessment include the following:

- Reflex response: involuntary motor response to sensory stimuli changes, which may appear before other signs or deficits
- Involuntary movement: movement that should not be seen in muscles at rest
- Muscle size (bulk): assessment parameter that is estimated or measured with a tape measure
- Muscle strength and grading: assessment method that localizes neurologic lesions
- Muscle tone: resistance encountered when the joint is moved for range of motion (ROM)

Upper Motor Neurons. Upper motor neurons (UMNs) consist of descending pathways that interface with the nuclei of the anterior horn cells of the spinal cord and the cranial nerve nuclei of the brainstem. UMN lesions are characterized by weakness, spasticity, hyperactivity of the tendon reflexes, and Babinski's sign, but minimal atrophy. The **clasp-knife reflex** is an abnormal sign in which a spastic limb resists passive motion and then suddenly gives way, like the motion of the blade of a jackknife. The UMN comprises two systems: the pyramidal and extrapyramidal.

The **pyramidal, or corticospinal,** tract is made up of central nerve fibers that arise from the motor cortex and travel down to the lower medulla, where they form a structure resembling a pyramid. Most of the fibers cross to the opposite (contralateral) side of the medulla and travel downward through the lateral corticospinal tracts of the spinal cord, where they synapse with anterior horn cells or with intermediate neurons. Most of these fibers are facilitatory; that is, they encourage the action of the lower motor neuron.[7] Lesions of the pyramidal system produce weakness with little or no atrophy, plus hyperactive reflexes, increased muscle tone, spasticity, and rigidity.

The **extrapyramidal system** is made up of all fibers, except for the corticospinal tracts, which influence movement. This includes the basal ganglia, nuclei of the brainstem, and cerebellum. The fibers of the extrapyramidal system are inhibitory, with the exception of the cerebellum. This system helps to maintain muscle tone and control movements, such as walking. Lesions in the extrapyramidal system produce movement disturbances, such as tremor, chorea, athetosis, dystonia, spasticity, and rigidity, without significant paralysis.

Working together, the pyramidal and extrapyramidal systems of the UMN provide a balance of facilitatory and inhibitory influences on the lower motor neuron pathways. Table 2-5 describes the clinical observations in each of these systems. It is often difficult to delineate a pyramidal from an extrapyramidal lesion during a clinical assessment.

Lower Motor Neurons. Lower motor neurons (LMNs) are defined as the anterior horn cells or cranial nerve nuclei, with their motor axons, neuromuscular junctions, and the muscle. Their cell bodies lie in the gray matter of the spinal cord. Muscle stretch reflexes, which are described later in this chapter, are a component of the LMN. LMN lesions produce loss of muscle tone and ipsilateral weakness, flaccidity, atrophy, weak or absent deep tendon plantar and abdominal reflexes, and fasciculations. Characteristics of upper and lower motor neuron syndromes are described in Table 2-6.

Reflex Responses. A reflex action is an involuntary function or movement in response to a particular stimuli occurring immediately without the involvement of will or consciousness. Three common types of reflexes are deep tendon, superficial, and pathologic.

A tendon reflex results from the stimulation of a stretch-sensitive afferent from a neuromuscular spindle, which, via a single synapse, stimulates a motor nerve leading to a muscle contraction.[2] A **deep tendon reflex (DTR)** is a brisk contraction of a muscle in response to a sudden stretch induced by a sharp tap by a reflex hammer on the tendon of insertion of the muscle. Absence of the reflex may be caused by damage to the muscle, peripheral nerve, nerve roots, or spinal cord at that level. A hyperactive reflex may indicate disease of the pyramidal system above the level of the reflex being tested. DTRs are checked and graded on a scale of 0 (absent) to 4+ (hyperactive). Reflex testing is very reliable because reflexes are involuntary. When approaching the patient, do not ask him or her to relax because this may further increase anxiety. Make the patient feel comfortable with general conversation or simple diverting questions.

Muscle stretch reflexes (MSRs), also known as deep tendon reflexes (DTRs), are a result of the reflex arc

TABLE 2-5	Pyramidal Versus Extrapyramidal Motor Syndromes	
	Pyramidal Motor Syndromes	**Extrapyramidal Motor Syndromes**
Unilateral movement	Paralysis of voluntary movement	Little or no paralysis of voluntary movement
Tendon reflexes	Increased tendon reflexes	Normal or slightly increased tendon reflexes
Involuntary movements	Absence of involuntary movements	Presence of tremor, chorea, athetosis, or dystonia
Muscle tone	General spasticity in muscles (e.g., clasp-knife phenomenon); hypertonia present in flexors of arms and extensors of legs	May have rigidity or intermittent rigidity (cogwheel rigidity)

From McCance KL, Huether SE: *Pathophysiology: the biological basis for disease in adults and children,* ed 3, St Louis, 1998, Mosby.

TABLE 2-6   Upper and Lower Motor Neuron Syndromes

	Upper Motor Neuron Syndromes*	Lower Motor Neuron Syndromes†
Distribution of affected muscles and brain	Muscle groups are affected; when movement is possible, the proper relationship among agonists, antagonists, synergists, and fixators is preserved	Individual muscles may be affected
	Synkinesias (residual movements) are present; attempts to move paralyzed part cause a variety of associated movements; movements of normal limb may cause imitative or mirror movements in the paralyzed limb	Individual muscles may be affected
Muscle tone	Increased muscle tone; hypertonia, specifically spasticity	Hypotonia, flaccidity
Tendon reflexes	Hyperreflexia with extensor plantar reflex present	Hyporeflexia; no abnormal reflexes present
Atrophy	Slight, caused by disuse	Pronounced atrophy
Fasciculations	Absent	May be present

From McCance KL, Huether SE: *Pathophysiology: the biological basis for disease in adults and children,* ed 4, St Louis, 2002, Mosby.
*Pyramidal motor syndromes.
†All are motor unit syndromes.

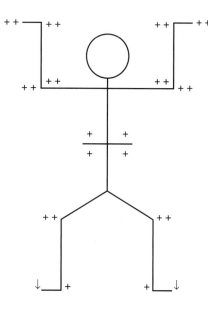

Scoring Deep Tendon Reflexes

Grade	Deep Tendon Reflex
0	Absent
±	Present only with reinforcement
1+	Present but depressed
2+	Normal
3+	Increased
4+	Clonus

Figure 2-2 The patient's reflex scores are recorded by entering the correct scores at the correct location on the stick figure.

(Fig. 2-2). The reflex arc is a simple neurologic unit of sensory neurons that carries a stimulus impulse to the spinal cord where it connects with a motor neuron that carries the reflex impulse back to an appropriate muscle. MSRs indicate the balance of inhibitory and excitatory impulses of the UMN as it interfaces with the LMN. Any LMN lesion usually results

in diminished or absent MSRs. UMN lesions facilitate the MSR and produce a hyperactive reflex. Table 2-7 lists the MSR, the muscle group involved, and the expected responses.

In performing reflex assessment, the absent reflex feels "dull." A generalized or bilateral absent reflex may indicate a peripheral neuropathy whereas an isolated absent reflex may indicate either a peripheral nerve or more commonly a root lesion or spinal shock in spinal injury. There are three types of reflexes: muscle stretch, superficial, and pathologic. Fig. 2-3 shows a scale of responses used to score and record DTR responses.

A **superficial reflex** is any neural reflex initiated by stimulation of the skin. Superficial reflexes may be abdominal, anal, or cremasteric. Superficial reflexes may produce a motor response when the cornea, skin, or mucous membranes are stimulated (Table 2-8). Superficial reflexes are usually present if the patient has LMN dysfunction but are absent with UMN dysfunction.

A **pathologic reflex** is any reflex that is caused by a lesion in or an organic disease of the nervous system. It results from an organic interference with the normal function of the nervous system. Pathologic reflexes result from UMN lesions either in the motor area of the brain or in the corticospinal tracts.

The best known of these reflexes is Babinski's reflex (Fig. 2-4, *C*). **Babinski's reflex** is the dorsiflexion of the big toe with extension and fanning of the other toes elicited by firmly stroking the lateral aspect of the sole of the foot. In adults it may indicate a lesion in the pyramidal tract. After explaining to the patient that you are going to stroke the bottom of his foot, gently stimulate with a blunt instrument up the lateral border of the foot and across the foot pad, firm enough to prevent a tickle sensation. Watch the big toe and the remainder of the foot.[2] This reflex, an extensor plantar response, involves the extension of the great toe, or dorsiflexion (upgoing toe) with fanning of the other toes.

Babinski's sign is normal in infants until approximately 2 years of age and is part of the defensive reflex called the

TABLE 2-7	Muscle Stretch Reflexes		
Muscle	**Reflex**	**Nerve Roots Involved**	**Peripheral Nerve**
Upper extremity brachioradialis	Brachioradialis	C5 to C6	Musculocutaneous
Biceps	Biceps jerk	C5 to C6	Radial
Flexor finger	Flexor finger jerk	C7 to C8	Median and ulnar
Triceps	Triceps jerk	C6 to C7	Radial
Patellar	Knee jerk (Patellar reflex) (Quadriceps reflex)	L2 to L4	Femoral
Achilles (gastrocnemius soleus)	Ankle jerk	L5, S1 to S2	Sciatic and tibial

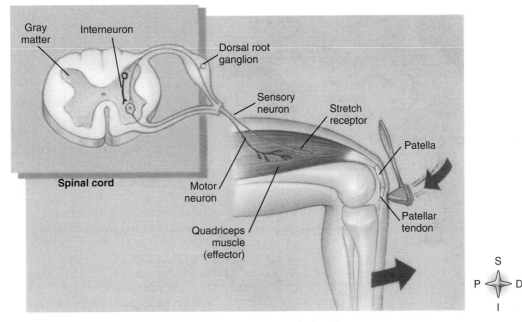

Figure 2-3 Patellar reflex. Neural pathway involved in the patellar (knee-jerk) reflex. *(From Thibodeau GA, Patton KT: Anatomy and physiology, ed 5, St Louis, 2003, Mosby.)*

TABLE 2-8	Superficial Reflexes	
Reflex	**Nerve(s) Involved**	**Normal Reaction**
Corneal	CN V and VII	Prompt closure of both eyelids when cornea touched with wisp of cotton
Pharyngeal	CN IX and X	Gagging response to pharyngeal stimulation
Upper abdominal	T8-T9-T10;	Contraction of abdominal muscle when upper abdomen or lower abdomen
Lower abdominal	T10-T11-T12	is stroked, so that there is a brief, brisk movement of umbilicus toward stimulus
Cremasteric	L1, L2	Elevation of testicle when inner aspect of thigh stroked
Bulbocavernosus	S3-S4	Pressure to glans penis with contraction of anus
Anal wink	S2-S3-S4	Stroke perianal area and contraction of external anal sphincter occurs
Bulbocutaneous	S4-S5	Contraction of anal ring as perineum is stroked or scratched
Anocutaneous	S5	
Plantar	L5, S1	Flexion of toes from stimulation of sole of foot

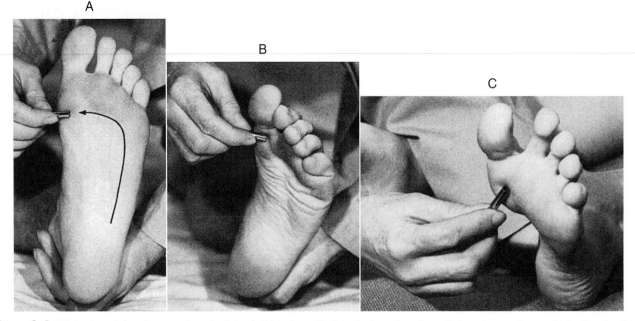

Figure 2-4 Elicitation of the plantar reflex. **A,** A hard object is applied to the lateral surface of the sole, starting at the heel and going over the ball of the foot, ending beneath the great toe. **B,** Normal response to plantar stimulation: flexion of all toes. **C,** Babinski's sign: dorsiflexion of the great toe and fanning of the other toes.
(From Malasanos L, Barkaushas V, Stoltenberg-Allen K: Health assessment, ed 4, St Louis, 1990, Mosby.)

flexion reflex. As cortical functions mature, the reflex becomes inhibited. In the face of cortical disease, there may be a reemergence of early reflexes. The loss of the inhibitory influences allows the reflex to resurface.[7]

Cerebellum. The cerebellum plays a key role in the coordination of muscle movement. Influences from the cerebellum are incorporated into the UMN system. Components of the cerebellar assessment are discussed later in this chapter.

Lateralizing Signs

In all components of motor and sensory assessment, it is essential to compare responses on one side of the body with those on the other side. Lateralizing signs are neurologic assessment findings on one side of the body only and include unilateral deterioration in motor movements and/or changes in pupillary response. Lateralizing signs help to localize the lesion to one side of the brain. For example, a patient who withdrew from painful stimuli with both arms at the last examination may now be posturing by withdrawing with the right arm but exhibiting abnormal flexion with the left arm. This change in response on the left side points to an expanding intracranial lesion on the right.

The occurrence of lateralizing signs indicates an emergency. Unilateral deterioration of motor movements and/or pupillary response may herald uncal or central herniation. Notification of the physician and immediate interventions are imperative.

Involuntary Movements

Movement disorders are not well understood. The act of any movement requires a change in the contractile state of the muscles, and anything that disrupts the CNS control of

muscle contraction could lead to involuntary motor movements. While observing the patient, the clinician should note any involuntary or abnormal movements. Examples of involuntary motor movements and their associated causes are listed in Table 2-9.

Abnormal Motor Responses

In the unconscious patient, noxious stimuli may elicit an abnormal motor response. These responses are identified as abnormal flexion or abnormal extension (Fig. 2-5).

The term **abnormal flexion** has replaced the term *decorticate posturing*. In response to painful stimuli, the upper extremities exhibit flexion of the arm, wrist, and fingers with adduction of the limb. The lower extremity exhibits extension, internal rotation, and plantar flexion. Interruption of the corticospinal pathways in the cerebral hemispheres or in the internal capsule may cause abnormal flexion.

The term **abnormal extension** has replaced the term *decerebrate rigidity* or *posturing*. When a patient is stimulated, the patient's teeth clench and arms extend stiffly in an adducted and hyperpronated position. The legs are stiffly extended, with plantar flexion of the feet. Extension is thought to be caused by a deep hemispheric lesion that descends into the midbrain and upper pons areas of the brainstem.

Because abnormal flexion and extension look similar in the lower extremities, the upper extremities are used to determine the presence of these abnormal movements. It is possible for the patient to exhibit abnormal flexion on one side of the body and extension on the other or to display these abnormal movements intermittently. Outcome studies indicate that abnormal flexion or decorticate posturing has a less serious prognosis than abnormal extension or decerebrate posturing.[8]

TABLE 2-9	Types of Involuntary Movements

Type	Characteristics	Causes
Chorea*	Nonrepetitive muscular contractions, usually of the extremities of face; random pattern of irregular, involuntary, rapid contractions of groups of muscles; disappears with sleep, decreases with resting; increases with emotional stress and attempted voluntary movement	Associated with excess concentration of or a supersensitivity to dopamine within basal ganglia
Athetosis*	Disorder of distal muscle postural fixation; slow, sinuous, irregular movements most obvious in the distal extremities, more rhythmic than choreiform movements and always much slower; movements accompany characteristic hand posture; slowly fluctuating grimaces	Occurs most commonly as a result of injury to the putamen of the basal ganglion; exact pathophysiologic mechanism is not known
Ballismus	Disorder of proximal muscle postural fixation with wild flinging movement of the limbs; movement is severe and stereotyped, usually lateral; does not lessen with sleep; ballism is most common on one side of the body, a condition termed *hemiballism*	Results from injury to subthalamus nucleus (one of the nuclei that comprise the basal ganglia); thought to be caused by reduced inhibitory influence in the nucleus, a release phenomenon; hemiballism results from injury to the contralateral subthalamic nucleus
Hyperactivity	State of prolonged, generalized, increased activity that is largely involuntary but may be subject to some voluntary control; not highly stereotyped but rather manifests as continuous changes in total-body posture or in excessive performance of some simple activity, such as pacing under inappropriate circumstances	May be caused by frontal and reticular activating system injury
Wandering	Tendency to wander without regard for environment	"Release" phenomenon; associated with bilateral injury to globus pallidus or putamen
Akathisia	Special type of hyperactivity; mild compulsion to move (usually more localized to legs); severe frenzied motion possible; movements are partly voluntary and may be transiently suppressed; carrying out the movement brings a sense of relief; a frequent complication of antipsychotic drugs	Dopaminergic transmission may be involved
Tremor at rest	Rhythmic oscillating movement affecting one or more body parts	Caused by regular contraction of opposing groups of muscles
Parkinsonian tremor	Regular, rhythmic, slow flexion-extension contraction; involves principally the metacarpophalangeal and wrist joints; alternating movements between thumb and index finger described as "pill rolling"; disappears during voluntary movement	Loss of inhibitory influence of dopamine in the basal ganglia, causing instability of basal ganglial feedback circuit within the cerebral cortex
Postural tremor		
Asterixis (tremor of hepatic encephalopathy)	Irregular flapping movement of the hands accentuated by outstretching arms	Exact mechanisms responsible unknown; thought to be related to accumulation of products normally detoxified by the liver
Metabolic	Rapid, rhythmic tremor affecting fingers, lips, and tongue; accentuated by extending the body part; enhanced physiologic tremor	Occurs in conditions associated with disturbed metabolism or toxicity, as in thyrotoxicosis (hyperthyroidism), alcoholism, and chronic use of barbiturates, amphetamines, lithium, amitriptyline (Elavil); exact mechanism responsible unknown
Essential (familial)	Tremor of fingers, hands, and feet; absent at rest but accentuated by extension of body part, prolonged muscular activity, and stress	Not associated with any other neurologic abnormalities; cause unknown

Continued

TABLE 2-9	Types of Involuntary Movements—cont'd	
Type	Characteristics	Causes
Intention tremor		
Cerebellar	Tremor initiated by movement, maximal toward end or movement	Occurs in disease of the dentate nucleus (one of the deep cerebellar nuclei responsible for efferent output) and the superior cerebellar peduncle (a stalk-like structure connected to the pons); caused by errors in feedback from the periphery and errors in preprogramming goal-directed movement
Rubral	Rhythmic tremor of limbs that originates proximally by movement	Results from lesions involving the dentatorubrothalamic tract (a spinothalamic tract connecting the red nucleus in the reticular formation and the dentate nucleus in the cerebellum)
Myoclonus	Series of shocklike, nonpatterned contractions of portion of a muscle, entire muscle, or group of muscles that cause throwing movements of a limb; usually appear at random but frequently triggered by sudden startle; do not disappear during sleep	Associated with an irritable nervous system and spontaneous discharge of neurons; structures associated with myoclonus include the cerebral cortex, cerebellum, reticular formation, and spinal cord

From McCance KL, Huether SE: *Pathophysiology: the biological basis for disease in adults and children*, ed 4, St Louis, 2002, Mosby.
*Choreoathetosis involves both chorea and athetosis; the precise pathophysiology unknown.

TABLE 2-10	Muscle Strength Grading Scale
Grade	Muscle Strength Term
0	Total paralysis, no muscular contraction detected Zero/Absent
1	Flicker, palpable or visible muscle contraction Trace
2	Active movement of muscle with gravity eliminated Poor
3	Active muscle movement against gravity Fair
4	Active muscle movement, against some resistance Good
5	Active muscle movement against full resistance Excellent/Normal

Assessment Techniques

When performing motor examinations, the clinician must assess bilateral extremities at the same time. This allows for comparison of function and identification of subtle differences.

Muscle Examination. Examination of the motor system includes the assessment of muscles for strength, bulk, atrophy, hypertrophy, tone, fasciculations, cramps, myokymia, pain, and fibrillation.

Muscle strength of the upper and lower extremities is assessed by having the patient perform a variety of functions against resistance applied by the clinician. Muscle strength or power is best graded with the use of some type of scale. Table 2-10 gives an example of such a scale. The actual scale used matters little. The important point is that all health care providers (clinician, physician, physical therapist, occupa-

tional therapist) should use the same scale. This enhances communication and reduces the potential for changes in the patient's condition to be missed completely. When the examiner places several fingers in the patient's palm and asks the patient to squeeze and release, the patient should let go. If the patient involuntarily grabs your hand without releasing, this primitive reflex may indicate frontal lobe pathology or diffuse encephalopathy.[2]

Muscle bulk is assessed together with muscle strength. Muscle mass is compared on both sides for similarity in size and shape. If muscle atrophy is noted, the distribution of the atrophy should be identified. The distribution and extent of the muscle atrophy provide important clues about the cause of the atrophy.

Hypertrophy is an increase in muscle size. The muscle may actually be normal in size when compared with atrophic muscle.

Muscle tone is also assessed during a motor examination. For this evaluation, the patient is asked to relax the extremity and allow the clinician to perform passive ROM. The clinician is assessing for the degree and quality of resistance to passive movements (i.e., spasticity, rigidity, or the reverse, flaccidity) (Table 2-11). Involuntary movement involving muscles should also be examined for evidence of **fasciculations:** the localized, uncoordinated, uncontrollable twitching of a single muscle group innervated by a single motor nerve fiber or filament that may be palpated and seen under the skin. Fasciculations may be seen in amyotrophic lateral sclerosis (ALS) or disorders such as dietary deficiency, cerebral palsy, fever, polio, sodium deficiency, tic, or uremia. **Cramps** may be a spasmodic and often painful contraction of one or more muscles (e.g., writer's cramp).

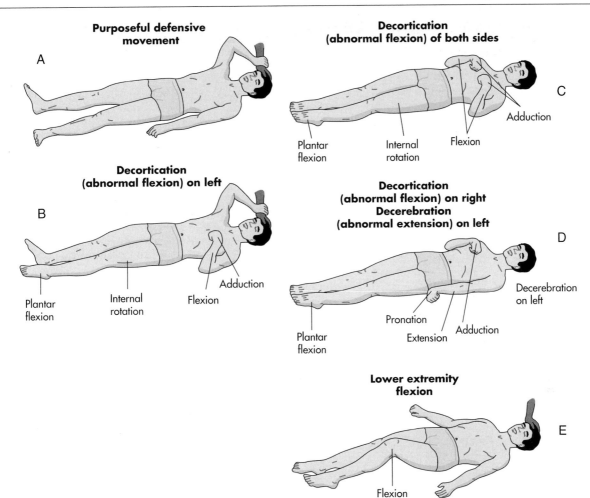

Figure 2-5 Abnormal flexion and abnormal extension. **A,** Purposeful defensive movement. **B,** Abnormal flexion response. Flexion of the arms, wrists, and fingers with adduction in the upper extremities. Extension, internal rotation, and plantar flexion in the lower extremities. **C,** Abnormal flexion response. Abnormal flexion of both arms and plantar flexion of the feet. **D,** Abnormal flexion response on the right side of the body and abnormal extension response on the left side of the body. **E,** Opisthotonic posturing.
(From Urden LD, Thelan LA, Stacy KM, Lough ME: Thelan's critical care nursing: diagnosis and management, *ed 4, St Louis, 2002, Mosby.)*

Myokymia is a condition manifested by spontaneous tetanic contractions, or muscle twitching. Such contractions noted in the face may indicate multiple sclerosis, a brain tumor, or cranial neuropathies.[1]

Muscle pain and tenderness can be elicited by squeezing the muscle or may be demonstrated when the muscle is in use or is being tested for strength.

Painful or Noxious Stimuli. After the clinician determines that the patient is incapable of comprehending and following a simple command, the use of noxious stimuli is required to determine the motor responses of the body. A variety of ways of administering painful stimuli are presented here. There are also several commonly used but less acceptable means of delivering noxious stimuli, which are also discussed. In all situations a variety of means should be used for serial assessments because repeated noxious stimuli to any part of the body will cause breakdown. It is important to document the type of stimuli, location, and duration. When the clinician finds it necessary to apply stronger stimuli for a longer period of time, the physician should be notified of a potential deterioration in the patient's neurologic condition.

There are two mechanisms of painful stimuli: central and peripheral. **Central stimulation** involves the trunk or central portion of the body and produces an overall body response. Central stimulation should be used for the initial introduction of pain. **Peripheral stimulation** is delivered more distally in the extremities and is important for the differentiation between hemispheric conditions and spinal cord injury. If the patient localizes to the stimuli, sensation is intact as the motor cortex gives a purposeful response. If the patient withdraws away from the stimuli, the cortex is not working as withdrawal occurs at the hypothalamus. Abnormal flexion occurs at the level of the upper brainstem, and abnormal extension occurs at the midbrain or pons. No response and flaccidity occurs at the level of the medulla. Assume that gross sensation is intact if the comatose patient responds to painful stimuli. Otherwise, the comatose patient's sensory status cannot be assessed.

TABLE 2-11   Alterations in Muscle Tone

Alterations	Characteristics	Cause
Hypotonia	Passive movement of a muscle mass with little or no resistance	Thought to be caused by decreased muscle spindle activity as a result of decreased excitability of neurons
Flaccidity	Muscles may be moved rapidly without resistance Associated with limp, atrophied muscles, and paralysis	Occurs typically when nerve impulses necessary for muscle tone are lost
Hypertonia	Increased muscle resistance to passive movement May be associated with paralysis May be accompanied by muscle hypertrophy	Results when the lower motor unit reflex arc continues to function but is not mediated or regulated by higher centers
Spasticity	A gradual increase in tone causing increased resistance until tone suddenly is reduced, which results in clasp-knife phenomenon	Exact mechanism unclear; appears to arise from an increased excitability of the alpha motor neurons to any input because of absence of the descending inhibition of the pyramidal systems
Gegenhalten (paratonia)	Resistance to passive movement, which varies in direct proportion to force applied	Exact mechanism unclear; associated with frontal lobe injury
Dystonia	Sustained involuntary twisting movement	Produced by slow muscular contraction
Rigidity	Muscle resistance to passive movement of a rigid limb that is uniform in both flexion and extension throughout the motion	Occurs as a result of constant, involuntary contraction of muscle
Plastic, or lead-pipe	Increased muscular tone relatively independent of degree of force used in passive movement; does not vary throughout the passive movement	Associated with basal ganglion damage
Cogwheel	The uniform resistance may be interrupted by a series of brief jerks resulting in movements much like a ratchet, "cogwheel" phenomenon	Associated with basal ganglion damage
Gamma and alpha	Characterized by extensor posturing (decerebrate rigidity)	Loss of excitation of extensor inhibitory areas by the cerebral cortex decreasing the inhibition of alpha and gamma motor neurons Loss of cerebellum input to lateral vestibular nuclei

From McCance KL, Huether SE: *Pathophysiology: the biological basis for disease in adults and children,* ed 4, St Louis, 2002, Mosby.

Central Stimulation

The clinician should always stand in a position to avoid being hit or kicked when applying a painful stimulus. The response may be unilateral or bilateral. Look for symmetry of response. Central stimulation includes the following:

- **Trapezius pinch:** This central noxious stimulus, which allows for observation of total-body response, is administered by squeezing the trapezius muscle. A trapezius pinch is often difficult to perform on large or obese adults.
- **Sternal rub:** This central noxious stimulus is administered by applying firm pressure to the sternum in a rubbing motion, usually with the clinician's knuckles. If this method were used repeatedly, the sternum could become bruised and excoriated. Open-handed firm patting of the sternal area to arouse the patient is a good method to use when a less noxious stimulus is needed to facilitate arousal of the patient.
- **Supraorbital pressure:** This central noxious stimulus is administered by pressing the thumb under the upper part of the patient's orbit. Patients with head injuries, frontal craniotomies, or facial surgeries should not be evaluated with this method because of

the possibility of an underlying fractured or unstable cranium. Bradycardia may result from pressure to the eye, and this method is contraindicated in patients with glaucoma; therefore the clinician should not develop the habit of applying supraorbital pressure to deliver a noxious stimulus.

- **Nipple and testicle pinch:** A health care provider should never use such noxious stimuli in the clinical setting. For obvious reasons, they are inappropriate, unnecessary, and unacceptable.

Peripheral Stimulation

Peripheral stimulation includes the following:

- **Nail bed pressure:** This peripheral noxious stimulus requires the use of an object such as a pen to apply firm pressure to the nail bed for 10 to 30 seconds. Pressure applied to each extremity allows for evaluation of individual extremity function. Although this pressure is classified as a noxious stimulus, if no response is elicited from nail bed pressure, other noxious stimuli should be used.
- **Pinching the inner aspect of the arm or leg:** This peripheral noxious stimulus is administered by firmly pinching a small portion of the patient's tissue on the

sensitive inner aspect of the arm or leg. Each extremity is evaluated independently. Although this form of noxious stimulus is most likely to bruise a patient, it is also the most sensitive for eliciting individual extremity responses.

Assessment of Sensory Function

The physiology behind the integration and interpretation of sensory stimuli is not fully understood. A sensory stimulus travels from its source at nerve endings into afferent nerve fibers, which travel up through the spinal cord and the thalamus into the contralateral parietal lobe of the cortex. The thalamus functions as the main sensory nucleus of the nervous system, and the cortex provides the refinement of fine sensory discrimination.

The sensory system has unusual decussation patterns. Touch, pain, and temperature cross to the contralateral side of the spinal cord shortly after entry, and position sense and vibration travel up the ipsilateral side until decussation occurs at the brainstem level. Because of this phenomenon, patients with incomplete spinal cord lesions often have unusual sensory patterns, which should be carefully assessed and monitored. The sensory component is one of the more difficult parameters to assess, and this assessment is easier when the patient is awake and alert. Because the sensory fibers are large, the sensory status may be symptomatic before the motor status. Patients' subjective complaints of tingling or decreased sensation therefore cannot be ignored.

Sensory System Components

Assessment of the sensory system evaluates **superficial sensation** and **deep sensation.** Explain the sensory tests to be performed, the stimulus used, and the response expected. The patient is expected to distinguish lateralization of stimulus, type of stimulus, and exact location of stimulus.[9] There are five basic modalities of sensation: vibration, joint position, light touch (large fiber—posterior tract), pinprick, and temperature (small fiber—spinothalamic tract). The posterior column remains ipsilateral up to the medulla, where it crosses over. The spinothalamic tract mostly crosses within one to two segments of entry. Vibration, joint position, and temperature senses are often lost without prominent symptoms. Light touch and pinprick loss is usually symptomatic.[2]

A sensory examination is done first with the patient in a comfortable position, eyes open to introduce the stimulus and then with the patient's eyes closed so that visual information does not influence the patient's ability to interpret sensations. When performing a sensory examination, the clinician should ensure that the patient can comprehend simple and complex commands and is cooperative. Explain each test and what is expected to allow the patient to concentrate and avoid the "startle reflex." Move from areas of sensory loss to areas of normal sensation or where sensation is expected to be **within normal limits (WNL).**
Superficial Sensation. Superficial sensation may involve lesions of the peripheral nerves, spinal roots, spinal cord, brainstem, thalamus, and cerebral cortex. The assessment includes light touch, pain, and temperature.

Light touch is assessed by stroking a wisp of cotton on the patient's skin while avoiding pressure or depressing the skin. Both sides of the body are tested, starting from the head and working down the body. The patient is asked to state where the sensation is felt and if the sensation is the same on both sides. A scale of 1 to 10 may be used.

Superficial pain is assessed by the use of a light pinprick on the skin. The clinician should begin the examination by demonstrating to the patient the items that will be used to produce sharp and dull sensations. Again, both sides of the body are evaluated at the same time by applying the lightest pressure needed for a response in random patterns. The patient should be able to define the sensation as sharp or dull. If an abnormality is identified, the area of abnormal or absent sensation should be mapped and further evaluated. In the case of a patient with spinal cord injury, the sensory level is frequently identified by marking on the patient's body. In this way subsequent clinicians can clearly see any changes in the sensory level.

Skin temperature is most frequently assessed with test tubes of hot and cold water applied in a random manner. Although seldom conducted with the hospitalized patient, temperature assessment may help further define a sensory deficit noted on superficial pain testing.
Deep Sensation. Deep sensation testing includes the assessment of vibration, position sense, and deep pain.

Vibration is evaluated with the use of a 128 Hz or 256 Hz tuning fork by striking it on the heel of the examiner's hand and holding the tuning fork by the stem to place over bony surfaces. Ask the patient to close his or her eyes and identify when the fork is vibrating and when it stops. The clinician starts distally on each extremity with the toe tips and distal parts of the body. If sensation is WNL, there is no need to proceed proximally.

Joint position sense is tested by the use of passive movement. The amount of movement normally detected is barely visible.[2] In the lower extremities the great toe is grasped and moved in an upward or downward motion. With the eyes open the patient is given a demonstration. With eyes closed, the patient is asked to indicate which way the toe was moved. The ankle, knee, and hip can be included in the tests. In the upper extremities the same procedure is done with the thumb, wrist, elbow, or shoulder. A minimum of three trials should be performed and, if the patient is successful, recorded as 3/3 position sense. If the patient is incorrect, the response is recorded as −1/3, −2/3, or −3/3, depending on the number of incorrect responses.

Deep pain is tested only when the other deep sensations are absent. It is assessed by increasing pressure or compression applied to various deep-lying structures with a motor response. Pressure is applied to the Achilles tendon, calf muscles, or upper arm muscles. Deep pain in muscles should be evaluated in several different planes to rule out sensitivity caused by a vein or artery instead of the muscle itself.[1] Of course, if phlebitis or deep vein thrombosis (DVT) is suspected, deep pain sensation should not be assessed in that extremity. The hypersensitivity or hyposensitivity of deep pain may indicate peripheral neuropathies, tabes dorsalis, spinal cord injury, or some muscle diseases. Slight variation of deep pain sense is difficult to assess, but it is the extremes of hypersensitivity or hyposensitivity that are most important diagnostically. **Dysesthesia** is a disagreeable sensation of burning pain, **hypalgesia** is diminished sensitivity to pain, **hyperalgesia** is increased sensitivity to pain, and **analgesia** is complete insensitivity to pain (see Chapter 23).

Other Tests of Sensation. Further refinement of the sensory assessment tests higher integrative sensory functions, including evaluation of two-point discrimination, stereognosis, and graphesthesia.

Two-point discrimination tests the ability to distinguish the separation of two simultaneous pinpricks. With the eyes closed, the patient is stimulated with two pinpricks at various distances and is asked to indicate when both pinpoints are perceived. The opposite side of the body is then compared for similarities. The normal distance of two-point discrimination varies in different areas of the body.

Stereognosis is the ability to distinguish common objects (e.g., coins, marbles, or safety pins) placed in the hand when the eyes are closed. The general testing of sensory perception should be performed before stereognostic testing is attempted. Generally, loss of sensory perception to light touch will alter the performance on this test. Astereognosis occurs in cortical disease, particularly of the parietal lobe.

Graphesthesia is the ability to recognize numbers or letters traced on the skin. As with stereognosis, general sensory perception should be intact before this test is attempted.

Assessment of the Pupils, Vision, and Eye Movement

Pupillary function, vision, and eye movement are important components of the neurologic assessment and can provide significant diagnostic information. Especially in the unconscious patient or the patient receiving neuromuscular blocking agents and sedation, pupillary response is one of the few neurologic signs that can be assessed. Because of the location of the third, fourth, and sixth cranial nerves (CNs III, IV, and VI) and the integration of the **medial longitudinal fasciculus (MLF)** for proper function, pupil and eye assessment provides valuable information about the function of the brainstem. Components of examination of the eye include the size and equality, shape, reactivity to direct and consensual light, acuity, visual fields, and accommodation. The examiner can evaluate the patient's vision and extraocular movements (EOMs), the cold caloric test (oculovestibular reflex), and assessment for doll's eyes (oculocephalic reflex). Serial evaluation, appropriate technique, recognition of abnormalities, and good documentation are all important. Funduscopic examination can be performed for advanced assessment of the eye to evaluate the optic disc, retina, and retinal vessels.

Pupils

The size, shape, and reaction of the pupils are functions of the autonomic nervous system. **Parasympathetic control** of pupillary reaction occurs through innervation of the oculomotor nerve (CN III), which exits from the brainstem in the midbrain area. When the parasympathetic fibers are stimulated, the pupil constricts. **Sympathetic control** of the pupil originates in the hypothalamus and travels down the entire length of the brainstem to the sympathetic chain in the cervical spine area and then back up to the pupil. When the sympathetic fibers are stimulated, the pupil dilates. Normally, sympathetic and parasympathetic innervation are equally balanced. Children usually have more widely dilated pupils, whereas the pupils of older adults are more constricted.

Changes in the pupils provide a valuable tool for assessment because of their pathway location. The oculomotor nerve lies at the junction of the midbrain and the tentorial notch. Papilledema may occur with swelling of the optic disc from increased intracranial pressure (ICP). Any increase in pressure that exerts force down through the tentorial notch compresses the oculomotor nerve (Fig. 2-6). Oculomotor nerve compression results in a dilated, nonreactive pupil. Sympathetic pathway disruption occurs with involvement in the brainstem. Pinpoint, nonreactive pupils are associated with loss of sympathetic control; loss of parasympathetic control leads to dilated, nonreactive pupils. Pupillary reactivity is also affected by medications, particularly sympathetic and parasympathetic agents, direct trauma, and eye surgery. Pupil reactivity is relatively resistant to metabolic dysfunction and can be used to differentiate between metabolic and structural causes of decreased levels of consciousness. The corneal reflex, or "blink" reflex, provides information about the trigeminal nerve (CN V) and the facial nerve (CN VII). Comatose patients may require a **tarsorrhaphy**, in which the

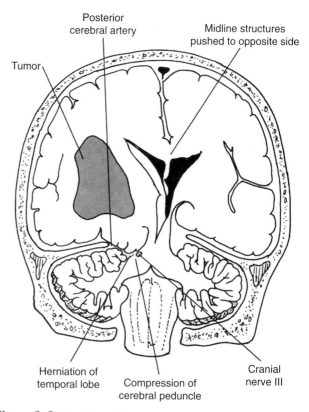

Figure 2-6 Uncal herniation with oculomotor nerve compression.

upper and lower eyelids are sutured together to protect the eye until the patient is responsive.

Evaluation of pupillary response includes assessment of the size, shape (round, irregular, or oval), and degree of reactivity of the pupils to light.

Pupil Size. Pupil size is best observed in the resting eye position with tangential lighting. The eyes should be midposition with normal pupil size varying from 2 to 6 mm. The two pupils should be compared for equality. Although most individuals have equally sized pupils, it is normal for some persons to have a discrepancy between pupil sizes of up to 1 mm. Inequality in the size of the pupils is known as **anisocoria** and occurs in 15% to 17% of the normal population. Document the size, shape, and symmetry of each eye before using the light. Devices called *pupillometers* are commercially available for precise pupillary assessment.

Changes or inequality in pupil size, especially in patients who have not previously had this discrepancy, could be the first sign of the impending danger of herniation and should be reported immediately (Table 2-12; see Fig. 2-11, *B*). With the close proximity of the oculomotor nerve (CN III) to the notch of the tentorium, assessment of the size and reactivity of the pupils plays a key role in the assessment of ICP changes. In addition to CN III compression, there are other possible reasons for changes in pupil size. Extremely small pupils could indicate narcotic overdose, lower brainstem compression, or bilateral damage to the pons. Large pupils could be a result of the instillation of cycloplegic agents, such as atropine or scopolamine.

Pupil Shape. Pupil shape is also noted in the assessment of pupils. Although the pupil is normally round, an irregularly shaped or oval pupil is not an infrequent occurrence in patients with elevated ICP. An oval pupil often indicates early CN III compression caused by transtentorial herniation (Fig. 2-7). An oval pupil may be associated with an ICP of 18 to 35 mm Hg. The oval pupil appears to represent a transitional pupil that will return to normal size if ICP can be controlled but that will go on to dilate and be unreactive if ICP is not treated or cannot be controlled.[6] The shape of a pupil may also be altered by previous ophthalmologic procedures, such as cataract surgery. Such findings should be noted in the initial assessment and confirmed through the patient's history.

Pupillary Reactivity. Pupillary reactivity to light is also part of pupil assessment. Pupillary reactivity is tested in each eye separately. The technique for evaluation of direct pupillary response involves the use of a narrow-beamed bright light shone into the pupil from the outer canthus of the eye and observes for reaction in both eyes. If the light is shone directly onto the pupil, glare or reflection of the light may prevent proper visualization by the assessor. The pupillary response should be graded using terms such as **brisk,**

TABLE 2-12 Pupillary Changes	
Pupillary Change	**Location and Pathogenesis**
Small (1 to 2.5 mm in diameter), reactive pupils	
Regularly shaped	Cerebral dysfunction, especially of metabolic origin
	Bilateral diencephalon dysfunction caused by sustained increased intracranial pressure
Irregularly shaped	Often found in encephalopathy, multiple sclerosis, and vascular disease, including diabetes mellitus
Midposition (4 to 5 mm in diameter or slightly larger, 5 to 6 mm in diameter), round, regular, but light fixed pupil that spontaneously fluctuates in size	Damage to dorsal tectum or pretectum of the midbrain interrupts the pupillary light pathways, but the accommodation pathways remain intact
	Hippus, alternating slight constriction and slight dilation of the pupils creating the impression that the pupils are bouncing, may be found
Dilated (greater than 5 mm in diameter), fixed pupil	Anoxia
	Atropine, scopolamine (large concentration), amphetamines, mydriatics, and cycloplegics
Midposition (4 to 5 mm in diameter), pupils fixed to light (may be slightly irregular or unequal)	Sympathetic and parasympathetic pathways that control pupil size and response in the midbrain are damaged most commonly by herniation but may be produced by tumors, hemorrhages, anoxia, and infarcts
	Drug effect: glutethimide (Doriden), atropine, scopolamine (large concentration)
Dilated (greater than 5 mm in diameter), fixed pupil with extraocular paralysis (usually bilateral)	Interruption of the oculomotor (CN III) tract between the nucleus and its point of exit from the brain
	Intrinsic midbrain damage
Sluggish-responding pupil that is gradually dilating (unilateral initially)	Temporal lobe herniation compressing the ipsilateral oculomotor nerve against the posterior communicating artery or tentorial notch as it passes through the tentorial notch en route to innervate the eye
Small, pinpoint pupils (less than 1 mm in diameter)	Dysfunction in the pons interrupts the descending sympathetic pathway
	Opiate effect
	In the absence of drugs, this is highly suggestive of a pontine hemorrhage

From Beare PG, Myers JL: *Adult health nursing,* ed 3, St Louis, 1998, Mosby.
CN, Cranial nerve.

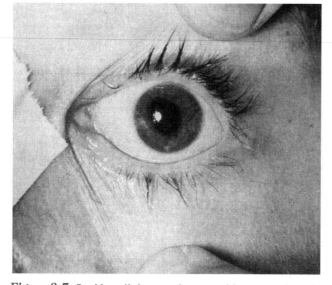

Figure 2-7 Ovoid pupil that may be seen with compression of CN III resulting from increased intracranial pressure and transtentorial herniation.

sluggish, or **nonreactive** with no change in response to light. In the older adult, pupils are often smaller and less reactive. Allow adequate time for the pupil response to occur. A slow or minimal pupil response can be difficult to detect.

Consensual pupillary response is constriction of the pupil in response to a light that is shone into the opposite eye. Because of this phenomenon, several seconds should elapse before testing the opposite pupil, which will be momentarily constricted. If the light is directed into a **blind eye,** there will be no direct or consensual response. If the light is directed into the opposite eye, which has vision, the sighted eye and the opposite, blind eye will both constrict. Accommodation is the process by which the eye adjusts and is able to focus and produce a sharp image at various changing distances from the object seen. The convexity of the anterior surface of the lens may be increased or decreased by contraction or relaxation of the ciliary muscle. Accommodation is tested by having the patient focus on an object held 1 to 2 feet in front of the face and then moving the object toward the face. As the object comes within 4 to 6 inches of the nose, the eyes will converge inward and the pupils will constrict. With aging, the lens become harder and less flexible and may result in loss of accommodation or the ability to focus on nearby objects. Table 2-13 discusses a variety of abnormal pupillary responses.

Vision

Assessment of vision evaluates the capacity for sight and the optic nerve (CN II) as it exits the eye, travels through the optic chiasm, and then courses back through the brain to the occipital lobes. The two most common types of testing are **visual acuity testing,** which evaluates central vision, and **visual field testing,** which evaluates peripheral vision. In the more advanced examination, the retina and optic disc are assessed. The clinician should also consider the age of the

patient when assessing vision. Table 2-14 lists the changes in vision that occur with age.

Visual Acuity. **Visual acuity** is a measure of the resolving power of the eye (e.g., recognizing letters or numbers at a given distance). Acuity is most easily tested by using standardized charts, such as the Near Vision Chart, Snellen chart, or handheld Rosenbaum chart. Ask the patient to read down from the largest letters to the smallest. Record results in distance from the chart and which letters were correctly read. Consideration of the patient's intellectual and educational level guides the selection of the type of standardized chart used. When standard charts are not available, visual acuity can be tested by reading various type sizes in a newspaper or by counting fingers. Visual acuity is assessed for each eye separately. If corrective lenses are worn, they should be worn during the test. The presence of normal visual acuity implies normal central vision.

Visual Fields. **Visual field** testing is the evaluation of peripheral vision. The field of vision is defined as that portion of space in which objects are visible during fixation of gaze in one direction.[7] Precise visual field testing is done by a neurophthalmologist, but gross visual field testing is possible during the routine examination. In gross visual field testing, the clinician stands a short distance in front of the patient. The patient is asked to close one eye and focus on the nose or forehead of the clinician. The clinician holds a pencil or finger outside of the patient's field of vision and slowly moves it into the field. The patient is instructed to indicate when the pencil becomes visible. All four quadrants—the upper, lower, nasal, and temporal quadrants—are assessed in the same manner. The same procedure is conducted for the other eye.

The visual fields of the eye depend on the visual pathways being intact from the retina through the optic nerves, chiasm, tracts, and radiations to the visual cortex in the occipital lobes (see Fig. 1-42).

Because lesions interrupting various parts of the pathway cause specific types of defects in the visual fields, it is frequently possible to determine the site of the lesion from the nature of the defect in the field.[7] Lesions of the eye and optic tract produce visual defects in one eye only. Optic chiasm lesions usually produce temporal defects in both eyes, and lesions occurring after the chiasm produce homonymous defects in both eyes.

The most common visual defects are (1) blindness in one eye, caused by damage to the eye, retina, optic disc, or track before entering the optic chiasm; (2) **bitemporal hemianopsia,** caused by a lesion at the optic chiasm that affects temporal vision on both sides (often seen when a pituitary tumor presses on the optic chiasm); and (3) **homonymous hemianopsia,** caused by damage to the optic fibers as they pass from the optic chiasm to the occipital lobes. As the optic fibers reach the occipital lobe, they form separations or radiations, which lead to inferior or superior quadrant homonymous hemianopsia with blindness or defective vision in the right or left halves of the visual fields of both eyes.

Retina and Optic Disc. The clinician inspects the patient's retina and optic disc through an ophthalmoscope. With the room darkened to allow for pupillary dilation, the patient is

TABLE 2-13   Abnormal Pupillary Responses

Condition	Characteristics	Causes
Amaurotic pupil (blind eye)	Both pupils same size; no response to direct light in blind eye; no consensual response to light in opposite eye; normal response to direct light in good eye; normal consensual response to light in blind eye; both eyes constrict on accommodation	Blindness in one eye is a result of injury or disease to retina or optic nerve before it reaches optic chiasm
Hippus	Pupil initially reacts briskly, followed by alternating dilation and contraction in response to light	May be normal (especially if viewing pupil under magnification); midbrain lesion; barbiturate toxicity; early uncal herniation with beginning pressure on CN III
Marcus Gunn pupil (swinging flashlight sign)	Pupils equal in size; slow direct-light reflex to affected eye; normal consensual reflex of affected eye; affected pupil constricts when light shone in normal eye but dilates when light shone in affected eye	Lesion anterior to optic chiasm Afferent pupil defect, optic atrophy, or retinal disease
Horner's syndrome	Unilateral small pupil (anisocoria); ipsilateral ptosis of eyelid; ipsilateral anhidrosis (loss of sweating)	Anterior root cord lesion at C8-T3 caused by trauma, vertebral disk compression, or vascular compromise; damage of hypothalamus
Adie's pupil (tonic pupil)	Unilateral in 80%; anisocoria with affected pupil larger than normal pupil; pupil slow to dilate in dark; pupil slow to constrict in light; more common in women	Loss of postganglionic parasympathetic fibers; after viral infection; hypersensitivity to cholinergic drugs
Argyll-Robertson pupil	Small, irregular, unequal pupils; absent response to light or ciliospinal reflex; reacts to accommodation; dilates minimally in dark	Neurosyphilis (tabes dorsalis); viral encephalitis; syringomyelia
Miosis	Pinpoint pupils that do not appear to constrict further with light; may observe constriction with magnification	Compromise of sympathetic pathway or parasympathetic irritation; pontine hemorrhage; opiate drugs; metabolic encephalopathies
Mydriasis Oculomotor nerve compression	Ipsilateral pupil dilated and nonreactive loss of visual field	Compression of CN III against tentorium as in uncal herniation or by posterior communicating artery from an aneurysm
Drug induced	Bilateral dilated pupils from amphetamines, glutethimide (Doriden), barbiturate overdose, ophthalmic mydriatics and cycloplegics (atropine sulfate, scopolamine hydrobromide, tropicamide)	Drug-induced pupillary dilation caused by sympathetic stimulants or parasympathetic blocking agents
Anoxia or death	Pupils bilaterally dilated and fixed in midposition	Transtentorial herniation, anoxia, death

CN, Cranial nerve.

TABLE 2-14   Changes in the Eye Caused by Aging

Structure	Change	Consequence
Cornea	Thicker and less curved	Increase in astigmatism
	Formation of a gray ring at the edge of the cornea (arcus senilis)	Not detrimental to vision
Anterior chamber	Decrease in size and volume caused by thickening of lens	Occasionally exerts pressure on Schlemm's canal and may lead to increased intraocular pressure and glaucoma
Lens	Increase in opacity	Decrease in refraction with increased light scattering and decreased color vision (green and blue); can lead to cataracts
	Increased firmness, loss of elasticity	Decrease in accommodation for near vision; presbyopia develops by age 50–55 years
Ciliary muscles	Reduction in pupil diameter, atrophy of radial dilation muscles	Persistent constriction (senile miosis); decrease in critical flicker frequency*
Retina	Reduction in number of rods at periphery, loss of rods and associated nerve cells	Increase in the minimum amount of light necessary to see an object

From McCance KL, Huether SE: *Pathophysiology: the biological basis for disease in adults and children*, ed 4, St Louis, 2002, Mosby.
*The rate at which consecutive visual stimuli can be presented and still be perceived as separate.

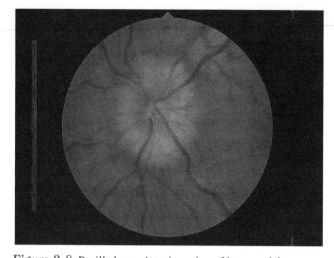

Figure 2-8 Papilledema. A serious sign of intracranial pressure.
(From Jarvis C: Physical examination and health assessment, ed 4, St Louis, 2004, WB Saunders.)

instructed to focus on a point in the distance. The normal optic disc, which is the termination of the optic nerve, is pink with sharply outlined disc margins. Retinal veins are also examined for pulsation, tortuosity, or hemorrhage. **Papilledema,** which characteristically indicates an elevated ICP, generally blurs the disc margins and decreases venous pulsations (Fig. 2-8). The optic disc may even appear to bulge. Papilledema is often a late sign in acute elevations of ICP, as may occur in head trauma, but may be the first sign of intracranial disease if elevated ICP has developed over time, as with a tumor.

Eye Movement

Eye movements are controlled with the interaction of three cranial nerves: oculomotor (CN III), trochlear (CN IV), and abducens (CN VI). **Conjugate eye gaze** is the normal movement of both eyes simultaneously in the same direction to bring something into view. It involves integrated functions of both the cerebral cortex and the brainstem. **Disconjugate gaze** is one eye deviated from the normal midposition at rest. In the cerebral cortex the frontal and occipital gaze centers control voluntary eye movements. The frontal gaze center controls rapid voluntary eye movement, and the occipital gaze center controls slow-tracking eye movement. In the brainstem, involuntary eye movement is integrated through the internuclear pathway of the MLF. The MLF provides coordination of eye movements with the vestibular and reticular formation, which leads to coordination of eye movement with head movement and position change.

Extraocular Movements. The **extraocular muscles** are the six sets of muscles that control movements of the eyeball. In the conscious patient, the function of the three cranial nerves of the eye and their innervation with the gaze centers in the cortex and the MLF in the brainstem can be assessed together. The patient should be asked to follow a finger through the full range of eye motions. If the eyes move together in all six fields, EOMs are intact (Fig. 2-9, *A*).

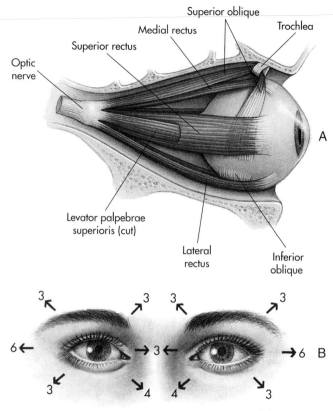

Figure 2-9 Extraocular eye movements. **A,** Extraocular muscles. **B,** Six cardinal directions of gaze used to test the function of the eye muscles together with the nerves that supply them. Numbers indicate the cranial nerve being tested by a particular eye movement.
(A, From Thibodeau GA, Patton KT: Anatomy and physiology, *ed 5, St Louis, 2003, Mosby. B, From Rudy E:* Advanced neurological and neurosurgical nursing, *St Louis, 1984, Mosby.)*

Injury to any of the three cranial nerves leads to paresis or paralysis of the muscles and causes dysconjugate gaze. Injury to the oculomotor nerve prevents the eye from moving inward and upward, inward and downward, or outward and downward. Also noted with oculomotor injury are **ptosis** (drooping eyelid) and a dilated pupil. Trochlear nerve injury, a rare injury, prevents downward gaze. Injury to the abducens nerve prevents the eye from looking outward. These nerve injuries may be either bilateral or unilateral. Although on physical examination the abnormal or absent eye movements are evident, the patient often is the first to notice the resulting **diplopia,** or double vision. For example, with right CN VI palsy, the patient experiences double vision with gaze to the right as the left eye moves inward under the control of the oculomotor nerve and the right eye remains midline because of the dysfunction of the abducens nerve. The abducens nerve is injured more frequently than the oculomotor or trochlear nerve because it has the longest course to travel from the pons in the brainstem to the eye.

Oculocephalic Reflex. To test the integrity of the brainstem function in the unconscious patient, eye movement and the

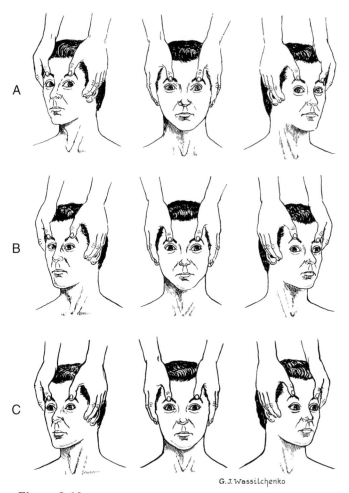

Figure 2-10 Test for oculocephalic reflex response (doll's eyes phenomenon). **A,** Normal response—the eyes turn together to the side opposite the turn of the head. **B,** Abnormal response—the eyes do not turn in a conjugate manner. **C,** Absent response—the eyes do not turn as the head position is changed. (*From Rudy E:* Advanced neurological and neurosurgical nursing, *St Louis, 1984, Mosby.*)

innervation of the MLF are assessed by eliciting the oculocephalic or doll's eye reflex. This procedure cannot be done on a conscious patient because cortical function will take over control of eye movements. In addition, the oculocephalic reflex is not routinely assessed on serial evaluations. If the patient is unconscious because of trauma, the clinician must ascertain that there is no cervical injury before performing this examination. Clearing the cervical spine (C-spine) by x-ray studies is usually performed in trauma settings.

To assess the oculocephalic reflex, while holding eyelids open, the clinician briskly turns the patient's head to one side while observing eye movements and then briskly turns the head to the other side and observes. If the oculocephalic reflex is intact, the eyes deviate to the direction opposite that of the head turn, and the doll's eyes reflex is present. If the oculocephalic reflex is not intact, the doll's eyes reflex is absent. This lack of response, in which the eyes remain midline and move with the head, indicates significant ipsi-

lateral lesion at the brainstem level. If the oculocephalic reflex is abnormal, the eyes rove or move in opposite directions. An abnormal oculocephalic reflex indicates some degree of brainstem injury (Fig. 2-10).

Oculovestibular Reflex. The oculovestibular reflex, or cold caloric test, is usually performed as one of the final clinical assessments of brainstem function. While the head is flexed at approximately 30 degrees, 20 to 50 ml of cold saline is injected into the external auditory canal after checking to see that the **tympanic membrane** is intact. The normal eye movement response is a rapid nystagmus-like deviation toward the irrigated ear. This response indicates brainstem integrity. This test is an extremely noxious stimulation and may produce an abnormal flexion or extension posturing response in the comatose patient. It is not recommended that this procedure be performed on a conscious patient; it is extremely painful and may also induce vomiting and vertigo. An abnormal response would be dysconjugate eye movements, which would indicate a lesion at the pontine level of the brainstem, or no response, which would indicate little or no brainstem function. Eye movements change in a rostral-caudal direction as dysfunction or injury descends (Table 2-15).

Assessment of Vital Signs

Because of the brain and brainstem influences on cardiac and respiratory functions, changes in pulse rate, respiration rate, blood pressure, and body temperature can be an indicator of deterioration in neurologic status. Abnormal vital sign changes may be late signs of neurologic pathology.

Cardiac Function

The brain's tremendous metabolic demand requires that an adequate supply of blood continually perfuse the brain. Evaluation of the cardiovascular system identifies inappropriate supply responses to the known cerebral demand. The balance of cerebral tissue supply and demand falls under the concept of cerebral autoregulation (see Chapter 1).

Decreased cardiac output, for whatever reason (e.g., vasodilation, bradycardia, tachycardia, hypovolemia, or inadequate pump), leads to **decreased cerebral perfusion pressure (CPP)** of cerebral tissue, hypoxia, and neurologic injury. In the presence of increased ICP, decreased cardiac output is even more detrimental because low blood pressure must overcome the additional resistance of ICP to provide blood to the brain.

Hypertension is a common manifestation of intracranial injury. Cerebral autoregulation, which is responsible for the control of cerebral blood flow, is frequently lost with any type of intracranial injury. After cerebral injury the body is often in a hyperdynamic state (increased heart rate, blood pressure, and cardiac output) as part of a compensatory response. With the loss of autoregulation, as blood pressure increases, cerebral blood flow increases, cerebral blood volume increases, and therefore ICP increases. Control of systemic hypertension should be managed carefully with precise orders for parameters to prevent hypoperfusion of the brain that could lead to infarction.

TABLE 2-15	Changes in Oculomotor Responses	
State	Resting and Spontaneous Eye Movements	Reflexive Eye Movements
Full consciousness	Eyes at rest, still (cortical gaze centers inhibit spontaneous roving eye movements)	Eyes move as the head turns Oculocephalic responses not elicited or inconsistently elicited (frontal gaze centers inhibit brainstem reflexes that fix gaze straight ahead) Oculovestibular (caloric) stimulation produces nystagmus
Cortical dysfunction or disruption of efferent pathways	Conjugate, horizontal, roving eye movements may be present (cortical gaze centers no longer inhibit these brainstem-generated roving eye movements)	Gaze fixed straight ahead regardless of head position—positive doll's eyes reaction (normal oculocephalic reflexes are no longer inhibited by frontal gaze centers)
Diffuse anoxic damage to cortex	"Ocular dipping"—slow, dysrhythmic downward movement followed by faster, upward movement	Nystagmus is no longer induced by caloric stimulation (normally a cold water stimulus produces deviation of the eyes opposite the irrigated ear; a warm water stimulus deviates the eyes to the same [ipsilateral] side) With an injury that depresses cortical gaze center function, the eyes (and often the entire head) will deviate, or appear to look toward the side of the injured hemisphere With an injury that irritates (stimulates) the neurons of the cortical gaze center, the eyes (and often the entire head) will deviate away from the injured hemisphere (all fibers from the frontal gaze centers decussate and therefore control the function of the contralateral pontine gaze center, which moves the eyes in the ipsilateral direction)
Mesencephalon dysfunction	Roving eye movements cease, and the eyes become immobile and directed ahead (roving eye movements require an intact brainstem) Eyes may turn down and inward	Oculovestibular reflexes become inconsistent and abnormal Loss of Bell's phenomenon (upward deviation of eyes on stimulation) (requires intact eye movement pathways from the mesencephalon to pons)
Pontine dysfunction	Loss of spontaneous blinking (requires an intact pons) "Ocular bobbing"—brisk, conjugate, downward movement of eyes with loss of horizontal eye movements	

From McCance KL, Huether SE: *Pathophysiology: the biological basis for disease in adults and children*, ed 4, St Louis, 2002, Mosby.

The medulla and the vagus nerve provide parasympathetic control to the heart. When stimulated, this lower brainstem system produces bradycardia. Increasing ICP frequently causes **bradycardia.** Abrupt ICP changes can also produce dysrhythmias such as premature ventricular contractions (PVCs), atrioventricular (AV) block, or ventricular fibrillation.

A condition observed in the presence of increased ICP that causes cerebral ischemia occurs when the cerebrospinal fluid pressure and the pressure within the intracranial arteries begin to equalize. This triggers a compensatory condition known as **Cushing's reflex.** As the cerebral arteries become more and more compressed, the arterial blood pressure rises to overcome the diminished blood supply to the brain.

Cushing's response is a set of three signs or symptoms (bradycardia, systolic hypertension, and widening pulse pressure) that are related to pressure on the medullary area of the brainstem. **Widening pulse pressure** is calculated by subtracting the diastolic blood pressure from the systolic blood pressure with 50 mm Hg normal. These signs are often in response to intracranial hypertension or a herniation syndrome. The appearance of Cushing's response is a late finding or may even be absent in neurologic deterioration. The clinician should pay attention to alterations in each component of the triad and initiate interventions accordingly.

Respiratory Function

The activity of respiration is a highly integrated function receiving input from the cerebrum, brainstem, and metabolic mechanisms. There is a close correlation in clinical assessment among altered LOCs, the level of brain or brainstem injury, and the respiratory pattern noted (Table 2-16). Under the influence of the cerebral cortex and the diencephalon, three brainstem centers control respirations. The lowest center, the medullary respiratory center, sends impulses through the vagus nerve to innervate muscles of inspiration

TABLE 2-16   Patterns of Breathing

Breathing Pattern	Description	Location of Injury
Hemispheric Breathing Patterns		
Normal	After a period of hyperventilation that lowers the arterial carbon dioxide pressure (PaCO$_2$), the individual continues to breathe regularly but with a reduced depth.	Response of the nervous system to an external stressor—not associated with injury to the CNS
Posthyperventilation apnea (PHVA)	Respirations stop after hyperventilation has lowered the PCO$_2$ level below normal. Rhythmic breathing returns when the PCO$_2$ level returns to normal.	Associated with diffuse bilateral metabolic or structural disease of the cerebrum
Cheyne-Stokes respirations (CSR)	The breathing pattern has a smooth increase (crescendo) in the rate and depth of breathing (hyperpnea), which peaks and is followed by a gradual smooth decrease (decrescendo) in the rate and depth of breathing to the point of apnea when the cycle repeats itself. The hyperpneic phase lasts longer than the apneic phase.	Bilateral damage to the hemispheres related to basal ganglia or dysfunction of the deep cerebral and/or diencephalic structures, seen with supratentorial injury and metabolically induced coma states
Brainstem Breathing Patterns		
Central neurogenic hyperventilation (CNH)	A sustained, deep, rapid but regular pattern (hyperpnea) occurs, with a decreased PaCO$_2$ and a corresponding increase in pH and increased PO$_2$ and may reflect midbrain or upper pons damage related to increased ICP.	May result from CNS damage or disease that involves the midbrain and upper pons; seen after increased ICP and blunt head trauma
Apneustic breathing	A prolonged inspiration (a pause at full inspiration) and a short expiratory phase. A common variant of this is a brief end-inspiratory pause of 2 or 3 seconds often alternating with an end-expiratory pause and may be related to an infarct, anoxia, or infection.	Indicates damage to the respiratory control mechanism located at the pontine level; most commonly associated with pontine infarction but documented with hypoglycemia, anoxia, and meningitis
Cluster breathing	A cluster of breaths has a disordered sequence with irregular pauses between breaths.	Dysfunction in the lower pontine and high medullary areas
Ataxic breathing	Completely irregular breathing occurs, with random shallow and deep breaths and irregular pauses. Often the rate is slow related to a deficit or injury to the medulla.	Originates from a primary dysfunction of the medullary neurons controlling breathing
Gasping breathing pattern (agonal gasps)	A pattern of deep "all-or-none" breaths is accompanied by a slow respiratory rate.	Indicative of a failing medullary respiratory center

From McCance KL, Huether SE: *Pathophysiology: the biological basis for disease in adults and children,* ed 4, St Louis, 2002, Mosby.
CNS, Central nervous system; *ICP,* intracranial pressure.

and expiration. The apneustic and pneumotaxic centers of the pons are responsible for the length of inspiration and expiration and the underlying respiratory rate.

Changes in **respiratory patterns** assist in identifying the level of brainstem dysfunction or injury. In respiratory assessment, the clinician must evaluate respiratory patterns, as well as the respiratory rate. All of the respiratory patterns listed in Fig. 2-11, *A,* except central neurogenic hyperventilation, could have a normal respiratory rate of 12 to 16 breaths per minute. Evaluation of the respiratory pattern must also include evaluation of the effectiveness of gas exchange in maintaining adequate oxygen and carbon dioxide levels. Hypoventilation is not uncommon in the patient with an altered LOC. Alterations in oxygenation or carbon dioxide levels can result in further neurologic dysfunction. The ICP increases with hypoxemia or hypercapnia. Evaluating per-

centage of oxygen saturation (O$_2$ sat) is another parameter for assessment of adequate breathing. The normal percentage of O$_2$ sat is 95% to 100%; mild hypoxia may occur at levels of 91% to 94%, with moderate hypoxia in the range of 86% to 93%; and severe hypoxia is usually considered below 85%.

Finally, assessment of the respiratory function in a patient with neurologic deficit must also include auscultation for adequate breath sounds, adventitious sounds, assessment of airway maintenance, and secretion control. Cough, gag, and swallow reflexes responsible for protection of the airway may be absent or diminished. Several respiratory patterns, such as **Kussmaul's respirations,** are also noted in metabolic disorders. These patterns are initiated in the cerebral cortex in response to metabolic alterations and are a compensatory mechanism. Respiratory patterns of metabolic disorders are

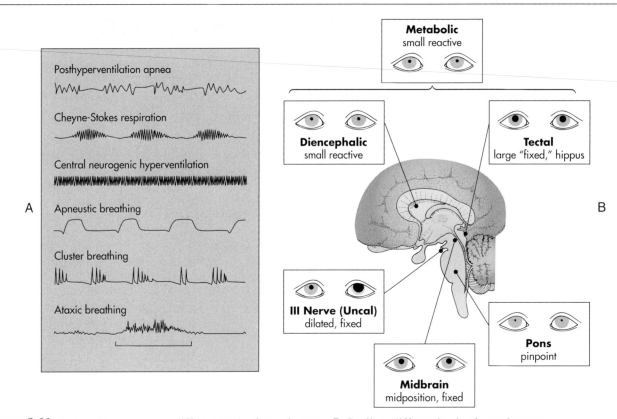

Figure 2-11 A, Breathing patterns at different levels of consciousness. **B,** Pupils at different levels of consciousness. *(From Beare PG, Myers JL: Adult health nursing, ed 3, St Louis, 1998, Mosby.)*

not identified in the same terms as the level of dysfunction of a structural injury. Patients receiving mechanical ventilation are assessed for ventilatory settings, FiO$_2$ and ventilatory parameters, arterial blood gases (ABGs) every 8 hours to adjust ventilation values, and chest x-rays as needed. Assessment is needed for proper placement and security of an endotracheal tube and patient's positioning to prevent aspiration.

Assessment of the Peripheral Nervous System

The cranial and spinal nerves, including their branches, constitute the peripheral nervous system (PNS). The characteristics of the peripheral nerve disorders may include paresis, paralysis, flaccidity, muscle atrophy, or loss of reflexes. If the affected peripheral nerve is the mixed type, the disorder may include pain and sensory disturbances. Therefore localized sensory loss with weakness usually implies involvement or a lesion of a peripheral nerve fiber. Assessment of the spinal nerves and peripheral branches is described in Table 2-17.

The 31 pairs of spinal nerves contain both sensory and motor neurons and are therefore called **mixed nerves.** They arise from the ventral and dorsal horn cells of the spinal cord, converge, and then divide into anterior branches or rami. Assessment focuses on the degree of motor/sensory function and deficits to include touch, pain, heat, cold, position, vibration, atrophy, paresis, paralysis, and loss of reflexes described in this chapter.

Cranial nerves may be purely sensory or motor, but most are mixed. Cranial nerve assessment will help determine if the structural and functional characteristics of the cranial nerves are intact.

Examination of the cranial nerves is essential to a complete study of the nervous system. The cranial nerve nuclei are located on the brainstem from the uppermost portion of the midbrain to the lowest portion of the medulla oblongata. Because of their location along the entire length of the brainstem, assessment of the cranial nerves provides valuable clues to the degree of injury or dysfunction that may be present in this area. The cranial nerves are a paired set of 12 nerves responsible for sensory and motor functions of the head and neck plus the modulation of a variety of visceral responses, such as salivation, heart rate control, and acid and digestive enzyme secretions of the stomach.

A complete cranial nerve examination is seldom done on a regular basis; portions of the cranial nerve examination are done with every neurologic assessment. Pupillary reaction and eye movement, cough and gag reflexes, facial movements in the stroke patient, and vital signs such as heart rate are all functions controlled by cranial nerves. Table 2-18 provides an overview of the 12 cranial nerves.

Cranial Nerves

Olfactory Nerve. The olfactory nerve (CN I) is a *sensory* nerve that relays information about smell. It monitors the intake of airborne agents into the respiratory system, helps

TABLE 2-17   Spinal Nerves and Peripheral Branches

Spinal Nerves	Plexuses Formed From Anterior Rami	Spinal Nerve Branches From Plexuses	Parts Supplied
Cervical 1 2 3 4	Cervical plexus	Lesser occipital Great auricular Cutaneous nerve of neck Anterior supraclavicular Middle supraclavicular Posterior supraclavicular Branches to muscles Phrenic (branches from cervical nerves before formation of plexus; most of its fibers from fourth cervical nerve)	Sensory to back of head, front of neck, and upper part of shoulder: motor to numerous neck muscles Diaphragm
Cervical 5 6 7 8 Thoracic (or dorsal) 1 2	Brachial plexus	Suprascapular and dorsoscapular Thoracic nerves, medial and lateral branches Long thoracic nerve Thoracodorsal Subscapular Axillary (circumflex) Musculocutaneous Ulnar Median Radial Medial cutaneous	Superficial muscles* of scapula Pectoralis major and minor Serratus anterior Latissimus dorsi Subscapular and teres major muscles Deltoid and teres minor muscles and skin over deltoid Muscles of front of arm (biceps brachii, coracobrachialis, brachialis), skin on outer side of forearm Flexor carpi ulnaris and part of flexor digitorum profundus; some of muscles of hand; sensory to medial side of hand, little finger, and medial half of fourth finger Rest of muscles of front of forearm and hand, sensory to skin of palmar surface of thumb, index, and middle fingers Triceps muscle and muscles of back of forearm and hand Sensory to inner surface of arm and forearm
3 4 5 6 7 8 9 10 11 12	No plexus formed; branches run directly to intercostal muscles and skin of thorax		
Lumbar 1 2 3 4 5 Sacral 1 2 3 4 5 Coccygeal 1	Lumbosacral	Iliohypogastric Ilioinguinal Genitofemoral Lateral cutaneous of thigh Femoral Obturator Tibial† (medial popliteal) Common peroneal (lateral popliteal) Nerves to hamstring muscles Gluteal nerves, superior and inferior Posterior cutaneous nerve Pudendal nerve	Sensory to anterior abdominal wall Sensory to anterior abdominal wall and external genitalia; motor muscles of abdominal wall Sensory to skin of external genitalia and inguinal region Sensory to outer side of thigh Motor to quadriceps, sartorius, and iliacus muscles; sensory to front of thigh and medial side of lower leg (saphenous nerve) Motor to adductor muscles of thigh Motor to muscles of calf of leg; sensory to skin of calf of leg and sole of foot Motor to evertors and dorsiflexors of foot; sensory to lateral surface of leg and dorsal surface of foot Motor to muscles of back of thigh Motor to buttock muscles and tensor fasciae latae Sensory to skin of buttocks, posterior surface of thigh, and leg Motor to perineal muscles; sensory to skin of perineum

*Although nerves to muscles are considered motor, they do contain some sensory fibers that transmit proprioceptive impulses.
†Sensory fibers from the tibial and peroneal nerves unite to form the medial cutaneous (or sural) nerve, which supplies the calf of the leg and the lateral surface of the foot. In the thigh the tibial and common peroneal nerves are usually enclosed in a single sheath to form the sciatic nerve, the largest nerve in the body, with a width of approximately $3/4$ inch. About two thirds of the way down the posterior part of the thigh, it divides into its component parts. Branches of the sciatic nerve extend into the hamstring muscles.

TABLE 2-18 | Cranial Nerves

Nerve*	Sensory Fibers†			Motor Fibers†		
	Receptors	Cell Bodies	Termination	Cell Bodies	Termination	Functions‡
I. Olfactory	*Nasal mucosa*	*Nasal mucosa*	Olfactory bulbs (new relay of neurons to olfactory cortex)			*Sense of smell*
II. Optic	*Retina*	Retina	Nucleus in thalamus (lateral geniculate body); some fibers terminate in superior colliculus of midbrain			*Vision*
III. Oculomotor	*External eye muscles except superior oblique and lateral rectus*	Trigeminal ganglion	Midbrain (oculomotor nucleus)	**Midbrain (oculomotor nucleus and Edinger-Westphal nucleus)**	External eye muscles except superior oblique and lateral rectus; fibers from Edinger-Westphal nucleus terminate in ciliary ganglion and then to ciliary and iris muscles	Eye movements, regulation of size or pupil, accommodation, *proprioception (muscle sense)*
IV. Trochlear	*Superior oblique*	Trigeminal ganglion	Midbrain	**Midbrain**	Superior oblique muscle of eye	Eye movements, *proprioception*
V. Trigeminal	*Skin and mucosa of head, teeth*	Gasserian ganglion	Pons (sensory nucleus)	**Pons (motor nucleus)**	Muscles of mastication	*Sensations of head and face,* **chewing movements,** *muscle sense*
VI. Abducens	*Lateral rectus*	Trigeminal ganglion	Pons	**Pons**	Lateral rectus muscle of eye	**Abduction of eye,** *proprioception*
VII. Facial	*Taste buds of anterior two thirds of tongue*	Geniculate ganglion	*Medulla (nucleus solitarius)*	**Pons**	Superficial muscles of face and scalp	Facial expressions, secretion of saliva, *taste*

TABLE 2-18 | **Cranial Nerves—cont'd**

| Nerve* | Sensory Fibers† | | | Motor Fibers† | | |
	Receptors	Cell Bodies	Termination	Cell Bodies	Termination	Functions‡
VIII. Acoustic a. Vestibular branch	*Semicircular canals and vestibule (utricle and saccule)*	Vestibular ganglion	*Pons and medulla (vestibular nuclei)*			*Balance of equilibrium sense*
b. Cochlear or auditory branch	*Organ of Corti in cochlear duct*	*Spiral ganglion*	*Pons and medulla (cochlear nuclei)*			*Hearing*
IX. Glossopharyngeal	*Pharynx; taste buds and other receptors of posterior third of tongue*	*Jugular and petrous ganglia*	*Medulla (nucleus solitarius)*	Medulla (nucleus ambiguus)	Muscles of pharynx	*Taste and other sensations of tongue,* **swallowing movements, secretion of saliva,** *aid in reflex control of blood pressure and respiration*
	Carotid sinus and carotid body	*Jugular and petrous ganglia*	*Medulla (respiratory and vasomotor centers)*	Medulla at junction of pons (nucleus salivatorius)	Otic ganglion and then to parotid gland	
X. Vagus	*Pharynx, larynx, carotid body, and thoracic and abdominal viscera*	*Jugular and nodose ganglia*	*Medulla (nucleus solitarius), pons (nucleus of fifth cranial nerve)*	Medulla (dorsal motor nucleus)	Ganglia of vagal plexus and then to muscles of pharynx, larynx, and thoracic and abdominal viscera	*Sensations and* **movements** *of organs supplied;* **for example, slows heart, increases peristalsis, and contracts muscles for voice production**
XI. Spinal accessory	Trapezius and sternocleidomastoid	Upper cervical ganglion	Spinal cord	Medulla (dorsal motor nucleus of vagus and nucleus ambiguus) Anterior gray column of first five of six cervical segments of spinal cord	Muscles of thoracic and abdominal viscera, pharynx, and larynx Trapezius and sternocleidomastoid muscle	**Shoulder movements, turning movements of head, movements of viscera, voice production,** *proprioception?*
XII. Hypoglossal	Tongue muscles	Trigeminal ganglion	Medulla	Medulla (hypoglossal nucleus)	Muscles of tongue	**Tongue movements,** *proprioception?*

Modified from Thibodeau GA, Patton KT: *Anthony's textbook of anatomy and physiology,* ed 5, St Louis, 2003, Mosby.

*The first letters of the words in the following sentence are the first letters of the names of the cranial nerves. Many generations of anatomy students have used this sentence as an aid to memorizing these names. It is "On Old Olympus Tiny Tops, A Finn and German Viewed Some Hops." (There are several slightly differing versions of this mnemonic.)

†*Italics* indicate sensory fibers and functions. **Boldface** type indicates motor fibers and functions.

‡An aid for remembering the general function of each cranial nerve is the following 12-word saying: "Some say marry money but my brothers say bad businesses marry money." Words beginning with S indicate sensory function. Words beginning with M indicate motor function. Words beginning with B indicate both sensory and motor functions. For example, the first, second, and eighth words in the saying start with S, which indicates that the first, second, and eighth cranial nerves perform sensory functions.

determine the flavor of foods, and serves as a protective mechanism against eating spoiled food and inhaling dangerous gases or smoke. Alterations in the ability to smell (**dysosmia**) may be an early indicator of Alzheimer's or Parkinson's disease. The olfactory nerve consists of sensory cells in the nasal mucosae, which are grouped together into bundles that pass through the cribriform plate of the ethmoid bone (part of the base of the frontal fossa) to the olfactory bulb. From the olfactory bulb these fibers form a tract that runs to the hippocampal gyrus and the temporal lobe on the same side. The sense of smell also integrates with other body systems and responses such as taste, salivation, peristalsis, and even sexual stimuli.

The olfactory nerve is tested by the use of a variety of odoriferous substances. With the patient's eyes closed, one nostril is occluded and the patient is asked to sniff a substance placed under the other nostril. Substances used may be coffee, mint, cloves, lemon extract, or vinegar. Highly volatile substances such as ammonia or alcohol should be avoided because they stimulate the pain fibers carried by the trigeminal nerve (CN V) and may interfere with the response. Commercially available tests can be used, such as the Smell Identification Test or Pocket Smell Test. The patient is asked to verify that an odor is perceived and then asked to identify the substance. Both nostrils should be tested separately. Although the patient may not always be able to accurately identify the substance, the perception of an odor excludes anosmia, or **hyposmia,** which is the loss of smell.

Common nonneurogenic reasons for a patient's inability to smell include obstruction of the nasal passages or allergic rhinitis, which may have to be relieved by a nasal decongestant before testing, sinus infection, tobacco smoking, and cocaine abuse. Evaluation of olfactory function for neurogenic causes is especially pertinent after trauma and fracture of the cribriform plate or ethmoid bone. Because of the relative fragility of the olfactory fibers as they run through the cribriform plate, these nerves are easily disrupted in head injury. **Anosmia** is the most frequent cranial nerve deficit seen after head injury.[6] Tumors, such as an olfactory groove meningioma, or abscesses at the base of the frontal lobe may also damage the olfactory nerve. These types of masses may cause atrophy of the olfactory and optic nerves on the ipsilateral side and often lead to a syndrome known as the **Foster Kennedy syndrome.** This syndrome is characterized by ipsilateral blindness and anosmia and contralateral papilledema.

Optic Nerve. The optic nerve (CN II) is a *sensory* nerve that is responsible for relaying visual input. The terminal organs of sight are the rods and cones, which are found in the deepest layer of the retina. The rods and cones relay impulses to the ganglion cells, which converge toward the optic disc and emerge from the eye as the optic nerve. The optic nerve then exits the orbit and enters the cranial cavity through the optic foramen. The two optic nerves join at the optic chiasm, where the fibers partially decussate before they continue to form the optic tract. Fibers of the optic tract continue to course posteriorly through the lateral geniculate body near the thalamus and on to the occipital lobes, where they terminate in the visual cortex.[7] The optic nerve is tested by

measuring visual acuity and visual fields and inspecting the retina and optic disc. These tests are discussed earlier in this chapter. **Amaurosis** is blindness or lacking vision resulting from a systemic cause (e.g., disease of the optic nerve or brain, diabetes, renal disease, or after acute gastric or systemic poisoning from excessive intake of alcohol or smoking tobacco). **Amaurosis fugax** is transient episodic blindness from decreased blood flow to the retina.

Oculomotor Nerves. CNs III, IV, and VI are usually tested together, since they all innervate muscles of the eye that allow for eye movement. These three motor nerves, working together, enable the eyes to move smoothly. The oculomotor nerve innervates the superior, inferior, and lateral rectus muscles and the inferior oblique muscle, all of which allow the eye to move upward, inward, and down and out. Assessment of CNs III, IV, and VI includes assessment of **EOMs,** which is described earlier in this chapter.

The third cranial nerve is a *motor* nerve and also has a parasympathetic component, which is responsible for pupillary constriction when stimulated. This function becomes particularly significant because of the location of the oculomotor nerve in the midbrain at the tentorial notch. Check for *nystagmus,* or involuntary, rhythmic movements of the eye that may be horizontal (common), vertical (rare), rotary, or mixed. Nystagmus may be an indicator of barbiturate intoxication or toxic levels of phenytoin. Assessment of the pupils, including pupillary reactivity, is also described in an earlier portion of this chapter.

Trochlear Nerve. This *motor* nerve comes from the lower midbrain area to innervate the superior oblique muscle of the eye. The trochlear nerve (CN IV) allows the eye to move downward and nasally. Of the three cranial nerves involved in eye movement, an isolated dysfunction of this nerve is the most difficult to identify. Patients with CN IV impairment may tilt their head away from the side of a fourth nerve lesion to compensate.[2] Conscious and alert patients may complain of difficulty climbing steps because they are unable to look down at their feet. Brainstem tumors, multiple sclerosis, head trauma, or stroke may cause CN IV palsy.

Trigeminal Nerve. The trigeminal nerve (CN V), the largest of the cranial nerves, is both a *sensory* and a *motor* nerve that controls ipsilateral facial sensation and mastication. The sensory portion of the trigeminal nerve has three divisions or branches: the **ophthalmic branch,** which innervates the conjunctiva, cornea, upper lid, forehead, and scalp; the **maxillary branch,** which innervates the cheek, nose, upper teeth, jaw, and mucosal surfaces of the hard palate, nasopharynx, and nasal cavity; and the **mandibular branch,** which innervates the lower jaw, pinna of the ear, side of the tongue, lower teeth and gums, and floor of the mouth. The motor portion of the trigeminal nerve runs with the mandibular division and supplies the muscles of mastication.

Before testing, ask if contact lens are worn (because they could inhibit the response) and look at the face for symmetry, nasolabial folds, abnormal movements (blinking), wasting, or a motionless appearance. The sensory and motor portions of CN V are tested separately. The sensory portion is assessed by evaluating touch, pain, and temperature in all three branches of the nerve. This should always be performed by comparing one side of the face with the other. The **corneal reflex,** which evaluates both CN V and CN VII, is also tested. The patient is asked to look up and away from the examiner. A small wisp of sterile cotton twisted to a point is gently touched to the cornea of the eye, avoiding the normal blink response. A normal response is a rapid and forceful bilateral closure of the eyelid. In the presence of CN VII palsy on the ipsilateral side, contralateral eye blink would indicate that the sensory portion (CN V) of the corneal reflex is intact. The motor portion of the trigeminal nerve is tested by asking the patient to clench his or her teeth, chew, and move the lower jaw from side to side against the resistance of the clinician's hand.

The most common disorder associated with the trigeminal nerve is **trigeminal neuralgia, or tic douloureux.** The pain of trigeminal neuralgia is described as shooting, stabbing, or electric in the affected zones. Pains generally shoot along one branch of this cranial nerve on one side. The mandibular and maxillary branches are most commonly involved. Tumors in the middle fossa and the cerebellopontine angle may also affect one or more portions of the trigeminal nerve. Such lesions impair sensory function more commonly than motor power.[7]

Abducens Nerve. The abducens nerve (CN VI) is the third of the three nerves that control eye movement for symmetry. This *motor* nerve arises from a nucleus in the pons and innervates the lateral rectus muscle of the eye, which allows the eye to move outward. Sixth nerve palsy is not uncommon, and the patient may first notice symptoms of diplopia as he or she attempts to look to the side. Abnormal findings may be detected in patients with pressure on CN VI from an aneurysm, a tumor, Chiari malformation, multiple sclerosis, or other conditions.

Facial Nerve. The facial nerve (CN VII) has a mixed function, which is primarily *motor,* with a *sensory* and *parasympathetic* component. This nerve provides motor innervation to the muscles of the face, taste to the anterior two thirds of the tongue, and general sensation to portions of the external ear. The facial nerve also carries some parasympathetic secretomotor fibers to the nose and mouth. The motor portion of the facial nerve arises from deep in the pons, travels through the internal auditory meatus with CN VIII, enters the facial canal, passes through the parotid gland, and reaches the muscles of the face. The sensory portion travels from the pons via the geniculate ganglion and ends on the taste buds of the anterior two thirds of the tongue. The parasympathetic fibers of the facial nerve arise from the superior salivary nucleus and innervate the maxillary and lacrimal gland and the mucous membranes of the palate, nasopharynx, and nasal cavity.[7] In patients with upper motor neuron (UMN) facial weakness, the forehead muscles are preserved; with lower motor neuron (LMN) facial weakness, all muscles are affected.[2]

Facial nerve testing begins with the initial observations of the patient at rest; asymmetry of facial expression during normal conversations or interpersonal interactions can be noted. Testing continues by asking the patient to raise the eyebrows, wrinkle the forehead, close the eyes tightly (examiner uses finger to try and open them), wink, purse the lips, whistle, show the teeth, blow out the cheeks, and wrinkle the nose and look up at the ceiling. Although not usually evaluated in a routine examination, taste can be tested by asking the patient to stick out the tongue and placing salt, sugar, or other similar substances on the anterior two thirds of the tongue.

Paralysis of the facial nerve results in complete loss of facial movement on the side with the cranial nerve deficit. Eating becomes difficult because the mouth droops. The cornea of the eye may be damaged because of the inability to close the eye. **Bell's palsy** is the term applied to an LMN lesion of the facial nerve (see Chapter 16). Bell's palsy, with its sudden onset, is often transitory and is believed to be caused by an inflammatory process and edema in the long, narrow facial canal that results in compression and, consequently, paralysis. LMN injury may also result from fractures of the base of the skull. A UMN lesion or central type of facial palsy results from damage to the portion of the motor cortex that controls facial movement.

Acoustic Nerve. The acoustic nerve (CN VIII) is a *sensory* nerve with two divisions: the cochlear or auditory division for the sense of hearing and the vestibular division for the sense of balance. The cochlear division travels from the ganglion of the cochlea in the temporal bone to the cochlear nucleus in the medulla oblongata and to both temporal lobes. The vestibular division travels from the internal auditory meatus to the vestibular portion of the labyrinth and to the medulla oblongata. In the medulla oblongata the fibers connect with the vestibulospinal tracts for reflex movements of the limbs and the trunk; with the medial longitudinal fasciculus for control of conjugate eye movement in relation to movements of the head; and with the cerebellum to assist in the control of muscle tone as it relates to postural adjustments.[7]

The cochlear division is tested after the external ear canal and tympanic membranes have been examined. A wide variety of more sophisticated hearing tests are available, but in the clinical setting some crude tests can be used. High-frequency hearing can be tested by masking the opposite ear and whispering in each ear, rubbing fingers together, or using a ticking watch. These hearing tests begin with the stimulus held away from the patient's ear and gradually moved closer. The patient is instructed to indicate when the sound is first heard. This type of hearing is frequently impaired in the older adult or in those exposed to a noisy environment.[7]

If the hearing in one ear is decreased, low-frequency hearing is tested using the Rinne or Weber tests. In the **Rinne test,** the clinician uses a tuning fork, placing it over the mastoid process (hearing through bone conduction). When the sound is no longer heard by the patient, the tuning fork is placed directly in front of the ear, where it should be heard for another 10 to 15 seconds (hearing through air conduction).

The **Weber test** consists of striking a tuning fork and placing it on the forehead. The vibrations should be heard equally in both ears. In deafness caused by dysfunction of the auditory nerve on one side, the vibration is better heard on the normal side.

The vestibular division of CN VIII is tested in a variety of ways. Balance is tested by observation of the patient's standing or sitting and gait assessment for wide-based ambulation. **Romberg's test** is performed with the patient's feet together and eyes closed and observed for swaying or falling to one side with the examiner ready to support the patient and prevent falling. In routine examinations the patient is asked to stretch his or her arms out to the side and touch the index finger to the nose, first with the eyes open and then with the eyes closed. The inability to accurately and rapidly perform this test is called **past-pointing.** A similar test asks the patient to touch the finger of the clinician, which is held midline in front of the patient. The eyes should also be observed for signs of nystagmus.

If the patient has clinical complaints concerning balance or vertigo, **caloric testing** may be done. This testing consists of stimulation of the semicircular canals by the slow instillation of cold normal saline (18° to 20° C) into the external canal. After introducing such cold saline, the clinician observes for nystagmus, past-pointing, and the development of vertigo, nausea, or vomiting. Caloric testing also involves interactions through the medial longitudinal fasciculus. Alterations of caloric responses are found in a wide variety of conditions, such as cerebellopontine angle tumors, intrinsic diseases of the brainstem, and labyrinthine diseases. In patients in deep coma, loss of caloric responses has a grave prognostic significance and is often used as one of the tests in the determination of brain death.

Glossopharyngeal Nerve. The glossopharyngeal nerve (CN IX) is a *sensory, motor,* and *parasympathetic* nerve for swallow and gag that is usually tested with the vagus nerve. The glossopharyngeal nerve provides for taste over the posterior one third of the tongue plus touch, pain, and temperature of the palate and pharynx. The parasympathetic fibers stimulate the salivary glands and the carotid reflex. The motor portion supplies innervation to the muscles used for swallowing. Because of the overlapping with other cranial nerves, CN IX is difficult to assess individually. The glossopharyngeal nerve arises from cells in the medulla oblongata. Fibers extend into the superior salivary nucleus to complete reflex arcs in salivation, and secretory fibers travel to supply the parotid gland. Motor fibers travel from a nucleus in the medulla oblongata to the stylopharyngeus muscle. To elicit the pharyngeal reflex, or **gag reflex,** touch the soft palate or posterior pharynx with a cotton-tipped applicator and watch the elevation of the palate, retraction of the tongue, and contraction of the pharyngeal muscles. This tests the afferent glossopharyngeal and the efferent vagus cranial nerves. Hoarseness, nasal speech, and problems with aspiration should alert the clinician to CN IX deficits.

Vagus Nerve. The vagus nerve (CN X), similarly to the glossopharyngeal nerve, has *motor* and sensory components; it also has *autonomic* function with afferents from the carotid baroreceptors and *parasympathetic* supply to and from the thorax and abdomen.[2] The vagus nerve is the primary motor and sensory nerve of the pharynx and larynx and is essential for swallow, phonation, cough, and gag. Other sensory fibers provide for visceral sensation from the esophagus, bronchi, and abdominal viscera. The autonomic functions of the vagus nerve are parasympathetic, and the nerve innervates the respiratory tract and the digestive tract, including peristalsis and secretion. The vagus nerve also plays a major role in the function of the carotid reflex and the sinoatrial node of the heart. When stimulated, the vagus nerve causes the heart rate to decrease. This complex nerve has cells that arise from a variety of nuclei and travel from the medulla oblongata to the end organs mentioned previously.

CNs IX and X, tested together, are assessed by listening for hoarseness when the patient talks and by observing for difficulty with swallowing. The patient is asked to open his or her mouth to inspect the soft palate—it should rise symmetrically when the patient says "ah" or when the back of the pharynx is stroked with a tongue blade and the uvula is midline. The autonomic portion of these nerves is difficult to assess. Damage to CNs IX and X can range from hoarseness to difficulty swallowing to loss of the airway protective mechanisms of cough and gag. Bilateral vagus nerve lesions are a medical emergency requiring emergent intubation.

Spinal Accessory Nerve. The spinal accessory nerve (CN XI) is a *motor* nerve that innervates the trapezius and sternocleidomastoid muscles to control shoulder elevation and head turning. It has also been suggested that a portion of this nerve, in conjunction with CNs IX and X, assists in swallowing and phonation. This nerve is unusual in that it arises from cells in the anterior gray matter of the first five spinal cord segments. These motor fibers unite along the upper cervical cord. They enter the skull through the foramen magnum and exit through the jugular foramen.

Assessment of CN XI at rest is focused on observations of atrophy, fasciculations, and asymmetry in motion. Look at the neck for atrophy, wasting, or abnormal head position. The spinal accessory nerve is tested in motion by asking the patient to shrug the shoulders to test the trapezius, or turn the head against resistance to test the sternocleidomastoid. The patient's inability to raise his or her head when in bed or raise a shoulder against resistance indicates damage on the ipsilateral side. The patient's inability to maintain a turned head against resistance indicates damage on the side opposite the head turn. Bilateral paralysis may cause the neck to fall backward.

Hypoglossal Nerve. The hypoglossal nerve (CN XII) is a *motor* nerve that supplies innervation to the muscles of the tongue. The nucleus of the nerve is in the floor of the fourth ventricle and emerges from the skull through the hypoglossal canal.

The hypoglossal nerve assessment includes observation, palpation, and percussion. The tongue is observed for atrophy with a scalloped look, fasciculations and involuntary movements, deviations, and limitations in strength and motion. CN XII is tested by asking the patient to stick out the tongue midline and check for deviations to either side. Then ask the patient to wiggle the tongue rapidly from side to side, up and down, and in and out rapidly, or to say "la-la-la." The patient is then asked to push the tongue into the cheek and resist the clinician's attempt to push the tongue back into the mouth. The tongue is palpated for atrophy. The clinician taps with a hammer to check for a myotonic response. Unless unsafe, provide a glass of water and ask the patient to swallow.

TABLE 2-19 Differences in Cranial Nerve Assessment Techniques and Findings in the Older Adult

Cranial Nerve	Adaptations in Test Techniques	Common Changes in the Older Adult
Olfactory	None	Progressive loss of smell
Optic	Use brighter light and place light sources behind patient when testing for visual acuity	Decreased visual acuity Presbyopia Diminished peripheral vision Funduscopic changes: arteriolar narrowing of vessels Increased tortuosity and silver-wire appearance of arterioles Retinal pallor Pupils smaller, with less brisk reaction to light and accommodation; may be unequal in size or irregular in shape
Oculomotor Trochlear Abducens	None	No expected changes in extraocular eye movements
Trigeminal	None	None
Facial	Sensory: Need to use more concentrated sweet and salt solution because absolute taste threshold is raised	Decreased perception of all taste modalities, especially sweet
	Motor: Test with dentures in place	May be facial asymmetry in edentulous patient unrelated to facial nerve function
Auditory	Test in a very quiet environment	Presbycusis—initially, increased loss of high tones; later, loss in all frequencies
Glossopharyngeal Vagus	None	Gag reflex should be present but may be sluggish
Spinal accessory	None	None
Hypoglossal	None	None

From Mezey MD, Rauckhorst LH, Stokes SA: *Health assessment of the older individual,* New York, 1980, Springer.

Damage to the hypoglossal nerve results in a tongue that points to the side of the damaged nerve when the tongue is protruded from the mouth.[6] Atrophy and fasciculations may be observed with the tongue resting in the mouth and may indicate bilateral LMN lesion. Patients with amyotrophic lateral sclerosis may exhibit fasciculations. Speech, swallowing, and respirations may be affected with CN XII lesions. **Dysarthria** and difficulty forming words should be noted.

ALERT: In the older adult, changes in assessment technique for the evaluation of cranial nerve function may be required. Do not assume that mental status changes are age related. Involve family members or others to validate assessment and determine if the older adult has hearing or visual impairment and is fluent in English. Bilingual older adults with English as a second language may be able to communicate only in their primary language after a cerebral insult. In general, the stimulus used to elicit the desired response needs to be enhanced or strengthened and the time allotted for normal response increased (Table 2-19).

Assessment of Cerebellar Function

The **cerebellum** is located dorsal to the brainstem and makes up part of the wall of the fourth ventricle. It is divided into two cerebellar hemispheres and a medial structure known as the vermis. The cerebellum is connected to the brain by three cerebellar peduncles.

The primary responsibility of the cerebellum is the integration of motor function, such as muscle coordination, maintenance of equilibrium coordination, and maintenance of muscle tone. Dysfunction of a cerebellar hemisphere results in a decrease in tone in the ipsilateral limbs; a deficit in the performance of rapid, alternating movements; and an inability to coordinate fine motor movements, such as those involved in locating a moving target. Lesions of the more central portion of the cerebellum, the vermis, tend to produce disturbances of gait, so that walking becomes broad based and unsteady.[6]

The most common coordination tests of the cerebellar system are the finger-nose test for intention tremor or past-pointing; testing of rapid alternating movement using pronation-supination for irregularity; the heel-to-shin test for irregularity; gait and station, including tandem, heel-to-toe gait; and the rebound test.

Upper Extremity Coordination Assessment

Finger-Nose Point-to-Point Testing. In the finger-nose test the patient is asked to touch the index finger of either hand to the nose. This should be performed smoothly and easily with eyes either open or closed. If there are any questions about the results of this test, the patient should be asked to repeat the finger-nose test several times in rapid succession.

Rapid Alternating Movements: Hands. Testing each hand separately with arms extended in front, the patient is asked to pronate and supinate rapidly, using the elbow as a fulcrum. The movements should be of equal amplitude, smooth, and even, with a well-maintained rhythm. This test may also be performed with the eyes open or closed, and there should be no arm drift.

- Patting test: The patient is asked to rapidly alternate patting the thigh with both the palm and the back of the hand; normally this test is performed briskly and with even amplitude and rhythm.
- Finger-finger test: The patient places his or her index finger on the clinician's index finger several times in rapid succession with the eyes open or closed.

Lower Extremity Coordination Assessment
Heel-Knee Point-to-Point Testing. Testing each leg separately while lying in the supine position, the patient is asked to put the heel of one foot on the opposite knee and slide the foot down the shin. This maneuver should be carried out smoothly and accurately and without tremor on each foot.

- Patting test: While lying in the supine position, the patient is asked to tap the clinician's hand as quickly as possible with the ball of each foot (one at a time); this maneuver should be carried out rapidly without awkwardness and in a coordinated manner, although alternating movements of the feet may be less well coordinated than hands as described previously.

Gait and Station
Gait and station are evaluated only in patients who are ambulatory. If there are any questions about the patient's ability to stand or move without falling, the clinician should have assistance to prevent injury.

Gait. Trunk coordination is also assessed by testing the gait. The patient is asked to rise from a sitting position and to walk briskly, first with the eyes open and then with the eyes closed, and to turn quickly. Observe for smooth rhythmic gait, erect posture, and arm swing. **Tandem gait** is assessed by asking the patient to walk heel-to-toe in a straight line; this can normally be done without a loss of balance. Any unsteadiness, lurching, or broadening of the base should be noted as indicators of abnormal function. **Truncal ataxia** is noted with lesions of the vermis of the cerebellum. Balancing is accomplished primarily from the ankles and secondarily from the hips. Abnormal gait patterns include the **scissor gait** associated with spinal lesions, **steppage gait** associated with peripheral nerve damage, **ataxic** or **cerebellar gait** associated with cerebellar disease, and **Parkinson gait** associated with diseases of the basal ganglia.[9]

Station. Station is tested by **Romberg's test** as described earlier. With feet together and arms extended in front, the patient should be able to stand erect and steady, first with the eyes open and then with the eyes closed. If the patient loses balance, this indicates a loss of position sense and could signify a significant problem. The clinician should always have one or more assistants at the patient's side to protect the patient from falling. If the patient has slight upper extremity weakness, it might be displayed with arm drift during the eyes-closed portion of Romberg's test.

Postural Adjustments
The ability to adjust to rapid postural changes can be assessed by asking the patient to walk around a chair, sit, and then rise quickly, or rise from a reclining position and walk across the room in a straight line.

Rebound Test
The rebound test is performed by observing the patient's response to sudden passive displacement of outstretched arms. Normally, such a movement is rapidly checked, and the displaced limb is returned to its initial position evenly and accurately. The ability to check movements quickly requires the coordinated action of agonists, antagonists, and synergists.

Dexterity Test
Dexterity and coordination of the hand are tested by asking the patient to perform fine motor movements, such as rapidly touching the fingertips with the thumb in sequential fashion. This should be done in a smooth, coordinated fashion.

Figure-of-Eight Test
While lying supine, the patient draws a figure-of-eight in the air with the great toe.

Assessment of the Autonomic Nervous System

The **autonomic nervous system (ANS)** regulates involuntary functions that include activities of cardiac muscle, smooth muscle, and glands. The ANS has two divisions: the sympathetic (**adrenergic**) and the parasympathetic (**cholinergic**). Assessment of the ANS may lead to the diagnosis of a neurologic disorder. Stimulation of the sympathetic (adrenergic) division assesses for tachycardia, dilation of the bronchi, release of adrenaline and noradrenaline that maintains blood pressure, decrease in bowel motility, inhibition of micturition, increased sweating, and dilation of the pupils. **Horner's syndrome,** caused by a brainstem lesion interrupting the descending sympathetic nerves, may be observed as a sympathetic defect with symptoms of ptosis of the upper lid, constriction of the pupil, and flushing of the face—ptosis, miosis, and anhidrosis of the affected side. Assessment for this syndrome should be performed in spine injuries at or above the first thoracic level to determine if the cervical sympathetic chair has been disrupted. Parasympathetic (cholinergic) division assessment checks for bradycardia, constriction of the bronchi, increase in salivation and lacrimation, increase in bowel motility, erections, initiation of micturition, and constriction of the pupil. The clinician should also be aware of and check for drugs that can interfere with autonomic function such as beta-blockers.[2] Other conditions to assess include the following:

- Sweating and skin temperature: Temperature impairment may be assessed to determine if the irregularity results from lesions in the hypothalamus; problems with sweating can be associated with syringomyelia and peripheral nerve injury.
- Cyanosis and pallor: Sudden changes in skin color should be assessed to rule out an autonomic response.
- Red and dry: Skin that is red and hot with impaired sweating indicates a sympathetic lesion.[2]
- Trophic changes: In patients with peripheral neuropathy and syringomyelia, the skin is assessed for evidence of changes (smooth, thick, or dry skin).

- Postural changes in blood pressure: The autonomic reflex controls blood pressure and may cause sudden changes that require immediate interventions.

Assessment of the Spinal Cord

Spinal Cord Function

The spinal cord serves as a pathway for transmission of sensory impulses from the peripheral nervous system (PNS) to the brain and for transmission of motor responses from the brain to the periphery. Thirty-one pairs of spinal nerves originate from the cord. Generally, spinal cord assessment is grounded in an understanding of the anatomy and physiology of the spinal cord (see Chapter 1). Most spinal cord disease can be diagnosed by the history, presenting symptoms, and initial assessment (see Chapter 12).

Thirty-three vertebrae surround the spinal cord and are connected by ligaments. When assessing for loss of spinal cord function, the clinician evaluates the patient for diffuse or generalized weakness, weakness of all four extremities, unilateral and bilateral weakness, patchy weakness, or variable weakness with a nonanatomic distribution. The clinician should determine the level of lesion for muscle or nerve damage and UMN versus LMN lesion versus mixed UMN and LMN.

Spinal Nerves

The 31 paired nerves without names that exit the spinal cord through adjacent vertebrae of the spine each have specific motor and sensory functions. The spinal nerves are divided into regions associated with the vertebral regions of the body and are numbered according to the level of the vertebral column at which they exit. There are 8 cervical nerves, 12 thoracic nerves, 5 lumbar nerves, 5 sacral nerves, and 1 coccygeal nerve (see Fig. 1-25).

Each spinal nerve innervates specific skin surface areas called dermatomes. Dermatome assessment is done to determine the level of spinal cord function, the level of spinal anesthesia for surgical procedures, and the level of postoperative analgesia when epidural local anesthetics are used. A dermatome chart traces the spinal nerves to their point of muscle innervation. When the clinician is assessing spinal cord function, a diagram of the dermatomes can provide anatomic clues to the level of injury or function (Fig. 2-12).

Motor Function

Whenever a motor examination is performed, the function of the spinal cord is being assessed. UMN control terminates in the anterior horn cells. The LMN and the reflex arc are integral to the spinal cord at the level each spinal nerve leaves

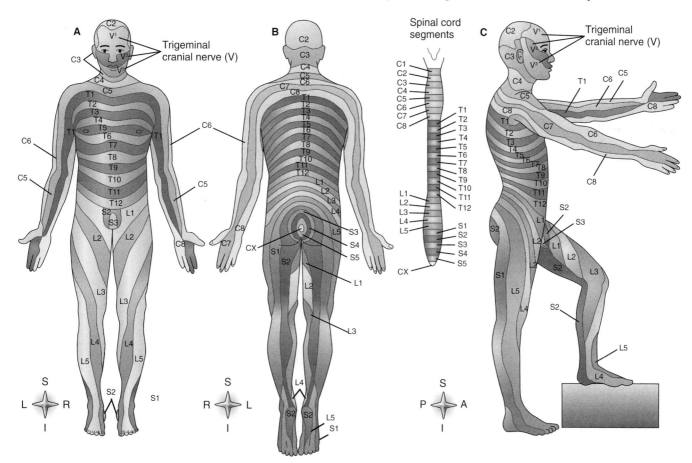

Figure 2-12 Dermatome distribution of spinal nerves. **A,** The front of the body's surface. **B,** The back of the body's surface. **C,** The side of the body's surface. The inset shows the segments of the spinal cord associated with each of the spinal nerves associated with the sensory dermatomes shown. *C,* Cervical segments; *T,* thoracic segments; *L,* lumbar segments; *S,* sacral segments; *CX,* coccygeal segment. *(From Thibodeau GA, Patton KT:* Anatomy and physiology, *ed 5, St Louis, 2003, Mosby.)*

the cord. Motor responses of the pyramidal system travel from the contralateral side of the brain, decussate in the medulla, and continue down the corticospinal tract of the spinal cord on the ipsilateral side to innervate with muscles for voluntary movement. Motor responses of the extrapyramidal system also begin in the contralateral side of the brain, decussate in the medulla, and travel through the rubrospinal, vestibulospinal, and anterior corticospinal tracts to provide control of fine movements and muscle tone.

Sensory Function

Sensory function levels in the spinal cord are more difficult to assess than motor function because of the unusual decussation patterns. The spinal cord relays pain, temperature, touch, vibration, and position senses, which enter from the periphery through the posterior root of the spinal nerve and travel to the brain. Pain and temperature enter the spinal cord, cross to the contralateral side at that level, and then traverse up the cord in the spinothalamic tract. Vibration and position sense enter the cord and travel on the ipsilateral side in the posterior or dorsal columns until they decussate in the medulla before proceeding to the thalamus on the contralateral side. These decussation patterns become particularly significant when evaluating a patient with a partial or incomplete spinal cord injury.

Assessment Techniques

A thorough spinal cord assessment involves evaluation of motor movement and strength, light touch and superficial pain, and position sense. In a patient with a new spinal cord injury, a thorough, well-documented baseline assessment is essential for comparison on serial assessments. This assessment should be documented on a spinal cord assessment flow sheet because the standard neurologic assessment flow sheet often does not include the level of detail required for ongoing spinal cord function evaluation.

The need for a complete evaluation of the spinal cord when new injury or damage is known or suspected cannot be overemphasized. Particularly in the cervical area, a slight change in motor or sensory parameters that goes unrecognized could have a devastating effect on the rehabilitation

potential and level of recovery. Any minor changes in spinal cord assessment should be considered significant and reported immediately. For example, with acute spinal cord injury (SCI), injury below T1 may produce paraplegia and injury above T1 may produce tetraplegia. Acute SCI produces **spinal shock** characterized by flaccid paralysis and complete loss of sensation at the time of injury. Injury that completely transects the cord results in permanent motor and sensory loss.

Motor Movement and Strength. When assessing motor function and strength in a patient with a spinal cord dysfunction, the clinician must assess and grade each of the major muscle groups. Table 2-20 describes the relationship between spinal nerves and muscle group movement and also indicates techniques to assess those muscle groups. After movement in each muscle group has been assessed in all four limbs, it is graded according to the scale found in Fig. 2-2. The resulting assessment determines damage to the corticospinal tract or main motor pathway (see Chapter 12).

Light Touch and Superficial Pain. Light touch and superficial pain testing begin the sensory component of the spinal cord assessment. The patient is asked to identify (1) if a touch is felt and where, and (2) whether the touch is sharp, dull, **hyperesthetic** (excessive sensation of pain in relation to stimuli applied), or absent. The test should be demonstrated first on the patient's cheek or some area above the level of dysfunction as the normal control.

The clinician charts variations in response to touch on a sensory assessment tool such as the American Spinal Injury Association (ASIA) Standard Neurological Classification of Spinal Cord Injury, which identifies key sensory points in **dermatomes** (areas of the body innervated by afferent fibers from one spinal root) (see Fig. 2-12 and Chapter 12).

Light touch and superficial pain testing is always performed with the patient's eyes closed or the patient's face screened from the body. The test is performed with a pinprick up and down all extremities and on the trunk. With a complete spinal cord injury, this assessment could indicate normal sensation above the level of injury, hyperesthesia or dull sensation around the level of injury, and absent sensation below the level of injury. In an incomplete

TABLE 2-20	**Spinal Nerve Innervation of Major Muscle Groups**	
Spinal Nerve	**Muscle Group Movement**	**Assessment Technique**
C5	Elbow flexors (biceps)	Arm is flexed; try to pull flexed forearm open.
C6	Wrist extensors	Fist is made with wrist cocked up with resistance when pushed down.
C7	Elbow extensors (triceps)	From the flexed position, the arm is straightened out against resistance.
C7	Thumb-index pinch	Index finger is held firmly to thumb against resistance to pull apart.
C8	Finger extensors	Middle finger is held firmly to thumb against resistance to pull apart.
C6-8	Hand grasp	Offer patient index and middle fingers to squeeze and let go to evaluate hand grasp.
L2	Hip flexors	Leg is lifted from bed against resistance.
L3	Knee extensors	From flexed position, knee is extended against resistance.
L4	Ankle dorsiflexion	Foot is pulled up toward nose against resistance.
L5	Long toe extensors	Long toe is pushed toward nose against resistance.
S1	Ankle plantar flexors	Foot is pushed down (stepping on the gas) against resistance.

Modified from Marshall SB et al: *Neuroscience critical care: pathophysiology and patient management*, Philadelphia, 1990, WB Saunders.

spinal cord injury, it is not uncommon to find patches of normal, abnormal, and absent sensation. The sensations of light touch and superficial pain are functions of the spinothalamic tract, as is temperature. Often, if a patient complains of **hyperesthesia,** the complaint includes a sensation of "burning" pain.

Specific nerves can also be assessed. For example, the clinician can use a sharp prick to assess the peroneal nerve by touching the web space between the great and second toe, or touch the medial and lateral surfaces of the side of the foot to test the tibial nerve. The radial nerve of the hand can be tested by touching the web space between the thumb and index finger, and the ulnar nerve by touching the distal fat pad on the inside tip of the small finger. In addition, the clinician can touch the distal surface on top of the index finger to assess the median nerve. Patient responses can be described as absent, impaired, or normal.

Pain. In response to the recent Joint Commission on Accreditation of Healthcare Organizations (JCAHO) standards of pain management, health care organizations are expected to develop policies and procedures so that all patients are systematically assessed for pain. A pain assessment includes the nature of pain, onset, duration, location, description, quality, alleviating or aggravating factors, and pain intensity (e.g., the use of a simple, standardized neuropathy pain scale from 0 to 10, with regular reassessment and follow-up). For patients unable to verbalize their pain, pain may be inferred by the observation of physiologic or behavioral indicators (e.g., withdrawal to touch, grimacing, and hemodynamics). Pain assessment, management, and formal documentation are discussed in Chapter 23.

Position Sense. Before beginning this test, the clinician demonstrates up-and-down movements to the patient to avoid any confusion in terminology. In order to test position sense, the patient's eyes should be closed or the face is screened from the body. The clinician grasps the patient's thumb or great toe and moves it up or down. The patient is asked to identify the movement. This test should be performed randomly, with the clinician moving the thumb or great toe in various patterns. Even with guessing, the patient has a 50% chance of correctly identifying the movement, so the results of this test should be carefully evaluated. Assessment of position sense evaluates the posterior or dorsal columns. These columns also carry sensations of deep pressure and vibration.

APPLICATION OF THE NEUROLOGIC ASSESSMENT

In the previous sections, the many components of the neurologic assessment are discussed in detail. When all of the assessment components are clearly understood, it is time to develop patterns of neurologic assessment that are needed for different patient conditions and levels of illness. A complete, comprehensive, detailed neurologic assessment would be unwieldy and unnecessary to perform on all patients at all times. It would be tragic, however, to eliminate an essential component of the assessment because of a lack of under-

standing of the necessary information. This section describes the components of the neurologic assessment used when assessing patients in a variety of situations. Although guidelines for component selection are described here, each patient's neurologic assessment should be individualized to provide the most accurate and complete information possible.

Emergent Assessment in the Field and During Transportation

One of the challenges of medical care today is to provide initial assessment of the urgently ill patient outside of the health care environment. This is a challenge because the spectrum of events that constitute an emergency can vary considerably with each patient. Patients seen in the field are often seriously or critically ill and require a rapid response. The first response is to stabilize ventilation and circulation. Known traditionally as the **ABCs** (airway, breathing, and circulation) of emergency care, these areas have particular importance for neurologically impaired patients. The brain requires a continuous supply of well-oxygenated blood to maintain minimum acceptable function. Any disruption or decrease in circulation or ventilation (oxygen and carbon dioxide exchange) may lead to serious secondary injury in an already-compromised neurologic system.

Although the degree of assessment and intervention differs with each patient, the process is dynamic; establishing management priorities is often of singular importance. Making correct decisions for action depends largely on whether the clinician uses an organized and systematic approach to the assessment process. The traditional tools of the neurologic examination may be helpful, but the initial observations that serve to focus the assessment require no equipment. During this period the most important tools are the senses of sight, touch, smell, and hearing. Much depends on the skill of the observer in interpreting what significance the information collected has in the clinical situation.

Components of Emergent Assessment
The rapid response time of emergency medical services (EMS) personnel in prehospital triage, assessment, and treatment has improved survival rates of patients during the **"golden hour"** following trauma. Standardized record keeping helps track patient assessment parameters from the scene through discharge and rehabilitation. After the initial assessment, prehospital providers determine the severity of the patient's condition and transport the patient.

Role of Level of Consciousness
The role that the level of consciousness (LOC) plays in the emergent assessment cannot be overemphasized. If the patient is conscious and able to communicate coherently, the caregiver must listen to what the patient says about the presenting symptoms and current illness. During transport the patient should be instructed to voice any changes in condition or sensation. "I'm feeling different or funny" is often a clue from the patient announcing deterioration or a change

in condition. In addition, deterioration may be occurring if the patient stops communicating or becomes less articulate.

When a patient is unconscious and can provide no verbal clues, the degree of observation and assessment must increase significantly. The LOC, pupils, vital signs, and breathing patterns should be reassessed frequently. Under the applicable city, county, or state guidelines for emergency medical services, interventions may be provided while the EMS team is in transport on the basis of deterioration in the patient's condition as evidenced by changes in breathing patterns or pupil size. The ability to perform early intubation and ventilation control or administer mannitol because of pupillary changes may decrease brain injury secondary to hypoxia or prevent increased ICP. Raising the head or elevating the head of the backboard may be necessary to prevent increased ICP. Suctioning equipment should be available with close observations for silent aspiration that could cause pneumonia and further complicate the patient's condition.

Emergency Department Assessment

The emergency department (ED) staff continues the patient assessment for airway, breathing, circulation, disability drugs (diabetic), symptoms of epilepsy, fever, GCS, and herniation syndromes. As soon as the ABCs are stabilized and the patient is exposed, a brief but rapid neurologic examination is performed to exclude focal neurologic abnormalities.[2]

The **primary survey** is the basis for all emergent interventions delivered in the care of patients. All factors assessed during the primary survey are of such a critical nature that any major deviation from normal requires immediate intervention. The assessment process does not continue until all life-threatening deviations in the primary survey receive appropriate intervention.[4]

Assessment parameters are incorporated into a standard emergency assessment tool and frequently include a record of the patient's Glasgow Coma Scale (GCS) score, as well as pupil and motor examination, until head injury is ruled out. Particular attention should be paid to readily available information on the immediate history of the patient's condition, such as the cause of the accident, mechanism of injury, and immediate response of the patient compared with the current response.

Any patient with a preexisting illness has a greater potential for deterioration. Outside of the hospital setting or during transport to the hospital, the potential for overlooking the deterioration is greater. Extra care is taken to observe and respond to subtle changes in the patient's condition, recording emergent field assessment as part of the ED report.

A **secondary assessment** follows the primary assessment and is brief. The goal of this assessment is to discover all abnormalities or injuries. The mnemonic often used in this survey is E (exposure), F (freezing/Fahrenheit), G (get vitals/history), H (head to toe), I (inspect posterior surface).[4]

A **focused assessment** is a detailed assessment of any area or organ system that has an abnormality or injury. Specialists are frequently involved in the focused assessment such as the neurosurgical team to treat life-threatening head or spinal trauma.[4]

Acute and Postacute Care Assessment

The initial hospital assessment for acute care is an essential component of a patient's clinical care. This initial assessment provides the basis for many diagnostic and therapeutic interventions. It is also the baseline for noting improvement or deterioration on serial assessments. When caring for a patient in the hospital, clinic, or home health care environment, the clinician must always be aware of the results of the initial baseline assessment for comparison.

Initial Assessment Components

Components of the initial assessment have been discussed previously in this chapter (see "Performance of the Adult Neurologic Assessment"). The clinician conducting the initial assessment must be thorough and careful to avoid missing important pieces of information. If the patient is acutely or critically ill, some components of the initial assessment may be delayed but should be evaluated as soon as the patient's condition warrants it.

Serial Assessment and Reassessment Components

Serial assessment of the patient is based on results of the initial baseline assessment. The serial assessment follows the basic neurologic examination with particular attention directed to the areas of abnormality noted on initial assessment. The role of serial assessment is to quickly identify any significant changes in the neurologic examination from the initial assessment. Because it is used for comparison, the serial assessment is less involved and less time-consuming than the baseline assessment; however, it is not less important.

More focused in nature, serial assessment requires the most organized, systematic approach. After the patient's neurologic deficits are known through the initial assessment, the clinician is tempted to assume that those deficits remain and to use that level for further assessment. However, each serial assessment should begin with the premise that the patient is neurologically intact and then quickly progress to identify the current deficits.

The conscious patient is assessed using the techniques described in this chapter. This systematic assessment takes 3 to 4 minutes and should be charted in the patient's record following the assessment. If the clinician finds an abnormality, that deficit must be evaluated in more detail and reported for further investigation by the treatment team. Significant deficits are reassessed and recorded until the physician arrives at the bedside for management of the patient's problems.

The Unconscious Patient

Patients with changes in LOC and associated neurologic signs and symptoms require close monitoring beginning with the history and time of onset, followed by immediate reporting of findings. In assessing the unconscious patient, the clinician should determine the LOC. First achieve maximal arousal of the patient to obtain the most accurate assessment.

Patients with alterations in the reticular activating system (RAS) may have altered consciousness. Assessment can also include blood glucose for hypoglycemia or hyperglycemia; blood gases for hypoxia/acidosis and hypercapnia; toxic screen for substance abuse; and imaging studies for stroke, head injury, or spine injury with increasing edema. After the patient has been stimulated, the clinician can proceed with the assessment, which includes the following:

- LOC: Perform the GCS assessment as a quick, reliable method to communicate with and describe the patient.
- Pupils: Perform pupil assessment with special attention focused on the size, reactivity, and shape of the pupil in comparison with the opposite eye and earlier assessments.
- Motor assessment: Evaluate each extremity; individually describe the stimulus required and the resulting motor response, particularly abnormal flexion and extension.
- Respiratory pattern: If the patient is not mechanically ventilated, observe respiratory patterns for any changes or irregularity.
- Vital signs: Vital signs should be compared with previous assessment for evidence of decreasing pulse rate or increasing systolic blood pressure; serial assessments should be accurately recorded in a timely manner with any changes noted, even subtle changes carefully considered and reported to the physician (e.g., increasing stimulation required to achieve the same response).

Special attention to alterations in consciousness require a thorough assessment and immediate reporting of possible causative factors: sudden elevation in temperature to rule out CNS infection (e.g., meningitis); purpuric rash for suspected meningococcal meningitis; needle marks for intravenous (IV) substance abuse; bitten and bleeding tongue indicative of seizure; multiple needle marks for unresponsive diabetic patient; sluggish and dilated pupil or small unreactive pupil, ptosis, or CN III palsy; sudden onset of weakness or hemiplegia; alcohol breath; or Cheyne-Stokes and other irregular or erratic respirations.

Rehabilitation Potential Assessment

The neuroscience clinician is a key health care professional responsible for identifying the patient's discharge needs for acute or home rehabilitation services. Appropriate assessment is determined by the outcome of the patient's neurologic illness, present status, and needs. Considerations are given to the patient's adaptation, adjustment and coping, degree of cognitive impairment, communication deficits, and functional abilities for self-care, as well as safety issues and family dynamics.

Rehabilitation assessment needs should be addressed at treatment team meetings or discharge rounds with the physiatrist to identify patients who are candidates for functional restoration or rehabilitation services (e.g., patients with disruption of motor, bowel, or bladder function; impaired ambulation and mobility; and speech disorders). In addition, it is recommended that rehabilitation concepts be initiated in the intensive care unit (ICU), throughout the acute care stay, and in conjunction with the attending physiatrist and rehabilitation professionals at the referral rehabilitation hospital or home care agency.[3]

Ideally, the physiatrist and clinician should be available before patient transfer to provide recommendations for the case manager or the life care planner, who will coordinate the rehabilitation focus or patient management after discharge. Certainly, neuroscience rounds in the acute care setting are an ideal forum in which to assess and, as a team, determine a plan of care for the patient. Referrals for rehabilitation (hospital unit, freestanding rehabilitation hospital, skilled nursing units, or outpatient rehabilitation services) should be discussed by the treatment team as soon as possible.

The guiding concept in rehabilitation is that "discharge or disposition begins at the time of admission." Every patient must be assessed for rehabilitation potential and functional restoration. Nursing rehabilitation interventions must be initiated in the acute care setting. In ICU and acute care units, rehabilitation interventions can be implemented to prevent secondary complications from the catastrophic illness or injury. Many long-term complications can be lessened and, in some cases, prevented with early rehabilitation intervention. For example, any patient in a prolonged immobilized state would benefit from referrals to physical therapy and occupational therapy for positioning recommendations, positioning aids (e.g., splints, edges, and cushions), range-of-motion (ROM) protocols, and activity tolerance assessment. The physical therapists, in conjunction with physicians and clinicians, are able to determine which patients are most likely to benefit from rehabilitation intervention (see Chapter 13).

NEUROLOGIC ASSESSMENT OF THE OLDER ADULT

Consideration for decreased ability to detect environmental stimuli is needed for the older adult assessment. Changes in vision and hearing and decreased response time may prevent the older adult from processing questions and information. As the U.S. population ages, including the 78 million baby boomers, health care professionals will be increasingly challenged to provide appropriate care to the older patient.

It is important to assess for impulsiveness and poor judgment, as well as muscle weakness, osteoporosis, impaired proprioception, cerebellar signs, basal ganglion dysfunction, and frontal lobe disease. In addition, assessment for risk of falling is essential along with awareness of any safety issues that could lead to falls, including podiatric and footwear problems. Muscle wasting, poor health status, painful arthritis, and polypharmacy are included in the assessment. The clinician should also be aware of myopathies and determine that muscle strength allows the individual to get up from a sitting position versus a neuropathy making it difficult to walk on the toes and heels. Ambulatory difficulty and balance problems may be related to orthostatic hypotension or dizziness from vascular disease or medications. Gait in the older adult who uses an assistive device should be observed with

TABLE 2-21	Age-Related Differences in Assessment of the Older Adult Nervous System	
Component	**Changes**	**Differences in Assessment Findings**
Central Nervous System		
Brain	Reduction in cerebral blood flow and metabolism	Alterations in selected mental functioning
	Decrease in efficiency of temperature-regulating mechanism	Decrease in body temperature, impairment of ability to adapt to environmental temperature
	Decrease in neurotransmitter content, disruption in integration as result of loss of neurons	Repetitive movements, tremors
	Decrease in oxygen supply, changes in basal ganglia caused by vascular changes	Changes in gait and ambulation (e.g., extra-pyramidal, Parkinson-like gait); diminished kinesthetic sense
Peripheral Nervous System		
Cranial and spinal nerves	Loss of myelin and decrease in conduction time in some nerves	Decrease in reaction time in specific nerves
	Cellular degeneration, death of neurons	Decrease in speed and intensity of neuronal reflexes
Functional Divisions		
Motor	Decrease in muscle bulk	Diminished strength and agility
	Decrease in electrical activity	Decrease in reactions and movement time
Sensory	Decrease in sensory receptors caused by degenerative changes and involution of fine corpuscles of nerve endings	Diminished sense of touch; inability to localize stimuli; decrease in appreciation of touch, temperature, and peripheral vibrations
	Decrease in electrical activity	Slowing of or alteration in sensory reception
	Atrophy of taste buds	Signs of malnutrition, weight loss
	Degeneration and loss of fibers in olfactory bulb	Diminished sense of smell
	Degenerative changes in nerve cells in vestibular system of inner ear, cerebellum, and proprioceptive pathways in nervous system	Poor ability to maintain balance, widened gait
Reflexes	Possible decrease in deep tendon reflexes	Below-average reflex score
	Decrease in sensory conduction velocity as result of myelin sheath degeneration	Sluggish reflexes, slowing of reaction time
Reticular Formation		
Reticular activating system	Modification of hypothalamic function, reduction in stage IV sleep	Increase in frequency of spontaneous awakening together with tiredness, interrupted sleep, insomnia
Autonomic Nervous System		
SNS and PSNS	Morphologic features of ganglia, slowing of ANS responses	Orthostatic hypotension, systolic hypertension

From Lewis SM, Heitkemper MM, Dirksen SF: *Medical-surgical nursing: assessment and management of clinical problems,* ed 5, St Louis, 2000, Mosby.
ANS, Autonomic nervous system; *PSNS,* parasympathetic nervous system; *SNS,* sympathetic nervous system.

the particular device to determine safe use and appropriateness. Physical and occupational therapists may be asked to participate in an assessment, especially when assistance is needed for evaluating strength, balance, transfers, and ambulation.

Sensory overload occurs with changes in the environment, especially toward night. Older patients may have a condition known as **sundowning,** in which they become confused and disoriented especially toward nightfall when visual cues and familiar stimuli are not easily apparent. In combination with dementia, sundowning can be a serious safety risk.

Neuronal loss clearly is a natural consequence of aging. Neurons do not divide; thus cell loss is permanent and inevitable. Brain weight decreases by 5% to 17% in older adults. Areas most affected by cell loss include the frontal and temporal lobes of the cerebral cortex. These are the areas that

determine personality, motor activity, and speech. Simple reaction time is also decreased with age because of several changes, including vision impairment, a decrease in the number of axons in nerves, and changes at the synapses that may slow conduction. Age-related changes that may be noted on physical examination of the older adult are described in Table 2-21.

Components of Older Adult Assessment

In addition to the other components of the initial neurologic assessment, an assessment of the older adult should include psychologic, psychosocial, and functional assessments. The clinician should listen carefully to everything the older patient describes. It is not uncommon for atypical or nonspecific complaints to be clues pointing to a chronic disease or even an acute illness. A change in the ability to remain in the same living environment or perform the same typical activities may be the only indications of deteriorating function.

General Examination Considerations for Older Adults

The difficulty in assessing the older adult involves distinguishing normal changes of aging from those of neurologic disorders (e.g., evidence of muscle wasting and atrophy, altered reflexes, vibratory changes, position sense). The clinician should be alert for asymmetric changes that may indicate a neurologic disorder in addition to an underlying chronic disease or injury. The clinician must also be alert for rapid changes in status and deterioration, since the older patient may lack reserves and display delayed or absent compensatory mechanisms. Sensory overload may occur with changes in the environment, especially at night. Older adults may display sundowning and become confused and disoriented at night, when visual cues and familiar stimuli are absent. In combination with dementia, sundowning can be a serious safety risk. Focusing on the following seven considerations during the examination often provides improved results:

1. Environment: Examinations should be conducted in a quiet area with reduced background noise and good but not bright illumination that keeps glare to a minimum. Chairs, examination table, and the bathroom should be accessible to older patients. Room temperature should be comfortable and adjustable as needed. Care should be taken to maintain the patient's privacy and dignity.
2. Communication: The patient's attention should be obtained before addressing with the patient's surname (e.g., Mr., Mrs., or Ms. Jones). The clinician should face the patient and use a low-pitched, soft voice with an unhurried manner and distinct pronunciation, especially when the patient is hearing impaired. Communication should be enhanced with prostheses as needed (e.g., glasses, hearing aids). The clinician should use visual and verbal communication plus touch and put suggestions in writing as needed. In addition, it is important to be aware that chronic disease may influence communication and history taking. Extra time should be allowed for history taking and the physical examination as needed.
3. Medications: The clinician should review the patient's regimen of prescription and over-the-counter (OTC) drugs at every encounter.
4. Physical, psychologic, psychosocial, and functional assessments: All components of the assessment should be addressed frequently.
5. Atypical or nonspecific presentations of chronic disease or acute illness: It is important to be aware that atypical presentations are common in older adults.
6. Pain: An older adult should always be queried about pain and discomfort. Older patients are usually reluctant to offer complaints, especially regarding chronic pain, because they have learned to accept ongoing pain as part of the normal aging process. In addition, the clinician should follow up on response to pain interventions and medications because older adults may respond differently.
7. Current laboratory findings: It is important to check all laboratory results for indications of infection, electrolyte abnormalities, dehydration status, and other significant variations.

CONCLUSION

A neurologic assessment is one component of a complete physical assessment. The techniques described in this chapter combine to structure the neurologic portion of the physical assessment, which, in turn, is incorporated into a complete assessment. Elements of all portions of the neurologic assessment, both normal and abnormal, are evaluated, analyzed, and documented. Taken as a whole, these assessment parameters are incorporated into the nursing process to diagnose and develop a list of actual and potential problems together with a plan of care. The goal is to help the patient recover quickly and safely. Expected outcomes can be achieved through expertise in performing an accurate neurologic assessment. The need for advanced assessment may be referred to other members of the treatment team with collaboration of findings for holistic management (e.g., physical therapists, speech pathologists, or physician).

RESOURCES FOR ASSESSMENT

American Association of Neuroscience Nurses: 888-557-2266, www.aann.org
Association of Rehabilitation Nurses: 800-229-7530, www.rehabnurse.org

REFERENCES

1. Bates BA, Bickley LS, Holkeman RA: *A guide to physical examination and history taking*, ed 9, Philadelphia, 2005, JB Lippincott.
2. Fuller G: *Neurological examination made easy*, ed 3, Philadelphia, 2004, Churchill Livingstone.
3. Hanak M: *Rehabilitation nursing for the neurological patient*, New York, 1992, Springer.
4. Jordan KS: *Emergency nursing core curriculum*, ed 5, Philadelphia, 2000, WB Saunders.
5. Lehman CA, Hayes JM, LaCroix M, Owen SV, Nauta HJW: Development and implementation of a focused neurological assessment system, *J Neurosci Nurs* 35(4):185–192, 2003.
6. Marshall SB: *Neuroscience critical care: pathophysiology and patient management*, Philadelphia, 1990, WB Saunders.
7. Mayo Clinic Department of Neurology: *Mayo Clinic examinations in neurology*, ed 7, St Louis, 1998, Mosby.
8. Plum F, Posner J: *The diagnosis of stupor and coma*, ed 3, Philadelphia, 1980, FA Davis.
9. Stewart-Amidei C: Assessment. In Bader MK, Littlejohn LR, editors: *AANN core curriculum for neuroscience nursing*, ed 4, St Louis, 2004, Saunders.

10. Teasdale G, Jennett B: Assessment of coma and impaired consciousness—a practical scale, *Lancet* 2:81, 1974.

SUGGESTED READINGS

Ackley BJ, Ladwig GB: *Nursing diagnosis handbook: a guide to planning care*, ed 5, St Louis, 2002, Mosby.

Adams RD, Victor M: *Principles of neurology*, ed 7, New York, 2001, McGraw-Hill.

Popp AJ, editor: *The primary care of neurological disorders*, Park Ridge, IL, 1998, American Association of Neurological Surgeons.

Ross RT: *How to examine the nervous system*, Stamford, CT, 1999, Appleton & Lange.

Rossi P: *Case management in healthcare: a practical guide*, Philadelphia, 1999, WB Saunders.

Selman WR, Benzel EC: *Neurosurgical care of the elderly*, Park Ridge, IL, 1999, American Association of Neurological Surgeons.

ALBERTO IAIA,
ELLEN BARKER

CHAPTER 3

Neurodiagnostic Studies

The impact of modern imaging technology on the clinical neurosciences has been called "revolutionary." Optimized imaging of the nervous system with speed, power, and simultaneous imaging in less time and with less exposure and data reconstruction without artifacts encompasses a wide variety of modalities that have undergone rapid evolution in the past few decades. It is anticipated that diagnostic brain imaging will become totally noninvasive.[15] The quality of image, safety, and timing for many studies have undergone major improvements with the ability to generate reports that can be read anytime, anywhere, within 10 minutes.

Neurodiagnostic studies are performed as adjuncts to a complete clinical examination. Clinicians can correlate information from the neurodiagnostic studies with clinical findings to assist in the determination of the type, extent, and location of neurologic disease. Using clinical examination findings, as well as the results from these studies, the clinician can plan an appropriate course of patient management.

Neurodiagnostic studies are also used to evaluate the effectiveness of various treatment modalities. Sophisticated studies are performed as outpatient procedures. This is more convenient for patients and helps to allay some of their fear and anxiety. Furthermore, new technology has expanded the scope of imaging studies so that they now have a place in the operating room.

This chapter focuses on current neurodiagnostic and laboratory studies used in patient evaluation. The discussion begins with an overview of the clinician's general responsibilities in neurodiagnostic testing. Individual studies, including an explanation of each technique, its rationale, associated complications, and other pertinent information, are then discussed. Brief sections on patient preparation and postprocedure patient care are included for easy reference.

PREPARATION FOR NEURODIAGNOSTIC TESTING

Patient Preparation and Education

The clinician has many roles in the care of patients undergoing neurodiagnostic studies. Because many of these tests are conducted on an outpatient basis, the clinician must consolidate patient and family teaching with patient preparation and with evaluation of potential complications. Some patients may not be prepared for detailed explanations of neurodiag-

nostic studies. Involving the family in early teaching is thus vital so that family members can later assist in patient teaching. The clinician should reinforce the rationale for each study with both verbal explanations and additional written information. Fear of the unknown can often impede the smooth completion of testing. Therefore preparatory teaching is essential to the success of neurodiagnostic studies.

The clinician can assist the patient in overcoming pretesting anxiety by facilitating an open discussion regarding the procedure, specific patient requirements (e.g., lying still), and any possible discomfort or unusual sensations. Some patients respond best to brief, simplified explanations, whereas others expect full details of all possible risks, benefits, complications, and alternative procedures. Patients with altered levels of consciousness or cognitive deficits usually require short, simple explanations. Providing explanations that are too detailed or technical may only serve to enhance patients' anxiety if they are unable to process the information. A fundamental challenge facing the clinician is to determine the appropriate level of information for each patient.

The clinician may be required to assist during the procedure itself, especially with patients who are confused or who have altered levels of consciousness. Constant monitoring of the acutely ill, unstable neurologic patient may be required, along with physical care, such as suctioning or respiratory management. Depending, of course, on the particular procedure, the patient may also need pretesting preparation, such as a surgical scrub or medication.

Following the neurodiagnostic study, the clinician assesses for any complications and discusses with the patient any postprocedure requirements, such as fluid intake or activity level restrictions. If the patient is to be discharged soon after the procedure, a verbal and written list of possible side effects and complications should be provided for the patient and family, as well as a phone number to call to report problems.

Documentation

Following each diagnostic procedure, the clinician documents the following:
- Name of the diagnostic study
- Preprocedure medications
- Time the patient left and returned to the nursing unit and the time the procedure began and ended
- Any adverse reactions from contrast dye or medications used in the study

- How the patient tolerated the procedure
- Postprocedure verbal and written instructions given to the patient and/or family

Informed Consent

Release forms are required by institutions for many neuro-diagnostic and laboratory studies. The patient's signature on the form means that the patient has received a thorough explanation and understands the purpose, risks, potential complications, and benefits of the test. Unless the patient understands this information, he or she will be unable to give informed consent. Although the patient's physician is responsible for providing the information, the clinician preparing the patient for the procedure can answer questions and make sure that the patient understands the information. A family member or guardian will be asked to complete the consent form if the patient is unable to give consent. If the patient or family member does not understand the information provided and has further questions, the physician must be notified to clarify any misunderstandings or incorrect assumptions before proceeding with the procedure. The signed release form becomes a part of the patient's permanent medical record (see Chapter 25).

RADIOGRAPHIC STUDIES

Skull Radiographs

Skull radiographs are not indicated for evaluation of closed head trauma because computed tomography (CT) is more efficient and effective for evaluation of intracranial injury, as shown by several publications in the mid-1980s. Currently, skull films are rarely used for evaluation of head trauma. Anteroposterior (AP), Townes', and lateral views are performed to determine the configuration, size, and shape of cranial and facial bones; unusual calcifications; evidence of a skull fracture; the integrity of the bony architecture; degenerative changes (e.g., bony erosion of the sella turcica); the position of the pineal body; or hyperostosis.

Pathologic findings on a skull film might include the presence of a fracture or bone erosion suggestive of intracranial or intraosseous lesions. Displacement of the normally calcified pineal body may also indicate a space-occupying lesion in the adult. Unusual calcification may indicate the presence of tumors or chronic subdural hematomas.

Patient Preparation

Patient preparation consists of patient teaching to help reduce anxiety about exposure to radiation. This is the only preprocedure preparation that is usually necessary.

Postprocedure Care

There are virtually no complications, and no specific post-procedure care is required.[14]

Spine Radiographs

Radiographs of specific regions of the spine are usually ordered in traumatized patients, those who have experienced spine injury, and those who have back or neck pain. Spine films may also be ordered for patients with motor or sensory impairment of the extremities. In the presence of significant spine trauma or neurologic deficits, however, spine CT is preferred to plain film radiographs, as CT has been shown to have higher sensitivity to detect osseous injury.

When plain films are obtained, AP, lateral, and oblique views are often not done in the emergency department but in the clinical setting. They are ordered for minimal evaluation. More complete evaluation would include oblique im-ages, cone-down images of the lumbosacral junction, and flexion and extension views. Pathologic findings may include vertebral fractures, traumatic dislocation, subluxation, lytic lesions, and collapsed vertebrae. Degenerative changes, such as scoliosis, spondylosis, spondylolisthesis, and foraminal stenosis, can also be identified. Flexion and extension views are helpful in evaluating possible segmental instability.

Patient Preparation

The clinician provides patient education to help reduce anxiety. In the patient with suspected cervical spine injury, the clinician must help the patient to maintain spinal precautions, including maintenance of head alignment and neck stabilization with a cervical collar. To obtain a clear image of C1 and C2, the radiograph needs to be shot through the patient's open mouth; C6 and C7 views may also be difficult to obtain because of body mass and may require downward traction on the patient's arms to obtain a clear view. Occasionally, swimmer's views or oblique views are needed for a clear C7 view.

Many hospitals with trauma facilities have specialized trauma radiology units with the capability of obtaining unusual angulations or views to avoid overlying artifacts or fixation. Most trauma centers currently bypass plain film radiographs, and evaluate the cervical spine with CT, in view of its proven higher sensitivity to subtle osseous injury.

Traumatized patients should receive spinal immobilization precautions until they are proved to be stable through a clinical examination and spine films.

Postprocedure Care

With spine precautions, the patient cannot be moved, be repositioned, be taken off the backboard, or have the hard collar removed until after being cleared, by x-ray studies and instructions from the physician in charge. There are no other special postprocedure preparations. Complications from obtaining spine films are rare. Of all the spine examinations involving radiation, plain film radiography gives the lowest dose, averaging 0.2 rad for the cervical spine and 0.7 rad for the lumbar spine.[7]

ALERT: The patient's neurologic status should be reassessed and documented after completion of spine radiographs.

Computed Tomography

With the introduction of **computed tomography (CT)** in the mid-1970s came many major advances in the diagnosis and treatment of patients with neurologic disorders. Direct visualization is possible when CT images are produced with the use of a computer to reconstruct images from the x-ray beam. Images in multiple sections are produced by measuring the various densities of the substances through which the x-ray beam passes. Cross-sectional, coronal, and sagittal images of the head and spine are produced. In dense structures, such as bone, x-ray beam penetration is lessened. These structures are light gray or white on a CT scan. Cerebrospinal fluid (CSF) and air, which are much less dense than bone, are nearly black on a CT scan. Brain tissue is various shades of gray on a CT scan (Table 3-1). Sections as thin as 0.5 to 1.3 cm are possible and can produce accurate images of very small abnormalities (Fig. 3-1).

There are no medical contraindications to performing CT; however, it is recommended that pregnant women undergo this examination only if there is a strong medical indication for it. During cranial CT in a pregnant woman, the amount

TABLE 3-1	Appearances of Tissues on Computed Tomography	
Tissue	Hounsfield Unit	Gray Scale
Air	−1000	Black (↓↓)
Fat	−100	Black (↓↓)
Cerebrospinal fluid	0	Black (↓)
Brain	30	Gray (−)
Extravasated blood	100	White (↑↑)
Contrast medium enhancement	100	White (↑↑)
Bone	1000	White (↑↑↑)

From Goetz CG, Pappert EJ: *Textbook of clinical neurology,* Philadelphia, 1999, WB Saunders.
↓↓↓, Marked hypoattenuation; ↓↓, moderate hypoattenuation; ↓, mild hypoattenuation; −, isoattenuation (to brain); ↑↑, moderate hyperattenuation; ↑↑↑, marked hyperattenuation.

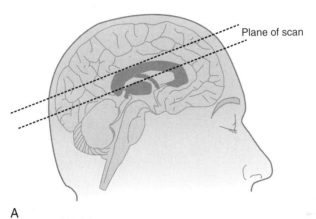

A

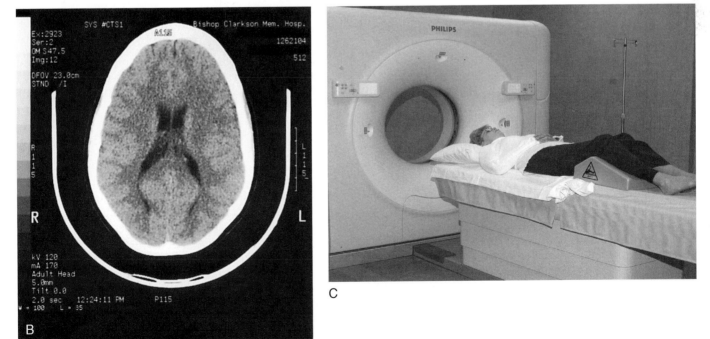

B

C

Figure 3-1 Computed tomography (CT) scans are taken at various cross sections of the brain. The image in **(A)** illustrates the cross section used for the scan shown in **(B). C,** Multidetector CT (MDT CT): These units allow acquisition of excellent quality CT angiography and imaging of the spine with multiplanar reconstruction (MPR).
(A and B, From Black JM, Hawks JH: Medical-surgical nursing: clinical management for positive outcomes, ed 7, St Louis, 2005, Elsevier Saunders. C, Courtesy of Neuroscience Imaging, Newark, DE.)

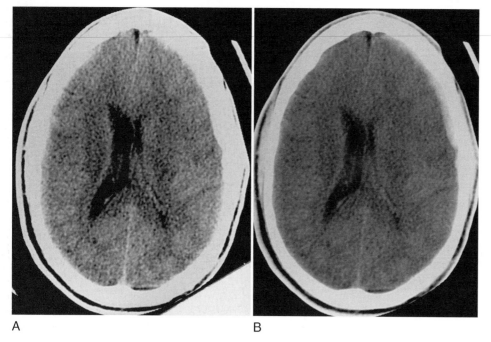

A   B

Figure 3-2 Computed tomography (CT) of a 23-year-old man after a motor vehicle accident. **A,** An acute frontal subdural hematoma causes compression of the left lateral ventricle, but it is difficult to see at routine brain windows (60). **B,** At subdural windows (1.50), the hematoma is identified subjacent to the calvaria. *(From Goetz CG, Pappert EJ: Textbook of clinical neurology, Philadelphia, 1999, WB Saunders.)*

of radiation exposure to the fetus is minimal because the x-ray beam is finely collimated and the mother can be shielded with front and back lead aprons. In the case of a nonemergent medical condition, however, it is prudent to wait until the patient is sure that she is not pregnant.[24]

The CT scan is used in neurologic patients to obtain non-invasive images of the brain and spinal canal; the cord per se is not well seen on CT. However, patients may be required to have an injection of a contrast medium to enhance lesions noted on noncontrast scans or if tumors are suspected. A noncontrast CT scan can usually be completed in 5 to 15 minutes, but the scanning time itself only lasts a few seconds. The recent introduction of helical CT and multidetector CT has further refined this modality such that many high-quality contiguous images can be obtained in a very short period of time to provide valuable information rapidly.[24] CT scanning is used to assist in the clinical evaluation of headaches, seizures, and trauma (Fig. 3-2).

The types of pathologic conditions seen on CT scans can include tumors, hemorrhage, edema, hydrocephalus, abscesses, foreign bodies (such as bullets), basilar skull fractures, strokes, atrophy, and congenital disorders such as Chiari malformation. Reformation of the CT images into sagittal and coronal planes is also helpful. Three-dimensional reformation of fracture fragments is also helpful in the evaluation of spine trauma and comminuted displaced fractures. For example, CT scanning provides evidence of the pattern and severity of structural brain damage after head injury, and its findings can be extensively related to the subsequent outcome. Other examinations, such as neuropsychologic testing and magnetic resonance spectroscopy, are also excellent tools for evaluating a patient following trauma.

Spiral CT, or **helical CT,** has been available for several years, and its advantages have been enhanced recently by the advent of multidetector (MDT) technology. The diagnostic

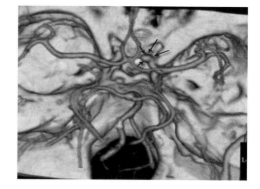

Figure 3-3 Computed tomography (CT) angiogram reveals the presence of an aneurysm *(arrows)* in the supraclinoid segment of the internal carotid artery (ICA). *(Courtesy of Alberto Iaia, MD, Neuroscience Imaging, Newark, DE.)*

capabilities differ from early-generation CTs in that multidetector scanners provide several axial images (up to 64) per individual gantry rotation, thus allowing imaging of a large continuous anatomic area in a very brief period of time (a few seconds). Advantages include speed of image acquisition, reduction of respiratory motion artifact, isotropic voxels, and superb quality of reconstruction of the axial data into sagittal and coronal planes (multiplanar reconstruction [MPR]). The main disadvantage of MDT CT is an overall increase in radiation exposure to the patient.

Helical CT angiography is used when a rapid collection of images is acquired after a bolus of contrast medium is injected.[23] It has been proven to have very high sensitivity for detection of aneurysms (Fig. 3-3), especially in the presence of subarachnoid hemorrhage (ruptured aneurysms) and for aneurysms greater than 3 mm in size.

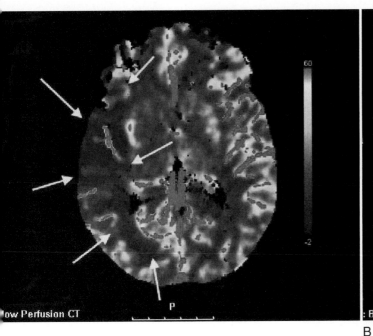

ow Perfusion CT

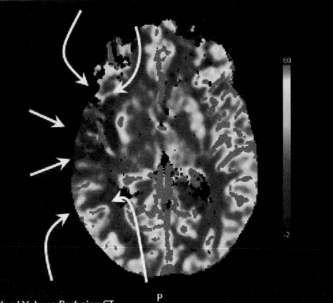

: Blood Volume Perfusion CT

B

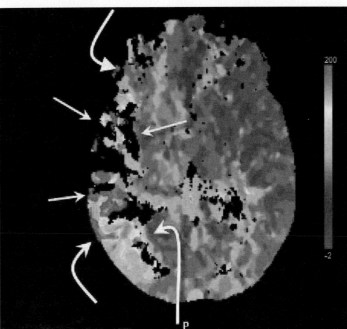

Time to Peak Perfusion CT

C

Figure 3-4 Perfusion head CT. **A,** Cerebral blood flow (CBF) map. **B,** Cerebral blood volume (CNV) map. **C,** Time-to-peak (TTP) map.
(Courtesy of Alberto Iaia, MD, Neuroscience Imaging, Newark, DE.)

Perfusion head CT is performed with MDT CT, in the presence of suspected acute ischemic injury, if the patient is presenting within 3 hours of onset of symptoms and is a candidate for reperfusion. An unenhanced head CT is performed initially to screen for the presence of hemorrhage. Subsequently, intravenous (IV) contrast is injected with a power injector via a large catheter (16 gauge) as MDT CT images are acquired repeatedly over an area of suspected ischemia. Based on the intravascular enhancement pattern, quantitative color maps can be derived that demonstrate the cerebral blood flow (CBF), cerebral blood volume (CBV), and time to peak (TTP) (Fig. 3-4). Perfusion CT and mag-

netic resonance diffusion-weighted images have become the leading technology in the diagnosis of acute stroke.

Figure 3-4 shows a perfusion head CT of a 43-year-old man with acute onset of left hemiparesis. In Fig. 3-4, *A,* the CBF color map reveals underperfusion in the right middle cerebral artery (MCA) territory *(arrows).* In Fig. 3-4, *B,* the CBV color map viable a region of infarct *(straight arrows)* and significant viable tissue (penumbra) in the periphery *(curved arrows).* In Fig. 3-4, *C,* the TTP color map shows a lack of blood flow in infarcted tissue *(straight arrows)* and delayed blood flow in the penumbra *(curved arrows).* Review of such parameters allows the clinician to establish two important diagnoses: first, if an infarct is indeed present, and second, if the infarct is complete or if there is reperfusable (viable) penumbra in its periphery. In the latter scenario, TPA may be administered to the patient.

Patient Preparation

In preparation for a CT scan, the patient is asked to lie on the CT table with the head immobilized for a head scan. The table is then moved into the gantry, a movable circular frame. The body part to be imaged (head or spine) is then centered in the machine. The gantry revolves around the part to be imaged and scans numerous times from many different angles. A clicking sound is heard as the gantry moves. If a contrast scan is performed, additional images are produced in a similar fashion after the IV injection of a contrast medium.

If the patient has a known contrast allergy, the clinician should document the type of reactions and inform the radiologist before the scan. Iodinated contrast agents are used to increase tissue density. Patients who are to have a contrast scan should be questioned about any history of allergy to iodine-based dye or shellfish because the contrast material may be iodinated. Patients may be instructed not to eat or drink for 2 to 3 hours before the scan. Some patients may experience flushing (a warm feeling), nausea, or a slight headache after the injection of the contrast; the clinician should therefore discuss these possibilities in preprocedure teaching.

Preprocedure preparation of the patient includes an explanation of the scan. The patient should also be prepared to lie flat and remain still during the scanning. The patient, or clinician, removes all objects from the hair. Some patients may experience claustrophobia from the CT scanner gantry. Those who are severely claustrophobic may require sedation 15 to 30 minutes before the scan. The most commonly used sedation is oral, intramuscular (IM), or IV diazepam (Valium) 5 to 10 mg. Although the patient will probably be alone in the CT room, he or she should be assured that the radiologic technologist is just outside the door and can see and hear the patient at all times. Communication can be maintained through a microphone from the patient to the control booth.

Patients who are acutely ill may require the presence of a clinician during the CT scan. The patient should be closely monitored for changes in vital signs, neurologic status, and airway patency. Patients with increased intracranial pressure (ICP) may experience additional problems because of the need to lie flat on the table, which further increases ICP. A hypo-osmolar agent (e.g., mannitol) can be administered before scanning to reduce the risk of herniation of the brain during the time the patient is not in the emergency department or intensive care area. A clinician should always remain with a critically ill patient, and emergency equipment for resuscitation and treatment should be close at hand.

Postprocedure Care

Following the CT scan, patients usually resume normal activities without restrictions. If a contrast scan is performed,

patients are usually encouraged to drink fluids to help the body rid itself of the contrast. Common reactions, which are not allergic, include nausea and vomiting and a sensation of heat. Patients should be monitored for signs of allergic reaction to the contrast medium, such as flushing, rash, and itching. The reported incidence is 1:40,000. Rarely, patients may experience an anaphylactic-like reaction with respiratory distress, a drop in blood pressure, and shock. However uncommon, this is a serious complication of the use of a contrast medium and can be life threatening.

Xenon Computed Tomography Quantitative Cerebral Blood Flow

Xenon computed tomography quantitative cerebral blood flow (Xe/CT/CBF) is a diagnostic technique that measures blood flow to various areas of the brain and defines the degree and extent of ischemia. The advent of perfusion CT and MR diffusion-weighted images has reduced the role Xe CT plays in the diagnosis of acute stroke. Xenon CT aids in the initial diagnosis of an acute ischemic stroke (AIS) and requires only an additional 15 minutes of time at the end of the regular CT scan. This procedure has proved to be useful in identifying and managing vasospasm, diagnosing brain death, and assessing the occlusion of major vessels in the treatment of cerebral tumors, aneurysms, and head injury.

Xenon gas is a natural component of air, is not radioactive, and after being inhaled by the patient is eliminated within 20 minutes. The gas, administered by a face mask, is safe, is odorless, and is allowed to reach levels of only 26% to 33%. Safety measures are built in, with alarms that protect the patient from inhaling unsafe levels or from becoming hypoxic. A high-speed computer with a color screen and printer displays color-coded results of 30 different areas of the brain with CBF measurements.

Patient Preparation

Adding the face mask at the end of the regular CT scan and explaining the procedure to the patient are the only additional patient instructions.[4] If the patient is unable to remain still, sedation may be necessary.

For patients undergoing outpatient CT, the individual should be informed that the procedure may take up to an hour. In addition, the individual should be accompanied by an adult who can drive and assist the patient, particularly if medication associated with the testing has been required. If the patient has diabetes mellitus (DM), the examination should be arranged so that his or her regular meal pattern and insulin administration schedules are maintained.

Postprocedure Care

After the procedure the patient should be observed closely for at least an hour for any adverse drug reaction and instability before discharge.[23] An emesis basin should be available in case the patient becomes nauseated. The patient should be instructed to increase fluid intake for the next 24 hours to help eliminate the contrast dye and to prevent dehydration.

Magnetic Resonance Imaging

Magnetic resonance imaging (MRI) gained widespread use after 1980, and its use continues to grow, with many institutions having multiple scanners. MRI does not involve any ionizing radiation. There is a magnetic field inside the bore of the magnet, with anywhere from 10,000 to 30,000 times the magnetic field of the earth.[24] The newer high-field MRI comes with software that is capable of perfusion imaging, advanced neurologic imaging packages, magnetic resonance spectroscopy, and high-strength gradients.[12] Quality images can be obtained for routine brain and spin imaging, magnetic resonance angiograms, and skull base imaging, as well as advanced applications including magnetic resonance spectroscopy, diffusion tensor imaging (DTI), and functional MRI.

MRI is the study of choice to evaluate most lesions in the brain and spine.[2] Like CT scanning, MRI uses computer technology to produce images of selected body parts. Unlike CT scanning, however, MRI relies on radiofrequency waves and a strong magnetic field rather than ionizing radiation to produce the images. MRI scans are images of hydrogen nuclei, the most abundant atom in human tissue. Hydrogen nuclei will uniformly align when placed in a powerful magnetic field.[9]

Radiofrequency waves are then introduced at right angles to the main magnetic field, producing a uniform spinning motion of hydrogen nuclei in human tissue. These nuclei are then tipped out of their previous alignment. This is referred to as **resonance.** When the radiofrequency waves are stopped, the nuclei will return to their previous alignment. This is often referred to as **relaxation time,** or the time it takes to relax back to uniform alignment. As the nuclei relax, radiofrequency signals are emitted. Each type of structure emits a different signal based on the hydrogen nuclei density and the time it takes to relax back to realignment. The MRI

computer then processes the radiofrequency signals, and high-resolution images are produced.[10]

MRI scans are often produced using two different types of imaging parameters: T1 and T2. T1 is the time it takes the proton to recover 63% of its longitudinal magnetization (spin-lattice relaxation time). T2 is the time it takes the proton to lose 63% of its transverse magnetization (spin-spin relaxation time). A **T1 image** is produced by measuring the relative proton density of the hydrogen nuclei. This is information about the water content of the structure. For example, brain edema is due to free water, which is an accumulation of hydrogen and oxygen. A T1-weighted image is used to differentiate normal structures from one another (e.g., differentiating CSF from brain tissue and gray matter from white matter). A **T2 image** is produced by measuring the relationship of the relaxation time of various hydrogen nuclei to other hydrogen nuclei. Selected tissues have different relaxation times, and even subtle differences can be picked up by MRI. A T2-weighted image is often used to identify subtle pathologic changes, such as tumors and small ischemic changes in the brain (Fig. 3-5).

Fluid attenuation inversion recovery (FLAIR) images are usually the most sensitive images for white matter pathology; they combine T1 and T2 effects and remove the effect of CSF on the image (Fig. 3-6).

Occasionally, IV contrast injection of gadolinium-chelated agents allows evaluation of the blood-brain barrier (BBB), enhancing lesions and vascular anatomy. MRI scans have made a tremendous contribution to neurologic evaluation, providing excellent details of normal anatomy not possible with other types of imaging, including CT. One of the advantages of MRI over CT is its superior contrast resolution with many tissues. Tumors, infection, edema, hemorrhage, vascular malformations, degenerative disorders, congenital disorders, and ischemic areas are just some of the types of pathologic conditions that can be imaged

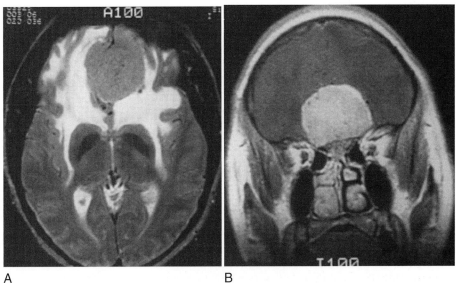

Figure 3-5 Magnetic resonance imaging: olfactory groove meningioma. **A,** Axial T2-weighted image shows a mass attached to the anterior falx (dural extension). Note relative low signal on T2WI and surrounding signal edema. **B,** Coronal T1-weighted image after contrast shows homogeneous enhancement of the dural-based extra-axial mass. *(From Goetz CG, Pappert EJ: Textbook of clinical neurology, Philadelphia, 1999, WB Saunders.)*

A   B

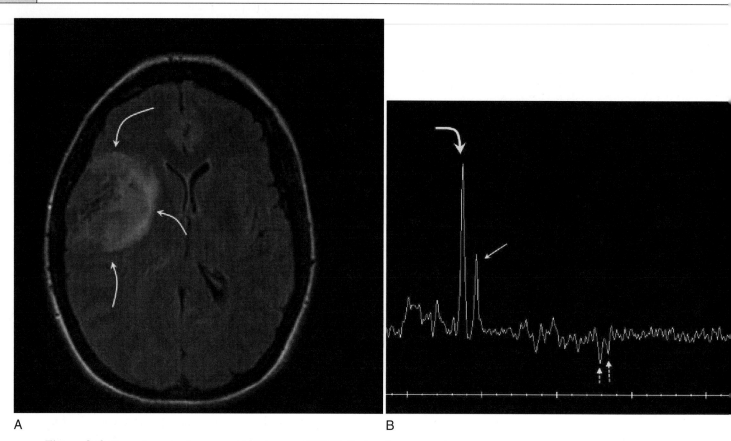

A   B

Figure 3-6 Dysembryoplastic neuroepithelial tumor (DNET) displayed on magnetic resonance spectroscopy (MRS). **A,** Axial FLAIR image shows a large right frontal mass *(curved arrows).* **B,** Graph of MRS PRESS technique marks elevation of choline peak *(curved arrow),* reduction in creatine *(straight arrow),* and lactic acid peak *(double dashed arrows);* these patterns are consistent with a high-grade neoplasm (DNET).
(Courtesy of Alberto Iaia, MD, Neuroscience Imaging, Newark, DE.)

with MRI. The advantages of CT and MRI are listed in Box 3-1.

ALERT: The Food and Drug Administration (FDA) notified radiology personnel and physicians in 2005 about the risk of serious injury or death associated with MRI in patients with implanted neurologic stimulators. The FDA advised careful review of an implant's safety labeling before MRI imaging. For questions, contact the Office of Surveillance and Biometrics (HFZ-510), 1350 Piccard Drive, Rockville, MD 20850.

Magnetic resonance (MR) diffusion-weighted imaging (DWI), or diffusion imaging, has become a valuable clinical tool in the evaluation of AIS. With its ability to detect ischemic diffusional changes earlier than CT or conventional MR signals, DWI is a valuable clinical diagnostic alternative. DWI is effective for noninvasive detection of early ischemic changes and traumatic brain injury. The sharp decline of the apparent diffusion coefficient (ADC) of water after cerebral ischemia is related to cellular swelling due to failure of ATP-dependent sodium/potassium pump at the membrane level, and it can occur as early as 2 minutes after the onset of ischemia.[5] The ADC map is actually more important than visually evaluating an area of restricted diffusion, because T2-weighted effects can falsely produce a bright area on the

BOX 3-1	Advantages of Computed Tomography and Magnetic Resonance Imaging

Computed Tomography (CT)
Can be used in patients with metal implants or fragments
Usually results in less claustrophobia than with MRI
Imaging time usually less than with MRI; good for the
  emergency/acute patient
May use nonionic or ionic contrast agents
Magnetic Resonance Imaging (MRI)
May use nonionic contrast agents
No radiation exposure
Improved differentiation between gray and white matter;
  good for white matter lesions (i.e., MS and lacunar
  infarcts)
Better views of the posterior fossa than with CT scans
  because of decreased bone artifact
Better visualization of the spinal cord, cord compression
Better visualization of acute infarction using diffusion-
  weighted imaging
Better noninvasive visualization of the arteries with MR
  angiography

MS, Multiple sclerosis.

diffusion-weighted examination. The diffusion changes may be related to the formation of cytotoxic edema as sodium and water shift from the extracellular to the intracellular compartment, leaving decreased extracellular water volume.[14]

In sharp contrast, a routine CT or MRI scan may be normal 50% to 60% of the time in the first 6 to 24 hours after the onset of stroke symptoms. If DWI is not done, the possibility of an acute cerebrovascular accident (CVA) remains, and a repeat CT or MRI scan is needed after 24 hours. DWI is now widely available, and it allows evaluation of vasospasm and neurovascular changes related to stroke immediately. DWI also shows an acute abscess as an intense increased signal from a focal collection. The advantages of early detection using DWI demonstrate reversible versus irreversible infarction that can improve patient selection for thrombolytic therapy or possibly extend the narrow "therapeutic window." The addition of a perfusion study based on the first pass of gadolinium diethylenetriaminopentaacetic acid (DTPA) contrast helps to evaluate the ischemic penumbra, which might be salvageable brain tissue after an acute infarction.

Functional MRI (fMRI) is another variant of MRI. It is a technique for imaging activity of the brain. A rapid succession of scans is taken to detect changes in oxygen consumption in the brain. Small changes in blood flow to various regions of the brain (blood oxygen level–dependent [BOLD] imaging) can identify active areas of the brain and localize important anatomic structures, such as Broca's area or the motor cortex. Such functional and anatomic information is of paramount importance during surgical planning for resection of tumors adjacent to eloquent cortex. In addition, increased activity in certain cells may help identify disease. For example, fMRI has been used to show clear distinctions in the putamen (the functioning area of the brain that controls movement) of individuals with attention-deficit/hyperactivity disorder before and after treatment with Ritalin.[8]

Intraoperative MRI in neurosurgery has increased rapidly and become more common because the surgical lesion can sometimes be seen only with MRI techniques. It is safe and has not been associated with intraoperative complications. This real-time imaging allows reliable updating of data with compensation for the brain shifting that typically occurs during tumor resection, and it significantly increases the extent of tumor removal. Images may be obtained during successive stages of a neurosurgical procedure, such as a tumor resection, arteriovenous malformations (AVMs), intracranial aneurysms, and skull base lesions. Along with the development of this new device has been the development of nonmagnetic instruments, such as retractors, aneurysm clips, microdissectors, life support systems, and the operating microscope.[21]

Intraoperative MRI is advocated to guide the surgeon to the lesion (allowing for a smaller craniotomy), to identify adjacent important structures that might be important to spare from resection, and to evaluate the postoperative appearance (intraoperatively). Real-time interventional procedures, such as cyst aspiration or needle-guided biopsy, are also possible.

All of the standard precautions for MRI apply, not only to the patient but also to the entire operating room staff, since they are all exposed to the high magnetic field. Exposure to a magnetic field has no known lasting biologic effects; it is considered safe, and there is no ionizing radiation. However, pregnant clinicians or patients should consult a physician as to whether or not an MRI study can be postponed until after the first trimester to protect the developing fetus.

A multidisciplinary Canadian group developed its own open MRI system as an intraoperative imaging system. The group used a conventional, biplanar, 0.2 Tesla (T) permanent magnet and built a fully equipped operating room suite around the magnet.[3]

Patient Preparation

Individuals undergoing outpatient MRI should be given instructions on the procedure and contraindications before the appointment to avoid cancellation of the scan. Any outpatient receiving medication must be accompanied by an adult who can drive and assist the patient after the imaging.

The primary role of the clinician in the management of patients who undergo MRI is patient education. The patient should first be assured that no ionizing radiation will be used. In some cases, however, the patient will receive an injection of a contrast medium, such as chelated salts of gadolinium, an agent that is used to enhance certain types of disease found on MRI. This contrast agent is known to cross the blood-brain barrier and enhance the imaging of many types of tumors. Approximately 10 to 15 ml of gadolinium (1 ml/5 kg) is injected intravenously, and the patient is imaged shortly thereafter.

Before the study, an assessment is performed to screen for any contraindications to MRI testing, such as the following: ferromagnetic objects in the body, aneurysm clips, cardiac pacemakers, heart valves, cardiac stent, embolization coil, medicine patches, intrauterine device (IUD), venous umbrella, artificial eye, artificial joint/prosthesis, hearing aid or other implants, spinal cord stimulator, implantable indwelling pump, shunts, tattoos, dentures or dental implant held by magnet, neurostimulators or transcutaneous electrical nerve stimulation (TENS) unit, bullets or shrapnel, surgical clips, and staples or wires. If in doubt, check with the manufacturer for specific guidelines of any implanted devices or ask if the patient has a special ID card with instructions.

In addition, the patient should be warned to remove items that may be rendered inoperable by the magnet, such as credit cards, tape recordings, and watches.

Box 3-2 lists many of the contraindications to MRI. The clinician should openly discuss the possibility of claustrophobia with the patient. In many centers videotapes of the MRI unit and the patient's responsibilities are used for teaching before the examination. Some patients may require sedation to combat the effects of claustrophobia, though open MRI imaging units are more becoming widely available. Chloral hydrate and diazepam (Valium) have been the most commonly used drugs. Patients should also be reminded that they will be required to remain still for 30 minutes to 1 hour while the scan is being performed, because motion produces artifact and interferes with image integrity. In addition, patients should be told that during imaging they will hear a

BOX 3-2	Magnetic Resonance Imaging Contraindications*

- Most known foreign bodies (e.g., metallic splinters or fragments) are safe if more than 6 weeks has elapsed so that fibrosis has occurred and as long as they are not in the eye or brain or close to the spinal cord.
- Metal prostheses/joint replacements are all safe; they are fixed in bone and will not move in the magnetic field. Interestingly, surgical stainless steel is nonmagnetic.
- Ferrous (iron) implants (e.g., aneurysm clips, intracranial, aortic) are generally contraindicated. A recent study showed that some nonferromagnetic clips display deflection in a magnetic field and therefore there is a small chance of unforeseen consequences when aneurysm clips are imaged. Generally, preoperative testing of the clips is required to make certain that they are safe for later MRI scans.
- Pacemakers and the epicardial pacemaker wires are unsafe for imaging. Because an electrical field can be produced in the varying magnetic and radiofrequency fields during MRI scans, the pacer wires can actually pace the heart during an MRI scan at rates similar to ventricular tachycardia. The pacemakers can also be deactivated or reprogrammed by the magnetic field.
- Metal heart valves are generally safe. If the patient has a very early Star Edwards valve series 1000 or less, the radiologist should be informed. Most intravascular stents are also safe.
- Intrauterine devices are safe.
- Intraventricular shunts are safe.
- Fractures treated with metal rods, pins, screws, and nails are safe. The rods are fixed into bones and therefore will not move during the scan.
- Harrington rods, although safe, may cause significant artifacts. Unfortunately, similar artifacts are also produced with CT imaging.

- In the case of shrapnel, which may be composed of various metals, the location and size are more important than trying to determine what type of metal is present. In general, as long as the shrapnel is not near the spine or in the orbits, it is likely to be safe as long as 4 to 6 weeks has elapsed for the body to form surrounding fibrosis. If the fragment is particularly large, the force exerted on the metal fragment is also proportionally large. When a patient with known shrapnel walks toward the magnetic field, he or she will slowly experience increasing force on the shrapnel. It is recommended that if the patient experiences pain or discomfort, the examination should not be performed.
- Vasectomy and fallopian tube clips are safe.
- Penile prostheses are generally unsafe because the spring valves are highly magnetic. The springs may become dislodged and the prosthesis unusable. MRI imaging is generally not recommended for these patients.
- Cochlear implants are generally unsafe because they are a neurostimulator that may be electrically stimulated by the pulse sequence and alternating radiofrequency and magnetic fields.
- Implanted pumps (insulin, opioid, or baclofen infusion devices) that may cause interference are contraindicated.
- Transcutaneous nerve stimulators are also not recommended because direct stimulation may occur as a result of the scan sequence.
- Spinal cord stimulators are contraindications.
- Elective scanning is generally not recommended during pregnancy, but it is possible to perform the scan if the study is medically indicated.

*NOTE: Depending on the part of the body being scanned, some of these items may not be contraindicated.
CT, Computed tomography; *MRI*, magnetic resonance imaging.

loud knocking sound. Earplugs may dull the noise, though some patients experience a headache because of this loud, repetitive sound.

For a head scan, the patient's head is placed in a head coil much like a helmet. The patient is positioned on the table, and the top of the head coil is pulled down over the patient's face. There is a large opening in the top of the coil for the face. Once the patient is inside the bore of the magnet, mirrors may be positioned on the unit so that the patient can see out the bottom of the magnet. This visual orientation is often helpful in reducing the effects of claustrophobia.

Patients undergoing a lumbar spine MRI are often placed feet first in the bore of the magnet with a surface coil on the area to be imaged. In such a situation, mirrors cannot be used, and patients frequently report increased claustrophobia. Regardless of which position they are in, patients can communicate through microphones and speakers with the radiologic technologist performing the scan. The use of television video glasses has also reduced the incidence of claustrophobia.

There are no dietary restrictions before an MRI. Before transporting the patient for an MRI, the clinician should be aware of any contraindications the patient may have that would interfere with the scan. In addition, the clinician should check for the following patient restrictions before scanning:

- Weight more than 300 pounds (check with technologists about the weight limit of the particular system, because some systems have a weight limit of 450 pounds)
- No jewelry, including hair clips, earrings, or bobby pins
- Body piercing(s) (these are discouraged but may not be a contraindication to the study)
- No sandbags that may contain metal filings used to stabilize the patient's head
- Permanent tattoo dyes sometimes contain iron

Not only can these items cause artifact on a scan, but also they can be pulled into the bore of the magnet, creating a projectile. Some institutions also require that an individual who has worked with metal have an x-ray of both eye orbits to rule out the presence of any small metal fragments in the eyes before MRI.

> **ALERT:** Metal objects can act as deadly projectiles in the MRI suite. News reports in July 2001 chronicled the death of a 6-year-old boy undergoing a postsurgical MRI following a brain tumor resection. The boy had received IV sedation and was receiving oxygen via a flowmeter from a wall unit when the anesthesiologist noticed that the oxygen was not flowing. When someone tried to pass a 6-pound oxygen ferrous cylinder, it flew into the bore of the magnet, crushing the child's skull. The child died from blunt trauma and a skull fracture 2 days later (see www.wcmc.com for a full incident review).

Because of the increase in the use of MRI scanners over the past several years, many types of equipment required for patient care are now made of nonferromagnetic material and can be used in the magnet room. Examples include specially designed ventilators and IV pumps. As a result, many more critically ill, unstable patients are being imaged with MRI. The clinician may be asked to stay with a patient while the MRI is being performed. There is no ionizing radiation and no known contraindication to remaining with a patient during the scan. Patients should be monitored closely for changes in neurologic status and vital signs. Some of the newer scanners allow patients to be connected to cardiac and respiratory monitors while in the scanner. Patients who have temporal lobe epilepsy may be at risk for developing seizure activity secondary to the repetitive auditory stimuli of the knocking sound and should be closely monitored for this possibility.

Postprocedure Care

There are no dietary or activity restrictions after an MRI. New computer software systems have greatly reduced imaging time as well, allowing a single sequence to be performed in 2 to 4 minutes. Generally, a complete set includes four to six different sequences, with additional time necessary only if the patient is to be scanned a second time after injection of gadolinium. Patients who receive sedative drugs or who have a history of asthma and receive contrast agent must be monitored during the MRI. There are pulse oximeters made especially for use in the MRI chamber.[24]

Open Magnetic Resonance Imaging

Hundreds of sites throughout the United States are now providing **open MRI.** The newer, open MRI machines have open sides with large magnets that are generally suspended 2 feet above the patient. These machines are less claustrophobic and quieter. The unit can accommodate patients weighing more than 300 pounds and is a welcome alternative for the 15% of patients who refuse an MRI procedure because of claustrophobia. Younger patients may be allowed to have a parent present. The child can see, touch, and talk to his or her parent during the examination, which helps keep the child calm.

For spine imaging, patients can see what is going on around them, and there is no sense of being trapped in a confined space. When the head or neck is being imaged, patients must be placed in the gap, and the open configura-

tion is not as helpful, since the head must face a wall only a few inches away. Field strengths generally are in the 0.2 to 0.3 T range, although higher-strength units have been introduced recently, up to 1 T. Closed MRI machines have higher-field magnets that are about four times the strength of open MRI magnets and scan faster. They also allow higher resolution and signal-to-noise ratio. Overall, the clinical utility of closed units remains significantly greater than that of open MRIs. In particular, visualization of subtle cord lesions and MR angiography remain grave handicaps of the open MRI systems. Thus, unless there are contraindications to a closed MRI study (claustrophobia or severe obesity), it is best to image the patient in a closed configuration system.

Blood Oxygen Level–Dependent Imaging

Instead of MRI images of brain anatomy, **blood oxygen level–dependent (BOLD) imaging** actually shows the precise location of increased neuronal activity in the human brain. Most important for researchers, the test is noninvasive, unlike the positron emission tomography (PET) scan, which can also image brain activity. BOLD imaging detects increases in blood flow to active areas in the brain by looking for pockets of highly oxygenated blood that may pinpoint, for example, areas of higher cognitive function, as well as disorders such as seizure activities. Localization of the motor cortex is accomplished by asking the patient to perform a finger tapping exercise during MR imaging; visual cortex and speech cortex localization can be obtained in similar fashion, employing paradigms that are specific for stimulation of such neurologic activity.

Magnetic Resonance Spectroscopy

Magnetic resonance spectroscopy (MRS) is a new technique that uses spectroscopy in combination with MRI. With conventional MRI it is often difficult to distinguish benign from malignant tissue or to identify areas of ischemia. Tissue metabolism in these different types of pathologic conditions varies greatly. MRS provides the opportunity to detect changes in tissue metabolism and to characterize the disease by its unique metabolic pattern.

There are several types of MRS, including phosphorous MRS and proton spectroscopy. Phosphorous MRS measures high-energy phosphates and adenosine triphosphate (ATP). The pH can also be calculated from phosphorous MRS. Pathologic processes, such as hypoxia and ischemia, are known to deplete ATP concentrations and inhibit cellular function, and such changes can be imaged using this technology.

The most commonly used MRS sequence is proton MR spectroscopy, which allows accurate determination of the nature of the lesion; namely, lesions greater than 1.5 cm in size can be categorized as being neoplastic or inflammatory in nature. In the presence of neoplasia, the clinician can often establish if the lesion is of low or high grade, based on its spectroscopic pattern (see Fig. 3-6).

MRS has also become very useful in distinguishing between the various types of dementias (human immunodeficiency virus [HIV] vs. Alzheimer's disease) and for diagnosis of hepatic encephalopathy. In children with white and gray matter disease, it is very effective in confirming the presence of mitochondrial disorders or other inborn errors of metabolism. Finally, the presence of lactic acid in the parahippocampal gyrus of children with seizure disorders has been shown to predict development of mesial temporal sclerosis.

MRS is performed by first producing an MRI image and then identifying a specific voxel (location) that the clinician is interested in. Spectroscopic imaging is then performed, which takes about 10 minutes. There is great promise for the future of MRS as clinical applications continue to increase. This is basically a noninvasive brain biopsy. It has no side effects and can provide additional information before treatment. Clinical management is the same as that for conventional MRI.

Diffusion Tensor Imaging

Echo planar imaging has been used for evaluation of the diffusion of water in the form of diffusion-weighted imaging (DWI), as a technique that allows detection of early infarct, vide supra. A newer application of diffusion studies is **diffusion tensor imaging (DTI)**, a technique that looks at directionality and strength (vector) of diffusion restriction, known as eigenvalues (or eigenvectors).

White matter tracts have known directionality and, as such, limit the random motion of unbound water in the direction of the white matter tract. Using sophisticated software, DTI allows the radiologist to image white matter bundles that have similar eigenvectors, thus grouping the fibers that share a direction and are part of a known connecting fascicle. Such technology is used for anatomic depiction of fibers that, until recently, could only be identified with myelin staining. More important, it allows visualization of the relationship of a mass to known fiber tracts. For example, the clinician is able to determine if a tumor has invaded a white matter tract or if it has simply displaced it (Fig. 3-7). A mass in the left insular region may involve the arcuate fasciculus, the white matter tract that connects Broca's and Wernicke's areas. If the mass has invaded the white matter tract, the patient will have conductive aphasia, and surgical resection is not likely to restore the neurologic deficit. DTI may show that the tumor has simply displaced the arcuate fasciculus, thus indicating that resection of the tumor is likely to successfully treat the patient's aphasia.

Patient Preparation and Postprocedure Care

Patient preparation and postprocedure care for this examination are the same as those for routine MRI; the sequence is acquired in approximately 8 minutes.

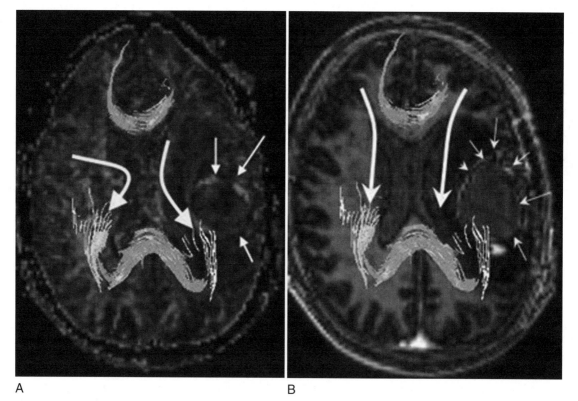

A   B

Figure 3-7 Diffusion tensor imaging (DTI) of a 65-year-old woman with left frontal glioma. **A,** Tractography, utilizing DTI, demonstrates a left posterior frontal mass *(straight arrows)* causing abrupt termination of white matter tracts along its postmedial aspect *(curved arrows)*. Interruption of white matter fibers and reduction of anisotropy suggests invasion of white matter tracts, rather than displacement. **B,** Anatomic data set reveals the interrupted fibers in posterior left frontal lobe, due to the enhancing mass *(small arrows)*; intact fibers are present in the posterior right frontal white matter *(curved arrows)*.
(Courtesy of Alberto Iaia, MD, Neuroscience Imaging, Newark, DE.)

Superconducting Quantum Interference Device

Research with a 100-channel **superconducting quantum interference device (SQUID)** to measure fluctuations in neuronal magnetic fields may hold promise for new levels of understanding of both healthy and injured brains. The device is used to enhance three-dimensional images of the brain constructed from MRI slices. SQUID can simultaneously monitor brain activity from several different sites, correlating disruptions caused by brain damage with abnormal patterns traced by the device.[1]

Magnetoencephalographic Mapping

Magnetoencephalographic (MEG) mapping is a completely noninvasive method of functional brain imaging that is akin to quantitative electroencephalography and complementary to other functional imaging methods, such as functional MRI or PET scanning. MEG mapping consists of recording, on the surface of the head, the magnetic flux associated with electrical currents in activated sets of neurons, estimating the location of such sets, and projecting them onto structural images of the brain, such as MRI images.[17] This technique allows for identification and visualization of the receptive language cortex in patients who have a brain tumor or epilepsy in the language-dominant hemisphere. In research studies these tests have been shown to concur with Wada's test in assessing hemispheric dominance for language.[20]

Magnetic Source Imaging

Magnetic source imaging (MSI) is a new technology that measures electrical activity in the brain and produces images that can identify the location of this activity. Both normal and abnormal electrical activity can be measured. On MSI images the electrical activity is indicated by small white dots. MSI uses a very weak magnetic field, in contrast to the strong fields used in MRI. The magnetic waves measure only electrical activity, not tissue and bone, so that clear images can be produced.

Patients undergoing MSI are first demagnetized to remove residual magnetism from their bodies. They are then secured on a special couch, which keeps them relatively still. Next, a wand is moved over the surface of the patient's head to produce a computer image of the skull. Stimulators are then placed on the lips and fingers of the patient. As these stimulators are activated, messages are sent to the brain and the MSI sensor records the electrical activity. Electrical brain activity is presented as small circles, with tiny white dots indicating the center of activity. MSI is currently being used for diagnosing migraine. As MSI technology improves and MSI images can be superimposed on MRI, the future possibilities of this technology seem endless.

ANGIOGRAPHY

Magnetic Resonance Angiography

Magnetic resonance angiography (MRA)—as well as **magnetic resonance venography (MRV)**—is used to study the flow in various vessels for vascular diseases. MRA techniques were introduced in 1990. The motion of blood flow in the presence of a radiofrequency pulse creates specific effects on the radiofrequency signals being emitted by moving protons. These effects can be manipulated to create vascular contrast on the MRI image. In general, the studies can be made to be sensitive to flow in a certain direction or in multiple directions. MRA is fast, but overlying tissue may obscure the underlying vessel. By using computers to remove the overlying and bright tissues, the technician can create a more accurate and sensitive MRA study.

Two-dimensional time-of-flight (2DTOF) techniques are based on gradient-echo (GRE) sequences and may overestimate the degree of stenosis; therefore correlation with three-dimensional time-of-flight (3DTOF) techniques or ultrasound may be needed to establish the real degree of stenosis. Some centers recommend contrast studies for carotid and neck imaging, but this is still not standard practice. With higher-field magnetic strengths and stronger gradients, the resolution is now approaching 0.5 mm and small-vessel detail is improving. Interventional MRA techniques are also being studied with MR fluoroscopy and image-guided catheters.

Patient Selection

Clinical applications seem to be the greatest for evaluation of carotid bifurcation and any atherosclerotic disease. Intracranial applications for MRA include large-vessel atherosclerotic disease, arteriovenous malformations (AVMs), and intracranial aneurysms without acute subarachnoid hemorrhage. This noninvasive method of angiography holds promise for the future as more sensitive head coils, stronger gradients, and sophisticated software are developed. Because of its noninvasive nature, it is quickly gaining popularity. However, it is not a study of the arteries alone.

Newer methods of three-dimensional contrast-enhanced MRA with subtraction techniques promise to extend the evaluation capacity of MRA to all vessels. Peripheral angiography is possible with specialized software and runoff studies, and aortograms can be routinely performed. This method is less invasive than digital subtraction angiography (DSA), and the gadolinium DTPA contrast used is less nephrotoxic. It is also less expensive and faster than a DSA study.

Patient Preparation and Postprocedure Care

Preparation and teaching is the same as with all MRI procedures and myelogram. The scan is painless, and there is little risk of complications. Contrast media can, of course, produce allergic reactions in some people.

Care is the same as with all MRI procedures, and most people can resume their normal activities following the examination.

Digital Venous Angiography

Digital venous angiography (DVA) is a computer-enhanced fluoroscopic technique used to visualize the arteries, most frequently the carotid and larger cerebral arteries. It is also referred to as digital vascular imaging (DVI). The technique is rarely used today, as the degree of detail it affords is much less than that of conventional angiography or CT angiography. It is much less invasive and has far fewer risks than cerebral angiography and therefore it was once used as part of an initial vascular evaluation. The IV DVA technique was limited, however, in that the low arterial iodine concentration resulted in low subject contrast because of natural dilution.[8]

The technique began with an initial image called a "mask," which was processed by the computer. The patient was then injected with radiographic contrast material. Following the injection, further images were taken. The computer then superimposed the contrast image on top of the mask image, and all similar structures, such as bone, were digitally subtracted. This process allowed visualization of only the vessels that were enhanced by contrast medium.

Patient Preparation

The role of the clinician is one of patient education and preparation. Patients should be assessed for allergies to iodine-based dye and for anticoagulants. An informed consent is required. Patients are asked to lie completely still during imaging. They may be asked to hold their breath at times. Swallowing and other minor movements can distort the images. Patients may experience a warm or hot, flushed feeling when the dye is injected. They should be told that this is to be expected and will pass within a few minutes. Usually patients are kept on nothing-by-mouth (NPO) status for several hours before the test or may be allowed clear liquids.

Patients are asked to lie on the x-ray table. An IV catheter may be placed in a peripheral or central vein. As the dye is injected, the area of interest is monitored with fluoroscopy and images are stored in the computer. After the dye is injected, the catheter is removed and a pressure dressing is applied to the site. Manual compression is generally superior to a pressure dressing. Manual compression of the venous site for 10 minutes after the procedure and for 15 to 20 minutes if the patient is anticoagulated is recommended. This procedure usually lasts 60 to 120 minutes.

Postprocedure Care

After the procedure the clinician must assess the patient's vital and neurologic status as ordered or every 15 minutes until the patient is stable. The site should be checked frequently for signs of bleeding or infection (over time). An ice pack may be ordered to combat local swelling. Fluids should be encouraged to assist the patient's kidneys with the excretion of the dye. The patient should be observed for a delayed reaction to the dye, which can occur 2 to 6 hours after the test. This is manifested by itching, rashes, hives, and dyspnea. The patient can resume normal activity 6 to 8 hours after the procedure. This test is often performed on an outpatient basis, so the family must be taught what to assess and to report any complications.

Cerebral Angiography

Cerebral angiography (digital subtraction angiography [DSA]) is an invasive radiographic technique used to evaluate cerebral vasculature. Because it is a direct intraarterial injection, it can provide information about the lumen of the vessels, vessel size, and the dynamic passage of contrast material, as in aneurysms, AVMs, AVFs, or occlusion (Fig. 3-8). It is often used to evaluate occlusive vascular disease in the carotid circulation. DSA can also be used to identify central nervous system (CNS) tumors, aneurysms, AVMs, and other vascular malformations. The technique has also been used postoperatively to evaluate the effectiveness of surgical vascular interventions. Vascular tumors can also be identified with the use of angiography. The volume of angiography has diminished as a result of noninvasive imaging techniques with MRA, MRV, and CT angiography. However, new interventional neuroradiologic procedures to embolize tumors or AVMs before surgery or to treat aneurysms or fistulas with balloons or coils deployed during angiography have been increasing in frequency.

Cerebral angiography may also be used intraoperatively and postoperatively to assess the effectiveness of vascular surgery, such as clipping feeding vessels of an AVM. Angiography remains the gold standard in the evaluation of cerebral aneurysms and AVMs and is considered to be the most accurate study in the evaluation of carotid artery stenosis.[10]

Patient Preparation

The role of the clinician in the management of the patient undergoing cerebral angiography is one of patient education, preparation, and intensive monitoring. The patient should be assessed for any bleeding disorders and for a history of allergy to iodine-based dye. The patient should be asked about any recent use of aspirin or anticoagulants. An informed consent is necessary. The entire procedure should be explained to the patient. Some patients may have heard stories about persons who have had bad experiences with angiograms. Such patients need to have their fears allayed. The patient is often kept on NPO status after midnight the night before the test; however, some patients may need to be well hydrated before the test to facilitate dye dilution and renal excretion. If the test is to be performed late in the day, the patient may be allowed clear liquids in the morning.

A complete baseline neurologic evaluation should be documented before and after the procedure. Peripheral pulses are also assessed and marked to facilitate later assessment. Pedal and radial pulses are marked. Dental prostheses are also removed. The patient is usually prepared with sedation (e.g., diazepam [Valium]) before being taken to the radiology area. Once in the radiology department, the patient is positioned supine on the x-ray table.

The most common site of catheter insertion is the femoral artery. The area is shaved and prepared with iodine and then draped with sterile drapes. An injection of local anesthetic is given, which produces local stinging. Once the area is

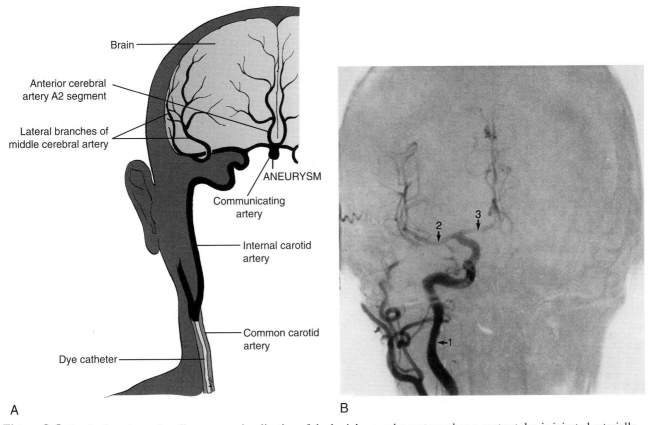

Figure 3-8 Cerebral angiography allows x-ray visualization of the brain's vascular system when a contrast dye is injected arterially. **A,** Insertion of dye through a catheter in the common carotid artery, subsequently outlining vessels of the brain. **B,** An angiogram using the subtraction technique. *1,* Internal carotid artery. *2,* Middle cerebral artery. *3,* Anterior cerebral artery A1 segment. *(From Black JM, Hawks JH:* Medical-surgical nursing: clinical management for positive outcomes, *ed 7, St Louis, 2005, WB Saunders.)*

anesthetized, the catheter is inserted into the femoral artery and passed up to the desired artery. The passage of the catheter with a radiopaque marking is followed with the use of fluoroscopy. Radiopaque contrast material is then injected. Patients usually experience an intense, hot, flushed feeling in the neck, face, and head. Rarely, a patient may describe it as feeling as though his or her head were about to explode; this is more often seen with direct vertebral artery injections. The patient should be told that this feeling is to be expected and will pass within minutes. It will, however, recur with each subsequent injection if more than one vessel is to be studied. Once the dye is injected, a series of radiographs is taken to follow the flow of the contrast through the vessels. After all injections, the catheter is removed, direct pressure is applied for 15 minutes or longer, and a dressing is applied. The procedure usually lasts 60 to 120 minutes, depending on the number of vessels to be imaged (one to four).

Postprocedure Care

The patient may be asked to flex his or her toes and feet following the procedure for a quick check for neurologic deficits.

The patient is then returned to the nursing unit. Vital signs and neurologic status, including peripheral pulse evaluation,

must be assessed as ordered or every 15 minutes for 1 hour or until the patient is stable, and every hour until a 12-hour period is complete and no complications have been detected. The patient should be encouraged to increase fluids after the test to help the kidneys clear the dye. A significant amount of dye is used in cerebral angiography and can create problems for patients with preexisting kidney problems or those who have received multiple tests using contrast material. Ice packs applied to the catheter site help reduce local edema. The site should be checked for signs of bleeding, hematoma, or infection (over time). The affected leg is assessed for coldness, cyanosis, pallor, numbness, and size as compared with the unaffected side. The extremity is usually immobilized for 6 to 8 hours after the test. The patient may be kept on complete bed rest for the remainder of the day. It is important to remind the patient to keep the extremity extended to prevent damage at the puncture site and to report any bleeding from the site. The patient should be observed for a delayed reaction to the dye, including itching, rashes, hives, or dyspnea.

Possible complications of angiography include hemorrhage from the puncture site, vasospasm or dissection secondary to catheter insertion, infection at the catheter site, and embolism secondary to trauma to the inside of the vessel wall during the procedure.[8] Atherosclerotic plaque may also become dislodged and embolized, resulting in a possible transient ischemic attack (TIA) or stroke. This procedure is still considered the gold standard in the evaluation of AVMs and AVFs because it is the only procedure that allows analysis of the dynamics of blood flow; hence, early filling of a venous structure, as seen in an AVM, can only be established by this technique. MRAs and CTAs can only provide a static image of the vascular anatomy, without the benefits of flow dynamics.

MYELOGRAPHY

Myelography is a diagnostic procedure using a lumbar puncture with injection of contrast medium into the spinal canal, and x-ray imaging (Fig. 3-9, *A* and *B*). The procedure allows for visualization of the lumbar, thoracic, or cervical thecal sac. Indications for the procedure include evaluation of herniated intervertebral disks, spinal stenosis, and congenital anomalies. Myelography is not used as commonly as in the past because MRI has become the technique of choice for evaluating the spine.[24] With the introduction of nonionic contrast agents, myelography has become a safer examination.

ALERT: Myelography should not be performed on patients with multiple sclerosis (MS), inflammation of the meninges, Pott's disease, or infections, or on patients with suspected bloody subarachnoid fluid or increased ICP.[24]

Patient Preparation

The role of the clinician is one of education and patient preparation to explain the procedure and to assess for allergies to any medicine, contrast dye, iodine, shellfish, or seafood. Report if the patient is pregnant or believes that she may be pregnant before the examination. An informed

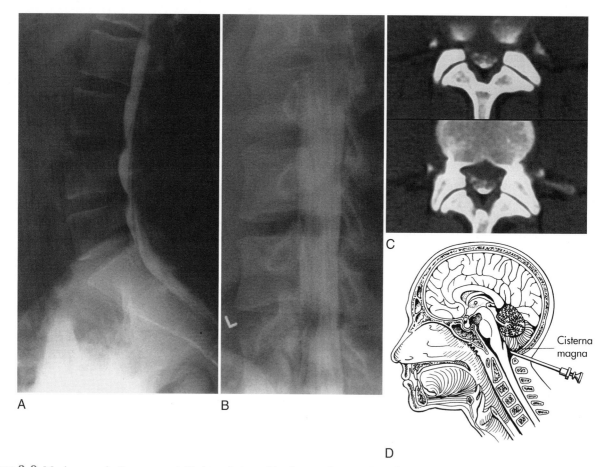

Figure 3-9 Myelogram. **A,** Prone cross-table lateral view of lumbar myelogram. Prominent ventral impressions on the contrast column are present at L3–4 and L4–5. Much milder ventral impressions are seen at L2–3 and L5–S1. A so-called double-density sign consistent with an eccentric posterior disk herniation is present at L3–4 and L4–5. **B,** Prone left anterior oblique view of lumbar myelogram. Left-sided filling defects are present at L3–4 and L4–5 secondary to eccentric posterior disk herniations at both levels. **C,** Axial computed tomography scans at and just below L3–4 disk space demonstrate moderately sized, broad-based central and left-sided posterior disk herniation extending into left lateral recess. This eccentric posterior disk herniation would account for the double-density sign seen in **(A). D,** Cisternal puncture.
(A–C, From Goetz CG, Pappert EJ: Textbook of clinical neurology, Philadelphia, 1999, WB Saunders. D, From Long BC, Phipps WJ: Medical-surgical nursing: a nursing process approach, ed 3, St Louis, 1993, Mosby.)

consent is usually required. Instructions to the patient may include the following guidelines before imaging:

- Increase clear fluid intake (nonalcoholic 24 hours before the examination) 4 hours before the myelogram; clear liquids may be given on the morning of the examination (e.g., coffee, tea, or juice).
- Omit solid food 4 hours before the examination so that the patient is well hydrated but will not become nauseated because of food in the stomach.
- Restrict food; restrictions may vary depending on the contrast agent used.
- Empty the bladder and bowels before the myelogram.
- Stop taking certain medications (per the physician's orders) before the myelogram: stop antiinflammatory medications the day of the examination; stop taking blood-thinning medications (Coumadin, Persantine, or aspirin); omit particularly drugs that may enhance the possibility of seizure activity (e.g., phenothiazines, tricyclic antidepressants, CNS stimulants, and amphetamines); check if monoamine oxidase inhibitors have to be discontinued 2 weeks before myelogram; stop muscle relaxants, depression medications, sleeping aids, antihistamines, or any medication for psychiatric treatment.

Special considerations include the following:

- Patients with diabetes mellitus (DM) who take metformin (Glucophage, Riomet, Glucovance, Avandamet, or Metaglip) must stop taking the medication 48 hours before the procedure. They must contact their health care provider and let him or her know that this medication must be stopped and have the health care provider prescribe an alternative medication to be taken during this period. The neuroradiologist must know what medication is going to be taken for replacement. Instructions must be provided by the clinician on how to prevent a hyperglycemic or hypoglycemic reaction before and after the procedure.
- In some institutions patients will have an IV started before the procedure to provide hydration and decrease postmyelogram headache.
- Patients prone to seizures may not be candidates for the procedure.
- Patients should be informed about where the procedure will be performed—in a radiology department or an outpatient imaging center.

The procedure is similar to a lumbar puncture (LP). The patient is prepared in the same manner as for a conventional LP, and the spinal needle is inserted into the lower lumbar area. The LP is frequently done under fluoroscopic control. The opening pressure may or may not be read. Approximately 5 to 10 mm of CSF may be removed, and the contrast medium is then instilled. Water-based contrast media, such as metrizamide (Amipaque), iohexol (Omnipaque), and iopamidol (Isovue), have replaced the use of oil-based contrast material, such as Pantopaque. Water-based contrast material is absorbed into the CSF fairly quickly and does not have to be removed. Water-based contrast material is also preferred because it flows more freely through narrow canals. This can help significantly if the clinician needs to differentiate between complete and partial blockage of the spinal canal. Oil-based contrast material, now no longer used, was associated with higher complication rates, and it required that patients be moved and tilted so that all of the contrast material could be removed at the end of the procedure. Residual oil-based contrast material often caused headaches, meningeal irritation, and possibly arachnoid adhesions.

Once the contrast material is injected, it is allowed to flow up to the area to be examined, and radiographic images are then taken to view the spinal sac, spinal cord, conus medullaris, and nerve roots. The patient may be tilted on a tilt table to allow the contrast to circulate. Patients are secured to the table to prevent sliding. Tilting may produce nausea, vomiting, dizziness, or vasovagal reactions. After the myelogram is completed, the needle is removed, pressure is applied for several minutes, and a dressing is applied. The patient is always examined with CT (Fig. 3-9, C) following myelography. Ideally, MDT CT is used, in order to acquire multiplanar reconstruction images. The need for myelography has diminished with the increased availability of MRI.

Postprocedure Care

Postprocedure care is similar to that for a conventional LP. Patients may experience possible complications, including nausea, vomiting, and headache, as a result of use of the dye. Some patients experience an increase in neck, back, or leg pain. Dizziness may also occur. If water-based dye is used, the patient should be encouraged to increase fluids to help remove the dye from the system. The head of the bed is elevated at about 45 degrees for 6 to 8 hours to prevent upward diffusion of the dye. Patients are encouraged to continue bed rest for approximately 12 hours. No alcoholic beverages should be consumed for at least 24 hours after the myelogram. No strenuous activity should be performed for 1 to 2 days after the procedure. Rarely, meningeal irritation with headache and possible seizures can result. Complications are similar to those for a conventional LP. The patient's vital signs and neurologic status should be monitored frequently or as ordered until the patient is stable. Delayed reactions to contrast media include dyspnea, tachycardia, rashes, and hives. These are usually easily treated with antihistamines.

In some cases myelography is performed via a cisternal puncture (Fig. 3-9, D). Patient management is similar to that for a cisternal puncture.

CISTERNAL PUNCTURE

A tap of the cisterns may be performed (1) if an LP cannot be performed because of a deformity or local infection or (2) to introduce a contrast medium, air, or carbon dioxide for myelography. Air cisternograms may be done in patients with severe contrast allergy when myelograms are needed. A cisternal puncture may be performed simultaneously with an LP to demonstrate a subarachnoid block. However, since the development of CT and MRI, the number of cisternal punctures being performed has significantly declined.

For a cisternal puncture, the patient is positioned on the side with pillows to align the head and spine. The chin is tucked down to the chest. The clinician may be asked to help the patient maintain this posture. Movement during the procedure can be very dangerous—even fatal—if there is significant injury to the medulla. The occipital area is shaved and prepared with an antiseptic solution, and the patient is draped. Several injections of a local anesthetic are given to numb the area. A short, beveled needle is inserted into the cisterna magna, immediately below the occipital bone (see Fig. 3-9, *D*). Once the needle is in place, the obturator is removed and the opening pressure is read with a manometer. CSF is then allowed to drip out of the needle to fill three to five small sterile vials. Closing pressure may be read with a manometer, and the needle is then removed. Manual pressure is applied to the puncture site for several minutes, and the area is covered with an adhesive bandage strip or sterile dressing. The entire procedure usually lasts 20 to 45 minutes.

CISTERNOGRAPHY

Cisternography can be preformed in three distinct ways. Cisternograms are performed in the radiology department with iodinated contrast, whereas radioisotope cisternography is performed in nuclear medicine department with radionuclide agents, vide infra. The third approach to cisternography is MRI cisternography.

Cisternogram

Cisternograms are performed by injecting iodinated contrast material into the subarachnoid space via a lumbar puncture, followed by head CT scan. **Cisternograms** are beneficial for evaluation of the patency of the CSF pathways. Because only a small amount of CSF normally enters the ventricles, flow of contrast material into the ventricles is minimal if the pathways are not constricted or blocked. This procedure is most useful in differentiating a mega cisterna magna from an arachnoid cyst. In the latter scenario, the contrast material injected does not immediately fill the cyst as it is separated by the subarachnoid space by a split layer of arachnoid membrane. With a mega cisterna magna, there is immediate opacification of the cistern on placement of contrast in the subarachnoid space.

Patient Preparation
Before the procedure an LP is performed. Then the iodinated contrast material is injected into the lumbar subarachnoid space; a head CT is performed immediately after the LP.

Postprocedure Care
After the procedure the patient is instructed to lie flat in the CT scanner. This test is contraindicated in patients who (1) have a deformity at the lumbar puncture site; (2) have an infection at the lumbar puncture site; (3) are pregnant; or (4) have increased ICP.

The patient should be reassured that the contrast material is usually excreted from the body within 24 hours. Drinking fluids will help expel the contrast. The injection site should be observed for redness and swelling. The patient should be kept with the bed flat for 2 to 4 hours to prevent an after-tap headache. Abnormal findings include cerebral neoplasm blocking the flow of CSF, pseudomeningoceles, mega cisterna magna, and arachnoid cyst.

Radioisotope Cisternography

Radioisotope cisternography may be performed with a lumbar puncture and, rarely, with a direct cisternal puncture. In this procedure, once the needle is in place, a radioisotope is instilled into the CSF. The isotope circulates, and scans are taken at regular intervals, such as 6, 12, 24, 48, and 72 hours after the injection. This is done to determine the path the isotope takes to clear the system. Cisternography may be performed to assess for hydrocephalus, CSF blockage, shunt patency, or CSF leakage. If, however, blocks in the CSF pathways prevent this reabsorption, some of the isotope may appear in the ventricles; in the setting of normal pressure hydrocephalus (NPH), for instance, there is abnormal CSF flow dynamics, causing radioisotope migration into the lateral ventricles, a finding that can confirm the diagnosis of NPH, in the correct clinical context. Cisternal scans may also be helpful in determining CSF leakage in patients with recurring meningitis or CSF rhinorrhea.

Patient Preparation
In addition to physical management during the tap, the clinician's primary role is one of education. If a lumbar puncture cannot be performed, a direct cisternal approach can be very frightening to most patients. The patient should be informed about the procedure, including what is expected of the patient and potential complications.

Following injection of the radionuclide agent, the patient is sent back to his or her room and asked to drink plenty of fluids. The patient is returned to the nuclear medicine department on serial times (vide supra) and placed supine; a radioactive counter is placed over the patient's head. These scans take approximately 45 minutes.

Postprocedure Care
Following the procedure, the patient should be kept with the bed flat for 2 to 4 hours to prevent an after-tap headache. If a direct cisternal approach was taken, the clinician must closely monitor the patient's vital signs and assess respiratory changes, which may indicate injury to the medulla. These respiratory changes may include respiratory distress and Cheyne-Stokes respirations. The patient's vital signs and neurologic status should be assessed as ordered or frequently, every 15 to 30 minutes, until the patient is stable. The puncture site should also be assessed for leakage or infection. The patient should be encouraged to increase fluid intake to help the body replace CSF.

Magnetic Resonance Cisternography

Magnetic resonance (MR) cisternography has been performed with a heavily T2-weighted two-dimensional fast spin-echo (FSE) technique. One such sequence is constructive interference in the steady state (CISS); this technique has provided detailed information about the topography of cranial nerves, blood vessels, and fine structural components to describe valuable landmarks with great accuracy. Phase-contrast flow-sensitive imaging allows for cine-phase imaging of the CSF surrounding the spinal cord. This is useful in patients suspected of having Chiari type I malformation or after surgery for such diagnosis. Patients with Chiari I have downward extension of the cerebellar tonsils, beyond the foramen magnum. This anomaly causes alteration of CSF flow dynamics, which can be visualized and measured on phase-contrast MRI of the cisterns. Conventional T1-weighted MRI with gadolinium enhancement is now able to visualize the nerve components in locations such as fine structures of the inner ear and cerebellopontine cistern. High-resolution three-dimensional imaging of the cochlea and internal auditory canals can be done with thin-section three-dimensional CISS or T2 DRIVE (driven equilibrium pulse sequence) techniques. Three-dimensional reconstruction of the cochlea and inner ear can also be produced.[20]

Diskography

In special circumstances a patient may require **diskography,** an invasive study for evaluation of questionable disk herniation. The study is often followed by CT. The intervertebral disk in question, usually cervical or lumbar, is injected with a radiopaque material. Since this can be accompanied by pain and discomfort, the clinician must prepare the patient to remain still and understand that there may be discomfort. Often, the diskogram will confirm the patient's diagnosis when other tests have failed. There is a great deal of controversy over the utility of diskography for evaluation of back pain.

CEREBROSPINAL FLUID EVALUATION: LUMBAR PUNCTURE

Lumbar puncture (LP) is a procedure that involves the introduction of a hollow needle and stylet between two vertebrae into the subarachnoid space of the lumbar part of the spinal canal below the level of the spinal cord, which ends at L1. It is commonly performed for either therapeutic or diagnostic purposes to evaluate CSF. Table 3-2 lists the characteristics and evaluation of CSF.

Patients undergoing an LP may be suspected of having a neurologic disorder (e.g., meningitis, Guillain-Barré syndrome, or multiple sclerosis [MS]). A contraindication to performing an LP is suspected increased ICP, which could result in herniation of the brainstem, coma, or death. Once strictly an inpatient procedure, LPs are now commonly performed in emergency departments and ambulatory care centers as well. Since the advent of CT and MRI, LPs are performed less frequently. Indications for an LP may include the following:

- CSF pressure measurement
- Withdrawal of CSF to reduce increased ICP
- Evaluation of the canal for the presence of CSF blockage or a tumor
- Injection of substances for visualization of the structures of the CNS
- Evaluation for signs of hemorrhage
- Removal of blood or pus from the subarachnoid space
- Laboratory analysis of CSF for infection (e.g., bacterial, fungal, or viral meningitis), neurosyphilis, or protein (which is often seen in demyelinating diseases)
- Therapeutic administration of drugs
- Placement of a small amount of the patient's blood in the epidural space to form an autologous epidural blood patch (AEBP) to prevent a CSF leak or to patch a leak
- Introduction of a local anesthetic to induce spinal anesthesia

Patient Preparation

The role of the clinician in the care of the patient undergoing an LP includes education, patient preparation, care, and follow-up. Education is a major factor because many people have misconceptions about LP. The clinician should complete a neurologic assessment and in some instances obtain a blood glucose level for comparison with the CSF glucose level. Many patients believe that the needle hitting their spinal cord will paralyze them. Although this is a remote possibility, it is extremely rare. The clinician can explain to the patient that often a level is chosen below the conus medullaris, where only nerve roots are present. Because of the size of the spinal needle, many believe that it will be excruciatingly painful. In fact, with the injection of a local anesthetic, most patients feel only pressure in the area of the procedure. Patients should empty their bowels and bladder before the test, if possible, for comfort. There are no dietary restrictions. It is important to have a baseline neurologic examination, especially of motor strength and sensation in the lower extremities. The clinician may be asked to help position the patient. There are two common positions for an LP. One position is a lateral recumbent position with the knees drawn up to the chest. The other position is sitting up flexed over an overbed table or tray with the head and arms resting on a pillow. Whichever position the physician prefers, the clinician assists the patient in becoming as comfortable as possible while remaining still. An assistant may also be asked to prepare the sterile field and the LP tray.

Once the patient is in position, the area of L4–5 is prepared with povidone-iodine or alcohol wipes and then covered with sterile drapes. An imaginary line is drawn from the tips of the iliac crest to help locate the site (Fig. 3-10). Several injections of a local anesthetic are given in the area. After a few minutes, when the local anesthetic has taken effect, the physician or qualified clinician inserts a spinal needle with an obturator through the skin just above or below the fourth lumbar verterbra (knowing the spinal cord ends an inch or more above that) into the subarachnoid space. Once the physician feels that the subarachnoid space has been entered, the obturator is removed. If pressure is being measured, a sterile

TABLE 3-2   Analysis of Cerebrospinal Fluid

Characteristic	Normal Findings	Abnormal Findings	Possible Causes/Comments
Pressure	Less than 200 mm H$_2$O	<60 mm	Faulty needle placement Dehydration Spinal block along subarachnoid space Block of foramen magnum
		>200 mm	Muscle tension Abdominal compression Bacterial meningitis Pseudotumor cerebri Brain tumor Subdural hematoma Brain abscess Brain cyst Cerebral edema (any cause) Hydrocephalus
Color	Clear, colorless	Cloudy/turbid	Cloudy as a result of microorganisms (e.g., WBCs) Turbid as a result of increased cell count
		Pale yellow or straw colored (xanthochromic)	Breakdown of RBCs with RBC pigments, high protein count
		Smoky	RBCs
Blood	None	Red blood cells: blood tinged	Traumatic tap—bloody in tube no. 1, less red in tube no. 2, and pale pink or CSF-like in tube no. 2 samples
		Grossly bloody	Traumatic tap—bloody in all three tube samples in subarachnoid hemorrhage
Volume	150 ml	Increase	Hydrocephalus
Specific gravity	1.007	Increase	Infection, presence of cells or protein, RBCs
White blood cells (WBCs)	0–5 mm^3	<500 mm^3	Bacterial or viral infections of meninges, neurosyphilis, subarachnoid hemorrhage, infarction, abscess, tuberculous meningitis, metastatic lesions
		>500 mm^3	Purulent infection
Glucose	50–75 mg/dl or 60%–70% of blood glucose	<40 mg/dl	Bacterial meningitis, tuberculosis, parasitic, fungal carcinomatous, subarachnoid hemorrhage
		>80 mg/dl	May not be of neurologic significance
Chloride	700–750 mg/dl	Decreased (<625 mg/dl)	Meningeal infection, tuberculous meningitis, hypochoremia
		Increased (>800 mg/dl)	May not be of neurologic significance; correlated with blood levels of chloride and not routine—done only on request
Culture and sensitivity	No organisms present	*Neisseria* or *Streptococcus*	Identify organisms to begin therapy; Gram stain for some cultures may take several weeks
Serology for syphilis	Negative	Positive	Syphilis
Protein (if CSF contains blood, this will raise the protein level)	15–50 mg/dl	Increased (>60 mg/dl)	Bacterial meningitis, brain tumors (both benign and malignant), complete spinal block, ALS, Guillain-Barré syndrome, subarachnoid hemorrhage, infarction, CNS trauma, CNS degenerative diseases, herniated disk, DM with polyneuropathy
		Decreased (<10 mg/dl)	May not be of neurologic significance
IgG	1–4 mg/dl		IgG and oligoclonal bands (abnormal protein bands associated with immunoelectrophoresis) may be present in multiple sclerosis and neurosyphilis
Oligoclonal bands	Absent		
Osmolality	295 osm/L	Increased	Protein, WBCs, microorganisms, RBCs
Lactate	10–20 mg/dl	Increased	Bacterial, seizure activity, fungal meningitis, CNS trauma, coma related to toxic or metabolic causes

ALS, Amyotrophic lateral sclerosis; *CNS,* central nervous system; *CSF,* cerebrospinal fluid; *DM,* diabetes mellitus; *IgG,* immunoglobulin G; *RBCs,* red blood cells; *WBCs,* white blood cells.

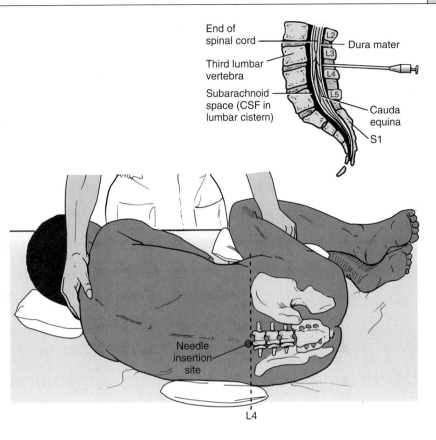

Figure 3-10 Patient position for lumbar puncture. An imaginary line can be drawn from the iliac crests. The fourth vertebra can be easily located because it lies on a line with the iliac crest.
(From Black JM, Hawks JH: Medical-surgical nursing: clinical management for positive outcomes, ed 7, St Louis, 2005, WB Saunders.)

manometer is attached to the spinal needle. CSF will flow up the manometer, and pressures are then read. Once the pressure has been recorded, the manometer is removed and the CSF is allowed to drip out into three to five small sterile tubes. CSF pressure may also be read and recorded at closing, before removal of the spinal needle. If the LP is being performed for therapeutic reasons, medication or dye may be instilled into the subarachnoid space. Depending on the size of the spinal needle and how quickly the spinal fluid drips out, the entire procedure usually takes only about 20 minutes.

Postprocedure Care

Once the procedure is completed, the physician removes the spinal needle, applies pressure to the area for several minutes, and puts a sterile cover over the puncture site. Some physicians or clinicians prefer that the patient be placed prone with a pillow under the abdomen to prevent CSF from leaking from the dural puncture site.

ALERT: The assistant should evaluate the color in each tube and may be asked to label the CSF tubes "No. 1," "No. 2," and "No. 3" and arrange for immediate delivery to the laboratory. CSF that is allowed to sit for extended periods of time or that is refrigerated may yield false results when tested.

Patients should be encouraged to keep their head flat for several hours and increase their fluid intake to raise the CSF volume. Keeping the head of the bed flat prevents downward traction on the meninges, which may occur if the patient sits or stands up too soon after the tap. It is possible that this pulls on the layers of the meninges and could result in a postspinal headache. Increased fluid intake will help hydrate the patient, and the body can then replace CSF removed during the tap. Patients may roll from side to side and use one pillow under their head for comfort.

The clinician should monitor the patient's vital signs and neurologic status as ordered or until the patient is stable after the LP. It is important to assess for signs of leakage, swelling, bleeding, infection (temperature >101° F [38.3° C]), inflammation at the site, and pain or headache. The clinician should observe for changes in the level of consciousness, motor changes (e.g., dysesthesias in the lower extremities), and problems voiding. Activity is usually restricted for 6 to 8 hours after an LP.

If the LP is performed on an outpatient basis, patients are usually discharged 60 to 90 minutes after the tap or when ordered by the physician. They are encouraged to lie in the car on the way home and remain flat in bed or on a couch for about 6 to 8 hours at home. Continued fluid intake is encouraged. Some physicians prefer to have the patient remain flat for up to 12 hours. The clinician is responsible for obtaining laboratory results, following up with the patient, and notifying the physician of any abnormal CSF findings (see Table 3-2).

Postdural puncture headache (PDPH) is a common complication of a dural puncture. It is thought that CSF leakage from the puncture site causes the headache, which is accompanied by nausea and vomiting. Several theories have been suggested, but there is no one accepted theory. PDPH seems to occur more commonly in women than in men. Classified as slight, moderate, or severe, most headaches can be treated with analgesics and subside in a day or so. Good hydration is recommended. A headache that is severe and lasts more than 3 days suggests that there is a persistent CSF leak from the LP. Referral to a neurosurgeon for an **autologous epidural blood patch (AEBP)** procedure may be helpful. Autologous blood (15 to 20 ml) drawn from the arm is injected slowly into the epidural space. The blood forms a gelatinous tamponade over the site of the CSF leak. Patients usually experience relief with few complications. In rare instances a surgical closure is required.

BIOPHYSICAL STUDIES

Carotid Doppler Imaging

Carotid Doppler imaging provides a noninvasive means for monitoring intracranial hemodynamics at the bedside. Christian Doppler first described this study in 1843. Doppler imaging uses ultrasonic technology to provide information about the patency of the carotid artery. Ultrasound depends on the presence of sonographic "windows," which allow sound wave propagation and detection of echo signals.[10] As a general rule, ultrasonography is indicated when visualization of the target object is not blocked by bone or air. Carotid ultrasonography consists of gray-scale imaging to assess the location and extent of plaque and Doppler to measure flow velocities and the degree of stenosis. Color may be added to the Doppler to improve visualization of the flow lumen and optimize the Doppler angle. The term **carotid duplex ultrasound** represents the union of the two.[10] This noninvasive test is used to detect the degree of stenosis or occlusion in the extracranial carotid artery. For example, before a carotid endarterectomy, the duplex ultrasound study can show abnormalities in the arterial diameter, pulsatility, intravascular echoes, and hemodynamic flow.

Patient Preparation

The role of the clinician is to educate the patient about the procedure. There is no special preparation.

The patient is asked to lie with shoulders relaxed and the head slightly extended away from the area to be imaged. Water-soluble acoustic gel is placed on the skin over the area to be imaged. The ultrasonic probe is then placed on the gel and run up and down over the course of the artery. The ultrasonic probe sends high-frequency sound waves to the vessels, and the echoes that are produced are measured to provide the image. Atherosclerotic fatty plaques and fibers are only faintly echogenic and can be missed if small. Plaque with calcification, however, is highly echogenic. Recordings of the blood flow are amplified and then documented. The test takes approximately 10 to 20 minutes, and there is no discomfort associated with it. Patients who are extremely obese and who have a great deal of fat in the neck area, as well as those with limited neck range of motion, may be difficult to image.

Postprocedure Care

The role of the clinician is one of patient education. There is no special preparation.

Cerebral Ultrasound

A cerebral ultrasound (previously known as **echoencephalogram**) is used to determine the size and position of cerebral structures. An ultrasonic beam is transmitted through the skull. (This study is of greatest value in the neonate who has an open anterior fontanelle, which serves as an excellent scan window.) The time needed for the cerebral structures to reflect the beam back to a transducer is then converted into an electrical impulse. When displayed and measured, this impulse helps determine the positions of the cerebral structures, especially the ventricular system. If the ventricles are significantly enlarged, additional tests may be useful, especially CT or MRI.

Doppler Ultrasound

Doppler ultrasound is a noninvasive device used to locate and assess patency of blood vessels, monitor pulses, or detect the movement of blood flow. Used with or without a headset, the Doppler device allows the clinician to hear characteristic alterations in blood flow and determine if the vessel is obstructed. Equipment required includes the Doppler flow detector, ultrasound conductive gel, and a stethoscope attachment and headset. After positioning the patient, the clinician selects the pulse point site and applies conductive gel. With the Doppler detector turned on, the clinician gently places the probe over the selected site at an angle, being careful to maintain contact with the gel without touching the patient's skin. The clinician listens until he or she hears the characteristic "whoosh" sound for the arterial flow and the howling sign that waxes and wanes for the venous flow. Sounds change above and below an obstruction (e.g., over the popliteal versus the pedal pulse points). Several attempts may be needed, the volume may need to be increased, or more gel may need to be added to locate the pulse point. Strong, consistent sounds are expected. Abnormal findings include diminished or absent pulse points and should be reported. After the assessment, all gel is removed from the patient's skin and from the device, the site is marked for future evaluations, and the findings are documented.

Transcranial Doppler Sonography

Transcranial Doppler (TCD) sonography is a diagnostic technique for noninvasive ultrasonic technique that measures local intracranial blood flow velocity and direction of key vascular structures.[13] No contrast agents are used. This technique has best results when used in certain segments of large intracranial vessels. TCD generally uses a 2 MHz pulsed Doppler transducer and is operator dependent in that it requires training and experience to perform and interpret. Vessel identification is based on the cranial window used, transducer position, and depth of sample volume.[10]

Candidates for TCD are those at risk for the following:

- TIAs related to arteriostenosis or with atherosclerosis
- Cerebrovascular disease (e.g., brain attack/stroke)
- Vasospasm secondary to subarachnoid hemorrhage following aneurysm clipping or coiling and following arteriovenous malformation (AVM) resection

Clinical settings include the bedside in the intensive care unit, where TCD can be used and repeated as needed, or applied for continuous monitoring, on a daily basis to measure blood flow velocities in patients with vasospasm, subarachnoid hemorrhage, or ruptured aneurysm. Brain death may be supported by TCD. In the operating room, TCD is used during carotid surgery. There may be a relationship between progressive increases in ICP and abnormal TCD waveforms. Other uses include evaluation of patients with migraine, venous diseases such as sagittal sinus thrombosis, arterial dissection, and flow reductions in AVMs; in the future TCD may play a role in brain death determination.[16]

Patients feel no discomfort during the procedure. Results of TCD are important clinically to determine treatment options and to detect or confirm the onset of vasospasm. Accuracy is dependent on the person performing the procedure, anatomic differences such as vessel size, and perfusion territory. Clinical decisions regarding patient care and treatment should never be based on a patient's TCD findings alone. Normal CBF velocities range from 30 to 80 cm/sec. Vasospasm is indicated with a CBF of 120 to 200 cm/sec or greater.[7]

Regional Cerebral Blood Flow and Perfusion Imaging

Many attempts have been made to quantify CBF. One technique that was used in the past is **regional cerebral blood flow (rCBF)** studies using the radioisotope xenon-133. The aim of these studies was to evaluate blood flow to the cerebral cortex and specifically to detect regions of increased or decreased local flow. This test was noninvasive. The patient had extracranial detectors placed around the head. The patient was then asked to breathe a mixture of oxygen and xenon-133 through a mask for 3 to 5 minutes. Xenon-133 is an odorless gas. As the xenon-133 entered the bloodstream and circulated up to the brain, the detectors picked up the flow and the computer then calculated the flow to the different areas. The procedure was occasionally used intraoperatively during aneurysm surgery to assess the effects of extreme hypotension.[2]

Currently, CBF is being studied with CT or MR perfusion techniques. Such studies are based on the dynamic passage of a nondiffusible tracer through the cerebral vasculature, injected via a large IV catheter (16 gauge) and a power injector. As contrast flows through the cerebral vasculature, the area of interest is imaged repeatedly, either with CT (iodinated contrast) or MRI (gadolinium). The passage of contrast causes a change in the appearance of the image; namely, there is increase of attenuation on CT, or reduction of signal intensity on echo planar MR imaging. Upon plotting a curve that measures the signal intensity (or Hounsfield Units [H.U.]) over time, the clinician can derive the cerebral blood volume (CBV), which is the surface area (integral) under the curve. Dividing the CBV by the mean transit time (MTT) yields the cerebral blood flow (CBF).

This technique has become essential in the diagnosis of acute infarction (CVA). A patient who presents with acute CVA within the first three hours will undergo CT perfusion in most centers and, rarely, MRI perfusion with DWI in other centers. A deficit on the CBV or on DWI indicates an area of irreversibly infarcted tissue. The CBF indicates the entire region of oligemia that is at risk. A mismatch between CBV and CBF or DWI and CBF indicates the presence of reperfusable tissue that is at risk of undergoing infarction (so-called ischemic penumbra) (see Fig. 3-4, *B*). When such a mismatch is seen, and if the clinical criteria are met, the patient receives thrombolytic therapy, in order to prevent the penumbra from undergoing infarction.

Patient Preparation

The role of the clinician is one of education to teach the patient about the procedure. Refer to Patient Preparation on p. 104. If the injection method is used, the clinician must be alert for such complications as hematoma or embolus formation.[6]

Postprocedure Care

As the patient has usually received iodinated contrast for the perfusion study, moderate hydration is encouraged in the 24 hours that follow the contrast administration.

ELECTROPHYSIOLOGIC STUDIES

Electroencephalography

Electroencephalography (EEG) has value for diagnosis, management, and prognosis. Patients may be scheduled to have a single-test 24-hour EEG monitoring, or EEG monitoring during treatment with an induced barbiturate coma. Therefore knowledge about EEG is essential.[18]

EEG is an electrodiagnostic technique to evaluate the frequency, amplitude, and special characteristics of the electrical impulses produced by the brain. EEG is indicated to investigate seizures, including the focus of seizure activity, spread of activity, and pattern of activity. Patients with seizures may have irritable areas of the brain that fire frequently but do not manifest themselves as clinical seizures. This, too, may be observed and recorded with EEG. EEG is sometimes performed in patients with cerebral tumors or dementia to identify areas of focal slowing of electrical activity. Trauma, drug and alcohol intoxication, and brain irritation secondary to infection can also be identified. EEG is also a valuable adjunct to the clinical determination of brain death.[23]

Patient Preparation

The role of the clinician in the management of the patient undergoing EEG includes patient education and preparation. The clinician should explain the procedure to the patient and reassure the patient that the electrical activity is being recorded from his or her brain. No electrical impulses will be delivered to the brain. The hair and scalp should be clean and free of oil, lotions, and spray.

Patients are told to refrain from caffeine and other stimulants for approximately 12 hours before the test. No other dietary restrictions are required. Stimulants can produce changes in the brain's electrical activity. Likewise, patients should not be sedated the night before the test because this, too, may produce erroneous information on the EEG recording. Patients are also asked to limit their sleep to 4 to 5 hours the night before the test. Patients are then encouraged to sleep during the EEG recording to evaluate changes during sleep. All medications should be given normally before the test unless otherwise ordered by the physician. Patients should also be told that they might be asked to hyperventilate during the test to stimulate certain brain activity. They will be asked to lie as still as possible because movement may interfere with the recording.[21]

EEG is usually performed in a specially equipped EEG room, which is designed to filter out outside activity, especially electrical activity, although portable monitoring may be done at the bedside. The patient is asked to lie in a bed or a reclining chair. Seventeen to 21 electrodes are attached to specific areas of the patient's scalp with a conductive paste. EEG signals are then picked up and recorded. The patient may be asked to perform activities such as opening and closing the eyes and hyperventilating, which may induce epileptogenic activity. Photostimulation, flashing a light in front of the patient, may also be performed to assess for seizure activity. The entire test may last 45 to 120 minutes.

EEG recording may also be performed with simultaneous video recording. This is done to evaluate the clinical manifestations of seizures at the same time as the EEG recording is being conducted. These video EEG recordings may last from 4 to 24 hours. Digital EEG recording is a new technology that is being used at some sites. This type of EEG recording uses computer technology to enhance EEG recording for more precise measurement of epileptogenic activity.

Postprocedure Care

After the test, the patient can resume a normal diet and activity. Patients who were sedated for a sleep evaluation should allow the sedative to wear off before resuming normal activity. Table 3-3 demonstrates classification of electrical brain activity.

Electromyography

Electromyography (EMG) is a neurophysiologic study performed to evaluate nerve conduction and subsequent skeletal muscle function. This assessment is performed with the skeletal muscle at rest and with voluntary muscle contraction. EMG is used to evaluate muscle disease, such as muscular dystrophy, amyotrophic lateral sclerosis (ALS), myasthenia gravis, myopathies, and inflammatory disorders of muscle such as polymyositis. It can be used to distinguish between primary muscle disease and lower motor neuron lesions. EMG is also used to evaluate neuropathies, spinal cord lesions, and peripheral nerve lesions. Although EMG will not indicate the cause of these lesions, it can help locate the structures involved and monitor the disease process over time. It is important, however, to remember that this diagnostic tool is helpful in only a small percentage of neurologic diseases.[24]

Patient Preparation

Patient preparation for EMG studies is primarily educational. Some patients complain of pain with the insertion of the EMG needles, and patients should be warned about this. The patient should be questioned about the use of anticoagulants or aspirin, which may lead to bleeding after insertion of the needle.

Postprocedure Care

There are no diet or activity restrictions before or after the test. After the test the patient is free to resume his or her normal activity.

Nerve Conduction Velocity

Nerve conduction velocity (NCV) studies may be performed along with EMG. Nerve conduction velocity is a study of the conduction time and amplitude of stimulation along the nerve.

The patient is taken to the EMG room and positioned to allow for access to the muscles involved. The muscles tested are determined on the basis of the patient's clinical examination. A ground lead is attached to the muscle that is being tested. A concentric needle electrode is then inserted into the muscle at rest. Rates of firing and the shape and dimension of potentials are recorded and displayed on an oscilloscope. A permanent record of the tracing can be made. With newer equipment the data can be stored for further evaluation. After

TABLE 3-3	Classification of Electrical Brain Activity	
Waveform	Duration	Description
Delta	1–4 cycles/sec	Normally seen in stages 3 and 4 of sleep (slow-wave sleep)
Theta	4–7 cycles/sec	Can be normal in drowsy adult; more common in children; can be characteristic of coma in brain-injured patient
Alpha	8–13 cycles/sec	Seen in occipital leads; normal in a relaxed individual with eyes closed
Beta	12–40 cycles/sec	Fast waves, indicating physical or mental activity or anxiety
Spike and slow waves	Variable	Irritable brain tissue such as seizure foci

recordings are taken at rest, the patient may be asked to slowly and progressively contract the muscle that is being tested. If NCV is being performed, two electrodes are placed, one proximally and one distally. The nerve is then stimulated by electrical current. The time that it takes an electrical impulse to travel between the two points and the time between the stimulus and muscle contraction are then recorded. Depending on the number of muscles studied and patient cooperation, EMG usually lasts 20 to 45 minutes. If NCV is performed, an additional 15 to 20 minutes is required.

Pathologic conditions seen on an EMG recording may include decreased amplitude of the waveform in such primary muscle disorders as muscular dystrophy, myopathies, and polymyositis. Myasthenia gravis presents a classic picture of progressively decreasing amplitude of the waveform. The muscles in the patient with myasthenia gravis may start off strong and progressively weaken with repeated use. This is evidenced on the EMG recording. Peripheral nerve injury is evidenced by a decrease in the number of muscle fibers contracting, as well as a slowing of conduction velocity.

Evoked Potentials

Evoked potential (EP) tests are electrodiagnostic studies to evaluate nerve conduction. They are a noninvasive, relatively painless way of gaining information about possible disturbances in conduction. EPs are used to diagnose disorders of the CNS, locate the site of CNS damage, evaluate treatment, and frequently monitor a patient intraoperatively. Three of the most common types of evoked potentials are **somatosensory evoked potentials (SSEPs), visual evoked potentials (VEPs),** and **brainstem auditory evoked responses (BAERs).**

Pathologic conditions identified with evoked potentials indicate the location of the problem but not necessarily the cause. The results of these tests always need to be correlated clinically. With SSEPs, slowed conduction may be seen in demyelinating disorders such as multiple sclerosis (MS) and many other degenerative conditions. VEPs may be abnormal in patients with optic neuritis, MS, or vitamin B_{12} deficiency. Patients with MS, as well as those with cerebellopontine angle and brainstem disorders, may have abnormal BAERs. Currently there is disagreement on the use of SSEPs in patients with spinal cord injury and the use of BAERs in patients with brainstem damage. With increased technology, EPs will continue to be used as a valuable adjunct to clinical evaluation. Testing for EPs is particularly useful in uncooperative, confused, or comatose patients.[9]

Patient Preparation
The role of the clinician in the care of the patient undergoing EP testing is one of education. The procedure, rationale, and expected patient cooperation should be explained to the patient. Patients are usually asked to shampoo their hair before the test and refrain from using lotions, oils, or sprays that might interfere with the recording electrodes. No dietary or activity restrictions are required before or after the test. Several electrodes are attached to various portions of the scalp with electrode gel or paste. A mild stimulus is given

that causes the nerve to react and transmit a message to the brain that is recorded by a computer for analysis.

For SSEPs, electrodes are placed on the skin over the median nerve in the wrist or over the perineal nerve near the knee. Electrical stimulation is then sent to these nerves and picked up by the electrodes on the scalp in the opposite hemisphere to check pathways from the nerves in the extremities to the brain.

Multiple electrodes are placed on the scalp along the vertex and occipital area for evaluation in VEPs to check the pathway from the eyes to the brain. Stimulation of the visual system is accomplished by using a checkerboard pattern, strobe lights, and retinal stimulation.

BAEPs are recorded using scalp electrodes placed along the vertex and on each earlobe. Patients are then subjected to bursts of tones or clicking heard via headphones. Patients who are evaluated are those individuals suspected of having damage to pathways from the ear to the brain, causing problems with balance or hearing. Depending on the patient's ability to cooperate, the test should take about 20 to 30 minutes. There are no aftereffects, and usually no special nursing care is required.

Postprocedure Care
Once the test is completed, the gel or paste is removed and the individual is usually allowed to resume his or her normal activities.

NUCLEAR MEDICINE TESTING

Brain Scan

A **brain scan** is a nuclear medicine imaging technique that has been used for many years. Its principle is based on the integrity of the blood-brain barrier (BBB).[19] A patient receives an IV injection of a radionuclide substance such as technetium-99m. This is allowed to circulate in the bloodstream for a period of time, usually several hours. Then, with the use of nuclear imaging devices, the head is scanned. Normally, this radioactive isotope would not cross the blood-brain barrier. In areas of localized disease, however, the blood-brain barrier is disrupted. This results in an increased uptake of the isotope and visualization on the brain scan.

Brain scan may be indicated in the evaluation of tumors, strokes, and headaches. However, newer technology, such as CT and MRI, has largely replaced it in acute evaluations. A brain scan cannot indicate the nature of the pathologic condition, only that the blood-brain barrier has been disrupted. For example, if a scan is performed soon after a cerebral infarct, the scan may be normal if the blood-brain barrier has not yet been disrupted. A follow-up scan several days later, however, is usually abnormal. The brain scan may also be used to evaluate cerebral blood flow. In that case a scan is done immediately following the injection of the isotope. Low flow would be expected in areas of occlusion versus high flow in areas of arteriovenous malformation (AVM). MRS is particularly useful in the evaluation of radiation necrosis versus tumor recurrence. When an MRI shows an abnormal enhancing area, nuclear medicine studies with PET are considered the most accurate, and specific tests confirm the diagnosis of radiation necrosis, which can look like a recurrent tumor on traditional imaging tests.

Patient Preparation

The primary role of the clinician in brain scanning is assessment and teaching. The patient should be questioned about any allergy to iodine. Confused or agitated patients may need to be sedated. The patient is asked to lie in several positions during the scan, including prone. This should also be explained. The scan generally lasts about 30 to 45 minutes.

Postprocedure Care

After the procedure the patient is encouraged to increase fluid intake to assist in excreting the isotope. Since only trace isotopes are used, no radiation precautions need be taken. The patient should also be assessed for signs of allergy to the isotope, such as itching, redness, and swelling.

Positron Emission Tomography

Positron emission tomography (PET) scanning is a nuclear medicine study that uses technology similar to that of CT. PET scans can assess perfusion and the level of metabolic activity in various organ systems, such as the brain. The purpose of PET scanning is to take CT images one step further and look at normal patterns of tissue metabolism. In the CNS, PET is used to evaluate oxygen and glucose metabolism, as well as CBF.

A cyclotron is used to constantly produce radionuclides that are positron emitting. These radiopharmaceuticals are then injected intravenously or inhaled. Once inside the body, these positrons combat electrons and are annihilated. This process of annihilation or destruction produces gamma rays. The patient's head is placed in a scanner, which consists of multiple crystal detectors that surround the patient. These crystals will scintillate, or give off light, when they pick up energy from the gamma rays. This scintillation is then coded by the computer and reconstructed to produce images. Deoxyglucose tagged with radioactive fluorine is one of the radiopharmaceuticals frequently used to evaluate the CNS.

Areas of pathology result in altered glucose and oxygen metabolism and altered CBF. An abnormal concentration of the radioactive isotope may be seen in patients with cerebral ischemia, stroke, or epilepsy. Abnormal metabolism of glucose in areas of contusion and in Alzheimer's disease are also identified on PET scans. In Alzheimer's disease there is decreased metabolism in the frontal, temporal, and parietal areas as compared with normal aging, which usually results in changes only in the frontal lobes. Malignant brain tumors will light up on a PET scan secondary to increased metabolism of glucose. Patients with seizures may show decreased metabolism in the epileptogenic areas with increased metabolism during and immediately after seizure activity. Oxygen use can be monitored in patients with cerebrovascular disease. PET also holds promise for evaluating diffuse axonal injury in the patient with head trauma and is currently being used to evaluate migraine, Parkinson's disease, and schizophrenia.

Patient Preparation

Several factors can interfere with PET results, including the use of caffeine, alcohol, and tobacco 24 hours before the scan or the use of tranquilizers or sedatives. These chemicals may stimulate or depress the CNS and alter the metabolism of glucose in the brain. Patients with severe anxiety may also show abnormally high metabolism of glucose on a PET scan.

The role of the clinician in the management of patients undergoing PET is primarily one of patient education. Explaining the procedure and what to expect is vital because the test is uncommon and may be frightening. The only food, fluid, or activity restrictions before or after the test are to omit caffeine, alcohol, and tobacco for at least 24 hours before the test. Before the procedure, one or two IV catheters may be inserted. One IV line is for the isotope injection, and the other is for drawing blood samples to determine the amounts of the isotope available in the blood at certain periods of time. The patient is sometimes asked to inhale a gas with a radioactive tag.

The patient's head is scanned much like it is in CT. The patient may be asked to perform various activities, such as thinking, reasoning, and remembering, to assess brain metabolism during these activities. Patients may be required to wear blindfolds and earplugs to eliminate extraneous stimuli. The procedure generally lasts about 60 to 90 minutes.

Postprocedure Care

After the procedure, patients are encouraged to increase fluids to help remove the isotope from the body. Normal activity and diet can be resumed.

TIP: PET is available in only a few centers across the country, although there is growing interest in its use. The cost of the cyclotron, radiopharmaceuticals, computers, and support personnel is prohibitive for most institutions. Recent advances in technology, however, are eliminating some of these barriers, and PET promises to be a significant diagnostic tool in the near future. For example, PET (versus invasive electrical stimulation or intraoperative cortical stimulation [ICS] recording of SSEPs) is an accurate method for mapping the primary somatosensory cortex before surgery. The need for ICS, which requires local anesthesia, may be eliminated with PET scanning to benefit patients with brain tumors, AVMs, or epileptogenic foci, where maximum resection during surgery could result in neurologic deficits.[4]

Single-Photon Emission Computed Tomography

Single-photon emission computed tomography (SPECT) is another nuclear medicine scan that uses radiopharmaceuticals and a standard gamma camera with computerized technology. The combination of these technologies results in the three-dimensional measurement of regional CBF. Radiopharmaceuticals such as iodine-1, -2, or -3–labeled amines produce gamma rays that are picked up by the rotating gamma camera. These radiopharmaceuticals are known to readily cross the blood-brain barrier. Areas of high flow receive increased perfusion of the radiopharmaceuticals, and low-flow areas emit less gamma radiation. After injection, the brain is imaged with the rotating gamma camera, and CT technology produces a detailed demonstration of the CBF. Blood flow to the cortical gray matter, basal ganglia, and thalamus is significantly higher than blood flow to the white matter; therefore gamma emission is far greater in the gray areas. The major clinical uses of SPECT are to detect cerebrovascular disease, seizures, and tumors. SPECT imaging frequently shows decreased perfusion to an area of infarction within 48 hours, whereas a CT scan may take much longer to become positive.

The boundary and extent of infarction are also more clearly delineated in SPECT than in CT. SPECT has also been used concurrently with EEG recording to evaluate CBF during and after seizure activity. Dramatic hyperperfusion during the ictal phase, as well as hypoperfusion interictally, has been demonstrated. SPECT is useful in outlining brain tumors because of the increased perfusion and therefore increased gamma uptake in the areas of the tumor.

SPECT has several advantages over PET scanning. The cost and ready availability of the radiopharmaceuticals are major advantages. Because SPECT uses equipment found in most nuclear medicine departments, it is not necessary to provide extensive additional equipment or personnel. No on-site cyclotron is required, which also helps to reduce the cost. SPECT has been called the "poor man's PET scan" because of the difference in cost. PET scans do provide higher spatial resolution (up to about 5 mm), whereas the resolution with SPECT is less (only about 8 mm).

There are many advances in SPECT, as well as in PET scanning. New computer software, imaging crystals in the gamma camera, and better radiopharmaceuticals are being developed. This type of neurodiagnostic study will probably gain popularity much faster than PET scanning because of the great difference in cost. For example, the ictal SPECT scan is one of the newer methods used to identify the epileptogenic seizure focus. Clinicians in some epilepsy centers have demonstrated excellent performance in the use of a video EEG epilepsy monitoring unit using SPECT.[11]

Patient Preparation

Patient preparation is similar to that in PET scanning. Patient education is vital to allay fears of the unknown. There are no known diet or activity restrictions before or following the scan. The patient will receive an injection of the radiopharmaceutical and will be scanned by the rotating gamma camera.

Postprocedure Care

Patients are encouraged to increase fluids to remove the radiopharmaceutical from the body.

SPECIAL SENSES TESTING

Electronystagmography

Electronystagmography is an electrodiagnostic test used to evaluate **nystagmus,** or involuntary eye movement, and the muscles controlling eye movement. This study measures changes in the electrical field surrounding the eye and makes a permanent recording of eye movement both at rest and as a result of various stimuli. Various procedures (e.g., pendulum tracking, changing head position, and caloric tests) are used to stimulate nystagmus, and recordings are made. Electronystagmography is used in the differential diagnosis of lesions of the vestibular system, brainstem, and cerebellum. It may also be beneficial to analyze unilateral hearing loss and vertigo.

The study is contraindicated in patients with perforated eardrums (who should not have water irrigation) and patients with pacemakers. Sedatives, stimulants, and antivertigo agents, as well as eye blinking, may alter results. The patient should be instructed not to apply makeup before the procedure, since electrodes will be taped around the eyes. Solid food should be avoided before the test, and caffeine and alcohol are generally not permitted for 24 to 48 hours before testing.

Abnormal findings may indicate brainstem lesions, vestibular system lesions, cerebellum lesions, congenital disorders, or demyelinating disease.

Caloric Testing

Electrodiagnostic caloric studies are used to evaluate the vestibular part of the eighth cranial nerve (CN VIII) by irrigating the auditory canal with warm or cool water. Normal findings include rotary nystagmus away from the side being irrigated with cold water. Hot water, conversely, induces nystagmus toward the side being irrigated. In abnormal test results, no nystagmus is produced. This may be caused by disease of the labyrinth or a dysfunction of CN VIII that is related to compression. Caloric testing is beneficial in the differential diagnosis of abnormalities in the vestibular system, brainstem, or cerebellum. If results are inconclusive, electronystagmography may be warranted. Electrodiagnostic tests are contraindicated in patients with perforated eardrums or acute disease of the labyrinth. Sedatives and antivertigo agents may alter results, and solid food should be avoided before testing to prevent vomiting. These studies are typically done as a series of tests to check cranial nerve/brainstem function to determine the presence of clinical "brain death."

Audiometric Studies

Audiometric studies are used to aid in diagnosis or rehabilitation. Individuals with injury to the auditory branch of CN VIII or hearing loss may be referred for a routine battery of audiologic studies. This may include pure tone air and bone testing, speech recognition and word discrimination, central auditory processing or brainstem testing, posturography, and rotary chair testing to discriminate between peripheral and central problems. The wide availability of audiometric testing allows for a much briefer bedside screening. For example, auditory perception is tested for acuity, perception of organized sounds, and rhythms. Tests evaluate levels of hearing loss in terms of loudness and clarity. They also help determine whether hearing loss is related to outer/middle ear dysfunction or inner ear disturbance (i.e., conduction delay versus neural loss).

Consideration is given to the patient's physiologic and psychologic condition, age, intelligence, and reaction time; the presence of tinnitus; and the patient's previous test experience. Any of these variables may require adjustment for test procedures and evaluation.

Visual Field Testing

Visual field testing is the evaluation of peripheral vision. Gross visual field testing may be performed by means of confrontation (see Chapter 2). For more precise testing, visual fields are evaluated by a neuro-ophthalmologist to include a perimeter and tangent screen. Visual field testing is used to detect scotomas that are a result of lesions of the retina or optic nerve; anopia, a rare condition characterized by loss of vision in the upper or lower half of the visual field; or hemianopia caused by the compression or destruction of the fibers of the optic tracts and their radiations.

Oculoplethysmography

Oculoplethysmography (OPG) is an important noninvasive test that indirectly measures blood flow in the ophthalmic artery. Because the ophthalmic artery is the primary major branch of the internal carotid artery, its blood flow reflects the alternative blood flow to the brain, as well as the carotid blood flow. This procedure measures eye pressure through suction cups placed on the eyes. OPG is indicated in patients who have symptoms of transient ischemic attacks (TIAs), cardiac bruits, or other neurologic symptoms such as dizziness or fainting. This test may be followed by cerebral angiography and is often performed after carotid endarterectomy. It is contraindicated in patients who have undergone eye surgery within the last 6 months, those who have lens implants or cataracts, and those who have had retinal detachments. It is also contraindicated in patients who are allergic to local anesthetics. Certain complications are also associated with OPG, including conjunctival hemorrhage, corneal abrasions, and transient photophobia.

OXIMETRY: OXYGEN SATURATION

Oximetry is a noninvasive method of monitoring arterial blood oxygen saturation (SaO_2) or oxygenation status at the bedside with a simple probe or sensor attached to the finger or ear. Pulse oximetry closely correlates with arterial blood gas (ABG) findings unless the patient has peripheral vascular disease and as long as the oxygen saturation is greater than 70%. The beam of light that passes through the tissue measures the amount of light that tissue absorbs. Before applying the disposable probe, the clinician determines if the skin is warm and has adequate circulation. The finger or earlobe is rubbed to increase blood flow, and the probe is attached for continuous recording. Alarm parameters can be set to alert clinicians to values that are lower than normal.

Inaccurate readings may result from severe anemia or abnormally low hemoglobin levels associated with carbon monoxide poisoning, cigarette smoking, nitroprusside, or lidocaine therapy. Pulse oximetry has accuracy limitations; therefore clinicians should be careful not to rely on the readings as absolute measurements of oxygen saturation. The ABG measurements are the gold standard. Sensor sites should be checked frequently and repositioned every 4 hours. Newer-generation models are designed to monitor pulse oximetry despite motion artifact and low perfusion.

Brain tissue oxygen and temperature ($PbtO_2$) can be measured by the insertion of a bolt into the white matter of the brain. This device can measure the difference between the supply and demand of oxygen at the cellular level with regional readings. Patients at risk can be identified with oxygen as an independent parameter that is directly correlated with patient outcome (see Chapter 12).

NEUROPSYCHOLOGIC TESTING

The availability of advanced neurodiagnostic studies provides the clinical treatment team with greater information to map the brain and to locate and identify pathologic lesions. At an appropriate time during recovery, selected patients with neurologic disorders (e.g., traumatic brain injury or stroke) may benefit from neuropsychologic testing. The testing is a method by which the patient's functional capabilities and emotional functioning are assessed after the cerebral injury. The referral may be to help answer questions about the patient's ability to return to work or school, or resume driving. Personality changes that occur after brain injury may be explained (e.g., disinhibition, lack of motivation, depression, or dysfunction in the executive system). The battery of interviews and tests can help the neuropsychologist delineate a patient's unique learning profile, specify strengths and weaknesses in learning strategies, provide data for developing a well-tailored program for cognitive remediation, and provide information to determine a patient's emotional and cognitive potential for recovery. Neuropsychologic assessment identifies and quantifies both cognitive strengths and deficits. Most referrals are made in six specific domains: (1) patient care, (2) rehabilitation, (3) educational planning, (4) forensic issues, (5) treatment outcome analyses, and (6) life care planning.[22]

Neuropsychologists (psychologists who specialize in understanding how brain dysfunction affects the cognitive, emotional, and behavioral performance of a patient) use standardized testing procedures and make an initial assessment. This evaluation is compared with later tests and can measure improvement that will affect ongoing recommendations regarding cognitive retraining. Tests are used to distinguish patients with psychiatric illness from those with neurologic illness. A full neuropsychologic examination requires 3 to 12 hours of testing and may need to be divided into several sessions because of patient fatigue, agitation, or other conditions. Over 700 tests are available, from which the neurophysiologist selects a battery of tests for an individualized evaluation. The testing battery may include the following well-known tests:

- Halstead-Reitan: Used to discriminate between normal individuals and patients with organic disease; includes six tests to measure parameters (e.g., abstract reasoning, tactile performance, memory, rhythm perception, speech intelligence, psychomotor speed, language function, sensory function, grip strength, personality)
- Luria-Nebraska: Tests items that discriminate brain-damaged patients from neurologically healthy individuals; consists of 269 individual items scored from 0 (no impairment) to 2 (impairment)[22]

A shorter neuropsychologic screening can be requested that requires less time but can offer valuable information regarding the patient's attention, orientation, short- and long-term memory, expressive and receptive language abilities, abstract reasoning, and intelligence. Results from the shorter screening may indicate that a full battery of tests is warranted. When referring a patient for neuropsychologic testing, the clinician needs to be as specific as possible concerning patient information such as the following:

- Current and past medical status
- Current medications
- Brief history of the present illness
- Brief review of the physical and neurologic examination results

Inpatient testing should be scheduled when the patient is alert and attentive and able to tolerate a block of time with the neuropsychologist without interruption.[22] Clinicians will find that the test results can be used to explain cognitive and behavioral changes to members of the family and other health care providers. Neuropsychologic reassessment helps track the so-called soft signs, such as patient improvement or lack of progress, which may not be as apparent to the patient and family as physiologic, or so-called hard, signs.

TELEMEDICINE

Telemedicine is the use of special telecommunication technology to provide clinical care to patients at distant sites. Telemedicine may enable full medical examination by specialists for patients in remote areas in a variety of real-life situations. In some regions of the United States, live, two-way interactive audio and video communications may be possible using technology capable of transmitting data (e.g., x-ray findings [teleradiology], laboratory analyses, and other diagnostic capabilities). Telemedicine also allows physicians to transmit diagnostic images from hospital to home or to major teaching institutions for review and advice.

Transmission of important patient and medical information in real-life situations may herald remote diagnostic testing where the patient and physician never meet face-to-face. Both parties are provided video equipment that allows participants to see and hear each other. Currently there are devices available that can transmit, for example, x-ray findings, laboratory reports, and close-up videoscopic pictures. This evolving technology holds promise for the future, when renowned specialists may be able to beam in on the patient at home from anywhere in the world for clinician consultation or teaching purposes or to provide clinicians with instant feedback; specialists may even be able to perform operative procedures by computerized robotics.

LABORATORY STUDIES

Urine Testing

Urine Specific Gravity

Urine specific gravity (SG) (1.005 to 1.303, usually 1.010 to 1.025) is a measure of waste and electrolyte concentration in the urine. A high specific gravity indicates highly concentrated urine, whereas a low specific gravity indicates dilute urine. Recent use of radiographic dyes will distort test results, as will dextran, sucrose, and diuretics.[16] No fasting is required. After the specimen has been taken, a urinometer or other device found in the nursing unit may be used or the specimen may be sent to the laboratory.

Abnormal findings include the following:

- Increased levels (>1.020) related to dehydration, pituitary tumor, or tumor that causes the **syndrome of inappropriate antidiuretic hormone (SIADH)**
- Increased levels (>1.030) related to decrease in renal blood flow and fever
- Decreased levels (<1.005) related to overhydration or diabetes insipidus (DI)
- Decreased levels (1.001 to 1.005) related to renal failure and hypothermia

Urine Osmolality

Urine osmolality (50 to 1200 mOsm/kg H_2O; average, 200 to 800 mOsm/kg H_2O) is a measure of the osmotic pressure of urine used to monitor electrolyte and water balance and to evaluate dehydration. It is more accurate than specific gravity in determining urine concentration. Osmolality testing is especially valuable in the workup of patients with renal disease, SIADH, or DI. No preparation is necessary for a random urine specimen; however, for a fasting specimen the patient should have a high-protein diet for 3 days before the test. Diuretics, radiocontrast dye, barbiturates, morphine, and anesthetics will all affect osmolality levels. Urine osmolality varies according to diet and hydration; therefore the urine osmolality should always be evaluated in relation to serum osmolality. The ratio of urine osmolality to serum osmolality should exceed 1.0 to 3.0 or more following a fast. Abnormal results include the following:

- Increased levels (>800 mOsm/kg H_2O) related to SIADH
- Decreased levels (<400 mOsm/kg H_2O) related to DI

Plasma Values: Serum Osmolality

A **serum osmolality** (280 to 300 mOsm/kg H_2O) test is an indicator of serum concentration. This test measures the number of dissolved particles (e.g., electrolytes, urea, or sugar) in the serum and is beneficial in analyzing fluid and electrolyte imbalance and in evaluating the serum for the presence of organic acids, sugars, or ethanol. Sodium contributes 85% to 90% of the serum osmolality; changes in osmolality are usually due to changes in the serum sodium concentration.[9] Doubling the serum sodium concentration gives an estimate of the serum osmolality. The hydration status of the patient is usually determined by calculating the serum osmolality. Lower than normal values may indicate fluid overload whereas higher than normal values may indicate dehydration. The administration of **hypotonic solutions** (e.g., 0.45% saline, 2.5% dextrose, and 0.33% saline) may decrease intravascular osmolarity or result in intracellular expansion. **Hypertonic solutions** (e.g., 5% dextrose in half saline, 5% dextrose in normal saline, or 5% dextrose in Ringer's lactate solution), may increase intravascular osmolarity and result in intracellular and interstitial dehydration. **Isotonic solutions** (e.g., normal saline, Ringer's lactate solution, or 5% dextrose in water) do not change osmolarity.

There are no food or drink restrictions for serum osmolality testing. It should be noted, however, that a cerebrovascular accident (CVA) or brain tumor might interfere with accurate test interpretation. Abnormal findings include the following:

- Syndrome of inappropriate antidiuretic hormone (SIADH): <250 mOsm/kg H_2O
- Diabetes insipidus (DI): >300 mOsm/kg H_2O

OLDER ADULT CONSIDERATIONS

Table 3-4 discusses special considerations of the older patient in diagnostic testing.

CONCLUSION

Clinicians may recognize the need for diagnostic studies and alert the treating team with recommendations. Other clinicians may or may not be responsible for ordering neurodiag-

TABLE 3-4 Older Adult Considerations: Diagnostic Tests	
Clinical/Diagnostic Interpretation	**Comments**
Electroencephalogram (EEG)	
Changes with age:	EEG abnormalities must be correlated with clinical data.
Alpha activity slows (slower in men than in women)	
Changes in sleep patterns (see Chapter 6)	
In delirium:	EEG can be useful in delirium to distinguish focal from nonfocal etiologies.
Alpha frequency slows (more than with "normal" aging)	
In dementia:	EEG can be useful in the dementia workup to rule out causes such as meningioma, metabolic disorders.
Alpha frequency slows (may be normal in up to 50% of cases)	
With severe dementia, EEG is severely slowed, may see loss of alpha and irregular delta activity	
Computed Tomography/Magnetic Resonance Imaging (CT/MRI)	
Changes with age:	Age-related changes are not necessarily an indication of a decline in intellectual function.
Increased prominence of sulci and fissures ("cortical atrophy")	
Ventricular enlargement, decreased brain size/weight	
In dementia:	Although cortical atrophy may be present, the clinical significance in predicting severity of dementia or distinguishing "normal from abnormal" is controversial.
Cortical atrophy (greater than with "normal" aging)	
Increased ventricular size	
In Binswanger's dementia: symmetric, deep white matter lucencies are present	
"General" considerations:	CT/MRI can be useful in the differential diagnosis to evaluate for brain injury, stroke, bleed, tumor, hydrocephalus, or vascular dementia causing the change in behavior, cognition, or function.
If memory impairment is preexistent, patients may have difficulty understanding test directions, significance, etc.	
Claustrophobia may occur during MRI	
Surfaces can be extremely uncomfortable (hard, cold), especially if older patients have kyphosis or osteoarthritis of spine	
Those with aneurysm clips, pacemakers, and other metallic substances must avoid MRI	
Lumbar Puncture (LP)	
None	LP can be useful in dementia workup to rule out infectious process.
	Procedure may be more difficult in those with osteoarthritis of spine.

MID, Multiinfarct dementia.

nostic studies. Advanced practice nurses may perform some of the actual procedures (e.g., an LP). Related to those procedures, however, patient preparation and monitoring of side effects to prevent complications are vital responsibilities. The bedside clinician is responsible for careful observation and close monitoring, and for making a rapid response to any decline in a patient's neurologic status following diagnostic testing.

Providing patient teaching and reducing test anxiety are other responsibilities of the clinician during hospitalization. It is therefore important to have firsthand knowledge of routine neurodiagnostic studies and to be able to demystify these studies, which are a vital part of the treatment regimen. Important, also, is the accurate documentation of any adverse reactions or patient complications, along with immediate notification of the physician and prompt intervention.

RESOURCES FOR TESTING

American Academy of Neurology: www.aan.com
American Association of Neurological Surgeons: www.neurosurgery.org
American Society of Neuroradiology: www.asnr.org

REFERENCES

1. Allison M: SQUID: latest innovation in neuroimaging, *Headlines,* Oct/Nov 1992, p 23.
2. Barker E: The xenon CT: a new neuro tool, *RN* 61(2):22–26, 1998.
3. Bernstein M, Al-Anazi AR, Kucharczy KW, et al: Brain tumor surgery with the Toronto open magnetic resonance imaging system: preliminary results for 36 patients and analysis of advantages, disadvantages, and future prospects, *Neurosurgery* 46(4):900–909, 2000.
4. Bittar RG, Olivier A, Sadikot AF, et al: Localization of somatosensory function by using positron emission tomography scanning: a comparison with intraoperative cortical stimulation, *J Neurosurg* 90(3):478–483, 1999.
5. Busch E, Beaulieu C, de Crespigny A, Moseley ME: Diffusion MR imaging during acute subarachnoid hemorrhage in rats, *Stroke* 29(10):2155–2161, 1998.
6. Falyar CR: Using transcranial Doppler sonography to augment the neurological examination after aneurysmal subarachnoid hemorrhage, *J Neurosci Nurs* 31(5):285–293, 1999.
7. Goetz CG, Pappert EJ: *Textbook of clinical neurology,* Philadelphia, 1999, WB Saunders.
8. Gould R: State of the art in digital imaging techniques. In Moss A, Ring E, Siggins C, editors: *NMR, CT and interventional radiology,* San Francisco, 1984, University of California Press.
9. Greenberg R, Ducker T: Evoked potentials in the clinical neurosciences, *J Neurosurg* 56(1):1–18, 1992.
10. Hershey BL: Neuroimaging. In Goetz CG, Pappert EJ: *Textbook of clinical neurology,* Philadelphia, 1999, WB Saunders.
11. Huntington NA: The nurse's role in delivery of radioisotope for ictal SPECT scan, *J Neurosci Nurs* 31(4):208–215, 1999.
12. Jones DK, Dardis R, Ervine M, et al: Cluster analysis of diffusion tensor magnetic resonance images in human head injury, *Neurosurgery* 47(2):306–314, 2000.
13. March K: Transcranial Doppler sonography: noninvasive monitoring of intracranial vasculature, *J Neurosci Nurs* 22(2):113, 1990.
14. Mason PJB: Neurodiagnostic testing in critically injured adults, *Crit Care Nurs* 12(6):64, 1992.
15. Mazziotta JC, Gilman S: *Clinical brain imaging: principles and applications,* Philadelphia, 1992, FA Davis.
16. Pagana KD, Pagana TJ: *Mosby's diagnostic and laboratory test reference,* ed 4, St Louis, 1999, Mosby.
17. Papanicolaou AC, Simos PG, Breier JI, et al: Magnetoencephalographic mapping of the language-specific cortex, *J Neurosurg* 90(1):85–93, 1999.
18. Rogers AE, Dykstra C: EEGs: a closer look at a familiar diagnostic test, *J Neurosci Nurs* 21(4):227, 1989.
19. Rudy E: *Advanced neurological and neurosurgical nursing,* ed 4, St Louis, 1984, Mosby.
20. Ryu H, Tanaku T, Yamamoto S, et al: Magnetic resonance cisternography used to determine precise topography of the facial nerve and three components of the eighth cranial nerve in the internal auditory canal and cerebellopontine cistern, *J Neurosurgery* 90(4):624–634, 1999.
21. Schulder M: Personal communication, Sept 19, 2000, Department of Neurosurgery, New Jersey Medical School, Newark, NJ.
22. Stebbins GT: Neuropsychological testing. In Goetz CG, Pappert EJ, editors: *Textbook of clinical neurology,* Philadelphia, 1999, WB Saunders.
23. Torres LS: *Basic medical techniques and patient care in imaging technology,* Philadelphia, 1997, JB Lippincott.
24. Wagle WA: Why and when radiological studies should be ordered for neurological disorders. In Popp AJ, editor: *The primary care of neurological disorders,* Park Ridge, IL, 1998, American Association of Neurological Surgeons.

PART TWO

Neurologic Disorders

Central Nervous System Infections

Infections of the central nervous system (CNS), primarily the brain and spinal cord, are often life threatening and as such represent distinct challenges to those diagnosing and treating them. Sometimes these conditions can be difficult to recognize and once recognized can also be difficult to treat, due to the location of the infection. Prompt diagnosis and the initiation of appropriate treatment are vital to resolve the problem. CNS infections such as bacterial meningitis require antibiotics with the ability to penetrate the spinal fluid in order to effectively kill the microorganisms.

This chapter discusses the fundamental chain of infection that is the basic infectious disease process.[74] A variety of infectious diseases are discussed, including meningitis (bacterial, viral, fungal), brain abscess, and surgical-site infections of the CNS. Insect-borne diseases such as Lyme disease, ehrlichiosis, and West Nile virus are reviewed as well.

It is to the advantage of the neuroscience clinician to have knowledge of fundamental infection control and the infections disease process. This knowledge significantly contributes to the clinician's ability to provide quality management to patients and truly be a patient advocate.

The diagnosis of and therapy for CNS infections is one of the most rapidly evolving and exciting areas in neuroscience. Infections of the CNS pose great challenges because these neuroinfective disorders often create acute, life-threatening situations. Prompt diagnosis and initiation of the appropriate therapies are imperative for an optimal neurologic outcome and recovery. Patient morbidity and mortality rates can be reduced with knowledge of the fundamental chain of infection and infection prevention strategies that affect disease transmission, neurologic assessment, and the implementation of acute supportive and rehabilitative interventions. Although there are many infections processes of the CNS, this chapter focuses on only the more common infections.

THE INFECTIOUS DISEASE PROCESS

The basic infectious disease process can be visualized as a chain formed of six links. In order for an infectious disease to reach the next host and cause disease, all of these links must occur in order without interruption. If even one of the six links is disrupted along the way, the infectious disease process stops and the next host will not acquire the pathogen. Figure 4-1 graphically illustrates this chain.

It is always helpful to think of this chain when considering any infectious disease process. One of the important roles of the neuroscience clinician is to be a true advocate for the patient. Implementing strategies to prevent infection burden in patients who are already very sick is one way nursing can make a significant reduction in a patient's morbidity and even mortality risk in some cases.

1. **Pathogen:** The pathogen is the potentially infectious microorganism. Microorganisms can be bacterial (e.g., *Haemophilus influenzae, Neisseria meningitidis*); viral (e.g., echoviruses, Herpes simplex virus); or fungal (e.g., *Candida albicans*), which manifest themselves as molds at ambient temperature and yeasts at body temperature. It should be noted that sometimes traditionally nonpathogenic microorganisms (i.e., those associated with "normal microbial flora" of certain parts of the body) can be pathogenic when introduced into an area of the body that should be sterile or where the organism does not normally inhabit. An example of this might be *Staphylococcus* species, coagulase negative (a normal component of human skin), which can cause disease when introduced into the normally sterile spinal fluid. This can happen in a motor vehicle accident, for example, when there is a traumatic injury with an open head wound. Some bacterial pathogens have special virulence factors to enhance their invasiveness and produce disease. They must be able to gain access to the host, find a unique niche, avoid normal host protective mechanisms, and multiply in the host. These capabilities make up the so-called pathogenic profile of the organism.[23] Predisposing factors may also make the host more vulnerable to CNS infections (e.g., chronic alcoholism, diabetes mellitus [DM], immunosuppression [such as that produced by steroid treatment], cancer immunotherapy, or even antirejection medications).

2. **Reservoir:** The reservoir is the habitat in which the microorganism exists peacefully. This is often the place in the human or animal host where the organism is "colonized." Examples of this in the human host would be the anterior nares, where methicillin-resistant *Staphylococcus aureus* (MRSA) colonizes, or vancomycin-resistant *Enterococcus* (VRE), which colonizes in the lower gastrointestinal (GI) tract and stool. These locales are the "reservoirs" for these organisms and cause no active infection for the host. The organisms remain

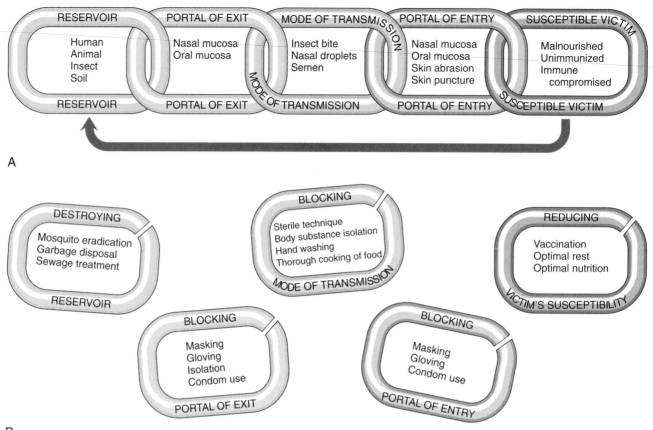

A

B

Figure 4-1 Breaking the chain of transmission of microorganisms from host to victim. *(From Copstead LC, Banaski JL:* Pathophysiology, *ed 3, St Louis, 2005, WB Saunders.)*

comfortable with sufficient nutrients and wait until the status of the host changes, which may encourage these organisms to grow and proliferate to a level and location(s) where an active infection begins.[69] Other examples of reservoirs include the skin and possibly contaminated inanimate objects such as bathroom doorknobs.

3. **Mode of escape:** This link represents how the microorganism gets out of its reservoir. An example is the same transient gram-negative microorganism that was acquired on the hand of a health care worker who has contact with a contaminated doorknob. Organisms can live for a significant amount of time on a fomite[55] (inanimate object) once placed there. The amount of time a microorganism can survive and be potentially infectious is characteristic of the individual microorganism itself.

4. **Transmission:** This link refers to the method the organism prefers or requires to be transmitted to the next host. Microorganisms want to survive, and they are preprogrammed to survive by spreading. Isolation practices in a health care facility are derived from knowledge of these methods. Microbes are transmitted by contact (i.e., touch) or by airborne droplets. Airborne microbes may be transmitted by mucous droplets small enough to travel long distances through the air, such as tuberculosis *(Mycobacterium tuberculosis)* and

chickenpox virus *(Varicella),* or larger mucous droplets that travel 3 to 6 feet from the host patient and drop due to their weight.[35] Examples of microbes that disseminate via droplet transmission are influenza virus and whooping cough *(Bordetella pertussis).*

5. **Mode of entry:** This refers to the way the infectious microorganism gets into the next host. For example, the organism may be transmitted by indirect contact (e.g., on the doorknob via dirty hands). Methods of hand hygiene are washing with soap and water at the sink or using an alcohol-based hand rub. It should be noted, however, that hands that are visibly soiled must be washed with soap and water. Steps 3, 4, and 5 can be thought of as a unit that fits together with the isolation practices generally used in health institutions. An example would be influenza virus, which can leave one host through the mouth via a cough, is transmitted through the air by large droplets of mucous, and then enters the next host's respiratory tract via the nostrils and breathing in the infectious droplets. To prevent this type of transmission, infection control would promulgate droplet precautions and a private room would be preferred. Table 4-1 lists a variety of infectious diseases affecting the CNS and recommended isolation practices.

6. **Host susceptibility:** This final link in the chain of infection revolves around how susceptible the host is to infection. Factors that come into play involve the

TABLE 4-1	Isolation Precautions Required for Infectious Diseases of the Central Nervous System

Disease or Condition	Recommended Isolation Precautions*	Comments
Diarrhea	Contact Precautions	This applies to antibiotic-associated *Clostridium difficile* as well; after active diarrhea is over, patient can go back to Standard Precautions.
Upper respiratory infection (cough, runny nose, fever, myalgia), especially during flu season (November–May)	Droplet Precautions	With the exception of diagnosed flu or RSV, patient can come out of Droplet Precautions when symptoms have resolved. It is possible for flu/RSV patients to still shed virus for 7 days in the former and 5 days in the latter after symptoms have resolved; those patients should be kept in Droplet Precautions for 7 and 5 days, respectively, even if respiratory symptoms have resolved.
Draining wound or abscess (cover if possible)	Contact Precautions	If the wound or abscess can be kept covered, Contact precautions may be suspended.
Arthropod-borne viral encephalitides (Eastern, Western, Venezuelan equine encephalomyelitis, St. Louis, California encephalitis, West Nile virus)	Standard Precautions; no added precautions	Rarely transmitted from person to person (by transfusion; and with West Nile virus via organ transplant, breast milk, or transplacentally). Install screens in windows and doors in endemic areas. Use DEET-containing mosquito repellants and clothing to cover extremities.
Cellulitis	Standard Precautions; no added precautions	No additional precautions necessary.
Closed-cavity infection	Standard Precautions; no added precautions	Category includes an open drain in place, limited or minor drainage, or no drain is in place; CSF leak also falls into this category unless a specific agent has been identified or there is a large amount of drainage or an abscess (see above).
Creutzfeldt-Jakob Disease, other prion-associated disease	Standard Precautions; no added precautions	ALERT: Special precautions are necessary when disposing of or disinfecting equipment and materials that had contact with the CNS of patients suspected of or having confirmed prion-associated diseases. See specific section in this chapter related to these precautions.
Dengue fever	Standard Precautions; no added precautions	Not transmitted from person to person.
Meningitis	Standard Precautions; no added precautions	Includes "aseptic" meningitis (i.e., viral or nonbacterial); bacterial meningitis (gram-negative enteric in neonates); fungal meningitis; *Listeria* meningitis; *Streptococcus pneumoniae* meningitis; tuberculous meningitis.
	Droplet Precautions	*Haemophilus influenzae* and known/suspected type B influenza: until 24 hours of antimicrobial drug therapy has been administered; then patient returns to Standard Precautions.
	Droplet Precautions	Meningococcal *(Neisseria meningitidis)* meningitis; use prophylaxis in those with *intimate* patient contact (erythromycin or a similar drug). After 24 hours of antimicrobial drug therapy, patient returns to Standard Precautions.
Multidrug-resistant organism	Contact Precautions	Generally patients infected with these organisms are placed in Contact Precautions; some hospitals have more stringent precautions depending on the microorganism(s) involved (organisms include MRSA, MDR-*Acinetobacter,* VRE, other drug-resistant gram-negative organisms). Contact facility's infection control epidemiologist.

*Reminder: Health care workers should use Standard Precautions with *all* patients. This is a set of work practices that puts a barrier between the health care worker and the patient. When the worker can reasonably anticipate splash or splatter of patient fluids, full face shield protection should be worn.
CNS, Central nervous system; *CSF,* cerebrospinal fluid; *MDR,* multidrug resistant; *MRSA,* methicillin-resistant *Staphylococcus aureus; RSV,* respiratory syncytial virus; *VRE,* vancomycin-resistant *Enterococcus.*

TABLE 4-2   **Possible Infection Control Interventions to Interrupt Disease Transfer to Another Host**

Link of Infectious Disease Chain	Possible Interventions
Pathogen	1. Use proper skin preparation on patient, including preoperative chlorhexidine gluconate baths the night before and the morning of the surgical procedure. 2. Let patient prep dry thoroughly before applying the drapes. 3. Administer appropriate antibiotic within 60 minutes of the incision.
Reservoir	1. Surgeon performs appropriate hand scrub, including cleaning under nails, before the case. 2. No participants in surgery should have artificial fingernails. 3. If the patient is in isolation of some sort, call infection control or look at any procedures you have for dealing with a surgical patient with that organism. 4. If surgical patient has a coexisting infection, be sure the operating team is aware of it; be prepared to reschedule the surgical procedure if necessary/possible to prevent the spread of that organism to the surgical site.
Mode of exit Transmission Mode of entry to next host	1. Wash your hands. 2. Use isolation precautions where appropriate. 3. Wear personal protective equipment as required including masks, gloves, gowns, etc. 4. Use aseptic technique. 5. Practice Standard Precautions. 6. When handling tissue during surgery be as gentle as possible, do not overcauterize, and always use careful sterile technique. 7. If sterile technique has been broken, move back from the table, go out and rescrub, regown, etc.
Host susceptibility	1. Encourage obese patient to lose weight before procedure. 2. Encourage patient to stop smoking before procedure (permanently if possible). 3. In patient who has diabetes, make sure condition as closely under control as possible. 4. Carefully have patient wash with chlorhexidine baths (usually 2%–4%) the night before and the morning of the surgical procedure.

general health of the next host. A cancer patient receiving chemotherapy is immunocompromised, as is a young child or an elderly patient or a patient with significant underlying disease (e.g., diabetes, asthma, peripheral vascular disease). Many factors affect the outcome of the infectious disease process.

In review, Table 4-2 divides the chain of infection into links and lists a variety of possible interventions, especially for the surgical patient, that can break this chain and prevent spread of the infection to others. It is helpful to think of this six-link process and how it relates to each of the infections discussed in this chapter. The clinician may not be able to intervene in all of the links of the disease process, but frequently can intervene in breaking at least one link, which subsequently protects the next host (i.e., other patients or health care workers) against infection. It is also important to realize that the use of these various interventions on a regular basis prevents the vulnerable neuroscience patient from acquiring a health care–associated infection during his or her stay. As patients in the hospital demonstrate increased acuity, the disease processes that the clinician is involved in will broaden.

INFECTIONS OF THE CENTRAL NERVOUS SYSTEM

The brain and spinal cord are relatively well protected from infective agents by the bones of the skull and vertebral column, the meninges, and the blood-brain barrier (BBB). This shield does have some weak points, however, such as the air sinuses and the thick bone of the mastoid process that covers the middle ear. It is also crossed by the emissary veins and by the diploic veins, which anastomose in the skull and have both external and internal venous connections.[21] Infections of the CNS often manifest as acute clinical situations. The infectious process may be straightforward and readily diagnosed, or the multidisciplinary team's expertise and experience may be needed to uncover the causative organism.

Infective culprits gain access to the CNS in a variety of ways, but the most common route of entry is hematogenous, or via the blood. Blood vessels within the choroid plexuses, meninges, and brain parenchyma are possible sites of invasion.[24] Organisms also enter the CNS by direct extension of nervous tissue via penetrating injuries that involve a defect in the dura at the base of the skull. This includes basilar skull fractures, missile injuries, fractures of the cribriform plate, and invasive neurosurgical procedures. Certain infections (e.g., parameningeal) may also result from an adjacent bony infection that involves the bones of the skull, face, and spine. Occasionally organisms invade the CNS along the peripheral nerves, such as with rabies. Creutzfeldt-Jakob disease may gain access to the CNS via corneal transplants, contaminated instruments, dura mater grafts, and natural growth hormone preparations that have been previously contaminated with this slow virus.

BACTERIAL MENINGITIS

Surrounding the brain and spinal cord are three protective membranes or meninges: the dura mater, the arachnoid membrane, and the pia mater.[67]

Bacterial meningitis primarily causes inflammation of the leptomeninges (pia mater and arachnoid) and involves the cerebrospinal fluid (CSF) in the subarachnoid space. Meningitis may result from four known causes: (1) bacteria, (2) viruses, (3) fungi, and (4) parasites. The infection can be acute, subacute, or chronic, with the patient's presentation dependent on the type of organism. Despite the introduction of effective bactericidal antibiotic treatment and the availability of preventive vaccine therapy, bacterial meningitis continues to be a serious cause of morbidity and mortality. Table 4-3 lists the available vaccines. The current meningitis vaccine is frequently recommended to college students via their new freshmen health packets and is mandated in some states.[46,75] It should be noted that this vaccine does not contain the type B meningococcal element. Type B is not generally found in the United States, occurring more often in other parts of the world.

Prevnar vaccine for pneumococcus (Streptococcus pneumoniae) is a conjugate vaccine for children, which is given by all pediatricians as a routine childhood vaccination.[26] The polysaccharide vaccine Pneumovax is not effective for children, but is quite effective in the elderly population with its activity lasting at least 5 years. It is currently recommended for all adults over 50 years of age and is frequently given during hospital stays to improve the level of immunity for the older adult. In addition, ProHIBIT for Haemophilus influenzae has been highly effective in protecting children from meningitis and other serious infections caused by this organism in the last 10 years. This vaccine is also routinely given to all children before school in the United States.

Etiology and Epidemiology

Bacterial meningitis is a common infectious disease that has been diagnosed throughout the world. In general, it affects the very young, the very old, and immunosuppressed persons; it favors males over females; and there is a higher incidence in the black versus the white population. However, these affinities are very pathogen specific. Patients with acute meningitis most often have fever, headache, meningismus, and altered mental status.[70] Approximately 2400 to 3000 cases of bacterial meningitis occur in the United States each year.[3,7] According to the Centers for Disease Control and Prevention (CDC), more than 300 people die each year from this disease. When this infection occurs, however, it has a significantly high case fatality rate in healthy adolescents.[27] This factor alone makes the disease frightening. Even those who survive can have horrific sequelae after this infection, including brain damage, organ failure, and multiple amputations from the toxin the meningococcal organism produces. When epidemics of bacterial meningitis, especially meningococcal meningitis, occur in a community, panic generally sets in and the public health system has to deal with the public's fears. This panic also occurs when health care workers are exposed to patients who are later diagnosed with bacterial meningitis. Prophylactic antibiotic treatment is warranted when intimate contact with the oral secretions of an infected person has occurred (see Table 4-3).

Before antibiotics came into use in the 1940s, mortality rates from bacterial meningitis were as high as 70%.[7,78] Although the mortality rate has improved with the use of antibiotics to 25%, this statistic has shown little improvement over the past 25 years.[45,78] In addition, the incidence of long-term sequelae in adults with bacterial meningitis is high. Some states, such as Maryland, have an increased number of cases among individuals younger than conventional college-age students.[72] This finding indicates the need to focus on earlier vaccination and education of physicians to recognize meningococcal meningitis in adolescents and young adults (ages 14 to 28). This will help to improve case fatality rates and possibly significant sequelae of this disease. Early administration of antimicrobial therapy in acutely ill patients lessens the risk of complications and sequelae.[63] The most common pathogens responsible for bacterial meningitis in the Unites States are included in Table 4-4. The overall annual incidence of bacterial meningitis has decreased and has been attributed to the widespread use of H. influenzae type B vaccine.

There has been an increase in nosocomial meningitis, especially in patients 16 years of age or greater.[72] In a study conducted by Massachusetts General Hospital between 1962 and 1988, accumulating all cases of meningitis in those patients older than age 16, 40% of the total cases (n = 493) were nosocomial in origin, with 38% of those being gram-negative rods.[17] The overall case fatality rate for patients with single episodes of nosocomial meningitis was 35% and did not vary significantly over the 27 years of this study. Acute meningitis syndrome can be caused by a wide variety of infectious agents and may also be a manifestation of noninfectious disease as well; causative agent and features are among the parameters to consider in making the differential diagnosis (see Table 4-4).

Pathophysiology

The bacterial pathogens that commonly cause meningitis reside in the nasopharynx (Box 4-1). Often an upper respiratory infection causes the bacteria to become blood-borne. Meningitis can be transmitted in one of four ways: (1) airborne droplets passed from infected individuals through sneezing, coughing, or kissing, or droplets passed along through saliva and transmitted via drinks, cigarettes, or utensils; (2) direct contamination, such as a penetrating head

BOX 4-1	Causes of Bacterial Meningitis

- *Streptococcus pneumoniae (S. pneumoniae)* (44%)*
- *Neisseria meningitidis (N. meningitidis)* (16%)*
- Group B streptococci (8%)
- Staphylococci (e.g., *S. aureus* and coagulase-negative organisms) (6%)
- *Haemophilus influenzae* type b (Hib) (5%)
- Gram-negative enteric bacilli (e.g., *E. coli, Enterobacter,* and *Serratia* species) (4%)

Modified from Roos KL: Nonviral infections. In Goetz CG, Pappert EJ: *Textbook of clinical neurology,* Philadelphia, 1999, WB Saunders.
*The most common bacteria that cause meningitis.

TABLE 4-3   Preventive Therapy for Meningeal Infections

Vaccines	Indications for Vaccine	Indications for Treatment After Exposure	Chemoprophylaxis
Meningococcal Meningitis Available: 1. Monovalent serogroup A 2. Monovalent serogroup C 3. Bivalent A–C 4. Quadrivalent A/C/Y/W-135	1, 2, and 3: Recommended for use in epidemics of serogroup A and C 4: Used for military personnel and travelers in epidemic areas Cannot be used as a substitute for chemoprophylaxis in documented exposures CDC can assist with determining epidemic status and with vaccine program planning	All close family contact and at-risk populations, military camps, and day care Those in crowded classrooms (with less than 30 inches distance between chairs) Those in frequent contact during lunch and breaks are also indications	Rifampin *Adults:* 600 mg bid or 10 mg/kg for 2 days
Pneumococcal Meningitis Pneumovax 23 includes 23 serotypes, yet does not prevent all infections	All those over age 2 who lack splenic function (as a result of surgery or sickle cell disease) Patients with diabetes Persons with chronic cardiorespiratory, hepatic, and renal disease Immunosuppressed patients Residents of chronic care facilities	Treatment with appropriate antibiotics is essential and must start as early as possible	Not recommended
Prenvar	Conjugate pneumococcal vaccine for children could reduce up to 95% of pneumococcal meningitis infections		
***Haemophilus* Influenzae** ProHIBIT *Children:* 18 months to 5 years; dosage is 0.5 ml IM given once	Children with chronic illness and all children over 18 months attending day care	All household contacts, especially those under 6 years of age Advised for those exposed or in close contact, such as in day care centers	Rifampin *Children:* 20 mg/kg (up to 600 mg) once a day for 4 days

Modified from Schwetz K: Nursing management of adults with infectious, inflammatory or autoimmune disorders. In Beare P, Myers S: *Principles and practice of adult health nursing,* St Louis, 1990, Mosby.

injury or surgical procedure; (3) the bloodstream, such as from pneumonia; or (4) direct invasion of the meningeal membranes, such as in a brain abscess. To survive and effectively penetrate the meninges, the bacteria must first be able to survive within the vasculature and overcome additional host defenses.

After successful bacterial invasion, the inflammatory response becomes widespread and involves the pia-arachnoid, CSF, and ventricles; it does not usually involve adjacent parenchymal brain tissue.[6] A purulent exudate forms and is circulated quickly throughout the CSF that surrounds the brain and spinal cord. This exudate is particularly attracted to the base of the brain, the sheaths of the cranial and spinal nerves, and the perivascular spaces of the cortex. The bacteria and exudate can create vascular congestion by plugging the arachnoid villi. This obstruction of CSF flow and decreased CSF reabsorption can lead to increased intracranial pressure (ICP), brain herniation, and death. Hydrocephalus also may be a late sequela.

Two defense processes that can alter the ability of the body to fight bacterial meningitis effectively are (1) deficient CSF complement levels, which directly interferes with opsonization and the efficient phagocytosis of bacteria, and (2) low serum immunoglobulin G (IgG) concentrations, which decreases the brain's ability to protect itself.[58] Both of these processes contribute to host deficiency at the outset of bacterial meningitis. The uncontrolled invasion of bacteria into the leptomeninges and subarachnoid space creates increased meningeal blood flow, with neutrophils coming to the defense and migrating into the subarachnoid space. After **phagocy-**

TABLE 4-4	Features of Infectious Meningitis

Causative Agent	Features
Acute Bacterial Meningitis Requiring Antibiotics	
Haemophilus influenzae	Most common meningitis (48%)
	Rarely seen in adults; 90% <5 years of age
	In children: follows upper respiratory infection or otitis media
	In adults: follows parameningeal infection, CSF leak, immunodeficiency
	Death rate 3%–8%; leading cause of acquired mental retardation, 30%–50% have neurologic sequelae
Neisseria meningitidis (meningococcal)	Common (20%) and rapidly progressive
	Children and young adults most often affected; 90% are <45 years of age
	Epidemics occur in winter and spring
	50% of those hospitalized die within 24 hours of onset of symptoms
	50% have petechial or purpuric rash
	Common toxic complications: DIC, adrenal infarction, pneumonia, and concurrent infections
Streptococcus pneumoniae (pneumococcal)	Less common (8%) but has severe consequences
	Seen in children, older adults, and those with predisposing factors: infections of lungs, ears, and sinuses; splenectomy; alcoholism; sickle cell disease; CSF leak; endocarditis; immunosuppression
	30%–60% die, some despite antibiotic treatment
	Common neurologic sequelae: deafness, mental retardation
Nosocomial infections (gram-negative)	Rarely seen except in hospitalized patients
	Associated with neurosurgery (50%), trauma (30%), entry of CSF, debilitated or immunosuppressed patients
	Onset of fever and low glucose in CSF are helpful in diagnosis
	May need intraventricular reservoir plus systemic therapy
Staphylococci	Associated with infected shunts, brain abscess, sinusitis, endocarditis, and septicemia
Streptococci	Group B seen in endocarditis, cellulitis
Acute Meningitis not Requiring Antibiotics	
Viral meningitis	Common in summer; self-limited illness
	Sequelae or need for hospitalization is rare
Chronic and Subacute Meningitis Treated With Antimicrobial Agents	
Mycobacterium tuberculosis	Rare except in areas of endemic primary infection, increased drug resistance, and coincidence in AIDS patients
	Active disease found elsewhere in body: lung, bone, or kidney
	Cranial nerve palsies common
	One third of patients die; one third have neurologic sequelae
Treponema pallidum (syphilis)	Meningitis may be asymptomatic (25%) or have typical meningitis symptoms plus cranial nerve palsies, seizures, and increased intracranial pressure
	Lack of treatment results in progressive illness and ultimately neuronal damage with paralysis, seizures, and aphasia
	General paresis (dementia plus the above) and tabes dorsalis (spinal cord involvement) occur 15–20 years after untreated infection
Fungal meningitis (coccidiomycosis, *Candida, Cryptococcus,* aspergillosis, mucormycosis)	Rare form of chronic meningitis
	More common as nosocomial infection in immunologically impaired hosts
	Coccidioidomycosis is endemic in southwestern United States
	Candida, Cryptococcus, aspergillosis are opportunistic and found throughout environment
	Typical symptoms of meningitis (headache, fever, and stiff neck) occur in 50%; focal neurologic deficits suggest mass lesion (microabscess or intravascular process)
Parasitic meningitis (*Toxoplasma gondii, Acanthamoeba*)	Although rare, toxoplasmosis has two presentations
	Congenital: with seizures, mental retardation, and blindness
	Acquired: most patients are immunosuppressed as a result of malignancy or autoimmune disease
Rickettsial meningitis	Subacute meningitis neurologic deficits
	Rocky Mountain spotted fever is most common form; easily treated and rarely fatal
	Carried by vector (lice, ticks, fleas); has typical rash, few focal neurologic deficits

From Beare PG, Myers JL: *Adult health nursing,* ed 3, St Louis, 1998, Mosby.
AIDS, Acquired immunodeficiency syndrome; *CSF,* cerebrospinal fluid; *DIC,* disseminated intravascular coagulation.

tosis, the process in which certain cells engulf and dispose of microorganisms and cell debris, neutrophils contribute to the exudate as they rapidly disintegrate and add to the purulent matter. The role of neutrophils in this process, however, is not yet completely understood.[73]

Assessment

The clinical assessment of adults with bacterial meningitis requires a thorough neurologic assessment. The clinical assessment often reveals a classic clinical presentation of the following:

- Altered level of consciousness (LOC) that ranges from confusion, combativeness, and drowsiness to coma
- Cranial nerve (CN) palsies (II, IV, VI, VII, VIII)
- Meningeal irritation: Kernig's sign, Brudzinski's sign, and photophobia
- Fever as high as 39.5° C (103° F) and chills, headache, and nuchal rigidity (the three most common symptoms)
- Nausea, vomiting, and irritability
- Photophobia, nystagmus, abnormal eye movement
- Rash in approximately 70% of patients (rash may not blanch when pressed)
- Seizures: generalized seizures can occur in all age-groups early in the course
- Rapid respirations or respiratory failure
- Shock, sepsis, hypotension; cool, clammy skin

The patient's history is important. Bacterial meningitis is a medical emergency that can progress rapidly, and therefore it demands rapid diagnosis and intervention to save the patient's life and prevent disability. Meningitis often presents a clinically diverse picture depending on the extremes of age and the causative organism.[41] A very uncomfortable, steady, or throbbing headache is a prominent early symptom. The headache may be intensified by sudden movement and results from stretching and irritation of the meningeal membranes. **Nuchal rigidity,** or resistance to flexion in the neck, is often an early sign of bacterial meningitis but is absent in 20% of patients, particularly the very young and the very old.

Signs of meningeal irritation include Brudzinski's sign and Kernig's sign. **Brudzinski's sign** is elicited by passively flexing the patient's head and neck onto the chest. A positive Brudzinski's sign results in involuntary flexion of the hips and legs (Fig. 4-2, *A*). **Kernig's sign** is the inability to extend the leg when the thigh is flexed onto the abdomen, which results from inflamed meninges and spinal roots. It is identified by flexing the patient's upper leg at the hip to a 90-degree angle and then attempting to extend the leg at the knee. Kernig's sign is present if the patient is unable to extend the leg or complains of hamstring pain (Fig. 4-2, *B*). The patient may also assume the tripod position with knees and hips flexed, back arched lordically, neck extended, and arms brought back to support the thorax.

Focal neurologic signs that include cranial nerve palsies can appear early or late.[58] Because of inflamed nerve sheaths, it is not uncommon to see dysfunction of CNs III to XII, with CN VII (facial) and CN VIII (acoustic) showing the greatest

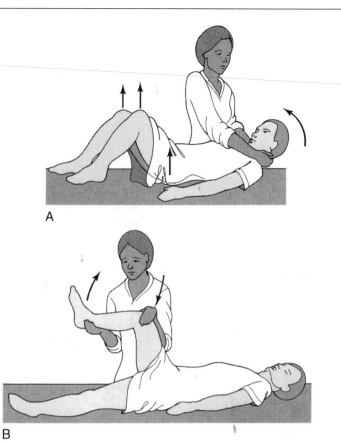

A

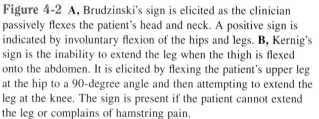

B

Figure 4-2 A, Brudzinski's sign is elicited as the clinician passively flexes the patient's head and neck. A positive sign is indicated by involuntary flexion of the hips and legs. **B,** Kernig's sign is the inability to extend the leg when the thigh is flexed onto the abdomen. It is elicited by flexing the patient's upper leg at the hip to a 90-degree angle and then attempting to extend the leg at the knee. The sign is present if the patient cannot extend the leg or complains of hamstring pain.

frequency of dysfunction (Table 4-5). Seizures are present in 50% of all cases.[31] Seizure frequency is 44% with *H. influenzae*, 25% with pneumococcal meningitis, and 10% with meningococcal meningitis.[31]

Alterations in LOC range from drowsiness to coma. Altered LOC results from increased ICP caused by cerebral edema, brain infarction, or obstruction of CSF flow.[73] Young adults with meningococcal meningitis may experience sudden alterations in consciousness that lead to rapid coma or manic behavior. The rash may initially be macular but may progress to petechiae and purpura, mainly on the trunk and extremities, and may be accompanied by signs of septic shock. Petechiae and purpuric lesions occur in approximately half of the patients with meningococcal meningitis (Figs. 4-3 and 4-4).

Neurodiagnostic and Laboratory Studies

Expedient diagnosis of bacterial meningitis is essential to successful patient outcome and can be based on the following studies:

TABLE 4-5	Cranial Nerve Involvement in Central Nervous System Infections		
Cranial Nerve(s)	**Anatomic Features**	**Significance**	**Consequence**
I	Traverses dura mater and ethmoid bone, surrounded by a cuff of arachnoid; terminates in free nerve endings within the nasal mucosa and nasopharynx	Is the only cranial nerve in direct contact with the external environment	May provide a route of direct CNS inoculation for neurotropic viruses
II	Develops as a part of the brain and is contained within the subarachnoid space up to its point of entry into the eye	Increased intracranial pressure causes papilledema; chronic increased pressure results in optic atrophy	Early signs are retinal vascular engorgement followed by blurring of the optic disc, with hemorrhages appearing later; initial visual change is enlargement of the physiologic blind spot; if intracranial hypertension persists, transient visual blurring and concentric constriction of visual fields occur; chronic papilledema progresses to optic atrophy and blindness; central scotomas may occur but are rare
	Myelin sheath is composed of central myelin	May be the target of immune response against central myelin in postinfectious encephalitis or encephalomyelitis	Visual field deficit (usually central or centrocecal scotoma)
III	Passes directly beneath the edge of the tentorium cerebelli below the uncus of the temporal lobe	Is almost always the first structure compressed by the uncus during transtentorial herniation	Paresis of CN III parasympathetic fibers causes pupillary dilation; interruption of nerve supply to all extraocular muscles except lateral rectus and superior oblique causes lateral deviation of the eye and ptosis
III, IV, V, VI	Travel together in the wall of the cavernous sinus	All may be affected by cavernous sinus thrombosis	Total ophthalmoplegia, midposition fixed pupil, corneal reflex and ipsilateral facial sensation
V, VI	Travel in close proximity to the tip of the petrous bone	May be injured in the course of chronic otitis media, especially where osteomyelitis of the petrous tip has developed	Abducens palsy (lateral rectus weakness) and ipsilateral facial pain or sensory loss (Gradenigo's syndrome)
IX–XI	Exit from the skull through the jugular foramen	May be injured by thrombosis of the internal jugular vein at the jugular foramen	Ipsilateral palatal weakness and diminished gag reflex; weakness of trapezius and sternomastoid muscles on the involved side (jugular foramen syndrome)
III–XII	Myelin sheaths composed of peripheral myelin	May be involved with peripheral nerves and spinal nerve roots in postinfectious polyneuritis (Landry Guillain-Barré syndrome)	Deficits of any cranial nerve except I or II may occur; CN VII most often involved

From Greenlee J: Anatomic considerations in central nervous system infections. In Mandell G, editor: *Principles and practice of infectious disease,* ed 3, New York, 1990, Churchill Livingstone.
CN, Cranial nerve; *CNS,* central nervous system.

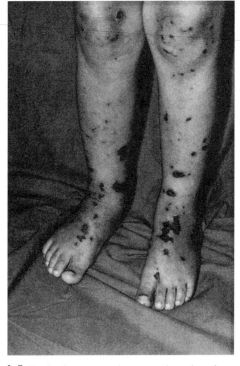

Figure 4-3 Rash of acute meningococcal septicemia or petechiae.
(From Farrar W, Keboli A: Meningitis due to Listeria monocytogenes *and other gram-positive bacilli. In Lambert H: Infections of the central nervous system, Philadelphia, 1991, BC Decker.)*

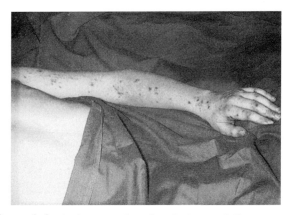

Figure 4-4 Meningococcal septicemia (purpura). Large ecchymoses beginning to resolve.
(From Farrar W, Keboli A: Meningitis due to Listeria monocytogenes *and other gram-positive bacilli. In Lambert H: Infections of the central nervous system, Philadelphia, 1991, BC Decker.)*

- Computed tomography (CT)/magnetic resonance imaging (MRI): Necessary before but should not delay a lumbar puncture.
- Lumbar puncture (LP): In patients with coma, if meningitis is suspected, a CT scan should be done as soon as possible followed by an LP to obtain CSF. CSF analysis is the most crucial diagnostic test and is

the gold standard for diagnosis. It includes measurement of above-normal opening pressure; observation of turbidity; cell count and differential (red blood cell count: negative); glucose, lactic acid, and protein concentration; Gram stain (usually positive); and cultures on blood agar, chocolate agar, and enriched broth. CSF abnormalities include polymorphonuclear leukocytic pleocytosis, decreased or absent glucose concentration, and increased protein concentration (Table 4-6). The serum blood glucose is obtained at the same time for comparison. The norm for the CSF glucose concentration is two thirds of the blood glucose concentration. Glucose is usually decreased (40 mg/dl) (see Chapter 2).

ALERT: Postpone the LP in certain patients, such as those in the acute phase of meningitis (i.e., those patients at great risk for bacterial shock syndrome, increased ICP, or brain herniation).[31] The initiation of rapid antibiotic therapy and blood cultures is warranted in all patients.[31]

- Two sets of blood cultures should be obtained before antibiotics are administered.
- Urine cultures.
- Arterial blood gases (ABGs).

Advances in the use of polymerase chain reactions (PCRs) to amplify specific areas of deoxyribonucleic acid (DNA) can also facilitate the diagnoses of several viral and bacterial diseases. Inquiry should be made to the clinical microbiology laboratory to determine what testing is done to help in prompt diagnosis of acute meningitis. Newer rapid PCR tests may be available in some centers.

Treatment

Emergency Department

Patients who present to the emergency department (ED) with suspected bacterial meningitis require immediate triage, diagnosis, and treatment. Patients or the family may report an acute onset of symptoms or symptoms that gradually developed over 1 to 2 days with headache, stiff neck, fever, and vomiting. Patients may have had a recent history of infection (e.g., ears, sinuses, or upper respiratory infection), illicit drug use, or foreign travel. Contributing or predisposing factors may include alcoholism, homelessness, infection with human immunodeficiency virus (HIV), spleen surgery (look for abdominal scar), recent neurosurgery for traumatic brain injury (TBI) with a fracture at the base of the skull, a CSF leak from the nose or ear, or an infected ventricular peritoneal (VP) shunt.

The urgent need for treatment in the ED is the first management priority for patients with bacterial meningitis. Antibiotic treatment should be started within 30 minutes of clinical presentation due to the rapidly progressive nature of this disease process. The treatment team should not wait for CT scan or LP results. If the LP must be delayed, blood cultures should be obtained and antibiotic therapy started immediately after.[12,45] After the administration of antibiotic therapy, the search begins for the offending organism via the patient's history, physical examination, and CSF and blood

TABLE 4-6	Typical CSF Findings in CNS Infection				
Infection	Cells	Percentage Neutrophils	Glucose	Protein
Bacterial meningitis	1000–10,000/μl	>50%	<40 mg/dl	>150 mg/dl
Aseptic meningitis	10–2000/μl	Early 2/3 > 50%	Normal	<100 mg/dl
Herpes simplex virus encephalitis	0–1100/μl	<50%	Normal	<100 mg/dl
Tuberculous meningitis	100–500/μl	Early >50% Late <50%	<40 mg/dl	>150 mg/dl

From Carpenter C et al: Infections of the nervous system. In Andreoli T, editor: *Cecil essentials of medicine*, ed 2, Philadelphia, 1990, WB Saunders.
CNS, Central nervous system; *CSF*, cerebrospinal fluid.

BOX 4-2	Potential Complications of Bacterial Meningitis

- Hydrocephalus caused by clogging and obstruction of the choroid plexus and arachnoid villi with purulent exudate
- Increased ICP caused by vasogenic edema with increased permeability of the blood-brain barrier (BBB)
- Cytoxic edema caused by the release of toxins from neutrophils and bacteria, leaky brain cell membranes, and increased secretion of antidiuretic hormone (ADH)
- Interstitial edema resulting from the obstruction of CSF circulation
- Vasculitis leading to thrombosis or hemorrhage
- Fibrous adhesions

---

cultures. Specific changes in antibiotic therapy based on the assessment findings should be made within 2 hours of initial patient contact. Droplet isolation is usually maintained for 24 hours after the initiation of the appropriate antimicrobial therapy.[37,57] In addition to controlling the infectious process, treatment goals must include preventing further brain insult from the possible complications of cerebral edema, hemorrhage, hydrocephalus, inflammation, and seizures (Box 4-2).

ALERT: Potential complications: The rapidly acting inflammatory infectious process of bacterial meningitis can produce a variety of associated complications, including hydrocephalus, increased ICP, and cytoxic edema.[73]

Acute Care

Once the ED protocols have been completed, the patient is transported to the intensive care unit (ICU) for acute care and close monitoring and observation. Comprehensive neurologic assessments are performed focused on the initial ED assessment described previously. During the acute phase of bacterial meningitis, therapy may include the following:

- Intravenous (IV) mannitol to treat rapid elevations in ICP
- IV fluids with intake and output (I&O)
- ICP monitoring and CSF drainage via external ventricular drain if ICP is elevated

- Bed rest with head of bed (HOB) elevated 30 to 45 degrees
- Intubation and hyperventilation to maintain the $Paco_2$ between 25 and 35 mm Hg
- Blood and CSF cultures (may be repeated as ordered)
- Administration of glucose for a low glucose concentration (less than 40 mg/dl) or for a CSF/blood glucose ratio less than 0.6
- Antibiotic therapy (based on specific organism identified)
- Dexamethasone (Decadron) therapy to decrease meningeal inflammation if ordered
- Seizure precautions and anticonvulsant therapy only if patient has seizures and may not be recommended prophylactically
- Private room with decreased lighting; a nonstimulating environment with respiratory isolation for 24 hours after the initiation of appropriate antibiotic therapy
- Pain assessment and appropriate pain management
- Fever management: antipyretics and cooling devices to control hyperpyrexia
- Induction of barbiturate coma if ICP continues to rise (see Chapter 10)

As the acute inflammatory period subsides, the patient requires close monitoring to prevent secondary complications. The clinician should observe and monitor closely for seizures, increased ICP, the syndrome of inappropriate antidiuretic hormone (SIADH) (see Chapter 5), disseminated intravascular coagulation (DIC), cerebral infarctions, pain and headache, GI bleeding, nutritional deficits, deep vein thrombosis (DVT), pulmonary embolus (PE), respiratory (pneumonia) or cardiac (endocarditis) complications, and septic shock. The drug of choice depends specifically on identification of the organism. Empiric therapy before organism identification is listed in Table 4-7; pathogen-specific therapy is listed in Table 4-8.

Because of increased capillary permeability during the acute inflammatory process, antibodies used during this time can easily pass through the blood-CSF barrier and effect greater penetration of the CSF. However, there is less capillary permeability as the inflammatory process improves, and this results in a decrease in the CSF antibiotic concentration. If there was a delay in treatment, the patient's condition may be a downhill course that leads to the loss of extremities, a vegetative state, or early death.

TABLE 4-7	Antimicrobial Therapy Based on Etiologic Organism		
	Antibiotic and Dose (Intravenous Unless Indicated)		
Organism	**Infants (>2000 g)**	**Children**	**Adults**
Group B streptococcus	Ampicillin 50 mg/kg q6h plus amikacin 10 mg/kg q8h or gentamicin 2.5 mg/kg q8h		
Neisseria meningitidis		Penicillin G 250,000–400,000 units/kg/day (divided q4h) plus (at end of therapy) oral rifampin; older than 1 yr: 10 mg/kg q12h for vdays; younger than 1 yr: 5 mg/kg q12h for 2 days	Penicillin G 20–24 million units/day (divided q4h) plus (at end of therapy) oral rifampin 600 mg q12h for 2 days
Streptococcus pneumoniae		Cefotaxime 225 mg/kg/day (divided q6h) or ceftriaxone x 40 mg/kg/day (in a once- or twice-daily dosing interval) *plus* vancomycin 40 mg/kg/day (q6h dosing interval)	Cefotaxime 8–12 g/day (divided q4h) or ceftriaxone 4 g/day (2 g q12h) *plus* vancomycin 2 g/day (in a 6 or 12 hr dosing interval)
Enteric gram-negative bacilli (except *Pseudomonas aeruginosa*)	Cefotaxime 50 mg/kg q8h plus amikacin or gentamicin	Cefotaxime or ceftriaxone (as above)	Cefotaxime or ceftriaxone (as above)
Pseudomonas aeruginosa	Ceftazidime 50 mg/kg q8h	Ceftazidime 150 mg/kg/day (q8h dosing interval)	Ceftazidime 6 g/day (q8h dosing interval)
Listeria monocytogenes	Ampicillin 50 mg/kg q6h plus amikacin or gentamicin for 3–5 days	Ampicillin 150–200 mg/kg/day (q4h dosing interval)	Ampicillin 12 g/day (divided q4h)
Haemophilus influenzae type b	Cefotaxime	Cefotaxime or ceftriaxone	Cefotaxime or ceftriaxone
Staphylococcus aureus, methicillin sensitive	Methicillin 50 mg/kg q6h	Oxacillin 200–300 mg/kg/day (divided q4h)	Oxacillin 12 g/day (divided q4h)
Staphylococcus aureus, methicillin resistant	Vancomycin 15 mg/kg q8h	Vancomycin 40 mg/kg/day (divided q6h)	Vancomycin 2 g/day (divided q6h)

From Goetz CG, Pappert EJ: *Textbook of clinical neurology,* Philadelphia, 1999, WB Saunders.

Postacute and Nonacute Care

Patients who are fortunate enough to be diagnosed and treated early may be transferred to the postacute or nonacute setting for follow-up. Therapies will be continued with close monitoring for potential complications (e.g., hydrocephalus). As the patient is stabilized, supportive therapy is continued in preparation for discharge, with explanations given regarding all treatments and medications and the need for absolute compliance.

Rehabilitation and Home Care

For patients requiring additional care, home health care and rehabilitation may be prescribed for neurologic deficits. Supportive therapies may include physical therapy (PT), occupational therapy (OT), speech therapy (ST), and rehabilitation

(see Chapter 13). Family support and education is provided to help the family cope with complications, particularly if one or more of the patient's extremities were amputated.

TUBERCULOUS MENINGITIS

Etiology and Epidemiology

Tuberculous (TB) meningitis is the most common and serious form of CNS tuberculosis. It is responsible for grave morbidity and mortality statistics in underdeveloped countries but until recently has not been a common cause for concern in developed nations. Currently the annual incidence is approximately 10 million worldwide.[4,68] Children under

TABLE 4-8	Pharmacology Summary: Meningitis, Encephalitis, and Parameningeal Disorders	
Infection	**Medication**	**Approximate IV Dosage**
Bacterial Meningitis		
Haemophilus influenzae	Ceftriaxone	4 g/day (qd or bid)
	Ampicillin	100 mg/kg/day
	Chloramphenicol*	100 mg/kg/day
Meningococcal	Penicillin G	15–24 million units/day (q4h)
	Chloramphenicol*	50–100 mg/kg/day
	Ceftriazone*	
Pneumococcal	Penicillin G	As above
	Chloramphenicol	50–75 mg/kg/day
	Ceftriaxone*	4 g/day (q6h)
Nosocomial Infection†		
Staphylococcus	Methicillin	10–12 g/day
Streptococcus group B	Penicillin G	As above
Gram-negative	Gentamicin (IV or intrathecal‡)	3–5 mg/kg/day
	Chloramphenicol	50–75 mg/kg/day
Pseudomonas	Third-generation cephalosporin	
	Gentamicin	As above
Tuberculous Meningitis	Isoniazid (INH)	10 mg/kg/day
	Rifampin	600 mg/day
Parameningeal Infection†		
Brain abscess	Penicillin G and chloramphenicol (or tetracycline*)	20 million units/day 1–1.5 g q4h
Epidural and subdural empyema	Methicillin/nafcillin and chloramphenicol	1.5–2 g q4h
Staphylococcus		1–1.5 g q4h
Encephalitis		
Herpes simplex	Vidarabine (Ara-A)	15 mg/kg/day
	Acyclovir	30 mg/kg/day

From Beare PG, Myers JL: *Adult health nursing,* ed 3, St Louis, 1998, Mosby.
*If allergic to penicillin.
†Dependent on sensitivity results.
‡Needs ventricular reservoir.

age 5 and adults under age 40 are most often affected, but TB meningitis may affect any age-group.[40,47] The incidence of TB meningitis is increasing in the United States due to the occurrence of neural tuberculosis in persons with acquired immunodeficiency syndrome (AIDS).[4,68] Patients may require prolonged hospitalization, and there is significant danger of death or irreversible brain damage.[68]

Pathophysiology

TB meningitis involves the basal meninges, cerebrum, and spinal meninges. It is nearly always preceded by the invasion of tuberculosis elsewhere in the body, often the lungs.[40,47] Brain or spinal subpial tuberculomas are the likely route through which tubercle bacilli enter the CSF.[40] When the tuberculomas erode the pia, mycobacteria enter the CSF, and meningitis follows.

The exudate that forms as a result of the bacterial invasion is located predominantly in the basilar cisterns and surrounds the cranial nerves and major blood vessels at the base of the brain. As the basilar cisterns become filled with the purulent exudate, the flow of CSF is blocked, and an obstructive hydrocephalus may develop. The exudate also blocks reabsorption of the CSF by arachnoid granulations, which results in communicating hydrocephalus.[23]

Assessment

Assessment of the individual with suspected TB meningitis may include the following:

- History: often uncovers a long history of symptoms, which may have been present for 2 weeks to 3 months before the onset of meningitis
- Comprehensive neurologic assessment
- Level of consciousness: confusion with significant behavioral changes that may progress to coma
- Pupils: large, sluggish
- Common initial symptoms: headache, fever, nausea/vomiting, irritability, difficulty sleeping, and fatigue
- Headache: may increase in intensity
- Significant behavioral changes: confusion that may progress to coma
- Motor status: involuntary movements not uncommon; may progress to hemiplegia
- Cranial nerve palsies: especially CNs III and VI
- Papilledema
- Increased ICP: with meningeal inflammation and advancing disease process
- Stiff neck (nuchal rigidity)
- Seizures

- Fever: may increase, with a temperature that ranges from a low-grade fever to (but not usually above) 39° C (102.2° F)
- Vital signs: possible increased pulse and irregular respirations

Neurodiagnostic and Laboratory Studies

Diagnostic studies for TB meningitis include the following:
- LP: Examine CSF for the TB organism, increased protein, decreased glucose levels, increased pressure, and a yellowish hue. Cultures and acid-fast stains by CSF are often negative, and moderate pleocytosis of 25 to 500 cells/mm³ occurs, with lymphocytes as the predominant cell. Polymorphonuclear leukocytes are present in increasing numbers, especially during the first 10 days of infection; thereafter lymphocytes predominate.[68]
- Chest x-ray.
- Tuberculin skin testing.
- CT/MRI to detect associated complications (e.g., areas of infarction, increased ICP, or hydrocephalus).[4,47]

The PCR research presently underway may also lead to a more rapid diagnosis of TB meningitis.[2,40,62]

Treatment

Acute Care

Depending on the severity of the patient's symptoms, the individual may be brought to the ED for emergency care. After treatment initiated in the ED, the patient is transferred to acute care to continue management. As with other bacterial infections of the CNS, the most significant factor in producing a favorable outcome depends on early identification of the offending tubercle bacilli and the rapid initiation of an effective antituberculous therapy. A 90% recovery rate is possible with early diagnosis and treatment.[4,68]

Medical Management

The literature cites some differences in the first-line drug approach and combination of recommended medication regimens.[9,47,68] Several drugs, each with special features, are used in the treatment of TB meningitis; variations in the medication regimen are presented in the following paragraphs (Table 4-9). After pharmacologic therapy, clinical improvement usually follows within 2 weeks. Research guidelines vary greatly in regard to the duration of effective treatment. Depending on the severity of the disease process, TB meningitis may require treatment for 6 months to 2 years.

Isoniazid, usually given in 300 mg/day dosages, is perhaps the most significant drug in the medication treatment program for TB meningitis. It has exceptional CSF penetration and low toxicity and is relatively affordable.[68] Pyridoxine is administered in 10 mg/day dosages along with isoniazid to prevent peripheral neuropathy because of the inhibitory effect that isoniazid has on the action of pyridoxine.

TABLE 4-9	Empirical Therapy for Tuberculous Meningitis	
	Dosage	
Drug	**Children**	**Adults**
Isoniazid (INH)	10 mg/kg/day once daily	300 mg/day
Pyridoxine		50 mg/day
Rifampin	10 mg/kg/day	600 mg/day
Pyrazinamide	30 mg/kg/day	30 mg/kg/day
Ethambutol*	15 to 25 mg/kg/day	15 to 25 mg/kg/day
Streptomycin†	20–40 mg/kg/day	
Corticosteroids Dexamethasone‡	0.15 mg/kg q6h	0.15 mg/kg q6h
Prednisone§	1 mg/kg/day	1 mg/kg/day

From Goetz CG, Pappert EJ: *Textbook of clinical neurology,* Philadelphia, 1999, WB Saunders.
*When antimicrobial resistance is suspected.
†The American Academy of Pediatrics recommends a combination of INH, rifampin, pyrazinamide, and streptomycin for tuberculous meningitis in children.
‡For altered consciousness, papilledema, focal neurologic signs, impending herniation, spinal block, hydrocephalus.
§For intractable headache, papilledema with otherwise normal neurologic examination.

Pyrazinamide is important in the treatment of TB meningitis because of its unique bactericidal activity. Pyrazinamide has a sterilizing effect on tubercle bacilli in acidic environments[68] and effectively penetrates the CSF. It is given in dosages of 35 mg/kg/day.

Rifampicin is used to prevent relapses because of its inhibitory effects on bacilli during spurts of metabolic activity.[62] However, adverse reactions to rifampicin are not uncommon, and the overall efficacy of rifampicin in TB meningitis treatment is currently uncertain.

Streptomycin, another drug used to treat TB meningitis, is usually limited to the first 2 to 3 months of treatment because its ability to penetrate the CSF depends on meningeal inflammation. Streptomycin, an ototoxic drug, is usually administered intramuscularly. Drug therapy with streptomycin continues for at least 1 year. It is discontinued if dizziness, tinnitus, or hearing loss occurs because of the possibility of permanent deafness.

Ethambutol at dosages of 15 to 25 mg/kg/day inhibits the growth of microbacteria. Often it is used as a second-line drug for situations in which other drugs cannot be prescribed. Ethambutol is used for the first 2 months of therapy because of its limited ability to maintain effective penetration of CSF after the initial inflammatory process. One potential side effect of ethambutol therapy is optic neuritis, which is manifested as impaired visual acuity and red-green color blindness and should be assessed weekly for the duration of treatment.[68]

Four-drug oral medication therapy that combines the bactericidal properties of isoniazid, rifampin, and pyrazinamide may be administered in conjunction with daily intramuscular doses of streptomycin.[4,68] Steroid therapy in the treatment of TB meningitis remains controversial. **Corticosteroids (dexa-**

methasone, prednisone) may be used to decrease inflammation and cerebral edema to prevent arachnoiditis in the acute stages of the disease. Patients are discharged when stable for close follow-up, and home health care is ordered as needed. Extensive education is needed for patient compliance with the medication regimen.

VIRAL MENINGITIS

In contrast to bacterial meningitis, patients with viral or aseptic meningitis may have similar symptoms. Viral meningitis is a nonpurulent inflammatory process that is confined to the meninges, choroid plexus, and other regions of the brain. Viral meningitis is caused by various viruses, such as the coxsackie viruses, mumps virus, and the virus of lymphocytic choriomeningitis. Characteristic symptoms may include malaise, fever (low grade), nausea, abdominal pain, and stiffness of the neck. Viral meningitis is more common in males than females and four times more common in children who are age 1 or older. The patient requires a comprehensive history and complete neurologic assessment.

The neurodiagnostic studies are the same as those used to diagnose bacterial meningitis described previously. When the laboratory results report viral antibodies, bacterial meningitis can be ruled out and supportive therapy provided. The CSF analysis from the LP usually reveals a characteristic normal glucose. Blood cultures are negative.

Nonacute and Home Care

Treatment is supportive, with pain relief for headache and the reassurance that most patients usually experience a benign clinical course that is short and uncomplicated with full recovery expected. If the patient experiences any motor deficits, rehabilitation can be prescribed and the patient discharged with instructions and follow-up clinic or office appointments.

LYME DISEASE

Lyme disease is the most common tick-borne disease in the United States. The incidence rate of Lyme disease has increased steadily since the first case was identified in 1982; it is a pathogen that has been seen worldwide. The United States has set up a systematic national surveillance system.[19,66] In 2001, 49 states reported 17,029 cases fulfilling the Centers for Disease Control and Prevention (CDC) surveillance case definition.[38,51]

Lyme disease primarily affects the skin, heart, joints, and CNS and is divided into early and late stages.[65,66] The first manifestation of the disease occurs on the skin and is called erythema migrans, which appears as an expanding erythematous papule or macule with central clearing at the site in the center of the deer tick bite.[51,64] It can resemble a bull's-eye target.

The organism, *Borrelia burgdorferi*, is a coiled spirochete. It can be cultured from the blood, skin lesion, synovial fluid, and CSF of infected patients. With the exception of skin biopsy specimens, the organism is very difficult to culture.[1,65,66,79]

Etiology

The bacterial spirochete that causes Lyme disease is introduced into the body by a tick bite. *B. burgdorferi* is carried in the feces or saliva of an infected tick. The Ixodes, or deer tick, is the main vector, the white-footed mouse the reservoir, and the white-tailed deer the intermediate host (Fig. 4-5). More than three fourths of cases occur from May to August, which is the peak time for questing (seeking of potential hosts) among nymphal Ixodes ticks. Ticks can thrive in moist, mild weather without heavy freezes. Infected ticks are endemic in some areas of the United States, most notably the Midwest, western wooded and coastal areas, and the northeastern coast.

The infection can cause disabling conditions such as joint pain and inflammation, arthritis, numbness and nerve complications, encephalopathy, chronic basilar meningitis, radiculitis, facial palsies, fatigue, and cardiac irregularities. In some cases, Lyme disease can be fatal.

The spirochete is passed to the tick during the larval stage as the ticks feed on the mice. The larval stage emerges in the spring 1 month after the eggs are deposited in the first year of tick life. Vegetation harbors the nymphal stage in the second year of tick life. Finally, the adult tick feeds on or is carried by the white-tailed deer or other feral or domestic animals. In either of the latter stages, a human may be an accidental host who becomes infected as the tick feeds (see Fig. 4-5). The tick must feed for 18 hours or more to implant the spirochete into the bloodstream, but because the tick is the size of a pinhead, most patients do not remember being bitten.

Pathophysiology

After the spirochete enters a human there is an incubation period of 3 to 32 days. At the end of incubation, the organism migrates to the skin and may cause a round, burning rash called erythema chronicum migrans (ECM). Immune complexes form when the patient develops antibodies. These complexes are deposited in the tissues and joints, where they contribute to the inflammatory response and rash. The organism also migrates to the lymph nodes and other body systems.

The pathophysiology of Lyme disease is best described by stages, with CNS involvement beginning as early as the initial rash stage (Table 4-10):

- Stage I: Occurs 3 weeks after the tick bite; characterized by ECM, general malaise, and flu-like symptoms. Neurologic symptoms include a stiff neck, headache, and fatigue.
- Stage II: Occurs 4 weeks to 6 months after the tick bite. Dissemination has occurred through blood and lymph, and the cardiac and neurologic systems are affected. Cardiac symptoms occur in 8% to 10% of patients and consist of palpitations, dizziness, shortness of breath, dysrhythmias, and, possibly, first-degree atrioventricular (AV) block. Neurologic

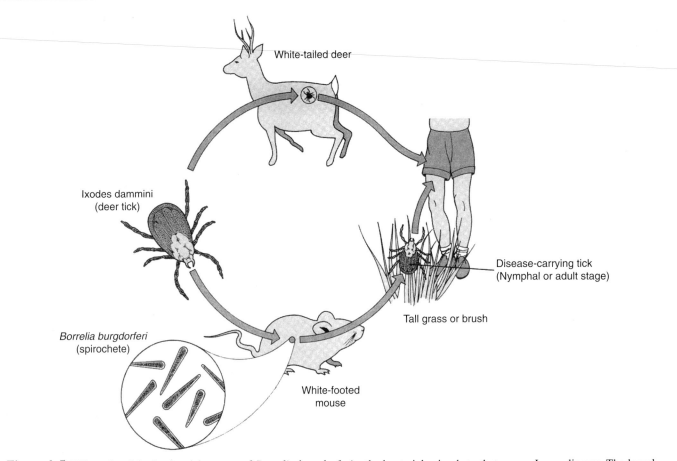

White-tailed deer

Ixodes dammini
(deer tick)

Disease-carrying tick
(Nymphal or adult stage)

Tall grass or brush

Borrelia burgdorferi
(spirochete)

White-footed
mouse

Figure 4-5 Life cycle of the Ixodes tick, vector of *Borrelia burgdorferi*—the bacterial spirochete that causes Lyme disease. The larval tick feeds on the white-footed mouse and becomes infected. When the larval tick molts into a nymph, it can inject the spirochete. Infected ticks at this stage can be in the grass, on humans, or on a pet or bird, or can be carried by a wild animal such as the white-tailed deer.

involvement may include chronic viral meningitis, Bell's palsy (CN VII), encephalitis, cranial neuritis, radiculitis (inflammation involving a spinal nerve root), and polyneuritis (an inflammation involving many nerves).[43]

- Stage III: Occurs a few weeks to 2 years after the bite. There is significant arthritis and evidence of invasion of brain parenchyma,[49] as well as chronic neuroborreliosis with parenchymal involvement (see Table 4-10).

In a patient who has not received the appropriate initial treatment, sequelae may occur 1 to 6 months after the onset of the disease. Those affected may develop monoarticular arthritis in the knees, CN VII palsies, carditis with heart block, viral meningitis, encephalitis, Guillain-Barré syndrome, mental changes with magnetic resonance imaging (MRI) abnormalities, transverse myelitis, and progressive neuropathy.[23,66]

In December 1998, the U.S. Food and Drug Administration (FDA) approved the world's first vaccine for the prevention of Lyme disease for individuals between 15 and 70 years of age. The vaccine contains an immunogenic recombinant protein of *B. burgdorferi*, outer surface protein A (Osp A) that has been lapidated for optimal immunity.[16,64] LYMErix

TABLE 4-10	Neurologic Manifestations of Lyme Borreliosis	
Stage I	**Stage II**	**Stage III**
Meningismus	Meningitis	Subacute encephalopathy
	Cranial neuritis	Polyneuropathy
	Peripheral neuritis	Encephalomyelitis
	Subtle encephalitis	Stroke
	Hemiparesis	
	Chorea	
	Cerebellar ataxia	

From Logigian EL, Steere AC: Lyme borreliosis. In Lambert H: *Infections of the central nervous system,* Philadelphia, 1991, BC Decker.

(SmithKline Beecham Biologicals) is an aluminum-adjuvant OspA vaccine. Three required doses of LYMErix (Osp A) within 12 months are needed to complete the full immunization. The second dose is given 1 month after the first dose and the third dose is given 11 months later. Immunization with Osp A vaccine stimulates the production of antibodies specific for Osp A. When a tick takes a blood meal from a vaccinated individual, it ingests these antibodies, which then bind to the surface of *B. burgdorferi* present in the tick midgut. Because of this unique mechanism, it is likely that high levels of circulating antibody will need to be maintained in vaccines to prevent against infection at the time of a bite from an infected tick.

Assessment

The first assessment should focus on the following:
- Complete health history

TIP: Specific questions should elicit information regarding the presence of a tick bite, a recent visit to a tick-infested area, and the details of the tick removal if the tick was removed.

- Neurologic assessment
- Cranial nerve palsies: especially CN VII
- Severe headache
- Skin examination: presence of a red macule or papule, malar rash, conjunctivitis, or urticaria
- Cardiac system: abnormal rhythms
- Palpation of the joints: pain and discomfort, signs and symptoms of arthritis
- Lymph nodes: regional lymphadenopathy
- Physical demeanor: assess appropriateness
- Malaise and profound fatigue

The symptoms of Lyme disease correlate with the stage of the disease. Neurologic assessment focuses on the signs and symptoms of meningitis. Because any nerve or nerve root may be involved, peripheral nerve function should be examined. Serial evaluation continues after admission and focuses on the aspects emphasized in the initial assessment. CNS function must also be evaluated because progression of the disease may produce encephalomyelitis.

ALERT: Pregnant women should seek medical care even in the absence of symptoms. Pregnant women and patients with a severe case of Lyme disease may require hospitalization and IV antibiotics. In addition, pregnant women with Lyme disease may be at risk for miscarriage, premature birth, stillbirth, and birth defects. Mothers who are promptly diagnosed and treated appear to have perfectly normal babies. It may be possible for the bacterium to pass from mother to fetus across the placenta, resulting in congenitally acquired Lyme disease.

Infectious disease and obstetric consultations should be requested to protect the mother and fetus. Breast-feeding mothers during active infection may want to discard breast milk during active infection and resume after treatment is completed when the mother is symptom free.

Neurodiagnostic and Laboratory Studies

Diagnostic and laboratory studies to identify Lyme disease include the following:
- MRI: Provides valuable data about brain involvement in the presence of nonspecific and sometimes confusing signs and symptoms.
- LP: A specific diagnosis is made by the PCR test using gene-splicing techniques to detect the bacterium itself and the presence of positive antibody titers in the serum and CSF. Immunoglobulin M (IgM) and

IgG Western blot analyses are considered confirmatory but may not be as sensitive as the enzyme-linked immunosorbent assay (ELISA). IgM titers peak between 3 and 6 weeks of onset, whereas IgG evolves more slowly over weeks to months. Specific IgG antibodies may appear in the CSF.[23] A negative titer in either does not, however, rule out Lyme disease, and false-positive results may occur with a number of other diseases (e.g., syphilis, Rocky Mountain spotted fever, and amyotrophic lateral sclerosis [ALS]).[44]
- Serum blood testing: For elevated erythrocyte sedimentation rate, leukocyte count, serum IgM, and serum glutamic oxaloacetic transaminase (SGOT); must be interpreted with caution.

If the patient seeks delayed treatment in the second or third stages, Lyme disease may manifest with the signs, symptoms, and radiologic manifestations of an intracranial mass lesion. In such cases, CT-guided stereotactic biopsy is necessary for tissue diagnosis to rule out the suspicion of a brain tumor. These studies are then confirmed by serologic testing.[49]

Treatment

Acute Care

Patients may or may not go to the ED following a suspected tick bite. Some individuals may still have the tick attached to their skin and request tick removal and testing for Lyme disease.

Lyme disease mimics many diseases, primarily chronic fatigue syndrome. The initial presentation and course of the disease may be highly variable. Initial symptoms may not initially be attributed to Lyme disease. Although Lyme disease most commonly affects the skin, nerves, and joints, any system (e.g., eyes, heart, lungs, and liver) may be involved.

Whether the patient with Lyme disease seeks emergency medical treatment or visits a family physician or health clinic with early symptoms, after diagnosis is suspected or established, the treatment of choice is antibiotic therapy (see Fig. 4-5). In the early stages, oral amoxicillin (Amoxil) 500 mg for 21 days is recommended and is prescribed for pregnant or lactating women, as well as children under 9 years of age. As with other CNS infections, early treatment is beneficial in preventing later complications.

Treatment with a high-dose IV medication is warranted when neurologic, cardiac, or arthritic signs appear. This treatment usually involves a third-generation cephalosporin such as ceftriaxone (Rocephin) at a dosage of 2 g every 8 hours for 30 days or cefotaxime (Claforan).[60] If IV therapy becomes necessary, successful treatment depends on the visual inspection and flushing of IV lines, verification of blood return every 4 hours to check patency of lines, and the changing of IV sites per hospital protocol during IV therapy. Ceftriaxone may precipitate calcium salts in adolescent girls, which causes gallbladder disease. Upper abdominal ultrasonography is recommended for patients who develop biliary colic while undergoing this treatment.

Approximately half of all patients with Lyme disease continue to experience minor recurring symptoms (i.e., headache, musculoskeletal pain, lethargy), even after antibiotic treatment. It remains unclear whether these symptoms result from a decreased number of live spirochetes (which would require further antibiotics) or from unresponsiveness to pharmacologic treatment.[44,53]

Patients with Lyme disease are infrequently admitted to a neuroscience critical care unit (NCCU) when rapid assessment of either CNS or peripheral nervous system (PNS) function is crucial. Assessment of central function focuses on LOC and on signs of acute infection, with careful determination of cranial nerve function. Rapid assessment of cardiac and respiratory systems is also essential if the patient is in acute distress.

ALERT: **Potential complications.** Bacteria may invade the brain and spinal cord early in Lyme disease. Complications occur in approximately 15% of those patients who undergo early treatment. Patients must be encouraged to comply strictly with the 10- to 21-day course of oral antibiotics. In some cases, 2 to 3 weeks of IV penicillin or ceftriaxone is required.

Surgical Management

In rare cases, the placement of temporary cardiac pacing devices may be required for a high degree of atrioventricular block.[44,53] Some patients may require a synovectomy or arthroscopic surgery to repair knee joints damaged by Lyme disease.

Postacute, Nonacute, and Home Care

Because Lyme disease is an acute recurrent inflammatory infection that is transmitted by a tick-borne spirochete, the affected areas may continue to cause problems. The knees, temporomandibular joint (TMJ), and other large joints are commonly affected with local inflammation and swelling. Range of motion (ROM) and hot or cold packs to the affected joints may relieve joint pain. Analgesics may be prescribed to relieve pain, and in some cases physical therapy may be needed.

Viral meningitis and Bell's palsy with paralysis of the facial nerve are examples of other conditions that may require time for recovery. The original symptoms last from one to several weeks and decline in severity over a 2- to 3-year period. There is no significant permanent joint damage. Medical follow-up may be required until symptoms subside. When symptoms linger, the clinician can reduce patient anxiety by explaining the disease process, course of treatment, and therapies to relieve symptoms.

Systems and symptoms that may become involved secondary to Lyme disease include the following:

- Cardiac: atrioventricular blocks, pericarditis, palpitations, syncope, myocarditis
- Neurologic: Bell's palsy, facial palsy that may be bilateral, meningitis, encephalitis, peripheral or cranial neuropathy, chorea, pseudotumor cerebri, mononeuritis multiplex, radiculopathy, memory loss, learning disabilities

---

| BOX 4-3 | Lyme Disease: Preventive Measures |

- Avoid tick habitats and, when visiting endemic areas, perform daily "tick checks"—especially along the hairline, around the ears, behind the knees, and in the armpits and groin.
- Empty water from birdbaths, containers, and anything that creates a breeding area.
- Use insect repellents and wear long-sleeved, light-colored shirts and long pants.
- Tuck the pants into socks or boots.
- Inspect pets for ticks and have them wear a tick collar.
- Remove ticks with fine tweezers; never use burning matches, petroleum jelly, or nail polish to remove a tick—do not crush the tick, which releases bacteria; apply alcohol to the spot, and save the tick in a small enclosed container for analysis because it is easier to test the tick for Lyme disease than a person.

- Others: joint swelling in one or a few joints followed by progressive or chronic arthritis, tendonitis, ECM, papilledema, conjunctivitis, and memory loss

Health Teaching

The prognosis is excellent for patients with Lyme disease who are appropriately treated, and there is a likelihood of full recovery. Education for the prevention of Lyme disease is a key role for clinicians[8] (Box 4-3). The patient should understand that early treatment of Lyme disease may abort the antibody response and thus the patient may be infected again if reexposed to *B. burgdorferi*—even within the same summer.[44,53]

Follow-up should include (1) observing for a rash or burning sensation, (2) strictly complying with the 10- to 21-day course of oral antibiotics, and (3) calling for medical advice. Post–Lyme disease syndrome (PLDS) has been observed in individuals who did not receive treatment with antibiotics. These individuals have complaints that included Lyme arthritis with knee pain, joint pain, sleep problems, facial nerve deficits, and other complaints. With greater public awareness and health teaching with more emphasis on the detection and treatment of Lyme disease with antibiotics, patients should expect few long-term neurologic or cognitive deficits.

OTHER TICK-BORNE DISEASES

Other tick-borne diseases include babesiosis, Q fever, Colorado tick fever, Rocky Mountain spotted fever, tick paralysis, and **human granulocytic ehrlichiosis (HGE).** HGE is a potentially fatal, tick-borne disease caused by a bacterium related or identical to *Ehrlichia phagocytophilia*. It is considered the second most common tick-borne infection in southeastern Connecticut, following Lyme disease. HGE can be transmitted by *Ixodes spinipalpis* ticks, which infect rodents. Of the residents in an area around Lyme, Connecticut, who sought treatment from their primary care physicians for acute febrile illness, 26% had laboratory evidence of HGE (by indirect fluorescent antibody staining or PCR testing). Patients with HGE are usually older and are more likely to have fever, chills, or dyspnea than are patients with Lyme disease. Campers and residents of rural areas are at greatest risk for HGE. Both Lyme disease and HGE should be considered in patients with a rash and fever. Antibiotic treatment is usually prescribed.

BRAIN AND SPINAL CORD ABSCESS

Infection processes that occur around the meninges, such as a brain abscess, subdural empyema, or extradural abscess, can be collectively considered parameningeal infections.[29] The majority of brain abscesses occur as the result of an extension of an infection arising from the frontal sinuses, mastoiditis, chronic otitis media, and dental or facial purulent foci.

Etiology and Epidemiology

A *brain abscess* is defined as an area of either encapsulated or free pus found in the brain parenchyma; this area varies in size and occurs either as a single lesion or as multiple lesions. Abscesses occur in approximately 1 out of every 100,000 hospital admissions. Men experience abscesses twice as often as women. The median age is 40 to 50 years, although they can occur at any age. Children under 15 years of age account for approximately 25% of all brain abscesses. Abscesses may develop after trauma, during neurosurgery, in association with other infections (specifically otitis media or paranasal sinusitis), from other sites such as abscessed teeth, from osteomyelitis, and from dirty needles.[34]

Osteomyelitis of the posterior wall of the frontal sinus may cause simultaneous epidural abscess, frontal lobe brain abscess, or subdural empyema. Streptococci, including anaerobic forms, are the most common bacterial agents, but fungi have also been found within CNS abscesses.[5] The infecting organisms may gain access to the brain by a hematogenous course from other foci in the body, but infection may also spread through sinus infection within the cranial cavity or from a penetrating head wound. Some patients give a history of headache and fever, but focal neurologic abnormalities are often absent. In other patients, somnolence, vomiting, and CN III or VI palsies can occur. Prompt head imaging and neurosurgical evaluation is imperative. The symptom course can last several weeks to months, but a fulminant course of even several days can erupt in very high fever and death in 2 weeks or less.

Although antibiotics and advanced neurodiagnostics and surgical techniques have improved the mortality and morbidity statistics in the past 10 to 15 years, some sources still report mortality rates as high as 33%.[13,71] Mortality rates differ according to the abscess location; an abscess is far more likely to be fatal if it is located in the thalamus, basal ganglia, or brainstem than in the cerebral hemispheres. Immunosuppressed patients and those with congenital heart disease are more susceptible to the development of a brain abscess.[3] Individuals who abuse drugs or who use contami-

nated needles are also at high risk for a brain abscess. In addition, patients with pulmonary arteriovenous malformations with right-to-left shunts are at greater risk because of the lack of filtration through the pulmonary capillary bed; the lungs normally filter out circulating bacteria.[3,38]

An **extradural abscess** is a collection of pus between the bone and the dura (e.g., mastoid infections) that results in pain and tenderness, elevated temperature, and discharge. Antibiotics remain the first-line treatment, and surgery may be indicated depending on the extent of the infection.

A **subdural empyema** or abscess most commonly follows sinusitis and usually develops over the convexity of the cerebral hemispheres within the subdural space.[3,38] A history of sinusitis or mastoiditis with a purulent discharge from the nose or ears usually precedes the current attack. Reports of severe headache and pain in and around the sinuses or mastoid area characterize an empyema. The diagnosis by CT or MRI can be missed if the collection is thin. These subdural effusions require the appropriate antibiotic therapy and may need surgical drainage. Cortical thrombophlebitis, which can result in focal epilepsy and hemiparesis, is particularly prevalent after a subdural empyema.

Spinal cord abscesses are classified as epidural or intramedullary. Individuals with diabetes mellitus (DM) show an increased incidence of **spinal epidural abscesses.** Debilitated individuals with sepsis more often develop **intramedullary spinal cord abscesses,** which may have originated as osteomyelitis in a vertebra. Spinal cord abscesses have four stages: (1) spinal aching, (2) severe root pain accompanied by spasms of the back muscles, (3) weakness caused by progressive cord compression, and (4) paralysis.

Intracranial epidural abscesses account for approximately 10% of all intracranial abscesses.[44] Before the advent of the human immunodeficiency virus (HIV) in the early 1980s, brain abscess accounted for approximately 1 in 10,000 general hospital admissions, with 1500 to 2500 cases treated in the United States each year.

Pathophysiology

The evolution of a brain abscess can progress through four stages: early and late cerebritis and early and late capsule formation. Initially, there is a **focal cerebritis** (inflammation of the cerebrum or brain) that may appear as a low-density area on a CT scan.[45] At least 10 days are necessary for this inflammation to mature from a "phlegmon" to an abscess. A brain abscess may take up to 14 days to form. A brain abscess acts either as a mass or as a destructive, space-occupying lesion. If left untreated, the abscess may enlarge and eventually rupture. Table 4-11 lists the predisposing conditions and likely pathogens in a brain abscess.

In general, a brain abscess may develop by one of four mechanisms:

1. The infectious organism reaches the brain from a nearby location such as nasal sinusitis or infections of the mastoid or middle ear.
2. The infectious organism reaches the brain by way of the hematogenous route from an infection in another location, commonly the lungs.

TABLE 4-11 Predisposing Conditions and Likely Pathogens in Brain Abscess	
Predisposing Condition	**Likely Pathogens**
Ear infection	Anaerobes, gram-negative aerobes *(Pseudomonas, Proteus)*, streptococci, *Haemophilus influenzae* (children)
Dental, sinus, mastoid, and pulmonary infections	Streptococci, anaerobes, staphylococcus, *Nocardia*
Trauma, surgery	*Staphylococcus aureus, Staphylococcus epidermidis*, gram-negative aerobes
Endocarditis, parenteral drug usage	*S. aureus, S. epidermidis*, streptococci, fungi, gram-negative anaerobes
Abdominal, pelvic infections	Anaerobes, gram-negative aerobes, streptococci
HIV/T-cell dysfunction	*Toxoplasma, Aspergillus, Candida, Nocardia*, mycobacteria, *Listeria, Salmonella, Cryptococcus* (and lymphoma mimicking abscess)
Neutrophil dysfunction	*S. aureus*, gram-negative aerobes, *Aspergillus, Zygomycetes, Candida*

From Johnson RT, Griffin JW: *Current therapy in neurologic disease*, ed 5, St Louis, 1997, Mosby.
HIV, Human immunodeficiency virus.

3. The infectious organism migrates to create a brain abscess by direct extension after a penetrating cerebral trauma or after a neurosurgical procedure.
4. Unknown: In approximately 20% to 25% of cases, no focus of infection is recognized.

Regardless of the infection focus, the infectious culprit is streptococci in more than 40% of abscesses. The infectious organisms can include *Staphylococcus aureus, Streptococcus viridans,* hemolytic *Streptococcus, Enterobacteriaceae,* and anaerobes.

Brain abscesses often begin near the cortical or cerebellar gray-white matter junctions. A majority occur in the cerebrum, and the remaining 20% are found in the cerebellum. Up to 20% of patients may have a brain abscess in more than one site. Initially, the infectious process begins as focal encephalitis and proceeds along a continuum of progressive encapsulation of pus toward the formation of an abscess. A pus-producing inflammation of the brain tissue leads to necrosis, perivascular cuffing, and cerebral edema. Defense mechanisms are then rallied, and microglia and fibroblasts attempt to begin capsule formation by surrounding the infected and necrotic site. During the next phase, granulation tissue and fibrous containment develop. Without treatment, the abscess slowly expands and eventually ruptures, resulting in brain herniation.

Assessment

A complete history is collected and a comprehensive neurologic assessment is performed. The assessment may reveal the following predominant signs and symptoms:
- Glasgow Coma Scale (GCS) score indicating altered LOC: confusion or drowsiness, coma, and ultimately herniation if left untreated
- Cranial nerve deficits: CN III, CN VI, or both
- Papilledema
- Nystagmus
- Focal neurologic deficit (e.g., hemiplegia)
- Neck pain with mild nuchal rigidity
- Headache: usually over the site of the abscess or paroxysmal headache (hemifacial or generalized, worsens with coughing or exertion)

- Seizures: focal or generalized
- Nausea and vomiting
- Fever: variable depending on the case
- Scalp tenderness: determined by palpating the head; symptoms often more related to the space-occupying properties of the abscess than to the infectious process
- Posture: especially head and neck position

The clinical presentation may vary widely according to the location of the abscess. Approximately 40% of patients may experience some impairment in their LOC. Seizures are a presenting sign in about one third of cases. About 75% of patients have focal findings related to the site of the abscess, the most common being hemiplegia.

Neurodiagnostic and Laboratory Studies

The following studies help lead to a diagnosis:
- CT: Computed tomography has revolutionized the diagnosis of brain abscess. Before CT, delays in diagnosis contributed significantly to the high morbidity and mortality rates in patients with brain abscess. Now diagnostic tests such as angiography, ventriculography, pneumoencephalography, and radionuclide brain scanning are virtually obsolete. CT is an excellent means of examining the brain parenchyma and is also the superior way of examining the paranasal sinuses, mastoids, and middle ear. Characteristically a brain abscess appears on contrast CT as a hypodense center with a peripheral uniform ring enhancement, surrounded by a variable hypodense area of brain edema (Fig. 4-6).
- Electroencephalogram (EEG): May reveal marked slowing at the site of the abscess; usually abnormal.
- LP: Not usually performed because of the potential risk of cerebral herniation.
- White blood cell (WBC) count and erythrocyte sedimentation rate may be mildly elevated.
- Culture and sensitivity will identify the organism responsible. A needle aspirate taken using meticulous aseptic technique is best, with an order for both

aerobic and anaerobic cultures. A fungal culture may also be considered.

- C-reactive protein (CRP): Distinguishes a tumor from an abscess. CRP is elevated in patients with a brain abscess, whereas patients with a brain tumor have low levels of CRP.
- Needle aspiration: If performed, allows for direct observation of the cavity contents and culture (as described previously) of the biopsied material.

Treatment

Acute Care

Patients or family members may recognize the need for emergency medical attention because the patient appears very ill. The presentation of a brain abscess, however, may be insidious because the primary source of the infection may

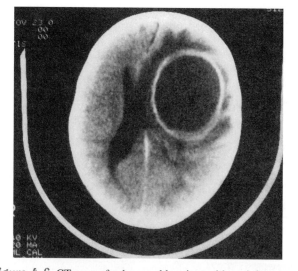

Figure 4-6 CT scan of a 1-year-old patient with an injury to the left orbit leading to osteomyelitis and a brain abscess in the frontal lobe. Contrast scan shows enhancement of thin rim. *(From Lambert H: Infections of the central nervous system, Philadelphia, 1991, BC Decker.)*

be resolved before the abscess becomes evident, particularly following antibiotic therapy.

After receiving emergency care, the patient is transferred to the ICU for close monitoring and critical care management. The patient's neurologic status is checked every 1 to 2 hours and documented for serial assessments to detect the first subtle signs of complications.

The location, age, and size of the abscess all have a bearing on the patient's outcome and response to management. In the early stages, diffuse cerebritis may be the forerunner to the formation of a discrete abscess.

Patients with a brain abscess may require the following:
- Intensive care with close monitoring
- Attention to neurologic status
- Steroid therapy to reduce edema, if ordered
- Strict I&O recordings
- ICP monitoring with precautions to prevent cerebral herniation
- Observation for signs and symptoms of meningitis

Patients receiving antibiotics, especially multiple antibiotic therapy, must receive administration using a rigid schedule. Because the infecting organisms multiply exponentially, the timing of administration is critical. Peaks and troughs often are ordered to gauge the effectiveness of antibiotic levels.

Medical Treatment

Appropriate antibiotic therapy that penetrates the blood-brain barrier (BBB) may successfully eradicate a subdural empyema (Table 4-12; also see Table 4-8). Mechanical ventilation may be required to support an altered respiratory status.

Brain abscesses measuring 3 cm or smaller are treated with antibiotics alone. Penicillin used concurrently with chloramphenicol and, more recently, with metronidazole maintains high drug concentrations needed for effective treatment. Parenteral antibiotics are usually given for 4 to 8 weeks with clinical evaluation and repeated CT scans to determine the clinical progress of abscess resolution.

Although the role of steroids continues to be controversial, they may be used when the patient deteriorates neuro-

Condition	Antibiotics
TABLE 4-12 Empirical Antibiotic Treatments for Brain Abscess	
Brain abscess	
Ear infection	Third-generation cephalosporin *and* metronidazole
Dental, sinus, mastoid, and pulmonary infections	Penicillin *and* metronidazole
Trauma and surgery	Vancomycin* *and* aminoglycoside *or* third-generation cephalosporin *or* imipenem
Endocarditis, parenteral drug usage	Vancomycin* *and* aminoglycoside
Abdominal and pelvic infections	Third-generation cephalosporin *and* metronidazole with or without aminoglycoside
Subdural empyema or cranial epidural abscess	See brain abscess
Spinal epidural abscess	Vancomycin* *and* aminoglycoside *or* third-generation cephalosporin *or* imipenem

From Johnson RT, Griffin JW: *Current therapy in neurologic disease,* ed 5, St Louis, 1997, Mosby.
*Vancomycin is used until sensitivity to nafcillin is established and in penicillin-allergic patients.

logically and experiences increased ICP. Steroids may inhibit the entry of antibiotics. They reduce the cerebral edema that surrounds brain abscesses but may also reduce the level of contrast enhancement around the abscess image on a CT scan.

Seizures may signal the abrupt onset of a brain abscess. In addition, they may be a potential problem throughout treatment or may appear several years after treatment. Therefore anticonvulsants should be prescribed until the patient is considered risk free.

Surgical Treatment

An **acute spinal epidural abscess** is managed with a laminectomy procedure with decompression of the spinal cord and drainage of the abscess. Intraoperative cultures determine the specific antibiotic therapy. Treatment must continue for weeks, with IV treatment followed after several months of oral therapy.

Abscesses that refuse to shrink in size or those that are large, accessible, or in close proximity to the ventricles are often treated surgically, usually in tandem with antibiotic therapy before and after surgery. Acutely ill patients admitted in a comatose state require immediate surgery. ICP is monitored and elevations are treated appropriately.

Surgical treatment may consist of stereotactic-guided drainage of the abscess. This procedure has minimal morbidity and mortality risks and should be considered for patients with small, multiple, or deep-seated abscesses; for those who are poor operative risks; or for those who have failed prior therapy. Intraoperative ultrasound may be used to target the abscess for precise localization. Stereotactic CT-guided aspiration, if available, is preferable to other surgical modalities because it allows for accurate drainage and installation of antibiotics directly into the cerebral abscess. IV therapy should continue postoperatively for 3 weeks, followed by oral therapy for approximately 6 weeks. The typical recovery period is 3 to 4 months, but some lesions can persist for up to 8 months. Follow-up imaging determines the long-term resolution.

A craniotomy is performed for well-formed abscesses. One option is direct aspiration of pus to drain the capsule, but this technique carries the possibility for abscess recurrence. A more risky option is craniotomy with removal of the capsule in total (see Chapter 8).

Appropriate clinical management depends on the location and age of the abscess and whether the abscess consists of one area or multiple areas.

Nonacute Care

Patients recovering from a frontal lobe, temporal lobe, or cerebellar abscess who have stabilized following surgical excision, aggressive antimicrobial emergency therapy, or intracranial pressure (ICP) monitoring will be transferred to the postacute setting for supportive care and observations to prevent or treat secondary infections in preparation for discharge. Patients will continue to receive treatments with ongoing close neurologic monitoring and assessment to include seizure precautions. For patients with a high acuity or who initially required ICP monitoring, the focus shifts to management of neurologic deficits from the initial insult, to include motor deficits, cranial nerve deficits, changes in cognition, memory loss, dementia, and dysphagia that affect many patients.

Rehabilitation specialists may be consulted to promote recovery of lost function and complications of immobility. Social services may be needed to prepare the patient and family for home care services with continuing IV therapy, PT, OT, and ST.

Home Care

Discharging patients on IV antibiotic therapy has become an alternative option in areas where this service is available. The home antibiotic therapy option depends on the neurologic and medical stability of the patient; the availability of health coverage for home care; the patient's level of education, visual acuity, gross-motor coordination, and personal hygiene; the patient's motivation and commitment to follow a rigid administration time schedule; home support or family; and the patient's ability to keep follow-up appointments. A verbal and written performance checklist or plan is needed to communicate patient-oriented goals. This plan includes all categories of care, beginning with the placement of a venous access device, wound care, infection monitoring, and concluding with troubleshooting techniques.

The home care nurse clinician who is monitoring the patient must have knowledge of brain abscesses, neurologic assessment, potential patient complications, and the side effects of antibiotic therapy. Arrangements must be made in advance for any potential emergencies.

ACUTE ENCEPHALITIS

Etiology and Epidemiology

Encephalitis is defined as an acute infection of the brain parenchyma and meninges that often is caused by herpes simplex or by any number of arboviruses. **Arbovirus** is a collective term that refers to the many arthropod-borne viruses, the majority of which belong to the Togaviridae, Flaviviridae, or Bunyaviridae families.[57] Other conditions known to cause encephalitis are enteroviruses, systemic viral disease (e.g., mononucleosis), and vaccinations for measles, mumps, and rubella. Infection by an amoeba **parasitic organism,** such as the one-celled *Naegleria fowleri* believed to be common across North America, can be contracted by swimming in infected water. All American freshwater lakes and streams may be infected; swimming in a drainage canal in Florida proved to be fatal for one 14-year-old boy.

Epidemiologists are unable to explain why the microbe affects some people but not others. The incidence of acute encephalitis is approximately 15 per 100,000 people. Many arboviruses that cause encephalitis occur in epidemics. The disease is fatal in approximately 20% of the patients hospitalized with viral encephalitis.[59] St. Louis encephalitis is the most commonly seen arbovirus encephalitis. Eastern equine encephalitis is less common but produces the most serious

TABLE 4-13	Classification and Characteristics of Viruses Causing Encephalitis			
Virus	Incubation Period (Days)	Location	Season	Affected Population
Eastern equine encephalitis	5–15	Atlantic, Gulf Coast, and Great Lake regions	Midsummer to early fall	Infants, children, and adults >50 years
Western equine encephalitis	5–10	All parts of United States, western two thirds of country	Summer to early fall	Infants and young children
Venezuelan equine encephalitis	2–5	Texas, Florida, Mexico; Central and South America	All year	Infants and young children
St. Louis encephalitis	4–21	United States and Canada, especially Mississippi River, Pacific Coast, Texas, and Florida	Summer and fall	Adults >40 years; older adults more often affected than younger ages
California encephalitis	5–15	United States, midwestern states, eastern seaboard, and Canada	Late summer and early fall	Children <15 years

Data from Davis L: St. Louis encephalitis. In Mohr J, editor: *Manual of clinical problems in neurology,* ed 2, Boston, 1989, Little, Brown; Jubelt B, Miller J: Infections of the nervous system: viral infections. In Rowland L, editor: *Merritt's textbook of neurology,* ed 8, Philadelphia, 1989, Lea & Febiger; Kennedy C: Acute viral infections excluding herpes simplex, rabies, and HIV. In Lambert H, editor: *Infections of the central nervous system,* Philadelphia, 1991, BC Decker; Peter G, editor: *Red book: report of the committee on infectious diseases,* ed 22, Elk Grove Village, IL, 1991, American Academy of Pediatrics; and Ray C, Minnich L: Viruses, rickettsia, and chlamydia. In Henry JB, Todd JC, editors: *Clinical diagnosis and management by laboratory methods,* ed 18, Philadelphia, 1991, WB Saunders.

problems. Table 4-13 summarizes the characteristics of viruses causing encephalitis.

Pathophysiology

Encephalitis may be mild or severe, with the degree of tissue destruction depending on the offending organism. The inflammation of encephalitis is nonsuppurant. After the virus gains entry into the CNS via the bloodstream or peripheral nerves, there is infiltration of polymorphonuclear leukocytes and mononuclear cells. This infiltration causes congestion and swelling, vasculitic lesions, myelin destruction, widespread nerve cell degeneration, necrosis, or hemorrhage.

Assessment

Assessment of LOC and a specific patient history are important and include the following:
- GCS: Assess for changes in LOC; confusion and, later, drowsiness that progresses to coma
- Cranial nerve palsies
- Motor changes, such as hemiparesis
- Neck stiffness
- Seizure activity
- Fever: high fevers
- Vomiting

Progression of these symptoms is common with Eastern equine encephalitis. Symptoms are often less severe with Western equine encephalitis and Venezuelan equine encephalitis. The neurologic symptoms of St. Louis encephalitis are usually preceded by a prodromal stage lasting 3 to 4 days. During this prodromal period, malaise, fever, headache, sore throat, and GI symptoms are common.[14] However, the signs of brain parenchymal dysfunction—changes in LOC, seizures, increased ICP, cranial nerve palsies, motor and sensory changes, speech changes—are not specific to the infecting agent.[39]

Acute Care

In acute cases, the patient should be seen in the ED. With acute encephalitis, the onset of the progressive symptoms discussed under Assessment may be abrupt.

The patient is transferred to the ICU for follow-up neurologic assessment, close monitoring, and supportive care. There is currently no specific antiviral treatment for encephalitis other than that used for the herpes virus. Priorities in treatment focus on symptomatic, supportive, and preventive care:
- Maintain a patent airway and respiratory status
- Control ICP, fever, and seizures
- Monitor fluid and electrolyte balance; syndrome of inappropriate antidiuretic hormone (SIADH) often occurs
- Promote adequate nutrition; monitor for high metabolic demand and positive nitrogen
- Establish a safe environment
- Prevent associated complications

The patient is discharged for follow-up at home after patient and family education. It is important for the patient to continue all medications and prescribed treatments.

HERPES SIMPLEX ENCEPHALITIS

CNS infections involving the herpes simplex virus (HSV) are among the most severe viral infections of the brain. **Herpes simplex encephalitis (HSE)** is one of several HSV infections including (1) acute encephalitis, (2) benign recurrent lymphocytic meningitis, (3) acute facial nerve paralysis, (4) recurrent ascending myelitis, and (5) neuritis localized to a single sensory nerve.

The patient may be treated in the ED following repeated seizures. Mortality rates of HSE-caused acute encephalitis are extremely high. The mortality rate for untreated patients is greater than 70%; fewer than 10% of survivors ever return to a normally functioning life.[18,21] It is unclear how the virus accesses the CNS, but it is apparent that both primary and recurrent HSV infections can cause CNS disease.[21] An LP with CSF analysis, MRI or CT scanning, and other diagnostic studies may be ordered to rule out other causes. Acyclovir IV given slowly is usually started promptly before the patient lapses into a coma and is continued for 10 days or more for maximum therapeutic benefit. Supportive therapy as described earlier for bacterial meningitis is instituted and maintained until the patient shows improvement. Fluid balance is important, and overhydration should be avoided.

WEST NILE VIRUS

Etiology and Epidemiology

The introduction of West Nile virus (WNV) into the United States in 1990s led to the largest **arbovirus epizootic** (animal outbreak) ever recorded in our history and had a significant effect on both humans and animals.[54] WNV was initially identified in Uganda in the 1930s, but had never been seen anywhere in the Western Hemisphere until it was first recorded in the United States in August 1999 in the borough of Queens, New York City. Members of the Corvid family of birds (includes crows and blue jays), as well as horses, seem to exhibit the most significant morbidity in the United States. The relative amount of an arbovirus present in the environment is the result of a complex relationship between the virus, the arthropod vector (mosquito), and the specific amplifying host (which is often a bird or a horse) (Fig. 4-7). Each arbovirus has specific species of hosts that become the primary reservoir of the host and amplify it to a large extent. There are also specific species of arthropods that are capable of transmitting the virus from the infected primary host reservoirs to naïve hosts (i.e., a host that has never seen the arbovirus before). These arthropods, in the case of WNV, are the mosquito primarily, but also can include ticks and midges. Factors

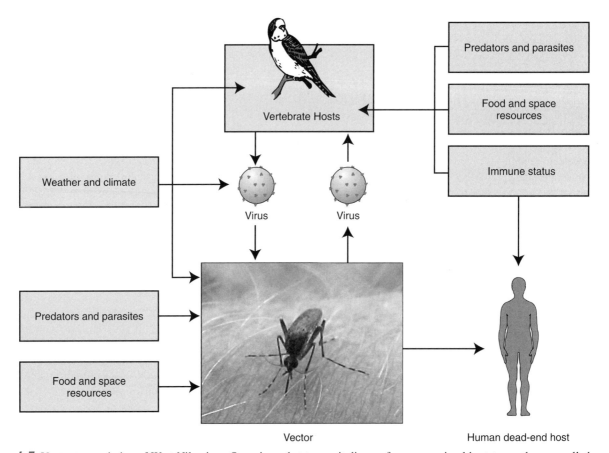

Figure 4-7 Vector transmission of West Nile virus. Organisms that transmit disease from one animal host to another are called *vectors*. Mosquitoes are vectors for the transmission of encephalitis from small creatures, usually birds and rodents, to humans. *(From Cuppett M, Walsh KM: General medical conditions in the athlete, St Louis, 2005, Elsevier Mosby, p 191.)*

that influence the amount of arbovirus in a certain environment include weather or climate changes, predators and parasites present, limitations on food and space resources, and the level of immunity in vertebrate populations.

Mosquitoes spread the virus from the birds to humans. The CDC is seeking answers to determine how the Aedes japonicus or the Culex mosquitoes (vectors) carry and transmit the virus. Intensive spraying for mosquitoes each summer is an attempt to control further outbreaks throughout the Western Hemisphere. The public should be vigilant and remove all outside containers that hold water after 5 to 7 days, where mosquitoes breed in the spring and summer (e.g., wading pools and bird baths). Some newly recognized modes of WNV transmission include organ transplantation. In fall 2002, four recipients of organ donations developed WNV infections shortly after transplantation. Because each patient had received organs from a single donor, the transplanted organs were identified as the route of acquisition of the infections. Further investigation of this case determined that the organ donor became infected after transfusion with WNV-contaminated blood products. Additional investigations determined that donation of blood and blood products by WNV-infected individuals before the development of symptoms has the potential to transmit the virus to the recipients of the products. As a result, FDA-mandated WNV screening of blood products began in July 2003.

Symptoms of WNV may include mild fever, headache, body ache, skin rash, and swollen lymph glands. Often the infection is subclinical and ignored. More severe infections are characterized by headache, a high fever, nuchal rigidity, stupor, disorientation, coma, tremors, seizures, muscle weakness, and paralysis. It has been estimated that about 1% of individuals who contract WNV will develop severe symptoms. According to the CDC, 25 people contracted WNV in 2001, and about 3% to 15% of those with severe infections may die from the disease.[76]

Fatality rates are highest in older adults and in immunocompromised patients (e.g., oncology patients, patients with HIV and herpes). Individuals may suffer only from the West Nile infection without CNS involvement. The spinal cord and brainstem (particularly the medulla) may be involved more extensively.[61] The virus multiplies in the blood and may cross the blood-brain barrier (BBB).

Assessment

In assessing for WNV, it is important to document the patient's history of exposure to mosquitoes and any evidence of mosquito bites up to 2 weeks before symptoms appear, as well as high fever, altered mental status, and coma. A comprehensive neurologic assessment is completed and includes the following:
- CNS changes with confusion
- Motor status: weakness, paralysis
- Sensory status: sensory changes from swelling of the brain
- Seizures
- Headache, muscle aches, and discomfort (e.g., stiff neck)

- Acute fever, conjunctivitis
- Lymphadenopathy, severe myalgias, roseolar rash

A diagnosis of WNV should be considered in patients with a history of potential exposure and a compatible clinical presentation of fever, headache, and myalgia, with or without GI symptoms, especially if the patients complains of neck stiffness, and has a change in mental status and if weakness is present. In severe cases, the assessment may reveal headache, high fever, nuchal rigidity, stupor, coma, tremors, seizures, muscle weakness, and paralysis.

Neurodiagnostic and Laboratory Studies

Diagnostic studies include the following:
- Blood studies
- LP: spinal fluid is tested and may reveal the presence of viral sequences in the CSF
- IgM capture ELISA (MAC-ELISA): the test of choice for rapid diagnosis; test advantage is high probability of accurate diagnosis when performed on the CSF during the acute phase
- MRI imaging: may demonstrate enhancement of the leptomeninges, the periventricular area, or both

Acute Care

Many individuals may have WNV with mild symptoms and never seek medical care. The very young and the very old are more vulnerable to WNV and may seek emergency care. In some cases WNV has been fatal for children and older adults.

There is no known vaccine or treatment for WNV, but current research is ongoing. For acutely ill patients, admission to the ICU is necessary to monitor for respiratory compromise and to initiate ventilatory support. Supportive management, IV fluids, nutrition, an indwelling urinary catheter, and close monitoring are provided to prevent secondary complications and infections. Motor changes may progress to flaccid paralysis. Although WNV can be fatal in severe cases, patients with less severe cases can be treated in the ED and released to their home with follow-up care. Supportive care may include airway management, ventilatory support, IVs, and prevention of complications (e.g., pneumonia). Corticosteroids and mannitol may be ordered for cerebral edema. Follow-up home care may be needed for those with slow recovery and chronic neurologic deficits.

SLOW VIRAL INFECTIONS OF THE CENTRAL NERVOUS SYSTEM

Creutzfeldt-Jakob disease (CJD), variant CJD (vCJD), Gerstmann-Straussler-Scheinker disease, kuru, fatal familial insomnia (FFI), and other diseases caused by prions make up a group of slow viral infections that affect the CNS.

Etiology

Creutzfeldt-Jakob disease (CJD) is one of several neurologically degenerative diseases caused by a group of protein particles called *prions*.[10,50] Prions are infectious due to their ability to replicate in the CNS and interrupt critical normal neuron function. CJD, variant CJD (vCJD), Gerstmann-Straussler Scheinker disease, kuru, and other prion diseases were originally called slow virus diseases because of the prolonged incubation period and initial designation as a viral condition. This group of fatal illnesses is characterized by a rapidly progressive dementia, myoclonus, psychiatric changes, often typical EEG changes, spongiform neuropathologic changes, and coma. These diseases all have an insidious onset with confusion, progressive dementia, and variable ataxia in patients ages 16 to over 80 years; more than 99% are over age 35 years. The long incubation period may become dormant after exposure and not cause symptoms for up to 40 years. However, after onset, the progressive dementia and total incapacitation associated with these diseases occur in a matter of weeks to months and are fatal. Death usually occurs within 3 to 12 months, but some patients survive 2 years or more after the onset of symptoms.

A spongiform illness called **scrapie,** similar to CJD in humans, has been known to affect sheep, goats, mink, cats, and cattle. The practice of manufacturing cattle feed from the carcasses of animals that have died from scrapie brought attention to the probability of beef contamination in Great Britain; this practice was banned in the 1980s and is no longer practiced. Human consumption of beef infected with bovine spongiform encephalopathy (BSE) has been linked to the increase in cases of a new and more deadly type of CJD, the so-called mad cow disease. There is further suspicion of a link between scrapie and CJD when the bones of animals that died of scrapie are used to fertilize pastures where beef cattle graze. Experts in Great Britain who have studied the disease suggest that the prion can move between species more easily than once believed. These issues are still being debated in the U.S. cattle industry.

An important factor in prion diseases is the resistance of these infectious protein particles to standard sterilization and disinfection. Information about appropriate sterilization and disinfection of items used in the hospital for procedures involving *any* CNS material from those suspected of or confirmed as having any of the prion diseases is extremely important. Clinicians can find information on www.cdc.gov, and the Communicable Disease Center refers to the World Health Organization (WHO) document, "WHO Infection Control Guidelines for Transmissible Spongiform Encephalopathies," dated March 1999.

It should be noted that standard precautions are sufficient for handling patients with these diseases, but extra care should be taken with direct handling of any CNS tissue (e.g., in the operating room [OR] during brain biopsy). If surgery involving the CNS is anticipated, it should be thoroughly discussed first with the infection control team. *Strict hospital policy* should be followed addressing CJD and other prion-producing diseases so that appropriate handling and cleaning of anything that has been in contact with the patient can be performed with strict adherence. Also, any laboratory studies anticipated should be discussed with the pathologist in the laboratory *before* sending materials to be tested.

Samples such as CSF need to be handled using special precautions.

Epidemiology

CJD occurs naturally in either of two forms: (1) the sporadic type (occurring at a rate of 1 case per 1 million people) and (2) because of inherited mutations of the prion protein gene. Genetic propensities and familial type due to genetic mutation that can be passed from generation to generation have been documented in geographic clusters in various parts of the world.[33] Possible transmission of vCJD via blood transfusion was recently published in *The Lancet*.[42] Epidemiologic evidence does not support that sporadic CJD is transmissible from person to person via blood transfusion, but this evidence does not apply to vCJD. This study revealed that 48 individuals were identified as having received a contaminated blood component from a total of 15 donors who later became vCJD cases. One of these recipients was identified as developing symptoms of vCJD 5 to 6 years after receiving a transfusion of red cells donated by an individual 3 to 5 years before the donor developed vCJD.

Pathophysiology

CJD seems to be contained in the CNS and is primarily a disease of gray matter, with the cortex and basal ganglia most often affected. The self-replicating protein, or *prion*, causes healthy proteins to die. Prions can have an incubation period of decades but may manifest earlier in some cases.

Characteristic CNS changes include diffuse brain atrophy, enlarged ventricles, and cerebellar atrophy with no inflammatory reaction. This disease may also create severe neuronal loss and astrocytic proliferation. Spongelike holes develop in the brain, and there is neuronal loss.[48]

Assessment

A history and complete neurologic assessment is needed to determine the phase of illness being experienced by the patient with CJD. Before experiencing a sudden downturn, about one third of the patients with CJD complain of symptoms for a period of weeks or months before seeking emergency medical care. The clinician should question the patient and family about

- Weight loss and anorexia
- Insomnia
- Malaise or dizziness

In addition, the following symptoms occur in the early stages of CJD:

- Progressive memory loss
- Mental deterioration with behavior changes
- Visual impairment
- Dysphasia

Patients may exhibit noticeable deterioration from week to week. Motor deficits develop in the next phase and include myoclonic jerks, an increased startle response from any stimuli, spasticity, and severe ataxia and dysarthria. Within a matter of months the patient rapidly enters the terminal third stage, in which dementia is severe, and the following symptoms are evident (see Fig. 4-7):

- Increased spasticity with myoclonus
- Muscle wasting
- Bowel and bladder incontinence
- Dementia

Neurodiagnostic and Laboratory Studies

Diagnostic studies include the following:

- CT/MRI: May document brain atrophy.
- EEG: Approximately half of the patients with CJD characteristically have abnormal EEG findings.
- LP: CSF studies are usually normal; an electrophoretic test on CSF is another useful laboratory examination that may show a sharp wave pattern.
- Brain biopsy: A definitive diagnosis is confirmed only by brain biopsy, either during hospitalization or at autopsy.

The brains of patients with CJD have a spongy appearance and show cortical atrophy. Extreme measures should be used to protect all OR staff who will have direct contact with collecting and preparing brain specimens for analysis.

Acute and Nonacute Care

When a patient with suspected CJD is seen in the ED, a comprehensive workup is quickly performed. There is no known treatment for CJD. Because the disease can spread iatrogenically, Standard Precautions should be taken to minimize transmission. In addition, special guidelines should be used in sterilization and washing procedures because of the virulence of this virus and its resistance to inactivation as discussed previously.

ALERT: In June of 2001, the Joint Commission on Accreditation of Healthcare Organizations (JCAHO) issued a Sentinel Event Alert that described two separate incidents at JCAHO-accredited hospitals in which a total of 14 patients were exposed to CJD through instruments used during brain surgeries. According to JCAHO, these incidents signal the need for renewed awareness of preventive measures and infection control in health care organizations, because regular sterilization techniques have not yet proven to be effective against CJD organisms.[36]

Acute or nonacute management begins by placing the patient in a private room using Standard Precautions. Although a private room is not necessary, it gives privacy for preparing the patient and family for the terminal course of the disease. Any invasive procedures performed on the patient should occur only after departments involved are knowledgeable about necessary precautions needed to protect their location, health care workers, and equipment. The hospital epidemiologist or infection control personnel should be consulted for specific advice before proceeding with any invasive procedures.

CJD progresses rapidly and almost daily. The patient's mental status declines, and the patient becomes bedridden and has problems of immobility. Acute care management focuses on the following:

- Impaired swallowing
- Inability to communicate
- Supportive therapy
- Good personal hygiene
- Nutrition with tube feedings
- Comfort or palliative measures with frequent turning and repositioning
- Seizure management
- Soft lighting with a quiet environment to decrease external stimuli
- Use of disposable materials
- Supportive care for the family
- Family conferences and frequent updates on the patient's condition (because of the potential for rapid deterioration)

The patient may be discharged to home or a long-term care facility, where death is usually the result of sepsis from respiratory, skin, or urinary infections or of aspiration when swallowing becomes difficult.[22] Organ donation is not an option for patients who die from CJD.

NOSOCOMIAL INFECTION

Nosocomial (health care–acquired) infection is extremely important in today's health care environment. Ten to fifteen years ago, many complex patients in ICUs were considered to have very high acuity, and health care costs soared. Those health care workers could not have anticipated the complexity of the patients routinely in the ICUs today, as well as the many devices attached to those patients. Modern medical practices allow many more opportunities for microorganisms to enter the body via tubes and other intrusions. The number and complexity of surgical procedures that patients undergo have increased as well. Patients having significant underlying diseases or advanced age are operated on with regularity. As stated earlier in the chapter, the chain of infection, host susceptibility, and opportunities for the entrance of microorganisms are important components of infection.[28]

SURGICAL SITE INFECTION

Until the end of the nineteenth century, infection was the greatest risk associated with any surgical procedure.[15,77] Widespread use of gloves did not occur until well into the 1900s. During the twentieth century, however, the standardization of aseptic techniques for use in the operating room greatly improved the outcome of operations involving basically clean procedures.[25] Box 4-4 defines the classifications of surgeries from clean to dirty procedures. A widely accepted system of classifying operative site by the degree of contamination was developed by the National Research Council for its cooperative study of the effects of ultraviolet irradiation of operating rooms on surgical site infections.[32,52]

Class I—Clean

An uninfected operative wound in which no inflammation is encountered and the respiratory, alimentary, genital, or uninfected urinary tract is not entered. In addition, clean wounds are primarily closed and, if necessary, drained with closed drainage. Operative incisional wounds that follow nonpenetrating (blunt) trauma should be included in this category if they meet the criteria.

Class II—Clean Contaminated

An operative wound in which the respiratory, alimentary, genital, or urinary tracts are entered under controlled conditions and without unusual contamination. Specifically, operations involving the biliary tract, appendix, vagina, and oropharynx are included in this category, provided no evidence of infection or major break in technique is encountered.

Class III—Contaminated

Open, fresh, accidental wounds. In addition, operations with major breaks in sterile technique (e.g., open cardiac massage) or gross spillage from the gastrointestinal tract, and incisions in which acute, nonpurulent inflammation is encountered are included in this category.

Class IV—Dirty Infected

Old traumatic wounds with retained devitalized tissue and those that involve existing clinical infection or perforated viscera. This definition suggests that the organisms causing postoperative infection were present in the operative field before the operation.

From Mangram AJ, Horan TC, Pearson ML, et al: Guideline for prevention of surgical site infection, 1999. Centers for Disease Control and Prevention (CDC) Hospital Infection Control Practices Advisory Committee, *Am J Infect Control* 27(2):97–132, 1999.

Most acute care hospitals have infection control professionals or epidemiologists whose role is to determine infection rates and also suggest interventions to decrease those rates when necessary. Infection control professionals generally benchmark their rates against the nationally gathered statistics. In the 1970s the CDC began the National Nosocomial Infection Surveillance Program (NNIS). The program consisted of 163 hospitals that sent their infection data to CDC so the latter could determine the "average" rate of different types of surgical procedures.[20,52] NNIS does this by obtaining rates of surgical site infections from many types of hospitals. All these hospitals divide their surgeries by *International Classification of Diseases*, ninth edition (ICD9) codes. All those surgical procedures having the same ICD9 codes are grouped together. Then the pooled mean of the rates is determined and published as a benchmark for other hospitals to compare to their own hospital rate. The case finding method must be the same, and 100% chart review is done by infection control professionals.

Many neurosurgical patients have operations such as craniotomies, laminectomies, and spinal fusions. Patients waiting for surgery should receive preoperative best practices to include chlorhexidine baths (2% to 4% solution) the day before and morning of surgery. The chlorhexidine removes the bulk of the endogenous bacteria on a surgical patient's skin and leaves a potent residual effect that will benefit the patient during the surgical process.[56] Chlorhexidine gluconate is an excellent and very effective skin preparation, but it has not been FDA approved for sites that may place it near the meninges, such as in neurosurgical surgery. The Healthcare Infection Control Practices Advisory Committee (HICPAC) Group has published a comprehensive manual about patient and facility preparation practices in the surgical setting.[30] Other important practices include the correct and timely (within 60 minutes of the incision) administration of preoperative antibiotic prophylaxis.

COMPREHENSIVE PATIENT MANAGEMENT

Care of the patient with an acute CNS infectious process requires finely tuned expertise in clinical management. The onset of symptoms can be very rapid, and arriving at an accurate medical diagnosis may be difficult. Patients in the acute stage of a CNS infection can be seriously ill and require frequent and thorough assessment of neurologic function to prevent complications. Supportive care and nursing interventions that foster optimal patient outcomes, as well as family coping and support, are necessary.

Assessment Considerations

The nursing assessment should include information obtained from the patient and family to identify possible risk factors that may have influenced the onset of the infectious process. The patient history should determine if a recent infection (e.g., upper respiratory, ear, sinus, mastoid, or dental), recent penetrating trauma, surgical procedure, or tooth extraction has occurred. Is there a history of tuberculosis, contact with another person with tuberculosis, or knowledge of anyone else—family member or friend—with similar symptoms? Because the symptoms of some CNS infections (e.g., encephalitis) are nonspecific before onset, it is important to determine whether the patient has been ill lately with the flu or has just not been feeling well. Has the patient had any recent viral infection, such as measles or mumps? Has he or she recently traveled out of the country? Known allergies or reactions to antibiotics also should be documented during the assessment.

Assessment of the patient with a CNS infection should also include the following:

- Notation of vital signs and temperature: Tachycardia and body temperatures ranging from 38° to 41° C (100° to 106° F) may be present. Rectal temperatures are preferred for accuracy and safety, because these patients are at risk for seizure activity. This can be easily completed when the patient is in a coma; otherwise oral, ear, or axillary temperatures are the norm.
- Airway protection and breathing patterns: These should be assessed immediately, because they may be affected if there is an altered LOC. LOC assessment data vary dramatically from patient to patient

depending on the causative organism, intensity of infection, and location of infection. The patient's LOC may range from awake and alert, to drowsy, to comatose.

In addition, neurologic testing includes the following:
- Orientation; confusion is often present.
- Pupillary size and response.
- Cranial nerve assessment: CNs III, IV, VI, and VIII are commonly involved in *H. influenzae* meningitis, and CNs III and VI are involved in TB meningitis.
- Speech patterns: Dysphasia can be present in the early stages of CJD.
- Motor function: Myoclonic jerks are present in 85% of patients with CJD.
- Sensory response and behavior: Personality changes and dementia are common signs of CJD.
- Meningeal irritation: Neck stiffness or nuchal rigidity, severe headache, Brudzinski's sign, Kernig's sign, and photophobia may be present.
- Nausea or vomiting.
- Seizures: 50% of all patients with *H. influenzae* meningitis may experience a seizure.
- Skin rashes: Meningococcal meningitis can cause a purpuric or petechial rash.

General Clinical Management Considerations

Interventions for the clinical management of patients with CNS infections in the acute phase involve monitoring neurologic function, preventing complications, administering antibiotic therapy (if ordered), providing supportive measures to promote comfort and recovery, and establishing therapeutic relationships that improve patient and family coping through the crisis.

Acute Care

During the acute phase, patients with a CNS infection are often managed in the ICU for ongoing assessment and hemodynamic monitoring; thus increases in ICP can be identified, managed, and minimized (see Chapter 10). The patient's neurologic status is carefully and frequently monitored as a priority on the care plan. The outcomes of patients with CNS infection often are directly related to LOC levels. Therefore the GCS or other assessment tools should be used to document neurologic function (see Chapter 2). Any alteration or change in LOC should be communicated to the physician immediately.

Some patients require endotracheal intubation with mechanical ventilation if there has been severe deterioration of neurologic function. Fluid volume requires careful assessment, monitoring, and regulation. Accurate monitoring of intake and output is essential, and IV fluids should be infused via a pump. Serum electrolytes should be monitored with attention toward serum sodium levels, because SIADH can occur with CNS infection. Symptoms of SIADH precipitated by an increased secretion of antidiuretic hormone (ADH) include a serum sodium level less than 126 mEq/L, an increase in urine sodium, and decreased urinary output (400 to 500 ml per 24 hours) (see Chapter 5). Fluid balance requires close monitoring because it relates to cerebral function.

Hyperthermia must also be controlled. Rectal temperatures are monitored, antipyretics are administered, and methods to control body temperature are used. Cooling blankets must be used with care to prevent shivering. Parenteral antibiotic therapy is usually ordered depending on the causative organism.

Meningeal irritation and headache are quite intense and are managed with analgesics, a darkened, quiet room, and a controlled environment. Other members of the team should be instructed to use care when assisting the patient to avoid quick, sudden movements. Patients often assume a fetal position to reduce the traction on nerve endings and decrease painful meningeal irritation. If pain can be managed successfully, patients have a better chance for rest, even if it is only short naps. Patient protection during this acute stage involves observing the patient frequently, initiating seizure precautions if the patient has seizure activity (see Chapter 24), and ensuring a safe environment. The patient's self-care needs (e.g., basic hygiene, bathing, toileting, and nutrition) also require supervision.

Postacute and Nonacute Care

After the acute phase of illness, patients with a CNS infection may recover completely, continue to experience mild to moderate residual neurologic deficits, or suffer devastating neurologic deterioration that results in total incapacitation and the need for long-term care. Recovering patients may need to be assessed for potential home antibiotic therapy to facilitate timely discharge. Patients with a mild to moderate residual neurologic deficit require assessment aimed at identifying patient strengths and abilities versus disabilities. In addition, these patients benefit from the collaborative establishment of a therapeutic program that facilitates recovery through rehabilitation. Patients who have experienced significant neurologic deterioration may need evaluation for long-term placement or home care (see Chapter 6).

Clinical management interventions depend on the functional level of the patient in the nonacute care stage. For the recovering patient, the nursing focus is on patient and family instruction, including home IV antibiotic therapy, and the coordination of discharge planning. Interventions for the patient with some residual neurologic deficit are planned by a multidisciplinary team, and clinicians collaborate with physical, occupational, and speech therapists to establish, deliver, and evaluate appropriate care plans to achieve a successful patient outcome.

Health Teaching Considerations

Extensive patient and family teaching may be required in the clinical management of patients with CNS infection. The families of patients with either meningococcal meningitis or *H. influenzae* meningitis, in particular, must be instructed in preventive prophylaxis. All household and daily care contacts require treatment according to the guidelines explained earlier in the section on meningitis.

During the acute phase of a CNS infection, patients and families are in crisis. They may be fearful, anxious, and irritable. The clinician's ability to direct and manage care and to establish trusting therapeutic relationships with both the patient and the family helps mobilize coping strategies and reduce the fear and anxiety that surround unknown situations. The clinician should remember that only a few days or weeks earlier the patient with a CNS infection was, in most cases, healthy.

Developing and tailoring the patient care plan should be a collaborative effort among all members of the health care team, the patient, and the family. Necessary teaching includes a careful explanation of the disease process, interventions, and outcome prospects. Questions from the patient and family should be encouraged, as should their participation in the patient's care. Family members should be introduced to key members of the nursing team, such as the primary nurse, clinical nurse specialist, and psychiatric nurse specialist.

TIP: The American College of Physicians–American Society of Internal Medicine (ACP-ASIM) has launched a national campaign to address the problem of emerging antibiotic resistance. They plan to develop clinical practice guidelines for diseases prone to overtreatment by antibiotics to ensure that important diseases (e.g., CNS infections) can be treated without fear of antibiotic resistance.

Nutritional Considerations

A nutritional assessment should include the unique needs of the patient with a CNS infection. This includes a neurologic assessment of the patient's level of cognition, impaired memory, and cranial nerve deficits that involve problems with chewing and swallowing (dysphagia). A swallowing screening test may be required in some cases. Nutritional requirements are determined both from the neurologic disease process and from nutritional needs to promote healing, combat malnutrition, and restore energy. The assessment should also include an evaluation of the patient's health history of diabetes or other major health concerns. Activities of daily living (ADLs), laboratory values (e.g., serum albumin), weight loss or gain, medications, renal status or disease, and the presence of pressure ulcers are important considerations. Of equal importance is the patient's past and current eating patterns, appetite level, psychosocial and mental health status (e.g., depression), and cultural and religious beliefs. The use or abuse of alcohol and drugs also factors into the nutritional evaluation.

Consultation with a nutritionist to review the nutritional assessment can help in formulating a dietary plan. It is important to have a plan that promotes nutrition and addresses safe eating and swallowing, the use of adaptive equipment, and the need for supplemental feedings. The care of the patient with dysphagia requires evaluation by the interdisciplinary team (and often a speech pathologist) and the development of a swallowing protocol for patients who require enteral nutrition. The feeding tube may include a nasogastric (NG) tube, a nasointestinal (NI) tube, percutaneous endoscopic gastrostomy (PEF), percutaneous endoscopic jejunostomy (J-tube), or gastrostomy (G-tube). Family and health care providers need special instructions in caring for, feeding, and administering medications to patients with feeding tubes.

Older Adult Considerations

Throughout hospitalization, older adults are at high risk for nosocomial infections. This risk increases with each invasive monitoring device, IV line, urinary catheter, drainage device, feeding tube, or mechanical ventilation. Line infections, skin and wound infections, pneumonia, and urosepsis can be minimized or prevented by the early removal or frequent changing of invasive devices, early detection, appropriate and aggressive antibiotic coverage, and adequate nutritional support.

The evaluation and treatment of older adult patients is often complex. Often they cannot accurately express their needs and feelings, and as a result milder problems may be undetected until the problem becomes advanced. They may experience confusion and delirium. Delirium can occur both before and after a seizure. Status epilepticus is also possible and can be fatal unless appropriately managed. Older patients may be febrile longer than younger patients, are at higher risk for thromboembolism, display agitation and cognitive changes, and have longer memory impairment. It has been suggested that demyelinating processes may be responsible for some of these symptoms. Some older adults show a rapid decline in independence following discharge. This requires home health care to assess the patient's home environment and to assess metabolic and neurologic deficits before discharge to ensure safe recovery at home.

Rehabilitation Considerations

Discharge options for patients with a CNS infection may include a transfer to a rehabilitation center for continued extensive therapy or a discharge to return home with assistance and continuation of patient rehabilitation. Patients with severe alterations in neurologic function or dementia may require long-term care. The patient should be encouraged to provide self-care as tolerated and to maintain seizure precautions, ambulation, and compliance with prescribed therapies.

Case Management Considerations

Families require much support and care after the patient has been discharged to home. They should be encouraged to express both their feelings regarding the reality of the situation and their fears and concerns. Family support groups are therapeutic forums in which families can share experiences with other families experiencing similar situations.

Hospital and agency-based case managers should perform a patient assessment as soon as feasible to determine the individual needs of the patient (Box 4-5). A comprehensive plan of action helps to coordinate the needed services, supports, and entitlements and includes measurable goals.

BOX 4-5	**Case Management Clinical Practice Protocol**

Acute

Patient identified on first day of admission by utilization log

Case manager (on site within 24 hours of admission):
- Review record/talk with inpatient treatment team
- Open chart
- Enroll patient in program

Patient offered/educated regarding case management program by case manager

Patient **accepts** program (if patient is deemed incompetent, is a minor, or has legal guardian or power of attorney, primary identified person will sign consent forms):
- Consent for services is reviewed and signed
- Patient's bill of rights is reviewed and signed
- Release of information is reviewed and signed
- Before discharge, baseline clinical measurements are completed and appropriate data gathered
- Follow-up home visit appointment is arranged by case manager
- Patient's physician(s), community case providers are notified by letter and telephone contact

Patient **refuses** case management program:
- Case manager will track patient
- If patient reappears at ED or is readmitted, program will be offered again by same case manager

Subacute/Stabilization

Case manager will be in contact with patient/family at least weekly (by telephone or home visits) for 8 weeks after discharge

Health Maintenance/Promotion/Prevention

A minimum of one monthly contact will occur, with comprehensive case map assessments (however, if at any time the patient requires more services or home visits, the case manager will adjust interventions to those specific needs)

At 4, 8, and 12 months—client will be contacted twice, with one home visit to complete on-site assessment and measurement tools

From Cohen EL, DeBack V: *The outcomes mandate: case management in health care today,* St Louis, 1999, Mosby.

Decreased use of emergency services and earlier identification of acute problems requires health teaching for increased health knowledge. A focus on health promotion and disease prevention is part of the patient and family education.

A case management patient follow-up after CNS infections focuses on the following:
- New or worsening neurologic deficits: reported immediately
- Physician and health provider: follow-up appointments
- Home health needs: nursing, rehabilitation, and health teaching
- Antiinfective therapy compliance: as prescribed

- Monitoring for enlarged ventricles and hydrocephalus with follow-up CT or MRI imaging and consultation with a neurologist
- Monitoring of temperature and WBC count: immediate response to first sign of infection
- Medications: name, dosage, frequency, purpose, and potential side effects
- Pain management: headache relief and discomfort using prescribed medications and comfort measures, such as heat or cold applications
- Seizure management: emphasis on full compliance with the anticonvulsant regimen, maintaining levels in therapeutic range, and education on first aid for breakthrough seizure activity
- Motor and sensory status: outpatient or home rehabilitation plan, need for assistive devices, evaluation of outcomes, and functional restoration goals
- Rest and nutrition to promote early recovery with measures to prevent rehospitalization
- Transportation to health care providers and therapy
- Patient and family coping

Case management documentation includes diagnostic-specific outcomes as part of the evaluation. The stated patient goals of the multidisciplinary team, either favorable or adverse, include (1) the patient's general health status; (2) patient satisfaction with health and with the care provided; (3) prevention of adverse factors such as medication errors, infection rates, and patient falls; (4) organizational effectiveness, such as cost and productivity; and (5) standards of care that reflect the practice of health care providers (e.g., home health care).[11] For information regarding average length of stay (LOS), patient outcomes, and hospital charges refer to the U.S. Agency for Healthcare Research and Quality (AHRQ) at www.ahrq.gov/data.

CONCLUSION

A CNS infection, meningitis or encephalitis, brain abscess, and other CNS disorders discussed in this chapter may be life threatening. Prompt recognition with appropriate studies for precise diagnosis is important because brain tumors, infarctions, or hematomas may mimic the appearance of an abscess. The treatments for these disorders are different and may not demand the same promptness of treatment as that required for a brain abscess. Clinical management must be tailored to the individual patient and the patient's specific treatment regimen to produce a positive patient outcome. Patient and family teaching to elicit participation in follow-up and home care is essential, because long-term antibiotic therapy is usually required.

The outcome for a patient with a CNS infection depends on rapid diagnosis of the offending organism, an effective treatment program, and an exceptionally knowledgeable clinician to direct and manage clinical care. All patients at high risk for CNS infection must be monitored closely and receive prompt treatment at the first sign of infection if the mortality and morbidity statistics for CNS infections are to be reduced.

RESOURCES FOR CENTRAL NERVOUS SYSTEM INFECTIONS

Centers for Disease Control and Prevention: Atlanta, GA 30333; 800-458-5231; www.cdc.gov/ncidod/dbmd/diseaseinfo

Creutzfeldt-Jakob Disease Foundation: PO Box 611625, North Miami, FL 33261-1625; www.cjdfoundation.org, www.mad-cow.org/

HCUPnet: Healthcare Cost and Utilization Project, Agency for Healthcare Research and Quality, Rockville, MD; www.ahrq.gov/HCUPnet/

The Lyme Disease Foundation: 1 Financial Plaza, Hartford, CT 06103; 800-525-2000, ext. 886; fax: 860-525-8425; e-mail: Lymefind@aol.com; www.lyme.org

Lyme Disease Network: www.lymenet.org

U.S. Agency for Healthcare Research and Quality (AHRQ): www.ahrq.gov/data/hcup/hcupnet.htm

REFERENCES

1. American Lyme Disease Foundation: Treatment, 2006. Available at www.aldf.com/Lyme.asp.
2. American Thoracic Society, CDC, and Infectious Disease Society of America: Treatment of tuberculosis, *MMWR Morb Mortal Wkly Rep* 52(RR-11), 2003.
3. Bell B, Britton J: Brain abscess. In Lambert H, editor: *Infections of the central nervous system*, Philadelphia, 1991, BC Decker.
4. Bonington A, Strang JI, Klapper PE, et al: Use of Roche AMPLICOR *Mycobacterium tuberculosis* PCR in early diagnosis of tuberculous meningitis, *J Clin Microbiol* 36(5):1251–1254, 1998.
5. Boss BJ, Farely JA: Alterations of neurologic function. In Heuther SE, McCance KL, editors: *Understanding pathophysiology*, ed 2, St Louis, 2000, Mosby.
6. Carpenter C et al: Infections of the nervous system. In Andreoli T, editor: *Cecil essentials of medicine*, ed 2, Philadelphia, 1990, WB Saunders.
7. Centers for Disease Control and Prevention: Bacterial meningitis statistics 2004 (last whole year completed). Available at www.cdc.gov.
8. Centers for Disease Control and Prevention: Lyme disease prevention, 2005. Available at www.cdc.gov/ncidod/dvbid/lymeprevent.htm.
9. Chambers H: Infectious disease: bacterial and chlamydial. In Papadakis M, Krupp M, editors: *Current medical diagnosis and treatment*, Norwalk, CT, 1992, Appleton & Lange.
10. Chin J, editor: *Control of communicable diseases manual*, ed 17, Washington, DC, 2000, American Public Health Association.
11. Cohen EL, DeBack V: *The outcomes mandate*, St Louis, 1999, Mosby.
12. Crossley K, Henry K, Thurn J: Meningitis and encephalitis. In Taylor R, editor: *Difficult medical management*, Philadelphia, 1991, WB Saunders.
13. Davis L: Brain abscess. In Mohr J, editor: *Manual of clinical problems in neurology*, ed 2, Boston, 1989, Little, Brown.
14. Davis L: St. Louis encephalitis. In Mohr J, editor: *Manual of clinical problems in neurology*, ed 2, Boston, 1989, Little, Brown.
15. Dellinger EP, Ehrenkranz NJ: Surgical infections. In Bennett JV, Brachman PS, editors: *Hospital infections*, ed 4, Philadelphia, 1998, Lippincott-Raven.
16. Dennehy P: Active immunization in the United States: development over the past decade, *Clin Microbiol Rev* 14(4):872–908, 2001.
17. Durand ML, Calderwood SB, Weber DJ, et al: Acute bacterial meningitis in adults: a review of 493 episodes, *N Engl J Med* 328(23):1712, 1993.
18. Emedicine from WebMD: Herpes simplex encephalitis, 2006. Available at www.emedicine.com/EMERG/topic247.htm.
19. Evans J: *Borrelia burgdorferi* (Lyme disease). In *APIC text of infection control and epidemiology*, ed 2, Washington, DC, 2005, Association for Professionals in Infection Control and Epidemiology.
20. Farr B, Scheld WM: Nosocomial meningitis. In Pankey G, editor: *Ochsner clinic reports on serious hospital infections* (an educational service provided by Wyeth-Ayerst Laboratories), 10(2), 1998.
21. Goldsmith SM, Whitley RJ: Herpes simplex encephalitis. In Lambert HP, editor: *Infections of the central nervous system*, Philadelphia, 1991, BC Decker.
22. Goetz CG, Pappert EJ: *The textbook of clinical neurology*, Philadelphia, 1999, WB Saunders.
23. Graham DI, Lantos PI: *Greenfield's neuropathology*, ed 6, London, 1997, Arnold.
24. Greenlee J: Anatomic considerations in central nervous system infections. In Mandell G, Douglass R, Bennett J, editors: *Principles and practice of infectious disease*, ed 4, New York, 2005, Churchill Livingstone.
25. Gruendemann B, Mangum S: *Infection prevention in surgical settings*, Philadelphia, 2001, WB Saunders.
26. Haiduven D, Poland G: Immunization in the healthcare worker. In *APIC text of infection control and epidemiology*, ed 2, Washington, DC, 2005, Association for Professionals in Infection Control and Epidemiology.
27. Harrison LH, Pass MA, Mendelsohn AB, et al: Invasive meningococcal disease in adolescents and young adults, *JAMA* 286:694–699, 2001.
28. Heymann DL: *Control of communicable diseases manual*, ed 18, Washington, DC, 2004, American Public Health Association.
29. Hickey J: *The clinical practice of neurological and neurosurgical nursing*, ed 4, Philadelphia, 1997, Lippincott-Raven.
30. HICPAC Group: Guideline for prevention of surgical site infection, 1999, *Infect Control Hosp Epidemiol* 20(4):247–278, 1999.
31. Hogan G, Ryan N: Bacterial meningitis. In Mohr J, editor: *Manual of clinical problems in neurology*, ed 2, Boston, 1989, Little, Brown.
32. Horan TC, Emori TG: Definitions of key terms used in the NNIS system, *Am J Infect Control* 25(2):112–116, 1997.
33. Hsaio K, Mainer Z, Kahana E: Mutation of the prion protein in Libyan Jews with Creutzfeldt-Jakob disease, *N Engl J Med* 324:1091–1097, 1991.
34. Huether SE, McCance KL: *Understanding pathophysiology*, St Louis, 2000, Mosby.
35. *Infection Control Today:* A clean sweep: surface cleaning in the healthcare environment, 2005. Available at www.infection-controltoday.com/articles.

36. Joint Commission on Accreditation of Healthcare Organizations (JCAHO): Sentinel Event Alert, issue 20, Exposure to Creutzfeldt-Jakob disease, June 1, 2001. Available at www.jointcommission.org/SentinelEvents/SentinelEventAlert/.

37. Johns Hopkins Medicine: Treatment recommendations for adult inpatients. Antibiotic guidelines, 2004. Available at www.hopkins-heic.org/amp/.

38. Kaplan K: Brain abscess. Symposium of infections of the central nervous system, *Med Clin North Am* 69:360, 1985.

39. Kennedy C: Acute viral infections excluding herpes simplex, rabies, and HIV. In Lambert H, editor: *Infections of the central nervous system,* Philadelphia, 1991, BC Decker.

40. Lin JJ, Harn HJ, Hsu YD, et al: Rapid diagnosis of tuberculous meningitis by polymerase chain reaction assay of cerebrospinal fluid, *J Neurol* 242(3):147–152, 1995.

41. Little JR: Central nervous system infections. In *APIC text of infection control and epidemiology,* ed 2, Washington, DC, 2005, Association for Professionals in Infection Control and Epidemiology.

42. Llewelyn CA, Hewitt PE, Knight RE, et al: Possible transmission of variant Creutzfeldt-Jakob disease by blood transfusion, *Lancet* 363(9407):417–421, 2004.

43. Logigian EL, Kaplan RF, Steere AC: Chronic neurologic manifestations of Lyme disease, *N Engl J Med* 232(21):1438, 1990.

44. Logigian EL, Steere AC: Lyme borreliosis. In Lambert H, editor: *Infections of the central nervous system,* Philadelphia, 1991, BC Decker.

45. McGee L, Baringer J: Acute meningitis. In Mandell G, Douglas R, Bennett J, editors: *Principles and practice of infectious disease,* ed 3, New York, 1990, Churchill Livingstone.

46. Mckinney W: Travel Health. In *APIC text of infection control and epidemiology,* ed 2, Washington, DC, 2005, Association for Professionals in Infection Control and Epidemiology.

47. Miller J, Jubelt B: Infections of the nervous system: bacterial infections. In Rowland L, editor: *Merritt's textbook of neurology,* ed 8, Philadelphia, 1989, Lea & Febiger.

48. Mocsny N: Precautions prevent the spread of Creutzfeldt-Jakob disease, *J Neurosci Nurs* 23(2):116, 1991.

49. Murray R, Morawetz R, Kepes J, et al: Lyme neuroborreliosis manifesting as an intracranial mass lesion, *Neurosurgery* 30(5):769–773, 1992.

50. Muto C, Pokrywka M: Creutzfeldt-Jakob disease and other prion diseases. In *APIC text of infection control and epidemiology,* ed 2, Washington, DC, 2005, Association for Professionals in Infection Control and Epidemiology.

51. Nadelman RB, Wormser GP: Management of tick bites and early Lyme disease. In Evans J, Rahn DW, editors: *Lyme disease,* Philadelphia, 1997, American College of Physicians.

52. National Academy of Sciences National Research Council: Postoperative wound infections: the influence of ultraviolet irradiation of the operating room and various other factors, *Ann Surg* 160(suppl 2):1–132, 1964.

53. National Center for Infectious Diseases: Tick borne diseases, 2006. Available at www.cdc.gov/ncidod/diseases/list_tickborne.htm.

54. Newton WN: West Nile virus. In *APIC text of infection control and epidemiology,* ed 2, 2005, Association for Professionals in Infection Control and Epidemiology.

55. Oliver D: Microbes and you: normal flora, *Science Creative Quarterly,* Sept-Nov 2006. Available at www.bioteach.ubc.ca/Biomedicine/normalflora.

56. Olsen M, Mayfield J, Lauryssen C, et al: Risk factors for surgical site infection in spinal surgery, *J Neurosurg* 98(2 suppl):149–155, 2003.

57. Peter G, editor: *Red book: report of the committee on infectious diseases,* ed 22, Elk Grove Village, IL, 1991, American Academy of Pediatrics.

58. Popp AJ, editor: *A guide to the primary care of neurological disorders,* Park Ridge, IL, 1998, American Association of Neurological Surgeons.

59. Purtillo D, Purtillo R: *A survey of human diseases,* ed 2, Boston, 1989, Little, Brown.

60. Rahn DW: Lyme disease: clinical manifestations, diagnosis, and treatment, *Semin Arthritis Rheum* 20(4):201, 1991.

61. Sampson BA, Ambrosi C, Charlot A, et al: The pathology of human West Nile infection, *Hum Pathol* 31(5):527–531, 2000.

62. Shankar P, Manjunath N, Mohan KK, et al: Rapid diagnosis of tuberculous meningitis by polymerase chain reaction, *Lancet* 337(8732):5–7, 1991.

63. Short WR, Tunkel AR: Timing of administration of antimicrobial therapy in bacterial meningitis, *Curr Infect Dis Rep* 3(4):360–364, 2001.

64. Sigal LH, Zahradnik JM, Lavin P, et al: A vaccine consisting of recombinant *Borrelia burgdorferi* outer-surface protein A to prevent Lyme disease, *N Engl J Med* 339:216–222, 1998.

65. Steere AC: Lyme disease, *N Engl J Med* 345:115–123, 2001.

66. Steere AC, Sikand VK, Maurice F, et al: Vaccination against Lyme disease with recombinant *Borrelia burgdorferi* outer surface lipoprotein A with adjuvant, *N Engl J Med* 339:209–215, 1998.

67. Sunderland P: Structure and function of the neurologic system. In Huether S, McCance K, editors: *Understanding pathophysiology,* ed 2, New York, 1996, Mosby.

68. Teoh R, Humphries M: Tuberculous meningitis. In Lambert H, editor: *Infections of the central nervous system,* Philadelphia, 1991, BC Decker.

69. Todar K: *Mechanisms of bacterial pathogenicity: colonization and invasion,* 2002, University of Wisconsin–Madison, Todar's Online Textbook of Bacteriology. Available at http://textbookofbacteriology.net/colonization.

70. Tunkel A, Scheld W: Bacterial meningitis: pathogenic and pathophysiologic mechanisms. In Lambert H, editor: *Infections of the central nervous system,* Philadelphia, 1991, BC Decker.

71. Tunkel A: Approach to the patient with central nervous system infection. In Mandell G, Douglass R, Bennett J, editors: *Principles and practice of infectious diseases,* ed 5, New York, 2005, Churchill Livingstone.

72. Tunkel A: Brain abscess. In Mandell G, Douglass R, Bennett J, editors: *Principles and practice of infectious diseases,* ed 5, New York, 2005, Churchill Livingstone.

73. Tunkel A, Scheld WM: Acute meningitis. In Mandell G, Douglass R, Bennett J, editors: *Principles and practice of infectious diseases,* ed 5, New York, 2005, Churchill Livingstone.

74. Tweeten SM: General principles of epidemiology. In *APIC text of infection control and epidemiology,* ed 2, Washington, DC, 2005, Association for Professionals in Infection Control and Epidemiology.

75. US Department of Health and Human Services, Centers for Disease Control and Prevention (CDC): Prevention and control of meningococcal disease and meningococcal disease and college students: recommendations of the Advisory Committee

on Immunization Practices (ACIP), *MMWR Morb Mortal Wkly Rep* 49(RR-7), 2000.

76. Varnell M: West Nile virus, *Advance for Nurses* 2(16):30, 2000.

77. Wangensteen OH, Wangensteen SD: *The rise of surgery: from empiric craft to scientific discipline,* Minnesota, 1978, University of Minnesota Press.

78. Wenger J, Broome C: Bacterial meningitis: epidemiology. In Lambert H, editor: *Infections of the central nervous system,* Philadelphia, 1991, BC Decker.

79. Wormser GP, Nadelman RB, Dattwyler RJ, et al: Guidelines from the Infectious Diseases Society of America, practice guidelines for the treatment of Lyme disease, *Clin Infect Dis* 31(suppl 1):S1–S14, 2000.

ELLEN BARKER

CHAPTER 5

Central Nervous System Metabolic Disorders: Syndrome of Inappropriate Antidiuretic Hormone and Diabetes Insipidus

The central nervous system (CNS) functions normally in a fluid environment with carefully balanced electrolyte concentrations and pH values. Multiple neurologic conditions (e.g., head injury, neurosurgery, and brain tumors) discussed throughout this book affect the relationship between the pituitary, hypothalamus, endocrine system, and hormones secreted by the endocrine glands, each of which can influence the fluid and electrolyte balance. The cells of the human body can survive only in a fluid environment with an electrolyte concentration and pH values that are maintained within a very narrow range.[19] If the brain is deprived of fluids and electrolytes essential to normal cerebral metabolism, cerebral function will be impaired, the patient's neurologic status will deteriorate, and complications or death may result.

Disorder of the sodium and water balance is a common complication following neurosurgery (e.g., aneurysmal surgery and surgery of the hypothalamus and surrounding structures) (see Chapter 18). Neuroscience patients must be continuously assessed and monitored for their response to therapy and their progress toward recovery. Early detection of disease-related impaired neuronal metabolism that interferes with function of the nervous system is critical to the protection and integrity of the brain.

This chapter focuses on critical parameters for the integrity of the nervous system that include fluid and electrolyte balance and osmolality in relationship to antidiuretic hormone (ADH) imbalances that result in the syndrome of inappropriate antidiuretic hormone (SIADH) or diabetes insipidus (DI). The various clinical conditions reviewed in this chapter can delay the patient's recovery and significantly add to the patient's morbidity and mortality risk. These metabolic topics are discussed with emphasis on clinical management and related pathophysiology and will be expanded on in other chapters (e.g., pituitary tumors in Chapter 7; neuroscience critical care management in Chapter 9; neurotrauma in Chapter 11; and aneurysms in Chapter 18).

PHYSIOLOGY OF FLUID AND ELECTROLYTE BALANCE

Total body water (TBW) accounts for approximately 60% of body weight. Under normal conditions, 20% of TBW is located in the extracellular fluid (ECF), and 40% is in intracellular fluid (ICF).[12] Intercompartmental fluid shifts can occur, depending on the concentration of various solutes (particles) on either side of the cell membrane. The movement of water down a concentration gradient to a lower concentration across a semipermeable membrane is a process called **osmosis.** Sodium, the principal extracellular **cation** (positively charged ion), and potassium, the principal intracellular cation, are the principal determinants of the osmotic gradient and influence the distribution of fluid.[7] Sodium plays a major role in maintaining the concentration and volume of ECF.[11]

Three properties of the blood can be manipulated for patients receiving intravenous (IV) fluids: (1) osmolality, (2) colloid oncotic pressure, and (3) hematocrit. **Osmolality** describes the molar number of osmotically active particles per kilogram of solvent. It is expressed in milliosmoles per kilogram of water (mOsm/kg), or as the concentration of molecules per weight of water.[17] **Osmolarity** measures the number of milliosmoles per liter of solution, or the concentration of molecules per volume of solution.[17] Normal serum osmolality is strictly maintained within a physiologic range of 280 to 294 mOsm/kg. Plasma osmolality greater than 294 mOsm/kg indicates that the concentration of particles is too great or that the water content is too little and the patient's condition is termed **water deficit.** A serum osmolality less than 275 mOsm/kg indicates that the amount of particles or solute is too small in proportion to the amount of water or that there is too much water for the amount of solute. This clinically significant condition is termed **water excess.**[11] Since the primary determinants of the plasma are sodium, glucose, and urea, a formula can be used to estimate the osmolality until the laboratory results are available by making the following calculations:

$$\text{Serum osmolality} = 2 \times (Na + K) + (BUN \div 2.8) + (Glucose \div 18)$$

where BUN is blood urea nitrogen.

A change in solute concentration on either side of the cell membrane can cause significant fluid shifts with resultant cellular dysfunction. For example, an increase in serum sodium concentration (to >150 mEq/L) causes serum hyperosmolality and cellular dehydration. Conversely, a decrease in serum sodium concentration (to >130 mEq/L) causes serum hypo-osmolality with resultant cellular edema. To maintain plasma or serum osmolality within the physiologic range, free water intake and excretion must balance. In conscious individuals, water intake is governed by the sensation of thirst. Water preservation/excretion by the kidney is regulated by ADH or vasopressin.[19,21]

Osmolality is approximately the same in the various body fluid spaces. Determining osmolality is important because it indicates the water balance of the body.[17] Common signs and symptoms of electrolyte disorders are listed in Table 5-1, and terms commonly used to understand fluid and electrolyte management are listed in Box 5-1.

| BOX 5-1 | Terms Commonly Used to Understand Fluid and Electrolyte Management |

Hydrostatic Pressure (HP)

The force within a fluid compartment. In the blood vessels HP is related to the dynamic force added to the fluid by the pumping of the heart and is the major force that moves water out of the vascular system at the capillary level. HP is about 40 mm Hg at the arterial end of a capillary and about 10 mm Hg at the venous end of the capillary.

Oncotic Pressure (OP) or Colloidal Pressure (CP)

The osmotic pressure exerted by a colloid in solution (a nondiffusible substance or a solute suspended in a solution; e.g., albumin, plasma, plasmanate, and dextran). Plasma OP is approximately 25 mm Hg. Dextran is a plasma expander and a colloidal solution.

Isotonic/Iso-Osmolar Fluid

Fluid with the same osmolality as the cell interior or isotonic crystalloid solution. A diffusible substance dissolved in solution (e.g., lactated Ringer's solution, 0.9% saline, or 5% dextrose in water) will pass through a selectively permeable membrane.

Hypotonic/Hypo-Osmolar Fluid

Solution surrounding the cells in which the solutes are less concentrated than the cells, with osmolality less than 280 mOsm/kg. The excess water can move into the cell, causing swelling of the cells. Distilled water is an example of a hypotonic solution.

Hypertonic/Hyperosmolar Fluid

Solution with solutes more concentrated than the cells, resulting in a water deficit and osmolality greater than 294 mOsm/kg. It can cause water to leave the cells, causing shrinking of the cells. An example of a hypertonic crystalloid solution is 3.0% saline.

Colloid oncotic pressure (COP) is the osmotic pressure generated by large molecules (e.g., albumin, hetastarch, or dextran). The COP becomes important where vascular membranes are permeable to small ions but not to large molecules. The **hematocrit** level of 30% to 33% gives the optimal combination of viscosity and O_2-carrying capacity, and may improve neurologic outcome. A reduced hematocrit of less than 30% exacerbates neurologic injury.

Fluid management can be challenging, particularly in those patients who receive diuretics such as mannitol (Osmitrol) or furosemide (Lasix) for the treatment of cerebral edema and increased intracranial pressure (ICP). It is important when administering IV fluids to recognize that crystalloid solutions (D_5W, lactated Ringer's, normal saline) do not contain any high-molecular-weight compounds and have an oncotic pressure of zero. In comparison, colloids (5% albumin, fresh frozen plasma) have an oncotic pressure similar to that of plasma.

Intravenous salt-free solutions containing glucose should be avoided in patients with brain and spinal cord pathology, because glucose is quickly metabolized leaving only free water that can reduce serum osmolality and increase brain water content. In contrast, hypertonic salt solutions have been found to decrease cerebral edema and lower ICP. When solutions (e.g., 1.5% sodium chloride or other hypertonic solutions) are ordered, they should be infused carefully to avoid hypernatremia. This current practice replaces past theories in which neuroscience patients with intracranial pathology were kept "dry." Research is underway to investigate the different percentages of sodium chloride solutions and determine if hypertonic saline solutions may be effective for patients with brain or spinal cord injury. The clinician must use caution in administering hypertonic saline to patients with brain injury and intracranial hypertension who also have cardiac conditions and electrolyte abnormalities.

ANTIDIURETIC HORMONE

Anatomy and Physiology

Antidiuretic hormone (ADH) or the neurohormone arginine vasopressin (AVP), also referred to as **vasopressin,** has a role in balancing sodium and water in the body and controls water conservation and concentrates the urine. Changes in the osmotic pressure of extracellular fluid trigger the release of AVP from the pituitary gland, which stores it, but AVP is actually synthesized in the hypothalamus. The release is coordinated with the activity of the thirst center, which regulates fluid intake. Vasopressin binds to receptor sites of the cortical collecting ducts of the kidneys resulting in increased free-water reabsorption.[26] ADH is synthesized in the paraventricular and supraoptic nuclei of the hypothalamus and is then transported down the axons of the infundibular stem and stored in the posterior pituitary or neurohypophysis (see Chapter 1). ADH's release is regulated primarily by osmoreceptors in the hypothalamus, and when released into the systemic circulation, ADH acts on vascular smooth muscle to cause vasoconstriction. Up to 10% of ADH may be

TABLE 5-1	Common Signs and Symptoms of Electrolyte Disorders	
Electrolyte	**Abnormality**	**Symptoms**
Sodium	Hyponatremia	Nausea/vomiting
		Abdominal cramping
		Weakness
		Headache
		Seizures
		Mild confusion
		Coma
		Respiratory depression
		Bizarre behavior
		Nystagmus
		Hallucinations
	Hypernatremia	Flushed skin
		Temperature elevation
		Mental confusion
		Seizures
		Coma
Potassium	Hypokalemia	Weakness
		Confusion
		Anorexia
		Nausea/vomiting
		Mental depression
		Flaccid paralysis
		Areflexic quadriplegia
		Respiratory insufficiency or failure, leading to death
	Hyperkalemia	Cardiac changes: tachycardia, bradycardia, cardiac arrest
		Loss of strength
		Loss of deep tendon reflexes (DTRs)
		Muscle weakness or cramping
		Paresthesias
		Focal neurologic signs
		Nausea
		Diarrhea
Calcium	Hypocalcemia	Tetany (tonic muscle spasms)
		Positive Chvostek's sign
		Positive Trousseau's sign
		Irritability
		Delirium
		Delusions
		Hallucinations
		Depression
		Dementia
		Seizures
	Hypercalcemia	Weight loss
		Cachexia
		Abdominal pain
		Muscle pain or weakness
		Stones formed of calcium in kidneys
		Anorexia
		Confusion
		Coma leading to death
Magnesium	Hypomagnesemia	Nausea/vomiting
		Muscle weakness and fasciculations
		Hyperreflexia
		Myoclonus
		Confusion
		Cardiac dysrhythmias
		Agitation
		Tremors
		Tetany
		Lethargy

Continued

TABLE 5-1	Common Signs and Symptoms of Electrolyte Disorders—cont'd	
Electrolyte	**Abnormality**	**Symptoms**
	Hypermagnesemia	Cardiac dysrhythmias
		Depressed DVTs
		Depressed respirations
		CNS depression
		Lethargy, leading to coma
		Muscle weakness, leading to paralysis or flaccid quadriplegia
		Dilated pupils

Data from Haas LB: Nursing management: endocrine problems. In Lewis SM, Heitkemper MM, Dirksen SR, editors: *Medical-surgical nursing: assessment and management of clinical problems,* ed 5, St Louis, 2000, Mosby; Horne MM, Bond ER: Fluid, electrolyte, and acid-base balance. In Lewis SM, Heitkemper MM, Dirksen SR, editors: *Medical-surgical nursing: assessment and management of clinical problems,* ed 5, St Louis, 2000, Mosby; and Huether SE: Fluids and electrolytes, acids and bases. In McCance KL, Huether SE, editors: *Pathophysiology: the biologic basics for diseases in adults and children,* ed 4, St Louis, 2002, Mosby.
CNS, Central nervous system; *DVTs,* deep venous thromboses.

excreted in the urine as an active hormone. In the presence of ADH, renal tubule permeability to water is increased, resulting in increased water reabsorption. Conversely, in the absence of ADH, renal tubule permeability to water is decreased, resulting in decreased renal excretion of large volumes of hypotonic fluid.[7,30] ADH is thought to cause vasoconstriction to raise the blood pressure in response to severe hypotension, such as after significant blood loss.

Control of Antidiuretic Hormone Secretion

The primary regulatory mechanism for the release of ADH is plasma osmolality, which is mediated by a delicate feedback mechanism. Osmoreceptors located in the supraoptic nuclei are sensitive to slight changes in plasma osmolality. For example, a 1% to 2% increase in plasma osmolality above 280 mOsm/L, secondary to an increase in extracellular sodium or a decrease in extracellular free water, can significantly increase ADH secretion. Increased ADH prevents free water loss from the renal tubules, restoring serum osmolality to normal levels. On the other hand, a decrease in serum osmolality will inhibit ADH release and promote free water loss, or diuresis.[19] Excessive or inappropriate ADH production predisposes to hyponatremia if water intake is not reduced in parallel with urine output.[14]

Hemodynamic factors also play a role in the regulation of ADH. Arterial baroreceptors, located in the carotid sinus and aortic arch, transmit information regarding changes in arterial pressure and blood volume via the glossopharyngeal and vagus nerves innervating the medulla. In turn, these medullary centers send impulses to the hypothalamic nuclei responsible for the production and secretion of ADH. A 10% decrease in the circulating blood volume stimulates these pathways and causes ADH release. Other factors that influence the release of ADH can be found in Box 5-2.[7,21]

Regulation of the Thirst Mechanism

The thirst mechanism plays an important role in the regulation of body water balance. The osmoreceptors that trigger the thirst mechanism are anatomically close to those that control ADH release. A serum osmolality greater than

BOX 5-2	Factors Affecting Antidiuretic Hormone Release

Factors Increasing ADH
Increased plasma osmolality
Trauma
Changes in the intravascular volume that are monitored by baroreceptors in the left atrium, carotid, and aortic arches
Decreased blood volume (shock, dehydration)
Nausea/vomiting
Emotional stress
Pain
Positive-pressure ventilation
Increased glucose levels (in the absence of insulin)
Nicotine
Pharmacologic agents
- Chlorpropamide
- Morphine
- Thiazides
- Carbamazepine
- Barbiturates
- Meperidine
- Anesthetic agents
- Vincristine

Factors Decreasing ADH
Decreased plasma osmolality
Ethanol ingestion
Lithium administration
Demeclocycline
Infusion of large volumes of hypotonic fluids
Hypertension

ADH, Antidiuretic hormone.

290 mOsm/kg triggers this mechanism. Individuals with an intact thirst mechanism who are able to ingest fluids can maintain normal hydration even with high urinary outputs. On the other hand, an individual with impaired antidiuresis who either cannot recognize the thirst stimulus or cannot ingest water, because of neurologic or mechanical deficits (e.g., the patient in a coma), is predisposed to a life-threatening condition.[19,21]

As stated previously, sodium is the principal determinant of serum osmolality. Physiologic mechanisms that regulate the excretion and reabsorption of sodium by the kidney include the renin/angiotensin system and aldosterone. **Renin,** a substance produced by the juxtaglomerular cells of the kidney in response to a decrease in extracellular fluid volume, converts angiotensin I to angiotensin II.

Angiotensin II stimulates the production of aldosterone by the zona glomerulosa cells of the adrenal cortex. The principal action of **aldosterone** is to increase sodium reabsorption by the distal convoluted tubules of the kidney. In addition, aldosterone increases the excretion of hydrogen ions and potassium. Simply stated: "Water follows sodium." Therefore by increasing the amount of sodium reabsorbed, water is conserved and extracellular fluid volume also is increased.[19]

Syndrome of Inappropriate Antidiuretic Hormone and Cerebral Salt-Wasting Syndrome

Syndrome of inappropriate antidiuretic hormone (SIADH) and cerebral salt-wasting syndrome (CSWS) are two potential causes of hyponatremia for the neuroscience patient.[5] SIADH is a volume-expanded state and CSWS is a volume-depleted state.[23] Distinguishing between the two syndromes and selection of the treatment of choice is critical to avoid untoward outcomes.

The **syndrome of inappropriate antidiuretic hormone (SIADH)** was first described in the 1950s by Schwartz and colleagues in a group of patients with oat cell bronchiogenic carcinoma. This syndrome is characterized by a persistent, abnormally high (inappropriate) secretion of antidiuretic hormone (ADH) in the absence of hemodynamic and osmotic stimuli.[4,27] SIADH is one of the rare diseases of the posterior pituitary, and the clinician should be alert to it as an abnormal condition that may alter the body's fluid and electrolyte balance. SIADH is sometimes referred to as **Schwartz-Bartter syndrome.** Various cerebral pathologic processes, mostly head trauma, can result in excessive release of ADH. SIADH can also result from overadministration of free water, or D_5W, in patients who cannot excrete free water because of excess ADH.

Cerebral salt-wasting syndrome (CSWS) is the most common cause of true or acute hyponatremia in neurosurgical patients (e.g., subarachnoid hemorrhage). It is characterized by a loss of sodium or urine sodium wasting, decreased plasma volume, decreased extracellular fluid volume, depressed uric acid levels, and decreased body weight. CSWS is thought to be due to failure of the CNS to regulate sodium absorption. The patient becomes hypovolemic from extracellular fluid volume depletion. In CSWS, serum uric acid levels are also unexpectedly low due to a tubular transport abnormality for uric acid.[18] It is important to understand the differences between CSWS and SIADH because while both may cause hyponatremia, the treatments are different.

With CSWS, albumin concentration, BUN/creatinine, and hematocrit may be elevated, serum potassium elevated or normal, and uric acid normal or decreased.[23] For example, hyponatremia in the case of a patient with a subarachnoid

hemorrhage may be due to CSWS, not SIADH. CSWS requires vigorous sodium and volume replacement. Fluid restriction could be harmful.

As a consequence of cerebral salt wasting, patients are both hypovolemic (volume contraction) and hyponatremic (natriuresis). Symptoms may be seen clinically about the tenth postoperative day. Patients may complain of increased thirst or headache. Assessment may reveal problems with orthostatic hypotension or tachycardia. The patient may appear to be lethargic with decreasing level of consciousness. Seizure precautions are recommended.

Treatment for CSWS includes volume replacement fluids with normal saline or hypertonic saline solutions, depending on the degree of hypovolemia.[13] Fludrocortisone (Florinef) 0.2 mg/day intravenously or orally may be given to promote the increased reabsorption of sodium.[2] A titrated dose is used to achieve the lowest effective dose. This prevents correction of the hyponatremia too quickly.

Etiology and Pathophysiology

The etiology of SIADH is thought to result from the following: (1) excessive activity of the neurohypophyseal system secondary to suprahypothalamic brain disease or processes that damage the supraoptic neurons; (2) abnormal reflex activity from baroreceptors (volume receptors); (3) ectopic secretion of ADH from neoplastic tissue; and (4) specific medications.[24] The rate of fall of the sodium level is thought to be more important than the magnitude of the fall in serum sodium. The main features of SIADH are water retention, or increases in TBW; solute loss (particularly sodium); and osmotic inactivation of cellular solutes.[12]

Nonmalignant pulmonary tissue also possesses the capability of triggering the secretion of ADH. In the presence of pulmonary disease, such as viral or bacterial pneumonia, ADH release can be traced to the stimulation of intrathoracic baroreceptors. Changes in intrathoracic pressure secondary to diffuse pulmonary disease and positive-pressure ventilation can also result in uncontrolled secretion of ADH.[24,30]

A common cause of SIADH is ectopic production of an ADH-like substance by various types of malignant tissue. The most common type of malignancy associated with this syndrome is bronchiogenic oat cell carcinoma. Other tumors include carcinoma of the duodenum and pancreas, leukemia, lymphoma, Hodgkin's disease, sarcoma, and squamous cell carcinoma of the tongue.[13] Other common causes of SIADH include several CNS diseases and various pharmacologic agents. A detailed list of these causes can be found in Table 5-2.[8,24]

The principal pathologic finding in SIADH is persistent, abnormally high levels of circulating ADH occurring without physiologic stimuli in the presence of normal renal and adrenal function. This "inappropriate" release implies that ADH is no longer regulated by plasma osmolality and volume. This imbalance upsets the fluid and electrolyte homeostasis of the body. Because the renal tubules continue to reabsorb free water regardless of the serum osmolality, hypo-osmolality of the extracellular fluid develops. Hyponatremia (serum sodium <135 mEq/L) results from both dilution reabsorption of free water and renal sodium excretion[3,28] (Fig. 5-1).

TABLE 5-2	Etiology of Syndrome of Inappropriate Antidiuretic Hormone (SIADH)
Condition	**Cause**
CNS trauma	Head trauma
General surgery	Pain, nausea
CNS hemorrhage	Subarachnoid hemorrhage, subdural hematoma
	Stroke
CNS neoplasms	Brain tumors
CNS infections	Brain abscess
	Meningitis
	Encephalitis
CNS diseases	Guillain-Barré syndrome (GBS)
	Multiple sclerosis (MS)
	Hydrocephalus
Pulmonary diseases	Pneumonia (bacterial or viral)
	Oat cell carcinoma of the lung
	Positive-pressure ventilation
	Tuberculosis
	Pulmonary abscess
Endocrine disorders	Addison's disease
	Hypopituitarism
Neoplastic disorders	Lymphoma
	Sarcoma
Hypovolemia	Blood loss and anemia
	Recumbent position
Pharmacologic agents	Barbiturates
	Bromocriptine (Parlodel)
	Carbamazepine (Tegretol)
	Chlorpropamide (Diabinese)
	Clofibrate (Atromid-S)
	Haloperidol (Haldol)
	Opiates (morphine)
	Phenothiazines
	Thiazide diuretics
	Tricyclic antidepressants
	Oxytocin (Pitocin)
	Vincristine, cisplatin, cyclophosphamide (Cytoxan)
Pain and stress	Secondary to intracranial or other causes

CNS, Central nervous system.

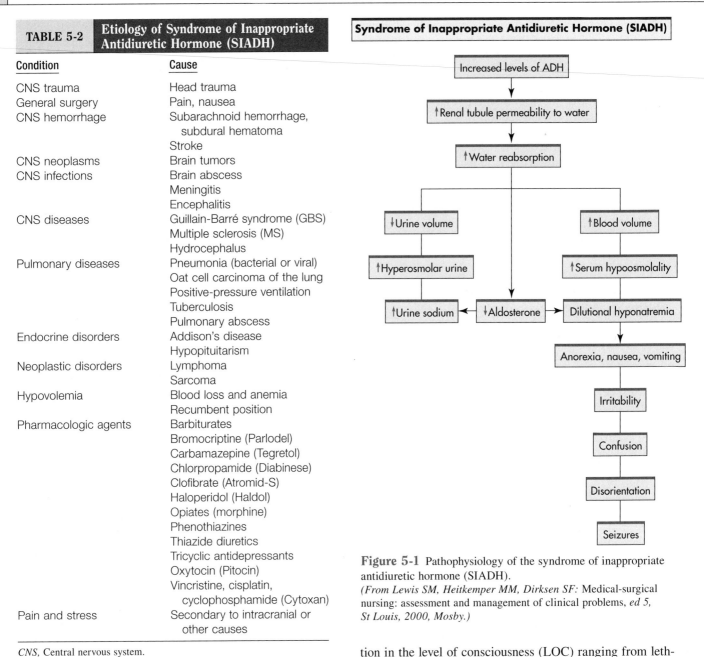

Syndrome of Inappropriate Antidiuretic Hormone (SIADH)

Figure 5-1 Pathophysiology of the syndrome of inappropriate antidiuretic hormone (SIADH).
(From Lewis SM, Heitkemper MM, Dirksen SF: Medical-surgical nursing: assessment and management of clinical problems, ed 5, St Louis, 2000, Mosby.)

As stated previously, ADH is produced in the hypothalamus and stored in the posterior pituitary. It is secreted in response to a delicate feedback mechanism that is governed by both serum osmolality and plasma volume. In SIADH this system breaks down, resulting in a continuous release and excessive blood level of ADH. This permits the collecting ducts of the kidney to reabsorb free water and results in an increased plasma volume. Because this free water retention is out of proportion to sodium reabsorption, dilutional hyponatremia develops and is compounded by renal **natriuresis,** the continued excretion of large volumes of sodium by the kidney. Despite these conditions, the patient exhibits no clinical symptoms of hypotension or volume depletion. CNS findings in SIADH are related to hyponatremia and resultant intracellular edema and include confusion, agitation, altera-

tion in the level of consciousness (LOC) ranging from lethargy to coma, headaches, anorexia, and muscle weakness.

ALERT: Seizures can occur with hyponatremia at or below 115 mEq/L.[30,32] Hyponatremia is the most common electrolyte disturbance in neurosurgical patients.

Assessment

SIADH is usually seen in critically ill patients in the intensive care unit following admission or postoperatively. Therefore the following patients should be assessed for SIADH: postoperative patients who have had pituitary surgery (ADH may increase for 5 to 7 days in response to surgery), patients with acute head injuries, patients with infection of the pulmonary system (pneumonia) or nervous system (meningitis), patients with psychiatric conditions (psychoses), and patients who are receiving specific pharmacologic agents that stimulate ADH (see Table 5-2).

In addition to the neurologic assessment, the clinician should investigate and assess patients who are suspected of having SIADH for the following signs and symptoms:

- Thirst and fluid status with accurate intake and output (I&O)
- Confusion
- Dyspnea
- Headache (monitor laboratory values and note that headache worsens as the sodium level decreases from 110 to 100 mEq/L)
- Fatigue (becomes more pronounced as the sodium level decreases)
- Weakness (progresses as the sodium level decreases)
- Increased body weight without edema
- Altered level of consciousness, lethargy
- Vomiting
- Muscle weakness and cramping
- Muscle twitching
- Convulsions and seizures (progress to coma and death as the sodium level decreases from 100 to 99 mEq/L or below)

Neurodiagnostic and Laboratory Studies

Specimens are collected for analysis. Laboratory findings of SIADH may include the following:[19,22,30]

- Serum sodium: dilutional hyponatremia with levels <135 mEq/L
- Urine sodium: >20 mEq/L
- Urine osmolality: higher than serum
- Serum osmolality: <275 mOsm/kg
- BUN/creatinine: renal function and values may be within normal limits (WNL) or decreased BUN/creatinine
- Urine specific gravity: >1.005
- Adrenal/threshold: WNL
- Serum potassium: <3.5 mEq/L

Treatment

Medical Management. Because SIADH may be the result of an underlying disease mechanism, initial treatment should be aimed at correcting the underlying cause and should include close monitoring of the neurologic status and the following considerations:

- Fluid restriction should be implemented for individuals with acute SIADH. Fluid restriction alone is usually sufficient to correct the hyponatremia associated with SIADH and result in loss of body weight and a steady rise in sodium levels and osmolality.[1] Such restriction of total fluid intake should be to less than the sum of insensible losses and urinary output and include the water derived from food (300 to 500 ml/day). Because insensible losses in adults usually approximate 500 ml/day, total discretionary intake (all water in liquid form) should be at least 500 ml less than urinary output. If achieved, this deficit usually reduces body water and increases sodium with a serum sodium increase of approximately 1% to 2% per day.[14]

- As the serum sodium begins to normalize, this restriction may be revised to a total daily fluid intake of 1000 ml.
- For severe hyponatremia (serum sodium <118 mEq/L) with associated neurologic deficits, an IV infusion of 3% hypertonic saline may be initiated.[14] The infusion must be titrated slowly at a rate of ≤0.05 ml/kg of body weight per minute because rapid infusion of this solution may cause congestive heart failure (CHF) secondary to rapid fluid retention or central pontine myelinolysis with flaccid quadriplegia. The effect should be monitored continuously by immediate laboratory analysis of serum sodium at least once every 2 hours, the infusion should be stopped as soon as serum sodium increases by 12 mmol/L or to 130 mmol/L, whichever comes first. Urinary output should also be monitored continuously since spontaneous remission of the SIADH can occur at any time and can result in an acute water diuresis that greatly accelerates the rate of rise in serum sodium produced by fluid restriction and 3% infusion.[14]
- Furosemide (Lasix) may be added as a diuretic; however, replacement of excreted potassium may be necessary. In severe cases of SIADH, IV saline is given along with diuretics to minimize the further expansion of the intravascular volume.
- For patients with an already-compromised cardiovascular system secondary to ischemia, a Swan-Ganz catheter may be inserted to monitor pulmonary capillary wedge pressure during the saline infusion.
- Pharmacologic agents that reduce renal tubule responsiveness to ADH may be used in chronic cases of SIADH to include demeclocycline (Declomycin).[20] These medications may take a week to reach maximum efficacy and are therefore not suitable for acute, rapid correction of SIADH-induced hyponatremia.[30,32]

Acute Care. Acute care of the patient with SIADH requires frequent and accurate assessments and management to minimize complications. Again, SIADH is usually a complication of an underlying disease process; therefore management priorities should be directed accordingly (see earlier discussion on assessment parameters). The following interventions should be an integral part of the clinical management of patients with SIADH.[2,8]

- Perform frequent neurologic assessments and assessments of mental status and LOC, which may be related to cerebral edema or increased intracranial pressure (ICP); carefully document findings to closely follow trends of improvement or deterioration.
- Perform a pulmonary assessment for early detection of pulmonary changes.
- Perform a cardiac assessment for dysrhythmias and blood pressure abnormalities.
- Monitor for seizure activity and institute seizure precautions as the serum sodium level decreases, with documentation of (1) duration, (2) type of seizure (focal versus generalized), (3) duration of loss of consciousness, (4) abnormal motor activity, (5)

characteristics of the postictal state, and (6) anticonvulsants administered.

- Measure accurately and record I&O to monitor for fluid retention (low urinary output) and dilutional hyponatremia.
- Restrict fluids (if mild/asymptomatic) to 800 to 1000 ml/24 hours; this intervention often is sufficient to correct the hyponatremia.[8]
- Monitor all medications that could increase the risk of SIADH (see Table 5-2).
- Obtain daily weights using the same scale, at the same time of day, with similar clothing (hospital gown) to monitor for sudden weight gain without edema.
- Reinforce dietary restrictions.
- Provide the appropriate oral hygiene.
- Collect and analyze specimens for urine and serum sodium osmolality to document SIADH and to rule out renal failure or other causes (see Neurodiagnostic and Laboratory Studies); monitor the rate of sodium decrease. Be aware of the serious side effects of hyponatremia; patients with a serum sodium level greater than 120 mEq/L are usually asymptomatic; therefore serum sodium levels should be checked daily or twice daily.
- Collect urine specimens to closely monitor specific gravity (may require hourly checks if severe).
- Position the bed either flat (supine) or elevate the head of the bed (HOB) no higher than 1 to 20 degrees.
- Teach the patient how to recognize and report adverse signs and symptoms of SIADH and hyponatremia.
- Report and document critical changes to the health care team for rapid interventions.
- Tailor assessments, interventions, and clinical diagnoses to the patient's response.

The underlying cause, if known, should be corrected (e.g., brain tumor removal, fluid restriction). However, interventions to reduce stress, pain, and discomfort; correct hypovolemia; and prevent vomiting should also be implemented.[8]

If fluid restriction does not correct the hyponatremia, pharmacologic therapy may be used to inhibit the action of ADH (see Medical Management). In extremely resistant cases or in instances of profound hyponatremia, 3% sodium chloride solutions must be administered slowly, with frequent reassessment of the patient's condition. Rapid correction of profound hyponatremia may result in permanent neurologic dysfunction caused by osmotic demyelination (e.g., central pontine myelinolysis with the development of profound brainstem impairment). Severe, untreated hyponatremia can also result in neurologic damage secondary to generalized tonic-clonic seizures or respiratory arrest.

Table 5-3 correlates various levels of hyponatremia with related clinical symptoms. Hypoglycemic medications, diuretics, synthetic hormone replacement, or any other drugs that may stimulate the release of ADH should be closely monitored or, if possible, discontinued during treatment for SIADH.[8,16]

The serum sodium level should gradually return to normal with appropriate interventions, and during this time the patient may experience weight loss and clearing of the sen-

TABLE 5-3	Correlation of Decreasing Sodium Levels and Symptoms
Serum Sodium Level	**Symptoms**
145–135 mEq/L	Normal concentration range; no symptoms
135–120 mEq/L	Generally no changes
120–110 mEq/L	Headache, apathy, lethargy, weakness, disorientation, thirst, anorexia, fatigue, seizures
110–100 mEq/L	Confusion, hostility, lethargy, or violence; nausea or vomiting, abdominal cramps, muscle twitching
100–95 mEq/L	Delirium, convulsions, coma, hypothermia, areflexia, Cheyne-Stokes respirations, death

Modified from Gray DP, Ludwig-Beymer P: Alterations of hormonal regulation. In McCance KL, Huether SE, editors: *Pathophysiology: the biologic basis for disease in adults and children*, St Louis, 1990, Mosby.

sorium. The clinician must closely observe for overtreatment and undertreatment response during the acute phase while keeping a high index of suspicion for the development of seizures.[24]

Gastrointestinal changes (i.e., diarrhea or constipation) must also be appropriately controlled. Explanations to the patient and family emphasizing strict adherence to treatment guidelines help reduce the anxiety and stress associated with frequent monitoring and neurologic assessment.[8,24]

Postacute Care. Ongoing assessment, including the previously mentioned parameters and related management priorities, should continue throughout the postacute care phase. Management priorities and health teaching regarding the primary disease process should also be carried out throughout this phase of care as the patient recovers and is prepared for discharge.

Rehabilitation and Home Care. Self-management for a chronic state of SIADH requires extensive health teaching. It is important for members of the health care team to validate the patient's ability to recognize the cause of SIADH, the treatment regimen, medications, and total compliance. Daily record keeping with a log of fluid restrictions and I&O can identify problems. Dietary instructions are needed that emphasize sodium and potassium balance. A weight log allows the patient to immediately recognize and report a sudden weight gain. The patient should wear medical identification at all times.

DIABETES INSIPIDUS

Etiology and Pathophysiology

Diabetes insipidus (DI) is characterized by **dehydration** (excessive loss of water from body tissue and imbalance of essential electrolytes: sodium, potassium, and chloride), **polydipsia** (excessive thirst), the inability of the renal tubules to conserve free water that results in **polyuria** (excretion of excessive amounts of pale, dilute urine), low urine specific gravity (1.001 to 1.005), serum hyperosmolality, and **hypernatremia** (a greater than normal concentration of sodium in the blood).[26] Central or neurogenic DI is related to a deficiency of vasopressin (Fig. 5-2).

DI may be either a temporary or a chronic disorder of the neurohypophyseal system when there is a deficiency of production or release of antidiuretic hormone (ADH). DI occurs when any lesion of the hypothalamus, infundibular stem, or posterior pituitary interferes with ADH synthesis, transport, or release.[9] Patients diagnosed with DI have a major problem in their inability to conserve water and the danger of dehydration or the inability to balance fluid intake with urinary output (I&O). Polyuria can exceed 5 ml/kg per hour of dilute

urine with a specific gravity of less than 1.010. Hypernatremia is evidenced by increased serum sodium (>145 mEq/L).[26] One example of potential dehydration or hypernatremia may be found in the patient who is receiving large doses of mannitol with resultant rapid diuresis.

DI may also occur during phenytoin use, in alcohol intoxication, and during bacterial meningitis. The two most common causes of hypernatremia in neurosurgical patients are iatrogenic (with osmotic diuresis due to mannitol) and DI. Destruction of the posterior pituitary gland from tumors or trauma, for example, results in a deficiency of vasopressin and the development of central DI. Replacement by consuming equal amounts of fluid is fatiguing, and nocturia interferes with sleep.

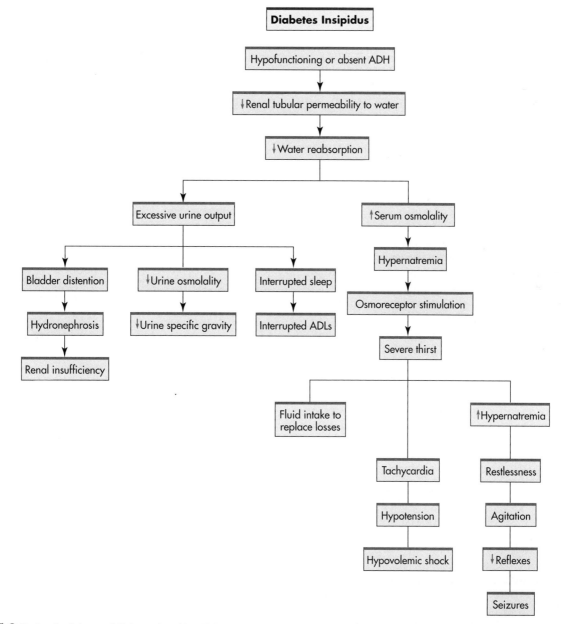

Figure 5-2 Pathophysiology of diabetes inspidus (DI). (*ADH,* Antidiuretic hormone; *ADLs,* activities of daily living.)
(From Lewis SM, Heitkemper MM, Dirsen SF: Medical-surgical nursing: assessment and management of clinical problems, *ed 5, St Louis, 2000, Mosby.)*

Primary polydipsia, characterized by **compulsive water drinking,** appears to have a higher female predisposition and can be distinguished from other forms of DI. An individual who drinks up to 15 L of water and produces an equal volume of urine output will suppress vasopressin secretion and have hypo-osmolar urine. Unlike DI, polyuria is decreased at night as polydipsia ceases with sleep.[30]

The pathophysiology of DI can be divided into two categories: neurogenic and nephrogenic. In **neurogenic** or **central DI** there is a decrease in ADH production or secretion secondary to an impairment of the hypothalamic neurohypophyseal system. **Nephrogenic DI** is characterized by impaired renal tubule responsiveness to the physiologic effects of ADH.[29] The cardinal clinical features of both types of DI include the following:[2,3,21]

- Urinary output greater than 200 ml/hr
- Urine specific gravity less than 1.010
- Plasma osmolality greater than 295 mOsm/kg
- Serum sodium greater than 135 mEq/L
- Severe polydipsia (occurs in a conscious individual and results in an output of 2 to 20 L/day)

Neurogenic DI may be the result of **primary DI** from a hypothalamic or pituitary lesion; **secondary DI** following injury to the hypothalamus or pituitary stalk; or **vasopressin-induced DI,** which is seen in the last trimester of pregnancy and is caused by an enzyme that destroys vasopressin (ADH).[30] A rare form of this condition occurs when an individual has **psychogenic DI** associated with compulsive water drinking of up to 6 L/day but usually no symptoms of nocturia.[30]

DI can result from a variety of lesions located along the neurohypophyseal axis. Destruction of the supraoptic nuclei of the hypothalamus results in total and permanent loss of the ability to secrete ADH, whereas a lesion below this landmark results in a partial and transient decrease in ADH production. Approximately 75% of the ADH-secreting neurons need to be destroyed before the patient develops the clinical symptomatology of the disease.[21,25]

The most common cause of neurogenic DI is disruption of the neurohypophyseal system. This disruption may be caused by surgical procedures in that area of the brain or by traumatic brain injuries. Closed head trauma that results from a rotational deceleration injury (e.g., the head striking the dashboard of a car) may cause DI secondary to the tearing or "shearing" of the small blood vessels that supply the hypothalamus and the pituitary stalk. This results in ischemia and necrosis of these structures and, consequently, a decrease in ADH secretion.[21,30]

Postsurgical DI occurs after procedures such as transsphenoidal hypophysectomies and removal of pituitary tumors, is usually transient, and typically follows a triphasic pattern:

- Approximately 12 to 24 hours after surgery, ADH release abruptly ceases, resulting in polyuria; this phase lasts for approximately 4 to 7 days.
- The second phase is characterized by an antidiuretic phase caused by the release of presynthesized ADH from ischemic and degenerating neurohypophyseal neurons. Free water is reabsorbed from the kidney, and serum hypo-osmolality and hyponatremia develop

(**transient syndrome of inappropriate antidiuretic hormone [transient SIADH]).**

- The third phase develops after the release of stored ADH is complete (there may be a delay in the development of this phase). After ADH stores are depleted, DI develops secondary to progressive neuronal degeneration.[6,19]

Vascular lesions of the brain can also result in the development of DI. Intracranial aneurysms, particularly those located on the **anterior communicating artery (ACA),** can cause DI either from a mass effect exerted on the hypothalamic supraoptic nuclei secondary to enlargement of the lesion or from rupture of the aneurysm with resultant subarachnoid hemorrhage. The hypothalamic nuclei may be damaged during the hemorrhagic insult or may become ischemic as a result of subarachnoid hemorrhage–induced vasospasm.[5]

Differentiated from neurogenic DI, the etiology of nephrogenic DI can be classified into two categories: congenital and acquired (Box 5-3). **Congenital nephrogenic DI** is a sex-linked (X chromosome) recessive genetic disease. Congenital nephrogenic DI is rare and accounts for less than 1% of all cases of this disease. **Acquired nephrogenic DI** is seen more commonly. It develops secondary to structural or pathophysiologic changes in the renal tubules. Causes of acquired nephrogenic DI include chronic hypokalemia, chronic hypercalcemia, polycystic kidney disease, obstructive uropathy, sarcoidosis, and chronic renal failure. Pharmacologic agents that can cause acquired nephrogenic DI include lithium carbonate, demeclocycline, amphotericin B, methoxyflurane, and furosemide.[6,21]

Box 5-4 summarizes the important differences between SIADH and DI.

BOX 5-3	Etiology of Diabetes Insipidus

Neurogenic Diabetes Insipidus
Head trauma
Postsurgery: hypophysectomy, pituitary tumors
Primary brain tumors: craniopharyngiomas, gliomas, meningioma
CNS infections: meningitis, encephalitis, intracranial abscess
Increased ICP
Idiopathic
Vascular: intracranial hemorrhage, stroke, brainstem hypoxia, aneurysm
Medications: phenytoin (Dilantin), clonidine (Klonopin); alcohol

Nephrogenic Diabetes Insipidus
Renal disease
- Pyelonephritis
- Obstructive uropathy
- Polycystic kidney disease
Hypokalemia
Hypercalcemia
Iatrogenic/pharmacologic agents
- Lithium
- Demeclocycline

ICP, Intracranial pressure.

BOX 5-4	Comparison of Syndrome of Inappropriate Antidiuretic Hormone and Diabetes Insipidus

Syndrome of Inappropriate Antidiuretic Hormone (SIADH)

Oliguria (<200 ml/hr in 2 consecutive hours)

Serum sodium: hyponatremia (<135 mEq/L)

Serum uric acid levels (<0.24 mmol/L) associated with an increased fractional excretion of urate

Elevated urine osmolality (>900 mOsm/kg H_2O)

Decreased plasma osmolality (<275 mOsm/L)

Urine sodium (<25–30 mEq/L)

Increased specific gravity (>1.030)

Normotension

No dehydration

Confusion, delirium, coma as sodium concentration decreases

Diabetes Insipidus

Polyuria (>250 ml/hr urinary output in 2 consecutive hours)

Serum sodium: hypernatremia (>135 mEq/L)

Decreased urine osmolality (<400 mOsm/kg H_2O)

Elevated plasma osmolality (>295 mOsm/L)

Urine sodium concentration decreased

Decreased specific gravity (<1.001–1.005)

Hypotension

Dehydration

Seizures, coma

Modified from Frost EAM: *Postanesthesia care unit—current practices,* St Louis, 1990, Mosby.

Assessment

Assessment of the patient with DI (neurogenic or nephrogenic) targets the clinical problems of hypernatremia and dehydration. A complete history and physical examination are needed to identify the cause. Patients who are awake and who are able to respond to their increased thirst stimulus can usually compensate for the excessive polyuria. With these patients, only mild hypernatremia may occur and is usually manifested by anorexia, nausea, and vomiting. The clinician should assess for the following:[28,32]

- Unquenchable thirst
- Preference for ice water or cold beverages
- Polydipsia
- Weight loss
- Constipation
- Polyuria (hourly urinary output >200 ml)
- Urinary frequency
- Nocturia
- Dry skin
- Poor skin turgor[31]
- Inability to respond to the increased thirst stimulus and compensate for the excessive polyuria
- Hypernatremia that becomes severe and is manifested by the following symptoms: confusion, irritability, stupor, coma, and neuromuscular hyperactivity progressing to seizures

Neurodiagnostic and Laboratory Studies

Serum calcium, glucose, creatinine, potassium, and urea levels provide clues to the diagnosis of DI. The following neurodiagnostic and laboratory studies may also be indicated:[2,3,22]

- Twenty-four–hour urine collection to quantitate polyuria
- CT/MRI: if acute DI results from increased ICP or to visualize the anterior and posterior pituitary glands and stalks and to demonstrate the presence of a suprasellar mass, cyst, hypoplasia, or an atopic lobe of the posterior pituitary
- Radioimmunoassay: to measure circulating ADH concentrations (not available at all facilities)
- Serum sodium: >135 mEq/L
- Urine osmolality: <200 mOsm/L (see Box 5-4)
- Serum osmolality: <300 mOsm/kg
- Urine specific gravity: of the first morning voiding (<1.010) for renal concentration capacity

Treatment

Medical Management

The medical management of DI is aimed at correcting the underlying cause of the polyuria and maintaining adequate fluid volume. Individuals with mild to moderate neurogenic DI who have an intact thirst mechanism can usually compensate for their fluid losses by increasing their oral intake. The polyuria that accompanies the polydipsia can be bothersome to the individual and can significantly interrupt sleep patterns to the point where pharmacologic therapy is warranted.[6,19]

Patients with acute neurogenic DI require the administration of IV fluids to replace urinary losses and prevent dehydration. Hormonal replacement should be initiated when polyuria greater than 6 L per 24 hours develops. The medication of choice in this situation for the initial management following head trauma or neurosurgery, or in an unconscious patient, is vasopressin (Pitressin). The peak onset of action is within 1 to 2 hours, and the duration of action is 3 to 6 hours. The usual dose is 5 to 10 units given subcutaneously, intravenously, or intramuscularly. Adverse effects of the administration of this medication include myocardial ischemia (secondary to the vasopressor effects of this medication), nausea, diarrhea, and abdominal cramping. In the acute care setting, aqueous vasopressin may be administered by continuous IV infusion. The initial dose is 2.5 units per hour and is titrated until a urinary output of 100 ml/hr is achieved.[6,19,25]

Individuals with chronic neurogenic DI require hormonal replacement therapy to reduce polyuria and polydipsia. For these patients the medication of choice is intranasal desmopressin acetate (DDAVP). Individuals with rhinitis or sinusitis may not be able to sufficiently absorb the nasal vasopressin. This synthetic analog form of vasopressin has a duration of action of 12 to 18 hours and is administered as a nasal spray.[20] The initial dose is 5 to 10 µg at bedtime, and the dose is increased in −2.5 to 5.0 µg increments until nocturnal polyuria is alleviated. The adverse effects of this type of therapy are rare and include nasal congestion and irritation,

TABLE 5-4	Drugs Prescribed for Diabetes Insipidus			
Drug	**Dose**	**Indication**	**Limitations**	**Side Effects**
Desmopressin (DDAVP)	Intranasally (5–40 µg (0.05–0.4 ml) in 1–3 doses/day; subcutaneously (2 to 4 µg/day in divided doses)	Central DI and vasopressin-resistant DI in pregnancy	High cost	Few (nasal congestion, headache, slight elevation of blood pressure, flushing of skin); severe hyponatremia may occur with overtreatment
Vasopressin (Pitressin)	5–10 units, 2–4 times/day subcutaneously/intramuscularly	Acute central DI, short-term management	Very short duration of action (1–2 hours)	Diaphoresis, paleness, headache, trembling, abdominal cramps, diarrhea, dizziness, nausea/vomiting; rare—angina, increased blood pressure, water intoxication

Data from *Mosby's 2005 drug consult for nurses,* St Louis, 2005, Mosby.
ADH, Antidiuretic hormone; *DI,* diabetes insipidus.

headache, nausea, and abdominal cramps. Table 5-4 summarizes the pharmacologic action and clinical indications for the various ADH preparations.[19,21]

Clofibrate (Atromid-S), carbamazepine (Tegretol), and thiazide diuretics may also be prescribed for symptomatic DI.[10] Supplemental ADH therapy has no clinical efficacy in cases of nephrogenic DI because the kidneys are unable to respond to ADH. In this clinical situation the use of a thiazide diuretic along with a sodium-restricted diet is the treatment of choice. The use of a thiazide diuretic (hydrochlorothiazide 50 to 100 mg daily) causes mild extracellular volume depletion with resultant increased proximal tubule reabsorption of sodium and water, leading to decreased water delivery to the distal nephron and decreased urinary output. The use of nonsteroidal antiinflammatory agents inhibits the synthesis of prostaglandins by the kidney, which in turn enhances renal responsiveness to ADH and thereby reduces polyuria. The drug of choice is indomethacin 100 mg daily.[19,21] Acute hypernatremia can be rapidly corrected. Chronic hypernatremia, however, should be corrected slowly as brain cells adapt to prolonged hyperosmolar states by solute accumulation. Rapid correction of TBW will result in fluid shift into the brain and cerebral edema.[13] There is no surgical management in the treatment of DI.

Acute Care
The patient with DI has polydipsia, polyuria, dilute urinary output, and a high plasma osmolality (see Neurodiagnostic and Laboratory Studies).

For patients who are awake and under constant supervision, a dehydration test may be administered to establish the diagnosis. Before the test, all drugs that influence the secretion or action of ADH should be discontinued. The patient should avoid tobacco and alcohol use for at least 24 hours before the test. The dehydration test procedure is as follows:
1. Obtain a baseline body weight, serum osmolality, serum sodium, and urine osmolality.
2. Allow patients who exhibit polyuria (urinary output >4 L/day) unrestricted access to oral fluids up to the initiation of the test. Put all other patients on nothing-by-mouth (NPO) status after midnight before the study.
3. Restrict IV/oral fluid intake to 7 hours.
4. Assess body weight and urine osmolality every hour or every 2 hours.
5. Achieve dehydration with either a 5% decrease in body weight, a serum osmolality greater than 295 mOsm/kg, or urine osmolality less than 800 mOsm/kg.
6. Administer 5 units of aqueous vasopressin subcutaneously, at this point, and measure urine osmolality 1 hour later.

The patient with *neurogenic DI* exhibits a response to the vasopressin, resulting in urine concentration. The patient with *nephrogenic DI* does not exhibit any response to the vasopressin and therefore continues to excrete high volumes of dilute urine.[6,19]

The clinician must be vigilant in performing continuous patient assessment and neurologic evaluations of the patient with acute neurogenic DI. If the patient is awake, alert, and able to respond to an increased thirst stimulus, the principal management priority is accurate measuring and recording of I&O. The patient with acute neurogenic DI who is not awake, alert and oriented, or able to respond is at risk for developing dehydration, hypovolemia, and shock. Acute management priorities for this group of patients include continuous assessments, careful documentation, and the following interventions:
- Assess and document LOC
- Maintain vital signs WNL and monitor for signs of tachycardia and hypotension
- Maintain strict I&O to determine fluid balance or loss and to balance fluid I&O
- Rehydrate for symptoms of extreme thirst
- Replace fluids (milliliter for milliliter, with a 10% increase to cover insensible water loss) using dextrose-in-water solutions; vasopressin may be added to the IV solution if output becomes excessive
- Measure and record daily weight using the same scales, at the same time, and with the patient wearing the same clothing (hospital gown)
- Monitor (in severe cases, hourly) and keep urine specific gravity WNL
- Assess mucous membranes and skin turgor and monitor for symptoms of dehydration and treat appropriately

- Evaluate for signs and symptoms of hypovolemic shock and treat appropriately
- Collect and analyze laboratory results (serum electrolytes, glucose, serum and urine osmolality) to determine abnormalities; report the patient's condition and response to treatment, as directed
- Collect and analyze reports of BUN/creatinine to evaluate renal function
- Provide adequate rest
- Provide safety measures to prevent injury secondary to dizziness and fatigue
- Monitor treatment outcomes and trends of improvement or deterioration
- Teach patients how to record I&O, the signs and symptoms of DI, and to alert the health care team members of problems of urinary frequency and extreme thirst that interfere with sleep and other activities

Postacute and Nonacute Care

Continual management priorities for patients with DI include completing an initial assessment, as well as the goals of prevention of severe dehydration and close monitoring of blood pressure to detect the early signs of hypotension and shock.

Health teaching is focused on the measurement and recording of accurate I&O and the cardinal symptoms of hypernatremia, including alteration in LOC, confusion, irritability, anorexia, nausea, and vomiting. Patient and family teaching must also include the expected results of pharmacologic hormone replacement therapy, as well as potential adverse effects.

Patients with transient DI usually are symptom free after a few days or weeks. The clinician should therefore stress the need for the patient to recognize the return of symptoms as a warning sign and to alert the clinician at the first sign of polydipsia and polyuria. Patients with chronic DI need to be prepared for the necessity of lifetime replacement therapy. After the medication and dosage have been determined, the clinician can plan a home program based on the patient's understanding of DI and its treatment. Patient responsibilities should be clearly explained verbally and with written instructions, including a number to call for emergencies. Prevention of dehydration with 2000 ml/day fluid intake is encouraged, with the goal being to balance I&O. The recognition of thirst as a protective mechanism is emphasized, along with the side effects of vasopressin overdosage and SIADH. Initially, a simple I&O flow sheet and a daily weight and medication record should be maintained. If the DI is found to be hereditary, genetic counseling and follow-up are important.

COMPREHENSIVE PATIENT MANAGEMENT

Health Teaching Considerations

Family members are encouraged to be active participants in home care until the patient is competent to manage independently. Nasal irritation, headache, and nausea may indicate overdosage of medication, whereas failure to improve may indicate underdosage.[15] Patients should be made aware that rhinitis and sinusitis can reduce intranasal absorption of DDAVP. Genetic counseling with follow-up is recommended for individuals with hereditary DI. Follow-up supervision of home care and return clinic or health care provider visits should be arranged to monitor temperature, appetite, and medication compliance at discharge.[13] Patients should be encouraged to always wear medical identification.

Older Adult Considerations

The complex mechanisms associated with water metabolism and balanced electrolytes cause frail older adults to be particularly vulnerable to age-related maladaptations and to the various disease processes and medical interventions that frequently occur with age.[15] The aging process may place older adults at higher risk for hyponatremia and water metabolism abnormalities. Symptoms may not occur until the serum sodium level is very low and becomes chronic, causing lethargy, confusion, and malaise. In addition to a thorough history and neurologic assessment of the older adult, the weight, I&O, nutritional status, and urinalysis are evaluated. It is essential to recognize and evaluate comorbid conditions, changes in or decreased thirst sensation, decreased urinary-concentration ability, changes in renal function, decreased cerebral blood flow, and salt/water imbalance. Dehydration, age-related decrease in TBW, and common electrolyte imbalances (e.g., hyponatremia or hypernatremia) can be seen in older adults exacerbated by the stress of hospitalization, changes in nutritional status, recovering from surgery or serious illness, receiving new or multiple medications, sleep deprivation, and pain.[33]

Clinical changes may be subtle and nonspecific requiring a high vigilance for close monitoring of symptoms, to include irritability, restlessness, lethargy, muscular twitching, spasticity, and hyperreflexia. Therapy for DI and SIADH requires close monitoring for overtreatment and undertreatment to avoid cerebral edema, CHF, and serious clinical complications.

CONCLUSION

Fluid and electrolyte balance and adequate oxygenation are integral to normal cerebral metabolism. Disruptions in this delicate balance can produce serious clinical symptoms ranging from mild confusion to coma or even death. The clinician must maintain a high level of suspicion for such disruptions in patients at risk for metabolic disturbance. Metabolic imbalance may be caused by a number of factors, including underlying primary pathologic conditions and surgical complications. Because metabolic disruptions may arise in a variety of clinical scenarios, specific assessment parameters must be followed for early detection of these conditions. Transient DI following neurosurgery may resolve spontaneously; however, patient outcome relates directly to appropriate and expedient treatment measures, which are derived from accurate assessment and diagnosis.

RESOURCES FOR MEDIC ALERT

Medic Alert Identification: 2323 Colorado Avenue, Turlock, CA 95382; 209-668-3333

REFERENCES

1. Asp AA: Alterations in endocrine control. In Copstead LC, Banasik JL, editors: *Pathophysiology,* ed 3, St Louis, 2005, Elsevier Saunders.
2. Bader MK, Littlejohn LR, editors: *AANN (American Association of Neuroscience Nurses) core curriculum for neuroscience nursing,* ed 4, St Louis, 2004, Saunders.
3. Barrow DL, Selman WR, editors: *Neuroendocrinology,* vol 5, Baltimore, 1992, Williams & Wilkins.
4. Bartter FC, Schwartz WB: The syndrome of inappropriate secretion of antidiuretic hormone, *Am J Med* 42(5):790–806, 1967.
5. Berry PB, Belsha CW: Hyponatremia, *Pediatr Clin North Am* 37(2):351–363, 1990.
6. Blevins LS, Wand GS: Diabetes insipidus, *Crit Care Med* 20(1):69–79, 1992.
7. Daniel TO, Henrich WL: Endocrine abnormalities and fluid and electrolyte disorders. In Kokko JP, Tannen RL, editors: *Fluids and electrolytes,* Philadelphia, 1990, WB Saunders.
8. Fitsch KL: Nursing management of adults with pituitary, hypothalamus and adrenal disorders. In Beare PG, Myers JL, editors: *Principles and practice of adult health nursing,* St Louis, 1990, Mosby.
9. Garcia JH, Conger KA: Ischemic brain injuries: structural and biomedical effects. In Grenvik A, Safar P, editors: *Brain failure and resuscitation,* New York, 1981, Churchill Livingstone.
10. Haas LB: Nursing management: endocrine problems. In Lewis SM, Heitkemper MM, Dirksen SR, editors: *Medical-surgical nursing: assessment and management of clinical problems,* ed 5, St Louis, 2000, Mosby.
11. Horne MM, Bond ER: Fluid, electrolyte, and acid-base balance. In Lewis SM, Heitkemper MM, Dirksen SR, editors: *Medical-surgical nursing: assessment and management of clinical problems,* ed 5, St Louis, 2000, Mosby.
12. Huether SE: Fluids and electrolytes, acids and bases. In McCance KL, Huether SE, editors: *Pathophysiology: the biologic basis for disease in adults and children,* ed 4, St Louis, 2002, Mosby.
13. Jellinek DA, Freeman R: Perioperative care. In Kaye AH, Black PM, editors: *Operative neurosurgery,* London, 2000, Churchill Livingstone.
14. Kasper DL, Braunwald E, Fauci AS, et al: Part 14. Endocrinology and metabolism. In Kasper DL, Braunwald E, Fauci AS, et al, editors: *Harrison's principles of internal medicine,* ed 16, New York, 2006, McGraw-Hill. Available at Harrison's Online, www.accessmedicine.com (accessed June 2, 2006).
15. Kugler JP, Hustead T: Hyponatremia and hypernatremia in the elderly, *American Family Physician.* Available at www.aafp.org/afp/20000615/3623.html (accessed March 30, 2006).
16. Marshall SB, editor: *Neuroscience critical care: pathophysiology and patient management,* Philadelphia, 1990, WB Saunders.
17. McCance KL: Structure and function of the hematologic system. In McCance KL, Huether SE, editors: *Pathophysiology: the biologic basis for disease in adults and children,* ed 4, St Louis, 2002, Mosby.
18. Millionis HJ, Liamis GL, Elisaf MS: The hyponatremic patient: a systematic approach to laboratory diagnosis, *Can Med Assoc* 166(8):1056–1062, 2002.
19. Morrison G, Singer I: Hyperosmolar states. In Maxwell MH, Kleeman CR, Narins RG, editors: *Clinical disorders of fluid and electrolyte metabolism,* New York, 1987, McGraw-Hill.
20. *Mosby's 2005 drug consult for nurses,* St Louis, 2005, Mosby.
21. Ober KP: Diabetes insipidus, *Crit Care Clin* 7(1):109–125, 1991.
22. Pagana KD, Pagana TJ: *Mosby's diagnostic and laboratory test reference,* ed 7, St Louis, 2005, Mosby.
23. Palmer BF: Hyponatremia in a neurosurgical patient: syndrome of inappropriate antidiuretic hormone secretion versus cerebral salt wasting, *Nephrol Dial Transplant* 15(2):262–268, 2000.
24. Piano MR, Huether SE: Mechanisms of hormonal regulations. In McCance KL, Huether SE, editors: *Pathophysiology: the biologic basis for disease in adults and children,* ed 4, St Louis, 2002, Mosby.
25. Reasner CA, Mueller GL: Hypothalamic and pituitary disease. In Civetta JM, Taylor RW, Kirby RR, editors: *Critical care,* Philadelphia, 1992, JB Lippincott.
26. Saborio P, Tipton GA, Chan JCM: Diabetes insipidus, *Pediatr Rev* 21(4):122–129, 2000.
27. Schwartz WB, Bennett A, Curelop S, Bartter FC: A syndrome of renal sodium loss and hyponatremia probably resulting from inappropriate secretion of antidiuretic hormone, *Am J Med* 23(4):529-542, 1957.
28. Sterns RH, Spital A: Disorders of water balance. In Kokko JP, Tannen RL, editors: *Fluids and electrolytes,* Philadelphia, 1990, WB Saunders.
29. Swearingen PL, Ross DG: *Manual of medical-surgical nursing: interventions and collaborative management,* ed 4, St Louis, 1999, Mosby.
30. Thibonnier M: Antidiuretic hormone: regulation, disorders, and clinical evaluation. In Barrow DL, Sellman WR, editors: *Neuroendocrinology: concepts in neurosurgery,* vol 5, Baltimore, 1992, Williams & Wilkins.
31. Tucker SM, Canobbio MM, Paquette EV, Wells MF: *Patient care standards: collaborative planning and nursing interventions,* ed 7, St Louis, 2000, Mosby.
32. Votey BR, Peters AL, Hoffman JR: Disorders of water metabolism: hyponatremia and hypernatremia, *Emerg Med Clin North Am* 7(4):749–769, 1989.
33. Wachtel TJ: The diabetic hyperosmolar state, *Clin Geriatr Med* 6(4):797–806, 1990.

ELLEN BARKER

CHAPTER 6

Altered States of Consciousness and Sleep

Coma and sleep disorders are conditions of decreased awareness and interaction with the environment. Because of the general similarity of these two states, they are presented together in this chapter. Information for the evaluation and treatment of the pathologic conditions of coma is presented first, followed by a discussion of the normal physiologic conditions of sleep and its associated disorders.

Management of an unresponsive state is one of the greatest challenges for neuroscience clinicians. The patient is totally dependent on caregivers for every need and is at high risk for significant complications. Early interventions result in a better outcome. The rapid identification and clinical management of altered or decreasing states of awareness and coma often mean the difference between death, disability, and recovery. All competent clinicians must have these skills because lacking such fundamental competence denies a critically ill patient an effective and timely review for treatment.

Coma is a very serious condition, often with a fatal outcome. Some patients die without ever regaining consciousness despite medical intervention. Others may recover from their initial insult and remain in states between consciousness and coma. Although increasing numbers of patients recover, those who do usually have deficits that require intense rehabilitation.[15,24] In the United States, facilities that provide coma rehabilitation have proliferated with the goals of stimulating arousal of comatose patients and rehabilitating them to a higher level of function. Coma arousal remains controversial and is considered by some to be investigational or not medically necessary. Others regard this therapy as beneficial with the potential to stimulate spontaneous recovery and improvement.

ALTERED STATES OF CONSCIOUSNESS

Consciousness may be defined as a state of awareness of one's self, one's environment, and others, and assessed through a set of responses to that environment.[10] Very little is known about the neural mechanisms that produce consciousness. We do know, however, that consciousness depends on excitation of cortical neurons by impulses conducted to them by a network of neurons known as the reticular activating system (RAS) (see Fig. 1-31). Drugs such as barbiturates

are known to depress the RAS, decrease alertness, and induce sleep. Amphetamines, on the other hand, are drugs that stimulate the cerebrum and enhance alertness and wakefulness probably by stimulating the RAS.[43]

Consciousness includes arousal and awareness. **Arousal** is the state of awakeness that is often called **level of consciousness (LOC).** It refers to the quality of vigilance and describes the degree to which an individual appears to be able to interact with the environment.[7] Dysfunction in the arousal system manifests as a decreased LOC or decreased awareness. **Awareness, or content of thought,** includes all cognitive (mental and intellectual) functions and affective states (mood). Awareness reflects the depth and content of the aroused state. It is dependent on arousal—an individual who cannot be aroused appears to lack awareness.[7]

Inattention and Confusion

A patient is often described as confused when unable to give the correct time or place or to name and answer questions appropriately. The term **confusion** lacks precision but in general denotes an inability to think with customary speed and clarity (Table 6-1). Failure may occur because of inattentiveness, disorders of language, forgetfulness, apathy, or abulia.[1] **Mild confusion** may be noted in patients who are oriented to time and place but are unable to remember that they are in the hospital. **Moderate confusion** may be found in patients who are disoriented to time and place, respond with a slowed verbal response, and are incontinent of bowel and bladder. **Severe confusion** may be observed in patients who are disoriented to person, place, or time and are unable to carry out more than the simplest command with few or no thought processes in operation. Such patients are unaware of much that goes on around them and often display bowel and bladder incontinence.[1]

Locked-in syndrome is total paralysis below the level of the nucleus of cranial nerve (CN) III with the ability to open the eyes and follow commands with the eyes. No other motor movement is possible. This syndrome is often a result of bilateral ventral pontine lesions or bilateral destruction of the medulla oblongata. It spares the somatosensory pathways and the ascending neuronal systems that are responsible for arousal and wakefulness, but it interrupts the corticospinal

TABLE 6-1	Levels of Acute Coma
State	**Definition**
Confusion	Loss of ability to think rapidly and clearly; impaired judgment and decision making
Disorientation	Beginning loss of consciousness; disorientation to time followed by disorientation to place and impaired memory; lost last is recognition of self
Lethargy	Limited spontaneous movement or speech; easy arousal with normal speech or touch; may not be oriented to time, place, or person
Obtundation	Mild to moderate reduction in arousal (awakeness) with limited response to the environment; falls asleep unless stimulated verbally or tactilely; answers questions with minimum response
Stupor	A condition of deep sleep or unresponsiveness from which the person may be aroused or caused to open eyes only by vigorous and repeated stimulation; response is often withdrawal or grabbing at stimulus
Coma	No verbal response to the external environment or to any stimuli; noxious stimuli such as deep pain or suctioning yield motor movement
• Light coma	Associated with purposeful movement on stimulation
• Coma	Associated with nonpurposeful movement only on stimulation
• Deep coma	Associated with unresponsiveness or no response to any stimulus

From Boss B: Concepts of neurological dysfunction. In McCance KL, Huether SE: *Pathophysiology*, ed 4, St Louis, 2002, Mosby, p 440.

BOX 6-1	Continuum of Descending States of Consciousness

Consciousness
↓
Wakefulness
↓
Arousal
↓
Drowsiness
↓
Confusion
↓
Inattentiveness
↓
Delirium
↓
Stupor
↓
Vegetative state
↓
Coma

pathways.[1] The patient is fully conscious because the reticular formation has been spared. A communication system can be established using eye movement and eye blinks. Electroencephalogram (EEG) and evoked potential studies are normal.[41]

There is a continuum between normal consciousness and coma. The continuum of brain activity may also range from confusion to deep coma (Box 6-1). The descent into the comatose state can be described in descending stages of consciousness.

The level of confusion may fluctuate between day and night and in response to medications, fatigue, and other factors. A condition sometimes referred to as **sundowning** can occur in older adults or in individuals with cognitive impairments. In this condition, individuals become confused or disoriented in the evening hours, when less light is available and visual cues are lost and when diminished visual or hearing capacity results in the loss of cues that help compensate for problems with cognition. Sundowning may be a result of decreased sensory stimulation and is not uncommon in dementia, in delirium, and in hospitalized older adults.

Delirium is an abnormal mental state characterized by confusion in which hyperactivity may be prominent. The patient is generally disoriented and may be restless and agitated and exhibit signs of illusion, hallucinations, and other characteristic disorders.[1] **Stupor** is a state in which mental and physical activity is decreased to a minimum. Patients appear to be asleep and can be roused only by vigorous and repeated stimuli.[1] **Obtundation** has been described as a mild to moderate reduction in alertness[41] (see Table 6-1).

A **vegetative state** is a physical condition in which a previously comatose patient continues to be unable to communicate or respond to stimuli despite giving the appearance at times of wakefulness. **Persistent vegetative state** terminology has been used for diagnosis, and **permanent vegetative state** is sometimes used as terminology for prognosis. These two terms are often misused and could have adverse influences. Therefore *vegetative state* is the terminology used in this chapter. Box 6-2 lists the responses that may be observed in patients who are in a vegetative state during assessment. Patients in a vegetative state may display the following characteristics:[1]

- Absence of any psychological meaningful adaptive response to the external environment
- Absence of any evidence of a functioning mind that is receiving or projecting information
- Inattentiveness; no purposeful behavior or signs of awareness of inner needs
- Appearance of prolonged periods of wakefulness
- Ability to blink to threat (menace) or light but appear not to be attentive
- Failure to signal appropriately by eye movement, although sometimes briefly follow moving objects in a slow intermittent pattern

- Roving eye movements or periods with the eyes open and closed after a variable time in the comatose state
- Inability to sense pain, stimuli, or hunger
- Reflex posturing
- Presence of nonvolitional "grasp reflex"
- Grinding of teeth, chewing and swallowing liquids and food placed in the mouth
- Initially the EEG may be isoelectric, but considerable activity and even rhythms may be found once the state has lasted for several months
- Inability to speak (verbalize) though may make sounds (vocalize) or respond to stimuli with grunting and groaning
- Inability of meaningful comprehension or response to the spoken word
- Meaningless movement of the trunk or limbs, occasional smile, shedding of tears
- Variable preserved pupillary, gag, spinal, and corneal and oculocephalic reflex
- Primitive postural and reflex movements of the limbs with fragments of coordinated movements (e.g., scratching or moving the hands toward a noxious stimulus)

- Total dependence, which requires bowel and bladder management for incontinence
- Intact hearing
- Results on an EEG that may approach normality with alpha rhythm or sleep patterns

Coma is the deepest form of unconsciousness, with no verbal response to the external environment or to noxious stimuli. Preliminary data seem to support the hypothesis that the absence of any response to external stimuli is indicative of an unfavorable outcome.[23]

Etiology

Structural Disorders and Metabolic Disorders

Disorders that can produce decreased arousal can be separated into the major groupings of structural disorders and metabolic disorders (Table 6-2). Further clinical distinction can be made between metabolic and structural coma (Table 6-3). The reticular activating system (RAS) in the brainstem maintains normal consciousness. Processes that disturb its function will lead to altered consciousness.[16] The mechanisms that produce coma are diverse and the clinical presentations vary. The mnemonic TIPS and the vowels AEIOU are a memory aid for the causes:

> T—Trauma
> I—Insulin and hypoglycemia
> P—Poisoning and psychogenic
> S—Shock
>
> A—Alcohol abuse
> E—Epilepsy/encephalopathy
> I—Infection of inborn errors
> O—Opiates and other central nervous system (CNS) depressants
> U—Uremia

Other Causes of Coma

If left untreated, **increased intracranial pressure (ICP)** can lead to decreased levels of consciousness from decreased cerebral perfusion pressure (CPP) and hypoxia. With severe hypoxia and acidosis, cerebral herniation syndromes can occur that must be treated to decrease the likelihood of permanent coma and death (see Chapter 10).

CNS **infections** and non-CNS infections can cause inadequate primary defense actions with stasis of body fluids, changes in pH secretions, and inadequate secondary body defenses that can cause alterations in consciousness. It is

---

BOX 6-2	Vegetative State Responses

- Eye opening, first in response to painful stimuli, and later spontaneously with increasingly prolonged periods; patient may intermittently move the eyes from side-to-side or follow a person or object but is incapable of "visual tracking"
- Blinking in response to a "threat" or to light
- Inattentiveness, with no signs of awareness of environment or inner needs
- Wakefulness accompanied by an apparent complete lack of cognitive functions
- Sleep-wake cycles or eyes that open spontaneously in response to external stimuli such as voice or touch
- Vegetative functions, with primitive posturing and reflex movements of the limbs
- Maintenance of intact brainstem reflexes, blood pressure, and breathing by the patient
- Intact pupillary, oculocephalic, chewing, and swallowing reflexes, but no discrete localizing motor responses
- No speech following of commands or speaking

TABLE 6-2	Comparative Coma Assessment: Structural Versus Metabolic Lesions	
Assessment Parameters	**Structural Coma**	**Metabolic Coma**
Symptom onset	Rapid, rostral-caudal deterioration	Progressive, variable dysfunction
Motor function	Coma onset follows motor abnormalities; may show focal findings	Coma onset precedes motor abnormalities
Reflex activity	May show focal findings	No focal findings
Pupillary reaction	Unilaterally nonreactive; bilaterally nonreactive later	Usually preserved

From Stewart-Amidei C: Assessment. In Bader MK, Littlejohns LR: *AANN core curriculum for neuroscience nursing*, ed 4, St Louis, 2004, Saunders.

TABLE 6-3   Clinical Manifestations of Metabolic and Structural Causes of Coma

Manifestation	Metabolically Induced Coma	Structurally Induced Coma
Blink to threat (cranial nerves II, VII)	Equal	Asymmetric
Discs (cranial nerve II)	Flat, good pulsation	Papilledema
Extraocular movement (cranial nerves III, IV, VI)	Roving eye movements; normal doll's eyes and calorics	Gaze paresis, nerve III palsy, medial longitudinal fasciculus (MLF) syndrome (internuclear ophthalmoplegia)
Pupils (cranial nerves II, III)	Equal and reactive, may be large (e.g., atropine), pinpoint (e.g., opiates), or midposition and fixed (e.g., glutethimide [Doriden])	Asymmetric and/or nonreactive; may be midposition (midbrain injury), pinpoint (pons injury), large (tectal injury)
Corneal reflex (cranial nerves V, VII)	Symmetric response	Asymmetric response
Grimace to pain (cranial nerve VII)	Symmetric response	Asymmetric response
Motor function movement	Symmetric	Asymmetric
Tone	Symmetric	Paratonic, spastic, flaccid, especially if asymmetric
Posture	Symmetric	Decorticate, especially if symmetric; decerebrate, especially if asymmetric
Deep tendon reflexes	Symmetric	Asymmetric
Babinski sign	Absent or symmetric response	Present
Sensation	Symmetric	Asymmetric

From Boss B: Concepts of neurological dysfunction. In McCance KL, Huether SE: *Pathophysiology*, ed 4, St Louis, 2002, Mosby, p 439.

frequently unclear if the initial fever and pleocytosis are related to CNS infection. Thus there should always be a search for other causes. CNS infections are serious and require blood, urine, sputum, and sometimes cerebrospinal fluid (CSF) cultures and treatment to be instituted immediately (see Chapter 4).

Ventilation that is insufficient to provide the lungs with air and support breathing adequate for support of life, as well as **hypoxia** can quickly lead to alterations in consciousness. Assessment may include pulse oximetry or arterial blood gas (ABG) analysis to document acid/base imbalance. Reversal of hypoxia and acid/base imbalances should be promptly addressed (see Chapter 9).

A **drug overdose (DO)** from the accidental or purposeful dose of a drug large enough to cause adverse reactions may also alter consciousness or induce coma or death. An opioid drug overdose can be emergently treated with an intravenous (IV) opioid antagonist such as naloxone (Narcan) every 5 to 10 minutes until consciousness returns. Treatment difficulties arise when patients have overdoses brought on by multiple and unknown recreational drugs.

Cerebral hemorrhage, brain tumors, metastatic tumors, cerebral abscesses, and infarcts may result in temporary or permanent alterations in consciousness. These conditions are associated with increased ICP and need to be emergently managed nonsurgically by treating the increased ICP; this is followed by appropriate treatment of the underlying cause (see Chapter 10).

Common Pathophysiology

Impairment of awakeness or arousal indicates bilateral frontal lobe dysfunction or dysfunction in the **ascending reticular activating system (ARAS).**[39] Regardless of etiology, the common pathophysiology for all impairment in arousability is either a reduction in cerebral metabolism or a reduction in cerebral blood flow (CBF).[39] The prognosis and physical signs vary and depend on the pathophysiology of the underlying cause of the coma or disease process and the location. This can result from diffuse encephalopathy, supratentorial lesions, or intratentorial lesions.

Outcome States

Irreversible coma occurs when there is an irreversible, permanent destruction of both cerebral hemispheres. The patient is no longer able to maintain external homeostasis (i.e., the ability to respond behaviorally in any major or appropriate way to the environment), although the brain continues to maintain the body's internal homeostasis. The **comatose** patient lies with eyes that do not open spontaneously or in response to stimulation and does not make an attempt to avoid noxious stimuli. Patients who lapse into a coma may be evaluated for whole brain death.[41] **Brain death, irreversible coma,** or **cerebral death** is the permanent absence of cerebral function.[1]

TIP: The cardinal findings in brain death are absence of any response to stimulation, absence of motor response, absence of brainstem reflexes (corneal, pupils, gag, or palpebral), absence of spontaneous respirations, relatively normal body temperature, and absence of any drugs that might impair consciousness.[41]

Few patients remain in a coma from trauma for more than 4 weeks.[39] After 4 weeks or more in a coma from trauma or other causes, the patient may experience a return of wakefulness in vegetative state. Long-term survival in a vegetative state is uncommon. Predicting which patient will enter a vegetative state is difficult during the first few days after the onset of coma. Clinical changes after the first week have more prognostic value than signs present during the first few days. Poor pupil reflexes, for example, may be an indicator of a poor outcome in some patients.

As mentioned earlier, locked-in syndrome describes quadriplegia and mutism with intact consciousness and the preservation of voluntary vertical eye movements and blinking. It may be due in some cases to a vascular lesion of the pars ventralis pontis. This is a rare, paralytic, neurologic condition in which an individual may be conscious and alert but unable physically to move any part of the body except the eyes. Patients may communicate by vertical eye movements and blinking to communicate—one blink for "yes," two blinks for "no." Bilateral destruction of the medulla oblongata or pons has rendered the individual unable to speak or move any of the extremities.[30] A communication board or other appropriate enhanced method of communication is essential for a patient with amyotrophic lateral sclerosis (ALS).

Diagnostic Studies

The following diagnostic and laboratory studies are considered initially:[38]
- Electrolyte panel including carbon dioxide, chloride, potassium, sodium
- Complete blood count (CBC) and differential
- Drug screen for toxicology
- Blood urea nitrogen (BUN) and creatinine (Cr)
- Computed tomography (CT) or magnetic resonance imaging (MRI) scan of the head may be ordered to rule out cerebral hemorrhage, mass, or structural causes

- Electrooculogram (EOG)
- Evoked potentials
- Lumbar puncture (LP) with CSF analysis for infection or other findings
- CBF studies as needed

Assessment

Assessment should include a description of the patient's level of consciousness and associated physical signs (Table 6-4). The neurologic evaluation of comatose patients involves a comprehensive examination performed on a regular basis. If the patient is unable to speak or fails to follow commands, the clinician should consider aphasias or lower cranial nerve dysfunction. In patients with an acute brain injury who are admitted and managed in an intensive care unit, the challenge is to find a tool that monitors the depth of coma but also, over time, pinpoints a deterioration or an improvement. A comprehensive assessment of neurologic function may not be practical to incorporate in routine neurologic checks. However, any assessment ideally should select clinical features that are tell-tale signs of a decreasing consciousness, increasing ICP, and brain herniation.

These signs can be summarized in the new **FOUR score** (Full Outline of Un-Responsiveness) coma scale that has been validated in a large study at the Mayo Clinic using a scoring pocket card included in the book.

The FOUR score is easy to learn, easy to use, and easy to teach, and it can be understood by all health care workers when used routinely. The gold standard tool has been the Glasgow Coma Scale (GCS) since its inception in 1974 (see Chapter 2). Shortcomings of the GCS involve inability to assess the verbal score after the patient has been intubated;

TABLE 6-4 Differential Characteristics of States Causing Coma	
Mechanism	**Manifestations**
Supratentorial mass lesions compressing or displacing the diencephalon or brainstem	Initiating signs usually of focal cerebral dysfunction
	Signs of dysfunction progress rostral to caudal
	Neurologic signs at any given time point to one anatomic area (e.g., diencephalon, mesencephalon, medulla)
	Motor signs often asymmetric
Infratentorial mass of destruction causing coma	History of preceding brainstem dysfunction or sudden onset of coma
	Localizing brainstem signs precede or accompany onset of coma and always include oculovestibular abnormality
	Cranial nerve palsies usually manifest "bizarre" respiratory patterns that appear at onset
Metabolic coma	Confusion and stupor commonly precede motor signs
	Motor signs usually are symmetric
	Pupillary reactions usually are preserved
	Asterixis, myoclonus, tremor, and seizures are common
	Acid-base imbalance with hyperventilation or hypoventilation is common
Psychiatric unresponsiveness	Lids close actively
	Pupils reactive or dilated (cycloplegics)
	Oculocephalic reflexes are unpredictable; oculovestibular reflexes are physiologic (nystagmus is present)
	Motor tone is inconsistent or normal
	Eupnea or hyperventilation is usual
	No pathologic reflexes are present

lack of assessment of respiration and brainstem reflexes; inability to assess a possible developing vegetative state; and inability to recognize pseudocoma (locked-in syndrome).

The FOUR score coma scale combines the most important neurologic signs into an easy-to-use scale with four components (eye response, motor response, brainstem reflexes, and respiration); the maximum score in each of these components is 4.

- *Eye response* (E0 to E4) involves noting eye opening to voice and pain, but also addresses horizontal eye tracking and vertical eye movements. When patients become drowsy, they first will fail to track finger movement (a command that requires some attention). With further neurologic change, patients then close their eyes when unstimulated, only to open to loud voice and finally only open eyes after a noxious pain stimulus or not at all. Patients in locked-in syndrome (mostly patients with a basilar artery occlusion causing a massive infarction of the pons) are able to blink and move eyes vertically while motionless, speechless, and appearing unconscious. Patients in a vegetative state who emerge from an eyes-closed coma within days to weeks will open their eyes, but with a vacant stare and no tracking of objects.
- *Motor response* (M0 to M4) involves a comprehensive evaluation of alertness and praxis, using a three-hand position test. Patients are asked to make a peace sign, a fist, and show thumbs up. This eliminates the often used "finger squeezing," which may be very difficult to distinguish from a grasp reflex. When patients lapse into a stupor, patients localize a pain stimulus (purposeful) but when deeper in a coma, only withdraw to pain, and develop extensor (abnormal extension) posturing. In deepest coma, patients show no response to pain after a pain stimulus is applied to the nail beds; leg withdrawal after pain may be a reflex such as the "triple reflex response." The **triple reflex response** could be explained as a spinal cord disinhibition consisting of a Babinski sign with flexion in the knee and hip. The recognition of myoclonus status epilepticus (constant brief muscle jerking in limbs and face) is important. This is seen typically in comatose patients with no motor response to pain, is a result of devastating ischemic brain injury after a cardiopulmonary resuscitation (CPR), and has a particularly poor outcome.
- *Brainstem reflexes* (B0 to B4) are very important in a coma and they become abnormal or disappear with significant brainstem displacement. The most important assessments are the pupil, corneal responses and the cough response, which measure the condition of the mesencephalon, pons, and medulla oblongata. Oculocephalic responses are important, but they are potentially dangerous to test in patients with a potential traumatic neck injury. Patients with a unilateral fixed pupil can be scored. When all three brainstem reflexes are absent the patient may be brain

dead and a more formal brain death examination should be undertaken.
- *Respiration* (R0 to R4) involves assessment of patients with an impaired consciousness who breathe differently. First when patients become sleepier, they may develop a Cheyne-Stokes breathing pattern (periodic breathing with building up of a rapid respiratory rate followed by apnea, only to be followed by the same cycle). Irregular breathing (gasping or apneic pauses) often indicate a deepening coma and inability to protect the airway with repeat obstruction of the pharynx. After intubation it is important to know whether the patient has a respiratory drive and is able to trigger the ventilator; therefore the respiratory component of this coma scale involves assessment of respiration in a nonintubated patient and triggering of the ventilator in the intubated patient.

These four components of the FOUR score were not meant to be totaled or summed, but a FOUR score of 0 would likely indicate that the patient could fulfill the criteria of brain death. The new score has shown good to excellent reliability, can be used to predict outcome, can be performed within 1 to 2 minutes, and requires very little training.

History of the patient's altered state of consciousness should be quickly obtained from family and witnesses. When removing clothing, observe for incontinence, Medic Alert jewelry, identification, and belongings in wallet or purse for clues. Inspect for head injury and assess stiff neck. Evaluate the following:

- LOC: use a standardized scale (e.g., GCS, FOUR score) and document using the intensive care unit (ICU) flow sheet (see Chapter 2)
- If unable to speak or follow commands, consider aphasia
- Respiratory: rate, rhythm, and pattern of breathing; Cheyne-Stokes respirations; erratic respirations
- Pupils: size, direct and consensual response to light, and accommodation; ipsilateral or bilateral dilated pupil may indicate signs of uncal herniation verus small reactive pupils[16]
- Cornea: protect if lids are not closed; corneal ulcerations may develop
- Eye positioning: at rest; voluntary response to eye movement; presence of roving eye movements and Bell's phenomenon, ptosis, CNs III, IV, and VI palsy, conjugate versus disconjugate movement
- Cranial nerve assessment: helps determine location of injury causing coma
- Oculocephalic reflex: a test for brainstem integrity to check for the doll's-eye reflex (if indicated by decreased LOC and if there is no suspicion of neck injury)
- Response to noxious stimulus: sternal rub, supraorbital or nail bed pressure if appropriate; presence of posturing spontaneously or to noxious stimulus
- Vital signs: blood pressure, respirations, pulse, temperature

- Skin integrity: breakdown at pressure points may develop early; pressure ulcers may already be present
- Bladder function: urinary catheter is inserted with strict intake and output (I&O)
- Pulmonary: lungs are auscultated to detect early signs of aspiration or atelectasis
- Motor status: voluntary motor movement to commands; strength in extremities on voluntary movement; spontaneous motor movement with abnormal flexion or abnormal extension (may be late signs); ipsilateral hemiplegia, tetraplegia
- Reflexes: deep tendon reflexes (DTRs) symmetric versus nonsymmetric, present or absent; presence or absence of gag and cough

After the health care team completes an assessment of airway, breathing, circulation, diabetes, drugs, seizures, fever, and GCS, a generalized assessment allows the clinicians to narrow the focus and offer guidelines or protocols for the appropriate diagnostic studies and treatments. A determination of the group in which to classify the patient can be made based on whether or not the patient has focal signs, brainstem signs, or other causes of coma. Additional diagnostic studies and treatments are described in the following sections according to the underlying cause of the altered state of consciousness.

COMA MANAGEMENT

Rapid and accurate identification of the underlying etiology of coma is critical at the same time that the patient is stabilized to prevent neurologic injury and cardiorespiratory or other complications. Treatment is based on the initial clinical history and signs. The diagnosis is established by clinical examination, laboratory results, and radiologic testing. The goal is to remove the cause, when possible; prevent secondary complications; and provide a multidisciplinary team management in the most appropriate clinical setting for optimal recovery and rehabilitation.

Initial Emergent Assessment and Management

The clinician needs to follow guidelines or a common protocol in assessing patients with impaired consciousness. The foremost consideration in the initial assessment is time; using a decision tree to think through the problems for quick evaluation and systematic treatment saves time (Fig. 6-1). In some emergency departments (EDs), a **"coma cocktail"** is administered for a very short-term intervention for coma reversal. Such cocktails include administration of a combination of thiamine (Batalin), glucose, naloxone (Narcan), and flumazenil (Romazicon). Acute withdrawal syndromes (e.g., hypertension and seizures) must be considered based on the balance of risks and benefits.

Emergency interventions take precedence over the general admission medical principles of history taking, physical examination, and investigational studies for diagnosis and treatment of a comatose patient. Box 6-3 lists the emergent medical management.

BOX 6-3	Emergent Medical Management of a Comatose Patient

- Institute emergency resuscitative measures to prevent hypoxia and brain damage.
- Determine the cause of the coma; this is a priority.
- Perform acute emergency medical treatment. These principles apply regardless of the etiology for the decreased arousal state.
- Maintain oxygenation and circulation, and establish an airway and supplemental oxygen.
- Intubate the patient with mechanical ventilation; this may be required for respiratory support and should not be delayed.
- Obtain arterial blood gas (ABG) analysis and pulse oximetry, and correct abnormal values.
- Threat shock, which may require the insertion of a central venous line, fluids, and blood.
- Draw blood immediately for routine analysis; many institutions include drug screening as part of the protocol.
- Insert intravenous (IV) lines for medications and fluids; maintain the patient on nothing-by-mouth (NPO) status.
- Treat hypoglycemia; this begins with the administration of IV glycogen or complex carbohydrates. The brain needs glucose for cerebral metabolism.
- Maintain the patient in the lateral position instead of the supine position to prevent aspiration.
- Prevent seizures with loading doses of anticonvulsants.
- Perform gastric aspiration and lavage if drug ingestion is suspected.
- Decompress the stomach by inserting a nasogastric (NG) tube to prevent vomiting.
- Insert an indwelling urinary catheter for strict intake and output (I&O).
- Maintain temperature control with a cooling/warming blanket; current research is investigating the use of forced hypothermia to decrease brain damage.

Additional Data

When a witness or family member can provide additional data concerning the patient's condition, an important timeline including when the first symptoms were observed and the amount of time that has elapsed may be established. Though not a formal history, data should be collected and documented from family, observers, police, or paramedics relating to the onset, early symptoms, and possible cause of the unresponsive state. In addition, it is important to gather information concerning the patient's history of previous or recent trauma, illness, medications, substance abuse, and psychiatric disorders.

Secondary Emergent Assessment and Management

After the initial triage and assessment, the secondary assessment can be implemented (Fig. 6-2). The health care team collaborates to determine whether the unresponsive state is the result of an **organic disease process** (e.g., brain tumor),

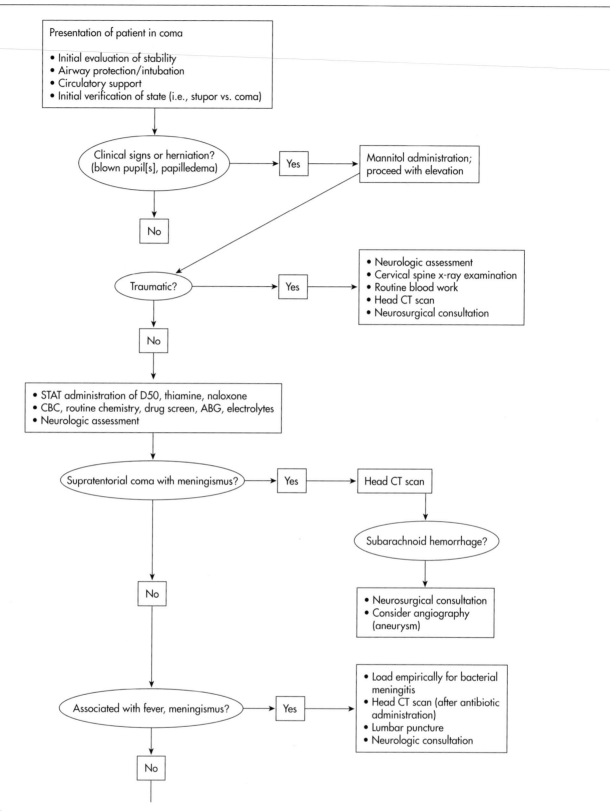

Figure 6-1 Coma evaluation and treatment algorithm.
(From Ritaccio AL: Stupor, coma, and brain death. In Popp AJ, editor: A guide to the primary care of neurological disorders, *1998, American Association of Neurological Surgeons.)*

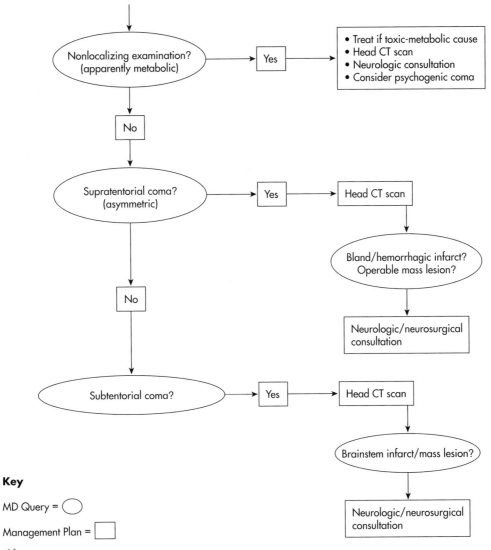

Figure 6-1, cont'd

a **psychogenic disorder** (e.g., catatonia), or **trauma.** If the etiology is organic, the cause must be identified as a **metabolic** problem, CNS infection, or a **structural** lesion (see Table 6-3). If the patient has a life-threatening metabolic problem, it must be treated emergently. The team determines as quickly as possible the history and etiology with a brief, focused assessment with particular attention to the brainstem functions.

Assessment and management for a coma includes the following:

- Airway, breathing, and circulation (ABCs); pulse oximetry; check for adequate ventilation and hypoxemia (blood oxygen) and/or anoxia or obstructed airway
- Upper airway and chest for oxygenation and ventilation; secure airway; adequate oxygenation (Po_2) and ventilation (Pco_2)
- Pulse, skin color, and capillary refill time for peripheral perfusion: in general, if the radial pulse is palpable, the systolic blood pressure will be above 80 mm Hg; if the femoral or carotid pulse is palpable, the systolic pulse will be above 70 mm Hg or 60 mm Hg, respectively
- Level of consciousness (LOC): a GCS score, FOUR score, and brief neurologic assessment to determine patient alertness, responsiveness to vocal stimuli or painful stimuli, motor function, and posturing
- Pattern of breathing
- Eyes (one of the most important assessments): pupil size and reactivity; funduscopic examination for papilledema, corneal reflex, eye position and extraocular movements (EOMs)
- Hypoglycemia: hepatic, ureic, endocrine causes
- Hyponatremia: fluid and electrolyte imbalances

The fundamental importance of pupillary reactivity cannot be overemphasized because the brainstem area that controls consciousness (i.e., the reticular formation) is adjacent to those areas of the brainstem that control pupillary constriction and dilation. It is important to delineate a

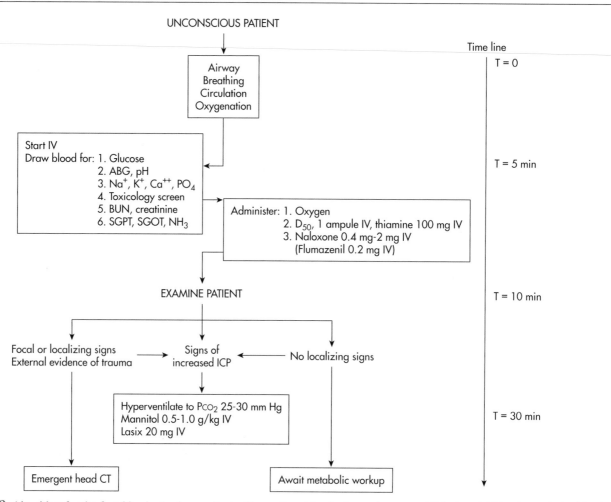

Figure 6-2 Algorithm for the first 30 minutes for a patient with an altered level of consciousness. *ABG,* Arterial blood gas; *BUN,* blood urea nitrogen; *SGPT,* serum glutamic pyruvic transaminase; *SGOT,* serum glutamic oxaloacetic transaminase; *ICP,* intracranial pressure; *CT,* computed tomography.
(From Johnson RT, Griffin JW: Current therapy in neurologic disease, ed 5, St Louis, 1997, Mosby.)

structural versus a metabolic cause of coma. Interruption of the sympathetic control of pupillary activity leads to a constriction (**Horner's pupil**). Bilateral interruption of descending sympathetic fibers at the pontine level leads to a bilateral Horner's pupil referred to as **"pontine pinpoint pupils."** Disruption of the parasympathetic pupillary innervation leads to an enlarged pupil, or **"blown pupil."** The presence of **"roving eye movement"** is important to observe because it implies that the brainstem connections for conjugate eye movement are intact.

> **TIP:** The ciliospinal reflex (CSR) is a self-limited pupillary dilation (6 to 8 mm) caused by noxious stimuli to the face, head, or upper trunk; this dilation is always bilateral and symmetric and occurs in seemingly nonreactive pupils.

Patients in a pentobarbital coma have a CSR that can mimic pathologic conditions. Recognizing a CSR can potentially lead to the reduction of unnecessary transport and medical interventions in critically neurologically ill patients in whom a pentobarbital coma has been induced.[3]

Potential Complications

A patient in a coma is at risk for complications that may include infections, metabolic alterations, skin breakdown and ulceration, and deep vein thrombosis (DVT) that may delay recovery from the coma.[13] Assessment is needed to evaluate the baseline status, with frequent reassessment to detect subtle, rapid, and significant changes that require emergency interventions. The possibility of hypoglycemia requires urgent blood glucose determination. An ampule of IV thiamine can be given before glucose to prevent Wernicke's encephalopathy in malnourished patients addicted to alcohol. Renal failure may cause uremia with fluid overload, electrolyte imbalance, or metabolic acidosis. Pulmonary complications include aspiration pneumonia with loss of protective reflexes. Sepsis can lead to multisystem organ failure, and stress ulcers may result in a gastrointestinal (GI) bleed.

Coma and Pregnancy

During the past 25 years, there have been approximately a dozen cases of female comatose patients who were pregnant and delivered. In the rare situation of a pregnant female, a multidisciplinary plan for the mother and infant should be available. A multidisciplinary team approach is needed to manage the care and complications of a comatose brain-dead patient on life support. The plan includes giving the fetus as much time as possible to develop for a reasonable chance for the baby to survive. Emotional support for the father and family members and the staff is very important. A multidisciplinary ethics committee should be consulted for ethical conflicts.

Acute Care Assessment

After resuscitation and any necessary lifesaving measures initiated in the ED, interventions are based on a priority as indicated by the results of the initial assessment (Box 6-4). The temperature regulating centers in the hypothalamus can be damaged by toxic agents, trauma, tumors, CNS infections, or vascular disease. Fever management is important with measures taken to keep the body temperature **normothermic.** Elevated temperatures may cause depression of the control mechanisms in the hypothalamus and result in increased cerebral metabolism and increased ICP with potential damage to brain cells or other body systems and decreased sweating. Somnolence and hypotension can accompany

hypothermia with cardiac dysrhythmias and other side effects depending on the core body temperature. Protocols or orders for temperature regulation should be individualized.

Some patients, however, may be considered candidates for new or experimental treatment protocols. A multicenter National Institutes of Health (NIH) grant to G. L. Clifton at the University of Texas also includes the Universities of Pittsburgh, California (Davis, San Francisco, and Los Angeles), Duke, St. Louis, and Mississippi. Researchers have studied the concept of cooling the body shortly after head injury to induce **hypothermia.** Earlier research showed that hypothermia with the use of cooling mechanisms and devices to reduce the core temperature to below 95° F or even 90° F for patients with a GCS of 5 to 7 causes no permanent disability and may speed recovery from a coma.[27] Current results may be considered less than optimal but seem to indicate that hypothermia can be safely applied as a useful adjunct to barbiturates and mannitol to control elevated intracranial pressure. More studies are needed to determine the optimal temperature, time from injury, and duration and rate of rewarming, with evaluation of newer technologies that protect the tissue and are affordable. Tests of systemic hypothermia as a neuroprotectant have been negative or equivocal.[11]

Shivering must be controlled with appropriate drugs, and intensive monitoring is required during the 24-hour

---

BOX 6-4   **Intensive Care Management for Coma**

- Position patient in lateral position if not intubated; if intubated, the head of the bed is generally elevated.
- Aspiration is a risk in the intubated; the stomach may be decompressed or an orogastric tube may be required.
- Institute measures to prevent deconditioning and iatrogenesis.
- Maintain normothermia and decrease fever with cooling devices.
- Induced hypothermia may be ordered to decrease brain damage.
- Sliding insulin scale may be ordered to prevent hyperglycemia.
- Institute measures to prevent DVT and PE (e.g., low-molecular-weight heparin, intermittent compression device).
- Establish a skin and eye care regimen to maintain skin and cornea integrity.
- Establish a regular bowel regimen and bladder programs. Some clinicians will maintain an indwelling urinary catheter until mobility is reasonable. The patient should be made catheter free if possible by the use of intermittent catheterization, an external catheter, or a bladder evacuation schedule. If an indwelling catheter must be maintained, a bladder care program is established to minimize the risk of infection.
- Maintain a passive range-of-motion (ROM) exercise program and positioning. Splints and other assistive devices may be used after evaluation by the rehabilitation team.

- Plan and implement an active exercise program for patients who have regained sufficient wakefulness based on the rehabilitation team's recommendation.
- Emphasize pulmonary hygiene.
- Establish a weaning protocol if the patient is receiving ventilatory support or oxygen therapy.
- Continue and provide consultations for appropriate support services (e.g., social services). Family members continue to be supported through the stages of grieving and their adaptation to the chronic illness. Referrals are made for support services that the family requires.
- Provide feedback to family members about their success in caring for a loved one who has altered consciousness; recognize their efforts, especially as time goes on and friends and other family members go about their lives.
- Use grief adaptation processes to assist family members in progressing through the grief, and assist them in developing or maintaining effective coping methods.
- Assess for caregiver fatigue. Help the primary caregiver integrate his or her personal, physical, psychologic, and social health care into the patient's plan of care.
- Identify options for assistance, and work with the caregiver to take advantage of all available options.
- Provide some assertiveness training, or take other measures to help the caregiver mobilize needed assistance.
- Mobilize resources, such as a respite care program, in conjunction with social services.

DVT, Deep vein thrombosis; *PE,* pulmonary embolus.

hypothermic state; approximately 12 hours is needed to rewarm the patient.[45]

> **ALERT:** **Hyperbaric oxygen (HBO$_2$)** therapy is the administration of 100% oxygen at more than three times the normal atmospheric pressure in a specially designed airtight chamber. The concept is to deliver high-dose oxygen (under increased atmospheric pressure) to neurons in order to speed the healing of injuries from hypoxia. Used primarily in emergency situations, HBO$_2$ therapy is available in some centers for enhancement therapy for patients in a coma.[37]

After transfer to the ICU, follow-up assessment and initial ICU documentation become the patient's baseline for serial assessments that continue as the patient's response is carefully monitored and evaluated:

- GCS score, FOUR score, or other coma scale scores to determine an increase or decrease in LOC
- Cranial nerve (CN) assessment
- Vital signs on a frequent basis for comparison and an analysis of an improvement or deterioration
- Reflex response: determine if reflexes are increased, decreased, or asymmetric
- Response to noxious stimuli: determine whether one side functions differently from the other
- Skeletal muscle motor responses
- CSF leak: check for rhinorrhea or otorrhea (especially if the patient has a history of recent head trauma)
- Nuchal rigidity: check cervical films before testing
- Note breath odor
- Skin: check for signs of trauma, needle tracks; Battle's sign and "raccoon eyes" for basilar skull fracture (24 to 48 hours after trauma)
- Complete cardiac, pulmonary, chest, and abdominal assessment; check ECG monitor

The goal of ICU multidisciplinary care is to stabilize the patient, manage medical interventions, and prevent complications through continuous observation and management. Surgical or bedside procedures may be necessary (e.g., surgical evacuation of a clot or insertion of a Foley catheter, nasogastric [NG] tube, and other monitoring devices). As soon as medically feasible, invasive lines and indwelling catheters should be removed and the patient evaluated closely for measures to prevent infection (see Chapter 9). Evaluations of the unresponsive patient in the ICU require an ongoing hourly assessment or more frequently if the patient's condition is unstable. Cardiac status should be continuously monitored, and, if warranted, ICP, CPP, brain tissue oxygen, or other monitoring should be performed. Otherwise, the routine serial assessments continue as follows:

- Neurologic assessment, with assessment of LOC using the GCS or other coma scales
- Cardiac status
- Pulmonary status: respiratory rate and pattern, lung sounds
- Chest x-ray examinations
- Laboratory tests: for example, electrolytes, osmolality, BUN, and hematologic studies
- Eye, skin, and corneal integrity
- Hourly I&O
- Measurements to assess renal and bladder function
- Bowel and bladder status
- Assessment for early, subtle signs of deterioration; assessment for complications
- Assessment of diagnostic, laboratory, radiology, and other test results

Removal of a hard cervical collar placed by the emergency medical services (EMS) providers for suspected cervical spine (C-spine) injury should be cleared by the treating physician in charge of the case before removal by the clinicians. The family's coping mechanisms also must be continually reassessed. The level of anxiety in family members may be particularly high when they cannot communicate directly with the patient. As diagnostic results are obtained and the cause and diagnosis are determined, information should be conveyed to the family along with explanations.

Because a coma is itself a symptom, the patient's data continue to be analyzed to determine the cause of unresponsiveness. Results of the assessment and of neurodiagnostic and laboratory studies suggest particular etiologies and guide treatment according to whether the etiology is a supratentorial or an infratentorial process or is metabolic or structural in origin (see Table 6-3).

Supratentorial Lesion

If the coma results from a supratentorial lesion, the patient's history and assessment will generally show a headache, prior head trauma, contralateral weakness and sensory loss, dysfunction progressing in rostral-caudal fashion manifesting eventually as bilateral third motor dysfunction, or deteriorating pupillary responses with cardiovascular abnormality.

Infratentorial Lesion

Patients with an infratentorial lesion often have a headache and vomiting or vertigo, diplopia or other signs of brainstem dysfunction, a sudden onset of coma, oculovestibular abnormalities (abnormal ice water caloric findings), cranial nerve palsies, or unusual cardiac or respiratory patterns.

Metabolic Coma

In patients with a metabolic coma, the history is usually positive for confusion and disorientation. Asymmetric motor signs are often absent.

Tremor and **asterixis,** an intermittent flapping movement of the outstretched hands, may be present in patients with a metabolic coma. Shocklike contractions of a group of muscles **(myoclonus)** may also be present with mild decreases in arousability. Most often, patients are flaccid and demonstrate no spontaneous movement. However, patients with metabolic coma may hyperventilate or hypoventilate. It is rare to see the irregular respiratory patterns that characterize an infratentorial structural disease process except when the disease progresses to affect the brainstem. Deep tendon reflexes and muscle tone are symmetric but may be increased or decreased.

Because the pupillary pathways are extremely resistant to metabolic insult, intact and symmetric pupillary and oculovestibular responses indicate a metabolic rather than a structural etiology.

Psychogenic Coma

A psychogenically induced coma is indicated by a failure to follow verbal input but with otherwise normal neurologic examination, EEG, and other investigations. These patients require an immediate consultation for psychiatric evaluation and care. A psychogenically induced coma is not discussed in this text.

Neurodiagnostic and Laboratory Studies

Studies are ordered based on the "index of suspicion" for the cause of the comatose state. The following are typical studies that help to discover the underlying cause of the coma and evaluate the effectiveness of ongoing treatment:[38]

- CT/MRI: Used to distinguish between supratentorial and infratentorial mass lesions; also to differentiate stroke verus tumor versus metabolic versus trauma causes

ALERT: There is a danger that the patient may aspirate during imaging, and therefore suction equipment should be readily available. Even when the lesion is not apparent, the shift in the ventricular system, the obliteration of cortical sulci, or the enhancement via contrast makes the differential diagnosis easier. An increase in ICP may occur during imaging, and the team must be prepared to treat such complications in the radiology suite.

- LP: when there is suspicion that the coma is a result of a CNS infection or intracranial hemorrhages, unless papilledema and CT suggest increased ICP, measure opening pressure; CSF can also be obtained from a ventriculostomy for analysis
- EEG: useful in detecting subtle seizure activity and distinguishing psychogenic unresponsiveness from an organic pathologic condition; also vital in establishing brain death (Fig. 6-3)

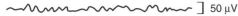

Alert wakefulness (beta waves)

Quiet wakefulness (alpha waves)

Stage 1 sleep (low voltage and spindles)

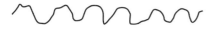

Stages 2 and 3 sleep (theta waves)] 50 µV

Stage 4 slow wave sleep (delta waves)

REM sleep (beta waves)

|← 1 sec →|

Figure 6-3 Electroencephalogram (EEG) stages of wakefulness and sleep.
(From Guyton AC, Hall JE: Textbook of medical physiology, ed 11, Philadelphia, 2006, Elsevier.)

- Cardiac study: 12-lead ECG; echocardiogram if the patient is hypotensive or the ECG suggests ischemia
- Analysis of gastric contents: with aspiration; may be requested if poisoning is suspected
- Blood: for electrolytes, blood counts, glucose, liver function tests (LFTs), BUN, toxicology, and evidence of infection
- Urinalysis: for specific gravity, glucose levels, acetone, and albumin
- Transcranial Doppler (TCD): to rule out vasospasm after the patient has been admitted to the critical care unit or relatively late in the course of the subarachnoid hemorrhage or as part of the screening for brain death

Treatment

Medical Management

In the ICU setting, clinical management of a coma is focused on maintaining an appropriate, "brain friendly" physiologic milieu, as well as prevention of secondary injuries, such as treatment of ICP, hyperglycemia, fever, hemodynamic instability, and hypoxia with low brain tissue oxygen concentration. The duration of the coma may be linked to long-term functional outcomes. A coma that lasts more than 6 hours may be indicative of severe cerebral dysfunction. In most cases, a coma lasts less than 1 month. Today, health care professionals are being encouraged to research and explore the possibility of implementing structured arousal stimulation programs as early as 72 hours after injury in the ICU. Starting early is of paramount importance to a patient's survival, quality of life, and overall long-term prognosis.[17]

Surgical Management

Immediate surgical evacuation is usually required for decreased arousal states caused by epidural and subdural hematomas. Treatment for hemorrhage, primary or metastatic tumors, cerebral abscesses, and infarcts may include surgical decompression. Partial or total resection may be indicated for some primary brain tumors; radiation therapy and chemotherapy may be indicated for primary and secondary brain tumors. Cerebral aneurysms may be surgically clipped or treated with stenting or endovascular coiling (see Chapter 18). Large hematomas of the cerebellum, subdural hematomas, and cerebellar infarcts are surgically evacuated (i.e., decompressed), and infarcted tissues are resected[28,39] (see Chapter 8). Surgical management is also useful in the management of acute hydrocephalus, which may occur with posterior fossa tumors or subarachnoid hemorrhage. Arteriovenous malformations (AVMs) may be treated surgically with the gamma knife, embolization, or other options (see Chapter 18).

Postacute Care and Assessment

Postacute care is a continuum of care based on continued nursing assessment:

- Reevaluate the patient every 6 to 8 hours
- Continue outcome of arousal stimulation program interventions

- Monitor pulmonary status for respiratory infections, aspiration pneumonia
- Check laboratory data in stable patients at least weekly
- Monitor for bladder and renal tract complications (e.g., urinary tract infection [UTI] or bladder stone); check urinary or external catheters in stable patients, usually every 4 to 8 hours
- Monitor nutritional status for malnutrition and evaluate swallowing, including the patient's ability to chew and swallow and gastroesophageal reflux; evaluate for percutaneous endoscopic gastrostomy (PEG) versus NG feedings for adequate protein and caloric intake; check weight gain or loss with frequent weights
- Monitor oral hygiene and ability to protect the airway and the return of swallowing and gag reflex
- Monitor bowel status daily for constipation or diarrhea
- Check skin for pressure ulcers; need for special bed with pressure-relieving coverings; evaluate 24-hour turning schedule, positioning and use of assistive devices, and out-of-bed wheelchair schedule and seating devices
- Monitor closely for DVT and pulmonary embolus (PE)
- Monitor for seizure activity and therapeutic levels of anticonvulsants
- Monitor for autonomic response with episodes of tachycardia, diaphoresis, hyperthermia, or blood pressure changes
- Assess for the risk of falls and injury as the patient becomes more alert and active
- Assess and document signs of improvement and evidence of recovery
- Assess family members with every contact, and encourage them to discuss their concerns with the health team; a support group for family members may be helpful
- Monitor verbal output and include orientation as appropriate
- Monitor ease of movement to assess spasticity, rigidity, increased muscle tone leading to contractures, and permanent deficits
- Monitor for the need of Multi-Podus boots or other devices that prevent contractures when performing range of motion (ROM) and exercises

Supportive care and measures to prevent secondary complications continue during postacute care. Improvement may be determined by a patient's increased spontaneous eye opening, motor activity, and wakefulness. Pictures from home, a clock and calendar for orientation, and comfortable sweatsuits or jogging clothes, a bathrobe, or other clothing items are positive reinforcement messages to the patient that recovery is expected.

During postacute care, little emphasis is placed on strategies that may potentiate early recovery.[13] Typically the comatose patient receives too little arousal stimulation and too much noxious stimulation from medical equipment attached to cardiac monitors, ventilators, feeding pumps, indwelling catheters, and venous and arterial lines. This equipment may have alarms and make monotonous noises. In addition, the patient is bathed daily, reassessed every 2 hours, and repositioned frequently, and, after evaluation by the physiatrist, has his or her joints put through ROM by physical therapists once or twice per day.

Early identification of potential complications of a coma prevents secondary brain damage and further disability. A sudden change in the patient's LOC requires an immediate response. Patients in a coma experience sensory deprivation because their ability to respond to stimuli is altered. Planning the therapeutic balance between the need to arouse the patient from the coma and to provide appropriate care is challenging.

Recovery Outcome

Recovery from a coma follows the normal hierarchic order in a sequential course from simple to complex, with the accomplishment of a simple skill occurring before the next, more complex skill. The anticipated order of response to stimuli is as follows:[19]

- Eye movement or tracking
- Head turning
- Leg movement
- Hand grasping
- Rolling
- Sitting
- Standing
- Complex cortical integration of movement

The differentiation between an arousable state, a vegetative state, or a slow-to-recover pattern may not be apparent in a patient in a coma. There is always the question of whether or not the patient can perceive sensory information. Bedside caregivers, family members, and visitors should assume that their conversations will be heard by the patient and act accordingly.

Outcomes to prevent secondary **brain injury** depend predominantly on the clinician's ongoing reevaluation of the patient's neurologic status to detect any subtle decreases in the level of brain function. Sudden changes that indicate a deterioration of neurologic status are followed by the initiation of more aggressive measures prescribed by the physician (e.g., increased hyperventilation, increased oxygenation, the appropriate administration of mannitol). The goal is further met by the diligent monitoring and managing of cardiac dysrhythmias, pulmonary atelectasis, pulmonary edema, acid/base imbalances, temperature alterations, and fluid and electrolyte imbalances (see Chapter 11).

Organ Donation

Despite the highest and most sophisticated nursing management, not every patient will recover. In cases where the family has decided on a death with dignity and to withdraw life support, organ donation can be discussed at the appropriate time with the family and information about the **organ donor** process provided with sensitivity and compassion.

Acute Rehabilitation

For patients in a coma, the **Rancho Los Amigos scale** is used to determine a level of cognitive functioning. Cognitive abilities are recorded from levels I to X, with I being the lowest. The Rancho level describes behavioral patterns of the various phases of recovery useful in developing a team plan of interventions for all disciplines, and in facilitating cognitive reorganization. For example, a patient who is unresponsive to any stimuli receives a Rancho Los Amigos (RLA) cognitive functioning level I (Box 6-5). Patients at levels other than level I typically fluctuate between three levels of cognitive function during the early phases of cognitive

BOX 6-5	**Rancho Los Amigos Cognitive Functioning Scale**

I: No response. Patient is unresponsive to any stimuli presented.

II: Generalized response. Patient reacts inconsistently and nonpurposefully to stimuli. Responses are the same regardless of the kind of stimulation applied.

III: Localized response. Responses are directly related to the type of stimulus presented but are inconsistent to specific kinds of stimulation. May follow simple commands inconsistently.

IV: Confused/agitated. Patient is in a heightened state of activity and has a severely decreased ability to process information; the individual is not aware of what he or she is doing.

V: Continued confused/inappropriate but nonagitated behavior. Patient appears nonagitated and alert and is able to follow simple commands; conversations may be confused.

VI: Continued confusion/emergence of appropriate behavior. Patient shows goal-directed behavior and follows simple directions consistently.

VII: Automatic/appropriate behavior. Patient appears appropriate and oriented within familiar settings (e.g., home or settings within the community).

VIII: Purposeful/appropriate behavior. Patient is consistently oriented to person, place, and time; alert and able to integrate past and recent events.

IX: Postacute. Patient independently shifts back and forth between tasks, uses assistive memory devices, is able to think about consequences of decisions/actions, is aware of disabilities, acknowledges others' needs, and may exhibit depression, irritability, and a low frustration tolerance.

X: Postacute. Patient is stable, can handle multiple tasks simultaneously, can create and maintain his or her own assistive memory device, anticipates the impact of impairments and takes actions to avoid problems, can recognize the needs of others and responds appropriately, and may exhibit periods of anger, depression, irritability, and low frustration tolerance when under stress.

Modified from Hagen C: Proper use of the Rancho levels of cognitive functioning, *Relearn Times* 8(1):1–6, 2001.

recovery. Such fluctuations may be in response to identified internal and external factors such as sustained or multisensory stimulation, time of day, sleep deprivation, and pain and discomfort.

Patients with an RLA level of I, II, or III; patients with a GCS score of 10 or less; patients with a stable ICP of 15 or less over a 24-hour period; and even patients receiving ventilation should be considered candidates for sensory stimulation.[13] In aggressive acute care settings, patients may have already been entered into a coma emergence program with coma recovery scale documentation. The rehabilitation team will be able to continue the sensory stimulation interventions with new goals for recovery.

With suitable candidates, the physiatrist and the rehabilitation team can initiate an early coma arousal regimen to help maintain the patient at his or her most functional level for the longest period of time, help move him or her to the next level, and prevent regression to a lower level of cognitive recovery from coma.

To prevent **deconditioning** (a multisystem decrease in functioning through disuse and immobility) and **iatrogenesis** (hospital-acquired injury and side effects of treatment), the clinician institutes the following:

- Skin care: activities to maintain or restore the skin, oral mucosa, and corneal integrity
- Pulmonary hygiene: turning, suctioning, and postural drainage; the ventilator is used to sigh or deliver larger volumes periodically
- Maintain vigilance for prevention of DVT and PE that may include low-molecular-weight heparin or other measures
- Positioning: maintain good alignment, frequent range-of-motion exercises, and assistive devices as needed with splints and other devices
- Bladder and bowel program (see Chapter 13)
- Eye care: measures to prevent the development of corneal abrasions or ulcers; instilling artificial tears or lubricants into the eyes and taping the lids shut are effective interventions
- Agitation: treatment using environmental control (e.g., providing an isolated, calm, quiet room and minimal stimulation)
- Safety: initial measures, such as a family member, sitter, or hospital policy after individualized assessment for the use of restraints and hospital policy to determine the least restrictive and most effective restraint, including mitts, waist belts, vests, and, last, the necessity of mechanical or chemical restraint

TIP: The need for use of physical restraints should be reevaluated and reordered daily according to hospital protocol considering restraints as a choice of last resort because they tend to increase agitation and restlessness.

- Minor or major tranquilizer or appropriate medications; may be necessary if the previous interventions are inadequate to control agitation
- Explanations to the patient regarding the care regimen, even when the patient does not respond

- Demonstrations of care and concern in the voice and touch and in therapeutic action
- Music, favorite television shows, tapes with familiar voices, objects from home, and fragrances used by the patient; may reduce agitation
- Nutrition and hydration: weight, calorie count, fluid I&O, and nutritional consultation within 24 to 48 hours to administer appropriate nutritional support via the appropriate route

The use of psychostimulants (e.g., methylphenidate [Ritalin] or dextroamphetamine [Dexedrine]) may be ordered. Dopaminergic stimulation may be used in patients recovering from traumatic brain injury. Brain injury is frequently associated with disturbance of dopamine transmission, and patients may be prescribed amantadine hydrochloride (Amantadine), bromocriptine (Parlodel), and levodopa (L-dopa). Anticonvulsants and antidepressants may also be used based on an individualized assessment and treatment plan. Modafinil (Provigil) has been used as a CNS stimulant to reduce the number of sleep episodes and increase daytime wakefulness.

Repeated and serial assessments help determine if stimulation therapy results in cognitive improvement. Such assessments include nursing interventions and observations and the manner in which the patient responds to and interacts with the family. Clinicians can incorporate stimulation techniques into the care of the coma patient and assess the patient's response.[19]

Comprehensive Patient Management at the end of the chapter includes health teaching, nutritional considerations, psychosocial considerations, and considerations for older adult patients.

Rehabilitation and Home Care

The primary goal of rehabilitation in coma patients is to increase the patient's level of responsiveness, regardless of whether this takes place in an acute care, a rehabilitation, or a home setting. A coma arousal program is the foundation of rehabilitation because a coma is viewed as a state of decreased responsiveness to the environment related to sensory deprivation. Caregivers, family members, and friends should be taught how to participate effectively in the coma arousal program once it has been implemented.[13]

Coma Arousal Plan

Joseph Giacino and Kathleen Kalmar[46] developed the **JFK Coma Recovery Scale,** which was revised in 2004 (CRS-R) with instructions and guidelines (see Appendix A). It consists of a set of tools for the coma emergence program with examples for multiple stimuli for the team of caregivers that can be continued by the family. Members of a coma emergence team (CET) can be trained to administer the program under the supervision of a physician. Physical therapy (PT), occupational therapy (OT), and speech/language therapy (ST) work together with the patient at the bedside to apply stimuli, which includes auditory, visual, motor, oromotor/verbal, communication, and arousal stimulation. Each assessment is documented on a numerical scale in each of these categories with

a total score of 25 points for the highest level on the CRS-R. For example, if the CRS-R score is 0 in each category for several weeks, the program may be discontinued. If, however, the individual's score from the stimulation guidelines progresses from 0 to the following: blink to noise (1), blink to light (1), abnormal extension (1), nonfunctional communication (1), and oral reflexive movement (1), stimulation that is maintained for 3 to 15 minutes (2), then the patient is exhibiting progress with a score of 7/25 and the program may be extended.

Repeated and serial assessments with tools such as the CRS-R will help determine if stimulation therapy results in cognitive improvement. Such assessments include nursing interventions and observations and the manner in which the patient responds to and interacts with the family. Clinicians can incorporate stimulation techniques into the care of the coma patient and assess the patient's response.[19]

An actual coma arousal plan considers the order of development of the CNS—auditory, visual, motor, oromotor/verbal, communication, and arousal. The clinician begins with the visual, for example, and attempts to get the patient to follow an object with his or her eyes, presents a noise to each ear and observes the response, performs ROM, and wipes or touches the face or arms. When purposeful and appropriate response is seen in a previously unresponsive or inappropriately responsive sensory system, the coma arousal program is extended. The evaluation of a program would assess if the patient stopped posturing on tactile stimulation or showed no evidence of neurologic deterioration. The cause for the cessation of posturing would determine if the coma arousal program is extended to include kinesthetic stimulation. If there is no posturing on turning, with range of motion, or with elevation of the head of the bed to a sitting position, olfactory and oral stimulation may be added. If the patient experiences increased tone in the oral structures, the coma arousal program may not extend to other later developing sensory systems.

Health care providers in both the rehabilitation and home setting monitor both the patient and family members through the grieving process and their adaptation to chronic illness. Reassessment is an ongoing process in the home setting because family situations are dynamic and change over time.

Chronic Conditions

The following detailed descriptions of chronic coma-related conditions are designed to educate family and providers. **Korsakoff syndrome,** also called Wernicke-Korsakoff disease, Korsakoff psychosis–amnesic dementia, or amnesic confabulatory psychosis, is an amnesic state caused by a thiamine (B_1) deficiency. This is often seen in alcoholics who have associated malnutrition. Symptoms of Korsakoff syndrome include impaired memory and judgment, a loss of social skills, signs of impaired intellect, and paranoid ideation. These symptoms develop gradually and persist as long as the thiamine deficiency continues. Thiamine replacement may help improve cognitive function and prevent the development of dementia, but once dementia has been established it may be permanent. Referral to a substance abuse counselor is appropriate.

Executive function deficits interrupt the mind's system of programming, verification, and correction. These overseer functions include anticipation, goal selection, planning, initiation, self-monitoring, and incorporation of feedback. The ability of an individual to start activities, sustain an activity, stop an activity, or shift from one activity to another, and to display self-awareness, has been described as the five important tasks of executive function. Initiation is described as starting and carrying out or sustaining activities or programming and involves the actual exhibition of the behavior, such as planning, initiating, and carrying out activities as productive activity and active thought. Self-monitoring and incorporation of feedback (self-correction), or knowing when to stop or suppress an activity, are described as effective performance. If something isn't working, making a shift is needed to try something else. As opposed to self-awareness (the ability to recognize one's own strengths and weaknesses), **anosognosia** (the inability to recognize illness in oneself) may be noted when the patient reports that nothing is wrong.

Characteristics

Executive system deficits result from pathologic conditions in the prefrontal areas. Based on an analysis of lesions, the dorsolateral prefrontal-subcortical circuit appears to be involved with executive function. This type of function includes the process of supervising other brain functions related to developing and implementing a plan. This region of the brain is also involved with motivation; consequently, lesions of these regions have been associated with apathy syndromes.

Patients with a severe deficit in motivation are motionless unless prompted externally or aroused to activity by extremely strong physiologic needs. In extreme situations, such patients do not even respond to hunger and thirst.

The patient with a motivation deficit appears to lack ambition, is often viewed as lazy, or is judged to be depressed. The patient with anergia often fails to appreciate his or her deficits and may even tend to minimize the importance of the cognitive problem or deny the deficits. The patient should be assessed for motivation, motion, awareness of feelings, safety concerns, and the presence of social graces.

Patients with a **goal formulation deficit** are unable to select or set a goal. Patients with a **planning deficit** are unable to produce a complete line of reasoning. **Programming deficits** may take the form of a failure to initiate, maintain, or discontinue a behavior. **Self-monitoring deficits** affect the inability to evaluate behavior by comparing it with the original task and goals. A self-monitoring deficit is manifested by the loss of "critical attitude" (i.e., the inability to use feedback relative to performance). A **feedback deficit** is the inability to change an action despite receiving feedback that the action is not correct.

The patient's executive system is reassessed on an ongoing basis. The frequency of assessment depends on the underlying pathologic condition and its effect on the arousal and vigilance systems. The patient's degree of instability and risk determines the frequency of assessment. Patients who are stable and have no risk for rapid neurologic deterioration may be reassessed frequently.

Management

With an executive system deficit, the etiologic factor is treated if possible. In some instances (e.g., minor head injury), the only treatment is time and cognitive retraining or coaching with feedback. Little research exists to clearly demonstrate the efficacy and cost-effectiveness of these therapies. Most data exist as anecdotal reports and clinically based evaluation studies.

Apathy and lack of motivation may be the clearest signs of executive system dysfunction. Motivation is assessed to some degree when orientation is examined, because orientation requires exercising sufficient motivation to identify relevant environmental cues. Family members and significant others need to be questioned regarding their knowledge of the patient's cognitive deficit, the cause of the condition, the therapeutic management of the cognitive deficit, and the prognosis for recovery. Level of anxiety and signs and symptoms of stress in family members and significant others should also be assessed. The coping skills of family members and significant others, which are evident during the early phases of the patient's hospitalization, also need to be evaluated.

Recovery of Consciousness

As patients recover consciousness, they pass through periods of confusion, disorientation, and memory gaps. Fall and injury prevention and safety are very important because the individual's judgment is still impaired. Agitated nonambulatory patients often benefit from the use of an enclosed bed on the floor (see Fig. 13-4). Rehabilitation goals focus on helping to regain strength mobility, speech, bowel/bladder control, cognition, and function to carry out activities of daily living (ADLs). Daily reassessment of the cognitive systems using observation techniques is appropriate. Assessment tools to measure orientation may include the GCS, Rancho scale, and **Galveston Orientation and Amnesia Test (GOAT)** (scored from 0 to 100). A GOAT score of greater than 75 is considered normal. The memory deficits are often best recognized in rehabilitation, in the home, or in the long-term care setting. Because the patient has become stable and other physiologic problems have been addressed, the memory deficit may show itself more clearly with less physiologic stress (see Chapter 13).

Initiative, goal selection, and planning emerge in familiar, flexible settings; therefore the clinician practicing on nonacute units or in home care is best able to assess executive functions during unstructured time in the evenings and at night. Executive systems are assessed by seeking information about the patient's performance of unstructured tasks or by observing unstructured task performance. Therapists, family, friends, and co-workers will be able to describe the patient's motivation and emotional tone following recovery. Observations include descriptions of what the patient does, step by step, from morning until night, when left alone, happy, under stress, or angry; coping abilities; and ability to make plans, learn, and remember.

COMPREHENSIVE PATIENT MANAGEMENT: ALTERATIONS OF CONSCIOUSNESS

Health Teaching Considerations

An individual who is discharged to home functioning at a Rancho level I to IV may continue to benefit from the coma emergence program that he or she was receiving during rehabilitation. Family and caregivers are given instructions not to provide too much stimulation that is too long in duration and too high in frequency at one time because it may cause "overload" (see Appendix B).

Regularly scheduled family conferences with the nursing staff, social worker, and other team members reinforce two-way communication and recognition of the family's needs. When patients who have been discharged and their families return weeks or months later to the nursing units where they recovered, it can be a morale booster to the treating team that was involved in the patient's care. Team members my find it amazing to see the recovered individual and feel the reward of knowing that they made a difference.

The burden of care for a family member who is unconscious presents a great emotional and financial burden for the family. The following teaching tips will help ease that burden:

- Explain what is being done for the patient and why it is being done; include the diagnostic tests required, the diagnosis, and the treatment.
- Teach the family about the patient's responses and what they mean; family members and significant others often misinterpret clinical signs (for example, they believe agitation is bad when in fact it indicates that the patient's coma is lighter, or they believe a hand grasp is in response to their touch when it is actually a reflex).
- Use crisis intervention techniques in some instances. All family members and significant others need to grieve, so facilitate this grief process by helping them recognize the need to grieve and accept normal grief reactions in themselves and in others.
- Help family members assess and mobilize their strength and resources; referral to social services and other hospital and community resources is often appropriate to deal with financial and other concerns.
- Show the family and significant others how to interact with the unconscious patient. Act as a role model with appropriate behaviors and explain how they should talk to and touch the patient while visiting.
- Involve the family members and significant others in patient care and teach them how to bathe, groom, turn the patient, provide ROM exercises, and carry out coma arousal protocols.
- Teach family members about the possible complications of altered levels of consciousness, possible changes in arousal states, possible reestablishment of a sleep-wake cycle, realistic hope, when and where to get help, how to alter the coma arousal program if the level of consciousness changes, and how to amend their responses to the patient in light of this alteration.
- Provide simple, specific information and directions to patients with cognitive deficits; provide information slowly, in small segments, and with frequent rest periods because the patient needs ongoing help to understand what has happened.
- Support family and friends in helping patients with retrograde amnesia to relearn episodic and sometimes semantic memories. Family and friends are essential in helping the patient relearn this information by recounting past events and sharing photographs, home movies, and souvenirs with the patient.
- Provide safety awareness teaching to the patient to the degree possible, as well as to the family and significant others.
- Provide updated information about the patient's condition, treatment plan, and prognosis; arrange for regular multidisciplinary meetings with the family.
- Teach the patient and family about the nature of cognitive deficits and how they influence behavioral responses, as well as the meaning of the behavioral responses to the deficits.
- Increase the effectiveness of interactions with the patient. Help the family and significant others learn how to teach the patient, allow ventilation of feelings, exhibit supportive behaviors, and decrease the patient's anxiety.
- Provide assistance on how to incorporate the lifestyle changes required by the patient's deficits while not unduly sacrificing their personal or family development.
- Encourage family members and significant others to join community support groups when possible.
- Consider end-of-life issues and the living will of patients who are not expected to recover (see Chapter 25).

Nutritional Considerations

A decreased level of arousal interferes with adequate nutrition, and a negative nitrogen balance develops because of the patient's inability to ingest foods and fluids by mouth and because of the limited caloric intake that can be achieved by an IV route. Calcium is also lost from the bones because of the lack of weight bearing. Additional calories are needed to compensate for the increased energy expenditures of patients who are posturing, restless, or agitated. Hypermetabolic states can increase catabolism to two and a half times the normal rate. The use of sedatives and relaxants may decrease this hypermetabolic state.

It must be determined whether the patient can be aroused sufficiently to safely and efficiently ingest foods and fluid orally; if the patient cannot be aroused, an alternative route for the delivery of nutrition and food is required. Enteral or parenteral feedings may be necessary if the patient is unable to ingest an adequate diet within a few days after loss of arousal. However, both have drawbacks: The parenteral route increases the risk of infection and hyperglycemia. A central line placement places the patient at risk for a pneumothorax during insertion. Decreased gut absorption resulting from decreased GI motility may present a problem with the enteral route, depending on the etiology of the coma state.

The following points about nutrition are important to remember for patients in a state of decreased arousal or coma:

- During the acute hospitalization stage, an early assessment of nutritional needs by the dietitian (within the first 24 hours of admission if possible) can help form a plan for appropriate nutrition therapy to prevent malnutrition and a negative nitrogen balance.
- A well-nourished patient with a negative nitrogen balance at the beginning of his or her illness can tolerate less than 1 week of catabolism.
- A poorly nourished patient or a patient in a hypermetabolic state can enter a negative nitrogen balance more rapidly and can experience rapid protein depletion.
- Inadequate nutrition with protein depletion compromises wound healing, predisposes the patient to decubitus development, increases the risk of infection and other complications, and prolongs recovery time.
- High-protein diets of 1.5 to 2.0 g/kg/day with 2000 to 5000 calories per day are needed for a negative nitrogen balance, but a better assessment of needs can be accomplished with indirect calorimetry.
- Supplemental vitamins and minerals are given to help minimize calcium loss, along with phosphorous and magnesium when patients are on steroids, diuretics, or hypovolemic therapy.
- Daily assessments of the skin, mucous membranes, and I&O are essential.
- Electrolytes, glucose, and protein (i.e., nitrogen balance studies) may be monitored weekly.
- Weight is assessed initially twice weekly and then weekly.
- Nutritional intervention adequacy is monitored through the collection of 24-hour urine samples for creatinine, BUN, and total nitrogen.
- Nutritional therapy may need to be adjusted during the postacute or nonacute phase of a coma as the patient's status changes.
- A patient's risk for aspiration must be evaluated by speech therapists and other health care providers.
- Oral suctioning equipment should always be available.
- Small, frequent meals are desirable if arousability is sufficient for the resumption of oral intake.
- Swallowing and feeding rehabilitation are part of the rehabilitation program.

Psychosocial Considerations

When a patient is totally unaware (i.e., in a comatose state), the psychosocial considerations shift entirely to the family and significant others:

- A devoted spouse or significant other may totally commit himself or herself to the patient and neglect his or her own health and personal needs to the point of exhaustion, or "caregiver burnout."
- The spouse may initially exhibit jealousy of the caregiver's intimacy with his or her loved one and resent such intrusions into the family's privacy.
- Family conferences that include a social services and spiritual counselor are helpful in overcoming these problems and supporting the spouse's ability to cope and manage this emotional and stressful period without guilt and resentment.
- Families may be overwhelmed, protective of their privacy, and very reluctant to allow friends, relatives, neighbors, or religious groups to share in the care of their loved one or to accept outside support.
- Professional counselors experienced in grief and bereavement or hospice care are effective in dealing with these issues.
- Financial strain and role reversals can add to the family's burden during this difficult time.
- Planned "time-outs" for family members should be arranged to give them "permission" to leave their loved one for "rest and recuperation."
- Legal counsel may be needed to advise family members about durable power of attorney, guardianship, advance health care directives, a living will, and insurance issues.
- Some patients may be discharged home where long-term care may fall to the responsibility of the family; involvement of the family at the earliest stages will help prepare them for this role.
- Inclusion of the family and significant other in supervised hands-on experiences at the bedside teaches them how to carry out ADLs while reinforcing the important role they serve as an integral part of the treating team.

Older Adult Considerations

Clinical manifestations often are more extreme in an older patient, and health problems with acute onset are often dismissed as senility or dementia. For example, a UTI might be a minor annoyance in a young adult but can cause significant delirium in an older adult. The presence of chronic illnesses may further complicate the medical management of coma and increase the difficulty in stabilizing older patients:

- The older patient in coma is at higher risk for medical complications and worse neurologic outcome.
- Deconditioning may delay recovery from coma; health care providers should focus on avoiding medical complications to prevent further deconditioning.
- Interventions aimed at recovery often must be instituted at a slower pace and with less aggressiveness in older patients.
- Older adults may demonstrate a serious decompensation in cognitive system function with even a minor illness or exacerbation of a chronic illness.

- Older adults may be very slow to recover function.
- Older patients may have more severe cognitive deficits in an unfamiliar setting with unfamiliar routines and are at higher risk for injury from falls when getting out of bed during the night for toileting.
- Medications are one of the most common cause of cognitive impairments in older adults; drugs that depress the CNS should be used with great caution or discontinued unless absolutely necessary.
- Older patients may be placed in an inappropriate facility because of a failure to recognize that cognitive functions may be only temporarily impaired.
- Normal age-related changes in the nervous system involve a slowing of information processing and a slight decrease in the efficiency of the recent memory system.
- Older adults can and do learn despite some impairment in the speed with which new information is processed.

Case Management Considerations

Patients who are in a comatose state or who have significant cognitive deficits require a case manager who has an in-depth understanding of the medical aspects of case, the treatment plan of care, potential patient complications, and medications. Input from the physician, the health care team, and the family is vital. After completing and documenting the preliminary screening and assessment, decisions on the anticipated level of care are made, payer approval is obtained, and the written case management plan is completed.

When recovery is not expected, plans for hospice care are needed during the final terminal phase. Many families may need help at some point in making decisions regarding long-term care placement when they are no longer able to provide 24-hour care in the home. The case management plan must be updated as goals are reached or as changes in the patient's condition show evidence of progression, regression, or failure to change.[40]

Specific outcome goals are based on the following considerations:

- Appropriate patient referrals, agencies, and follow-up with the health care team (e.g., physiatrist, physical therapist, occupational therapist, and social services)
- Family support and a team of caregivers to facilitate a smooth transition from acute care to rehabilitation and to home (e.g., preparation of the room for equipment and supplies)
- Ordering and checking of equipment to ensure good working order (e.g., feeding pumps, suction, oxygen, hospital bed, special mattress, IV poles); an assurance that family and caregivers know how to operate and troubleshoot equipment
- Written instructions for incontinence care: bowel and bladder management
- Written instructions for feeding tube and delivery system with adequate supply of nutritional supplements

- Written instructions for administration and the potential side effects of medications prescribed and available in the home; medications must be reviewed judiciously because of the issues of polypharmacy in older adults
- Considerations for planned respites and community support for family
- Review of handwashing and other techniques with family and caregivers for prevention of infections
- When and how to call 911 and respond to a medical emergency

CONCLUSION: COMA

Disorders of consciousness may involve either a loss of arousal or responsiveness (e.g., coma) or loss of one or more cognitive functions (e.g., attention, memory, and executive activities). Various types of trauma, brain attack or stroke, tumors, infections, degenerative conditions, and metabolic imbalances may produce a decrease in arousal or cognition. The patient's age, severity, and site of the pathologic condition often determine whether arousal is decreased or only cognitive functions are impaired. The onset of decreased arousal or impaired cognitive function may be abrupt and sudden, subacute and develop over a few days, or slowly progressive over weeks to months. Older patients are particularly at risk for impaired cognitive function. Many patients do not recover from coma. Helping the family and significant others cope with the devastating illness and comatose state of a loved one, which may end in death, requires the resources of the multidisciplinary neuroscience team.

SLEEP

Sleep can be defined as an altered state of consciousness from which a person can be aroused by sensory or other stimuli, which distinguishes it from coma. Sleep is restorative, vital to the proper functioning of the nervous system, and essential for survival. Both our physical and mental health depends on approximately 8 hours of sleep as our brain is designed to be awake for about 16 hours maximum.[34] The amount of sleep we need depends on multiple factors, including metabolic regulation, neuronal restoration, and memory consolidation.

Sleep requirements change from infancy through adulthood. Infants require approximately 16 to 20 hours of sleep daily, adolescents need an average of 9 hours, and most adults require 7 to 8 hours of sleep. Many adults claim as few as 5 hours of sleep while others need 10 hours. During the first 3 months of pregnancy, women often sleep several more hours than usual.[34] With advancing age, adult sleep becomes less efficient. While total sleep requirement changes little, many older adults may nap during the usual waking period to compensate. Individuals who suffer from sleep disorders may also experience fatigue, irritability, lost work productivity, and inability to concentrate, creating a cycle that becomes difficult to break.

An estimated one third of adults in the United States have trouble sleeping, and about 10% may have sleep disorders more serious than simple loss of a night's usual amount of sleep. Americans are becoming a society in which sleep deprivation is the norm, with chronic "sleep debt." Chronic insomnia has been labeled a major public health problem because sleep deprivation is dangerous in many situations (e.g., driving). Indeed, the biologic drive to sleep may be so powerful that the brain may actually shut down or cause a "sleep attack" when experiencing sleep deprivation. The National Sleep Foundation has estimated that driver fatigue or drowsiness is responsible for an estimated 100,000 motor vehicle crashes each year.[36] Nearly 32 million drivers admit to falling asleep behind the wheel. Some states such as New Jersey have made fatigued driving a criminal offense with "Maggie's Law." The law was enacted following a crusade by parents whose daughter was killed by a man who fell asleep at the wheel.

Awareness that sleep deprivation in health care providers leads to medical errors and impaired judgment has changed the rules for medical residents' hospital rotations and shifts. Recognition that drowsiness is the brain's last step before falling asleep is an important step to ensuring safe work practice in any environment, particularly fields such as mass transit and commercial hauling by rail and truck.

In addition, research suggests that sleep deprivation can be a health hazard that can affect the immune system in detrimental ways.[25,26]

The first sleep laboratory was founded in 1970 by William C. Dement, MD, called the "father of sleep," and Christian Guilleminault, MD. Today, sleep medicine specialists use sophisticated laboratories to study sleep patterns and identify and treat sleep disorders that cause distress and discomfort. Many neuroscience clinicians, however, are not aware of the signs and symptoms of sleep disorders. It is important to develop the expertise to query patients about sleep patterns in order to identify individuals who may be experiencing impaired function or the serious complications of a sleep disorder. Getting less than the recommended 7 to 8 hours of sleep over a cumulative period of time may lead to an increased risk of hypertension, stroke, and other health problems. The International Classification of Sleep Disorders identifies over 80 sleep disorders.[14]

Neuroscience clinicians often care for patients who experience sleep disturbances resulting from primary neurologic diseases or injuries, such as sleep-related epilepsy, sleep-related headaches (migraines), and degenerative disorders such as Parkinson's disease and Alzheimer's dementia. Selection of the best treatment for a sleep disorder is based on age, presence of relevant concomitant diseases, evidence of drug abuse, whether the sleep disturbance is a primary disorder or merely a symptom, and severity. Transient and persistent sleep problems each require different treatment. The goal of therapy is to improve the quality of sleep to allow the patient to be alert and functioning at a high level during waking time.

This section provides an overview of sleep physiology and then outlines the most common sleep disorders, including disorders of excessive somnolence, disorders of initiating and maintaining sleep, and parasomnias.

NORMAL SLEEP PATTERNS

Normal sleep consists of a cycle that lasts about 90 minutes and is repeated four to six times during the night. The physiologic state of sleep is marked by the following:
- Reduced consciousness or relative unconsciousness
- Diminished activity of the skeletal or voluntary muscles
- Depressed metabolism

Humans have a need for sleep periodically, usually in a predictable circadian (Latin meaning "around a day") rhythm. **Circadian rhythms** are regular changes in mental and physical characteristics that occur in patterns during the course of a 24-hour cycle. Circadian rhythms are changes affecting the repetition of certain physiologic activities (e.g., sleeping, eating, breathing), which are controlled by a pinhead-sized area of the hypothalamus that contains about 20,000 neurons.[34] Sleep impairs breathing efforts and alters both the volume of ventilation and the stability of breathing patterns. The tone in the pharyngeal muscles that open the airway falls with sleep onset, causing the upper airway to become more collapsible.[34]

Sleep is divided into non–rapid eye movement (NREM) and rapid eye movement (REM) sleep. NREM sleep is further divided into four stages. The stages are defined by the brain's EEG or electrical activity, eye movements, and muscle tone (Fig. 6-4):
- Stage I (2% to 5% of sleep time): light sleep with low arousal threshold; **myoclonia,** or sudden muscle spasm or contraction, may occur similar to a "jump" felt when startled; eye movements change from rapid while awake to slow
- Stage II (45% to 55% of sleep time): still light sleep with a mix of **sleep spindles** and high-voltage slow waves called K-complexes; eye movements stop during stages II to IV
- Stage III (10% to 20% of sleep time): slow wave sleep (SWS) characterized by frequent high voltage
- Stage IV: extremely slow wave activity called **delta waves** with high arousal[20,34]

Sleep cycles progress from stage I to stage IV to REM sleep several times a night with a complete cycle lasting about 90 to 110 minutes. The first REM period generally occurs after an individual has been asleep for 80 to 100 minutes and may last for 5 to 30 minutes.[18] REM sleep begins with signals from the pons that are carried to the thalamus, which relays them to the cerebral cortex. REM sleep is characterized by low-voltage EEG, rapid eye movements, and further decrease in muscle tone. Because eye movements and EEG results resemble waking activity, REM sleep has been called "paradoxic sleep." Other characteristics of REM sleep are listed in Box 6-6. As adults age, the amount of SWS progressively declines; between ages 60 and 65, normal adults may experience little or no SWS while the amount of REM sleep decreases only slightly.

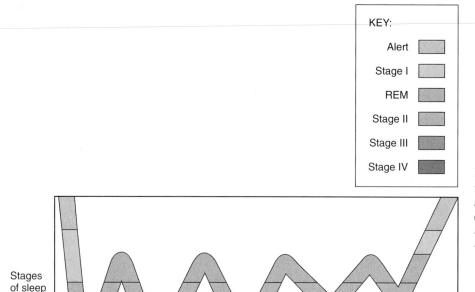

Figure 6-4 Stages of sleep: three to five 90-minute sleep cycles that include a sequence of five sleep stages. *(From Solomon EP, Schmidt RR, Adranga PJ: Human anatomy and physiology, ed 2, Philadelphia, 1990, Saunders College.)*

KEY:

Alert
Stage I
REM
Stage II
Stage III
Stage IV

Stages of sleep

Hours of sleep

BOX 6-6   Characteristics of REM Sleep

- Episodic bursts of rapid eye movement (REM); the cycle may last from a few minutes to half an hour and increases in length during sleep as deep sleep decreases
- Most dreaming occurs; adults spend more than 2 hours each night dreaming
- Loss of tone in antigravity muscles
- Loss of temperature regulation
- Heart rate and blood pressure are altered; respirations are irregular
- Loss of temperature regulation
- Loss of tone in the chest wall muscles causes lung volume to fall, making breathing more dependent on the diaphragm
- Obstructive sleep apnea is often more pronounced
- Regulation is primarily at the level of the brainstem*
- Penile erection in men; clitoral engorgement in women[†]
- Cerebral blood flow increases
- Intracranial pressure (ICP) may increase

*Commele CL, Walters AS, Heming WA: In Goetz CG, Pappert EJ, editors: *Textbook of clinical neurology,* Philadelphia, 1999, WB Saunders.
[†]Huether SE: Pain, temperature, sleep and sensory function. In McCance KL, Huether SE: *Pathophysiology: the biological basis for disease in adults and children,* ed 4, St Louis, 2002, Mosby.
REM, Rapid eye movement.

Physiologic changes that occur during NREM sleep include the following:

- Breathing pattern becomes very regular
- Breath volume and rate decrease slightly, which is associated with a mild increase in blood carbon dioxide (pCO_2) and a decrease in blood oxygen content (pO_2)
- Decreased muscle tone, which makes the upper airway more prone to collapse and increases resistance to breathing, thus causing snoring
- Decreased basal metabolic rate and corresponding decrease in body temperature by 0.5° to 1.0° C (0.9° to 1.8° F)
- Decreased heart rate and blood pressure
- Pupillary constriction and reduced deep tendon reflexes

NEUROCHEMICAL ANATOMY OF SLEEP

Sleep is influenced by various mechanisms, but the brain's electrical processes responsible for sleep are complex and incompletely understood. The primary physiologic structure that generates circadian rhythm is located in the hypothalamus. Hormones such as cortisol and thyroid-stimulating hormone are influenced by the circadian clock. In addition, the pineal gland is a neuroendocrine gland that secretes melatonin, which is released in response to decreased environmental light and promotes drowsiness, though there are no proven indications for melatonin. Important neurotransmitters involved in sleep include acetylcholine, gamma-aminobutyric acid, serotonin, glutamate, and norepinephrine.

Growth hormone is secreted during SWS. Thus disrupted sleep may inhibit growth in children. Therefore sleep deprivation is an important consideration for young adults who have not achieved their full growth potential.[12]

Reduced cognitive function has been correlated with sleep deprivation in normal adults. Some experts believe that sleep gives neurons used during waking hours a chance to repair themselves and exercise important neuronal connections that might deteriorate from lack of activity.[34] It is important that health care providers recognize that patients with impaired cognition from neurologic disorders need planned periods of restorative sleep to regain and maintain the critical balances of the nervous system.

COMMON SLEEP DISORDERS

Sleep disorders are commonly divided into **disorders of initiating and maintaining sleep (DIMS), disorders of excessive somnolence (DOES),** and parasomnias. Each is characterized by a specific set of criteria. DIMS includes insomnia and sleep-wake schedule disorders with the following patient symptoms:

- Difficulty falling asleep (more common in young adults)
- Early-morning awakenings
- Waking during the night (more common in older adults) or early in the morning
- A transient/situational or persistent pattern
- An association with mental illness; use of or withdrawal from certain drugs, including alcohol; sleep-related respiratory and nervous system changes; and medical illnesses

DOES includes narcolepsy with symptoms characterized by the following:

- A tendency toward sleep when the patient should be awake
- A major complaint that daytime sleepiness occurs at undesirable times
- Inappropriate episodes of sleep during the day
- Possible disturbance of nighttime sleep
- Poorly refreshing sleep

Insomnia and Other Sleep-Wake Disorders

Insomnia refers to the subjective complaint of difficulty falling asleep or staying awake and has been described as the most common sleep complaint, affecting from 6% to 12% of adults. It is included in the DIMS category. Individuals may complain of poor quality of sleep with a sense that sleep is inadequate, insufficient, or interrupted. It is subjective because sleep requirements vary and because the restorative aspect of sleep is difficult to measure. For some, insomnia may occur night after night for months or years and yet only a few will actually seek medical care. Yet, insomnia today is associated with impaired function and considered a disorder verus a symptom of other medical

disorders. Clinicians may find that in some individuals, insomnia does not disappear when medical disorders improve. Many people experience disrupted sleep with complaints of difficulty falling asleep, difficulty staying asleep, and poor quality sleep. Causes of insomnia include emotions and thoughts that interfere with sleep, medications, substance abuse, external stimuli, personality, age, stress, anxiety, poor sleep habits, and pain.

Chronic insomnia is the term used for individuals who have trouble falling asleep or staying asleep night after night. Treatment is based on identifying and treating the underlying cause of the symptoms. All patients will benefit by practicing good sleep habits and behavior, or "sleep hygiene." The clinician can educate individuals and family members using a take-home handout as illustrated in Box 6-7. Occasionally some individuals are prescribed hypnotic medications to help initiate and prolong sleep.

The National Center on Sleep Disorders Research has estimated that 70 million Americans suffer from a sleep problem and nearly 60 million have a chronic disorder.[32] The condition is underreported, with women and older adults more commonly affected. Psychiatric symptoms and medical symptoms are often risk factors. A survey by the National Sleep Foundation (NSF) suggests that sleep is sensitive to hormonal changes in women, which can inhibit them from getting enough quality sleep.[35] The menstrual cycle, pregnancy, and menopause—biologic events unique to women—cause sleep deprivation in 56% of women. Insomnia, or difficulty falling and staying asleep, is a significant problem during all three events.

Individuals with insomnia may suffer from depression and have other health problems that disrupt sleep; some are related to orthopedic problems, arthritis, fibromyalgia, irritable bowel problems, or gastroesophageal reflux. These individuals should be diagnosed and treated for insomnia but also referred to appropriate health care professionals for treatment of these conditions. Establishing regular patterns of waking up and light therapy are recommended. For example, morning light exposure is recommended for individuals with delayed sleep phase and evening light exposure is recommended for individuals with advanced sleep phase.

Sleep-wake schedule disorders (SWSDs) include cataplexy and sleep apnea. **Cataplexy** is a condition marked by sudden muscular weakness, which may be triggered by emotions, and hypotonia, in which a person falls into the deepest stage of REM sleep immediately and without warning. The usual duration is less than 2 minutes. The individual may experience knee or leg buckling, jaw sagging, and head drooping. The criteria for diagnosis are to identify appropriate triggering events and sites of muscle weakness with five or more episodes over the individual's lifetime.

Etiology

Insomnia is frequently associated with psychologic conditions such as anxiety and depression. More than one sleep disorder may contribute to the sleep problem, and without appropriate treatment of all of the disorders, sleep quality may not significantly improve.

BOX 6-7	Recommendations for Sleep Hygiene

Increase Natural Drive for Sleep
- Avoid naps; if you have to take a nap, take a brief 10–15 minute nap
- Restrict sleep period to an average number of hours you have actually slept per night in the past few days
- Quality of sleep is important—too much sleep in bed can decrease quality the next night
- Get regular exercise; when possible 40 minutes of activity is beneficial but avoid exercise activities at least 6 hours before bedtime
- Take a 30 minute warm shower or bath within 2 hours of bedtime
- A warm or hot drink may promote relaxation

Work With Your Own Internal Daily Cycles
- Get out of bed (OOB) at the same time each day; maintain regular and appropriate sleep-wake times
- Regulate the amount of time in bed
- Seek maximum light exposure during the day and minimize light exposure at night
- Do not expose yourself to bright light if you get OOB during the night

Drug Effects
- Do not smoke to get yourself back to sleep
- Minimize nicotine: do not smoke after 7:00 PM (heavy smokers sleep often sleep very lightly and have reduced amounts of REM sleep, also smokers may wake after 3–4 hours of sleep due to nicotine withdrawal)
- Stop smoking or arrange for a smoking cessation program
- Try to avoid caffeine entirely for a 4-week period; afterward limit yourself to a maximum of 3 cups per day and none after 10:00 AM because caffeine's half-life may be 10–12 hours for some individuals
- Alcohol may seem to help you fall into light sleep but disrupts sleep; it robs you of REM and deeper sleep; may result in sympathetic overdrive

Avoid Being Aroused in Your Sleep Setting
- Keep your clock face turned away, and do not find out what time it is when you wake up at night
- Avoid strenuous exercise after 6:00 PM
- Do not eat or drink heavily for 3 hours before bedtime; a light bedtime snack may help sleep
- If you suffer from heartburn, avoid heavy and spicy evening meals; elevate head of bed with 3–4 inch blocks under the legs
- Do not go to bed too full or too hungry
- Keep the room where you sleep dark, quiet, well ventilated, and at a comfortable temperature during the night
- Use ear plugs and eye shades if needed
- Light reading at bedtime may help; avoid work-related reading
- Set aside a "worry time" before bedtime; make a list of one-sentence problems and worries with a brief way you will deal with it tomorrow
- Forgive yourself and others
- Learn relaxation and deep breathing techniques (ask your clinician for instructions) to help you enjoy the pleasant sensation of relaxation
- Use "stress management" strategies during the day
- Avoid a mattress that is too firm or too soft and pillows that are not a comfortable height
- The need for prescription sleep aids should be discussed with your health care provider
- Use the bedroom area for sleep only; do not perform work activities in the bedroom that lead to prolonged arousal
- If possible, make arrangements for caregiving responsibilities for children, pets, or other family members with a responsible person

SWSDs may result from an irregular sleep-wake schedule, such as that caused by rapid time zone changes, shift or night work, and self-imposed sleep-wake schedule disruptions. During hospitalization, the need for monitoring and treatments, as well as the presence of lighting throughout the entire night, may induce an SWSD.

Delayed-phase and advanced-phase syndromes and non–24-hour sleep-wake syndromes arise from the following:
- An intrinsic abnormality in the **circadian pacemaker,** the biologic clock of wakefulness and sleep
- An abnormality in the pacemaker's capacity to respond to external synchronizing cues
- An impairment in the reception or transmission of synchronizing cues

Pathophysiology

Patients with insomnia suffer from poor sleep and disturbances in the wake or sleep system, which produces excessive wakefulness. Abnormalities are detectable in sleep duration, in the architecture of sleep (sleep stages and progression of sleep cycles through the night), and in the physiology of sleep.

Assessment

A detailed history of the sleep complaint and interview is the most important element in the evaluation of an individual with a sleep disorder. Some individuals may be asked to keep a "sleep diary." It is important to identify the triggering events and the duration. A sleep partner or roommate may be given the **Pittsburgh Sleep Quality Index** to complete (see Appendix C). Questions are structured to identify the areas in which patients may have difficulty:
- Falling asleep
- Staying asleep
- Waking up too early, feeling unrested
- Snoring, gasping, or choking; or periods when the person stops breathing during sleep
- Dreaming vivid dreams in which the person "acts out"
- Jerking of the legs or arms that interrupt sleep

In addition, the patient should fill out a detailed individual assessment as follows:[45]
- Height, weight, and vital signs
- Detailed sleep history, including hour in and out of bed

- Severity of the complaint
- Duration of the sleep problem
- Characteristics of the patient's lifestyle, work, home, school, and recreational activities
- Number of actual hours spent sleeping
- Symptoms that occur during sleep
- Symptoms that cause nocturnal awakenings
- Degree to which daytime functioning is impaired
- History from spouse, sleep partner, or significant other of events that are observed during sleep
- Detailed description of abnormal events
- General health history, including a medication/drug history
- Results of a thorough physical and neurologic examination
- Pulmonary studies results
- Blood work results
- Psychologic test: may include the Minnesota Multiphasic Personality Inventory (MMPI), the Beck Depression Inventory, the State-Trait Anxiety Inventory
- Caffeine intake (e.g., coffee, tea, cocoa, cola drinks)
- Alcohol consumption
- Tobacco use
- Nighttime habits, such as performing anxiety-provoking activities before bed
- Nighttime rituals, including bathing versus showering, having a snack, watching television, reading, lowering the room temperature, using air-conditioning, and using a certain type of heat (dry versus moisture added)
- Living conditions, such as living in one room, activity level of household
- Ability to stay awake when relaxed, stressed, anxious, ill, or upset
- Patient's perception of the cause(s) of sleep problems
- Measures patient has used to relieve sleep disorders (and effectiveness)
- Abnormalities of the upper airway, enlarged tonsils, oral cavity abnormalities (e.g., enlarged tongue, low palate, throat infection)

A sleep specialist may also complete the **Epworth Sleeping Scale (ESS)** for individuals with a sleep disorder. The scale measures the chance of dosing using a scale of 0 to 3. Total score ranges from 0 to 24. A score of 10 or greater usually indicates a sleep problem, and a score of 13 or greater indicates a serious sleep problem.

ALERT: A seizure disorder must be ruled out if unusual events occur during the night and especially if they occur at random times throughout the night. Even if a waking EEG is normal, a nocturnal seizure disorder should be suspected when there is an extreme disturbance of bedclothes, bedwetting, and blood on the pillow and bedclothes.

Neurodiagnostic and Laboratory Studies
Neurodiagnostic and laboratory tests include the following:
- **Nocturnal polysomnogram (NPSG):** criteria for ordering such a typical sleep study include a

---

BOX 6-8	Sleep Study

In preparation for an overnight **sleep study** in the sleep clinic, the participant is asked to do the following:
- Avoid napping and drinking any caffeinated or alcoholic beverages
- Take a shower, avoid using any body lotions, shampoo hair without applying hair conditioner or hairspray
- Eat dinner before arriving at the sleep clinic
- Bring a snack to the clinic if that is the usual nightly routine
- Bring usual nightclothes to wear and own pillow

Once at the clinic:
- A technician will apply scalp sensors that are attached to monitoring equipment
- Participants will be advised of the camera and other equipment in the room that will continuously record their sleep and body movements throughout the study
- Monitors will record brain waves, eye movements, heart rate, muscle activity and body motion, respirations, and snoring
- Continuous positive airway pressure (CPAP) is usually available for those who require it
- Technicians are available by intercom and will inform the participant when the study is completed and he or she is free to leave the clinic
- After analyzing the study results, the physician will meet with the participant to review the findings and offer the appropriate interventions

---

significant sleep problem that has persisted for 6 months to 1 year (Box 6-8 and Fig. 6-5)
- EEG
- Electrooculogram (EOG): for eye movements
- Electromyogram (EMG): using the chin muscle
- Thoracic and abdominal respiratory effort
- Nasal and oral airflow
- Blood oxygen saturation
- ECG
- Unobtrusive videotaping: may be used to capture abnormal behavior

Treatment
Pharmacologic interventions include sleep-promoting medications such as hypnotics, antidepressants (trazodone), and antipsychotics. Hypnotics may include Lunesta, zolpidem (Ambien), and the benzodiazepines (e.g., triazolam [Halcion] or clonazepam [Klonopin]). Zolpidem is also a popular drug for insomnia. Triazolam at excessive doses has been found to cause memory deficits and hallucinations.

In general, not all of the benzodiazepines are useful as hypnotic agents for sleep disorders and their popularity has waned as new drugs have become available.[29] Three commonly prescribed benzodiazepines for sleep disorders may include long-acting flurazepam (Dalmane), intermediate-acting temazepam (Restoril), and short-acting triazolam (Halcion).[31] Benzodiazepines tend to alter the gamma-aminobutyric acid (GABA) neurotransmitter to inhibit brain cells from firing and counter a state of hyperarousal that

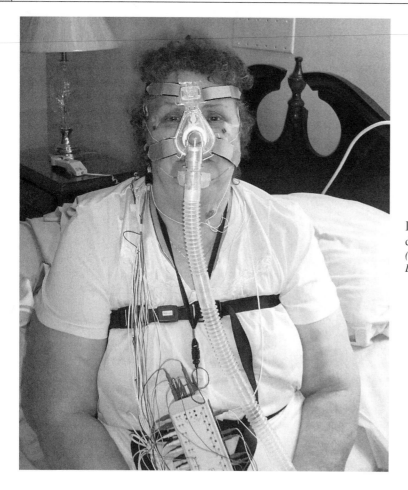

Figure 6-5 Patient with positive airway pressure device.
(Courtesy of Lee Dresser, MD, St. Francis Hospital Sleep Lab, Wilmington, DE.)

interrupts sleep. An antipsychotic such as quetiapine (Sero-quel) may be effective in promoting sleep onset.[31]

The treatment program for DIMS combines several behavioral elements that include the following:

- Improve general sleep hygiene and modification of lifestyle patterns
- Treat underlying sleep disorder
- Support insight-oriented and behavioral psychotherapeutic techniques, adjunctive use of hypnotic medications, use of antidepressant medications, and treatment of other conditions that interrupt sleep (e.g., nocturia)
- Treat associated medical problems as appropriate

Transient insomnia caused by stress, anxiety, and tension may respond to deep breathing exercises and progressive muscle relaxation training. Medical problems interfering with sleep, such as painful arthritis or gastroesophageal reflux, should be treated appropriately. Selected individuals will benefit from hypnotic medications, including zolpidem tartrate (Ambien) and temazepam (Restoril). Temazepam is a benzodiazepine that produces a hypnotic effect and is one of the older, sedating therapies that may offer benefits for about 2 weeks and has side effect of daytime drowsiness and rebound insomnia.[29]

Irregular sleep-wake patterns are generally treated with behavioral therapy. A regular sleep-wake cycle is reestablished by limiting the number and duration of daytime naps and by restricting sleep to conventional sleep periods. Physical activity and exercise during the daytime are encouraged but should be avoided for several hours before bedtime.

Chronotherapy and phototherapy have emerged as treatments for sleep-wake schedule disorders. **Chronotherapy,** a behavioral technique in which bedtime is systematically delayed by 3-hour increments each day until the desired bedtime is reached, is used to treat a delayed sleep phase syndrome. The conventional 24-hour day is then maintained by a rigid bedtime and morning rising schedule. In contrast, an advanced sleep phase syndrome is treated with a systematic delay of bedtime until the desired bedtime is achieved.

In **phototherapy,** or bright light therapy, a patient with a delayed sleep phase sits in front of bright lights after awakening. Phototherapy has been found to stabilize the sleep pattern and increase afternoon alertness. In patients with advanced phase or dampened circadian rhythms, evening light therapy may prove useful in delaying sleep onset. This approach may prove helpful to shift workers and to patients suffering from jet lag. The optimal duration of exposure and time of day for phototherapy are individually determined. Investigators concluded that 2 days of bright light therapy over 4 hours while the subjects watched television experienced fewer days of feeling depressed and longer total sleep time. The bright light therapy was effective in insomniacs who primarily had difficulty with early-morning awakenings.[22]

Acute Care. Sleep disturbance is a significant stressor in the ICU as a result of frequent monitoring and treatment. It contributes to impaired cognition and possibly affects recovery.[3] The primary goals are to minimize sleep loss, produce only a transient and easily reversible sleep disturbance, and prevent the development of a persistent sleep disorder. Interventions vary based on diagnosis, age, symptom severity, and patient response.

When possible, prepare a schedule that balances nursing care, medical rounds, therapies, visitation, and bedside interventions with blocks of uninterrupted bulk periods for sleep to prevent sleep deprivation. Assess for pain and provide adequate pain management. Establish cycles of darkness and sleep-wake cycles with a "Do Not Disturb" sign on the patient's door. Avoid waking a patient during the night for nursing procedures such as a bed bath, daily weights, or routine diagnostic studies. Use central monitoring versus entering a patient's room for vital signs and hemodynamic monitoring. Review all medications for side effects affecting sleep.

Nonacute Care. During nonacute care the identity of the sleep problems often has been established. Assessment parameters include the following:

- Ask the patient relevant information about sleep, sleep deprivation, and activities affecting sleep since his or her hospital admission
- Identify current medications and the potential adverse side effects affecting sleep
- Record information related to pain, respiratory status, cardiovascular status, weight, neck appearance, the presence of abnormal motor movements, and cognitive status
- Review the patient's history of chronic illness and physical conditions that disrupt sleep, such as chronic obstructive pulmonary disease (COPD), asthma, bronchitis, arthritis, nocturnal angina, hyperthyroidism, hypertension, duodenal ulcer, reflux esophagitis, nocturia, and seizure disorders
- Inquire about the presence of preexisting sleep problems

The goal in the nonacute care setting is to prevent the development of a persistent sleep disorder and reverse any transient sleep disorder. Poor sleep hygiene practices may need to be eliminated. Careful assessment and monitoring are continued with vigilance to prevent sleep-related complications. To treat transient psychophysiologic DIMS, the clinician promotes sleep in a nonacute setting based on the individual's needs.

Sleep Apnea

Sleep apnea (SA) is a common sleep disorder characterized by periods in which respiration is absent and can be dangerous. Because the individual with sleep apnea is momentarily unable to contract respiratory muscles or to maintain airflow through the nose and mouth, it is easily recognized.

Apnea is derived from the Greek word "without breath." It is defined as the absence of spontaneous respiration.[30] It can also be described as cessation of airflow that lasts for ≥ 10 seconds during sleep. It is a common yet dangerous condition that clinicians should easily recognize and treat. The patient is momentarily unable to contract respiratory muscles or to maintain airflow through the nose and mouth. It is characterized by recurrent apneic and hypopneic episodes. SA produces a drop in oxygen that can occur every night and can cause polycythemia, pulmonary hypertension, right-sided heart failure, and systemic hypertension. It is associated with increased risk of stroke, motor vehicle crashes, depression, and workplace accidents.

This serious, potentially life-threatening condition affects approximately 18 million Americans and is more common among males and individuals who are overweight. Approximately 4% of women and 9% of men have sleep apnea in their working years.[4] The use of alcohol or sleeping aids can make sleep apnea worse.

There are several types of sleep apnea, and its high prevalence and serious associated morbidity is a major medical problem. It has been shown to precipitate high blood pressure, heart problems, and brain attacks/strokes. Any neurologic condition that affects the brainstem has the potential to affect ventilation during sleep.

Pickwickian syndrome, also known as **obesity-hypoventilation syndrome,** is an abnormal condition characterized by obesity, decreased pulmonary function during sleep, CO_2 retention, hypoxia, somnolence, and polycythemia.[30]

Hypopnea is described as decreased airflow ≥ 10 seconds associated with arousal and oxyhemoglobin and characterized by an abnormally shallow and slow respiration. Obstructive hypopneas can result in a 30% reduction in airflow and can last up to 10 seconds. This can trigger a reduction in oxygen saturation. It is associated with a reduction in airflow and a decrease in oxygen saturation described as oxyhemoglobin desaturation.

Obstructive apneas and hypopneas during sleep are usually tallied together to yield the Apnea-Hypopnea Index (AHI).[30] This index is used to determine the severity of SA by measuring the average number of apnea events per hour of sleep. As the AHI increases, so does the severity of the symptoms. An AHI of less than 5 is normal. An AHI of 5 to 30 events per hour is considered mild SA, 15 to 30 events is moderate SA, and greater than 30 events is commonly regarded as severe SA.[30] The consequences of sleep apnea can result in fragmented sleep patterns with hypoxia and hypercapnia that can lead to cardiovascular complications and the individual experiencing excessive daytime sleepiness. Daytime sleepiness often leads to increased motor vehicle crashes and work-related injuries with poor performance on the job. The individual may complain of depression and a decreased quality of life.

Obstructive sleep apnea (OSA) is the most common form of apnea and is one of the most common sleep disorders seen in sleep disorder clinics. During normal sleep, the muscles of the throat relax, which can narrow the airway. In OSA the airway narrows and closes. The negative pressure created by expansion of the chest with inspirations cause collapse of soft tissue in the upper airway. Apnea occurs when airflow is absent in spite of continued thoracic breathing movement and exaggerated inspiratory efforts. An elongated soft palate, large tongue, obese neck, large tonsils, and abdominal obesity predict the potential for OSA. Apnea typically lasts 10 to 90 seconds; the sleeper snorts, gasps, takes a few breaths, and awakens momentarily. Symptoms of OSA include CO_2 retention, hypoxia, loud snoring, poorly refreshing sleep, excessive daytime sleepiness, and morning headaches. Individuals with OSA may wake hundreds of times during the night without remembering it. There is clear evidence that OSA has adverse effects on blood pressure, cardiovascular status, and probably cardiovascular mortality risk. Effective therapy with continuous positive airway pressure (CPAP) can improve blood pressure and cardiac function in adults with OSA. CPAP has been shown to improve cardiac function and quality of life.[5]

Mixed apnea is a combination of central sleep apnea (CSA) and OSA. It starts as brief periods of CSA and becomes an OSA with both obstructive and central apneic events. A mixed apnea begins with an absence of respiratory effort and airflow and then develops into an obstructive sleep apnea. It is a form of OSA.

Central sleep apnea (CSA) is a form of SA resulting from decreased respiratory output. It is fairly rare and may, for example, involve primary brainstem medullary depression resulting from a tumor of the posterior fossa. CSA occurs when the airways stay open and the diaphragm and chest muscles stop working. The cause of CSA is not understood but is thought to arise from alterations in the functioning of chemoreceptors that monitor the hypoxic and hypercapnic influences on respiration. In some individuals, CSA may follow a period of chronic hyperventilation.

Etiology and Pathophysiology

Increased age, male gender, obesity, family history, the use of alcohol or sedatives, smoking, and a short upper airway cause individuals to be at increased risk for developing SA. Patients with underdeveloped muscles, neuromuscular disease causing weakness of respiratory muscles, and anatomic narrowing of the upper airway are also at increased risk for OSA. CSA is associated with heart failure and various CNS diseases (e.g., stroke and multiple-system atrophy).

Assessment

SA is more common in males and in overweight, middle-aged, or older individuals. Obese males may have increased neck thickness. A sleep and health history is obtained from the individual, family, or sleep partner regarding alcohol intake, obesity, nocturnal gasping and choking, snoring that is loud and chronic, witnessed apnea, excessive daytime sleepiness, sleeping at inappropriate times (e.g., work), morning headache, and the use of any medications, sleeping pills, and stimulants. Significant others may report personality or cognitive changes, sleeping in inappropriate settings, and automobile and other injuries. The following characteristics are also assessed:

- Presence of tonsillar hypertrophy or enlarged neck (≥17 inches in males, ≥16 inches in females) or airway abnormality

- Blood pressure (hypertension) and respiratory status: breath sounds, chest movement, thoracic deformities
- Episodes of falling asleep during the day or while working or driving
- Behavioral changes: fatigue, irritability, difficulty concentrating, and personality changes
- Decreased libido and declining interest in sexual activity
- Oropharyngeal assessment: nasopharyngeal narrowing
- Level of alertness and awareness
- Skin color changes related to low oxygen saturation

Neurodiagnostic and Laboratory Studies

After a thorough history and physical, the following studies may be required:[38]

- Blood: routine
- Pulmonary function tests (PFTs)
- **Multiple Sleep Latency Test (MSLT):** a measure of the individual's ability to sleep during a series of structured naps; this test is typically done in the morning
- NPSG: The gold standard diagnostic study; conducted in a specially constructed overnight sleep laboratory (see Fig. 6-5 and Box 6-8)

The NPSG is explained to the patient in detail. The individual is asked to avoid caffeine for several days before testing. The study is usually completed in one night and performed by a certified sleep technologist. The signs and symptoms may not be good predictors of the disease severity. Electrodes are applied, monitors are connected, and the lights are turned off. The individual is allowed to sleep per normal routine. This study may include chin and leg muscle movement (electromyography), eye movements (electro-oculography), nasal and oral airflow (airflow monitors), EEG, chest wall movement and respirations (chest impedance), abdominal movements, and oxygen saturation (pulse oximetry). Sound sensors may be used to document snoring, and audiovisual recordings may be performed to document restless motion and fitfulness. A physician trained in sleep disorders interprets the data. In certain situations, sleep studies can be performed at home with portable equipment.

Treatment

Medical Management. Once an accurate diagnosis has been determined, treatment goals are to reduce the morbidity and mortality risks and reduce the excessive sleepiness in order to give the individual a better quality of life. For OSA, overweight patients or those with morbid obesity are encouraged to lose weight. Others are encouraged to avoid alcohol and sedatives, and avoid sleep deprivation. Some patients are helped by avoiding the supine position during sleep, smoking cessation, and using oral or dental appliances that help ensure airway patency. The mouth guard helps to lift up the soft palate and hold the tongue forward.

Treatment of OSA depends on the severity. In moderate to severe cases, CPAP with a nasal mask is used to keep the airway open and maintain positive intraluminal pressure in the upper airway. CPAP is quite successful at relieving the snoring and apnea, and it also helps normalize blood pressure. CPAP prevents sleep disruption and hypoxemia associated with sleep apnea and restores the normal sleep architecture. Many patients find it difficult to comply with CPAP therapy because they must wear a small mask on the nose and mouth during sleep. Reassurance is needed to emphasize the positive benefits compared to the minor discomfort. Bilevel positive airway pressure (BiPAP) provides different pressures during inspiration and expiration and may be better tolerated for individuals with OSA.[2] An example of a BiPAP protocol is listed in Box 6-9.

Medications that may aid in the treatment of ISA include decongestants and nasal sprays to ensure patency of the airways. Some individuals may need oxygen therapy in conjunction with CPAP and BiPAP. Occasionally respiratory stimulants such as acetazolamide (Diamox) or theophylline (Theo-Dur) are prescribed.[29]

| **BOX 6-9** | **Bilevel Airway Pressure Protocol** |

- Consider when patient does not tolerate continuous positive airway pressure (CPAP) or when apneas or hypopneas or snoring persist despite CPAP pressure of 16 cm H_2O
- Start with an inspiratory positive airway pressure (IPAP) of 8 cm and an expiratory positive airway pressure (EPAP) of 4 cm
- If snoring or apneas/hypopneas persist after 5 minutes, increase IPAP and EPAP by 2 cm each and continue until snoring, apnea, and hypopneas are eliminated
- If pressure reaches an IPAP of 16 cm and an EPAP of 12 cm without elimination of any respiratory events, lower the IPAP to 10 cm and the EPAP to 4 cm; continue the upward titration of pressure as needed in increments of 2 cm every 5 minutes
- If pressure reaches an IPAP of 16 cm and an EPAP of 10 cm without control of events, decrease the IPAP to 12 cm and the EPAP to 4 cm and continue upward titration
- If events are not controlled at an IPAP of 16 cm and an EPAP of 8 cm, increase the pressure no further and notify the physician
- Further upward titration of pressure may be necessary during REM sleep
- If central apnea or oxygen desaturations of 5% or greater persist after elimination of snoring and obstructive events, raise the IPAP pressure by 1 cm every 5 minutes until these events are eliminated
- If central events or desaturation persist despite an IPAP of 16 cm, begin lowering the EPAP by 1 cm every 5 cm until these events are eliminated
- If snoring or obstructive events reappear at any time, raise the EPAP by 1 cm every 3 minutes until these events are eliminated; if persistent desaturations continue to less than 89%, notify the physician

---

Surgical Management. Several surgical procedures, including septoplasty and removal of the tonsils and adenoids, have been helpful in treating sleep apnea. A uvulopalatopharyngoplasty (UPP) to remove the uvula, portions of the soft palate, and pharyngeal tissue can significantly improve OSA and reduce snoring. Laser-assisted uvulopalatoplasty (LAUP) can be performed as an office procedure and excises only part of the uvula and part of the soft palate. Maxillofacial surgery that enlarges the airway at the base of the tongue is called **genioglossal advancement.** A tracheostomy is an invasive procedure and is reserved for extreme cases but will eliminate OSA. Gastric bypass may be considered in extreme cases for the ultimate treatment of OSA.

ALERT: According to the American Sleep Apnea Association (ASAA), the risk of administering a general anesthetic to patients with sleep apnea is increased. When a general anesthetic suppresses upper airway muscle activity, it may impair breathing by allowing the airway to close. The ASAA advises that attention to sleep apnea continue into the postanesthesia period because the lingering sedative and respiratory depressant effects of anesthesia can pose difficulty, as can some analgesics. After the last dose of anesthetic and opioids or sedative has been administered, the ASAA recommends monitoring for several hours and possibly through one full natural sleep period. Because of these concerns, same-day surgery may not be appropriate for individuals with OSA.

Sleep apnea has been recognized for its impact on cardiovascular health. Selected cardiac patients, or older adults with coexisting cardiac problems in association with SA, may have an implantable pacing device. Individuals with an implanted cardiac device should provide full disclosure concerning their history of cardiac disease, sleep disorder, and contact information of treating providers for consultation. A higher vigilance of observation and monitoring may be required.

Potential Complications. Complications associated with SA include right-sided heart failure, peripheral edema, hypertension, cardiac dysrhythmias, memory loss, emotional disturbances, and strokes. These complications are progressive if the SA is left untreated. Individuals with a history of myocardial infarction (MI), hypertension, heart failure, stroke, COPD, smoking, diabetes, alcoholism, obesity, daytime sleepiness, snoring, and observed apneas should be assessed for SA.

Narcolepsy

Narcolepsy is a disorder of excessive somnolence (DOES). It is a disabling syndrome of unknown etiology characterized by sudden sleep attacks, sleep paralysis, and visual and auditory hallucinations at the onset of sleep. Excessive daytime sleepiness (EDS) creates numerous problems for an individual. Narcolepsy is typically associated with cataplexy and other REM sleep disorders and is treatable. The affected individual may complain of frequent napping, memory lapses, visual disturbances, and other conditions. An estimated 135,000 Americans have narcolepsy.

Etiology

Disease states produce many common sleep disorders. The most common causes of sleep disorders are circadian rhythm disorders. Long thought to have genetic or familial influences, narcolepsy has recently been tied to the loss of a few neurons that produce the neuropeptide hypocretin in the hypothalamus of the CNS.

Pathophysiology

The onset of narcolepsy typically occurs in early adulthood and may consist of a variety of symptoms; however, cataplexy (an abrupt, bilateral loss of skeletal muscle tone) is most specific to narcolepsy. Narcolepsy is characterized by a dysfunction in the ascending reticular activating system (RAS) resulting in insufficient activation of higher brain centers. Work related to the pathophysiology of narcolepsy with animal models and with neurotransmission and neurotransmitters has shown that a chemical in the brainstem, known as hypocretin or orexin, is responsible for maintaining wakefulness. In narcoleptics, this chemical is present in only minute amounts or is missing entirely.[6,9,42]

Assessment

Specific questions on the Pittsburgh Sleep Quality Index that apply to individuals with narcolepsy include the following topics:

- Falling asleep at inappropriate times, driving, and traveling in a car, plane, bus/train
- Falling asleep suddenly without warning
- Napping during awake hours

Neurodiagnostic and Laboratory Studies

Diagnostic tests specific to narcolepsy include the following:

- MSLT: a measure of the tendency to fall asleep
- **Maintenance of Wakefulness Test (MWT):** measures ability to remain awake
- Fatigue Severity Scale (FSS): self-report
- Fatigue Impact Scale (FIS): self-report
- Drug screens: detect substance abuse
- Genetic tests: help confirm diagnosis of narcolepsy

Treatment

Although there is no known cure for narcolepsy, it can be treated symptomatically. CNS stimulants such as methylphenidate (Ritalin) 5 to 100 mg per day, dextroamphetamine (Dexedrine), and modafinil (Provigil) 200 to 800 mg per day can be effective in compensating the excessive somnolence, as well as pemoline (Cylert) 37.5 to 300 mg per day. Modafinil (Provigil) is indicated for excessive sleepiness and sleep disorders associated with narcolepsy, obstructive sleep apnea/hypopnea syndrome (OSAHS), and shift work sleep disorder.[29]

Tricyclic antidepressants and, more recently, selective serotonin reuptake inhibitors (SSRIs) such as fluoxetine hydrochloride (Prozac)[29] have been used to treat the cataplexy and narcolepsy successfully. A significant recent advance came when sodium oxybate received regulatory approval as a treatment for cataplexy and narcolepsy because it effectively treats cataplexy and shows promise for the treatment of excessive sleepiness and for improving sleep quality in patients with narcolepsy.[44]

Education about narcolepsy is paramount for the patient, family, and significant others. Because short naps provide many patients with considerable relief from sleepiness, individuals may benefit from scheduled naps coinciding with times when they are most sleepy.

OTHER SLEEP DISORDERS

Restless Leg Syndrome

Restless leg syndrome (RLS) is a common benign condition first described in the 1940s that is underdiagnosed and treatable. RLS is characterized by an irritating sensation of uneasiness, tiredness, and itching deep within the muscles of the leg, especially the lower part of the limb. It is sometimes accompanied by twitching and sometimes by pain. There is an irresistible urge to move the legs due to disagreeable leg sensations.[33] Symptoms worsen later in the day. There seems to be a strong genetic component, and about half of the individuals with RLS have a family history or consider it an inherited disorder. RLS is a common cause of insomnia. Symptoms are made worse by holding still and better by movement. This condition is more common in patients with a history of disease or iron deficiency and during pregnancy. In an older adult hospitalized patient, it may cause agitation. It is important to recognize this since tranquilizing agents used to treat agitation, such as haloperidol (Haldol), make RLS worse.

The condition is identified through the individual's account of symptoms and ruling out other disorders with similar symptoms. Diagnostic studies are recommended to rule out conditions such as iron deficiency and peripheral neuropathy. Kidney function tests and ferritin levels are ordered to rule out kidney disease. Individuals with mild RLS may not require medication. Therapy for RLS is individualized according to age, severity, symptom frequency, existing medical conditions, and medications the patient may be using (see Chapter 19 for detailed discussion of RLS). The exact cause is unknown, but RLS may be associated with dopamine function. There is no cure and the condition may be ongoing. Physical activity can relieve symptoms, and individuals are encouraged to have a routine exercise regimen. Individuals with RLS should be instructed on the benefits and side effects given the following options that may be prescribed for the pharmacologic treatment of RLS:[33]

- Dopaminergic agents (e.g., carbidopa/levodopa, ropinirole) are the first-line drugs for RLS. However, carbidopa/levodopa should not be used daily for RLS because it can lead to eventual worsening of symptoms.
- Opioids (e.g., codeine) or methadone hydrochloride can be used for RLS, especially when there is associated pain.
- Benzodiazepine (e.g., clonazepam); tolerance is a problem.

- Anticonvulsants (e.g., gabapentin) can be considered, especially when there is associated pain with RLS symptoms.
- Iron or ferrous sulfate is used for patients with serum ferritin levels less than 50 μg.[21]

Periodic Limb Movement Disorder

Individuals with RLS may also have **periodic limb movement disorder (PLMD),** or repetitive movements that usually occur in the lower limbs approximately every 20 to 40 seconds. This idiopathic disorder is generally considered benign other than for its potential to disrupt sleep and cause excessive daytime sleepiness. An abnormality of the mu opiate receptor has been postulated in this condition. The exact pathophysiologic basis for both RLS and PLMD is not known. There is evidence of reduced dopaminergic activity, and there is a high incidence in patients with degenerative disorders (e.g., Parkinson's disease).[29] It is important to recognize PLMD and not attribute it to the Parkinson's disease process. RLS and PLMD are evaluated and managed in similar ways according to their severity and associated sleep disruptions.

Parasomnias

Parasomnia is a category of sleep disorders in which abnormal physiologic behavioral events occur during sleep. Examples of parasomnias are nightmare disorders, sleep terror disorder, sleepwalking disorder, and REM behavioral disorders. Some parasomnias appear in certain sleep stages (e.g., cluster headaches that occur during REM sleep). The patient may be difficult to arouse during a parasomnia and have poor recall of the parasomnia events in the morning when fully awake. Over 23 different forms of parasomnias are recognized, and more than one form may occur in the same patient.

Sleep-Provoked Disorders or Conditions

Sleep disorders can cause significant problems because of the importance of sleep for restorative and integrative purposes. Sleep deprivation for even short periods can produce decreased physical and cognitive functioning and can compromise recovery from illness. Clinicians need to be aware that some conditions or diseases are aggravated by sleep. Such problems may develop or become exacerbated during sleep. Medical conditions that may be aggravated during sleep are listed in Box 6-10.

COMPREHENSIVE PATIENT MANAGEMENT: SLEEP DISORDERS

Health Teaching Considerations

Patients with sleep disorders and their family or significant others, or those at high risk for developing sleep disorders, benefit from education about the problems associated with

---

| BOX 6-10 | **Medical Conditions Affected by Sleep** |

- **Intracranial pressure** may elevate during periods of REM sleep
- Patients with degenerative diseases such as **parkinsonism** may experience restless leg syndrome (RLS), periodic leg movement disorder (PLMD), or REM behavior
- Review the patient's history for **nocturnal seizure activity,** and check the anticonvulsant medications
- Monitor for symptoms of **coronary artery disease (CAD),** which is most often affected during REM sleep
- Observe for **asthmatic attacks** that may occur during REM sleep at night, which may cause the patient to lose stage IV sleep
- In patients with **chronic obstructive pulmonary disease (COPD),** lowered PO_2 occurs most dramatically during REM sleep (when voluntary neuromuscular control is reduced); this can result in pulmonary hypertension
- Assess patients with diabetes for hypoglycemia; patients with **uncontrolled diabetes** may need their glucose levels monitored during the night, because glucose levels vary considerably at night

REM, Rapid eye movement.

| BOX 6-11 | **Teaching Tips for Sleep Problems** |

- Review of all equipment, purpose, application: apnea monitor or CPAP
- Medications: drug-drug interactions, side effects and importance of compliance
- If surgical intervention is prescribed, preoperative and postoperative teaching and preparation
- Patient, family, and caregiver written and verbal information concerning dual diagnoses of the underlying neurologic disorder and the diagnosed sleep disorder that could create increased disease burden for the patient and caregivers
- Pain management to prevent pain from disrupting sleep
- Educate about the importance of good sleep hygiene (see Box 6-7)
- Weight reduction strategies, if needed that can improve obstructive sleep apnea

CPAP, Continuous positive airway pressure.

---

sleep deprivation. Appropriate items for teaching include those listed in Box 6-11.

Nutritional Considerations

Patients with a sleep disorder who are affected by particular foods and beverages will benefit from a dietary consultation. In general, foods and beverages that contain caffeine or other stimulants should be eliminated from the diet; hot and spicy foods that may irritate the GI system should also be eliminated. Overeating and drinking before retiring also interferes with sleep. Obese patients with obstructive apnea benefit from enrolling in a weight reduction program and being supported to set realistic goals, such as losing approximately 2 pounds per week.

Psychosocial Considerations

Sleep disorders may cause an individual to experience irritability, fatigue, concentration difficulty, disorientation, and negative moods. Interpersonal relations with family, friends, and others may be adversely affected, and poor job performance, marital discord, and low self-esteem may be seen. Injuries may occur related to sleep problems. Severe sleep disorders coupled with mental health problems may lead to suicide attempts in stressed and anxious patients. Appropriately recognizing and diagnosing sleep disorders and providing medical, psychologic, and supportive treatment will allow individuals to live more productive and enjoyable lives.

Older Adult Considerations

The quality of sleep deteriorates in older adults. As sleep cycles become less efficient, older adults may experience some of the changes listed in Box 6-12.

Older adults are particularly vulnerable to transient sleep disorders that, if not therapeutically managed, develop into a persistent DIMS, or sleep cycle phase shift. This in turn can impair individuals' cognitive function and overall health

BOX 6-12	Sleep Changes in Older Adults

Marked decreases in slow wave sleep
Frequent awakenings during the night and early awakening in the morning
Reduced REM time and markedly decreased or absent stage 4 NREM sleep
More time in stage 1
  • Total sleep time is decreased and older adults take longer to fall asleep, awaken earlier in the morning and more frequently during the night
  • Older adults are less able than younger individuals to tolerate sleep deprivation
Reaction to noise and activity in the acute care settings; high risk for developing an ICU psychosis and phase shifts while hospitalized
Higher incidence of restless leg syndrome (RLS), sleep apneas, and psychophysiologic insomnias
Chronic illnesses that impair sleep, such as arthritis, chronic obstructive pulmonary disease, congestive heart failure (CHF), diabetes mellitus, and depression
Overuse of sleep medication with the potential for undesirable side effects
A need to nap during the day
Sleep problems of the spouse, which affect patient's sleep

From Huether SE: Pain, temperature, sleep and sensory function. In McCance KL, Huether SE: *Pathophysiology: the biological basis for disease in adults and children*, ed 4, St Louis, 2002, Mosby.
ICU, Intensive care unit; *NREM,* non–rapid eye movement; *REM,* rapid eye movement.

status. Therefore the initial problems of a sleep disorder must be aggressively managed.

Persons with dementia often experience a phase shift because the external cues that maintain the 24-hour sleep-wake cycle have become meaningless to them. Such patients need a strong sleep hygiene program and may need a resynchronizing program if they experience a phase shift.

Rehabilitation and Home Care Considerations

Rehabilitation focuses on the medical or mental health therapies appropriate for the etiology of the sleep disorder. The interventions and patient and family teaching previously discussed are used in the rehabilitative stage of care (see Chapter 13).

Assessment of Home Environment

In addition to the assessment features already discussed, the home environment and especially the sleep environment should be assessed. Family situations that increase stress, tension, or family dysfunction and could contribute to sleep disturbances are evaluated. After completing a thorough assessment, the clinician can teach the patient and family to perform the following interventions.

Interventions After Discharge

  • Identify and maintain habits and lifestyle patterns that minimize sleep cycle disruptions, including structuring and reinforcing the efforts to modify behavior
  • Develop positive attitudes, make changes in the home sleep environment, and develop desirable health habits
  • Establish bedtime habits that allow a sleep period of 7 to 8 hours (unless the patient knows from experience that his or her sleep needs are greater or less than this)
  • Establish regular schedules by developing a routine of going to bed and arising at regular times every day
  • Learn to avoid sleeping excessively and "resting" in bed on weekends and holidays while maintaining some flexibility in the bedtime schedule
  • Learn techniques to wind down from the day's activities before going to bed, and avoid stress and mental stimulation just before bedtime
  • Maintain an environment conducive to sleep, which may include a specific type of bed, mattress, and pillow; sleeping alone or with a partner; and controlling the room temperature and monitoring the amount of light and noise in the room
  • Avoid caffeine and alcohol
  • Evaluate with the treating health care team if alternative therapies with herbs and acupuncture should be used; report outcome and any side effects

Case Management Considerations

A case manager may be assigned to an individual with complex and serious sleep problems that cause disability and affect breathing, overall general health, safety, and quality

BOX 6-13 Case Management Guidelines: Sleep Disorders

- Complete patient assessment; review diagnosis, cause, treatment, medications, evidence of depression and potential serious social and economic difficulties that interfere with physical activities and cause social withdrawal
- Identify barriers to periods of restful and restorative sleep; never blame patient for snoring
- Develop a treatment plan after consultation with the treatment team; the plan should contain appropriate goals and measurable expected outcomes
- Provide support for treatment compliance
- Coordinate prescribed therapies, health care providers, and special equipment (e.g., bed, CPAP machine, or supplemental oxygen)
- Identify follow-up appointment dates and mode of transportation if patient is unable to drive due to sleep attacks
- Research and identify community resources and support groups
- Determine if patient and family have adequate funds for medications and required supplies
- Provide 24-hour telephone contact number for questions and problems

From National Heart, Lung, and Blood Institute: *Restless leg syndrome: detection and management in primary care*, NIH pub no 00-3788, Bethesda, MD, March 2000, US Department of Health and Human Services, Public Health Service.
CPAP, Continuous positive airway pressure.

of life. Special equipment may be needed in the home with health teaching, medications, and evaluations. Case management guidelines are provided in Box 6-13.

CONCLUSION: SLEEP

Sleep is a complex state that inhibits neuronal stimulation. The disruption of sleep patterns can disrupt mental and physical health. Sleep patterns can change with advancing age, hormonal changes, and psychologic and neurologic disorders. Continued research is needed for scientists to better understand the cause of insomnia and to develop better treatments.

Neuroscience clinicians should include sleep assessment and interventions in their patient plan of care of CNS disorders that can cause sleepiness or fatigue, including Parkinson's disease, myotonic dystrophy, multiple sclerosis, dementia, amyotrophic lateral sclerosis (ALS), intracerebral tumors, stroke, head trauma, narcolepsy, and RLS. Patients with the following diagnoses may exhibit sleep disorders in association with neurologic disorders that include dementia, Alzheimer's disease, Parkinson's disease, epilepsy, traumatic brain injury, stroke, and spinal cord injury (SCI).[8] Other neurologic patients at risk are those who are overweight or have enlarged necks or medical conditions (e.g., diabetes or thyroid disorders).

During the initial patient assessment, the clinician can determine if the patient has a specific sleep disturbance. The sleep environment can be assessed and appropriately modified. A follow-up assessment will allow monitoring of the effectiveness of interventions for sleep disorders. Health teaching will help patients and their families understand and deal with their sleep disorders. Careful monitoring of sleep patterns will detect and prevent complications during neurologic recovery.

Acknowledgments

The author would like to acknowledge the contribution for this chapter from Lee Dresser, M.D., with Wilmington Neurology Consultants, Newark, Delaware, and Director of the St. Francis Hospital Sleep Lab, Wilmington, Delaware.

RESOURCES FOR COMA

Agency for Healthcare Research and Quality, Department of Health and Human Services: www.ahcpr.gov
Albert Einstein Healthcare Network: Coma and severe brain injury information: www.einstein.edu/efront/dll?durki=8115
Coma Recovery Associates Support Group: South Nassau Communities Hospital, 2445 Oceanside Road, Oceanside, NY 11431
Coma Recovery Association, Inc.: www.comarecovery.org
National Institute of Neurological Disorders and Stroke: Coma and severe brain injury information: www.ninds.gov/healthandmedical/disorders/comadoc.htm

RESOURCES FOR SLEEP

American Academy of Sleep Medicine: www.aasmnet.org
American Narcolepsy Association: PO Box 5846, Stanford, CA 94305
American Sleep Apnea Association: www.sleepapnea.org
Association of Sleep Disorders Center: 604 Second Street SW, Rochester, MN 55902
Help for Insomnia: www.iris-publishing.com/sleep.html
Mayo Clinic Sleep Disorders Center: www.mayohealth.org
Narcolepsy Network, Inc.: www.narcolepsynetwork.org
National Center for Sleep Disorders Research: www.nhlbi.nih.gov
National Sleep Foundation: www.sleepfoundation.org

REFERENCES

1. Adams RD, Victor M: *Principles of neurology,* ed 7, New York, 2001, McGraw-Hill.
2. Aldrich MS: Sleep disorders. In Goetz CG, Pappert EF, editors: *Textbook of clinical neurology,* Philadelphia, 1999, WB Saunders.
3. Andrefsky JC, Frank JI, Chyattie D: The cliospinal reflex in pentobarbital coma, *J Neurosurg* 90(4):644–646, 1999.
4. American Sleep Apnea Association: www. sleepapnea.org/info/index/html.
5. Ballard RD: Sleep disordered breathing and the heart, *MedSci Update* 22(2)1–8, 2005.
6. Baumann CR, Bassetti CL: Hypocretins (orexins) and sleep-awake disorders, *Lancet Neurol* 4(10):673–682, 2005.

7. Bleck TP: Levels of consciousness and attention. In Goetz CG, Pappert EJ, editors: *Textbook of clinical neurology,* Philadelphia, 1999, WB Saunders.

8. Blissitt PA: Sleep and sleep disorders. In Tucker SM et al: *Patient care standards: collaborative planning and nursing interventions,* ed 7, St Louis, 2000, Mosby.

9. Blouin AM, Thannickal TC, Worley PE, et al: Narp immunostaining of human hypocretin (orexin) neurons: loss in narcolepsy, *Neurology* 65(8):1189–1192, 2005.

10. Boss BJ: Concepts of neurologic dysfunction. In McCance KL, Huether SE: *Pathophysiology: the biologic basis for disease in adults and children,* ed 4, St Louis, 2002, Mosby.

11. Clifton GL: Is keeping cool still hot? An update on hypothermia in brain injury, *Curr Opin Crit Care* 10(2):116–119, 2004.

12. Commele CL, Walters AS, Heming WA: In Goetz CG, Pappert EJ, editors: *Textbook of clinical neurology,* Philadelphia, 1999, WB Saunders.

13. Davis AE, White JJ: Innovative sensory input for the comatose brain injured patient, *Crit Care Nurs Clin North Am* 7(2):351–371, 1995.

14. Diagnostic Classification Steering Committee: *International classification of sleep disorders: diagnostic and coding manual (revised edition),* Rochester, MN, 1997, American Sleep Disorders Association.

15. Fakhry SM, Trask AL, Waller MA, et al: Management of brain-injured patients by an evidence-based medicine protocol improves outcomes and decreases hospital charges, *J Trauma* 56(3):492–499, 2004.

16. Fuller G: *Neurological examination made easy,* ed, 3, New York, 2004, Churchill Livingstone.

17. Gerber CS: Understanding and managing coma stimulation: are we doing everything we can? *Crit Care Nurs Q* 28(2):94–108, 2005.

18. Guyton AC, Hall JE: *Textbook of medical physiology,* ed 11, Philadelphia, 2006, Elsevier.

19. Helwick LD: Stimulation programs for coma patients, *Crit Care Nurse* 14(4):47–52, 1999.

20. Huether SE: Pain, temperature, sleep and sensory function. In McCance KL, Huether SE: *Pathophysiology: the biological basis for disease in adults and children,* ed 4, St Louis, 2002, Mosby.

21. Kryger MH, Roth T, Dement WC: *Principles and practice of sleep medicine,* Philadelphia, 1989, WB Saunders.

22. Lack L, Wright H, Kemp K, Gibbon S: The treatment of early-morning awakening insomnia with two evenings of bright light, *Insomnia and Sleep Health* 28(5):616–623, 2005.

23. Lippert-Gruner M, Wedekind C, Ermestus RI, Klug N: Early rehabilitation concepts in therapy of the comatose brain injured patients, *Acta Neurochir* 79(suppl):21–23, 2002.

24. Lu J, Marmarou A, Choi S, Maas A, et al: Mortality from traumatic brain injury, *Acta Neurochir Suppl* 95:281–285, 2005.

25. Majde JA, Krueger JM: Links between the innate immune system and sleep, *J Allergy Clin Immunol* 116(6):1188–1198, 2005.

26. Malik SW, Kaplan J: Sleep deprivation, *Prim Care* 32(2):475–490, 2005.

27. Marion DW, Penrod LE, Kelsey SF, et al: Treatment of traumatic brain injury with moderate hypothermia, *N Engl J Med* 336:540–546, 1997.

28. McCance KL, Heuther SE: *Pathophysiology: the biological basis for disease in adults and children,* ed 4, St Louis, 2002, Mosby.

29. *Mosby's 2005 drug consult for nurses,* St Louis, 2005, Elsevier Mosby.

30. *Mosby's medical nursing and allied health dictionary,* ed 6, St Louis, 2002, Mosby.

31. Mycek MJ, Harvey RA, Champe PC, et al: *Lippincott's illustrated reviews: pharmacology,* ed 2, Philadelphia, 2000, Lippincott Williams & Wilkins.

32. National Heart, Lung, and Blood Institute: *Problem sleepiness,* NIH pub no 97-4071, Bethesda, MD, March 1997, US Department of Health and Human Services, Public Health Service.

33. National Heart, Lung, and Blood Institute: *Restless leg syndrome: detection and management in primary care,* NIH pub no 00-3788, Bethesda, MD, March 2000, US Department of Health and Human Services, Public Health Service.

34. National Institutes of Neurological Disorders and Stroke: *Brain basics: understanding sleep,* NIH pub no 04-3440-c, Bethesda, MD, 2004, National Institutes of Health, US Department of Health and Human Services.

35. National Sleep Foundation: The women and sleep poll. Press conference, Oct 22, 1998, Washington, DC.

36. National Sleep Foundation: Drowsy driving: "the silent killer" facts and stats. Press conference, Nov 20, 2002, Washington, DC.

37. Neubauer RN, Gottlieb SF, Miale A: Identification of hypometabolic areas in the brain using brain imaging and hyperbaric oxygen, *Clin Nucl Med* 17(6):477–481, 1992.

38. Pagana KD, Pagana TJ: *Mosby's diagnostic and laboratory test reference,* ed 7, St Louis, 2005, Elsevier Mosby.

39. Plum F, Posner F: *Diagnosis of stupor and coma,* Philadelphia, 1982, FA Davis.

40. Rossi P: *Case management in healthcare: a practical guide,* ed 2, Philadelphia, 2003, WB Saunders.

41. Stewart-Amidei C: Assessment (editor). In Bader MK, Littlejohns LR: *AANN core curriculum for neuroscience nursing,* ed 4, St Louis, 2004, Saunders.

42. Swick TJ: The neurology of sleep, *Neurol Clin* 23(4):967–989, 2005.

43. Thiibodeau GA, Patton KT: *Anatomy and physiology,* ed 5, St Louis, 2003, Mosby.

44. Thorpy MJ: Cataplexy associated with narcolepsy: epidemiology, pathophysiology and management, *CNS Drugs* 20(1):43–50, 2006.

45. Tucker SM, Canobbio MM, Paquette EV, et al: *Patient care standards: collaborative planning and nursing interventions,* ed 7, St Louis, 2000, Mosby.

46. Personal communication from Giacino J, October 4, 2005.

EILEEN M. BOHAN, GARY L.
GALLIA, HENRY BREM

CHAPTER 7

Brain Tumors

The term *brain tumor* (neoplasm) is generally used to describe any tumor arising within the cranial vault. Tumors may originate within the brain tissue itself (intraaxial) or may develop from outside the brain tissue (extraaxial). A variety of different tumor types are discussed in this chapter, but there are some features common to all brain tumors. As tumors grow, they displace normal brain tissue, cause surrounding edema, and increase intracranial pressure. Symptoms of tumor growth may be temporary and relieved with medical or surgical management or permanent and irreversible. Without treatment, brain tumors are potentially fatal because of their location within the rigid cranium. For these reasons, timely diagnosis is crucial to maximize survival benefit, as well as quality of life.

The patient diagnosed with a brain tumor faces an array of concerns regarding treatment choices, follow-up care, and risk of recurrence. There are additional questions about the effects of the tumor and treatments on the patient's quality of life, ability to work, and overall survival. During the course of treatment, the patient is likely to be seen by physicians, clinicians, rehabilitation specialists, social workers, and numerous other staff. Because a multidisciplinary approach is so often necessary, it is crucial that the patient have a clear understanding of who is managing the plan of care. This ensures that communication and information between the team and the patient and family is comprehensive and consistent.

Whether a patient is cured of the brain tumor with surgery alone or must undergo multiple treatments over many months, the impact of the diagnosis of a brain tumor on the patient and family members is overwhelming. An understanding of the process, as well as acceptance of the vital multidisciplinary aspect of treatment, aids the patient, members of the family, and staff in accomplishing their therapeutic goals in the least disruptive manner possible.

This chapter focuses on the classification of and grading systems for brain tumors, presenting signs and symptoms, diagnostic studies, management and treatment modalities, rehabilitation, and case management issues. A section is also devoted to research initiatives underway for new systemic and local therapies for malignant brain tumors.

INCIDENCE AND ETIOLOGY

Brain neoplasms constitute approximately 95% of all central nervous system (CNS) tumors, with spinal cord tumors accounting for 5%. Brain tumors are the second leading cause of death from a neurologic cause after stroke.[10] These tumors are divided into two distinct categories: primary and secondary. **Primary tumors** originate in the brain. Estimates of frequency for benign and malignant tumors are greater than 40,000 new cases in the United States each year.[18] The most common primary adult brain tumors are located in the cerebral hemispheres (Fig. 7-1, *A*) and are discussed in detail later in this chapter.

Secondary, or **metastatic, tumors** originate in other organs and disseminate to the brain. Metastatic tumors have been underestimated in the past. Currently, it is estimated that there are more than 150,000 new cases in the United States each year, making them the most common adult brain tumors.[17,88] Although there are widely varying estimates of occurrence by primary site in the literature, lung and breast cancers have the highest incidence of metastases to the brain, followed by malignant melanoma, renal malignancies, and gastrointestinal malignancies (Fig. 7-1, *B*).

Because the brain does not have a lymphatic system, it is unlikely that brain tumors will disseminate systemically.[98] However, with more sophisticated diagnostic tools and improved tumor treatments, seeding to the leptomeninges (pia mater and arachnoid membrane) is increasing in frequency. This occurs through direct extension from a primary brain tumor or through spread from systemic tumors. Estimates of leptomeningeal metastasis (LM) are approximately 5% of patients with cancer. Treatment is dependent on histology but generally involves chemotherapy or radiation. Doses are limited because of the risk of neurotoxicity, and the median survival is 3 to 6 months with treatment.[19]

Over the past several decades there has been an increase in the incidence of brain tumors. In part, this increase can be attributed to improvements in diagnostic tools. More advanced and sophisticated imaging techniques have been used, as discussed later in this chapter and in more detail in Chapter 3. Tumor occurrence is influenced by the following:

- Age (e.g., occurrence rates for meningiomas increase with advancing age)
- Gender (e.g., gliomas are more common in men, and meningiomas are more common in women)
- Ethnicity (e.g., African Americans are more likely to be diagnosed with a meningioma than with an astrocytoma)
- Geographic location (e.g., brain tumor rates are higher in developed countries)

Other presumed risk factors are genetic and familial influences, environmental factors, previous exposure to ionizing

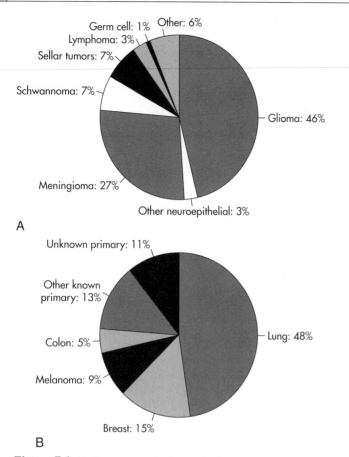

A

B

Figure 7-1 A, Percentage of primary brain tumors by histologic type. **B,** Percentage of metastatic brain tumors by site of origin. (*A, Modified from Central Brain Tumor Registry of the United States (CBTRUS): Statistical report: 2004–2005 primary brain tumors in the United States, 1997–2001 years data collected, Hinsdale, IL, 2004, CBTRUS. B, Modified from Burger PC, Scheithauer BW, Vogel FS: Surgical pathology of the nervous system and its coverings, ed 4, New York, 2002, Churchill Livingstone.*)

radiation, exposure to electromagnetic fields,[49] nutrition, and personal habits. Although there has been discussion of the relationship between cellular phones and brain cancer, current data do not support this.[55] No clear-cut etiology has yet been identified, and it is evident that more extensive research is needed.[4,134]

PROGNOSTIC FACTORS

The tumor type and degree of differentiation are significant factors affecting the patient's prognosis. Another important variable relates to the patient's age at diagnosis. The younger patient, regardless of tumor histology, has a better outcome. Early detection and minimal neurologic deficits are also associated with improved quality of life and enhanced survival. The anatomic tumor location may affect overall prognosis. Tumors that are deep, involve eloquent areas of the brain, or are located in the brainstem may be less accessible. In these cases the tumors may be inoperable or surgery may lead to permanent neurologic deficits.[98]

PATHOPHYSIOLOGY

Brain neoplasms have disparate cellular types and biologic characteristics. They originate from various areas of the brain and body and can be either slow growing or behave aggressively. Although they make up a diverse histologic group, brain tumors are remarkably similar in their clinical impact on the brain. Many tumors cause blood-brain barrier (BBB) disruption, with consequent cerebral edema and increased intracranial pressure (ICP). Computed tomography (CT) and magnetic resonance imaging (MRI) are obtained to evaluate the extent of brain edema and to assess the level of BBB disruption. Contrast uptake at the site of many tumors is a consequence of BBB disruption.[25,28]

As tumors grow, they displace or invade normal brain tissue. Rapidly growing tumors can quickly cause significant neurologic deficits. Some very slow growing tumors, however, can grow to be quite large as a result of the brain's plasticity, which allows the brain to be slowly compressed and deformed over time. Figure 7-2 shows a preoperative MRI view of a convexity meningioma, intraoperative tumor resection, and an MRI taken postoperatively.

Although the incidence of symptomatic intracranial hemorrhage caused by a tumor (or hemorrhage within a tumor) is low, these situations can be acute and devastating. The frequency of a hemorrhage is dependent on the tumor histology. Some metastatic lesions, such as melanomas, are more likely to hemorrhage than primary tumors.[64]

Tumor growth can also lead to obstruction of the flow of cerebrospinal fluid (CSF), leading to hydrocephalus. ICP increases as the tumor enlarges and can lead to herniation and rapid neurologic deterioration.

Edema, ICP, hemorrhage, and herniation syndromes are extensively discussed in Chapter 10.

CLASSIFICATION

Brain tumors have a number of different characteristics that define their uniqueness. They can be classified by the following:
- Biologic behavior: benign versus malignant
- Location of origin: primary versus secondary (metastatic)
- Histology: cell type

These characteristics are discussed in the following sections.

Benign Tumors Versus Malignant Tumors

Brain tumors are classified not only by their cell type, but also by their degree of differentiation. Many brain tumors are well differentiated and are referred to as "benign." **Benign** tumors that are completely resected during surgery may in fact be cured and require no further therapy. There are also many well-differentiated tumors that cannot be completely removed because of their anatomic location. Deep tumors, brainstem lesions, and those that blend with normal brain tissue may not be cured with surgery. Although

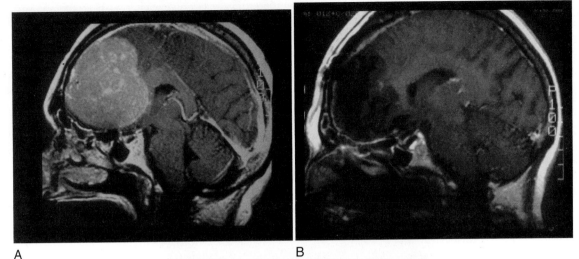

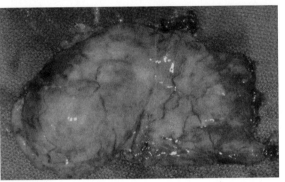

Figure 7-2 Meningioma resection. **A,** Preoperative enhanced sagittal MRI. **B,** Postoperative enhanced sagittal MRI. **C,** Meningioma after surgical removal.

these are classified histologically as low grade or benign, they are considered by many neuro-oncologists to be **malignant** because of their ability to recur, cause neurologic deficits, and even cause death. Many benign brain tumors recur in spite of multiple treatment modalities. In addition, low-grade tumors can become histologically high grade or malignant over time.

Primary Tumors Versus Secondary Tumors

Tumors that originate in the brain are considered primary brain tumors. They are derived from cells found in the CNS. They do not seed or spread outside of the CNS, although some brain tumors, such as medulloblastomas and ependymomas, can spread within the CNS along CSF pathways.[98]

Secondary (metastatic) brain tumors originate outside the CNS and seed to the brain, typically through the lymphatic system or blood vessels. They are considered malignant because of the ability to spread to multiple areas of the body.

Histology

From the time that brain tumors were described and categorized in a publication by Cruveilhier in 1829, there have been multiple modifications of the classification system used to describe microscopic (histologic) and macroscopic features of CNS tumors. These tumors had previously been described solely on the basis of their cellular features. In the early twentieth century a distinction was made between the structure of different brain tumors (classification) and the varying degrees of differentiation or malignancy within the tumor type (grading). A number of grading systems have been established over the past century to clarify the differences in behavior between tumors of similar cellular structures.[43] Table 7-1 outlines the similarities and differences among these systems.[111]

In this chapter, tumors are described according to cell type. Table 7-2 reviews the most common tumors in each of the seven World Health Organization (WHO) histologic classifications: (1) neuroepithelial; (2) peripheral nerve; (3) meningeal; (4) lymphoma and hematopoietic; (5) germ cell; (6) sellar; and (7) metastatic. It includes information about clinical and radiographic features, as well as typical treatment regimens. Based on data from the Central Brain Tumor Registry of the United States (CBTRUS), of primary brain tumors, more than 42% are gliomas and approximately 30% are meningiomas, with schwannomas and pituitary tumors making up 8% and 7%, respectively.[18] Although there are more than 100 different WHO tumor types, these four

TABLE 7-1   Comparison Grading for the Diffuse Astrocytomas

Grading Systems	Grade 1	Grade 2	Grade 3	Grade 4
Kernohan	Cells: no anaplasia	Cells: most appear normal, anaplasia in small numbers Cellularity: mild	Cells: anaplasia in half of cells	Cells: extensive anaplasia, few "normal" appearing
	Cellularity: mild Mitoses: none Vessels: minimal endothelial or adventitial proliferation	Mitoses: none Vessels: as in grade 1	Cellularity: increased Mitoses: present Vessels: more frequent endothelial and adventitial proliferation	Cellularity: marked Mitoses: numerous Vessels: marked proliferation
		Transition zone: less broad	Necrosis: frequent, regional	Necrosis: extensive
	Transition zone to normal brain: broad		Transition zone: narrowed	Transitional zone: may be sharply demarcated
WHO	Pilocytic astrocytoma	Astrocytoma: tumor composed of astrocytes (fibrillary, protoplasmic, gemistocytic, giant cell, and combinations thereof); atypia evident, but no mitoses	Anaplastic astrocytoma: astrocytoma showing mitotic activity; such tumors are not difficult to distinguish from glioblastoma	Glioblastoma: anaplastic tumor, usually astrocytic, with high cellularity, endothelial proliferation, or necrosis with pseudopalisading
St. Anne–Mayo	None of the following four criteria: Nuclear abnormalities Mitoses Endothelial proliferation Necrosis	One criterion	Two criteria	Three or four criteria
Ringertz	Astrocytoma: tumor showing infiltrative growth pattern and mild to moderate hypercellularity; cytologic features resembling normal astrocytes with only mild nuclear abnormalities	Anaplastic astrocytoma: cellular infiltrative astrocytic tumor containing astrocytes with moderate pleomorphism; mitoses and moderate vascular proliferation may be seen, but necrosis is absent		Glioblastoma multiforme: markedly pleomorphic astrocytic tumor with high cellularity, frequent mitoses, increased vascularity and necrosis; may show limited infiltration

From Shaw EG et al: Low-grade hemispheric astrocytomas. In Black PM, Loeffler JS, editors: *Cancer of the nervous system,* Oxford, 1997, Blackwell Science.

account for more than 85% of primary brain tumors. A more in-depth discussion of the management of these most common primary tumors is presented in this chapter with representative MRI scans. A section is also included on brain metastases, with occurrence estimates between 24% and 45% of patients diagnosed with systemic tumors.[15]

TYPES OF BRAIN TUMORS

Primary Brain Tumors

Gliomas

Gliomas are the most common primary brain tumor (Fig. 7-3). They occur in all age-groups, with 75- to 84-year-olds having the highest incidence and individuals under 20 years

of age the lowest. However, frequency is also associated with histology. For example, pilocytic astrocytomas are more often seen in children.[18] Gliomas are divided into grades by features of aggressiveness. The WHO grading system divides astrocytic tumors into four grades:[133]

- Grade I: pilocytic astrocytoma
- Grade II: astrocytoma
- Grade III: anaplastic astrocytoma
- Grade IV: glioblastoma multiforme

Unfortunately, the most malignant glial tumor, glioblastoma multiforme (GBM), is also the most common.

In addition to grading, the neuropathologist evaluates tumors by their degree of cell proliferation. Different labeling methods have been used to measure cells in varying phases of cell proliferation: Ki-67/MIB-1, bromodeoxyuridine (BUdR), and proliferating cell nuclear antigen (PCNA),

TABLE 7-2   Common Brain Tumors by Classification

Tumor	Definition/Histology	Clinical Features (Signs and Symptoms, Radiographic Appearance)	Treatment/Comments
Neuroepithelial *Gliomas*			
Astrocytic	Many neoplasms fit into this category; tumors have varied histologic features, invasiveness, and clinical outcome Diffusely infiltrating tumors may be WHO grade II, III, or IV	Varies with grade and tumor location	
WHO grade I: pilocytic astrocytoma	Most common pediatric glioma; 85% cerebellar Circumscribed; slow growing; cystic; low cellularity	Increased ICP or focal neurologic signs Well circumscribed; contrast enhancing; often cystic	Surgical removal can be curative Can be associated with type 1 neurofibromatosis
WHO grade II: diffuse astrocytoma	Cellular differentiation; slow growth; infiltration of brain structures Composed of well-differentiated fibrillary or gemistocytic astrocytes; increased cellularity; typically no mitoses	Symptoms subtle or acute; seizures are common initial sign Typically do not enhance on CT/MRI scan	Biopsy or craniotomy; gross total resection and young age are positive prognostic indicators; radiation for residual tumor in some cases
WHO grade III: anaplastic astrocytoma	Anaplasia and cellular proliferation Hypercellularity; nuclear atypia; mitoses	Recent history of symptoms; may manifest similar to lower-grade tumors Ill-defined low density; some tumors enhance; likely to have brain edema	Biopsy or craniotomy; RT with or without chemotherapy Young patients with good Karnofsky Performance Score (KPS) have better prognosis
WHO grade IV: glioblastoma multiforme	Poorly differentiated; cellular pleomorphism; highly mitotic; microvascular proliferation; necrosis	Recent clinical history; increased ICP; neurologic symptoms; ring enhancing; central area of necrosis	Biopsy or craniotomy; RT with chemotherapy; investigational protocols Gross total resection and young age have more favorable outcome (controversial)
Oligodendroglial WHO grade II	Well differentiated; diffusely infiltrative	Long history of symptoms; often seizures and headaches	Biopsy or craniotomy; or RT for residual or recurrent tumor Treatment decisions based on pathologic evaluation of 1p 19q deletion
	Moderately cellular; occasional mitoses; calcification	Well demarcated; calcification common; cortically based; little edema	
WHO grade III/anaplastic	Significant mitoses; vascular proliferation or necrosis		Radiation/chemotherapy Treatment decisions based on pathologic evaluation of 1p 19q deletion
Mixed glioma (oligoastrocytoma)	Features of astrocytoma and oligodendroglioma		Varying estimates of frequency; prognosis dependent on age, KPS, surgical result, and use of RT

Continued

TABLE 7-2   Common Brain Tumors by Classification—cont'd

Tumor	Definition/Histology	Clinical Features (Signs and Symptoms, Radiographic Appearance)	Treatment/Comments
Ependymoma	Slow-growing tumor of children and young adults; originates from wall of the ventricles Moderately cellular gliomas; rare mitoses; perivascular rosettes	Symptoms are location dependent; may manifest with signs of hydrocephalus; posterior fossa most common site	Surgical resection recommended and correlates with improved prognosis Craniospinal radiation: in general, not currently given without evidence of tumor dissemination
		Well circumscribed; some contrast enhancement; hydrocephalus, ventricular, or brainstem displacement may be noted	
	May be anaplastic/WHO grade III		
Embryonal Medulloblastoma			
Also described as primitive neuroectodermal tumors	Malignant; invasive; cerebellum; tendency to metastasize within the CSF Largely pediatric tumors	Gait disturbance; symptoms related to CSF obstruction Intense enhancement on MRI	Surgery, radiation, chemotherapy Leptomeningeal metastases results in poor prognosis About one third of patients have CSF metastases; craniospinal RT
Tumors of the Peripheral Nerves			
Vestibular schwannoma ("acoustic neuroma")	Benign; usually encapsulated; composed of differentiated neoplastic Schwann cells Composed of spindle-shaped cells	Schwannomas of CN VIII cause decreased hearing or tinnitus Well circumscribed; enhancing; sometimes with bone erosion	Slow growing; benign; curable with treatment Surgery or radiosurgery High incidence in type 2 neurofibromatosis Although curable with surgery, cranial nerve deficits (usually temporary) affect body image and quality of life
Tumors of the Meninges			
Meningioma	Slowly growing; usually benign; attached to dura mater; composed of neoplastic meningothelial (arachnoid) cells Several subtypes; occasional mitoses *Atypical meningioma:* Increased mitotic activity and other aggressive features *Malignant meningioma:* High mitotic index; malignant cytologic features; infiltrative	Symptoms related to compression of brain structures; may elicit headaches or seizures Enhancing dural masses; possible calcification; "dural tail;" may have edema, particularly in atypical and malignant types	Involvement of skull may lead to hyperostosis Convexity, sphenoid ridge, parasagittal, cerebellopontine angle, olfactory groove, parasellar, optic nerve Amount of tumor resection may be influenced by location and is correlated with favorable prognosis
Lymphomas and Hemopoietic Neoplasms			
Malignant CNS lymphoma	Arises in CNS in absence of systemic lymphoma Diffusely infiltrates brain Most often supratentorial Often periventricular and may extend to leptomeninges	Causes neurologic or neuropsychiatric symptoms Solid lesions; diffuse enhancement; solitary or multiple	Typically diagnosed through stereotactic biopsy or CSF Temporarily sensitive to steroids; if possible, withhold steroids until tissue diagnosis is obtained High-dose methotrexate appears effective as single agent in non-AIDS CNS lymphoma; less neurotoxicity; RT may be deferred Radiation alone associated with 1-year median survival; often combine chemotherapy and radiation; associated with significant neurotoxicity Recent increased incidence in immunocompetent patients; may be decreasing in AIDS patients

TABLE 7-2	Common Brain Tumors by Classification—cont'd		
Tumor	**Definition/Histology**	**Clinical Features (Signs and Symptoms, Radiographic Appearance)**	**Treatment/Comments**
Germ Cell Tumors	Arise in gonads and extragonadal sites Often of mixed histologic types; germinoma and teratoma most common Children and young adults	Symptoms location dependent; diabetes insipidus is classic for suprasellar germinoma Germinomas appear solid and enhance; teratomas have cysts, calcification, and fat	Germinomas respond to radiation therapy; curable Totally resected teratomas have improved prognosis Chemotherapy used for some germ cell tumors
Sellar Tumors Craniopharyngioma	Benign, partly cystic Composed of multistratified squamous epithelium; calcification	Visual disturbance; endocrine abnormalities; cognitive and personality changes; increased ICP Cyst capsule; contrast enhancement; calcification	Tumor size and extent of surgical resection affect outcome Radiation may be used for residual tumor
Pituitary Adenomas	Benign, epithelial; originating from the adenohypophysis Radiologic classification Microadenoma <1 cm Macroadenoma ≥1 cm Pathologic classification by hormonal content; structure; cell derivation	*Hypersecretion* Prolactin: galactorrhea, amenorrhea GH: acromegaly ACTH: Cushing's syndrome TSH: Hyperthyroidism (rare) *Hyposecretion* Hypopituitarism caused by large tumors that compress the gland and impair secretory capabilities *Pituitary apoplexy* Acute hemorrhage or infarction; can also cause hypopituitarism *Neurologic symptoms* Visual loss (bitemporal hemianopia); headache; cranial nerve deficits; hydrocephalus	*Pharmacologic* Dopamine agonists for prolactinomas Somatostatin analogs for GH-secreting tumors *Surgical* Transsphenoidal/transnasal microsurgery for approximately 95% of surgical cases; less morbidity than transcranial, which is used for patients with extensive intracranial involvement *Radiation* Used for hypersecretory states refractory to medical management and for residual/recurrent tumor
Metastatic Tumors	Originate from primary systemic neoplasms Anaplasia Many metastases have well-defined borders and displace rather than infiltrate brain	Symptoms typically occur over a short time period Discrete, rounded, ring enhancing; solitary or multiple lesions	Prognosis dependent on number of metastases; location; systemic dissemination; age Resection of solitary metastasis and RT results in improved prognosis Common sites of origin include lung, breast, melanoma, renal (unknown primary: 10%)

Data from references 15, 17, 18, 20, 41, 43, 68, 73, 76, 97, 133.
ACTH, Adrenocorticotropic hormone; *AIDS*, acquired immunodeficiency syndrome; *CN*, cranial nerve; *CNS*, central nervous system; *CSF*, cerebrospinal fluid; *CT*, computed tomography; *GH*, growth hormone; *ICP*, intracranial pressure; *MRI*, magnetic resonance imaging; *RT*, radiation therapy; *TSH*, thyroid-stimulating hormone; *WHO*, World Health Organization.

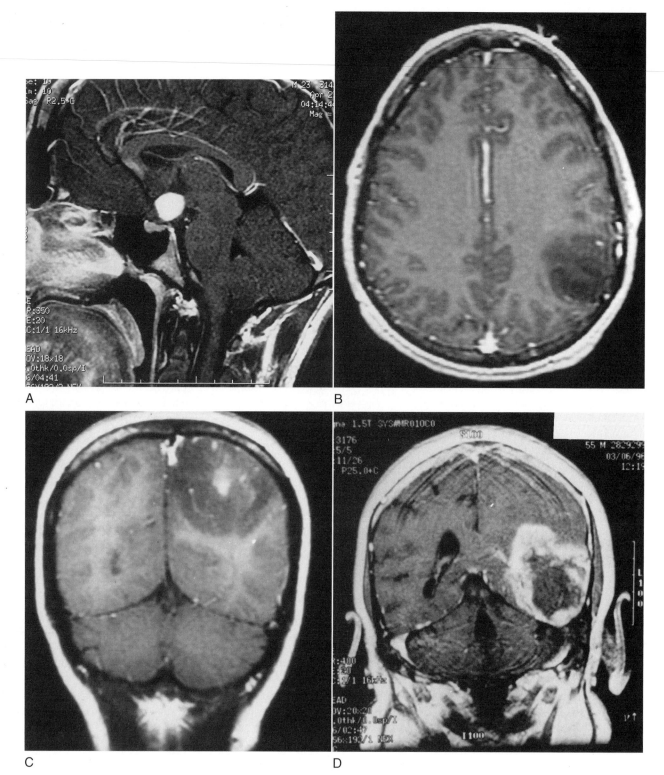

Figure 7-3 Enhanced MRI studies of gliomas. **A,** Sagittal view of pilocytic astrocytoma (grade I). **B,** Axial view of astrocytoma (grade II). **C,** Coronal view of anaplastic astrocytoma (grade III). **D,** Coronal view of glioblastoma multiforme (grade IV).

for example. Studies have shown that a higher labeling index is associated with a higher tumor grade. Survival is correlated with a low labeling index. Of the low-grade astrocytomas, those having a lower labeling index are associated with increased survival.[87,109]

Depending on the tumor location and the patient's overall neurologic/medical status, gliomas may be treated by stereotactic biopsy or debulked through an open craniotomy. With the exception of **grade I pilocytic astrocytomas,** which can be cured with surgery, gliomas cannot be completely resected.

Grade II astrocytomas may be aggressively treated with craniotomy for tumor debulking. Some centers recommend adjuvant radiation therapy (RT) postoperatively, whereas other institutions observe the patient with follow-up MRI scans until there is evidence of recurrence. Several factors are considered in this decision: extent of surgical resection, histology, tumor size, and patient age. Although several studies suggest that 5-year overall survival is similar regardless of the timing or dosing of RT, or the addition of chemotherapy,[112] this issue remains controversial and further studies are underway to help define the optimal therapy. Some experts believe that the long-term risks of RT may be significant enough to warrant a conservative approach, especially in younger patients.[67] These risks, however, must be weighed against the potential neurologic sequelae of tumor progression.

Grade III anaplastic astrocytoma and **grade IV glioblastoma multiforme** require an aggressive approach in order to slow recurrence. Surgical biopsy or debulking is followed by a therapy program that includes RT in combination with chemotherapy or investigational drugs, as described later in this chapter. A postoperative baseline imaging study (CT or MRI) within the first 48 hours after surgery is recommended.

Most malignant gliomas recur and continue to require aggressive intervention, often with investigational protocols. There is evidence that surgical reduction of tumor bulk, if possible, improves both the duration and the quality of survival,[69] although this remains a somewhat controversial issue. Patients with recurrent malignant gliomas are offered multiple treatment options with no guarantee of survival benefit. These include reoperation, additional forms of radiation and chemotherapy, and investigational protocols for which there are no survival statistics and for which side effects are unknown. Patients may be treated for recurrence more than once.

Oligodendrogliomas

Oligodendrogliomas make up a relatively small percentage of gliomas (10% to 15%)[17] and are considered slower growing than astrocytomas. They can be either low grade or malignant.[70] Low-grade oligodendrogliomas that have undergone aggressive surgical resection are often followed with serial MRI scans before considering adjuvant treatments. Many of these tumors are highly chemosensitive, and some oncologists recommend chemotherapeutic agents before considering radiation. Recent studies have shown that when these tumors have a genetic change identified as loss of heterozy-

gosity (LOH) of chromosomes 1p and 19q, they are more responsive to treatment and have lower rates of recurrence.[76,118] Therefore pathologic evaluation of oligodendrogliomas may include testing for these chromosomal deletions. The two most commonly used chemotherapeutic approaches are temozolomide and combination procarbazine, CCNU, and vincristine (PCV).[11,119,120] It is not unusual for the pathologist to return a histologic diagnosis of mixed oligoastrocytoma with features of both tumor types.

Tumors of the Peripheral Nerves: Vestibular Schwannomas

Vestibular schwannomas are histologically benign tumors that are generally slow growing (Fig. 7-4); however, they may have periods of inactivity alternating with periods of more rapid growth.[89] The most common presenting signs of this tumor type include unilateral hearing loss, tinnitus, facial numbness or weakness, and disequilibrium, or vertigo. Tumors that are small and asymptomatic may be followed with serial MRI scans and audiograms. Radiographic or clinical signs of tumor progression necessitate intervention.

Because there is increased surgical morbidity associated with increased tumor size, surgery should be planned accordingly. Significant improvements in intraoperative technologies that have reduced overall postoperative morbidity include facial nerve and auditory monitoring, improved microsurgical equipment, and advances in neuroanesthesia.[63] The surgical procedure may be performed by a neurosurgeon in conjunction with an otolaryngologist. Three surgical approaches can be used, depending on the tumor size and location and the patient's degree of functional hearing. The advantages and disadvantages of each approach are given in Table 7-3.[45]

The surgical procedure also involves risks. Patients may have postoperative hearing loss, facial nerve paralysis, head-

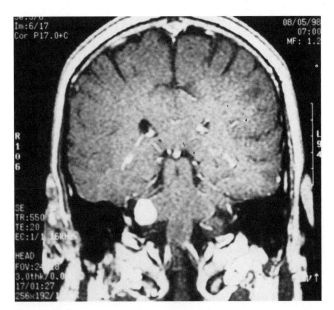

Figure 7-4 Enhanced coronal MRI of vestibular schwannoma.

TABLE 7-3	Surgical Approach to Tumors of the Cerebellopontine Angle
Approach	**Rationale**
Suboccipital (retrosigmoid)	Excellent exposure of CPA and brainstem for large tumors
	Preferred approach for nonacoustic CPA tumors (i.e., meningioma, epidermoid)
	Favorable hearing conservation in small tumors (<2.0 cm) situated in the medial IAC
	Limited lateral dissection to remove tumor in distal IAC
	Limited anatomic exposure in patient with posterior course of sigmoid sinus or high jugular bulb
Translabyrinthine	Excellent exposure of facial nerve at lateral end of IAC
	Limited retraction of the cerebellum
	Hearing always sacrificed
	Limited anatomic exposure in patients with anteriorly placed sigmoid sinus or high jugular bulb
Middle fossa	Excellent exposure of distal IAC and facial nerve for small intracanalicular tumors
	Poor exposure of CPA
	Retraction of temporal lobe necessary for exposure
	Favorable hearing preservation in small tumors (<2.0 cm)
	Less headache (possibly)

Data from references 8, 17, 32, 45, 63, 108.
CPA, Cerebellopontine angle; *IAC,* internal auditory canal.

TABLE 7-4	Vestibular Schwannoma: Selected Complications
Complication	**Discussion/Management**
Unilateral hearing loss	Larger tumors more likely to be associated with increased risk of hearing loss
	Preoperative audiometry as baseline
	Intraoperative auditory nerve monitoring
	Appropriate surgical procedure to minimize risk
Facial nerve paresis/plegia	Protection of cornea because of inability to completely approximate the eyelids
	Artificial tears and lubricating ointments (especially at bedtime)
	Moisture chamber applied to provide both lubrication and protection
	Dietary changes to accommodate facial weakness
	Tarsorrhaphy to suture eyelid margins to prevent keratitis
	Gold weight sometimes placed in the upper eyelid to prevent keratitis
	House-Brackmann facial nerve grading scale used to evaluate improvement in facial function over time
Dysequilibrium	May be a transient result of manipulation of the vestibular nerve
	Typically recovers with or without rehabilitation, although possible to have mild permanent balance compromise
	Recommended that all patients undergoing surgical removal of vestibular schwannoma be evaluated by a vestibular rehabilitation professional after surgery
Headaches	Not uncommon, especially following suboccipital and translabyrinthine approaches
	MRI/CT obtained to evaluate for bleed or hydrocephalus
	Exact etiology unknown
Cerebrospinal fluid leak	Assessment for rhinorrhea, otorrhea, or salty taste
	May require lumbar drain or surgical repair
	Patient teaching to recognize symptoms after hospital discharge

Date from references 29, 45, 56, 106, 116.
CT, Computed tomography; *MRI,* magnetic resonance imaging.

aches, or balance difficulties. In addition, CSF leak occurs in 5% to 15% of cases.[8,32,108] Table 7-4 outlines selected postoperative complications,[29,45,56,106,116] which are often temporary but may be permanent. The most important variables affecting the patient's outcome are the tumor size and location, the surgeon's expertise, and intraoperative monitoring.

Endoscopy is also being used in some centers as an adjunct to or as a replacement for the microscope. The advantages of this approach include high magnification of vessels and cranial nerves, flexibility of the scope to better visualize the anatomy, and less invasiveness. The disadvantages of this approach include decreased visualization secondary to blood on the endoscope, limited view of the operative bed, and potential for injury from the heat-generated light source. Therefore many surgeons currently use this tool in conjunction with the microscope, not as a replacement.[124]

Radiosurgery, which is discussed later in this chapter, is playing an increasing role in the management of vestibular schwannomas and other brain/skull base tumors. It has the goals of controlling tumor growth and reducing tumor size.

Several studies have shown high tumor control rates and low morbidity, which includes preserved cranial nerve function.[74,84]

When considering the options for the patient with an acoustic neuroma, the role of the surgeon and radiation oncologist is to evaluate the patient's clinical and radiographic data and discuss treatment options, including the following: conservative observation, with serial MRIs and office visits; surgical intervention; and radiosurgery. To ensure that the patient can make an informed consent, appointments should be scheduled with both disciplines to adequately understand the risks and benefits of each approach.[125]

Tumors of the Meninges: Meningiomas

30%

Meningiomas arise from the arachnoid covering of the brain (Fig. 7-5). Although they occur in all age-groups, there is a greater incidence in patients between 50 and 70 years of age. Meningiomas are seen more often in women than in men, and they are apt to increase in size during pregnancy, presumably because they have hormone receptors. Although they are most often benign (>90%), some meningiomas may be more aggressive. Meningiomas can also occur in association with neurofibromatosis. They occur in numerous locations, and extent of surgical resection is correlated to location.[20,79]

Because they generally grow slowly, meningiomas may become quite large before causing symptoms. The clinical presentation depends on tumor location. Peritumoral edema is associated with increased morbidity, particularly in older individuals.[48] Asymptomatic meningiomas may be managed conservatively with serial imaging. Many meningiomas can be completely resected, and neurologic function often improves postoperatively. Recurrence rate is thought to be linked to the extent of surgical resection. Some histologic features are also associated with more aggressive behavior and a higher rate of recurrence.[94] Atypical, malignant, and anaplastic meningiomas are much more likely to recur, and multimodality forms of treatment may be required.[81]

In the past, RT has been used for patients who are not surgical candidates, for surgically inaccessible meningiomas, for more aggressive meningiomas, or for residual or recurrent tumors. In some studies the recurrence rate was significantly reduced when subtotal resection was combined with RT.[79,117] Currently, some patients are opting for fractionated radiotherapy to the tumor and surrounding brain as an alternative to surgery. Radiosurgery delivered as a single high dose to the tumor is increasingly being used, given recent published data on long-term results.[36,65] It may be used for tumors causing minimal edema or mass effect, small tumors, residual disease, and tumors that are surgically challenging, such as skull base meningiomas. The goal of surgery is to resect the entire tumor, if possible. RT is used for tumor control.

The results of studies using pharmacologic management of aggressive meningiomas have been published. RU486, an oral preparation that is a progesterone receptor antagonist, has been used in the treatment of unresectable meningiomas.[21] Hydroxyurea has been used in patients with recurrent meningiomas, sometimes in combination with radiotherapy.[50] Alpha-interferon has been used for histologically malignant tumors, as have some combination chemotherapeutic regimens.[21] These modalities are currently being used in selected cases, particularly meningiomas that are refractory to other treatments.

Tumors of the Sellar Region: Pituitary Tumors

7%

CBTRUS estimates that tumors of the sellar region make up 7% of primary brain tumors.[18] Other estimates are as high as 17%, based on radiographic and autopsy data.[30] **Pituitary tumors** have a presentation unlike that of other brain tumors and are managed differently, both medically and surgically. This uniqueness warrants the separate discussion that follows.

The anterior pituitary gland (adenomas rarely originate in the posterior portion of the gland) is responsible for secreting specific hormones that provide control of growth, reproduction, and lactation, as well as thyroid, adrenal, and gonadal functions. When these pituitary cells proliferate, adenoma formation is possible[92] (Fig. 7-6, *A*).

Adenomas are benign tumors that are diagnosed more often in women. Secretory tumors are most common and display symptoms that are based on the specific cell type,[78,97,122] as outlined in Table 7-2. Tumors in the pituitary

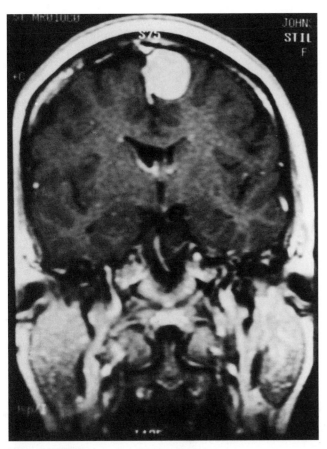

Figure 7-5 Enhanced coronal MRI of meningioma with a dural tail.

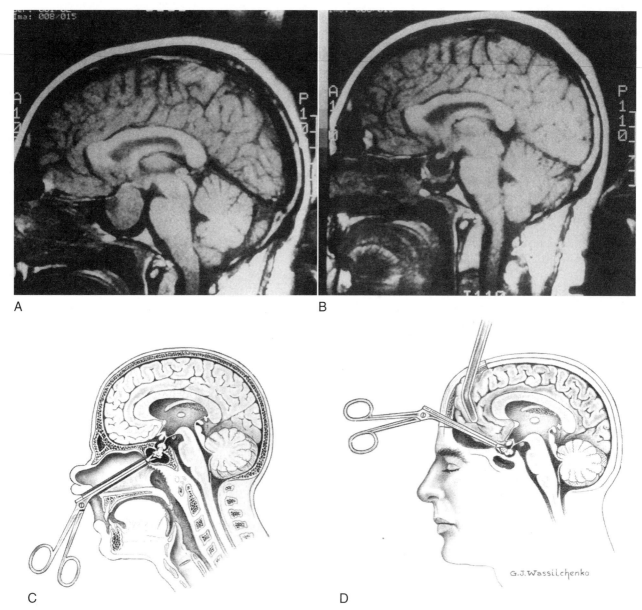

Figure 7-6 Pituitary tumor and surgical approaches for removal. **A,** Preoperative sagittal MRI with gadolinium of pituitary adenoma. **B,** Postoperative sagittal MRI with gadolinium showing status following resection of pituitary adenoma. **C,** Transsphenoidal surgical approach. **D,** Transcranial surgical approach.
(*C* and *D, From Rudy E: Advanced neurological and neurosurgical nursing, St Louis, 1984, Mosby.*)

region are overwhelmingly benign, with carcinomas making up approximately 0.2% of pituitary tumors.[59] If adenomas expand in size, they can compress the pituitary gland and surrounding structures. Symptoms are gradual in onset and may initially be ignored or attributed to other causes. Lateral tumor growth may impinge on the cavernous sinus and affect cranial nerves III, IV, V, and VI. Upward extension may cause compression of the optic chiasm, resulting in the classic bitemporal visual field cut. In some cases, continued upward expansion results in hypothalamic or ventricular involvement. Some tumors are asymptomatic, particularly microadenomas (<1 cm)[30] and those that grow downward into the sphenoid sinus.

Patients are emergently evaluated for pituitary apoplexy—hemorrhage or infarct within the tumor or the sellar region—if they have or develop severe headache, nausea and vomiting, or visual acuity or field loss. Although acute onset of apoplexy is seen in only 5% of pituitary tumors, it is a life-threatening situation requiring immediate attention. This condition may also be associated with cranial nerve palsies and hormonal abnormalities. Hypothalamic and brainstem compression may lead to altered temperature regulation, cardiac and respiratory symptoms, pupillary changes, and changes in mental status.[60,73]

Once there is radiographic confirmation of apoplexy, steroids are initiated and emergency surgery may be warranted.

If treated quickly, devastating symptoms may be completely reversible. Some pituitary tumors bleed but are asymptomatic. In these cases, hemorrhage is recognized radiographically or at the time of histologic diagnosis.

There are a number of approaches to managing pituitary adenomas, depending on the tumor size and extension, the patient's symptoms, and the cell type. Small, asymptomatic microadenomas are often followed radiographically. Some secretory adenomas are medically managed. Nonfunctioning, large, or symptomatic lesions require surgical intervention, and the vast majority are treated by the transsphenoidal or transnasal approach (Fig. 7-6, *C*). The less invasive endoscopic approach previously described has also been employed recently.[93,104] In those cases where there is extensive intracranial involvement, a transcranial approach is used[136] (Fig. 7-6, *D*). In some instances RT is recommended.

The treatment of pituitary adenomas requires a multidisciplinary approach. On radiographic confirmation of the tumor, endocrinology, neuro-ophthalmology, and neurosurgery consultations should be obtained. A treatment plan is developed only after endocrine blood and urine tests have established that medical management is not indicated, and visual fields and acuity have been assessed. A surgical plan (when warranted) is then developed.

A multidisciplinary team approach is indicated for the postoperative management of the patient who has undergone transsphenoidal/transnasal surgery. The neurosurgeon, otolaryngologist, endocrinologist, and neuro-ophthalmologist are equally involved in monitoring the patient's progress or complications. In addition to standard neurosurgical assessment as outlined in Chapter 2, additional assessments are made:

- Monitor intake and urinary output; assess urine specific gravity; obtain daily weights; obtain electrolytes to assess for diabetes insipidus (DI)
- Monitor nasal drainage to evaluate for a CSF leak
- Evaluate visual acuity, visual fields, and extraocular movements for deficits or improvements from preoperative examination

In cases of residual tumor, tumor recurrence, or hypersecretory states refractory to medical management, RT may be recommended. With improvements in imaging (MRI), patients may be followed for evidence of tumor progression. Although radiation is an effective adjuvant treatment for persistent or recurrent pituitary adenomas, the possibility of side effects—panhypopituitarism requiring hormone replacements, optic nerve damage, and radionecrosis—warrant careful consideration,[71] particularly in young patients of childbearing potential. Stereotactic radiotherapy and radiosurgery are also being used in appropriate cases.[58]

Metastatic Brain Tumors

Metastatic brain tumors have recently increased in incidence, partly as a result of better imaging and staging of these tumors, improved survival in patients with control of the primary site, and a growing older population (Fig. 7-7). Brain metastases occur most often in patients with lung, breast, melanoma, renal cell, and colorectal primary sites.

These tumors are likely to be diagnosed after discovery of the primary lesion, but in some cases a primary site is unknown at the time of surgical removal. Metastases are most often found in the cerebral hemispheres, with a smaller percentage in the cerebellum and brainstem. Metastatic lesions are often well circumscribed, centrally necrotic, and associated with edema.[15,68]

The signs and symptoms, diagnostic workup, and surgical treatment typically follow the same pattern as for primary brain tumors. However, histologic confirmation of a metastatic lesion necessitates a full systemic workup (staging). Solitary tumors are usually surgically accessible and are associated with increased survival. When multiple intracranial lesions are present, a biopsy may be necessary to establish a diagnosis. In some situations histology from the primary site obviates the need for a neurosurgical procedure. RT, with or without surgery, is often the treatment of choice, as discussed later in this chapter.[5] To date, systemic chemotherapy for brain metastases has not shown significant improvement in survival, although it is being used in selected patients who have chemosensitive systemic tumors.[53] Additionally, multimodality treatments with surgery, radiation therapy, chemotherapy, or novel investigational agents are being attempted.[5,68] After treatment is completed, follow-up MRI or CT scans are necessary as a baseline and then every 2 to 4 months to evaluate for recurrence.

Assessment

The diagnosis of a brain tumor is based on a comprehensive history and physical examination, as well as radiographic studies to localize the lesion. Symptoms are related to elevated ICP (general) or to the tumor location (focal). A comprehensive neurologic assessment and patient history may reveal that patients with increased ICP exhibit one or more of the following signs:

- Papilledema (swelling of the optic discs)
- Headaches (experienced by over 50% of patients with brain tumors)
- Nausea and/or vomiting

These three symptoms are referred to as the triad of symptoms in patients who have a brain tumor and are experiencing increased ICP. Left untreated, increased ICP may lead to brain herniation and, eventually, to brain death.[41,72,98]

Changes in Mental Status. Mental status changes can be subtle or severe, depending on the degree and location of brain compression or destruction. Mental status changes are not a direct result of increased ICP but develop as the brain is affected by shifting or herniation. Patients complain of a wide array of symptoms, which may resolve if they are caused by pressure rather than destruction. Although mental status changes may be caused by frontal lobe tumors and aggressive neoplasms (e.g., GBM), they also occur from mass effect caused by the tumor or from hydrocephalus.[7,44,54]

Seizures. Approximately one third of patients with brain tumors have seizures as an initial symptom, but during the course of their disease, more than 50% of patients experience some type of seizure. Adults with no previous history of epilepsy will immediately undergo radiographic imaging to

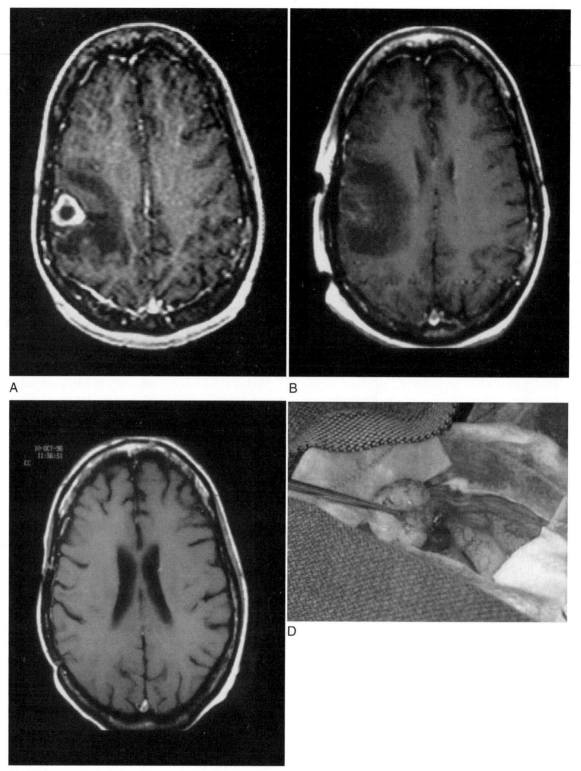

Figure 7-7 Metastatic adenocarcinoma from a primary lung tumor. **A,** Preoperative enhanced MRI. **B,** Postoperative enhanced MRI. **C,** One-year postoperative enhanced MRI. **D,** Intraoperative tumor resection.

| TABLE 7-5 | Neurologic Deficits and Clinical Management in Relationship to Tumor Location |

Deficits	Assessment*	Interventions
Frontal Lobe		
Contralateral paresis/plegia; motor aphasia; intellectual impairment; emotional lability; personality changes; urinary frequency, urgency, incontinence; seizures; impaired sense of smell	Motor examination Mental status: observe patient; interview family; assess orientation, general knowledge, spelling, and short-term memory	Physical and occupational therapy consultations Neuropsychiatric/cognitive therapy Speech therapy Pharmacologic management
Temporal Lobe		
Temporal lobe seizures; dysnomia; receptive aphasia; memory problems; perceptual/spatial disturbances; vision	Interview of patient regarding seizure history Assessment of ability to follow one-, two-, and three-step commands	Seizure prophylaxis/precautions Teaching regarding items such as seizure diary, driving restrictions Cognitive therapy
Parietal Lobe		
Sensory deficits (position, vibration, touch, temperature); calculations; left-right discrimination; visual fields; language; seizures	Test sensation, position, vibration	Occupational therapy for safety and cognitive retraining
Occipital Lobe		
Contralateral homonymous hemianopia (e.g., left lesion leads to loss of vision on right side of each eye); visual hallucinations; seizures	Visual examination to include fields, visual perception, and spatial relationships Interview to include visual hallucinations	Neuro-ophthalmology evaluation Occupational therapy for visual retraining
Cerebellum		
Ipsilateral ataxia; incoordination; nystagmus; increased intracranial pressure (ICP)	Coordination testing (finger to nose; rapid alternating movements); evaluation of intention tremor or ataxia	Physical and occupational therapy for balance and coordination Assistive devices Teaching regarding signs of increased ICP
Brainstem		
Cranial nerve deficits; sensory/motor impairment; vomiting; breathing; heartbeat	Cranial nerve testing	Therapy appropriate to cranial nerve deficit Pharmacologic management
Intraventricular		
Increased ICP; hydrocephalus (gait disturbance; cognitive deficits; urinary incontinence); sudden death	Gait testing	Teaching regarding possible shunt Patient/family education regarding obstruction and emergency surgery

Data from references 3, 7, 41, 44, 54, 72.
*Each examination is recorded only once, but there are many areas of overlap.
ICP, Intracranial pressure.

assess for a space-occupying lesion in the brain. Certain tumor types (e.g., low-grade gliomas) and those in specific locations are more likely to be associated with seizure activity. Of supratentorial tumors, frontal and temporal lobe tumors are more likely to be epileptogenic. A presentation with seizures is a good prognostic sign because it leads to early detection and treatment, as well as prevention of neurologic deficits.[3,52,130] Seizure management is discussed in Chapter 24.

Focal Neurologic Signs. Focal neurologic signs represent tumor compression or destruction that is location dependent. Table 7-5 outlines the most common neurologic deficits by location and appropriate nursing interventions.

Neurodiagnostic and Laboratory Studies
When a patient has specific symptoms raising suspicion of an intracranial lesion, the following studies may be obtained:

- CT: used as a screening study to determine whether a lesion is present (often at presentation to an emergency department); also used to evaluate bone, blood, and calcification
- MRI: localizes the lesion and assesses the amount of edema and mass effect on surrounding structures; preferred over CT because it evaluates tumors in three planes: axial, coronal, and sagittal; in addition, it provides greater anatomic detail than CT, is superior in showing hemorrhage or a cyst within a tumor, and demonstrates the relationship of a tumor to blood vessels[1]
- Magnetic resonance angiography (MRA): provides a noninvasive method of assessing vascular anatomy and identifying vessels that supply blood to the tumor (feeding vessels);[16] there are occasions when an MRA may obviate the need for an arteriogram, though

arteriogram is still used to identify and perform embolization of feeding vessels with the use of glue preparations to enhance the safety of the upcoming surgical procedure

- Functional MRI (fMRI): a type of imaging that detects physiologic changes during the performance of certain tasks and aids in the preoperative assessment of language, motor and sensory function, and tumor location[131]
- Positron emission tomography (PET): measures brain metabolism and cerebral blood flow and is used to differentiate low-grade from high-grade tumors or radiation necrosis from active malignant lesions; PET/CT is now able to image tumor metabolism[26]
- Magnetic resonance spectroscopy (MRS): uses magnetic resonance to assess the metabolic activity of abnormal areas on MRI and likewise is used to differentiate treatment necrosis from active tumor, as well as high-grade from low-grade tumors[47]

These and other imaging tools are discussed in detail in Chapter 3.

Treatment

Medical Management. In cases where tumors are asymptomatic, are incidentally found, and appear radiographically low grade or benign, it is reasonable to follow with serial MRI or CT. Once the natural history of a particular tumor is established, less frequent imaging and evaluations can be coordinated. Although many tumors may ultimately require surgical intervention, some benign lesions that do not cause symptoms or show patterns of growth do not require treatment. Those tumors that require treatment may receive the interventions described in the following paragraphs.

Corticosteroids are an efficient means of decreasing ICP and neurologic symptoms. Once a tumor has been discovered and the extent of edema is assessed, steroid therapy is initiated. Symptoms caused by pressure, as opposed to destruction, are typically improved with steroid treatment. Dexamethasone is used in the perioperative period. Although there is no universally prescribed formula for dexamethasone use, 4 mg four times a day is commonly initiated several days before surgery (or sooner with radiographic or clinical signs of edema and mass effect). In cases of severe neurologic deterioration, urgent medical management includes hyperventilation, fluid restriction, osmotic agents, diuretics, and possibly CSF drainage.[41,42] These measures may be essential to reverse a herniation syndrome.

Steroids can be tapered once postoperative edema has decreased. Peak swelling postoperatively is approximately 72 hours. It should be noted that steroid tapers are modified to patient tolerance and will be different in each case.

Antacids or H2 blockers are used to prevent the gastrointestinal side effects of steroids. Some physicians do not prescribe these drugs for short courses of steroid therapy.

Anticonvulsants are ordered when a patient has seizures or when an intracranial neoplasm has been discovered. In addition to the one third of patients with seizures, patients with supratentorial lesions are typically given prophylactic anticonvulsant therapy perioperatively, even in the absence of a seizure disorder. This is a subject of some controversy, and studies have had varying results. One study showed that when patients were randomly placed into groups receiving anticonvulsants or groups receiving no treatment, the seizure incidence was identical postoperatively, suggesting that anticonvulsants may be unnecessary in the patient without a seizure disorder.[35] Further studies are underway.

Multiple antiepileptic drugs (AEDs) are used for seizure management of brain tumor patients, depending on seizure type and patient drug tolerance and response. Neurosurgeons often use phenytoin perioperatively because it can be administered intravenously and therapeutic serum drug levels can be obtained.

Some anticonvulsants may interact with certain chemotherapeutic agents. Drugs such as phenytoin can increase the activity of the P450 system in the liver, so that higher doses of chemotherapy are needed in order to attain the maximum tolerated dose (MTD). Some chemotherapy drugs may decrease the effectiveness of anticonvulsants, thus increasing the risk of seizures. Anticonvulsants may affect other drugs and drug levels (e.g., dexamethasone and warfarin).[3,96] Further discussion of seizures and anticonvulsants can be found in Chapter 24.

If steroids and anticonvulsants are necessary in the perioperative period, they may be required on a long-term basis during treatments and following tumor recurrence. Potential side effects are discussed in Table 7-6.

Surgical Management. If a decision is made to proceed with surgical intervention, a baseline neurologic evaluation is obtained and will be crucial in determining true neurologic deterioration in the postoperative period. With managed care and shorter hospital stays, patients are leaving the hospital within a few days of surgery. They are left with a feeling that they have received too much information too soon and that they and family members will not be able to manage emergency situations as they arise. Therefore written information given to the patient before the hospital admission should attempt to anticipate questions and problems that may arise and should include appropriate telephone numbers for easy reference. A preoperative teaching sheet, sent to patients as early as possible before surgery, alleviates a number of questions and fears (Box 7-1). Written instructions should include

---

| BOX 7-1 | Preoperative Teaching Sheet |

- Name of planned procedure, date, and surgeon's name
- Required preoperative testing and schedules
- Perioperative medications and number to call for questions about dosage or side effects
- General information about hospital stay (e.g., ICU stay, IV lines and catheters, dressings, average length of stay)
- Postoperative appointment schedule (i.e., staple removal, postoperative visit, imaging schedule)
- Helpful telephone numbers: scheduling secretary, clinician, surgeon, emergency numbers

ICU, Intensive care unit; *IV,* intravenous.

TABLE 7-6 Side Effects of Medications		
Selected Side Effects	**Symptoms**	**Comments**
Steroids (to Treat Edema and Increased Intracranial Pressure)		
Immunosuppression	Predisposition to infection	Glucocorticoids are most commonly used.
Antipyretic side effects	Masking of infection	Steroid tapering is empiric and depends on amount of edema, extent of neurologic symptoms, and length of use.
Steroid-induced diabetes	Hyperglycemia	Other treatments (e.g., radiation, chemotherapy, local therapies) may increase the need for and duration of steroid therapy.
Mental status changes	Decreased attention, emotional lability, psychosis	Adrenal suppression is common; avoid too quick a taper.
Skin changes	Easy bruising, striae	Symptoms should be reversible once steroids are discontinued.
Cushing's-type symptoms	Moon facies, increased appetite, weight gain, hump back, hirsutism, hypertension	
Bone changes	Osteoporosis, joint pain	
Myopathy	Proximal muscle weakness	
Anticonvulsants (for Seizure Disorder and Prophylaxis)		
Fatigue	Inability to adequately perform ADLs; mental slowness	Monitor serum levels when appropriate; EEG and drug taper as soon as medically indicated.
Interactions with other drugs (chemotherapy, antibiotics, anticoagulants, steroids)	Variable serum levels and inconsistent seizure control	There is ongoing research regarding need for anticonvulsants perioperatively in patients who have never had a seizure.
Allergic reactions	Skin rash, fever, possible Stevens-Johnson reaction	

Data from references 3, 35, 41, 42, 96.
EEG, Electroencephalogram.

as much information as possible presented in a clear, concise manner.

For the majority of cases requiring surgical intervention, there are two distinct surgical approaches.

Stereotactic Biopsy

Stereotactic biopsy is used for diagnostic purposes only, specifically for tumors that are located in deep or eloquent areas of the brain. In some cases, histology will have previously been established and tissue is necessary only to confirm the diagnosis of recurrent tumor rather than treatment effect and necrosis. Although PET and spectroscopy studies may be used for this purpose, there are occasions when tissue is required before a new therapy is initiated. Investigational studies, for example, require tissue diagnosis before patient enrollment.

The surgeon generally obtains a number of specimens from different areas within the lesion to minimize the risk of sampling errors. Frame-based and frameless stereotactic biopsies can be performed. Figure 7-8 shows the apparatus used for frame-based tissue sampling under CT stereotactic guidance and shows an MRI study of metastatic lesions, with the coordinates. Frameless biopsies are also performed using fiducials that correspond to specific MRI or CT locations.[2,132,140] These procedures are discussed in greater detail in Chapter 8.

Craniotomy

Craniotomy has a twofold purpose: it provides tissue for diagnosis, and it provides treatment through tumor removal.

It is used for lesions that are surgically accessible, have surrounding edema causing mass effect, or require debulking to allow for other therapies. (Radiation and chemotherapy can cause additional edema and mass effect.) In many cases tumor resection relieves increased ICP and helps to reverse or stabilize neurologic deficits. Chapter 8 discusses cranial surgery, awake surgery, neuroanesthesia, and intraoperative monitoring/equipment in detail. Ultrasound, frameless stereotaxy (Fig. 7-9), cortical mapping, intraoperative MRI, and endoscopic neurosurgery are discussed. These advances have greatly enhanced the safety and efficacy of brain tumor surgery.[80,86,127,129]

Implantable Devices for Delivery of Local Therapy

There have been recent advances in the treatment of primary malignant brain tumors and metastatic lesions with the use of local therapies introduced at the time of tumor removal. Biodegradable chemotherapy wafers, radiation-filled balloons, and catheters able to deliver chemotherapeutic agents, immunotherapy, and other substances are discussed later in this chapter. However, it is important to have an in-depth discussion of these options with the patient preoperatively and to include these options in the informed consent when appropriate.

Acute Care. Postoperative management of the patient who has undergone craniotomy or stereotactic biopsy for a brain tumor focuses on assessment and intervention for a number of potential complications. In the immediate postoperative period patients may be slow to respond because of the effects

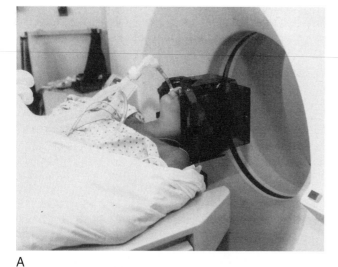

A

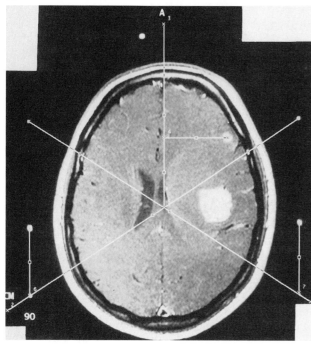

B

Figure 7-8 Stereotactic biopsy. **A,** Apparatus for CT-guided biopsy. **B,** Enhanced MRI of two metastatic lesions with coordinates for biopsy.
(Courtesy of Dr. Alessandro Olivi, Johns Hopkins University, Baltimore, MD.)

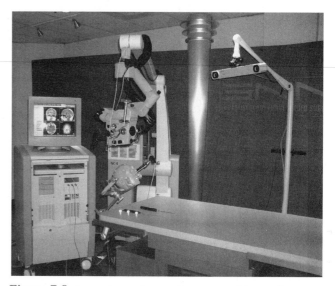

Figure 7-9 Apparatus and computer-generated image for frameless stereotaxy.
(Courtesy of Surgical Navigation Specialists, Ontario, Canada.)

of general anesthesia. Temporary changes in mental status or new focal neurologic signs should resolve rather quickly in this situation. If there is a significant change from the baseline examination, a CT or MRI study is obtained to rule out postoperative hemorrhage or cerebral edema. Edema is expected and can often be treated with corticosteroids. Significantly increased ICP requires medical management in an intensive care environment with the patient under close observation. Occasionally, surgical intervention is required for acute postoperative hemorrhage. Table 7-7 outlines a surgical treatment plan for patients with brain tumors. See

Chapter 9 for a discussion of neuroscience critical care management.

Postacute and Nonacute Care. It is useful to have knowledge of the resources—both in the hospital setting and in the community—available to staff, the patient, and family members. Figure 7-10 shows a screening sample and discharge planning tool to be used by the multidisciplinary team. It should be implemented as soon as the patient has been transferred from the neuroscience critical care unit to the neuroscience nursing unit. Completion of this tool allows the team members to assess and prepare for specific needs at the time of discharge. For example, the following questions should be considered: Does the patient live alone? Will there be specific dietary needs? Is the home environment conducive to recovery? Will transportation to follow-up therapy be needed? If inpatient rehabilitation is needed, what center is appropriate for specific neurologic needs and for family convenience? What consultations will be needed postoperatively, and can they be obtained during the inpatient stay?

Before discharge, a physiatrist and rehabilitation medicine consultation should be obtained for most patients following surgery for a brain tumor. The physical and occupational therapists will evaluate the patient and provide a baseline assessment of any cranial nerve, motor, sensory, speech, or cognitive deficits. They will also make recommendations for further therapy if necessary. Plans are made before discharge for the appropriate level of therapy.

At the time of discharge, written instructions should again be given to the patient for his or her particular situation, with information on medication dosages and schedules, "do's and don'ts," and appropriate phone numbers for routine or emergency situations. It is virtually impossible to answer every question and predict all problems and side effects that the patient might experience. The clinician (i.e., registered nurse [RN], physician's assistant [PA], or nurse practitioner [NP])

TABLE 7-7	Surgical Treatment Plan of Care for Patients With CNS Tumors

Evaluation	Management/Care	Considerations
History and physical	Baseline evaluation to include the following: • Neurologic examination • Medication review • Review of medical and surgical history; history of present illness • Discussion of surgical risks and benefits • Preoperative laboratory studies/other testing/consults	Discuss same-day care process; most patients are admitted on surgery day and undergo preoperative testing as outpatients before admission. Develop teaching pamphlet or provide multiple phone conferences or office appointments.
Medications (steroids; anticonvulsants; discontinue warfarin, aspirin, or NSAID; continue other previously prescribed medications)	Provide information about medication schedules, side effects, expected duration of medications.	Individual steroid needs vary. Provide medical/hematology consults as needed.
Neuroimaging/testing	Identify tumor, provide comparison to previous imaging studies, assist in surgical planning.	Obtain preoperative MRI or CT shortly before surgery date. (MRA, fMRI, other testing when appropriate.) Perform EEG as needed. Perform ECG and chest x-ray examination. Perform other testing as needed.
Surgical procedure	Establish diagnosis, tumor removal.	It is preferable to discuss surgical consent with patient **and** family.
Intraoperative Management		
Neuroanesthesia	Ensure patient safety. Decreased risk of increased ICP, seizures.	Risks and benefits of anesthesia per physician. Family will be updated during the procedure.
Equipment/monitoring	Minimize intraoperative complications through tumor localization, safe tumor removal, more complete tumor resection, and protection of eloquent areas of the brain.	Specific intraoperative equipment depends on tumor type/location and institutional availability.
Postoperative Care		
Neurologic critical care	Perform complete neurologic examination (vital signs, level of consciousness, cranial nerves; motor; sensory; coordination). Evaluate and manage increased ICP.	Diet is resumed, activity is resumed as tolerated within 24 hours of surgery. MRI/CT scan is performed after surgery as baseline.
Inpatient monitoring	Prevent complications. Perform medical/surgical management of hemorrhage, infection, increased ICP, etc.	Encourage increased activity. Maximum brain edema during first 72 hours. Steroid taper usually begins during hospitalization.
Consultations/testing	Assess need for physical/ occupational therapy, radiation oncology, medical oncology.	Histology is available several days after surgery; therapy may begin 2–3 weeks after surgery. Ensure that appropriate referrals are in place before discharge, if possible. Discuss goals, duration, and possible side effects of therapy.
Discharge planning	Provide organized plan for home care and outpatient therapy. Supply information regarding community resources/support groups.	Discharge planning should be initiated on discharge from ICU. In some cases, hospice services may be necessary.

Modified from Bohan E, Glass-Macenka D: Surgical management of patients with primary brain tumors, *Semin Oncol Nurs* 20(4):240–252, 2004.
CT, Computed tomography; *ECG,* electrocardiogram; *EEG,* electroencephalogram; *ICP,* intracranial pressure; *ICU,* intensive care unit; *MRI,* magnetic resonance imaging; *NSAID,* nonsteroidal antiinflammatory drug.

Screening Information

Demographics	Name, date of birth, address, phone number, occupation.
Admission information	Include date of admission; patient ID number; ID bracelet applied; admission from home, emergency department, etc.; family spokesperson; admission information supplied by patient, family member, medical record, etc.
Diagnosis	
Medications	
Allergies	
Removable devices*	This section should include glasses, dentures, etc., and their disposition.
Personal habits	Alcohol, cigarettes, other.
*Sample: Removable Devices	_X_ Dentures _X_ Glasses ___Prosthesis(es) ___Hearing aid ___Contact lenses ___Other **Disposition:** *locked in safe at nurses station; patient to OR. EB*

Completed by _____   Initials _____   Date _____

Planning Tool

	Patient Information	Plan	Date Completed/ Initials
Nutrition*	Dietary restrictions, preferences		
Rehabilitation medicine needs	Deficits: mobility, activities of daily living		
Social work	Social and financial support, placement needs		
Consults	Other diagnoses requiring intervention		
Cultural	Native language and interpretive services needed		
Pastoral	Religious affiliation: does patient request chaplain?		
Discharge plan	Anticipated equipment or services needed at home; placement other than home		
*Sample: Nutrition	*Diabetes mellitus*	*1800 ADA diet* *Nutrition consult*	**12/22/07** **12/23/07** *EB*

Completed by _____   Initials _____   Date _____

Figure 7-10 Screening and discharge planning tool.

should encourage the patient to report any symptoms and to ask questions. It is also important to be reliable and consistent in returning phone calls. Because patients have a tendency to sit by the phone, waiting for a response, they should be told in advance when they should expect a call back. If their needs are more urgent, they should be given an emergency number to call. Certain events require a call to the local emergency medical system. Patients and family members should know when to use this number (e.g., acute change in mental status or loss of consciousness).

From the time a patient is treated for the first symptoms of a brain tumor, through the diagnostic workup and treatment phases—and even after therapy is completed—the knowledge that a tumor exists in the brain is frightening and overwhelming. More than with any other medical or surgical problem, an abnormality in the brain is a threat to the patient's individuality. Fear that this abnormality may change the processes of thinking or behaving or may actually render the patient incapable of understanding or communicating becomes a burden to the patient and to loved ones.

Although the role of the interdisciplinary medical team is important in the treatment of any medical problem, adequate care of the patient with a brain tumor depends on absolutely every member of the team. There are a number of individuals who coordinate patient care activities, as outlined in the following section. The clinician, however, is generally responsible for teaching and reinforcing previous teaching by other team members, documenting demographic and treatment planning information, carrying out specific patient treatments, and preparing the patient and family for follow-up care. The clinician is often asked to interpret information presented by other members of the treatment team. Therefore, in addition to having expertise in the areas of perioperative patient care, the clinician should have a clear understanding of the patient's classification and grade of tumor, tumor location and symptoms, medications and side effects, tests that may be required, postoperative therapies, and recent developments in the care of brain tumors.

Rehabilitation

In some cases a short outpatient therapy plan is initiated either in the home or at a rehabilitation facility 2 to 3 days per week. Occasionally an inpatient stay is required to speed recovery and to ensure maximal safety, quality of life, and independence. Neurologic deficits are dependent on the size and location of the tumor, as well as its invasiveness. Temporary deficits that may resolve independently of formal rehabilitation improve more rapidly with intensive, professional intervention.[85] A physiatrist and team of physical, occupational, and speech therapists work with clinicians, social workers, physicians, nutritionists, clergy, and the family to provide a comprehensive plan of care.[37] Traumatic brain injury units are often invaluable in addressing the postoperative needs of the patient after surgery for a brain tumor.

For patients who have undergone gross total removal of a benign brain tumor, no further therapy is required. Close observation for tumor recurrence is recommended indefinitely. The remainder of patients require one or several treatments for residual tumor. In the brain, even benign tumors may require adjuvant therapy to treat residual disease that cannot be aggressively removed without devastating neurologic consequences.

BOX 7-2	Use of Radiation in Brain Tumors

- Tumors stereotactically biopsied for diagnosis only
- Residual tumor after craniotomy
- Recurrent low-grade tumors
- Malignant, highly invasive tumors
- Brainstem lesions considered too dangerous for safe biopsy
- Brain metastases
- Symptom management (e.g., hypersecretory states in patients with pituitary adenomas)

Therapies

Radiation Therapy. Because many brain tumors cannot be resected completely, it is essential to provide therapy for residual neoplastic cells. The goal of radiation is to kill tumor cells by damaging their deoxyribonucleic acid (DNA) while protecting the surrounding normal tissue.[101] See Box 7-2 for situations where radiation is traditionally used.

Conventional Radiation Treatment

The goal of RT is to allow for the highest dose of radiation to the target area while minimizing effects to normal brain tissue. This is accomplished by producing enough energy to damage DNA just before the process of cell division. Because tumor cells are dividing rapidly, they are more sensitive to the radiation. There is a maximum tolerated dose from which normal cells are able to recover. Thus treatment planning is the key to ensuring protection of the normal brain while providing local control of tumor.[101] Simulation takes place before therapy, with imaging studies and measurements being taken while the patient is in the treatment position. This provides for localization of the tumor and precise treatment delivery. Treatment planning takes into account the preoperative tumor volume in cases where the tumor has been debulked or resected. The radiation oncologist assesses this information in combination with tumor histology to identify the fields to be treated. A facemask is typically used to prevent movement and decrease the risk of injury.

Conventional RT has been used effectively for many years. Current treatment typically uses fractionated (divided dose)[33] radiotherapy daily, 5 days a week, for approximately 6 weeks. Total doses vary with the tumor type but are generally in the range of 6000 centigray (cGy) for primary brain tumors. Studies have been conducted to establish if a lower dose would be appropriate and to dose escalate in the hope of increasing survival with higher doses. Results have indicated that survival data diminish with decreasing doses and doses greater than 6000 cGy provide no survival benefit.[107,126]

For brain metastases, particularly multiple metastases, shorter courses of radiotherapy are generally used. Whole brain RT, typically 10 treatments totaling 3000 cGy, is used in some institutions to provide palliation while improving neurologic status and minimizing toxicity.[113] Whole brain radiation, however, is no longer exclusively the treatment of choice for multiple metastases. The radiation oncologist discusses with the patient the risks and benefits of both whole brain radiation and stereotactic radiosurgery to individual lesions with the option of using whole brain at a later date if necessary. In patients with a single metastasis or controllable disease, combinations of surgery, higher-dose RT, stereotactic radiosurgery (SRS), and chemotherapy may be used to increase the likelihood of local control in the brain.[75,90]

Three-dimensional conformal radiation therapy (3DCRT) techniques (shaping of the radiation beam to conform to the shape of the entire tumor volume) are regularly used.[33] Machines designed to perform radiosurgery, such as the linear accelerator and gamma knife, are being used to administer stereotactic external beam conformal radiotherapy, with the goal of increasing the radiation dose but more accurately targeting the dose to decrease the volume of normal brain tissue receiving radiation.[61]

Intensity-Modulated Radiation Therapy

Intensity-modulated radiation therapy (IMRT) uses three-dimensional imaging as a planning technique for giving extremely focused radiation. It maximizes 3DCRT by using nonuniform radiation beams delivered in unique patterns. Its goal is to distribute a uniform dose to the tumor while minimizing the dose to surrounding normal tissue. IMRT provides greater control of the radiation dose distribution by allowing not only shaping of the beams in three dimensions to conform to the target, but by providing a means to vary the intensity of different parts of an individual beam to protect normal tissue within that beam or to escalate the dose to an area of tumor.[33,95]

Stereotactic Radiosurgery

An advance in the treatment of some types of brain lesions has come in the form of radiosurgery, which is able to locate the lesion in a three-dimensional plane and provide a single large dose or a small number of fractionated doses to a specific target. The principle is the same as that for a stereotactic biopsy. A frame is used, and coordinates are obtained, usually under MRI guidance. Varying doses of ionizing radiation may be given in extremely focused beams. There are currently several types of radiosurgery.

- Gamma knife: spherical dose distribution
- Linear accelerator: arc treatments using circular collimators
- Cyber knife: linear accelerator with robotic arm
- Tomotherapy: mounted linear accelerator rotates around the patient

Patients with relatively small (≤3 cm), solitary, fairly discrete lesions are good candidates for this therapy, but the use of radiosurgery varies by institution. Its use is being expanded to more infiltrative and larger lesions as techniques improve. The advantage of stereotactic radiosurgery is that it can give a high dose of radiation to a well-defined target while providing substantial protection to nearby normal tissue.[95,137,138]

Brachytherapy

Brachytherapy uses a radioactive material introduced into the tumor or the tumor resection cavity to provide high doses of radiation to a small area. It is also used in cases where external beam radiation therapy has previously been used.

The radioactive isotopes may be implanted on either a temporary or a permanent basis, delivering a dose within a 1 to 2 cm distance from the seeds.[123] Brachytherapy may be delivered by implantation of seeds or balloons for local delivery of high doses of radiation into the tumor or tumor resection cavity. One form of brachytherapy uses liquid iodine-125 introduced into a balloon that has been placed at the time of surgical resection. Once the brachytherapy is completed, the balloon may be removed. Figure 7-11 demonstrates preoperative enhanced MRI of GBM, a postoperative skull x-ray film, and MRI with the balloon in place, taken 1 day after balloon placement.[22,77]

Radiosensitizers

Substances are being evaluated for their ability to enhance the effects of RT. It is thought that the addition of certain agents may increase destruction of tumor cells while preserving the integrity of normal cells. Multiple substances have been used in other solid tumors to potentiate the effects of radiation.

Several recent studies are based on the hypothesis that tumors are hypoxic and that hypoxia decreases the effectiveness of RT. Introducing a substance that improves the uploading of oxygen to the hypoxic tumor tissue will enhance the effectiveness of RT. One such sensitizer, efaproxiral (RSR13), has been administered in conjunction with RT in phase I and II studies. Safety and drug dosing have been established, with evidence of survival benefit.[62,110]

Boron Neutron Capture Therapy

The basic premise of boron neutron capture therapy (BNCT) is to use atomic energy and nuclear fission to treat human subjects with various types of tumors. Reactors have been used to produce particles that concentrate in and kill tumor cells. BNCT is a promising type of indirect nuclear therapy. BNCT uses a carrier (boronated compounds), most commonly given intravenously, followed by radiation (neutron beams) delivered from a nuclear reactor. The boronated compounds capture the neutrons to yield high-energy radiation particles that are deposited in and treat a very localized area, while sparing normal tissue. Only selected centers are using this highly specialized therapy for certain types of brain tumors—most commonly glioblastoma and melanoma.[6,82,121]

Chemotherapy. Many brain tumors are benign and do not require further intervention beyond surgical removal. Some low-grade tumors cannot be removed in their entirety because of their diffuse and infiltrative characteristics and may require additional treatment with RT or chemotherapy.[76] Malignant neoplasms are often treated with multimodality therapy, including surgical debulking, radiation, chemotherapy, and investigational approaches.

Malignant gliomas—the most common primary brain tumors—are notoriously resistant to chemotherapy. A number of drugs are being used alone or in combination with other therapies in the hope of improving survival. Recent results of studies using the alkylating agent temozolomide have shown that low-dose use concurrently with RT and higher doses continuing after RT increase survival compared with RT alone. Once RT is complete, temozolomide is given orally for 5 days in 28-day cycles.[115] The nitrosoureas are administered as carmustine (BCNU) in an intravenous (IV) form and

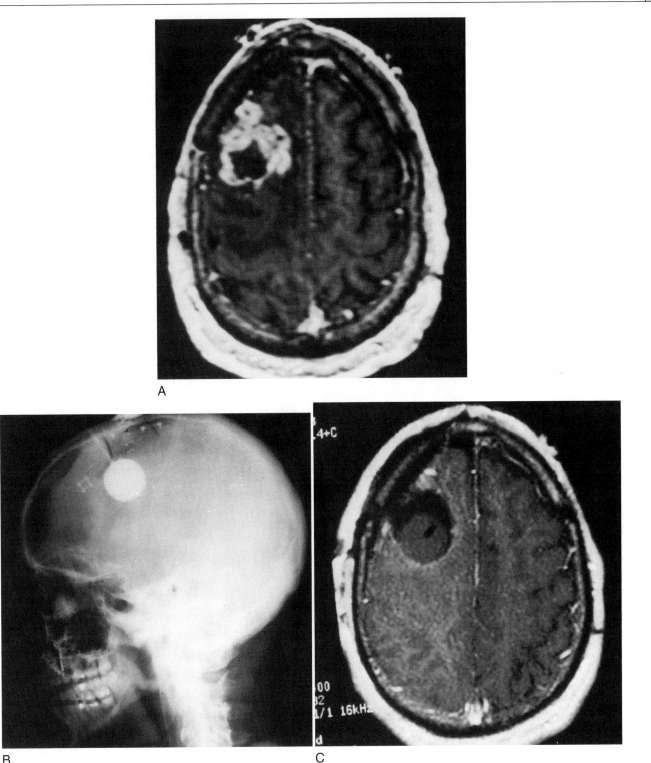

A

B   C

Figure 7-11 Liquid iodine-125 brachytherapy. **A,** Preoperative enhanced axial MRI of recurrent glioblastoma multiforme. **B,** Postoperative skull x-ray film with balloon in place. **C,** Postoperative enhanced axial MRI of tumor resection cavity with balloon in place.
(Courtesy of Dr. Alessandro Olivi, Johns Hopkins University, Baltimore, MD.)

Figure 7-12 A, Chemotherapy-impregnated polymers being removed from sterile packaging at the time of surgery for malignant glioma. **B,** Intraoperative view of polymers implanted in the tumor bed after tumor resection. **C,** Polymers appear black on the axial T_1-weighted MRI.

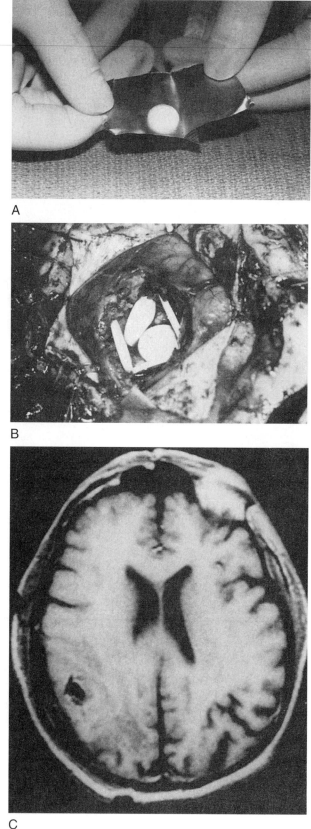

A

B

C

lomustine (CCNU), the oral preparation. They are typically given approximately every 6 weeks. Dosing of CCNU may be difficult if the patient has vomiting as a side effect. A combination therapy using procarbazine, lomustine, and vincristine (PCV) has been used for malignant gliomas. Procarbazine is also administered as a single agent to treat recurrent malignant gliomas (Table 7-8).

In an effort to bypass the problems presented by the BBB and to avoid systemic toxicities associated with IV or oral chemotherapeutic agents, a biodegradable polymer impregnated with BCNU was developed.[13,14,128] The polymers are implanted at the time of surgery and release the drug over 2 to 3 weeks. They can be used at the time of initial diagnosis and at recurrence. They are commercially available as Gliadel (GMI Pharma, Inc., Minneapolis, MN). Studies have also been completed showing the safety of higher-dose BCNU wafers,[91] and efficacy studies are forthcoming. Figure 7-12 shows the appearance of a wafer as it is being removed from the sterile foil wrap, intraoperative placement of wafers, and the postoperative appearance of the wafers on an MRI scan.

Table 7-8 presents a more detailed description of the commonly used drugs for malignant gliomas with doses and side effects. Multiple other drugs and combination therapies are also being used for malignant brain tumors because there is currently no one approach that provides acceptable survival benefit. These approaches include new drugs or drugs that have been effective in the treatment of other solid tumors; chemotherapeutic agents administered before or concurrently with radiation; chemical BBB disruption before or in conjunction with chemotherapy; and chemotherapy given intraarterially.[41,115]

Investigational Therapies. Despite the advances made in neuroimaging, neurosurgery, radiation therapy, and medical oncology, the prognosis for most patients with malignant brain tumors remains poor. Therefore attempts are being made to use aggressive new approaches to the treatment of these tumors. Innovative techniques for delivering radiation and chemotherapy, which have been approved by the U.S. Food and Drug Administration (FDA), have been discussed previously in this chapter. In addition, many new approaches are under development.

New therapeutics must establish that they are safe and effective before they are approved for marketing. This process is the responsibility of the FDA. Although beyond the scope of this chapter, the process of developing a new drug requires approximately 10 to 15 years and is estimated to cost almost 900 million dollars. In addition, only one out of 5000 to 10,000 compounds that enter preclinical testing is approved

TABLE 7-8 Selected Chemotherapeutic Agents for the Treatment of Malignant Gliomas

Drug	Description	Dose	Side Effects	Nursing Implications and Comments
Carmustine (BCNU)	Nitrosourea Alkylating agent Lipid soluble	150–200 mg/m^2 IV every 6–8 weeks	Myelosuppression Gastrointestinal Fatigue Pulmonary fibrosis	Teaching re: need for blood tests/office visits. Serum blood counts at 3 and 6 weeks. See Table 7-9. Seen after multiple (+6) cycles. Pulmonary function tests suggested.
Lomustine (CCNU)	Nitrosourea Alkylating agent Lipid soluble Has a short half life	130 mg/m^2 orally at bedtime every 6 weeks _SE = N/V_	Same as BCNU Bone marrow toxicity may be more cumulative than BCNU	Teaching re: need for blood tests/office visits. Serum blood counts at 3 and 6 weeks.
Temozolomide _used alone in combo. for malignant gliomas_	Methylating agent	150–200 mg/m^2 for 5 days in a 28-day cycle (lower doses used during RT)	Myelosuppression Gastrointestinal Fatigue Rash	Blood tests before next dosing. Teaching re: need for blood tests/office visits. Studies in adjuvant use in GBM with RT; recurrent grade III astrocytoma. Approximately 10% of patients suffer extended periods of low platelets or other blood count abnormalities, requiring transfusions. Once counts recover, lower doses may be used.
Procarbazine, CCNU, vincristine (PCV)	Triple-drug therapy	42-day cycle; procarbazine = 60 mg/m^2 from day 8–21 CCNU = 110 mg/m^2 orally on day 1 Vincristine = 1.4 mg/m^2 on days 14 and 29	Myelosuppression Gastrointestinal Fatigue Pulmonary symptoms Peripheral neuropathy Irreversible myelosuppression possible with multiple nitrosourea regimens	Serum blood counts at 3 and 6 weeks (some oncologists obtain weekly levels). No survival benefit of PCV over single-agent BCNU. Vincristine has been eliminated because of side effects (neuropathy) combined with inability to cross BBB.
Procarbazine	Alkylating agent	56 day cycle; 125–150 mg/m^2 for 28 days; no drug for 28 days	Myelosuppression Interactions with some drugs (e.g., MAO inhibitors)	Serum blood counts. Occasionally used as single agent for recurrence.
Gliadel chemotherapy wafers	Carmustine wafers Biodegradable over 2–3 weeks	Implanted at the time of tumor surgery Eight 7.7 mg wafers Stored at −20° C	Local brain edema May cause treatment necrosis Studies showed no systemic side effects	Steroids may be required in larger amounts or for longer duration to decrease edema.

Data provided by Michel Zeltzman, CRNP, Department of Medical Oncology, Johns Hopkins, Baltimore, MD.

for marketing.[83] In general, therapeutic development can be divided into phases. The first phase is the preclinical phase, which involves testing (both in vitro and in animal model systems). If successful, an application for an investigational new drug (IND) must be submitted to the FDA. If approved, clinical trials begin with phase I studies that focus on human safety and pharmacology of the agent tested. Phase II studies examine the effectiveness of a therapeutic agent. Phase III studies are larger clinical trials and the final step before submitting a new drug application to the FDA. Some of the current investigational approaches being developed in the laboratory and being tested in phase I to III trials are described here.

As described earlier, Gliadel wafers are approved for use in patients with newly diagnosed high-grade malignant gliomas as an adjunct to surgery and radiation, and in patients with recurrent GBM as an adjunct to surgery.[38] The success of Gliadel wafers has led to the development of numerous other polymer-based antineoplastic treatment approaches utilizing other conventional chemotherapeutic compounds, angiogenesis inhibitors, and immunomodulators. For more detailed information regarding the preclinical analysis of these polymer-based treatment approaches for patients with brain tumors, the reader is referred to the work of Raza and colleagues (2005).[102]

In recent years, much research has focused on various tumors' resistance to chemotherapy. A major mechanism of resistance to alkylnitrosoureas such as BCNU is the DNA repair protein, O6-alkylguanine-DNA alkyltransferase (AGT). This enzyme enables tumors to resist the effects of many chemotherapeutic agents. In brain tumor patients treated with BCNU, higher AGT levels correlated with poorer survival.[9,57] The substance O6-benzylguanine (O6-BG) binds to and inactivates AGT, diminishing the cells' ability to repair the DNA and thus potentiating the cytotoxic effects of BCNU.[40] The combination of systemic BCNU and O6-BG, however, results in severe bone marrow toxicity. To minimize this toxicity, preclinical models evaluated the efficacy of locally delivered BCNU after pretreatment with O6-BG. They demonstrated improved survival without significant toxicities.[103] Phase I and phase I/II clinical trials of Gliadel BCNU polymers (implanted at the time of surgery for recurrent malignant glioma) combined with IV administration of O6-BG have been completed,[100] and a phase II clinical trial is currently underway.

Another strategy to overcome the limitations of the BBB is through convection-enhanced delivery (CED). CED is a drug delivery method that uses positive pressure infusion to generate a pressure gradient that optimizes distribution of macromolecules within the brain. This method is currently being explored in the targeting of tumor cell surface proteins. More specifically, the interleukin-13 receptor alpha 2 (IL-13Rα2) chain is expressed on a majority of GBMs, but not in normal brain tissue. IL13-PE38 is a protein in which interleukin-13 is conjugated with the enzymatically active portion of *Pseudomonas* exotoxin A.[24] Thus this strategy selectively brings a toxin to tumor cells expressing IL-13Rα2. Numerous phase I and II trials demonstrated that CED of IL13-PE38 can be safely administered to patients.[66] A phase III randomized study testing the efficacy of IL13-PE38 CED is ongoing.

An alternative mechanism to increase the intracranial dose of chemotherapeutics is via disruption of the BBB. Although this can be accomplished with several agents, mannitol is most commonly used. With this protocol, the BBB is transiently opened allowing enhanced intracranial delivery of antineoplastic agents. Several clinical trials incorporating this strategy are ongoing.[34]

Viral-based gene therapy strategies have also been developed to treat patients with malignant gliomas. In general terms, the basis underlying this methodology is the selective destruction of neoplastic cells by the introduction of a specific gene via a virus. The introduction of several genes via different viruses (including retroviruses, adenoviruses, and herpes viruses) has been used in phase I and II clinical trials.[23]

Tumor vaccination is also under development for patients with malignant gliomas. In this modality, the patient's tumor is exposed, in vitro, to either autologous immune system cells such as dendritic cells or to an immunostimulant and subsequently readministered to the patient. These activated immune cells, once readministered to the patient, induce an antitumor response within the brain. Several phase I trials have been completed demonstrating that this is a safe strategy.[105,114,135,139] Additional studies will be necessary to evaluate efficacy.

These and other approaches to the treatment of primary malignant gliomas are being explored in experimental studies at numerous institutions. Both systemic and local therapies are being used, and patient outcomes are being assessed.

Data collection and interpretation must be precise. Patient and family understanding and informed consent are necessary both ethically and legally. Eligibility requirements are highly structured and are mandated for each protocol participant. It is often difficult for a patient to learn that he or she is not eligible for a study that may be perceived as the only logical avenue for treatment of a recurrent malignant neoplasm. It is crucial for the multidisciplinary team to provide reasonable, viable alternative treatments.

Several studies have assessed patient understanding of informed consent. Patients who had received additional information from a research clinician, a booklet, or an interactive computer program were more likely to be knowledgeable about the details of the clinical trial, voluntary nature of the trial, and availability of other treatments than those who had been given the standard interview alone.[27]

Several brain tumor consortia and cooperative groups have been organized to facilitate the process of exploring new treatment modalities and to maximize patient participation in clinical trials. The consortium approach makes it possible to consolidate the resources of a number of brain tumor treatment centers. They are able to provide multiple clinical trials that test new treatments for both newly diagnosed and recurrent tumors.[46]

Side Effects of Therapy

Although the surgical and medical management of patients with all classes of brain tumors has become increasingly more sophisticated, accurate, and effective over the past several decades, these treatments are often associated with a number of side effects. Some of the side effects are short-lived and mild, whereas others may be life threatening or greatly compromise quality of life. The effects of tumor growth on ICP are discussed earlier in this chapter. Tumor treatments may also increase ICP. The medications used to treat ICP and seizures are not without consequence for many patients.

A significant number of patients with brain tumors (35%) develop thromboembolic disorders, such as deep vein thrombosis and pulmonary embolus. Patients may have various symptoms ranging from leg swelling and pain to shortness of breath and respiratory distress.[39,41]

Combining chemotherapy, anticonvulsants, anticoagulants, or other medications can alter the effectiveness of one or more of these drugs by activating the P450 enzyme in the liver, increasing metabolism, and accelerating drug clearance.[41] Patients may suffer significant cognitive compromise from these treatments.[7] Some treatments affect the immune system, rendering the patient more susceptible to other illnesses (e.g., steroid-induced *Pneumocystis carinii* pneumonia [PCP]).[99] Side effects necessitate withholding or discontinuing treatment, thus increasing the risk of tumor recurrence. Finally, return to work or other activities of daily living (ADLs), such as driving, housekeeping, or sports, may be delayed during treatment and for a period of time after therapy. Further discussion of the side effects of treatments, symptom management, and patient and family teaching is presented in Table 7-9.

COMPREHENSIVE PATIENT MANAGEMENT: BRAIN TUMORS

Nutritional Considerations

A nutritional assessment for patients with a brain tumor should include the unique needs of the individual. This includes a neurologic assessment of the individual's level of cognition, impaired memory, and any cranial nerve deficits that involve problems with chewing and swallowing, or dysphagia. Nutritional requirements are determined both from the neurologic disease process and from nutritional needs to promote healing, combat malnutrition, and restore energy. The assessment should also include evaluation of the individual's health history (e.g., diabetes or other major health concerns). ADLs, laboratory values (such as serum albumin), weight loss or gain, medications, renal status or disease, and the presence of pressure ulcers are important considerations. Of equal importance are the individual's past and current eating patterns, appetite level, side effects of medications/treatments, and psychosocial and mental health status (such as the presence of depression), as well as cultural and religious beliefs. The use or abuse of alcohol and drugs also factors into the nutritional evaluation. Consultation with the nutritionist to review the nutritional assessment helps to formulate a dietary plan that will promote nutrition and provide safe eating and swallowing,

the use of adaptive equipment, and the need for supplemental feedings.

The care of individuals with dysphagia requires the interdisciplinary team's evaluation, often with a speech pathologist's evaluation, and the development of a swallowing protocol for individuals who require enteral nutrition. The feeding plan may include a nasogastric (NG) tube, nasointestinal (NI) tube, percutaneous endoscopic gastrostomy (PEG) tube, percutaneous endoscopic jejunostomy tube (J-tube), or gastrostomy tube (G-tube). Family and health care providers need special instructions for the care of (and methods of feeding and administration of medications to) individuals with feeding tubes.

Older Adult Considerations

As American culture prepares for the increased population of older adults in all aspects of culture, there is ongoing discussion about how to best provide for their physical, financial, and emotional needs. Therefore the health care of older individuals is currently a major priority. The incidence of some tumor types (e.g., meningioma) increases with age, and many of these patients are in otherwise extremely good health. Advances in brain tumor imaging have led to accurate and early diagnosis. Intraoperative monitoring and instrumentation have improved outcomes for all age-groups. Adjuvant therapies are being developed and improved. All of these factors are encouraging for continued improvements in survival.

Although many older patients are able to tolerate medical and surgical brain tumor treatments, they also require closer monitoring in the hospital setting and improved resources in the community. Family members increasingly find themselves in the role of caregiver. It is necessary to closely monitor medication schedules and be vigilant for drug side effects and interactions. Older patients are more quickly susceptible to the complications of immobility and require increased levels of activity as tolerated. Moreover, some older patients experience temporary cognitive impairment or exacerbation of preexisting cognitive problems during and after treatment.

The multidisciplinary neuro-oncology team is faced with the challenge of providing a level of care that enhances not only survival but also quality of life for the older population. A plan of care that provides for treatment of the tumor with a maximal degree of independence is a challenge that faces the entire medical team.

Case Management Considerations

Once the patient has been diagnosed with a brain tumor, how can an organized and effective plan of care be put into place? How can it be ensured that the plan is implemented? As has been indicated, this is not a solitary event that begins and ends on a preplanned schedule. It involves a series of activities, some unplanned and unanticipated. Although there is no formula for a positive patient experience, the outline in Box 7-3 describes a comprehensive plan of care for the patient being treated for a brain tumor.

TABLE 7-9 Side Effects of Treatments

Selected Side Effects	Symptoms	Symptom Management Patient/Family Teaching
Surgery (for Biopsy or Tumor Removal)		
General		
Anesthetic reaction	Nausea, vomiting	Antiemetics, comfort measures—goal to reduce straining, which increases ICP.
Hemorrhage	Headache, changes in mental status, neurologic deterioration	May require reoperation.
Infection	Wound erythema, drainage	Antibiotics; possible reoperation.
Neurologic		
Increased ICP	Headache, nausea, vomiting; mental status changes	Modify steroids.
Seizures	Related to tumor location	For more in-depth discussion of increased ICP, seizures, and craniotomy, see Chapters 10, 24, and 8, respectively.
Focal signs	Related to tumor location	
Chemotherapy (Attempt to Destroy Residual Tumor Cells)		
Effect on dividing cells	Anemia	Doses and schedules may need to be modified to adjust for side effects.
	Thrombocytopenia (increased risk of intracranial hemorrhage)	Transfusions/medications when indicated.
	Neutropenia (predisposition to infection)	
	Fatigue	Plan events and rest periods accordingly.
	Gastrointestinal: nausea and vomiting	Antiemetics before treatment and as needed; dietary changes to include bland/favorite foods; small, more frequent meals.
	Alopecia	Volunteer organizations in many communities to help with scarf tying, wig styling, makeup, etc.
Interactions with other drugs	See anticonvulsants (see Table 7-6)	
Emboli (DVT/PE)	Leg swelling; shortness of breath or agitation	Seen in patients with brain tumors, especially high-grade gliomas; can occur at any point during course of illness; also occurs in patients who have never received chemotherapy.
		Associated with decreased mobility.
		Ultrasound or venogram for diagnosis.
		Treat with anticoagulation or IVC filter placement.
		Brain CT before anticoagulation.
Radiation Therapy (Attempt to Destroy Residual Tumor Cells)		
Increased ICP (discussed above)		
Other symptoms related to area of treatment (e.g., endocrine changes after treating pituitary gland)	Headache, nausea, vomiting; mental status changes; neurologic deterioration	Symptoms are treated with the addition or modification of glucocorticoids.
	Alopecia	In the first 3 months after RT, CT/MRI may show increased contrast enhancement secondary to blood-brain barrier breakdown rather than tumor progression/recurrence.
Local Therapies (e.g., Chemotherapy, Radiation Placed Into Tumor or Tumor Resection Cavity)		
Increased ICP caused by high-dose therapy into the tumor	Discussed above	
Tumor necrosis	Symptoms related to increased ICP	Necrosis may require reoperation.
		An increase in glucocorticoid dose and/or duration may be necessary.
		Necrosis has a radiographic appearance similar to malignant tumor; PET or MRS may be used to differentiate necrosis from recurrent tumor.
Experimental/Investigational Protocols		
Side effects are unknown at time of treatment		Make clear in the informed consent that specific side effects are unknown and that patient's participation in the study may lead to new information.

Data from references 3, 35, 39, 41, 42, 48, 52, 67, 69, 70, 72, 76, 99, 126.
CT, Computed tomography; *DVT/PE,* deep vein thrombosis/pulmonary embolism; *ICP,* intracranial pressure; *MRI,* magnetic resonance imaging; *MRS,* magnetic resonance spectroscopy; *PET,* positron emission tomography; *RT,* radiation therapy.

BOX 7-3 Case Management for Patients with Brain Tumors

Clinical presentation: complete an assessment, chart review, and interviews with the health care team.

Diagnostic workup: review all diagnostic test results and orders for continuing studies, including the following:
- History and physical examination
- Results from MRI or CT and other diagnostic studies as indicated

Treatment:
- Administer medications, including steroids, antacids, and anticonvulsants, when indicated; continue patient teaching regarding medication dosage, time and frequency of administration, potential side effects, and importance of strict compliance.
- Discuss stereotactic biopsy or craniotomy results and the need for follow-up appointments with the health care team.
- Explain the inpatient or outpatient rehabilitation plan; patient may have orders for home rehabilitation therapy and a plan for independent exercises.
- Outline the radiation therapy program and potential side effects; if patient has completed radiation, discuss the outpatient plan, including scheduled appointments.
- Review chemotherapy and potential side effects. Local therapy (implantable sustained-release chemotherapy wafers or local radiation therapy).
- Systemic chemotherapy with treatment schedule and side effects.
- If patient has completed treatments, discuss the outpatient follow-up schedule.

Plan for follow-up:
- Serial MRI or CT scans with frequency based on the histologic diagnosis and clinical status.

Multidisciplinary team:
- To include neurologists, neurosurgeons, medical oncologists, radiation oncologists, neuroradiologists, clinicians, social workers, and neuropathologists.
- Follow-up appointments with appropriate team members.

Community resources:
- Contact national and regional brain tumor associations.
- Enroll patient in a support group if available and based on patient preference.

Individual needs:
- Discuss specific patient care issues, such as the following: driving restrictions; patient needs to notify Department of Motor Vehicles; wig for treatment-related alopecia; physician may submit prescription to insurance company for possible reimbursement.

Recognize signs and symptoms of tumor recurrence:
- Discuss possible reoperation for debulking of tumor to decrease ICP and facilitate further therapies.
- Discuss additional radiation or chemotherapy (systemic or local therapies) when appropriate.
- Screen patient for experimental protocols.
- Teach the patient about the potential risks, unknown benefits, and alternative treatment options.

Hospice:
- Before patient's enrollment in home hospice, assess family supports.
- Provide respite care/inpatient hospice as patient or family needs warrant it.

CT, Computed tomography; *ICP,* intracranial pressure; *MRI,* magnetic resonance imaging.

The majority of patients diagnosed with brain tumors die of the disease or treatment-related complications. Yet there is very little in the literature regarding quality-of-life and end-of-life issues. Patients and family members find it difficult to prepare for death, particularly in the setting of such aggressive approaches to treatment. It is the responsibility of the multidisciplinary team not only to recommend appropriate treatment modalities but also to acknowledge the time when comfort measures are warranted. The neuro-oncology clinician plays an integral role in this process.[31] Hospitals are increasingly initiating palliative care services for inpatient care and discharge planning.[12,51]

Hospice

Resources vary by community, but most locales have home **hospice** services. This enables the patient to die at home with family members providing comfort measures and participating in terminal care. Medical professionals make regular, planned visits to the home to administer medications and treatments and to provide information and family support. Many hospice facilities have special services for children of terminal patients.

Hospice also includes inpatient services for patients whose needs are too great for the home environment. Respite care is also offered in many institutions. The patient is admitted to the hospice facility for a short stay (approximately 2 weeks) while the family attends to other important matters or takes a much-needed rest. Insurance plans vary, but many offer excellent hospice benefits.

CONCLUSION

Brain tumors, both benign and malignant, are diagnosed in children, as well as in adults; in men and women alike; in all communities; and in all races and ethnic groups. Some tumors are followed conservatively and never need treatment. Others are completely removed surgically and require no further therapy. However, the majority of brain tumors require multimodality therapy, including surgery, radiation therapy, and chemotherapy. Often these tumors recur, and the patient is subjected to further treatment. Investigational protocols, with unknown benefit, may be offered. The most aggressive (and most common) primary brain tumors are not associated with long-term survival. Patients may require rehabilitation, and eventually, many patients with brain tumors require the support of inpatient or home hospice services. Family members may experience difficulty adjusting to a loved one's diagnosis and be unprepared for the caregiver role.

In an effort to adequately treat primary and metastatic brain tumors, new surgical and medical techniques have been developed that have shown promise. Intraoperative equipment and monitoring techniques have continued to develop, with new ways of identifying and mapping brain function in order to enhance surgical safety and accuracy. Advances are being made in the delivery of both radiation and chemotherapy. Moreover, new genetic and biologic approaches are being explored. Multi-institutional consortia have been developed to explore new drugs and new delivery systems. These significant advances in diagnosis and treatment of brain tumors, combined with an improved multidisciplinary approach, have the goals of increasing survival and quality of life for patients with brain tumors and their families.

Acknowledgments

The authors would like to thank Dr. Lawrence Kleinberg and Michel Zeltzman, CRNP, Johns Hopkins University, Baltimore, Maryland, for their advice and expertise.

RESOURCES FOR PATIENTS AND CAREGIVERS

Acoustic Neuroma Association: 600 Peachtree Plaza, Suite 108, Cummings, GA 30041-6899; 770-205-8211; fax: 770-205-0239; www.anausa.org; e-mail: ANAUSA@aol.com

American Brain Tumor Association: 2720 River Road, Suite 146, Des Plaines, IL 60018-4110; 800-886-2282; fax: 847-827-9918; www.abta.org; e-mail: info@aBTA.org

American Cancer Society: 800-227-2345; www.cancer.org

Musella Foundation: 1100 Peninsula Boulevard, Hewelett, NY 11557; 516-295-4740; www.virtualtrials.com/btlinks; e-mail: musella@aol.com

National Brain Tumor Foundation: 22 Battery Street, Suite 612, San Francisco, CA 91111-5520; 800-934-2873; www.braintumor.org; e-mail: nbtf@braintumor.org

National Cancer Institute, National Institutes of Health: 800-422-6237; www.cancer.gov

New Approaches to Brain Tumor Therapy (NABTT): www.NABTT.org

Pituitary Tumor Network Association: 16350 Ventura Boulevard, Suite 231, Encino, CA 91436; 805-499-9973; www.pituitary.org

T.H.E. Brain Trust: 186 Hampshire Street, Cambridge, MA 02139-1320; 617-876-2002; www.braintrust.org; e-mail: info@braintrust.org

The Brain Tumor Society: 124 Watertown Street, Suite 3H, Boston, MA 02472-2500; 800-770-8287; www.tbts.org; e-mail: info@TBTS.org

The Health Resources, Inc.: 564 Locust Street, Conway, AR 72032; 501-329-5272

Vestibular Disorders Association: PO Box 4467, Portland, OR; 800-837-8428; fax: 503-229-8064

REFERENCES

1. Akella NS, Twieg DB, Mikkelsen T, et al: Assessment of brain tumor angiogenesis inhibitors using perfusion magnetic resonance imaging: quality and analysis results of a phase I trial, *J Magn Reson Imaging* 20(6):913–922, 2004.

2. Amundson EW, McGirt MJ, Olivi A: A contralateral, transfrontal, extraventricular approach to stereotactic brainstem biopsy procedures, *J Neurosurg* 102(3):565–570, 2005.

3. Armstrong TS, Kanusky JT, Gilbert MR: Seize the moment to learn about epilepsy in people with cancer, *Clin J Oncol Nurs* 7:163–169, 2003.

4. Armstrong TS: Introduction, *Semin Oncol Nurs* 20(4):221–223, 2004.

5. Bajaj GK, Kleinberg L, Terezakis S: Current concepts and controversies in the treatment of parenchymal brain metastases: improved outcomes with aggressive management, *Cancer Invest* 23(4):363–376, 2005.

6. Barth RF, Coderre JA, Vicente MG, Blue TE: Boron neutron capture therapy of cancer: current status and future prospects, *Clin Cancer Res* 11(11):3987–4002, 2005.

7. Baumgartner K: Neurocognitive changes in cancer patients, *Semin Oncol Nurs* 20(4):284–290, 2004.

8. Becker SS, Jackler RK, Pitts LH: Cerebrospinal fluid leak after acoustic neuroma surgery: a comparison of the translabyrinthine, middle fossa, and retrosigmoid approaches, *Otol Neurotol* 24(1):107–112, 2003.

9. Belanich M, Pastor M, Randall T, et al: Retrospective study of the correlation between the DNA repair protein alkyltransferase and survival of brain tumor patients treated with carmustine, *Cancer Res* 56(4):783–788, 1996.

10. Bohnen NI et al: Descriptive and analytic epidemiology of brain tumors. In Black PM, Loeffler JS, editors: *Cancer of the nervous system*, Cambridge, MA, 1997, Blackwell Science.

11. Brandes AA, Tosoni A, Vastola F, et al: Efficacy and feasibility of standard procarbazine, lomustine, and vincristine chemotherapy in anaplastic oligodendroglioma and oligoastrocytoma after recurrent radiotherapy, *Cancer* 101:2079–2085, 2004.

12. Braunack-Mayer THN, Beilby J: The impact of the hospice environment on patient spiritual expression, *Oncol Nurs Forum* 32(5):1049–1055, 2005.

13. Brem H, Langer R: Polymer-based drug delivery to the brain, *Sci Med* 3:2–11, 1996.

14. Brem H, Piantadosi S, Burger PC, et al: Placebo-controlled trial of safety and efficacy of intraoperative controlled delivery by biodegradable polymers of chemotherapy for recurrent gliomas, *Lancet* 345:1008–1012, 1995.

15. Brem S, Panattil JG: An era of rapid advancement: diagnosis and treatment of metastatic brain cancer, *Neurosurgery* 57(5 suppl):5–9, 2005.

16. Bullitt E, Zeng D, Gerig G, et al: Vessel tortuosity and brain tumor malignancy: a blinded study, *Acad Radiol* 12(10):1232–1240, 2005.

17. Burger PC, Scheithauer BW, Vogel FS: The brain—tumors. In *Surgical pathology of the nervous system and its coverings,* ed 4, New York, 2002, Churchill Livingstone.

18. Central Brain Tumor Registry of the United States (CBTRUS): *Statistical report: 2004–2005 primary brain tumors in the United States, 1997–2001 years data collected,* Hinsdale, IL, 2004, CBTRUS.

19. Chamberlain M: Neoplastic meningitis, *J Clin Oncol* 23(15):3605–3613, 2005.

20. Chamberlain MC, Blumenthal DT: Intracranial meningiomas: diagnosis and treatment, *Summary Expert Review of Neurotherapeutics* 4(4):641–648, 2004.

21. Chamberlain MC: Intracerebral meningiomas, *Curr Treat Options Neurol* 6:297–305, 2004.

22. Chan TA, Weingart JD, Parisi M, et al: Treatment of recurrent glioblastoma multiforme with GliaSite brachytherapy, *Int J Radiat Oncol Biol Phys* 62(4):1133–1139, 2005.

23. Chiocca EA, Aghi M, Fulci G: Viral therapy for glioblastoma, *Cancer J* 9(3):167–179, 2003.

24. Debinski W, Obiri NI, PastanbI, Puri RK: A novel chimeric protein composed of interleukin 13 and *Pseudomonas* exotoxin is highly cytotoxic to human carcinoma cells expressing receptors for interleukin 13 and interleukin 4, *J Biol Chem* 270(28):16775–16780, 1995.

25. Doolittle ND, Abrey LE, Bleyer WA, et al: New frontiers in translational research in neuro-oncology and the blood-brain barrier: report of the tenth annual blood-brain barrier disruption consortium meeting, *Clin Cancer Res* 11:421–428, 2005.

26. Ell PJ: PET/CT in oncology: a major technology for cancer care, *Chang Gung Med J* 28(5):274–283, 2005.

27. Ellis PM: Attitudes towards and participation in randomized clinical trials in oncology: a review of the literature, *Ann Oncol* 11:939–945, 2000.

28. Engelhard HH: Brain tumors and the blood-brain barrier. In Bernstein M, Berger MS, editors: *Neuro-oncology: the essentials,* New York, 2000, Thieme.

29. Enticott JC, O'leary SJ, Briggs RJ: Effects of vestibulo-ocular reflex exercises on vestibular compensation after vestibular schwannoma surgery, *Otol Neurotol* 26(2):265–269, 2005.

30. Ezzat S, Asa SL, Couldwell WT, et al: The prevalence of pituitary adenomas: a systematic review, *Cancer* 101(3):613–619, 2004.

31. Fairbrother CA, Paice JA: Life's final journey: the oncology nurse's role, *Clin J Oncol Nurs* 9(5):575–579, 2005.

32. Fishman AJ, Marrinan MS, Golfinos JG, et al: Prevention and management of cerebrospinal fluid leak following vestibular schwannoma surgery, *Laryngoscope* 114(3):501–505, 2004.

33. Fiveash JB, Spencer SA: Role of radiation therapy and radiosurgery in glioblastoma multiforme, *Cancer J* 9(3):222–229, 2003.

34. Fortin D, Desjardins A, Beuko A, et al: Enhanced chemotherapy delivery by intraarterial infusion and blood-brain disruption in malignant brain tumors, *Cancer* 103(12):2606–2615, 2005.

35. Foy PM, Chadwick DW, Rajgopalan N, et al: Do prophylactic anticonvulsant drugs alter the pattern of seizures after craniotomy? *J Neurol Neurosurg Psychiatry* 55:753–757, 1992.

36. Friedman WA, Murad GJ, Bradshaw P, et al: Linear accelerator surgery for meningiomas, *J Neurosurg* 103(2):206–209, 2005.

37. Gabanelli P: A rehabilitative approach to the patient with brain cancer, *Neurol Sci* 26:S51–S52, 2005.

38. Gallia GL, Brem S, Brem H: Local treatment of malignant brain tumors using implantable chemotherapeutic polymers, *J Natl Compr Canc Netw* 3(5):721–728, 2005.

39. Gerber DE, Grossman SA, Streiff MB: Management of venous thromboembolism in patients with primary and metastatic brain tumors, *J Clin Oncol* 24(8):1310–1319, 2006.

40. Gerson SL: MGMT: its role in cancer aetiology and cancer therapeutics, *Nat Rev Cancer* 4(4):296–307, 2004.

41. Gilbert M, Loghin M: The treatment of malignant gliomas, *Curr Treat Options Neurol* 7:293–303, 2005.

42. Gomes JA, Stevens RD, Lewin JJ 3rd, et al: Glucocorticoid therapy in neurologic critical care, *Crit Care Med* 33(6):1214–1224, 2005.

43. Gonzales MF: Classification and pathogenesis of brain tumors. In Kaye AH, Laws ER Jr, editors: *Brain tumors: an encyclopedic approach*. New York, 1995, Churchill Livingstone.

44. Gottwald B, Wilde B, Mihajlovic Z, Mehdorn HM: Evidence for distinct cognitive deficits after focal cerebellar lesions, *J Neurol Neurosurg Psychiatry* 75:124–131, 2004.

45. Grant GA, Mayberg M: Vestibular schwannomas. In Bernstein M, Berger MS, editors: *Neuro-oncology: the essentials*. New York, 2000, Thieme.

46. Grossman SA, Fisher JD, Piantadosi S, Brem H: The new approaches to brain tumor therapy (NABTT) CNS consortium: organization, objectives, and activities, *Cancer Control* 5:107–114, 1998.

47. Gujar SK, Maheshwari S, Bjorkman-Burtscher I, et al: Magnetic resonance spectroscopy, *J Neuroophthalmol* 25(3):217–226, 2005.

48. Gurkanlar D, Er U, Sanli M, et al: Peritumoral edema in intracranial meningiomas, *J Clin Neurosci* 12(7):750–753, 2005.

49. Gurney JG, van Wijingaarden E: Extremely low frequency electromagnetic fields (EMF) and brain cancer in adults and children: review and comment, *Neurooncol* 1:212–220, 1999.

50. Hahn BM, Schrell UM, Sauer R, et al: Prolonged oral hydroxyurea and concurrent 3D-conformal radiation in patients with progressive or recurrent meningioma: results of a pilot study, *J Neurooncol* 74:157–165, 2005.

51. Hanley E: The role of palliative care services, *Care Manag J* 5(3):151–157, 2004.

52. Hildebrand J, Lecaille C, Perennes J, Delattre JY: Epileptic seizures during follow-up of patients treated for primary brain tumors, *Neurology* 65(3):212–215, 2005.

53. Hwu WJ, Lis E, Menell JH, et al: Temozolomide plus thalidomide in patients with brain metastases from melanoma: a phase II study, *Cancer* 103(12):2590–2597, 2005.

54. Inskip PD, Tarone RE, Hatch EE, et al: Laterality of brain tumors, *Neuroepidemiol* 22:130–138, 2003.

55. Inskip PD, Tarone RE, Hatch EE, et al: Cellular telephone use and brain tumors, *N Engl J Med* 344:79–86, 2001.

56. Isaacson B, Kileny PR, El-Kashlan HK: Prediction of long-term facial nerve outcomes with intraoperative nerve monitoring, *Otol Neurotol* 26(2):270–273, 2005.

57. Jaeckle KA, Eyre HJ, Townsend JJ, et al: Correlation of tumor O6 methylguanine-DNA methyltransferase levels with survival of malignant astrocytoma patients treated with bischloroethylnitrosourea: a Southwest Oncology Group study, *J Clin Oncol* 16(10):3310–3315, 1998.

58. Jane JA Jr, Vance ML, Woodburn CJ, Laws ER Jr: Stereotactic radiosurgery for hypersecreting pituitary tumors: part of a multimodality approach, *Neurosurg Focus* 14(5):e12, 2003.

59. Kaltsas GA, Nomikos P, Kontogeorgos G, et al: Clinical review: diagnosis and management of pituitary carcinomas, *J Clin Endocrinol Metab* 90(5):3089–3099, 2005.

60. Kamboj MK, Zhou P, Molofsky WJ, et al: Hemorrhagic pituitary apoplexy in an 18-year old male presenting as non-ketotic hyperglycemic coma (NKHC), *J Pediatr Endocrinol Metab* 18(6):611–615, 2005.

61. Khatua S, Jalali R: Recent advances in the treatment of childhood brain tumors, *Pediatr Hematol Oncol* 22(5):361–371, 2005.

62. Kleinberg L, Grossman SA, Carson K, et al: Survival of patients with newly diagnosed glioblastoma multiforme treated with RSR13 and radiotherapy: results of a Phase II New Approaches to Brain Tumor Consortium safety and efficacy study, *J Clin Oncol* 20(14):3149–3155, 2002.

63. Koerbel A, Gharabaghi A, Safavi-Abbasi S, et al: Evolution of vestibular schwannoma surgery: the long journey to current success, *Neurosurg Focus* 18(4):e10, 2005.

64. Kondziolka D, Bernstein M, Resch L, et al: Significance of hemorrhage into brain tumors: clinicopathological study, *J Neurosurg* 67:852-857, 1987.

65. Kreil W, Luggin J, Fuchs I, et al: Long term experience of gamma knife radiosurgery for benign skull base meningiomas, *J Neurol Neurosurg Psychiatry* 76:1425–1430, 2005.

66. Kunwar S: Convection enhanced delivery of IL13-PE38QQR for treatment of recurrent malignant glioma: presentation of interim findings from ongoing phase 1 studies, *Acta Neurochir Suppl* 88:105–111, 2003.

67. Laack NN, Brown PD: Cognitive sequelae of brain radiation in adults, *Semin Oncol* 31(5):702–713, 2004.

68. Langer CJ, Mehta MP: Current management of brain metastases, with a focus on systemic options, *J Clin Oncol* 23(25):6207–6219, 2005.

69. Laws ER: Surgical management of intracranial gliomas—does radical resection improve outcome? *Acta Neurochir* 85(suppl):47–53, 2003.

70. Lebrun C, Fontaine D, Kamaioli A, et al: Long-term outcome of oligodendrogliomas, *Neurology* 62:1783–1787, 2004.

71. Levy A: Pituitary disease: presentation, diagnosis, and management, *J Neurol Neurosurg Psychiatry* 75(suppl 3):47–52, 2004.

72. Lovely MP: Symptom management of brain tumor patients, *Semin Oncol Nurs Neurooncol* 20(4):273–283, 2004.

73. Lubina A, Olchovsky D, Berezin M, et al: Management of pituitary apoplexy: clinical experience with 40 patients, *Acta Neurochir* 147(2):151–157, 2005.

74. Lunsford LD, Niranjan A, Flickinger JC, et al: Radiosurgery of vestibular schwannomas: summary of experience in 829 cases, *J Neurosurg* 102(suppl):95–99, 2005.

75. Martin JJ, Kondiolka D: Indications for resection and radiosurgery for brain metastases, *Curr Opin Oncol* 17(6):584–587, 2005.

76. Mason W: Oligodendroglioma, *Curr Treat Options Neurol* 7:305–314, 2005.

77. Matheus MG, Castillo M, Ewend M, et al: CT and MRI imaging after placement of GliaSite radiation therapy system to treat brain tumor: initial experience, *Am J Neuroradiol* 25:1211–1217, 2004.

78. Melmed S, Vance ML, Barkan AL, et al: Current status and future opportunities for controlling acromegaly, *Pituitary* 5:185–196, 2002.

79. Mendenhall WM, Friedman WA, Amdur RJ, Foote KD: Management of benign skull base meningiomas: a review, *Skull Base* 14(1):53–60, 2004.

80. Meyer FB, Bates LM, Goerss SJ, et al: Awake craniotomy for aggressive resection of primary gliomas located in eloquent brain, *Mayo Clin Proc* 76:677–687, 2001.

81. Modha A, Gutin PH: Diagnosis and treatment of atypical and anaplastic meningiomas: a review, *Neurosurgery* 57(3):538–550, 2005.

82. Moore C, Hernandez-Santiago BI, Hurwitz SJ, et al: The boron-neutron capture agent beta-d: -5-o-carboranyl-2'-deoxyuridine accumulates preferentially in dividing brain tumor cells, *J Neurooncol* 74(3):275–280, 2005.

83. Moore SW: An overview of drug development in the United States and current challenges, *South Med J* 96(12):1244–1255, quiz 56, 2003.

84. Muacevic A, Jess-Hempen A, Tonn JC, Wowra B: Results of outpatient gamma knife radiosurgery for primary therapy of acoustic neuromas, *Acta Neurochir Suppl* 91:75–78, 2004.

85. Mukand JA, Blackinton DD, Crincoli MG, et al: Incidence of neurologic deficits and rehabilitation of patients with brain tumors, *Am J Phys Med Rehabil* 80(5):346–350, 2001.

86. Nakao N, Nakai K, Itakura T: Updating of neuronavigation on images intraoperatively acquired with a mobile computerized tomographic scanner: technical note, *Minim Invasive Neurosurg* 46:117–120, 2003.

87. Neder L, Colli BO, Machado HR, et al: MIB-1 labeling index in astrocytic tumors—a clinicopathologic study, *Clin Neuropahtol* 23(6):262–270, 2004.

88. Nussbaum ES, Pjalilian HR, Clio KH, Hall WA: Brain metastases: histology, multiplicity, surgery, and survival, *Cancer* 78:1781–1788, 1996.

89. Nutik SL, Babb MJ: Determinants of tumor size and growth in vestibular schwannomas, *J Neurosurg* 94:922–926, 2001.

90. O'Neill BP, Iturria NJ, Link MJ, et al: A comparison of surgical resection and stereotactic radiosurgery in the treatment of solitary brain metastases, *Int J Radiat Oncol Biol Phys* 55:1169–1176, 2003.

91. Olivi A, Grossman SA, Tatter S, et al: Dose escalation of carmustine in surgically implanted polymers in patients with recurrent malignant glioma: a new approach to brain tumor therapy. CNS Consortium Trial, *J Clin Oncol* 21(9):1845–1849, 2003.

92. Oyesiku NM: Assessment of pituitary function. In Rengachary SS, Ellenbogen RG, editors: *Principles of neurosurgery*, ed 2, Philadelphia, 2005, Elsevier Mosby.

93. Oyesiku NM: Nonfunctioning pituitary adenomas. In Rengachary SS, Ellenbogen RG, editors: *Principles of neurosurgery*, ed 2, Philadelphia, 2005, Elsevier Mosby.

94. Ozen O, Demiran B, Altinors N: Correlation between histological grade and MIB-1 and p53 immunoreactivity in meningiomas, *Clin Neuropathol* 24(5):219–224, 2005.

95. Pang LJ: Radiation oncology update, *Hawaii Med J* 62(5):109–110, 2003.

96. Phuphanich S, Baker SD, Grossman SA, et al: Oral sodium phenylbutyrate in patients with recurrent malignant gliomas: a dose escalation and pharmacologic study, *Neurooncol* 7(2):177–182, 2005.

97. Pickett CA: Update on the medical management of pituitary adenomas, *Curr Neurol Neurosci Rep* 5(3):178–185, 2005.

98. Pignatti F, van den Bent M, Curran D, et al: Prognostic factors for survival in adult patients with cerebral low-grade glioma, *J Clin Oncol* 20(8):2076–2084, 2002.

99. Pruitt AA: Treatment of medical complications in patients with brain tumors, *Curr Treat Options Neurol* 7(4):323–336, 2005.

100. Quinn JA, Desjardins A, Weingart J, et al: Phase I trial of temozolomide plus O6-benzylguanine for patients with recurrent or progressive malignant glioma, *J Clin Oncol* 23(28):7178–7187, 2005.

101. Rakesh RP, Wolfgang AT, Mehta MP: Radiation therapy for central nervous system tumors. In Rengachary SS, Ellenbo-

138. Yu C, Shepard D: Treatment planning for stereotactic radio-surgery with photon beams, *Technology in Cancer Research and Treatment* 2(2):93–104, 2003.

139. Yu JS, Liu G, Ying H, et al: Vaccination with tumor lysate-pulsed dendritic cells elicits antigen-specific, cytotoxic T-cells in patients with malignant glioma, *Cancer Res* 64(14): 4973–4979, 2004.

140. Zonenshayn M, Rezai A: Stereotactic surgery. In Rengachary SS, Ellenbogen RG, editors: *Principles of neurosurgery*, ed 2, Philadelphia, 2005, Elsevier Mosby.

SUGGESTED READINGS

Burger PC, Scheithauer BW, Vogel FS: The brain—tumors. In Burger PC, Scheithauer BW, Vogel FS: *Surgical pathology of the nervous system and its coverings*, ed 4, New York, 2002, Churchill Livingstone.

Entire issue. *Semin Oncol Nurs* 20(4), 2004.

Entire issue. *Neurosurgery* 57(suppl 5), 2005.

Rengachary SS, Ellenbogen RG, editors: *Principles of neurosurgery*, ed 2, Philadelphia, 2005, Elsevier Mosby.

gen RG, editors: *Principles of neurosurgery,* ed 2, Philadelphia, 2005, Elsevier Mosby.

102. Raza SM, Pradilla G, Legnani FG, et al: Local delivery of antineoplastic agents by controlled-release polymers for the treatment of malignant brain tumours, *Expert Opin Biol Ther* 5(4):477–494, 2005.

103. Rhines LD, Sampath P, Dolan ME, et al: O6-benzylguanine potentiates the antitumor effect of locally delivered carmustine against an intracranial rat glioma, *Cancer Res* 60(22): 6307–6310, 2000.

104. Rudnik A, Zawadzki T, Wojtacha M, et al: Endoscopic transnasal transsphenoidal treatment of pathology of the sellar region, *Minim Invas Neurosurg* 48:101–107, 2005.

105. Rutkowski S, DeVleeschouwer S, Kaempgen E, et al: Surgery and adjuvant dendritic cell-based tumour vaccination for patients with relapsed malignant glioma, a feasibility study, *Br J Cancer* 91(9):1656–1662, 2004.

106. Ryzenman JM, Pensak ML, Tew JM: Headache: a quality of life analysis in a cohort of 1,657 patients undergoing acoustic neuroma surgery: results from the Acoustic Neuroma Association, *Laryngoscope* 115(4):703–711, 2005.

107. Scott CB et al: Long-term results of RTOG 90-06. A randomized trial of hyperfractionated radiotherapy to 72Gy and carmustine vs. standard RT and carmustine for malignant glioma patients with emphasis on anaplastic astrocytoma patients, *Proc ASCO* 17:401a, 1998.

108. Selsnick SH, Liu JC, Jen A, Newman J: The incidence of cerebrospinal fluid leak after vestibular schwannoma surgery, *Otol Neurotol* 25(3):387–393, 2004.

109. Shaffrey ME, Farace E, Schiff D, et al: The Ki-67 labeling index as a prognostic factor in grade II oligoastrocytomas, *J Neurosurg* 102(6):1033–1039, 2005.

110. Shaw E, Scott C, Suh J, et al: RSR13 plus cranial radiation therapy in patients with brain metastases: comparison with the Radiation Therapy Oncology Group recursive partitioning analysis brain metastases database, *J Clin Oncol* 21(12): 2364–2371, 2003.

111. Shaw EG, Scheithauer BW, Dinapoli RP: Low-grade hemispheric astrocytomas. In Black PM, Loeffler JS, editors: *Cancer of the nervous system,* Cambridge, MA, 1997, Blackwell Science.

112. Shaw EG, Tatter SB, Lesser GJ, et al: Current controversies in the radiotherapeutic management of adult low-grade glioma, *Semin Oncol* 31(5):653–658, 2004.

113. Soffietti R, Costanza A, Laguzzi E, et al: Radiotherapy and chemotherapy for brain metastases, *J Neurooncol* 75:31–42, 2005.

114. Steiner HH, Bonsanto MM, Beckhove P, et al: Antitumor vaccination of patients with glioblastoma multiforme: a pilot study to assess feasibility, safety, and clinical benefit, *J Clin Oncol* 22(21):4272–4281, 2004.

115. Stupp R, Mason WP, van den Bent MJ, et al: Radiotherapy plus concomitant and adjuvant temozolomide for glioblastoma, *N Engl J Med* 352:987–996, 2005.

116. Trang RR, Megerian CA: I cannot smile or wink anymore: facial nerve weakness after acoustic neuroma surgery, *Curr Surg* 62(2):156–161, 2005.

117. Uy NW, Woo SY, The BS, et al: Intensity modulated radiation therapy (IMRT) for meningioma, *Int J Radiat Oncol Biol Phys* 53:1265–1270, 2002.

118. van den Bent MJ, Chinot O, Boogerd W, et al: Second-line chemotherapy with temozolomide in recurrent oligodendroglioma after PCV (procarbazine, lomustine, and vincristine)

chemotherapy: EORTC brain tumor group phase II s 26972, *Ann Oncol* 14:599–602, 2003.

119. van den Bent MJ, Looijenga LH, Langenberg K, et al: Cl mosomal anomalies in oligodendroglial tumors are correla with clinical features, *Cancer* 97:1276–1284, 2003.

120. van den Bent MJ, Taphoorn MJ, Brandes AA, et al: Phase study of first-line chemotherapy with temozolomide in recurrent oligodendroglioma tumors: the European organizati for research and treatment of cancer brain tumor group stud 26971, *J Clin Oncol* 21:2525–2528, 2003.

121. van Rij CM, Wilhelm AJ, Sauerwein WA, van Loenen AC Boron neutron capture therapy for glioblastoma multiforme *Pharm World Sci* 27(2):92–95, 2005.

122. Verhelst J, Abs R: Hyperprolactinemia: pathophysiology and management, *Treat Endorinol* 2(1):23–32, 2003.

123. Vitaz TW, Warnke PC, Tabar V, Gutin PH: Brachytherapy for brain tumors, *J Neurooncol* 73:71–86, 2005.

124. Wackym PA, King WA, Meyer GA, Poe DS: Endoscopy in neuro-otologic surgery, *Otolaryngol Clin North Am* 35(2):297–323, 2002.

125. Wackym PA: Stereotactic radiosurgery, microsurgery, and expectant management of acoustic neuroma: basis for informed consent, *Otolaryngol Clin North Am* 38(4):653–670, 2005.

126. Walker MD, Strike TA, Sheline GE: An analysis of dose-effect relationship in the radiotherapy of malignant gliomas, *Int J Radiat Oncol Biol Phys* 1725–1731, 1979.

127. Weingart J, Brem H: Basic principles of cranial surgery for brain tumors. In Winn HR, editor: *Youmans neurosurgical surgery,* ed 5, Philadelphia, 2003, Saunders.

128. Westphal M, Hilt DC, Bortey E, et al: A phase 3 trial of local chemotherapy with biodegradable carmustine (BCNU) wafers (Gliadel wafers) in patients with primary malignant gliomas, *Neurooncol* 5(2):79–88, 2003.

129. Whittle IR: Surgery for gliomas, *Curr Opin Neurol* 15:663–669, 2002.

130. Wick W, Menn O, Meisner C, et al: Pharmacotherapy of epileptic seizures in glioma patients: who, when, why and how long? *Onkologie* 28(8–9):391–396, 2005.

131. Wilkinson ID, Romanowski CA, Jellinek DA, et al: Motor functional MRI for preoperative and intraoperative neurosurgical guidance, *Br J Radiol* 76:98–103, 2003.

132. Woodworth G, McGirt MJ, Samdani A, et al: Accuracy of frameless and frame-based image-guided stereotactic brain biopsy in the diagnosis of glioma: comparison of biopsy and open resection specimen, *Neurol Res* 27(4):358–362, 2005.

133. World Health Organization: Classification of tumours. In Kleihues P, Cavenee WK, editors: *Pathology and genetics of tumours of the nervous system,* Lyon, France, 2000, IARC Press.

134. Wrensch MR, Minn Y, Bondy ML: Epidemiology. In Bernstein M, Berger MS, editors: *Neuro-oncology: the essentials,* New York, 2000, Thieme.

135. Yamanaka R, Abe T, Yajima N, et al: Vaccination of recurrent glioma patients with tumour lysate-pulsed dendritic cells elicits immune responses: results of a clinical phase I/II trial, *Br J Cancer* 89(7):1172–1179, 2003.

136. Youssef AS, Agazzi S, van Loveren HR: Transcranial surgery for pituitary adenomas, *Neurosurgery* 57:168–175, 2005.

137. Yu C, Jozsef G, Apuzzo ML, Petrovich Z: Dosimetric comparison of cyberknife with other radiosurgical modalities for an ellipsoidal target, *Neurosurgery* 53(5):1155–1163, 2003.

ALLYSON DELAUNE, ANIL
NANDA, ELLEN BARKER

CHAPTER 8

Cranial Surgery

Cranial surgery today is sophisticated and highly technical. Neurosurgeons perform cranial surgery to treat patients with brain tumors, head injury and trauma, epilepsy, aneurysm and arteriovenous malformations (AVMs), and Parkinson's disease, as well as for pain relief, for improved functional operations (e.g., deep brain stimulation [DBS] and various other disorders), and to include cerebrospinal fluid shunts for hydrocephalus. Neuroscience clinicians manage these patients perioperatively, helping them to recover as quickly and as safely as possible while implementing measures to prevent perioperative complications.

Despite all the advances and improved outcomes in brain surgery, it is still a frightening experience for patients. As patients and their families go through the steps of examinations, diagnostic studies, the potential diagnosis of a brain lesion, and the prospect of cranial surgery, open and honest communication and compassion are needed. This chapter briefly describes neurosurgical history, perioperative considerations, patient teaching, neurodiagnostic investigations, anesthesia considerations, and operative positioning. The chapter explains the fundamental concepts and management of a patient undergoing craniotomy and craniectomy procedures, hydrocephalus and shunting procedures, neuroendoscopic third ventriculostomy, and stereotactic radiosurgery. Perioperative management and management of potential complications are also reviewed.

BRIEF HISTORY OF CRANIAL SURGERY

Cranial surgery dates back to the Neolithic period, when humans used a procedure called *trepanation* in which tools made of stone or bone were used to remove pieces of the cranium. In prehistoric times, this procedure was performed for a variety of indications such as correction of skull fractures or the release of evil spirits. It is impressive that many of these patients survived, considering that these procedures were performed without anatomic knowledge, antisepsis, or anesthesia.[27]

The practice of neurosurgery has evolved throughout history. The hallmarks of neurosurgical advances include advanced knowledge of anatomy and function, invention of the operative microscope, development of imaging modalities, computer-assisted surgery, operative neurophysiologic monitoring systems, and the advent of radiosurgery. Despite these advances in knowledge and technology, a vast amount of mystery remains within the neurologic system.[27]

FUNDAMENTAL CONCEPTS OF NEUROSURGERY

There are common terms used for neurosurgical procedures (Table 8-1) and four important fundamental perioperative concepts unique to neurosurgery that must be considered in the management of the neurosurgical patient.[19]

1. *Etiology of the lesion.* Advances in technology provide diagnostic tests and intraoperative imaging that demonstrate the precise location and characteristics of the lesion (see Chapter 3). These tests help neurosurgeons plan the surgical approaches that are least disruptive to the brain and provide the best postoperative outcome. Patients may require emergency testing (e.g., computed tomography [CT] scans) during the immediate postoperative course to differentiate between an expanding lesion, edema, or a hemorrhagic lesion to determine appropriate medical treatment.

2. *Dynamics of cerebrospinal fluid (CSF) homeostasis.* Careful observance of intraoperative and postoperative CSF dynamics helps prevent postoperative complications (e.g., hydrocephalus and increased intracranial pressure [ICP]) that could lead to cerebral herniation and death.

3. *Control of cerebral blood flow (CBF).* CBF that is compromised from an intraoperative retraction or postoperative edema can result in ischemic brain damage. Techniques are used, therefore, to closely monitor and evaluate the effects of CBF intraoperatively and postoperatively for timely treatment (see Chapters 9 and 10).

4. *Regulation of water and sodium homeostasis.* Hypovolemia and hypervolemia, as well as sodium electrolyte imbalances, are major concerns associated with neurosurgery. Failure to recognize and treat the early signs and symptoms of problems with water and sodium homeostasis could lead to seizures, coma, or death.

It is important to consider these four important neurosurgical concepts and to integrate them into clinical practice and the management of neurosurgical patients.

INDICATIONS FOR CRANIAL SURGERY

The cause or indication for cranial surgery may be related to the following conditions:
- Brain neoplasm (tumor): partial or complete tumor excision[43]

TABLE 8-1	Terminology for Common Neurosurgical Procedures
Term	**Definition**
Burr hole	Small opening in the skull made with a drill. A burr hole can be used to drain and remove localized fluid collection beneath the dura.
Craniotomy	Surgery involving an opening into the skull with lifting of a bone flap and opening of the dura to remove a lesion, repair a damaged area, drain blood from a hemorrhagic area to control bleeding, or relieve increased intracranial pressure (ICP). *Supratentorial* (see Fig. 10-1, *A*) means above the tentorium, involving the cerebrum. Multiple burr holes may be drilled, with extensions of burr holes for craniotomy.
Craniectomy	Excision into the cranium with tongue forceps to cut away a portion of the bone (e.g., for posterior fossa surgery) infratentorially (see Fig. 10-1, *B*), with lesions located below the tentorium, involving the brainstem or cerebrum with no replacement of the cranial bone. Some surgeons repair cranial defects at the time of surgery with a cranioplasty.
Cranioplasty	Repair of a skull defect or deformity resulting from trauma, malformation, or a previous surgical procedure using artificial material to replace damaged or lost bone. Repair prevents secondary injury to the underlying brain and has a cosmetic effect.
Stereotaxis	Precision localization of a specific area of the brain using a frame or a frameless system based on three-dimensional coordinates. This procedure may be used for biopsy, radiosurgery, or dissection.
Intracranial shunting	Provision of an alternate pathway to redirect the cerebrospinal fluid (CSF) from one area (e.g., the ventricles) to another (e.g., the peritoneal cavity), using a tube or device implanted to perform this function. Ventriculoperitoneal shunt placement, lumbar-peritoneal shunt placement, and Ommaya reservoir placement are common neurosurgical procedures.

- Central nervous system (CNS) infection or abscess: drainage of the abscess
- Vascular abnormalities (e.g., AVMs or aneurysms with intracranial hemorrhage): clipping of the aneurysm or excision of the AVM
- Craniocerebral trauma (e.g., skull fractures, hematoma, cranial bone defect): repair of the fracture or excision of the hematoma
- Epilepsy and functional disorders (e.g., movement disorders): excision of seizure foci, insertion of a vagus nerve stimulator, or a lesion-producing procedure to relieve involuntary movements
- Intractable pain: insertion of stimulators to relieve pain, neurolysis, neuroablation, neural blockade, or nerve root decompression
- Congenital or postoperative disorder (e.g., hydrocephalus): shunting or ventriculostomy

Refer to the appropriate chapters for comprehensive discussions of these disorders, their particular pathophysiologic conditions, and neurosurgical procedures.

PREOPERATIVE CONSIDERATIONS

Patient Teaching

Patients preparing to undergo cranial surgery experience fear and anxiety related to an uncertain diagnosis and surgical outcome. Patients fear potential life-altering deficits in motor function, speech, and cognition following surgery. Although these emotions are to be expected, an effective preoperative educational program can help alleviate some of these fears and provide reassurance to the patient. Studies have reported that effective preoperative education can improve patient outcomes and reduce length of stay.[13] A reduced length of stay decreases costs for the patient and facility. In today's age of increasing health care costs, attention to cost containment measures cannot be disregarded.[8,12,38]

A combination of verbal and printed material is most effective in preparing patients for surgery. Patients may retain less than half of the verbal information provided to them.[1] A comprehensive preoperative educational patient packet enables a review of information not retained in the verbal preoperative meeting. Some institutions have initiated interdisciplinary preoperative education programs for patients and their families/caregivers in classroom settings. Clinicians, clinician anesthetists, physical therapists, and other members of the treating team provide patients with information pertaining to the preoperative period, surgical day, and recovery period.[2] These classes encourage patient involvement and enable practitioners to foresee potential needs in individual patients.

Current research has yet to elucidate the most effective time period to present patients with preoperative education. It should be noted that patients have access to a plethora of information and misinformation via the Internet. Information provided soon after the surgical plan is established might prevent patients from using unreliable sources of education.

Preoperative printed and verbal education specific to cranial surgery should contain the following:

- Information about the patient's diagnosis, need for surgery, and other alternatives
- List of reliable information resources
- Craniotomy procedure
- Surgical risks and benefits
- Preoperative instructions: nothing by mouth (NPO; Latin, *nil per os*), surgical scrub on the evening before surgery, medication instructions

- Step-by-step information about the surgical day: admission, day surgery, anesthesia, operating room (OR), OR holding room, recovery room, intensive care unit (ICU)
- Description of postoperative period
- Information about recovery: physiotherapy (PT), occupational therapy (OT), rehabilitation
- Discharge instructions: medications, activity, diet, wound care, follow-up schedule, progress expectations
- Facility map
- Emergency contact phone numbers

General Preoperative Assessment

Medical History and Neurologic Assessment

The preoperative neurologic assessment is used to identify medical problems that may negatively affect the surgical outcome. The patient's medical history is obtained and a physical examination is performed by the neurosurgeon, neurosurgical resident, or midlevel practitioner (e.g., neuroscience clinician practitioner, advanced practice clinician, or clinical specialist). The admitting clinician incorporates this information and also obtains a history and records it into the nursing database. Institutional policy regarding the time frame that the nursing history, neurologic assessment, and nursing database must be obtained is established by hospital policy and by the Joint Commission on Accreditation of Healthcare Organizations (JCAHO).

The medical history should include information pertaining to the patient's general health status (see Chapter 2). A review of systems records any preexisting medical conditions. Information specific to cardiac, respiratory, and endocrine systems is collected, since preexisting conditions place the patient at a greater risk during anesthesia, surgery, and recovery. A review of family history identifies potential problems that might place the patient at greater risk but are not physically evident with the assessment. A strong family history of coronary artery disease (CAD) and other cardiac problems might require more thorough investigation in asymptomatic patients. A neurologic examination is performed by the physician to identify and document existing neurologic deficits before surgery.

Evaluation of past medical history includes previous illnesses and prior injuries. Potential problems in the perioperative period can be identified and prevented by a thorough evaluation. Previous surgical history is obtained. Prior spinal surgery requires a meticulous approach during surgical positioning.

Current medication history is relevant. Patients on anticoagulants, antiplatelet drugs (e.g., aspirin, clopidogrel [Plavix]), and antiinflammatory drugs may be instructed to discontinue these medications before surgery. Collaboration with the patient's internist may be necessary due to their familiarity with the patient's current medical status and potential risk of discontinuing them. Patients on diabetic drugs are typically instructed to hold their morning doses of oral (PO) drugs or insulin. The medical history provides an opportunity to instruct patients regarding medication usage before surgery. Limited understanding may cause patients to discontinue necessary medications before surgery, placing them at risk for exacerbation of preexisting medical conditions.

A thorough social history evaluation provides information regarding tobacco, alcohol, and drug addiction. Knowledge of these habits aids in preventing complications of withdrawal in the postoperative period. Awareness of cigarette use alerts the clinician to ensure aggressive pulmonary conditioning in the postoperative period to prevent complications such as atelectasis and pneumonia.

A thorough head-to-toe neurologic assessment is performed to identify and document a baseline condition of the patient. The assessment may also identify potential problems requiring further workup and treatment by the treating team before surgery. It is imperative that a neurologic examination is performed and deficits documented. This information is useful for comparing the patient's preoperative and postoperative neurologic status.

Special Assessment Considerations. It is recommended that every patient have an individualized proactive plan for **postoperative pain management** that is based on the type of cranial surgery, the expected severity of postoperative pain, underlying medical conditions, and the patient's preference based on past positive or negative experiences with postoperative pain (see Chapter 24). The unique features of the older patient should be considered, including reductions in dosages of drugs that may cause CNS depression (Tables 8-2 and 8-3).

Herbal Product History

The use of herbal products is prevalent. Current literature reports that up to 32% of patients use herbal or dietary supplements.[28] Lack of a Food and Drug Administration (FDA) approval process for herbal therapy combined with an attitude that herbals are "natural" and therefore harmless has resulted in underreporting of usage by patients. The literature reports that 53% to 70% of patients fail to report the use of herbal medications.[28] Herbal marketing campaigns focus on potential attributes but fail to alert the public of the potential risks of product usage. The effectiveness and action of prescribed medications may be altered when combined with herbal products.[7]

Failure to report usage can result in potentially lethal complications for the neurosurgical patient. Ginkgo biloba and garlic supplements have been found to inhibit platelet aggregation and subsequently increase bleeding and clotting times, placing the patient at risk for intraoperative hemorrhage.[28,42] Identification of herbal product usage should be addressed during the medication history.

Preexisting or High-Risk Medical Conditions

Special consideration must be given to patients with preexisting or high-risk medical conditions that could affect surgery, such as the following:

- Obese individuals store anesthesia in fatty tissue.
- Cigarette smokers require a greater depth of anesthesia to obtund the cough reflex and are more susceptible to postoperative complications.
- Trauma patients may have other injuries that will impair effective breathing, and with increased age, surgical risks increase.

TABLE 8-2   Normal Age-Related Changes and Their Significance

System	Age-Related Changes	Significance
Body composition and weight	Between ages 25 and 75, body fat doubles, size and weight of organs decrease, and body water decreases from 61% to 53%. Male weight increases and then declines after mid-50s. Female weight increases and then declines after mid-60s.	Increased lipid drug toxicity, dehydration, increased drug toxicity, prolonged drug effects. Functions vary, some decline. For both sexes, increased risks associated with obesity or malnutrition.
Integumentary system	Dermis thins, collagen decreases, skin is less elastic. Decrease in eccrine and apocrine glands, epidermal growth and division, and subcutaneous fat in legs and arms. Hair thins and grays. Adipose tissue redistributes to waistline and thighs.	Increased wrinkling, potential for infection, and risk of pressure ulcers. Impaired heat and cold regulation. Decreased wound healing, skin barrier capability, and microbial protection. Alteration of body image.
Musculoskeletal system	Decreased bone density, altered bone modeling. Bones become thin and porous. Lean body mass decreases. Spine becomes flexed.	Osteoporosis, fractures, bone pain, height loss, and arthritic changes common. Poor balance, function, and mobility; muscle strength and endurance decrease. Changes in height and posture.
Neurologic system	Some cortical atrophy, and brain weight decreases. Blood flow decreases 15% to 20%. Lipofusion accumulates in the brain, and abnormal proteins increase. Increase in reaction time and slowed movements. Impaired coordination. Decreased vibratory sense in lower extremities. Decreased sensation to light touch, pain, joint position. Sluggish tendon reflexes (e.g., some may be absent). Decreased metabolic activity, muscle vasodilation. Inability to get rid of excess heat, mass, skin sensors. Less efficient shivering, impaired sweating, and Deterioration of baroreceptor responses. Beta-receptor response decreases, alpha-receptor response remains unchanged. Smell and taste discrimination and papillary and salivary flow decrease.	Decrease in short-term memory. Response time slows. Intelligence, personality, long-term memory unchanged. Increases in time to fall asleep and nocturnal wakening, decreased REM and deep sleep. Increased risk of falling. Reflexes absent in 50% to 70% of normal people 65 years of age and older. Decreased heat production and loss. Changes in Valsalva response and postural hypotension. Less efficient cardiac muscle, arterial tone, and response to beta-adrenergic medication. More peripheral resistance. Decreased interest in food, reduced ability to discern odors and scents.
Hearing	Atrophy of external auditory canal, decreased and thickened cerumen. Stiffening of the ossicular bones, decreased hair cells in organ of Corti.	Bilateral and symmetric presbycusis, sensorineural hearing loss. Loss of high frequencies, difficulty with consonant/sibilant discrimination.
Immune system	Thymus gland involution, impaired T-cell function.	Increased risk for infection and malignancies. Reduced antigen response.
Respiratory	Mechanics of ventilation altered. Loss of elastic recoil, stiffening of chest well, increased ventilation/perfusion mismatch. Decreased response to hypercapnia. Decreased airway clearance and cough and laryngeal reflexes, decline in mucociliary clearance.	Airway closure, decreased vital capacity and pulmonary reserve. Diaphragmatic breathing increases. Arterial hypoxemia. Greater risk for respiratory failure under anesthesia. Increased risk of aspiration and infection.
Renal system	Nephron loss. Glomerular filtration rate (GFR) and creatinine production declines. Delayed response to sodium deficiency. Reduced capacity to excrete water and salt. Increased renal threshold for glucose. Other renal functions impaired. Nocturia, nonrenal in origin. Bladder capacity decreases approximately 50%. Detrusor muscle weakens. Prostate hypertrophy.	Prolonged half-life of drug clearance, potential for toxicity. Diminished GFR despite "normal" serum creatinine. Increased risk of volume depletion and dehydration, fluid overload, and hyponatremia. Urine glucose less reliable. Vitamin D production impaired. Hormones and erythropoietin production impaired. Sleep disturbances, stress incontinence, frequency, nocturia, decreased urinary stream, and urinary retention.

TABLE 8-2	Normal Age-Related Changes and Their Significance—cont'd	
System	**Age-Related Changes**	**Significance**
Gastrointestinal system/stomach	Parietal cell loss and decrease in gastrin secretion, some delay in gastric motility and emptying.	Pernicious anemia may develop. Reduced use of acid-preferring medication. May have little significance.
Intestine	Decrease in blood supply, slowed transit time, atrophy of the colon mucosa.	Impaired synthesis of calcium and B and fat-soluble vitamins.
Liver	Decrease in liver mass, blood flow, and microsomal oxidation.	Prolonged half-life of some drugs.
Endocrine	Decreased secretion and action of insulin. Other pancreatic secretions remain adequate.	Hyperglycemia in response to glucose loads in nondiabetics.
Hematopoietic	Decline in active bone marrow. Numbers of red blood cells (RBCs), platelets unchanged. Reduced ability to accelerate RBC production. White blood cell numbers unchanged. Neutrophil and monocyte activity decreases.	Anemia in older adults not a normal process of aging. Slight decline in chemotaxis and phagocytosis.
Vision	Limited upward conjugate gaze, slowed pupillary constriction, impaired accommodation, corneal reflexes, lens opaqueness, arcus senilis (i.e., white arc around cornea).	Presbyopia, delayed light-to-dark adaptation, poor night vision, decreased acuity, distortion of blue-green color spectrum, problems with night glare.
Cardiovascular	Degeneration and fibrosis of pacemaking and conduction tissue. Impaired early diastolic filling due to prolonged isovolume relaxation and decreased vascular compliance. Decreased arterial compliance. Impaired compensatory mechanisms. Decreased baroreceptor sensitivity. Decreased target organ response to beta-adrenergic stimulation, decreased renin, angiotensin, and aldosterone. Resting cardiac output is maintained. Exercise maximum achievable heart rate decreases but exercise cardiac output maintained by increased stroke volume.	Increased risk for conduction disturbances, hypotension with dehydration, tachyarrhythmias, and vasodilators. Presence of a fourth heart sound. Systolic hypertension and ventricular hypertrophy. Decreased heart rate response to stress. Increased risk for hypotension. Cardiac risks increased more with disease than by age.

From Bailes BK: Perioperative care of the elderly surgical patient, *AORN J* 72(2):186–207, 2000.
REM, Rapid eye movement.

- Older patients may require lower dosages for drugs that cause CNS depression (see Tables 10-2 and 10-3 for older adult considerations).
- Pregnant patients may have subarachnoid hemorrhage (SAH) from a ruptured AVM or aneurysm, or from head or spine trauma, that will require immediate consultation with the patient's obstetrician and a high-risk neonatologist.
- Obstructive sleep apnea is underdiagnosed in approximately 80% of patients.[6] Obese patients (body mass index >30), male sex, and alcohol use are considered risk factors. Patients with sleep apnea may pose challenges during intubation and are at greater risk of developing postoperative respiratory depression and cardiac complications[6] (see Chapter 6).

Day-of-Surgery Assessment. The majority of patients scheduled for elective surgery have typically had a preadmission appointment for completion of all surgical tests and preparation. The patient is scheduled for admission to the hospital facility the morning of surgery. Delays in the admission or day surgery process can potentially alter the scheduled surgery. Collaboration from all involved services is required to prevent delays. A tight schedule should not be allowed to cause a hasty preoperative assessment as this is the last checkpoint that may identify potential risks for the patient undergoing surgery.

Although patients may have undergone a history and physical examination when they were initially evaluated by the neurosurgeon, a neurologic reassessment must be completed on the surgical day to detect changes that may have occurred in the interim period between preadmission evaluation and surgery. Individual facility policy dictates the allowable amount of time between the history and physical examination and the actual operative procedure. A preopera-

TABLE 8-3	Assessment and Nursing Interventions for the Older Patient

Patient Assessment	Nursing Interventions
General	Do not use patient's first name unless invited to do so. Provide as much privacy as possible. Supply extra blankets for warmth (especially of the feet). Assess and document respiratory effort, skin warmth, and color. Note verbal and nonverbal clues about pain. Note vital signs and report significant abnormalities. Review American Society of Anesthesiologists or cardiac risk index (if available). Review medical history for presence and number of chronic diseases. Older patients often will answer yes to questions even when they do not understand them. Instructions will need to be repeated. Reassurance is needed as older patients often have many fears regarding the hospital setting (e.g., falling from narrow stretchers). Have an adequate number of staff members available to help with transfers.
Integumentary system	Inspect as much of the patient's body surface as possible. Note and document all bruises, sores, tears, abrasions, rashes, pressure ulcers, or other lesions. Note nutritional status. Check weight and height. Seek nutritional information from family members or other caregivers. Plan for and use padding and other positioning devices to protect bony prominences. At the end of the procedure, inspect body surfaces for any abrasions or burns, and assess bony areas for redness or blanching. Document findings and communicate to other peers. Follow up postoperatively. Review risk factors for pressure ulcer development.
Vision and hearing	Older adults may not be able to read your name tag without eyeglasses unless they have intraocular lens implants. You must tell them who you are. Check the chart regarding the presence and location of eyeglasses and hearing aids. People with hearing deficits often read lips. If possible, talk to the patient without a mask. Talk slowly and distinctly. Repeat or restate as often as needed. Try pitching your voice up or down to determine which range the patient can hear better. Do not shout.
Mental status/ cognition	Ask patients questions from the Short Portable Mental Health Questionnaire to establish a baseline cognitive status. Another option is to give the patient three things to remember (e.g., apple, watch, pencil), have the patient repeat the items, and then ask him or her to repeat the items to you several minutes later. Inability to do so indicates some cognitive deficit; however, people suffering from chronic illness, pain, lack of sleep, nutritional deficiencies, depression, anxiety, hearing impairment, and speech difficulties may have reduced cognitive status that improves as their health improves. Assess for symptoms of depression, acute delirium, or other psychosocial issues that may affect recovery. Do not label a patient with a diagnosis of dementia unless it has been established with appropriate testing. Review common causes of delirium.
Laboratory and diagnostic tests	Review, document, and report significant abnormal findings. Due to age-related "dampening" of the immune system, white blood cells and differential may not reflect the presence of infection. Review age-related changes in laboratory values.
Chronic disease states	*Rheumatoid arthritis:* Has the patient been on or is the patient currently on steroid therapy? Patients on steroids will need steroids during and after the surgery to prevent a severe "Addison-type" crisis. They will have impaired immune response and are at risk for surgical infections. Blood glucose levels usually are elevated. *Cerebrovascular accident:* Patient may have weakness or flaccidity, and some speech impairment, or inability to communicate may be present. Assess carefully for the ability to move and be positioned for surgery. *Parkinson's disease and other movement disorders:* Assess for rigidity, mobility, and tremors. Assess and document condition of skin and presence of pressure ulcers; document medication administration. *Cardiovascular:* Review chart for 12-lead electrocardiogram or echocardiogram. Older people experiencing cardiac ischemia may complain of dyspnea, not pain. Systolic murmurs are common in people older than 65 years of age. Note regularity or irregularity of heartbeat; arrhythmias are common in otherwise healthy older people. Older people with no documented heart disease often have a fourth heart sound. The presence of the third heart sound is always abnormal. Assess blood pressure; document if and when medications were taken. Review age-related changes of the cardiovascular system and review cardiac risk index. *Diabetes mellitus:* Review chart for blood glucose levels. Assess and document medication and when taken. Review how insulin will be provided to the patient during surgery. Assess patient for neuropathy and skin condition and document.
Medications	Ask patient, family members, or significant others about medications, over-the-counter medications, vitamins, nutritional supplements, and herbal preparations. Document and report any that may interfere with coagulation or anesthesia. Ask about use of alcohol, benzodiazepines, "nerve pills," and sleeping pills (withdrawal from these substances without appropriate medical supervision can result in seizures, possibly death). The anxiety that the patient may be showing may not be related to the planned surgery but to withdrawal symptoms. Document and report immediately.
Functional status	Ask patient or family members about physical limitations. If possible, have patient move about to demonstrate ability to move and turn. Check chart for activities of daily living assessment or comments. Prepare OR bed with appropriate support materials. Document and communicate data to other peers.

From Bailes BK: Perioperative care of the elderly surgical patient, *AORN J* 72(2):186–207, 2000.
OR, Operating room.

tive assessment should include a physical and neurologic examination and pain assessment. A review of pertinent scans (magnetic resonance imaging [MRI], CT), electrocardiogram (ECG), chest x-ray, and laboratory work is necessary to identify potential problems before surgery. Surgical and postoperative complications can be decreased by a thorough review of preoperative laboratory work. Abnormalities in coagulation place the patient at risk for hemorrhage during surgery and in the postoperative period. Anticonvulsant

levels in the nontherapeutic range place the patient at risk for seizures. Information specific to the patient's physical and neurologic status immediately before the surgery is useful to compare the preoperative and postoperative conditions.

A preoperative checklist is a helpful tool to ensure that all necessary tests have been performed and reviewed in order to ensure patient safety (Fig. 8-1).

Anesthesia Assessment. It is reported that greater than 70% of surgery performed is either on an outpatient basis or on

Figure 8-1 Example of a neurosurgery preoperative note.

Patient Name/MR#

NEUROSURGERY
Pre-Op Note

Date of this Note:	Time of this Note:	Attending Surgeon performing procedure:

Procedure-related diagnosis:

Procedure planned:

OPERATIVE CONSENT
☐ Completed
   by: _____
☐ On chart

BLOOD CONSENT
☐ Completed
   by: _____
☐ On chart

ANESTHESIA PRE-OP
☐ Anesthesiology paged & notified (if inpatient)
☐ Anesthesia consent on chart
☐ Anesthesia pre-op done
☐ Name of Anesthesia person responsible for preop:_____
☐ Sent to Anesthesia pre-op clinic
☐ History of anesthesia problems? Y/N
☐ Family history of anesthesia problems?
☐ Allergies:_____
☐ Medications affecting coagulation (Aspirin, Ticlid, Plavis, Coumadin)?
☐ Problems requiring visit to doctor in past?

BMP	CBC	OTHER TESTS	BLOOD PRODUCTS
Na_____	WBC_____	ECG: Done OK N/A (for Age >50 y.o., or w/problems)	☐ T & C (within 30 days) ☐ T & C ___units PRBCs ☐ T & C ___units FFP ☐ T & C ___units Platelets
K_____	Hct_____		
BUN_____	Platelets_____	CXR: Done OK N/A (for Age >50 y.o., or w/problems)	
Cr_____	COAGULATION	UPT: Done OK N/A (for all females > 7 y.o.)	Medication allergy:
Glc_____	INR_____		☐ Pre-Op Antibiotics ordered
	PTT_____	U/A: Normal N/A UTI Present	☐ NPO after midnight order written

ADDITIONAL CHECKLIST
Y   N
☐   ☐   This operation has been posted in the operating room.
☐   ☐   Pre-operative antibiotics have been written for (on call to O.R.)
☐   ☐   An ICU bed/floor bed has been reserved for this patient for the post-operative period.
☐   ☐   Acquisition of special vendor items (including instrumentation) for this case has been
            arranged, and the specific representative has been contacted.
☐   ☐   This patient has been medically cleared for surgery (if reason exists for acquiring clearance),
            and a clearance note is in the chart from the primary team.
☐   ☐   If this patient is seen in consultation and will be transferred to the primary team after the peri-
            operative period, transfer arrangements have been discussed with the primary team.
☐   ☐   All films have already been printed for this case.
☐   ☐   For shunt cases, is there an order to clamp the drain and notify if change/ICP too high?
☐   ☐   Are any films needed immediately pre-operatively such as STEALTH or CT?
☐   ☐   Do culture results preclude operation?
☐   ☐   Does the patient have any of the following which may need Cardiology or Pulmonary consult
            prior to O.R.: Shortness of Breath with mild exertion/Asthma/Diabetes/Orthopnea? _____
☐   ☐   Special considerations (per O.R. posting template) have been addressed while pasting this case.
☐   ☐   IS the correct OPERATIVE SIDE MARKED WITH A SHARPIE (X with a circle around it) on the tragus?
            (DO NOT MARK either side for a midline procedure)

DATE OF SCHEDULED CASE: _____/_____/_____

_____   _____   _____
Physician Signature   Printed Last Name   Pager#

| BOX 8-1 | **Goals of Anesthetic Preoperative Assessment** |

- Establish rapport with patient and family
- Educate patient about anesthesia during surgery and postoperative management, including pain management
- Establish baseline record of medical/surgical history, anesthetic history, and current medications
- Interpretation and evaluation of significant laboratory data
- Development of anesthetic plan
- Obtain signed informed consent

From Findlay JM: Cerebral vasospasm, In *Youmans neurological surgery,* ed 5, Philadelphia, 2004, Saunders, pp. 1839–1867.

elective patients being admitted the morning of the procedure.[10] This trend has decreased the time available for the anesthesiologist to perform preoperative anesthesia assessments. Time constraints limit the assessment to immediately before the surgery. Research indicates that preoperative condition is predictive of mortality and morbidity rates following surgery. Considering this fact, a thorough preoperative assessment is imperative to minimize patient mortality risk.[10]

Implementation of anesthesia preoperative assessment clinics has decreased surgical cancellations significantly and proven to be cost effective by alleviation of some standard preoperative tests that are deemed unnecessary (Box 8-1). An estimated 30 to 40 billion dollars is spent on preoperative tests each year, with a potential 50% savings by "selective ordering of tests."[10]

General Preoperative Management

Patient Consent

The patient's attending neurosurgical team is responsible for explaining the procedure in language that can be understood by the patient, and for obtaining full informed consent. Patients' and family members' questions must be referred back to the neurosurgeon. Written records for surgical consent must be signed and dated and placed in the patient's chart. The clinician must ensure that the informed consent process has been completed and witness the patient's signature, if this has not been completed (see Chapter 25).

The informed consent process is often viewed by health care providers as a procedure taken to ensure against potential liability. In actuality, it is an opportunity to ensure that the patient is well informed regarding the goal of his or her surgery, as well as the risks and benefits. Patients should be informed regarding their surgery and realize that while the neurosurgeon makes recommendations, it is their decision to undergo surgery. Patients should be encouraged to actively participate in the consent process by thoroughly reading the consent form and clarifying information that they do not understand.

Informed consent forms often include terminology and explanations that are not understood by the patient. It is estimated that one quarter of Americans have low literacy

skills with, half reading under an eighth-grade level.[34] This fact should be considered when consent is obtained. The practitioner obtaining consent should assess the patient's understanding of the consent. Lack of understanding of information provided in the consent form can lead to confusion in the postoperative period if patients experience complications that they did not understand were possible. The clinician should alert the surgeon if questions arise.

Patient Identification

In 2004, the JCAHO received 70 reports from accredited facilities of surgical procedures performed on the wrong site. Erroneous communication was cited as the root cause for surgery performed on the wrong site.[41] To decrease wrong site events, JCAHO established a universal preventive protocol. This protocol requires a patient verification process, marking of the operative site, and a required "time-out" before the procedure. During the patient verification process, the patient is identified while all of his or her tests, imaging, and other pertinent information are gathered, checked, and corroborated by the surgical team. The operative site should be marked by the surgeon or an informed member of the surgical team. Marking should preferably be done before patient sedation and transport to the OR. The patient should be involved in the marking process when possible. A time-out is performed by the surgical team before the procedure, during which the patient and procedure are verified again (Fig. 8-2).[41]

Patient Preparation

The neurosurgical team will evaluate the presurgical diagnostic studies and laboratory test results to identify surgical risk factors. If the studies are all within normal limits, the patient is prepared for surgery. The patient's records are reviewed for completeness, including preoperative teaching, test results, consent forms for signatures, and completion of physical examination as required by JCAHO.

Medications. Depending on the individual patient, the following medications may be ordered as part of the surgical hospitalization:[19]

- Antibiotics: to prevent infections
- Anticonvulsants: to prevent seizures in high-risk groups (e.g., patients with a cerebral abscess, meningioma, or glioma in close proximity to the primary motor cortex; patients with a past or recent history of seizures)
- Steroids (e.g., dexamethasone): to reduce neural tissue swelling secondary to malignant disease or sepsis with a parenteral IV loading dose of 4 mg every 6 hours
- Anticoagulants: to minimize the risk of deep vein thrombosis (DVT) and pulmonary embolism (PE); an estimated 30% to 45% frequency of DVT and PE in neurosurgical patients may be prevented by using standard heparin to treat thrombolic complications and low-molecular-weight heparin for DVT prophylaxis, with the administration of 5000 units subcutaneously followed by 5000 units every 12 hours postoperatively

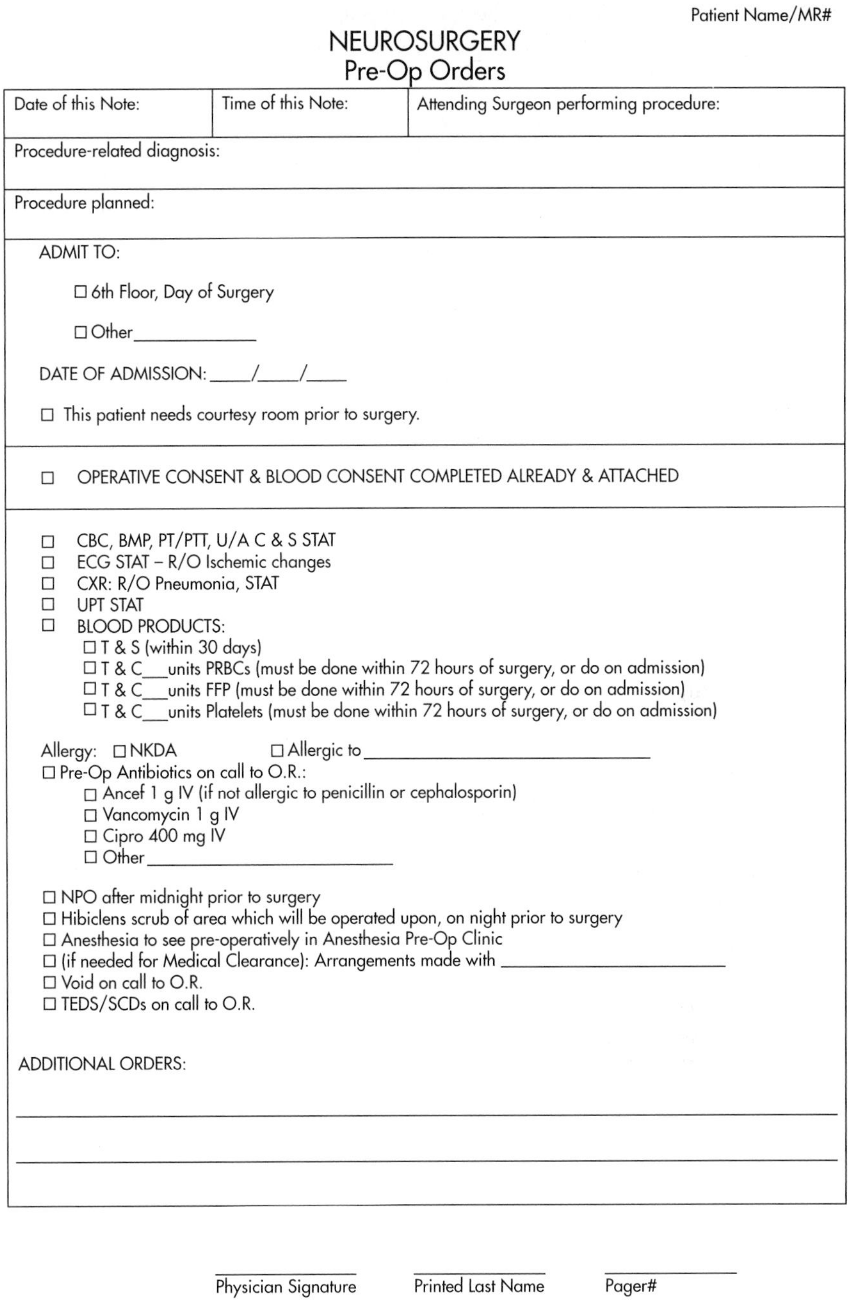

NEUROSURGERY
Pre-Op Orders

Date of this Note:	Time of this Note:	Attending Surgeon performing procedure:

Procedure-related diagnosis:

Procedure planned:

ADMIT TO:

    □ 6th Floor, Day of Surgery

    □ Other_____

DATE OF ADMISSION: ____/____/____

□ This patient needs courtesy room prior to surgery.

□   OPERATIVE CONSENT & BLOOD CONSENT COMPLETED ALREADY & ATTACHED

□   CBC, BMP, PT/PTT, U/A C & S STAT
□   ECG STAT – R/O Ischemic changes
□   CXR: R/O Pneumonia, STAT
□   UPT STAT
□   BLOOD PRODUCTS:
    □ T & S (within 30 days)
    □ T & C___units PRBCs (must be done within 72 hours of surgery, or do on admission)
    □ T & C___units FFP (must be done within 72 hours of surgery, or do on admission)
    □ T & C___units Platelets (must be done within 72 hours of surgery, or do on admission)

Allergy: □ NKDA   □ Allergic to_____
□ Pre-Op Antibiotics on call to O.R.:
    □ Ancef 1 g IV (if not allergic to penicillin or cephalosporin)
    □ Vancomycin 1 g IV
    □ Cipro 400 mg IV
    □ Other_____

□ NPO after midnight prior to surgery
□ Hibiclens scrub of area which will be operated upon, on night prior to surgery
□ Anesthesia to see pre-operatively in Anesthesia Pre-Op Clinic
□ (if needed for Medical Clearance): Arrangements made with _____
□ Void on call to O.R.
□ TEDS/SCDs on call to O.R.

ADDITIONAL ORDERS:

_____

_____

_____

Physician Signature	Printed Last Name	Pager#

Figure 8-2 Example of neurosurgery preoperative orders.

Preoperative Holding Unit. Once the initial baseline assessment is complete, further assessment is done on a periodic basis as determined by the patient's medical status until the patient is transported to the OR. A perioperative clinician must identify the patient and closely monitor the patient for any change in respiratory and neurologic status. Vital signs are recorded, minor procedures may be performed (e.g., line insertions), and all measures are taken to ensure patient safety until the patient is transported to the OR suite.

Neurodiagnostic and Laboratory Studies

In addition to the routine tests, the following general diagnostic and laboratory tests may be ordered before cranial surgery:

- Electrolytes: particular attention should be paid to sodium and potassium, which are important for cardiac stability
- Prothrombin time/activated partial thromboplastin time (APTT), international normalized ratio (INR),

thrombin clotting time: screen for coagulation disorders and clotting deficiencies (for example, a single dose of aspirin may impair platelet function for 7 to 10 days)
- Arterial blood gas (ABG) studies: done if oxygenation problems are suspected
- ECG: records the electrical impulses of the heart and indicates how well the heart is functioning (if there is evidence of coronary artery disease, myocardial infarction, or abnormalities of the heart rate or rhythm or other abnormalities, the patient's surgery may be delayed until the problem is corrected; or if the brain lesion is contributing to the cardiac dysrhythmias, surgery may be the best treatment to remove the lesion or pressure and restore normal cardiac function)

TIP: Patient guidelines for the indication of a 12-lead ECG include the following:[19] age over 50, ischemic heart disease (dysrhythmia/angina), hypertension, cardiomyopathy, diabetes mellitus in a patient over 40 years of age, electrolyte imbalance, and thyroid disease.

- Typing and crossmatching for blood products: patients scheduled for elective surgery may have previously elected to donate blood for intraoperative autologous blood replacement
- CT, MRI, arterial angiography, x-ray study, other neurodiagnostic studies: may be required; films and documents usually accompany the patient to the OR (see Chapter 3)

CRANIOTOMY

A **craniotomy** is any operation that involves an incision into the cranium. In general, patients undergo a craniotomy for the purposes of diagnosis and treatment of their underlying condition.

Preoperative Preparation

Preoperative Patient Instructions

Patient preparation and instructions may include the following:
- Do not wear any jewelry, makeup, or nail polish to the hospital
- Do not take aspirin or aspirin products for 1 week before surgery

Admission preoperative orders for the clinician may include the following:
- Have the patient shower and shampoo the hair with antibacterial shampoo the night before surgery
- Maintain the patient on NPO status (nothing by mouth) after midnight
- Adherence to all hospital policies and procedures, CareMap, or clinical pathways for the selected cranial procedure

Operating Room Preparation

The perioperative clinician prepares the OR and makes preparations for receiving the patient into the neurosurgical suite. Attention to patient comfort and reassurance can be offered as the patient is removed from the stretcher and placed on the operating table (see operative textbooks for details).

Patient Positioning

There are numerous factors considered to position the patient for cranial surgery. Age and patient condition, location of the lesion, access to operative area, head position in relation to the heart, accessibility to imaging equipment, and anesthesia monitoring are all evaluated before deciding on a surgical position.[14] Each position has unique advantages and disadvantages and may be modified accordingly (Fig. 8-3).

Supine Position The supine position is the most basic and common position used for cranial surgery. In this position, care is taken to ensure that the head is held in alignment with the body axis to prevent cervical spine injury or compression/obstruction of vessels. The head is positioned on a head-

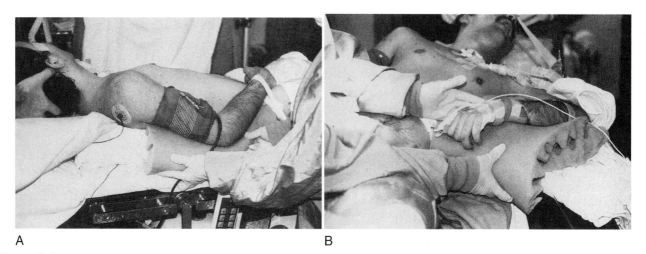

A   B

Figure 8-3 Perioperative clinician padding bony prominences to prevent nerve injury to a patient with contractures. **A,** Under elbow and shoulder. **B,** Under wrists and to elevate hand to prevent dependent edema during surgery.

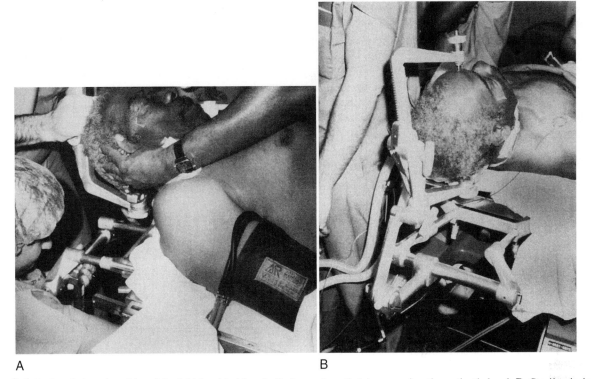

A   B

Figure 8-4 Patient being placed in a Mayfield head holder. **A,** Perioperative clinician securing the patient's head. **B,** Sterile pin in the outer table of the skull to secure the head during cranial surgery.

rest or by skeletal fixation (Fig. 8-4). Positioning the head above the heart increases venous return. If the head is rotated, padding is used to raise the shoulder to maintain body alignment. Arms are positioned at the sides ensuring that shoulders are not abducted greater than 90 degrees to prevent peripheral nerve compression. Positioning the knees in a slightly flexed position prevents sciatic nerve stretch. Ankles are padded to decrease heel pressure and tendon injury. Sequential compression devices with or without compression stockings should be placed to increase venous return and prevent deep vein thrombosis.[14]

Prone Position. The prone position is used to provide exposure for posterior fossa and suboccipital approaches. The head is positioned using skeletal fixation. Once the head is positioned, the face is checked to ensure that the eyes are protected and that there is no compression on the chin. The breasts, especially in females, should be separated and padding placed around if necessary. Arms are placed at the patient's sides with the palms adducted. Abdominal pressure should be decreased. Genitalia, especially male, should be checked to ensure there is no compression and that the Foley catheter is not crimped. Padding is placed at the shoulders, elbows, hands, groin, and knees. Once positioned, lower extremity peripheral pulses are checked. Complications are more common in the prone position and are related to anesthesia, compression of the chest and abdomen, nerve palsy, pressure injury, and air embolism.[14]

Lateral Position. Lateral positioning provides exposure for temporal, skull base, and posterior fossa approaches. The head is positioned using skeletal fixation or a ring-shaped pad. The dependent arm is placed in a hanging or ventral position. Axillary rolls are placed below the armpit to prevent nerve injuries. The upper arm can be secured along the torso or positioned with pillows or a rest. The torso is supported and secured in place. Padding is placed under the hip and between the knees. The dependent lower extremity is flexed.

ALERT: To prevent brachial plexus stretch, place an axillary roll four fingerbreadths below the armpit to prevent compression of thoracic nerve.[14]

Sitting Position. The sitting position allows for exposure in posterior fossa and subtemporal approaches (Fig. 8-5). Current literature cites advantages to the sitting position, including improved access to midline lesions, improved cerebral venous drainage, decreased intracranial pressure, and improved drainage of blood and CSF. Although the advantages are significant, the potential complications are of such significance that this position is rarely used today. Potential complications include **venous air embolism,** hypotension, postoperative **tension pneumocephalus,** and subdural hematoma.[14]

Positioning Complications
Careful positioning is supervised by the circulating nurse and operating team to prevent intraoperative complications, including the following:
- **Venous air embolism**
- Hypotension
- Postoperative **tension pneumocephalus**

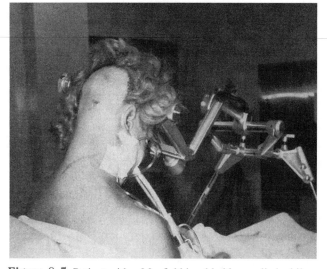

Figure 8-5 Patient with a Mayfield head holder applied while in a sitting position. Patient intubated in final position with a central venous pressure (CVP) catheter and IV lines in place.

- Subdural hematoma
- Tension pneumocephalus
- Subdural fluid collection[14]

Tension Pneumocephalus and Subdural Fluid Collection. Tension pneumocephalus, defined as "gas under pressure," is a complication that occurs more frequently in the sitting position and is infrequently reported in other positions. Gas may become trapped in the dural spaces, in the intraventricular spaces, or intraparenchymally. Tension pneumocephalus requires evacuation as it produces symptoms and sequelae of other space-occupying lesions.[17]

The same contributing factors (decreased brain volume due to intraoperative mannitol, decreased intravascular volume and loss of CSF) that result in tension pneumocephalus also contribute to the formation of subdural hematomas.[14]

Air Embolism. Air embolism is a serious complication that occurs when air enters a "noncollapsible" vein due to negative pressure in the vein created by positions that place the head above the heart. Once air enters the vein, it becomes trapped in the right atrium, potentially resulting in decreased venous return, hypotension, and cardiac arrhythmias. This complication can occur in any position where the head is positioned above the heart but occurs most frequently in the sitting position.[17]

Skin Pressure Injury. A thorough nursing assessment performed in the perioperative period can alert the treating team to patients who are at increased risk for pressure injuries. These at-risk patients may include the following: (1) vascular disease or circulatory problems; (2) decreased mobility due to arthritis, injuries, or other skeletal issues; (3) older adult patients with decreased skin integrity; (4) poor health due to known disease states such as cancer, cardiac disease, or respiratory disease; and (5) pediatric patients, who may require special positioning equipment. Current literature states that increased age, a diagnosis of diabetes or vascular disease, and patients undergoing vascular surgery are the most significant predictors for developing pressure ulcers.[18,39]

Peripheral Nerve Injury. Improper positioning creates tension or compression of nerves, resulting in postoperative nerve injury. Preexisting conditions such as diabetes and other factors such as hypotension, hypothermia, and use of tourniquets during surgery also contribute to nerve injury.[14]

Head Fixation Complications. Head fixation complications include the following:

- Scalp necrosis
- Vessel puncture
- Skull fracture
- Scalp laceration
- Pin site infection
- Bleeding
- CSF leak

Patient Head and Skin Local Preparation

Shaving of the operative site was once considered standard procedure. Research now demonstrates that this is an unnecessary procedure, which may be performed if the surgeon indicates that the hair may interfere with surgery. If necessary, hair should be removed by either clipping or depilatory. If a surgeon deems that shaving is necessary, it is best to remove hair immediately before surgery as greater intervals between shaving and surgery increase surgical site infection rate.[11,24]

Scrubbing of the surgical site should be performed by gloved personnel according to the policy of the facility. Most hospitals require that the patient shampoo with antibacterial soap the night before surgery. The site is then typically scrubbed in the OR with a chlorhexidine solution. The surgical site should be scrubbed beginning at the site of incision, moving peripherally. Sponges should be discarded once used, ensuring the usage of fresh sponges at the incision site. Once scrubbing is complete, the site is dried with a sterile cloth and the adhesive drape is placed over the site creating a barrier between the patient's skin and the surgeon and OR staff.[11]

Anesthesia Preparation

Information pertaining to the patient's diagnosis and complexity of the operative procedure is evaluated in the preoperative period. Anesthetic procedure for the patient undergoing cranial surgery can present challenges due the varied pathology requiring unique monitoring and anesthesia.[35]

Intraoperative Preparations and Imaging

Standard oral endotracheal intubation is used for the cranial procedure. After general anesthesia has been induced, an indwelling urinary catheter is inserted and connected to a straight drainage system to record output. If necessary, a site on the thigh is shaved to apply a grounding safety pad that must be attached to the patient if an electrocoagulation unit is used. To prevent venous stasis, improve circulation, and prevent DVT and pulmonary embolism PE, antiembolic stockings and/or an intermittent compression device (ICD) is applied for thrombosis risk assessment. After the sterile draping is completed and suctions and electrosurgical cords are attached, the patient is ready for cranial surgery. The surgical team can then proceed.

Intraoperative imaging includes ultrasonography (USG), transcranial Doppler (TCD), MRI, CT, and angiography. Intraoperative image guided systems provide visual data used by the neurosurgeon to aid in surgical resection of brain lesions. **Fluoroscopy** provides serial x-ray images immediately available for the surgeon to view. **Ultrasound,** once used frequently for intraoperative imaging, is now used less frequently since the advent of more sophisticated equipment. With the advent of frameless stereotactic navigational equipment (Fig. 8-6), it was feared that USG would become obsolete.[4] However, this technology continues to be expanded and redefined, providing significant intraoperative contributions to real-time lesion localization and cerebrovascular flow dynamics.[4] **Three-dimensional stereotactic navigational systems** provide surgeons with an intraoperative tool that greatly increases the accuracy of lesion localization. Although these systems have significantly advanced, they are still limited in that most rely on preoperative images for localization of the lesion. Anatomic changes can occur during surgery due to opening of the dura, increased ICP, and fluid volume changes. Such changes are not accounted for with systems that rely on preoperative images. The advent of intraoperative MRI systems has enabled the surgeon to view the progress of the surgery throughout the operative period. Accurate targeting can be verified with real-time images during the procedure, preserving nearby critical structures.[22]

A special OR suite is dedicated to **intraoperative MRI (IOMRI).** The IOMRI team undergoes specialized training before using the equipment due to safety considerations of working within the magnetic field. Team members are screened for any physical conditions such as pacemakers/noncompatible implants that would prevent them from working in the suite. There are numerous safety considerations specific to the unit. Operative equipment, tools, and anesthesia equipment must be checked for compatibility. Some facilities have instituted a color coding system for tools compatible with IOMRI. This system alleviates compatibility questions. The magnetic field has the potential to create electrical currents within cables or wires that are looped or crossed, placing the patient at risk for burns. All cords should be padded when they are in close contact with the patient. Looping or crossing of wires should be prevented.[37]

IOMRI is a significant technologic advance. However, it requires its own physical suite, special operative equipment, and trained staff. As a result, this equipment is cost prohibitive for many facilities.

Craniotomy Procedure

Several important factors require deliberation before starting the craniotomy procedure. Careful positioning of the patient's head, taking into consideration the location of the surgical target, is important to alleviate potential intraoperative complications. Improper positioning can cause a change in surgical trajectory, potentially altering the accuracy and goal of the resection.[5] Positioning the patient's head with the operative site parallel to the floor is recommended. A tilt in the operative site forces the surgeon to work at an angle, increasing difficulty of the procedure, thereby causing discomfort and fatigue for the surgeon.[5]

The exposures used in craniotomies are chosen for their unique surgical advantage (Fig. 8-7). The decision for the approach is made with careful consideration by the surgeon. Knowledge of cranial topography, landmarks, and anatomic location of the lesion is incorporated into this decision.[5] The six most common approaches used for craniotomy are detailed in Table 8-4.

Craniotomy incisions are planned based on location of the lesion. The patient is positioned to provide optimum access.

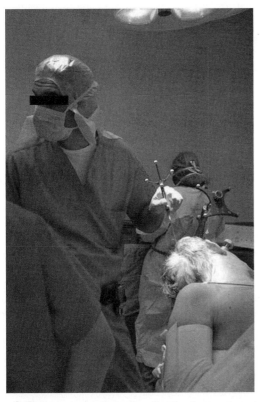

Figure 8-6 Preoperative lesion localization by neurosurgeon using frameless stereotaxy.

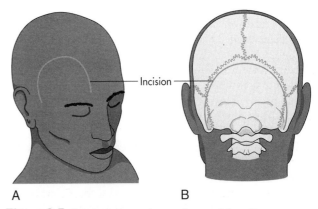

Figure 8-7 Surgical approaches to the cranial cavity. **A,** Supratentorial approach. **B,** Infratentorial approach. *(From Beare PG, Meyers JL: Adult health nursing, ed 3, St Louis, 1998, Mosby.)*

TABLE 8-4	Six Common Approaches Used for a Craniotomy Procedure	
Approach	**Indication**	
Frontosphenotemporal	Anterior and posterior circulation aneurysm	
	Parasellar, sphenoid, anterior skull base tumors	
Subtemporal	Posterior cavernous sinus	
	Petroclival region	
	Basilar artery lesion	
Anterior parasagittal	Lateral and third ventricle parasagittal convexity	
	Parafalcine tumors	
	Distal anterior cerebral artery aneurysms	
Posterior parasagittal	Medial parietal and occipital lesions	
	Posterior corpus callosum	
	Trigone	
Midline suboccipital	Cerebellar vermis, fourth ventricle, pineal region tumor	
Lateral suboccipital craniectomy/ far-lateral transcondylar extension	Posterior fossa, cerebellopontine (CP) angle tumor	

From Clatterbuck RC, Tamargo RJ: Surgical positioning and exposures for cranial procedures. In Winn HR, editor: *Youmans neurological surgery,* ed 5, Philadelphia, 2004, Saunders.

The incisional size is formed by considering the exposure required for bone and brain dependent on the indication for treatment. Tumor resections may require a larger incision and exposure than other procedures such as microvascular decompressions. Once the assessment on positioning and incision size is made, and the patient is properly prepared and draped, the incision site is infiltrated with local anesthetic containing a vasoconstrictive agent such as epinephrine.

An incision is made into the skin and **galea aponeurotica,** or epicranial aponeurosis (Fig. 8-8, *A* and *B*). This is a fibrous membrane that covers the cranium between the occipital and frontal muscles of the scalp. Bleeding is controlled as the soft tissue is peeled off the periosteum, and a scalp flap is turned and clips applied. A **burr hole** (or holes) (Fig. 8-9) is drilled, and a saw is used to connect the holes to release the bone flap. Liberal application of bone wax may be used to control bleeding from the edges of the extremely vascular bone. The bone can be turned back or removed and wrapped in saline-moistened sterile sponges to be replaced during closure or at another time.

The dura mater is opened circumferentially (Fig. 8-8, *C*), and the surgeon begins the tedious task of controlling bleeding from major dural vessels. Bleeding can be interrupted using bipolar coagulation as the surgeon works deep into the brain toward the lesion. An operating microscope may be brought into the field to magnify the site. Microsurgical instruments are used for delicate work. As the lesion is removed (Fig. 8-8, *D*), a cavity may be left that the surgeon

can pack with Gelfoam or another surgical agent for hemostasis and to retain the edges of the brain structure surrounding the site. Hemostasis is established, and the surgical bed is inspected and closed with the dura closed in a watertight fashion to prevent CSF leakage (Fig. 8-8, *E*). If the dura is part of the surgical lesion, a **dural graft** may be applied.

Closing Process
The cranial plate or bone flap previously removed for a cranial procedure is wired or sutured, the periosteum and muscle are approximated, and the galea is closed. Skin closure can be achieved with staples or sutures (Fig. 8-8, *F*). A portable, self-contained closed-wound drainage tube may be inserted through a separate small incision or stab wound to prevent development of deep wound infections. A ventriculostomy or bolt may also be placed during surgery (see Chapter 12 for a complete discussion of ICP monitoring).

Once the dura is closed, preparation should be made to ensure that the patient awakens from anesthesia smoothly and without coughing in response to the endotracheal tube. Administering small doses of thiopental or succinylcholine immediately before bandaging the head may allow smooth emergence and extubation. Suctioning of the mouth and pharynx should be carried out before reversing the muscle relaxant.

The cranial wound may be treated with an antibacterial ointment, and a head dressing is applied with cotton balls behind the ears to prevent bending the ears back too tightly. The neurosurgical team slides the patient onto the stretcher with the head elevated while the anesthesiologist attaches portable oxygen, a cardiac monitor, and all other equipment that must accompany the patient to the postanesthesia care unit (PACU) or the neuroscience critical care unit (NCCU) as quickly and safely as possible.

Acute Postoperative Management
The immediate postoperative period in the PACU or NCCU following craniotomy is a precarious period requiring meticulous nursing assessment to identify complications. The decline of neurologic function in the postoperative period warrants emergent action. Risks are individualized to the patient, and any complication is immediately treated. It is difficult to generalize complications as each indication carries its own risks related to lesion location and functionality of the anatomic location.

Postoperative Assessment
Possible causes of postoperative decline include routine neurologic assessment and monitoring with particular attention for signs and symptoms of (1) hematoma formation, (2) cerebral infarction, (3) seizure activity, (4) increased ICP, (5) acute hydrocephalus, (6) pneumocephalus, (7) postoperative edema causing increased ICP, and (8) vasospasm.[17]

Craniotomy Complications

Hemorrhage
Current literature reports postoperative hemorrhage rates between 0.8% and 1.1% with a mortality rate of 32%. The risk

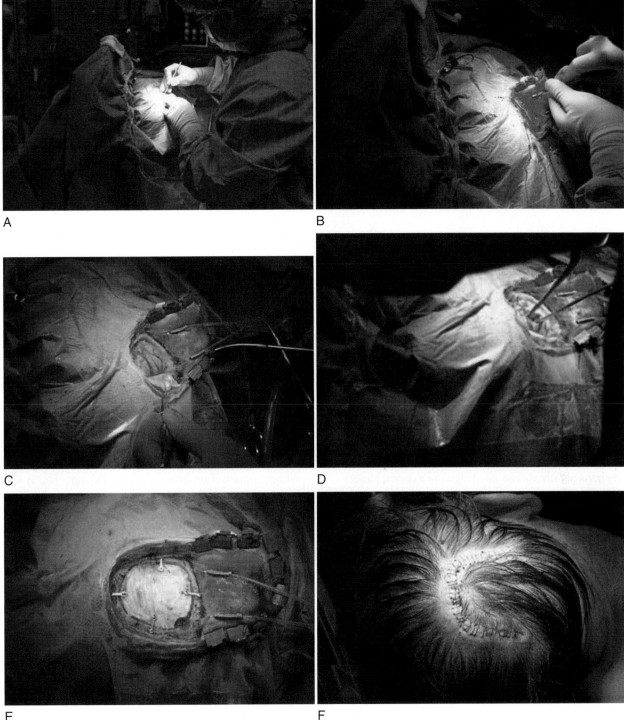

Figure 8-8 Craniotomy procedure: From skin cut to staple closure. **A,** Skin cut. **B,** Galea. **C,** Opening of dura. **D,** Resection of tumor. **E,** Bone flap is replaced. **F,** Skin incision is closed with staples.

factors associated with postoperative hematoma include increased intraoperative blood loss and ICP, use of antiplatelet and anticoagulant agents, disorders that affect clotting, coagulopathies, hypertension, preoperative use of mannitol, and preoperative alcohol consumption. A majority of hematomas develop within the 24-hour period following surgery and have a greater mortality rate than those developing past that time.

ALERT: The most common clinical manifestation of postoperative hematoma is a decrease in level of consciousness (LOC) and requires the notification of the neurosurgeon. The most frequently cited indication for postoperative hematoma formation is meningioma.[16,44]

Cerebral Infarction

Postoperative cerebral venous infarction can occur from sustained venous hypertension, a disruption of cortical draining

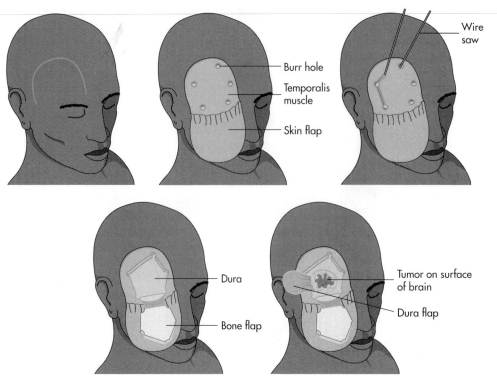

Figure 8-9 Stages of craniotomy. *(From Beare PG, Meyers JL:* Adult health nursing, *ed 3, St Louis, 1998, Mosby.)*

veins with thrombosis caused by intraoperative injury to a cerebral sinus, especially the superior sagittal sinus.[16] There is an increased risk for venous infarction during the resection of parasagittal falcine meningiomas due to their close relation to venous structures.[20] Postoperative arterial infarction occurs following intraoperative occlusion or injury to a cerebral artery.

Seizure Activity

Current literature reports a 4% to 19% seizure incidence in the early postoperative period, with lesions in the supratentorial compartment responsible for the majority.[20] Propensity for postoperative seizures is determined by numerous factors, including influences such as diagnosis, patient condition, and preexisting epilepsy.[29] Several operative factors influence seizures, including (1) cerebral hypoxia, (2) intraoperative brain tissue manipulation, (3) hematoma formation, and (4) cerebral edema.[20] Patients with the following diagnoses are at greater risk for seizures: brain abscess, tumor, AVM, or aneurysm.[20] Preoperative subtherapeutic anticonvulsant levels are strongly correlated to postoperative seizure occurrence.[26]

ALERT: Seizures can be deleterious for patients, raising the risks of increased ICP, cerebral damage, and altered cerebral blood flow[20] (see Chapter 24).

Acute Hydrocephalus

Acute hydrocephalus can develop from obstruction of the ventricular system as a result of intraventricular bleeding or postoperative hematoma. The incidence of acute hydrocephalus is greater in surgeries involving the posterior fossa. The literature reports a 20% incidence of hydrocephalus in pediatric patients following posterior fossa tumor resections.[15]

Pneumocephalus

Pneumocephalus occurs when air is present in the intradural or extradural spaces. This is a common finding on postoperative CT scans. Patients with minimal pneumocephalus are usually asymptomatic and this condition typically resolves without intervention. However, if the amount of air continues to increase, patients will develop the neurologic consequences of an enlarging space-occupying lesion. Patients undergoing skull base surgery and those who undergo surgery in the sitting position are at greater risk.

ALERT: Tension pneumocephalus, which is a more serious complication, is defined as air under pressure and requires rapid identification and surgical evacuation.[20]

Edema and Increased Intracranial Pressure

Postoperative cerebral edema typically occurs within 5 hours following surgery and peaks at between 48 and 72 hours.[20] Surgical retraction of brain tissue, impaired venous drainage, and use of bipolar coagulation are identified causes of postoperative formation of edema.[20] Prolonged edema results in decreased intracranial compliance with a subsequent increase in ICP. Patients who do not undergo ICP monitoring require early identification of signs of increased ICP (change in LOC, headache, nausea/vomiting, pupil changes, change in motor function, change in sensory function, incisional bulging, cranial nerve deficit) (see Chapter 10) in order to provide essential intervention. The goal of treatment is to maintain cerebral perfusion (CPP) pressure between 55 and 60 mm Hg while reducing the ICP.[20] Interventions to reduce ICP include increasing arterial pressure, hyperventilation, surgical removal of space-occupying lesions, dexamethasone, diuretics, sedation, and maintaining head-of-bed elevation between 30 and 45 degrees[20] (see Chapter 10).

Vasospasm

Cerebral vasospasm described as cerebral arterial narrowing typically occurs following subarachnoid hemorrhage (SAH) but may also occur as a result of cranial surgery. Vasospasm is radiologically evident following SAH in approximately 50% of cases. Clinical manifestations of vasospasm occur in 20% to 30% of patients after SAH. A delayed neurologic decline can be indicative of vasospasm. After clinical, laboratory, and imaging studies have ruled out other possible causes of neurologic decline, vasospasm may be investigated by the use of transcranial Doppler, CT, MRI, or angiography.[9,23]

A thorough neurologic assessment is performed on postoperative admission to the PACU or NCCU. Postoperative orders following craniotomy vary between facilities. An acute care order guideline for the first 24 hours following craniotomy is outlined in Box 8-2.

Serial assessments must continue throughout the length of the hospitalization regardless of the postoperative time period (acute, intermediate, and late). The assessments identify the following: CSF leak, infection, fever, venous thromboembolic disorder (DVT/PE), pulmonary abnormalities, cardiac abnormalities, renal abnormalities, gastrointestinal (GI) abnormalities, musculoskeletal abnormalities, pain, alterations in sleep, the need for medication management, abnormal activity, and psychosocial needs.

Intracranial Pressure. Patients with ICP or CPP monitoring will have the waveform pattern and the ICP evaluated and documented as part of the PACU or NCCU routine. The upper limit for ICP is 15 mm Hg. Increased ICP above 20 mm Hg may indicate postoperative swelling, edema, or bleeding. CPP is the difference between the mean arterial pressure (MAP) and ICP. If the brain is not adequately perfused in the immediate postoperative period, when the risk of edema is greatest, the patient can suffer an infarction and

brain damage. CPP can be calculated by using the following formula:

$$CPP = MAP - ICP$$

CPP serves as a measure of the adequacy of cerebral oxygen needs. The normal range for CPP is 60 to 110 mm Hg. A value less than 50 mm Hg is associated with cerebral ischemia and is to be avoided through the use of therapeutic interventions (see Chapter 10).

Dressing and Drains. If a surgical drain is required, the surgeon will insert the drain with a stab wound as described earlier. A bright red bloody drainage may fill the drainage container for a few hours postoperatively and gradually diminish in volume until the drainage becomes thick and dark before finally ceasing. The drain is usually removed 24 to 48 hours postoperatively by the surgeon. Physician preference or unit protocols for wound care should be followed. The gauze or cling turban dressing should not be too tight and should allow one finger to be easily inserted at the edge.

Scalp necrosis, wound infection, and bulging or swelling at the site are rare complications that must be reported immediately. Close observation is essential to detect significant changes, such as redness, drainage, or any signs of infection.

Bleeding. Hematoma formation and hemorrhage are conditions that require an immediate response and reporting to the physician. The amount and characteristics of the bleeding must be described accurately. The patient may have to be returned to the OR on an emergency basis. Changes in the LOC, ICP/CPP, and pupils may be early indicators of oozing, bleeding, or massive hemorrhage.

Cerebrospinal Fluid Leak

Cerebrospinal fluid (CSF) leaks manifest as rhinorrhea, otorrhea, or incisional leaks. **Rhinorrhea** is CSF drainage from the nose caused by loss of integrity of the frontal, ethmoid, or sphenoid bones following trauma or surgery. **Otorrhea** is drainage from the ear that typically results from trauma or surgery involving the temporal bone. Transsphenoidal approaches and skull base surgery create an increased risk of developing CSF leaks.[2] A characteristic sign of a CSF leak is a **"halo" sign** (see Chapter 10) appearing on clothing or bedding as a darkish bloody stain with a surrounding yellow-tinted ring. Patients with CSF leaks are at an increased risk of developing meningitis and must be closely monitored. Treatment for CSF leaks includes head-of-bed elevation and in some cases a lumbar puncture (LP). Most CSF leaks resolve spontaneously and rarely require surgical intervention.

Infection

Although surgical site infections (SSIs) occur in only 1% to 4% of craniotomy procedures, they can cause significant morbidity. The clinician must remain vigilant in assessment of this complication, taking into consideration any known risk factors that cause the patient to have a higher possibility of developing infection.[20,25] Surgical site infections can be confined to the incision, involve the bone flap, or manifest as meningitis or a brain abscess. Predictive risk factors for

BOX 8-2	Acute Postoperative Neurosurgical Orders

- VS q15min × 4, then q1h
- Neurologic checks q1h
- Activity: bed rest, head of bed elevated 20–30 degrees
- DVT protection: sequential compression device/TED hose
- Input and output q1h
- Incentive spirometry q2h while awake
- Diet: NPO except ice chips/medications
- NS + 20 mEq KCl/L at ___ml/hr
- O_2 2L/NC for O_2 saturation <95%
- Medications:
- Laboratory results:
- Notify neurosurgeon of neurologic deterioration or outside specified VS parameters

DVT, Deep vein thrombosis; *NPO,* nothing by mouth; *NS,* normal saline; *VS,* vital signs.

SSI include emergency surgery, clean-contaminated or dirty surgery, and surgery lasting longer than 4 hours. Postoperative risk factors include CSF leak and reoperation.[25] Patients continue to be at risk for infection postoperatively due to the use of invasive monitoring equipment (ICP) and invasive lines. Patients in a deconditioned state or with known systemic diseases such as diabetes or cancer are also at greater risk of postoperative infection (see Chapter 4).

> **ALERT:** *Staphylococcus aureus* is the organism responsible for the largest percentage of SSIs. An analysis of published studies revealed that use of prophylactic broad-spectrum antibiotics significantly reduces the SSI rate.[1]

Fever

Fever is defined as a body temperature above 38° C that is produced in response to inflammatory cytokines. Inflammation, in the form of tissue injury incurred during surgery, can invoke the production of inflammatory cytokines and induce a febrile response. Although fever typically provokes the suspicion of infection, they are not necessarily correlated. Fifty percent of fevers in the NCCU are not related to infection. Noninfectious fevers typically occur as single episodes. Evaluation is warranted in fevers, in particular recurrent febrile episodes.[31]

Causes of the fever should be explored, and the signs and symptoms carefully documented. During the first 48-hour postoperative period, fever usually originates from the respiratory tract (i.e., atelectasis or pneumonia), from the renal tract (i.e., urinary tract infection), or from invasive lines or catheters. After 48 hours, more complex causes may precipitate fever and may be more difficult to diagnose and treat. These include meningitis, sinusitis, brain abscess, PE, sepsis, and multisystem organ failure (MSOF) leading to delirium, lethargy, and coma.

> **ALERT:** Immunosuppressed patients receiving steroids may not exhibit the classic "fever profile"; therefore even minor increases in temperature should be explored.

Hospital guidelines or physician orders should be followed when the following three cultures (triple culturing) are required: (1) respiratory, (2) blood, and (3) serum cultures, or in some cases, CSF specimens. After triple culturing and changing of invasive lines and catheters, a broad-spectrum antibiotic may be ordered until an investigation can uncover the specific organism and cause.

Acetaminophen (Tylenol) may be ordered in addition to hyperthermia blankets or devices, cold packs, removal of most of the patient's bedclothes, and lowering of the ambient temperature. Shivering may be controlled with small doses of chlorpromazine hydrochloride.

Venous Thromboembolic Disorder

Neurosurgical patients have a 25% risk of developing a DVT; 1.5% to 5% of these patients develop a PE, which will prove to be fatal in 9% to 50% of incidences. **Virchow's triad** describes the contributing factors related to thromboembolism formation. The triad includes venous stasis, vascular injury, and a hypercoagulable state due to decreased levels of antithrombin III lasting between 5 and 7 days postoperatively.[6,32]

The morbidity associated with venous thromboembolism has sparked debate regarding the best preventive method available. The use of anticoagulants such as heparin and low-molecular-weight heparin are known to reduce the incidence of thrombus formation but are also known to place the patient undergoing craniotomy at risk for postoperative intracranial hemorrhage. Recent research indicates that the use of mechanical prophylaxis such as an **intermittent sequential compression device (ICD)** may provide adequate protection without the risks associated with anticoagulants.[6]

Deep vein thrombosis (DVT) results from immobilization or venous stasis from thrombosis of the deep leg veins. The thrombus may be in one of the iliac or femoral deep veins of the lower extremities. The exact incidence of DVT in neurosurgical patients is difficult to determine; estimates range from 9% to 50%. Common signs and symptoms of DVT may include the following:

- Pain that may exacerbate with exercise but not disappear with rest
- Tenderness
- Warmth of the affected area
- Sudden swelling of leg in the affected area
- Homan's sign (although this sign—discomfort in the calf muscles on forced dorsiflexion of the foot with the knee straight—may be suggestive of DVT, it is not consistently present in all patients)
- Venous distention and redness or discoloration of the skin
- Low-grade fever
- Tachycardia

In most patients, DVT is clinically silent. In other cases, no single physical symptom or sign is sufficiently accurate to establish a diagnosis of DVT. When symptoms are apparent, their intensity and variety are directly related to the degree of obstruction of venous outflow and inflammation of the vessel wall. Contrast venography, Doppler studies, impedance plethysmography (IPG) scan, iodine fibrinogen uptake scan, and duplex ultrasound studies help to diagnose DVTs. Prevention of DVTs consists of ICDs and getting the patient out of bed (OOB) as soon as possible. Treatment may include one or more of the following options:

- Heparin 5000 units intravenously (IV) with subsequent infusions of 1250 units per hour; dose is adjusted to an APTT of 1.5 to 2 times the control
- Warfarin (Coumadin) tablets initiated on the first day of treatment and titrated to an INR of 2 to 3
- Heparin is discontinued when the therapeutic level of warfarin (Coumadin) has been confirmed for 2 days; most patients continue Coumadin therapy for approximately 3 months

> **ALERT:** It is recommended that a bag of IV solution to which heparin has been added be repeatedly agitated or inversed every few minutes to keep the heparin thoroughly dispersed and to prevent drug pooling during patient administration in order to ensure even distribution and drug delivery.

- Early ambulation
- Mechanical methods: methods include a foot pump, intermittent pneumatic compression (IPC), and graduated elastic antiembolic stockings
- Low-dose heparin 5000 units subcutaneously two to three times per day or according to the physician's order or protocol
- Low-molecular-weight heparin (LMWH):
  - Tinzaparin sodium (Innohep)
  - Enoxaparin (Lovenox): subcutaneously at a weight-based dosage of 1 mg/kg every 12 hours
- Concurrent warfarin (Coumadin) is begun either immediately or within the first 2 days and may be continued for up to 6 months; enoxaparin is continued until a therapeutic level of warfarin is reached
- Thrombolytics: alteplase (Activase) or streptokinase (Streptase) for prompt resolution; however, this therapy does not inhibit development of additional thrombi and includes the risk of fatal intracerebral hemorrhage
- Surgical placement of a vena caval umbrella filter (e.g., the Greenfield) in the inferior vena cava
- Surgery to remove a large thrombus

Pulmonary embolism (PE) is a life-threatening situation if the formation of an embolus blocks a major pulmonary vessel. PE can cause cardiogenic shock followed by circulatory failure and death. More than 60% of PEs may be clinically undiagnosed. Death may occur in as little as 30 minutes if undetected and not treated emergently. Signs and symptoms may include the following:

- Sudden dyspnea and shortness of breath (SOB)
- Chest pain
- Sweating and dizziness
- Hemoptysis
- Hypotension
- Peripheral circulatory failure
- Rapid, shallow breathing
- Tachycardia
- Extreme anxiety

If measures to prevent clotting fail, the dislodged clot can travel from the extremities until it lodges in either the pulmonary artery or one of the branches. The blood flow becomes obstructed, the pulmonary vessels constrict, and the result is a ventilation/perfusion (V/Q) mismatch. The LOC may deteriorate unless the patient receives immediate interventions. The head of the bed (HOB) is elevated, oxygen is administered, and pain is relieved. The following testing is used to confirm the diagnosis:

- V/Q lung scan
- Spiral CT scan
- Chest x-ray study
- Pulmonary angiogram
- ABG studies and ECG

The diagnosis should be quickly confirmed, and treatment initiated as soon as possible to prevent further clots and to dissolve the clot with anticoagulant or thrombolytic therapy as described earlier for DVTs.

Cardiac Assessment and Management

The intraarterial catheter, cardiac monitor, cuff blood pressure readings, and other devices used to monitor the patient's heart provide indicators of cardiovascular status. These parameters provide feedback that allows rapid interventions in response to subtle or life-threatening changes. Cardiac care guidelines apply to the patient recovering from cranial surgery, with an emphasis on maintaining blood pressure within the normotensive range and preventing hypotension or hypertension, cardiac dysrhythmias, and conditions that decrease cardiac output. A 12-lead ECG on admission will document a baseline record that can be compared with previous records and later trends.

Cardiac complications occur when the location of a lesion or ICP affects the cardiac regulatory areas and provokes changes in the cardiac status. Complications may include the following:

- Hypertension or hypotension
- Dysrhythmias
- **Cushing's response** (a late response characterized by a rise in systolic blood pressure, slowing of the pulse, and irregular respirations)

Renal Assessment and Management

Disorder of sodium and water balance is a common complication after neurosurgery. Most patients will have an indwelling urinary catheter inserted perioperatively with orders for strict recording of intake and output (I&O) every 2 hours to assess for volume, color, odor, consistency, and specific gravity. Data to evaluate alterations in renal function can be obtained from the assessment of daily weights, accurate calculation of 24-hour I&O, and observation for the presence of edema. Daily laboratory results are obtained to monitor blood urea nitrogen (BUN), creatinine, and electrolytes.

If the urinary output falls below 30 to 40 ml/hr or rises above 200 ml/hr for 2 consecutive hours, the patient may be exhibiting early signs of the **syndrome of inappropriate antidiuretic hormone (SIADH)** or **diabetes insipidus (DI)** (see Box 5-3 and Chapter 5 for a complete review of these two conditions). A routine urine specimen should be collected and sent for analysis on the first postoperative day and as needed.

Gastrointestinal and Nutritional Assessment and Management. Patients may vary in their ability to take nourishment postoperatively, depending on the type and location of their cranial lesion. Initially, the patient will be on NPO status until a positive gag and swallowing reflex are determined and the patient is awake and alert enough to take nourishment by mouth. Bowel sounds must also be present. Clearing the oral cavity and offering ice chips is comforting for the patient, who may have a sore throat from intubation and a dry mouth from lack of nourishment since the night before surgery.

Following physician orders or by unit protocols, the patient's diet can be advanced to clear liquids, soft foods, or whatever the patient can tolerate during recovery and as appetite returns. There are patients who will be unable to take nourishment by mouth postoperatively and may require the insertion of a feeding tube and supplemental feedings.

Potential GI complications include gastric and duodenal ulceration, or Cushing's ulceration. GI ulcers occur postoperatively from increased secretion of hydrochloric acid and pepsin, which can cause mucosal damage. Cushing's ulcers result from hypersecretion of acid caused by overstimulation of the vagal nuclei. An imbalance between the sympathetic and parasympathetic components of the autonomic system at the hypothalamic level of control of the digestive system may be responsible. Also, the patient's medications may contribute to stress ulcers (e.g., corticosteroids, anticonvulsants, and antibiotics).

Acid secretions damage the mucosa, can cause gastric bleeding, and can cause perforation of small vessels. Bright red hemorrhage or "coffee-ground" secretions may produce bloody stools that are guaiac positive. The bleeding may be significant enough to cause gastric distress, a drop in blood pressure, and a decrease in hemoglobin. Attempts to prevent GI bleeding include a regimen to control gastric pH, administration of antacids, and the use of H2-receptor antagonists.[30] Tube feedings also help neutralize gastric acidity.

ALERT: If there are symptoms of frank bleeding, an immediate response is needed and the physician should be notified. Gastric lavage or other means may be required to stop the active bleeding. The prevention of hypotension will stop a sudden drop in hemoglobin levels that can compromise cerebral perfusion.

A temporary **paralytic ileus** is a condition characterized by a decrease or absence of intestinal peristalsis that may occur postoperatively. The patient will experience abdominal tenderness and distention, absence of bowel sounds, lack of flatus, and nausea and vomiting. Close monitoring, making the patient comfortable, and instructing the patient to avoid swallowing air are helpful interventions.

If paralytic ileus does not resolve spontaneously, a flat-plate abdominal x-ray film will be required. A nasogastric (NG) tube, connected to intermittent suction, can be ordered for decompression. The amount and description of the drainage are recorded.

Return to a full diet may include fluid restrictions based on the patient's recovery status. A nutritional consultation to determine caloric intake and postoperative nutritional requirements should be arranged to provide optimal protein, carbohydrates, fats, and other essentials for wound healing. Malnutrition and starvation with diarrhea and poor absorption are to be avoided; however, a patient with an altered LOC, motor deficits, and impaired gag and swallowing reflexes may develop nutritional deficits.

Monitoring GI status includes the following:
- I&O
- Electrolytes
- Daily weight or as needed
- Skin turgor
- Edema
- Oral cavity changes
- Weekly 24-hour urinalysis for nitrogen analysis
- Laboratory studies
- Urinalysis

Musculoskeletal and Skin Assessment and Management

The assessment of muscle strength, tone, atrophy, abnormal movements, tremors, or fasciculations immediately after surgery alerts the surgical team to postoperative complications (e.g., excessive brain swelling, hemorrhage, or increased ICP).

Peripheral nerve injuries can occur at any time during the perioperative period. The long-term disability that results may have serious consequences for a patient. Nerve lesions are more common in diabetic patients than in the general population. The ulnar, peroneal, and femoral nerves are especially vulnerable in patients who are thin. A high incidence of postoperative neuropathies has been reported after induced hypothermia. Neurosurgery and the use of the sitting position for approaches to the posterior fossa are associated with nerve injuries. Laryngeal nerve injury may result from the large size of the probe, tracheal intubation, and excessive neck flexion. The brachial plexus, ulnar, radial, sciatic, and peroneal nerves are commonly injured during surgery. Padding can alleviate pressure injuries, and abduction of the arm should be limited to 90 degrees or less. The elbow should not be fully extended. External rotation should be avoided. Patient transfer should not involve pulling of the arms.

Although rare, if a head-holding device was applied intraoperatively, the patient's scalp should be checked at the pin sites for redness, swelling, hematoma (a rare complication), or a CSF leak. These sites are cleaned with soap and water. Crusting should be removed with alcohol and a cotton-tipped applicator. An antibacterial ointment can be applied at these sites.

Surgery of long duration increases the likelihood of pressure areas and skin breakdown. Cases of skin burns from electrical equipment are rare but may be discovered during a thorough assessment of the skin integument.

An occasional skin reaction from allergies to intraoperative medications (e.g., phenytoin sodium and antibiotics) is not unusual. At the first appearance of a red, itching, or unusual skin reaction, and before the next dose, the physician must be notified. Close monitoring of the patient's reaction is needed, and the problem investigated and recorded along with any new orders.

Pain

The patient recovering from cranial surgery will experience pain, which should not be undertreated out of fear that medications will mask the neurologic assessment or depress respirations (see Chapter 23). Pain management is a high priority. A pain assessment should lead to interventions that prevent or control pain. The patient's pain should be defined in such a way that the clinician can understand the patient's subjective suffering and develop an appropriate treatment plan (see Chapter 23). Compared with other types of surgery, most patients report minimal pain following cranial surgery (with the exception of patients who have had a frontal craniotomy). Assessment and documentation of pain and treatment allow for frequent evaluations to detect early trends of "breakthrough pain" or excessive drowsiness and to make necessary adjustments for successful pain management.

Even though patients who have undergone cranial surgery may report less pain than patients recovering from general or other types of surgery, prolonged positioning, stretched neck muscles, and head-immobilizing devices may cause extreme patient discomfort on awaking from anesthesia. Restlessness and agitation may be early indicators of discomfort. Complaints of headache may range from moderate to severe in the immediate postoperative period. Analgesics from the following three categories can be considered:[19]

- *Opioids.* Morphine, codeine, and fentanyl act at the opioid receptors and have properties that may produce sedation, respiratory depression, cardiovascular depression, nausea and vomiting, pupillary effects, pruritus, and constipation.
- *Nonsteroidal antiinflammatory drugs* (NSAIDs). Ibuprofen and a large number of other NSAIDs act by inhibition of prostaglandin synthesis and can produce bronchospasm in patients prone to airway obstruction, renal failure in patients with renal disease, GI bleeding by gastric erosion, and hypocoagulability by interfering with platelet function.
- *Local anesthetics* that act to block pain in a particular location.

The right analgesics should be prescribed and administered at the right time to the right patient in the right amount via the right route after a pain assessment that may include the 0-to-10 pain severity scale. Close observation and frequent monitoring of the patient's response to medications and other interventions should guide postoperative pain relief.

ALERT: Aspirin products, anticoagulants, or any medications containing aspirin or ingredients to prolong bleeding time are to be avoided to prevent the risk of postoperative bleeding.

Despite research that supports the use of morphine, some clinicians continue to administer only codeine, which may be ineffective. Severe postoperative pain is most commonly treated with opioid analgesics (e.g., morphine 1 mg IV every 5 to 10 minutes) so that analgesia can be carefully titrated against sedation in the patient in whom analgesia is difficult to achieve.[19] Patient-controlled analgesia (PCA) pumps are self-administered with settings to control the amount and frequency. Close patient monitoring is required to assess for side effects, including nausea and vomiting, and to determine if the patient is awake and alert enough to operate the controls.

There is current interest in the safety, efficacy, and practicality of **nebulized morphine** as an alternative. Nebulized morphine can deliver effective pain relief medication when the morphine is quickly absorbed in the lungs. A new delivery method has already been reported to successfully relieve breathing difficulties in patients suffering from lung cancer. The nebulizer device discharges a fine mist of medication through a mouthpiece or mask worn over the patient's mouth. The morphine mist, which is diluted with 3 ml of saline, enters the lungs as the patient breathes in and out for 5 to 10 minutes. Codeine (which is metabolized to morphine) 30 to 40 mg given intramuscularly or orally every 4 to 6 hours is considered a weak opioid and is appropriate for less severe pain. Acetaminophen (Tylenol), codeine, or a combination of these two drugs may relieve the headache. Morphine sulfate (MS) 1 mg IV bolus is often prescribed for a severe headache and may also decrease ICP (see Chapter 23).

Sleep

The patient's sleep-wake cycle is disturbed for several days postoperatively. The frequency of assessments and close patient monitoring contribute to sleep interruption and deprivation. Medications that interfere with rapid eye movement (REM) sleep and the noise of an ICU setting are very disruptive and annoying. When a patient's pain is being evaluated, these factors should be considered.

To avoid repeated interruptions that add to patient discomfort, physician and clinical assessments can be performed together during rounds. Planned quiet periods can be scheduled and a "do not disturb" sign put on the door. Excessive noise is eliminated and intrusions minimized as much as possible (see Chapter 8).

Nausea and Vomiting

Postoperative nausea and vomiting (PONV) is a typical reaction to general anesthesia and surgery. The patient's comfort is maximized, and increased ICP can be prevented using routine care. Antiemetics are routinely ordered and administered according to the patient's level of PONV and may include droperidol (Inapsine), prochlorperazine (Compazine), cyclizine (Marezine), and ondansetron (Zofran).

Activity

The patient is restricted to bed, with bed rest maintained for the prescribed hours with the HOB usually elevated 20 to 30 degrees. The patient should be repositioned every 2 hours. When turning or repositioning the patient, one clinician should support the head in a neutral position to avoid flexion, eliminate pain, and reduce the risk of elevated ICP as other clinicians complete the turn or reposition. A "lift" sheet or device to logroll the patient also reduces skin friction and shearing of skin. Assistive devices (e.g., a thin polyethylene board, a mechanical moving device) are also very useful for moving heavy patients. Patients who have been maintained on steroid therapy are at high risk for skin breakdown and reduced wound healing.

After the prescribed hours on bed rest, the patient may be able to sit on the side of the bed with assistance, sit in a chair, or ambulate. The patient's acuity will determine recovery. Evaluation by the neurosurgical team and input from the patient help establish the rate and type of ambulation. As soon as the patient's medical condition has stabilized and is free of complications, transfer to a step-down unit is possible.

Postacute Care

Discharge and Patient Education

After transfer to the step-down unit, the patient is generally more responsive and aware of his or her environment, the period of high-risk complications is over, body strength and functions that may allow the patient to be out of bed are returning, and there are extended patient-family interactions. Monitoring is less frequent; however, even a subtle deterioration in the patient's condition requires notification of the surgical team with frequent assessments until the cause is determined and appropriately treated. Patient teaching with a review of detailed verbal and written discharge instructions prepares the patient to recover at home with family support and home health care if needed. Appointments for follow-up care include wound care, activity, diet, medications, and potential complications to report immediately at the onset.

If a visiting home health team is ordered, communication and arrangements should be established to plan a smooth transition to the patient's home. The family should be prepared to deal with transient cognitive changes postoperatively that can be expected to resolve over 3 to 6 months. The family can address any changes in personality, intellect, and behavior (e.g., lack of interest, decreased motivation, and fatigue) with patience and tolerance. The patient and family should be provided with coping strategies and referrals to appropriate resources. The patient's and the family's positive attitude toward recovery will be affected by the positive, caring attitude of the clinical team and staff at the time of the patient's discharge.

Perioperative Psychosocial Considerations

The day of neurosurgery is one of extreme stress and anxiety for the family, yet there are often few opportunities for clinician contact until the patient is returned to the designated nursing unit for recovery. Hospitals are becoming more aware of family isolation during this period. Families of same-day surgery patients may be asked to report to a designated waiting room that is staffed with a receptionist and has telephone connections to the OR suite. OR staff may provide updates to the receptionist during the surgery to keep the family informed and to tell them where the patient can be visited postoperatively.

As soon as possible after the patient has settled into the assigned nursing unit after surgery, the family must be allowed a short visit with a brief report of the patient's condition and an explanation of the equipment and ICU care.

The ongoing psychosocial assessment of the patient's response to the surgery and the recovery process will identify distress and ineffective coping mechanisms. Physical symptoms predominate in the first 24 to 48 hours, but as the discomfort diminishes, the patient's awareness of any deficits or disabilities may cause expressions of alarm and fear. Presurgical teaching prepares patients and their families for some of the side effects of surgery (e.g., swollen eyes, facial swelling, weakness, nausea and vomiting, and headache). Patients should be reassured that these effects are temporary. For patients who need additional supportive help with recovery, consultations should be arranged with the psychiatric clinical specialist or other appropriate consultants.

CRANIECTOMY

A **craniectomy,** which is done to remove a tumor, hematoma, scar tissue, or infected bone tissue, differs from a craniotomy, in which a bone flap is removed for access to the brain and replaced at the end of the procedure. Routine preoperative procedures and preparation are similar to those described

---

| BOX 8-3 | **Potential Hazards for Patients During a Craniectomy** |

Venous air embolism (VAE), which is a serious concern with posterior fossa surgery and may trigger a cascade of events:[17]

Air entering the heart (air and blood in the right ventricle may prevent effective cardiac output and produce a "millwheel murmur")

Pulmonary edema and reflex bronchoconstriction, which may result from air in the pulmonary circulation

Hypotension

Tachycardia

Dysrhythmias

Neck vein congestion

Cyanosis

Death secondary to acute cor pulmonale and anoxia from obstruction of the pulmonary circulation

Vital sign changes due to brainstem manipulation

Airway obstruction

Position-related brainstem ischemia

Use of a precordial Doppler ultrasonic transducer will detect changes in the signal to alert the surgeon to occlude the sites where air can enter. Air can be recovered by aspiration of the central venous or pulmonary artery catheter. A chest x-ray study may be performed for documentation of catheter placement.

---

in the previous section. For a craniectomy, a rongeur is used to remove small pieces of bone, bit by bit, versus turning a large bone flap. Postoperatively, therefore, there is no large bone flap to cover and protect the wound. The posterior fossa approach may be used with the patient positioned in the prone or sitting position (see Fig. 8-5). Included in the indications for posterior fossa surgery are lesions involving the cerebellum, pons, medulla, and lower cranial nerves. Although the sitting position causes less tissue retraction and damage to cranial nerves, cranial nerve stimulation may be used throughout the procedure to immediately alert the surgeon to potential nerve impairment or damage. Evoked potentials are used most commonly in posterior fossa surgery, brainstem auditory evoked potential (BAEPs) are used when the neural pathways for conductive hearing may be jeopardized, and visual evoked potentials (VEPs) are helpful during resection of pituitary tumors and craniopharyngiomas.

Special precautions are taken by the anesthesiologist with the patient in the sitting position because of the possibility that air may come from the puncture of the three-point head holder site, the soft tissue, the dome, the dural edge, the dural sinuses, or the bridging veins over the cerebellum. Box 8-3 includes hazards of the sitting position during craniectomy.

Acute, Postacute, and Discharge Care

Most craniectomy patients will be recovered overnight in an ICU or NCCU. During the immediate postoperative period the patient requires frequent neurologic assessment and monitoring. Acute postoperative assessment and interventions include the following:

- LOC and sudden unresponsiveness from brainstem compression
- Hypertension from brainstem edema
- Bradycardia, or irregular respirations, which may indicate a cerebral hemorrhage
- Signs of brainstem infarction if an air embolism is suspected or was detected intraoperatively
- Dehydration and syncope are to be avoided postoperatively
- Respiratory and cardiac changes that could result in cardiopulmonary arrest
- Increased ICP from brain edema, hematoma, hydrocephalus, or infection
- Cushing's ulcer: related to the stress of surgery
- Lower cranial nerve deficits (e.g., vagus) and other cranial nerve deficits due to surgical manipulation
- Monitoring for deafness, visual changes, and other conditions that require special attention and interventions from cranial nerve compression or edema
- CSF leak
- Vertigo, nausea, and vomiting
- Headache
- Careful repositioning with support of the head and logrolling of the patient every 2 hours
- Careful movement: the removal of large tumors prohibits turning onto the operative side until the brain has compensated
- Eye care with artificial tears and lubricant, eye patching, or tarsorrhaphy to temporarily suture the eyelids and protect the cornea if the corneal reflex is diminished or absent
- Early ambulation: helps prevent problems of immobility; however, the patient's gait and balance could be affected and assistance needed with instructions to move and rise slowly to avoid hypotension, nausea, and vertigo

In complicated cases or for prolonged surgery, the ICU stay may be longer than 24 hours because of nausea and vomiting, cranial nerve deficits, and problems with elevated ICP. Gag and swallowing reflexes must be intact and ICP controlled before the patient is ready for transfer from the NCCU. The remainder of the recovery is the same as for patients recovering from a craniotomy, with awareness of the wound precautions, protection of the craniectomy site, and problems with headache, which may persist, causing discomfort for a longer period of time as compared with craniotomy. In uncomplicated cases, patients are transferred to the post-acute unit within 24 hours with special precautions for the surgical site, which has no bone flap for protection, and prepared for discharge after a short stay.

HYDROCEPHALUS AND SHUNTING PROCEDURE

Hydrocephalus is a neurologic condition marked by dilation of the cerebral ventricles. Hydrocephalus most often occurs secondarily to obstruction of the CSF pathways accompanied by abnormal or excessive accumulation of CSF in the brain that results in dilated ventricles. Congenital hydrocephalus is present at birth and usually traced to a birth defect of brain malformation. Acquired hydrocephalus develops at birth or at some point afterward from conditions that cause an increase in the resistance to drainage of CSF. It occurs when the rate of CSF absorption is less than the rate of production. The CSF is usually under increased pressure. Hydrocephalus can be communicating when CSF is blocked after it exits from the ventricles and is not absorbed or noncommunicating when the flow of CSF is blocked along one or more of the pathways connecting the ventricles. Idiopathic normal pressure hydrocephalus (NPH) is a syndrome seen on older adults characterized by the triad of gait impairment, cognitive decline or dementia, and urinary incontinence. The CT or MRI scan demonstrates ventriculomegaly. The CSF tap test involves a lumbar puncture to check opening pressure and removal of 40 to 50 ml of CSF to see if the removal of a large volume of CSF improves symptoms for an indication that shunting will be effective. A hospital admission with prolonged external CSF drainage is performed on a limited basis and has the potential for infections and other complications.

In older patients the arachnoid villi may have calcified, further reducing the flow of CSF. Surgical diversion of CSF around an obstructive intracranial mass usually involves ventriculoperitoneal (VP) shunting. Most shunt procedures are performed to provide an alternative pathway for CSF. Some of the causes are (1) increased production of CSF (from a choroid plexus papilloma), (2) obstruction of CSF flow (a tumor in the aqueduct of Sylvius or SAH, or noncommunicating hydrocephalus), and (3) a communicating interference in absorption of CSF by the arachnoid villi caused by infection (meningitis) or hemorrhage. Unless measures are taken to provide an alternate pathway for CSF circulation, the patient will eventually lapse into coma, suffer brain herniation, and die. Shunts used to initially be set at low, medium, or high pressure. With advancing technology, commercial shunts are now available that can be adjusted and programmed according to the level of drainage required.

Caution must be taken if the shunt can be accidentally readjusted in strong magnetic fields (e.g., an MRI scan) or even relatively weak magnetic fields found in the home. The newer adjustable ProGav Miethke shunt ball-on-spring valve unit contains an integrated overdrainage compensating and gravitational device known as a "shunt assistant." This brake system is intended to prevent changes in the valve's performance level in a magnetic field to prevent accidental readjustment. In addition, the anti-siphon reduces posture-related overdrainage and flow remains constant as shunt performance is not affected by the body posture.

Medical and Surgical Management

Treatment of hydrocephalus consists of a temporary ventriculostomy as described in Chapter 10. Medications may include acetazolamide (Diamox), a loop diuretic (e.g., Lasix), and seizure medications as needed.

The primary surgical treatment is shunting of the CSF, with the VP shunt being the most commonly used system.

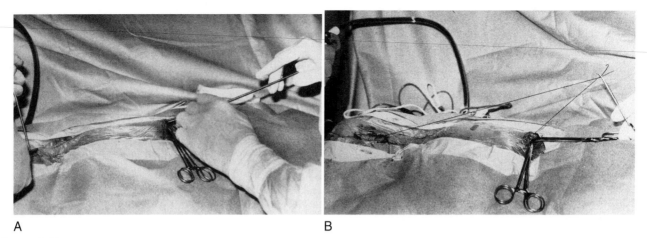

A   B

Figure 8-10 Shunt procedure. **A,** Trocar is tunneled under the skin. **B,** Silk suture is tunneled under the skin to pull the peritoneal catheter through.

After routine preoperative preparation the patient is taken to the OR for the 30- to 45-minute procedure, in uncomplicated cases. The VP technique with pressure-controlled valves under the scalp is a short procedure that allows ease of insertion and revision, has few complications, and shunts CSF into the peritoneal cavity.

A VP shunt is performed with the patient under general anesthesia and placed in a supine position with a shoulder roll for support and the head turned to the nonoperative side. After routine preparation from the head to the abdomen, a small scalp incision is made, a burr hole is drilled into the cranium, and a small abdominal incision is made. The shunt components consist of a proximal catheter (plastic or silicon), a reservoir, a valve (to regulate the flow of CSF), and a distal/terminal catheter. The ventricular catheter is placed, usually in the right ventricle. As CSF escapes, specimens may be collected for analysis, and the valve is connected and sutured. The valve pressure flow control and design type are based on the clinical picture and diagnosis. The peritoneal catheter is introduced through the trocar sleeve, and the sleeve is removed. After a cervical incision is made, the tunneling device is passed under the subcutaneous layer of skin from the cervical incision to the peritoneal area (Fig. 8-10). Connections are made to ensure a closed system, and the reservoir and shunt are checked for leaks or malfunctions before the wounds are sutured closed. Sterile dressings are placed on the small incision sites (Fig. 8-11), and the patient is returned to the PACU or NCCU for postoperative recovery. An x-ray or intraoperative ultrasound study may be used to check catheter placement.

Postoperative Management

Postoperative clinical management involves the following:
- Position the patient supine and elevate gradually as ordered, or as tolerated; avoid positioning on the site of the cranial incisions
- Monitor for overshunting, which could collapse ventricles and cause bleeding from bridging veins causing headache or subdural hematomas

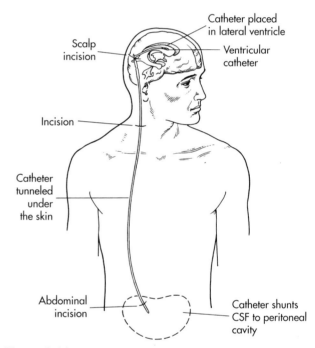

Figure 8-11 Patient with a ventriculoperitoneal (VP) shunt.

- Monitor for underdrainage: symptoms of hydrocephalus recur
- Monitor for elevated ICP
- Observe strict monitoring of I&O
- Perform frequent neurologic checks and monitor for change in LOC
- Observe for wound infection, hematoma, hemorrhage, peritonitis, and meningitis
- Monitor for shunt failure and catheter occlusion
- Monitor for headache, and provide analgesics
- Monitor for seizures, and provide ordered anticonvulsants

Patient recovery is dictated by the type of anesthesia used and the potential complications expected by the health care team who performed the procedure. Postoperative clinical management with comprehensive verbal and written patient and family teaching is critical for patients with a permanent shunt. Potential complications may include the following:

- *Mechanical.* Shunt malfunction may cause increased ICP with headache, lethargy, and vomiting; overshunting with collapsed ventricles may be present with headache that is relieved when the patient is recumbent; perforation of the abdominal cavity with the tip of the catheter leads to pain and distention.
- *Infections.* These are often caused by *Staphylococcus aureus* and may result in fever, ventriculitis, or meningitis; seeding of the infection may occur from the brain to the drainage site in the peritoneal cavity with resultant peritonitis or peritoneal cysts. Fever, soreness of neck and shoulders, or redness along the shunt tract should be reported immediately.
- *Functional.* Occlusion of the catheter openings may occur with plugging by the choroid plexus, clots, or tissue; mechanical failure may occur from detachment of the system at connecting sites or from kinking of tubing.
- *Subdural or intracerebral hematoma.*
- *Seizures.*

Emphasis on shunt failure and infection must be stressed in all cases to prevent serious side effects and neurologic deficits. The hospitalization is short, but the need for long-term follow-up is emphasized. Immediate reporting of fever, headache, irritability, and signs of increased ICP are reviewed, as well as the benefits of having a VP shunt. Patients are taught that the supine position will temporarily relieve symptoms until medical help is available. Faced with the problems of an obstructed shunt, the patient may seek treatment at the emergency department, where an emergency tap can be performed. Patients are admitted and observed after an emergency shunt tap to complete diagnostic studies to fully investigate the complications or for surgery to replace the shunt. Shunt revisions may be necessary over time.

NEUROENDOSCOPIC THIRD VENTRICULOSTOMY

Neuroendoscopic third ventriculostomy (NTV) has gained more widespread use with the introduction of new endoscopic technology. It is used today for the primary therapy of hydrocephalus and as an alternative to shunt replacement for aqueduct stenosis or noncommunicating hydrocephalus. The goal is to maintain normal ICP and to eliminate the need for extracranial shunts by reestablishing CSF pathways. The procedure bypasses the blockage at the level of the aqueduct or the exit foramina of the fourth ventricle by fenestrating the floor of the third ventricle to enable communication between the basilar cisterns and the third ventricle. It is contraindicated for patients with communicating hydrocephalus.[21]

Patient selection includes individuals over the age of 6 months. Anatomic considerations are that the lateral ventricle should be of adequate size for access, the foramen of Monro and the third ventricle should be adequate to permit passage of the ventriculoscope, and the floor of the third ventricle should be attenuated and bulging downward.[21] A CT scan, ultrasound study, CT ventriculogram, or MRI is performed to determine the location of the CSF blockage and position of the basilar artery and other vessels.

General anesthesia is used, avoiding anesthetic agents that could raise the ICP, since most patients have some degree of increased ICP. The dura is opened, and a rigid or flexible camera is carefully maneuvered and passed through the foramen of Monro until the floor of the third ventricle is visualized. An intraoperative ventriculogram can be obtained for verification. The floor of the third ventricle is perforated with the tip of the endoscope and other instruments to create an opening. Balloon catheters can be placed in the opening and inflated to enlarge the site. Various methods (e.g., lasers or bipolar diathermy) have been used to burn a permanent hole at the site, with care being taken not to damage or cause hemorrhage of nearby vessels.[21]

Vascular injuries with intraventricular hemorrhage, cerebral bleeding from damage to adjacent cerebral vessels, cranial palsy (e.g., of cranial nerve III), traumatic basilar artery aneurysms, SAH causing hydrocephalus, and death are rare but potential problems with NTV. The use of intraoperative Doppler ultrasound with small probes passed through the endoscope has been reported.[3]

The flow of CSF must adjust to the new pathway, and ICP may be elevated postoperatively. Patients may be allowed out of bed (OOB) the first postoperative day. Postoperative headache, papilledema, nausea, and vomiting are not uncommon patient complaints. Potential complications include the following:[21]

- Disability and/or death from bleeding of the basilar artery
- Hypothalamic damage
- Infections
- Blockage and overdrainage
- Reclosure of the penetrated site
- Failure of technique, resulting in increased ICP

Long-term follow-up is needed to monitor patients for future blockage; an excellent prognosis is expected. There are few reports in the literature regarding complications of NTV, such as hemorrhage.[3]

STEREOTACTIC RADIOSURGERY

Definition and Forms

Lars Leksell, a Swedish neurosurgeon, invented the first stereotactic system for intracranial use, known as the gamma knife, in 1967.[4] This form of radiosurgery uses cobalt 60 as its energy source. Initially used in the treatment of trigeminal neuralgia and functional disorders, this technology now has wide applicability for the treatment of intracranial pathology. Today, numerous forms of stereotactic radiosurgery exist and are used for the treatment of intracranial lesions. Linear accelerators are used for more traditional forms of fractionated radiation treatments and can be converted to perform intracranial radiosurgical procedures. Linear accelerator–

TABLE 8-5	Success Rates of Gamma Knife and Linear Accelerator Radiosurgery for Tumor Control and Arteriovenous Malformation Obliteration	
Indication	Leksell Gamma Knife	Linear Accelerator Radiosurgery
Metastasis	85%-94%	85%-96%
Acoustic neuroma	89%-94%	>90%
Meningioma	89%-96%	94%-98%
Arteriovenous malformation <4 cm	71%-80%	80%-87%

From Winn HR, editor: *Youmans neurological surgery,* ed 5, Philadelphia, 2004, Saunders.

based systems use x-rays as the source of energy. A healthy debate between radiosurgeons pertaining to the superiority of radiosurgical modalities has contributed to significant research in the field. The Leksell Gamma Knife Society maintains a worldwide database that currently reports approximately 200,000 procedures performed.[40] Despite the chosen modality of treatment, the radiobiology remains the same. A high dose of ionizing radiation is precisely focused on an intracranial target causing alterations in cell DNA, primarily from the formation of free radicals secondary to ionization of the water content of the cell.[4] Once damaged, cells die over time through a genetically programmed process termed *apoptosis,* or programmed cell death.

Indications

Before the advent of radiosurgery, intracranial lesions were surgically resected, treated with fractionated radiotherapy, or deemed inoperable. Numerous neurosurgical indications are now treated with radiosurgery, sparing the patient from a craniotomy and subsequent lengthy recovery (Table 8-5). The most frequently treated conditions are tumors (benign and malignant), arteriovenous malformations, functional disorders (Parkinson's disease and essential tremor), and trigeminal neuralgia.

Radiosurgery has alleviated the need for craniotomy in many patients. However, not all patients with intracranial pathology are considered candidates for the procedure. Lesion size is a recognized limitation in gamma knife surgery, with treatment of lesions smaller than 3 cm being standard. Treatment of lesions larger than 3 cm increases the risk of known side effects (i.e., cerebral edema and radiation necrosis). Another advantage to radiosurgery is that multiple lesions, such as multiple intracranial metastases, can be treated in one sitting.

Procedure

Patients are typically admitted to day surgery or a radiosurgical suite. Following completion of necessary forms, patients receive IV lines. Placement of a stereotactic head frame is the only invasive part of the radiosurgery procedure. Frames are placed by neurosurgeons under conscious sedation and local anesthesia. Head frame placement is quick and should cause little discomfort to the patient. Following application of the head frame, patients are transported for imaging studies (MRI, CT, or angiography). Images are transported to the radiosurgery computer where localization is performed by neurosurgeons, radiation oncologists, medical physicists, or a combination of all. Patients are then positioned on the treatment table with their head stabilized within the unit. Treatment times vary according to the size and location of the lesion being treated. As with other forms of radiation, the treatment is painless. Depending on the facility, patients are discharged following the procedure or admitted for observation for 24 hours. Follow-up consists of serial scans (MRI, CT, or angiography) and physician visits. Patients may experience a transient headache following the procedure.

COMPREHENSIVE PATIENT MANAGEMENT

Rehabilitation Considerations

Cranial surgery and shunting may leave some patients with short-term temporary deficits that respond to a prescribed period of rehabilitation. The rehabilitation team consisting of a physiatrist, an occupational therapist (OT), a physical therapist (PT), and a speech and language therapist (ST) (see Chapter 13) can evaluate the patient for outpatient or home care, visit the home, and develop a plan of safe rehabilitative care.

Older Adult Considerations

Admission for cranial surgery presents a host of special considerations for older adults (Box 8-4). Changes in body weight composition and actual weight are part of the normal aging process. The older adult with increased weight or obesity has the capacity for prolonged drug and anesthesia storage effects. Skin thins with age, particularly with steroid use, and can result in the potential for pressure ulcers and poor wound healing, especially with prolonged immobility. Bones and joints undergo degenerative changes with the potential for pain and dysfunction from arthritis or osteoporosis. Problems with balance and mobility require supervision and care in positioning, transferring to and from bed or chair, and ambulation. Comprehensive pain assessment and management for preexisting pain issues in addition to pain-related neurosurgical procedures is challenging.

Age-related changes in the special senses (vision and hearing) can create safety issues, problems with "sundowning," and confusion during an acute hospitalization. The administration of new drugs, IV medications, and fluid administration may lead to renal problems, incontinence, or patients attempting to get out of bed to use the bathroom, which may result in falls and injury. Refer to Chapter 2 for additional assessment of the older adult.

Close observance of mental status changes and monitoring of cardiac, respiratory, and GI status are necessary to

| BOX 8-4 | Cranial Surgical Considerations in the Older Patient |

Preoperative Phase
- Assessment of preexisting conditions, social situation; atypical presentation/nonspecific symptoms; medication history; patient outlook regarding surgery; acute/chronic confusional states
- Stabilization of acute emergencies; preexisting conditions
- Teaching regarding perioperative course; importance of mobility, functional status; safety; acute confusional states (potential for); spouse and family teaching
- Informed consent, including physician's legal responsibilities; nursing role as a liaison; assessment of mental status, competency
- Preoperative medications, including age-associated alternations in pharmacokinetics and pharmacodynamics; necessity for altered dosages

Intraoperative Phase
- Anesthesia, including potential for acute confusional states (secondary to drugs, decreased CBF, hypoxia and/or hypercarbia); age-associated changes requiring smaller doses and shorter time to induction
- Attention to positioning to prevent pressure sores; hypothermia secondary to thalamic age-associated changes, drugs, past history

Postoperative Phase
- Prevention of iatrogenic complications: these include impaired function; medication side effects, infection, pressure sores, delirium, depression, urinary incontinence, pulmonary complications, constipation, and DVTs or PE
- Unrelieved pain: older adults are more susceptible and may develop pneumonia or respiratory complications related to inadequate deep breathing, coughing, and repositioning related to unrelieved pain
- Underreporting of pain: closely observe for behavioral signs (e.g., moaning, restlessness, agitation, changes in mental status, grimacing, refusal to eat, inability to sleep) and failure to report pain and request medication, which may be overcome by the use of the visual analog scale or the face scale for pain assessment (see Chapter 23)
- Discharge planning: determine the patient's social situation, including spouse and family/friend support, as well as community services available

CBF, Cerebral blood flow; *DVTs,* deep vein thromboses; *PE,* pulmonary embolism.

detect early signs and symptoms of complications for prompt interventions. Psychosocial support and allowing extra time for questions and activities of daily living (ADLs) are effective measures to decrease fear and anxiety and promote recovery and return to home and family.

Case Management Considerations

There is nothing as frightening to a patient and his or her family as "brain surgery." Depending on the patient's age, prognosis, and level of function, case management may be required to coordinate individualized, comprehensive services. Neurologically impaired patients constitute a large portion of any caseload.[36] The goal is to help the patient return home, recover, or adapt to a life with temporary or permanent functional alterations without complications or the need for rehospitalization. Assessment and planning include the following:

- Interview: includes information from the clinical team concerning background information of the preoperative condition requiring neurosurgery and presurgical deficits
- Neurologic assessment: includes LOC, Glasgow Coma Scale (GCS) score, mental status, motor and sensory function or deficits, cranial nerve function or deficits, cerebellar function or deficits, and neuropsychologic function or deficits
- Rehabilitation: requires rehabilitation physician consultation for a plan that may include physical therapy, occupational therapy, speech and language therapy, and neuropsychologic testing that includes evaluation of cognition and executive functioning
- Special services: include services of specialists in the areas of nursing, nutrition, recreation, social work, vocational/educational services, and prosthetics
- Medical care: includes return appointments and visits to the clinic, neurosurgeon, neurologist, psychologist, or other specialist with arrangements for transportation
- Pain: requires management of headache and discomfort related to the surgery
- Late onset of hydrocephalus with a decreased LOC, changes in gait, onset of incontinence, or other behavioral changes: requires reevaluation by the neurosurgeon, who will probably order a CT scan to confirm or rule out enlarged ventricles and noncommunicating hydrocephalus that may require a shunt procedure
- Support: provided by family, significant others, or community or religious associations
- Home: includes assessment of living arrangements to determine barriers to ADLs, potential for injury and harm, and equipment needs (e.g., special bed or toileting needs)
- Plan of care: includes measurable and realistic goals for the patient and family
- Plan approval: by government or private payer, the patient and family, and the clinical team
- Budget: addresses cost containment measures that will ensure services for the duration of need, sources for payment, and alternative funding
- Implementation of plan: includes health teaching and identification of significant changes or complications, with instructions for emergency care, wound and skin care, medication review with dosage and side effects, schedule of services, list of providers, and emergency numbers for contact[33]
- Frequent reassessment: provides review for the patient and family; assesses clinical team and payer satisfaction with progress and outcomes

Case management may be needed for only a short period of time, or it may be needed for the lifetime of a patient with severe neurologic problems. Case management helps afford the patient the best possible quality of life and the ability to function at his or her highest level of care for that patient's life expectancy.

CONCLUSION

The practice of neurosurgery has undergone significant advances in anatomic and functional knowledge, equipment and technology, imaging modalities, and surgical technique. Despite these advances, it remains a frightening prospect for the patient who fears potential loss of function and independence. Highly educated and skilled clinicians provide comprehensive management and invaluable services to patients and their families. Patient and family education and support throughout all phases of the neurosurgical experience is needed as part of the multidisciplinary neurosurgical team. Perioperative and rehabilitative management is a significant role for the clinician in identifying risks, responding early and appropriately to the earliest indications of complications, and intervening immediately on behalf of the patient and his or her family to recover the patient as safely and quickly as possible.

RESOURCES FOR CRANIAL SURGERY

American Association of Neurological Surgeons: www.aans.org

American Association of Neuroscience Nurses: 888-557-2266; www.aann.org

American College of Surgeons: www.facs.org

Hydrocephalus Association: 415-732-7040

National Hydrocephalus Foundation: e-mail: hydrobrat@earthling.net

REFERENCES

1. Barker FG: Efficacy of prophylactic antibiotics for craniotomy: a meta-analysis, *Neurosurgery* 35(3):484–492, 1994.
2. Buchanan RJ, Brant A, Marshall LF: Traumatic cerebrospinal fluid fistulas. In Winn HR, editor: *Youmans neurological surgery,* ed 5, Philadelphia, 2004, Saunders.
3. Buxton N, Punt J: Cerebral infarction after neuroendoscopic third ventriculostomy: case report, *Neurosurgery* 46(4):999–1000, 2000.
4. Chang SD, Adler JR, Steinberg GK: General and historical considerations of radiotherapy and radiosurgery. In Winn HR, editor: *Youmans neurological surgery,* ed 5, Philadelphia, 2004, Saunders.
5. Clatterbuck RC, Tamargo RJ: Surgical positioning and exposures for cranial procedures. In Winn HR, editor: *Youmans neurological surgery,* ed 5, Philadelphia, 2004, Saunders.
6. Danish SF, Burnett MG, Ong JG, et al: Prophylaxis for deep venous thrombosis in craniotomy patients: a decision analysis, *Neurosurgery* 56(6):1286–1292, 2005.
7. den Herder C, Schmeck J, Appelboom DJ, deVries N: Risks of general anesthesia in people with obstructive sleep apnea, *BMJ* 329(7472):955–959, 2004.
8. Dunbar C: Making cents: what patient education can do, *Nurs Spectrum* 2002. Available at http://community.nursingspectrum.com (accessed Sept 2005).
9. Findlay JM: Cerebral vasospasm. In Winn HR, editor: *Youmans neurological surgery,* ed 5, Philadelphia, 2004, Saunders.
10. Fletcher S, Lam AM: Anesthesia: preoperative evaluation. Winn HR, editor: *Youmans neurological surgery,* ed 5, Philadelphia, 2004, Saunders.
11. Fogg DM: Infection prevention and control. In Rothrock JC, editor: *Alexander's care of the patient in surgery,* ed 2, St Louis, 2003, Mosby.
12. Garretson S: Benefits of pre-operative information programs, *Nurs Stand* 18(47):33–38, 2004.
13. Gilmartin J: Day surgery: patient's perceptions of a nurse-led preadmission clinic, *J Clin Nurs* 13(2):243–250, 2004.
14. Goodkin R, Mesiwala A: General principles of operative positioning. In Winn HR, editor: *Youmans neurological surgery,* ed 5, Philadelphia, 2004, Saunders.
15. Greenberg MS: Hydrocephalus. In Greenberg M: *Handbook of neurosurgery,* ed 5, New York, 2001, Thieme Medical Publishers.
16. Greenberg MS: Operations and procedures. In Greenberg M: *Handbook of neurosurgery,* ed 5, New York, 2001, Thieme Medical Publishers.
17. Greenberg MS: Skull fractures. In Greenberg M: *Handbook of neurosurgery,* ed 5, New York, 2001, Thieme Medical Publishers.
18. Heizenroth PA: Positioning the patient for surgery. In Rothrock JC, editor: *Alexander's care of the patient in surgery,* ed 2, St Louis, 2003, Mosby.
19. Jellinek DA, Carroll T: Surgical physiology. In Kaye AH, Black PM, editors: *Operative neurosurgery,* London, 2000, Churchill Livingstone.
20. Jenkins AL, Deutch H, Patel NP, Post KD: Complication avoidance in neurosurgery. In Winn HR, editor: *Youmans neurological surgery,* ed 5, Philadelphia, 2004, Saunders.
21. Jones RFC, Vonau M: Endoscopic third ventriculostomy. In Kaye AH, Black PM, editors: *Operative neurosurgery,* London, 2000, Churchill Livingstone.
22. Kanan A, Gasson B: Brain tumor resections guided by magnetic resonance imaging, *AORN J* 77(3):583–588, 2003.
23. Kassell NF, Sasaki T, Colohan AR, et al: Cerebral vasospasm following aneurysmal subarachnoid hemorrhage, *Stroke* 16(4):562–572, 1985.
24. Kjonniksen I, Anderson BM, Sondenaa VG, Segadal L: Preoperative hair removal—a systematic literature review, *AORN J* 75(5):928–938, 2002.
25. Korinek AM: Risk factors for neurosurgical site infections after craniotomy: a prospective multicenter study of 2944 patients, *Neurosurgery* 41(5):1073–1081, 1997.
26. Kvam DA, Loftus CM, Copeland B, Quest DO: Seizures during the immediate postoperative period, *Neurosurgery* 12(1):14–17, 1983.
27. Liu CY, Apuzzo ML: The genesis of neurosurgery and the evolution of the neurosurgical operative environment: part I—prehistory to 2003, *Neurosurgery* 52(1):3–19, 2003.
28. MacKichan C, Ruthman J: Herbal product use and perioperative patients, *AORN J* 79(5):948–959, 2004.
29. Manaka S, Ishijima B, Mayanagi Y: Postoperative seizures: epidemiology, pathology, and prophylaxis, *Neurol Med Chir* (Tokyo) 43(12):589–600, discussion 600, 2003.

30. Marshall SB, editor: *Neuroscience critical care: pathophysiology and patient management,* Philadelphia, 1990, Saunders.

31. Marino PL: The febrile patient. In *The ICU book,* ed 2, Baltimore, 1998, Williams & Wilkins.

32. Marino PL: Venous thromboembolism. In *The ICU book,* ed 2, Baltimore, 1998, Williams & Wilkins.

33. Mordiffi SZ, Tan SP, Wong MK: Information provided to surgical patients versus information needed, *AORN J* 77(3):546–562, 2003.

34. Paasche-Orlow MK, Taylor HA, Brancati FL: Readability standards for informed-consent forms a compared with actual readability, *N Engl J Med* 348(8):721–726, 2003.

35. Prestigiacoma CJ, Quest DO: Neurosonology. In Winn HR, editor: *Youmans neurological surgery,* ed 5, Philadelphia, 2004, Saunders.

36. Rossi PA: *Case management in health care: a practical guide,* Philadelphia, 1999, Saunders.

37. Russell L: Intraoperative magnetic resonance imaging safety considerations, *AORN J* 77(3):590–592, 2003.

38. Scott A: Managing anxiety in ICU patients: the role of preoperative information provision. British Association of Critical Care Nurses, *Nurs Crit Care* 9(2):72–79, 2004.

39. Schultz A: Predicting and preventing pressure ulcers in surgical patients, *AORN J* 81(5):985–994, 2005.

40. Stieber VW, Bourland JD, Tome WA, Mehta MP: Gentlemen (and ladies), choose your weapons: gamma knife vs. linear accelerator radiosurgery, *Technol Cancer Res Treat* 2(2):79–85, 2003.

41. JCAHO: Universal protocol for preventing wrong site, wrong procedure, wrong person surgery. Available at www.jointcommission.org (accessed Sept 2005).

42. Vale S: Subarachnoid hemorrhage associated with ginkgo biloba, *Lancet* 352(9121):36–37, 1998.

43. Weingart J, Brem H: Basic principles of cranial surgery for brain tumors. In Winn HR, editor: *Youmans neurological surgery,* ed 5, Philadelphia, 2004, Saunders.

44. Zetterling M, Ronne-Engstrom E: High intraoperative blood loss may be a risk factor for postoperative hematoma, *J Neurosurg Anesthesiol* 16(2):151–155, 2004.

CYNTHIA BLANK-REID,
LEWIS J. KAPLAN,
THOMAS A. SANTORA

CHAPTER 9

Neuroscience Critical Care Management

The management of the critically ill neuroscience patient requires the greatest amount and complexity of knowledge, technical skills, and expertise of any specialty in nursing.[4,5] There is little room for clinical error in the management of intracranial pressure, fluids and electrolytes, respiratory function, cerebral circulation, nutrition, and neuropharmacologic interventions. Through independent study, special classes, and other educational opportunities, clinicians can acquire knowledge of the principles of neuroscience critical care management that they need in order to function with competence and confidence in this specialty intensive care environment.

This chapter provides information for the management of the neuroscience patient in an intensive care unit (ICU) by the neuroscience clinician working with a multidisciplinary team. Successful management draws on the expertise of each member of the team to formulate and implement a unified, physiologically sound treatment plan for each patient. Aggressive application of intensive neuroscience clinical management techniques is needed in order to decrease "secondary injuries," minimize complications, maximize outcomes of central nervous system (CNS) insults and injury, and restore homeostasis.[4,5] Specific areas to be covered include monitoring devices, ventilator support, pharmacologic support, goals of therapeutic intervention, therapeutic procedures, nutritional therapy, rehabilitation, nutrition, and case management. The chapter also explores general critical care issues that are applicable to the neuroscience critical care unit (NCCU) patient population, including end-of-life decisions.

NEUROSCIENCE CRITICAL CARE NURSING

Neuroscience critical care nursing, at its best, matches professional skills and health care resources with patient need at a moment when life appears to hang in the balance. In these circumstances, the likelihood of patient survival is dependent on the quality and appropriate utilization of the health care provider's skills and resources. The role of the clinician in managing a patient in the **neuroscience critical care unit (NCCU)** is complex, challenging, and rewarding.

Neuroscience critical care nursing is an evolving specialty that combines a mastery of intellectual and technical skills that promote clinical actions based on appreciation and determination of physiologic clinical data. It is the clinicians' role to determine the correct mixture of science and art for each individual patient. As the patient responds, be it positively or negatively, the clinician must be able to adjust his or her clinical actions appropriately.

Neuroscience critical care nursing is a subspecialty of critical care practiced in a setting where neuroscience patients are grouped together for direct observation and close monitoring using innovative and sophisticated equipment for rapid and lifesaving interventions. The foundation for successful patient management in an NCCU is dependent on clinicians with a strong scientific background based on the material listed in Box 9-1.

Multidisciplinary Team Management

NCCUs were originally designed to concentrate on three specific parameters: (1) critically ill neuroscience patients, (2) complex monitoring and therapeutic devices, and (3) properly educated staff with expertise in neuroscience patient care and mastery of neuroscience-specialty device utilization. The goals of the specialty NCCU are improving the efficiency and outcome of patient care while reducing costs. A multidisciplinary NCCU team is essential for optimal patient therapy. No single health care provider can meet every need of a critically ill neuroscience patient at all times. Each member of the team contributes a unique and specialized skill that in combination may allow for the best possible outcome for the patient. In the current era of cost containment and limits on resource availability, a multispecialty team approach may enhance the effectiveness of patient care by application of evidence-based pathways of care, early recognition and timely interventions for pathway deviations, and expert management of invasive procedures/devices. This multispecialty approach may decrease complications, length of stay in the NCCU, and health care expenditures. The multidisciplinary NCCU team is patient focused—a structure that allows personnel to respond directly and promptly to the needs of patients.

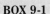

BOX 9-1	Prerequisites for Neuroscience Critical Care Nursing

- In-depth knowledge of neuroanatomy and neurophysiology (see Chapter 1)
- Competent neurologic assessment skills and interpretation of findings (see Chapter 2)
- Hemodynamic monitoring, including cardiac, interpretation of dysrhythmias, and fluid pressure-volume relationships
- Excellent knowledge base of neurodiagnostic and laboratory studies, with the ability to analyze and interpret test results (see Chapter 3)
- Clinical expertise in postoperative neurosurgical management (see Chapter 8)
- Broad-based knowledge and proficiency in specific neurologic diseases and disorders, and emergency interventions treated in the particular NCCU
- Critical care skills for acute patient monitoring and rapid clinical decision-making responses
- Knowledge and experience in setting up and operating sophisticated emergency and monitoring equipment and therapeutic devices (see Chapter 10)
- Cardiopulmonary and cerebral resuscitation
- Neurologic rehabilitation theory and principles of practice (see Chapter 13)

NCCU, Neuroscience critical care unit.

Essentials of a Neuroscience Critical Care Unit

Standards and Policies for Neuroscience Critical Care

The establishment of hospital **critical care guidelines** and protocols, as well as the policies, protocols, and procedures for the NCCU, should be consistent with guidelines set forth by national professional and health care organizations. Unit-based protocols, critical pathways, and standing orders based on standard-of-care guidelines from these organizations and the scientific literature serve as guides for the health care team and permit rapid interventions for life-threatening neurologic emergencies.

Admission Criteria

Patients who are admitted to an NCCU demonstrate a need for monitoring, intervention, or advanced levels of care that cannot be readily delivered on the general nursing unit. To facilitate optimal utilization of this specialized hospital resource, most NCCUs have written criteria for both admission and discharge.

Patient selection criteria may be conveniently broken down into five categories:

1. **Hemodynamic indicators:** Patients who display hemodynamic compromise, defined as follows: systolic blood pressure (SBP; >180 or <60 mm Hg), heart rate (HR; >120 or <60 beats/min), respiratory rate (RR; <10 or >30 breaths/min), and arterial oxygen saturation (SaO$_2$; <92%). These patients may require ongoing volume expansion, vasoactive infusions, and endotracheal intubation with mechanical ventilation and supplemental oxygen. In addition, systemic hypoperfusion with cool extremities, oliguria, narrow pulse pressure, metabolic acidosis, and acidemia indicate the need for NCCU admission.

2. **Physiologic indicators:** Rather than demonstrating hemodynamic instability indicated by abnormal vital signs as have been outlined, these patients demonstrate the sequelae of inadequate organ perfusion. Each organ system displays characteristic signs and symptoms of organ dysfunction. The CNS manifestations of organ dysfunction include a diminished level of consciousness (LOC), coma, posturing (flexor or extensor), seizures, intracranial hypertension, thermodysregulation, coagulopathy requiring blood product administration, autonomic dysfunction, new onset of paralysis, and incipient brain death.

3. **Structural indicators:** This category stems from the need for NCCU care of patients without hemodynamic instability or physiologic dysfunction, but who have sustained injuries or undergone procedures that require monitoring for untoward events (e.g., a patient who has undergone a stereotactic brain biopsy and requires close monitoring for 24 hours).

4. **Comorbid indicators:** These indicators can exert devastating influences on patient outcomes. Important comorbid conditions include symptomatic coronary artery disease or cardiomyopathy, pulmonary hypertension, chronic obstructive pulmonary disease, renal failure, liver failure with cirrhosis, malnutrition, type 1 (insulin-dependent) diabetes, solid-organ transplantation, severe endocrinopathy, substance abuse, and malignancy.

5. **Institutional policies:** Every institution has its own set of unique polices that may direct NCCU admission for certain diagnoses, care requirements, or medications (e.g., epidural catheters, vasopressor or cardiac drugs).

Discharge Criteria

As important as entry criteria are in prioritizing NCCU admissions, discharge criteria facilitate the timely transfer of patients to less acute nursing units. Discharge criteria vary among institutions and are influenced by the presence of nonacute or intermediate care units, as well as nursing and physician staffing patterns, clinician patient ratios, and clinical expertise. The ultimate authority for discharge rests with the primary service, but as more NCCUs move to a closed format, discharge authority may reside with the **critical care intensivist** (the physician who has expertise in caring for patients who are critically ill). Examples of discharge criteria are given in Box 9-2.

PATIENT MONITORING

General Monitoring

In the NCCU setting, **hemodynamic monitoring** is governed by the unique needs of the patient, as well as by a minimum standard of care (SOC) that has been formulated by the Society of Critical Care Medicine. Monitoring devices may be classified as noninvasive or invasive. As technology

BOX 9-2	Neuroscience Critical Care Unit Discharge Criteria

- Reasons justifying admission and stay in the unit have been resolved.
- Appropriate care can be rendered in a medical/surgical floor bed.
- The patient is no longer considered salvageable.
- Continued stay in the unit is deemed more detrimental to the patient psychologically than beneficial physiologically (i.e., ICU psychosis).
- Vital signs are stable on the basis of trends established in the NCCU, and the patient is not receiving vasopressors.
- End-organ function is stable.
- The patient does not require hemodynamic monitoring, or the monitoring required can be continued in another unit with telemetry.
- Beds in other units are not available, or there is a limited number of nursing staff and/or other patients with a greater need for the extensive or specialized monitoring and treatment available in the unit.

ICU, Intensive care unit; *NCCU*, neuroscience critical care unit.

progresses, more noninvasive devices will supplant their invasive counterparts. At a minimum, patients admitted to an NCCU should have the following processes monitored:

- Neurologic assessment: LOC, Glasgow Coma Scale (GCS) score, FOUR score, pupillary response, and motor strength
- Hemodynamic assessment: devices to measure and record vital signs (temperature, HR, RR, and blood pressure)
- Continuous electrocardiography (ECG)
- Continuous arterial pulse oximetry
- Urinary output

NCCU Monitoring Tools

Noninvasive Methods

Temperature. Temperature can be taken via the oral or rectal route, tympanic membrane, or bladder by means of an indwelling urinary catheter. When a brain tissue oxygenation ($pBtO_2$) probe or a pulmonary artery catheter (PAC) is used, core temperature can be measured along with brain and systemic blood flow parameters, respectively. Temperature regulation is an essential part of the management of neuroscience patients, since hyperthermia increases the brain's metabolic rate of oxygen consumption and hypothermia may affect cardiac status.

Heart Rate and Electrocardiography. Many institutions monitor patients using a four- or five-lead system with an automatic lead switch button and lead simultaneous analysis features. The device must have modifiable alarms with settings that can be prescribed (preferably audible, visual, and time trackable) with printable data and monitors for ECG data, as well as radio frequency noise.

Blood Pressure Measurement. Blood pressure measurement can be done with a standard, manually inflatable sphygmo-

manometer. Despite the widespread prevalence of automated noninvasive blood pressure (NIBP) monitoring systems, a manual cuff is essential in conditions of systolic hypotension when the blood pressure must be determined by manual means using Doppler auscultation.

Pulse Oximetry. Pulse oximetry allows for continuous monitoring of oxygen saturation. This technology compares the absorption of two infrared light waves (wavelengths of 960 nm and 680 nm, the frequency of maximal absorbance of oxyhemoglobin and deoxyhemoglobin, respectively) while continuously eliminating the absorption caused by all the other tissues as blood is "pulsed" into the region at the monitoring probe. **Hypoperfusion** will artificially diminish the readings from a pulse oximeter because of decreased pulse volume or insufficient change in optical density to register accurately. In general, when no reading is obtainable or the readings do not correlate with the patient's heart rate as determined by the ECG, the problem rests with the patient's perfusion status and not with the arterial saturation per se or the site chosen to apply the oximeter probe. Severe anemia (hemoglobin [Hgb] <5 g%) will also depress the readings because of a lack of change in optical density.[24]

In conditions of hypothermia, hypoperfusion, acidosis, alkalosis, and other severe metabolic derangements (i.e., severe sepsis), pulse oximeter values in the low range (90% to 93%) may not correlate with standard values of the partial pressure of oxygen (PaO_2). In this instance, arterial blood gas (ABG) determinations should be performed to aid in assessing the arterial oxygen content.

Capnometry, Capnography, and End-Tidal Carbon Dioxide Measurement. **Capnometry** (quantitative measurement of carbon dioxide in expired gas) is a continuous, noninvasive method for evaluating the adequacy of carbon dioxide exchange in the lungs. The principle behind capnometry is that the carbon dioxide measured at the end of a tidal exhalation ($PetCO_2$) will approximate the alveolar carbon dioxide level and thus the partial pressure of dissolved carbon dioxide (PCO_2) in the blood.

Capnometry helps ensure that the ventilator is connected to the patient and allows determination of the adequacy of alveolar ventilation. Under normal pulmonary conditions, the $PetCO_2$ underestimates the $PaCO_2$ by 5 to 7 mm Hg. Changes in minute ventilation that are designed to produce a certain $PaCO_2$ may therefore be followed without the need for ABG determination.

Cerebral Blood Flow Monitoring. Cerebral blood flow (CBF) monitoring is useful in select patient populations (e.g., cerebral aneurysm). CBF velocity (see Chapter 3), which usually but not always reflects CBF, can be easily performed at the bedside study using a **transcutaneous Doppler device (TCD).** CBF can be evaluated with stable xenon (Xe) computed tomography (CT), perfusion CT, CT angiography, or traditional four-vessel angiography; these latter studies require transportation to diagnostic areas outside of the NCCU.

Electroencephalogram Monitoring. Electroencephalogram (EEG) monitoring is needed for certain patient populations at risk for seizures or to closely monitor seizures during hospitalization for treatment interventions (see Chapter 24).

Invasive Methods

Arterial Catheters. The majority of NCCU patients may be safely managed with noninvasive measurement and recording of arterial blood pressure. There are, however, specific subsets of patients whose care may not be safely undertaken without beat-to-beat measurement of arterial pressure. Such patients include those who require the following:

- Vasoactive infusions
- Therapy for elevated intracranial pressure (ICP) or active therapy for maintenance of adequate cerebral perfusion pressure (CPP)
- Monitoring for significant acid-base disturbances requiring frequent ABG studies to obtain pH/PCO_2 determinations in patients in whom the clinician is unable to noninvasively measure the blood pressure (e.g., patients with proximal musculoskeletal injury, patients with limitations due to dialysis access)

A written procedure (e.g., critical care procedure manuals) should be consulted regarding the insertion technique, preferred sites, and care for arterial catheters.

Pulmonary Artery Catheter. A pulmonary artery catheter (PAC) is inserted into a pulmonary artery to measure cardiac output, pulmonary arterial pressure, and pulmonary occlusion pressure (also called capillary wedge pressure). It is an extremely useful diagnostic tool that can be used to manage critically ill patients. Numerous critical care procedure manuals can be consulted as to the insertion technique, preferred sites, and care of PACs, as well as normal hemodynamic values. The key concept regarding the use of a PAC is that it allows for bedside hemodynamic measurement of intracardiac pressures and cardiac output; these measurements allow derivations of various cardiac parameters (stroke volume, systemic vascular resistance, ventricular work indices) to assess myocardial contractility or cardiac efficacy. Invasive hemodynamic monitoring allows for direct measurement of pulmonary artery and arterial pressures for fluid management and for assessment of cerebral perfusion. Various catheters are available, with different types of "access" ports. The different ports can be used for transvenous pacing, mixed venous oxygen saturation measurements, and additional fluid and medication administration.

Jugular Vein Oxygen Measurement. Analyzing the arterial–jugular vein oxygen difference (AVJDO$_2$), jugular bulb venous oxygen pressure (PjO$_2$), and jugular vein saturation (SjO$_2$) is thought to provide assessment of cerebral blood flow. Some critical care units have the ability for placement of a fiberoptic catheter into the jugular bulb that allows for continuous recording of jugular venous oxygen saturation and intermittent sampling of venous blood gases. When venous and arterial blood gases are analyzed simultaneously, the values can be used to calculate the arteriovenous oxygen difference (AVJDO$_2$) and, in conjunction with CBF measurements, determine the cerebral metabolic rate of oxygen (CMRO$_2$) consumption (Table 9-1).

The internal jugular vein is cannulated, and the catheter is inserted in a retrograde fashion using the Seldinger technique. A confirmatory lateral neck x-ray study should be done to ensure that the catheter tip is at the level of the mandibular ramus-body junction. Catheter care is the same as for any central venous catheter.

TABLE 9-1	Clinical Interpretation of SvO$_2$ Measurements	
SvO$_2$ Measurement	**Physiologic Basis for Change in SvO$_2$**	**Clinical Diagnosis and Rationale**
High SvO$_2$ (80%–95%)	Increased oxygen supply	Patient receiving more oxygen than required by clinical condition
	Decreased oxygen demand	Anesthesia, which causes sedation and decreased muscle movement
		Hypothermia, which lowers metabolic demand (e.g., with cardiopulmonary bypass)
		Sepsis caused by decreased ability of tissues to use oxygen at a cellular level
		False high positive because PA catheter is wedged in a pulmonary capillary
Normal SvO$_2$ (60%–80%)	Normal oxygen supply and metabolic demand	Balanced oxygen supply and demand
Low SvO$_2$ (less than 60%)	Decreased oxygen supply caused by:	
	Low hemoglobin	Anemia or bleeding with compromised cardiopulmonary system
	Low arterial saturation (SaO$_2$)	Hypoxemia resulting from decreased oxygen supply or lung disease
	Low cardiac output	Cardiogenic shock caused by left ventricular pump failure
	Increased oxygen consumption (VO$_2$)	Metabolic demand exceeds oxygen supply in conditions that increase muscle movement and increase metabolic rate, including physiologic states such as shivering, seizures, and hyperthermia

From Thelan LA: *Critical care nursing: diagnosis and management,* ed 3, St Louis, 1998, Mosby.
PA, Pulmonary artery; *SvO$_2$,* oxygen saturation of mixed venous blood.

TIP: This catheter is never used for infusion therapy. When calibrating this catheter, slow aspiration must be undertaken so that a mixture of all brain venous blood is sampled.

A normal PjO_2 is 35 to 40 torr, and a normal SjO_2 is 62% to 70%. Saturation below 55% is indicative of global brain ischemia and warrants treatment. A brain sustaining an unrelenting injury may manifest progressively falling SjO_2 levels; rescue therapy may reverse such a trend. In fact, it has been demonstrated that a falling SjO_2 will accurately track cerebral ischemic episodes and that the number of SjO_2 values lower than 50% correlates directly with poor neurologic outcome. In addition, the desaturation pattern can be correlated with the appearance of infarction evidence on brain CT scanning.

TIP: The clinician must also be aware that up to 50% of "desaturations" may be inaccurate (catheter impinging on the wall of the internal jugular vein [IJV]; low light intensity reading evident). Low SjO_2 values should be confirmed by PjO_2 measurement; if values are artifactual, head repositioning to neutral may correct the wall artifact.[10]

Jugular venous oxygen monitoring is not used as a measure of cerebral metabolism. First, like SvO_2 (oxygen saturation of mixed venous blood), SjO_2 is reflective of flow and the $AVDO_2$ from all portions of the brain, but what the clinician really wants is a local descriptor of how an injured portion of brain is using oxygen. Dead brain tissue does not use oxygen and may provide a spuriously elevated SjO_2 in the face of significant devitalization. Therefore the catheters have little utility in the face of massive brain injury but may be helpful in the management of patients whose traumatic brain injury (TBI) is significant enough to warrant ICP monitoring (i.e., Glasgow Coma Scale [GCS] score <8) or operative therapy. In these situations the goal is to prevent secondary brain injury by optimizing brain blood flow. Furthermore, since the catheters are typically placed in the right internal jugular vein (RIJV), where flows are larger and faster, the values may not reflect left-sided metabolism; left-sided placement for left-sided lesions may be preferred. Regardless of the side of insertion, the values must be integrated into a coherent evaluation of the patient's status before they are acted on.[22]

ICP Monitors. Intracranial pressure monitoring is discussed later in this chapter. For further details, see Chapter 10.

Neurodiagnostic and Laboratory Testing

Laboratory studies for NCCU patients include frequent and ongoing monitoring of numerous studies. Because of the different preferences of physicians, the different needs of patients, and institution-specific protocols, this topic is not covered in depth. Many NCCUs have protocols that include standing orders for laboratory tests. Examples of this include a protocol where the clinician analyzes the patient's electrolyte values and responds to a decreased potassium level with a standing order for intravenous (IV) potassium replacement. There should be protocols regarding the timing and urgency of diagnostic tests after the order is placed, the level of monitoring required during transport, and the level/number of hospital personnel required to safely transport a patient from the critical care setting to other areas in the hospital for diagnostic studies. Some critical care clinicians, for example, have emergency keys to quickly access elevators for rapid transportation when testing is ordered on a "stat" basis.

Neurodiagnostic and laboratory studies may include the following (see Chapter 3):

- *Computer tomography (CT):* Frequently used to assess the potential for worsening intracranial mass effect, especially in postoperative craniotomy/craniectomy patients or in management of CNS-injured patients. Portable CT, which is available today in select centers, allows brain imaging without the need for transportation out of the NCCU. In the near future, this modality will be more widely available.
- *Magnetic resonance imaging (MRI):* Used to provide fine anatomic detail of mass effects or status of stroke victims.
- *Electroencephalography (EEG):* May be used as an intermittent test or continuous study of patients that have potential seizure disorders or diminished brain function due to electrical disturbances.
- *Transcranial Doppler:* Bedside analysis of blood flow velocities used frequently to assess cerebral blood flow; increased velocities in patients with cerebral aneurysm indicate vasospasm.
- *Xenon CT or CT angiography:* Used to measure cerebral blood flow.
- *Fluoroscopy:* Used to assess potential spine instability in trauma patients with diminished LOC, or adequacy of spine reduction following traction and/or halo fixation of spine fracture/dislocation.
- *Chest x-ray study:* To rule out atelectasis, pneumonia, lung disease, and pneumothorax, and for endotracheal (ET) tube placement.
- *Complete blood count (CBC):* To determine if infection is occurring and how much oxygen-carrying hemoglobin is present.
- *Electrolyte panels:* Important to follow trends in the neurologically impaired; the injured brain is susceptible to worsened swelling in the presence of hyponatremia (e.g., cerebral salt wasting due to release of brain natriutic protein) and hyperglycemia; diabetes insipidus may result from brain injury and can lead to rapid changes in serum electrolytes, especially resulting in hypernatremia.[21]
- *Coagulation assays:* Brain injury may induce a coagulopathy due to release of tissue thromboplastin; therefore the prothrombin time (PT)/activated partial thromboplastin time (APTT), fibrinogen level and measures of fibrin degradation (i.e., fibrin split products [FSP], or D-dimers) should be assessed.
- *Bronchoscopy/bronchoalveolar lavage (BAL):* To assist in obtaining appropriate sputum specimens, as well as open up congested airway passages.
- *ABG studies:* To evaluate ventilation ($PaCO_2$), oxygenation (PaO_2), and acid-base status.
- *Cultures:* These studies may include sputum, blood, urine, CSF, and wound cultures (if indicated) to rule out infection.

- *Ultrasound (US):* Used as a deep vein thrombosis (DVT) surveillance tool; US surveillance of the lower extremities has become common in the neurologically impaired patient because of the high risk for thromboembolic events due to stasis, potential vascular intimal injury, and coagulopathy.
- *Lung scans:* To assess perfusion capabilities and look for mismatching conditions (e.g., pulmonary embolism [PE]).

CARE OF THE NEUROLOGICALLY IMPAIRED PATIENT

Hemodynamic Drug Therapy

The use of hemodynamic drug therapy is common with NCCU patients. In fact, the use of hemodynamic drug therapy and respiratory issues are common reasons why patients are admitted to an NCCU. The list of pharmacologic agents available is extensive, with each one having its own indications for use, dosing requirements, and unique side effects. Because of the in-depth discussion needed for the topic of hemodynamic drug therapy, the reader is encouraged to read one of the numerous texts on advanced cardiac life support drug therapy.

Complications of hemodynamic drug therapy with neuroscience patients must be considered during agent selection. An example of this problem is drugs that may increase weakness in patients with myasthenia gravis (MG) who require admission to an NCCU. Examples of such drugs include quinidine, lidocaine, propranolol (Inderal), and phenytoin (Dilantin). In patients with TBI, it is common to require the use of **inotropic agents** for elevation of the mean arterial pressure (MAP) to maintain the **cerebral perfusion pressure (CPP)** at levels of 60 to 70 mm Hg or greater. The clinician also needs to be facile at altering the MAP with afterload-reducing agents, as well as treating dysrhythmias in order to maximize the CPP.[10,23,33]

Prevention of Secondary Brain Injury and Complications

The traumatized brain is very sensitive to secondary hypoxia, ischemia, and hypotension. One important goal of the NCCU staff following neurosurgery, brain attack/stroke, or severe traumatic brain injury (STBI) is to decrease secondary brain injury (see Chapter 11). Prompt management of **secondary brain injury** will affect mortality and long-term morbidity rates after TBI. Some important strategies are described in the following sections.

Hypotension and Hypoxemia

Both hypotension and hypoxemia function as independent predictors of poor neurologic outcome following TBI. Furthermore, prehospital hypotension is associated with increasingly difficult intracranial hypertension management. In an effort to improve outcome from TBI, both physician-directed field resuscitation and improved neuroscience critical care enhanced neurologic outcome in two independent studies. Despite increasing awareness of the effects of secondary brain injury by health care providers, secondary brain injury has been documented at an alarming frequency in the ICU. It is important to note that greater numbers of cerebral desaturation episodes (measured with a brain tissue oxygenation [pBtO$_2$] probe or brain PO$_2$) also correspond to delayed infarction patterns on cerebral CT imaging. Certainly, aggressive therapy of both hypotension and hypoxemia is warranted.[10]

The concept of **euvolemia** as a goal for cerebral resuscitation has been recently challenged. There is mounting evidence that achieving the unstressed volume (normal intravascular volume) for a traumatically injured system results in inadequate perfusion and that hypervolemic resuscitation should be pursued and balanced with ICP and CPP measurements. Unmonitored hypervolemic expansion may promote intracranial hypertension and cerebral edema. Therefore some investigators have explored the use of hypertonic saline (3% NaCl solution) as a resuscitation fluid. A study in patients with severe head injury (GCS score <8) described improved neurologic outcome following a single bolus of 250 ml of hypertonic saline administered before reaching the hospital. Hypertonic saline (HS) is thought to increase microvascular flows while decreasing white cell–vascular wall adherence (decreasing inflammation). However, HS can increase ICP in the face of injury; therefore routine use of hypertonic resuscitation fluids awaits randomized, prospective controlled trials with a documented survival benefit.[10]

In evaluating volume expansion, one must examine the physical determinants of CBF. Clearly, vessel diameter exerts profound influence over CBF, whereas CPP and blood viscosity exert less influence. In fact, maximal arteriolar vasodilation (200% to 300% increase in diameter) can augment cerebral blood volume (CBV) by up to 900%, based on the large cross-sectional area of the cerebral arterioles. Under normal circumstances, changes in CPP and/or viscosity are offset by the reciprocally altered vessel diameter and thus keep the CBF matched to the cerebral metabolic rate of oxygen (CMRO$_2$) demands. These seemingly coupled phenomena are known respectively as **pressure and viscosity autoregulation.** The complementary and diametrically opposed roles of nitric oxide and endothelin, in addition to other vasoactive mediators, are currently being investigated in maintaining cerebral vasoregulation. The important role of **toxic oxygen metabolites** in disrupting vascular reactivity and membrane stability is discussed later.

Close hemodynamic monitoring to control blood pressure and oxygenation is essential to prevent even one episode of hypotension or hypoxemia during the patient's admission in the NCCU. Written standing orders, guidelines, or protocols provide the necessary tools for quick intervention and prevent delays in treatment.

Intracranial Pressure and Cerebral Perfusion Relationships

Despite complex monitoring schemes, a major complication of unresolved intracranial hypertension is **cerebral herniation** (see Chapter 10). One of the commonly monitored indicators of the adequacy of cerebral resuscitation and cerebral homeostasis is ICP (see Chapter 10). When a cerebral lesion has been treated surgically and an ICP monitoring device has been inserted, measurement of ICP and CPP can be monitored and controlled.

The premise that underlies ICP monitoring and control of ICP elevation is that intracranial hypertension is a marker of disordered pressure-volume relationships and that restoration of a normal balance enhances neurologic recovery. Data from the Traumatic Coma Data Bank indicate that the longer the period of time and the greater the number of times that a patient's ICP exceeds 20 mm Hg, the worse the neurologic outcome. Aggressive ICP management is needed with patients at high risk for elevated ICP.

Normal ICP in a supine patient is less than 15 mm Hg; values greater than 20 mm Hg indicate intracranial hypertension (see Chapter 12). Intracranial hypertension stems from a number of etiologies that include, but are not limited to, increased amounts of CSF, increased CBF, increased blood volume, increased cerebral parenchymal volume, and intra-axial or extraaxial mass lesions.

The "gold standard" for measurement of ICP is the **external ventricular drainage (EVD)** described in Chapter 10. The American National Standard for Intracranial Pressure Monitoring Devices has specified parameters to which ICP monitoring devices must conform. These are as follows:

- Pressure monitoring capability of 0 to 100 mm Hg
- Inaccuracy ±2 mm Hg when monitoring pressures between 0 and 20 mm Hg
- A 10% maximum allowable error during pressure monitoring between 20 and 100 mm Hg

Fluid-coupled external strain gauge monitoring devices easily conform to these standards, using disposable arterial pressure transducers that are readily recalibrated. Ventricular catheters may also use tip strain gauge or fiberoptic tip pressure transduction technology.

ICP values are used to calculate CPP using the following formula:

$$CPP = MAP - Mean\ ICP$$

CPP values below 60 mm Hg have been associated with worsened neurologic recovery following TBI. Maintenance of CPP above 50 or 60 mm Hg is needed to improve neurologic outcome on the basis of enhanced cerebral perfusion and the avoidance of cerebral ischemia.

Surgeon preference will determine the type and location of monitoring device. These devices may be placed in the brain parenchyma or subarachnoid, subdural, or epidural spaces. Depending on the system selected, the ICP monitoring device may transduce ICP via an external strain gauge, catheter tip strain gauge, or fiberoptic technology.

TIP: Unlike the ventricular catheters with a catheter tip strain gauge or fiberoptic technology, all of the other devices are calibrated *before* insertion and cannot be recalibrated once in place. The ICP values are therefore subject to drift.

Unlike a fluid-coupled system, the fiberoptic or catheter tip strain gauge can measure ICP independently of head position or elevation. Obviously, it is important to ensure accurate ICP measurement so that appropriate interventions may be undertaken to manage intracranial homeostasis.

Complications. The more invasive ICP monitoring systems increase the risk of complications that include five categories:

1. Hemorrhage
2. Infection
3. Malposition of catheter
4. Obstruction of the system
5. Malfunction

The risk-benefit analysis may be a factor in the decision to insert a monitoring device, with most NCCUs reporting low and acceptable complication rates.[4,5] Decisions that could increase the complication rate, such as irrigation of EVD systems with medication (e.g., urokinase), require protocols and staff trained in the procedure. Irrigation may be needed to promote dissolution of intraventricular clots that could cause hydrocephalus; however, irrigation markedly increases the likelihood of colonization in a manner analogous to multiple access central venous pressure (CVP) catheters. Catheter malposition may occur with EVD systems, but they have a smaller rate of malposition compared with fiberoptic systems. When an EVD cannot be placed, a parenchymal fiberoptic catheter tip system may be used because of its ease of insertion, minimal cost, and acceptable complication rate.

Insertion of an ICP Monitoring Device. Insertion of an ICP monitoring device may be performed in the NCCU under strict sterile conditions (see Chapter 10). A sterile dressing is placed and closely observed for dryness and intactness. Dressing changes and the duration of monitoring are determined by unit protocol. Placement of a monitoring device early, before the intracranial hypertension elevates above 15 mm Hg, has been found to correlate with a reduced mortality rate from neurologic causes, particularly in patients who are heavily sedated or pharmacologically paralyzed.

Data Collection. Data collection begins with the measurement and analysis of ICP at the time of insertion. Once the EVD is in place, the waveform should be assessed as a means of verifying accurate placement and monitoring (see Chapter 10). Trends can be evaluated to guide treatment of ICP. The most ominous sign identified by ICP monitoring and waveform analysis is an ICP value higher than 20 mm Hg that is associated with an "A" plateau waveform. This combination indicates sustained intracranial hypertension and mandates therapy to reduce ICP and an investigation into its cause (e.g., low blood pressure).

Therapy for Intracranial Hypertension

Therapy for intracranial hypertension is based on the cause, as well as available therapeutic interventions (see Chapter 10). Options include neutral head positioning, head elevations, induced hypocapnia, isovolemic dehydration (furosemide and mannitol), CSF drainage (EVD catheter), viscosity reduction (hypertonic saline), sedation and/or paralysis, metabolic rate reduction (i.e., barbiturate coma), hypothermia, cerebral debridement, or decompression craniotomy/craniectomy. Clinical measures are initiated with prescribed medical therapy, and each level of treatment is evaluated.

The next level of therapy is generally instituted when the previous level has failed to control the ICP (see Chapter 10). When ICP elevation is sustained, CT scan of the head is frequently helpful to delineate the precipitating cause. If available, the use of a portable CT scanning device for critically ill neuroscience patients, who are at risk for herniation and too unstable to transport, offers a safer means for diagnosis.

Analgesia, Sedation, and Neuromuscular Blockade.

In general, analgesics and sedatives are administered in combination in critically ill patients. In neuroscience patients who are mechanically ventilated and invasively monitored, both classes of medications are warranted to allow for smooth performance of routine care (e.g., suctioning, bathing) and for control of blood pressure, CBF, and cerebral oxygen utilization. Administration of analgesics and sedatives together is known to potentiate each other's effect and allow for smaller doses of each agent. The most commonly used analgesics are morphine sulfate and fentanyl sulfate.

Neither fentanyl nor morphine significantly affects CBF, $CMRO_2$ consumption, or ICP in standard doses; larger doses that result in hypotension or a decrease in MAP may lead to increased ICP. It is important to note that both of these agents are associated with substantial respiratory depression. Furthermore, morphine has been associated with histamine-induced hypotension, and fentanyl may cause acute chest rigidity syndrome with the inability to ventilate the patient without pharmacologic relaxation. Both morphine and fentanyl may be safely used as continuous and titratable infusions in critically ill patients. Meperidine is avoided because of the common side effect of dysphoria and, with prolonged use, accumulation of the metabolite normeperidine, which reduces the seizure threshold.[28,32]

The most commonly used sedatives are benzodiazepines. The choice of agent depends on the planned duration of administration, intended effect, therapeutic response, personnel time cost, and local pharmacy directives. It is important for the clinician to recognize that analgesics and sedatives may influence blood pressure by vasodilation and, occasionally, myocardial contractility depression.[28,32]

All of the commonly administered benzodiazepines are also anticonvulsants and bind to a nonspecific benzodiazepine receptor in the CNS. Incidentally, this receptor is closely related to the gamma-aminobutyric acid (GABA) receptor. All three of the most commonly used agents (lorazepam, midazolam, and diazepam) can cause prolonged respiratory depression following prolonged use regardless of the method of administration (bolus or continuous infusion). It is our practice to deliver an initial loading bolus and then initiate a continuous infusion to avoid "peaks and valleys" of drug effect and ICP.

An alternative to benzodiazepines is propofol, a lipid-based sedative/hypnotic with rapid onset and offset of activity; despite these desirable pharmacokinetic actions, prolonged effects may be seen in patients with renal failure. Since it is lipid based, it has a vast volume of distribution. It is known to reduce MAP, CBF, ICP, and $CMRO_2$ in a dose-dependent fashion and has anticonvulsant properties as well. Furthermore, propofol has a safety and efficacy profile similar to that of benzodiazepines in patients with TBI.[32] There are a number of deleterious side effects, which limit the usefulness of this agent, including hyperlipidemia, hypotension, myocardial depression, urine and hair discoloration (frequently turns urine green), and promotion of bacterial or fungal sepsis from the lipid-based, preservative-free solution. Nonetheless, sedative choice remains a matter of individual and institutional preference. Interestingly, propofol is rapidly becoming the agent of choice for acute management of delirium tremors and **status epilepticus;** both of these entities are relatively common in trauma patients.

> **TIP:** Propofol is devoid of analgesic properties and therefore requires the concomitant delivery of an analgesic agent in patients with traumatic injury.[27]

The safe and appropriate use of sedatives is essential. Adjustments in sedative agent administration should follow a well-conceived scheme. To that end, a sedation algorithm is an ideal tool for identifying a stepwise progression for sedation using single- or multiple-agent therapy. A good clinical algorithm should also identify when changing to an alternative agent is indicated. These schemes are derived by a multidisciplinary team, activated by physician order, but implemented by the bedside clinician without minute-to-minute physician attention. The key feature of these management pathways is a patient who is able to interact enough for the clinician to obtain objective evaluation of the patient's neurologic condition. When that evaluation is not possible or is unreliable, bispectral index (BIS) monitoring is useful and can be readily employed.[24,33]

Neuromuscular blocking agents are used to induce muscular paralysis for a variety of reasons, including, but not limited to, the following: reducing peak airway pressures during mechanical ventilation, reducing total-body oxygen consumption and metabolic rate, protecting life-sustaining indwelling devices (e.g., pulmonary catheters), placement of an artificial airway, and controlling ICP. Neuromuscular blocking agents are classified as either nondepolarizing or depolarizing, depending on the pharmacologic properties.

Agent selection entails consideration of factors identical to those surrounding analgesic and sedative selection. Commonly used agents include pancuronium, vecuronium, and *cis*-atracurium. All may be given by bolus or continuous infusion. All of these drugs are nondepolarizing agents. Nondepolarizing agents act as competitive inhibitors to acetylcholine at the neuromuscular junction. The paralytic effects can be reversed by the administration of cholinesterase inhibitors such as neostigmine.

Pancuronium frequently causes tachycardia and may result in prolonged paralysis when given in conjunction with steroids or aminoglycosides.[28] Vecuronium is also a nondepolarizing agent and is considered an ideal neuromuscular blocking agent because it does not have many of the problems associated with pancuronium. The onset of action is relatively brief, and there is an absence of cardiovascular side effects or histamine release. Vecuronium use in renal failure will result in prolonged neuromuscular blockade. Both pancuronium and vecuronium have active metabolites and are reported to result in prolonged neuromuscular blockade in some patients following cessation of drug therapy. Since *cis*-atracurium is cleared by plasma elimination independent of either hepatic or renal function, protracted neuromuscular blockade will not occur with its use in patients with multiple organ failure.

It is important to remember that the patient's corneas need to be protected when neuromuscular blocking agents are being used. The eyes need to be kept moist, which can be accomplished by instilling artificial tears and taping the eyelids shut or applying a moisture chamber.

Iatrogenic paralysis (from pharmacologic agents) is commonly titrated to an effect monitored by a peripheral nerve stimulator applied over the ulnar or other peripheral nerve distribution. Using the "train of four" algorithm of the stimulator, no motor endplate blockade results in four twitches of the adductor pollicis muscle resulting from four supramaximal triggering stimuli applied to the ulnar nerve; complete blockade yields no muscular response. A common goal of blockade is enough medication to result in two twitches out of a "train of four." The goal of twitch monitoring is to avoid overparalysis to diminish the risk of prolonged neuromuscular blockade following withdrawal of the agent. In addition, if feasible, many clinicians allow patients to emerge from paralysis once each 24-hour period to perform a neurologic assessment and help ensure return of neuromuscular function following cessation of drug therapy. There are no data to support this practice as a preventive measure, but it seems to make intuitive sense. There is a growing trend to avoid chemical relaxation throughout the United States; chemical relaxation is rare in the European Union for patient management in the critical care arena.

Complications of Neuromuscular Blockade. The myriad of potential complications of neuromuscular blockade are described in detail in Chapter 10. However, two important complications deserve mention: **postparalysis syndrome** and the **polyneuropathy of critical illness.** The postparalysis syndrome is diffuse motor weakness associated with elevated creatine kinase (CK) levels and preserved sensory nerve function on electromyography and nerve conduction velocity testing. By comparison, critical illness polyneuropathy involves both sensory and motor nerves and is less frequently associated with neuromuscular blocking agents as an etiologic cause. Polyneuropathy of critical illness is believed to be related to the underlying disease and carries a less favorable prognosis for recovery than postparalysis syndrome. There are some data implicating the amino-steroid structure of vecuronium and pancuronium in the pathogenesis of both of these complications; a parallel can be drawn between the neuromuscular blockade polyneuromyopathies of postparalysis syndrome and critical illness polyneuropathy and the neuromuscular block polyneuromyopathies identified in patients on long-term steroid regimens.

Patients with severe TBI and intracranial hypertension may require analgesia and sedation, as well as neuromuscular blockade, to help limit ICP and control CPP, and because they still feel pain. Since it is impossible for the NCCU team to perform a complete neurologic examination on a paralyzed patient, an ICP monitor is also essential. In addition, reducing **total-body oxygen utilization** by abolishing muscular activity may make more oxygen available for cerebral oxygen consumption. This effect may be monitored by jugular vein saturation (SjO_2) or near-infrared spectroscopy (NIS) techniques. In addition, since the use of pharmacologic paralysis presents the external appearance of a quiet, restful patient, it is important to have some means of titrating sedation to an appropriate level. Recommendations may include using a modified single-lead EEG montage known as the **bispectral index (BIS).** This device integrates a power spectrum of the coherence of electrical activity of the monitored areas of the brain and translates the information into an analog value ranging from 0 to 100. Lower numbers indicate deeper levels of sedation. This device has been successfully used in the operating room (OR) to monitor and titrate the level of benzodiazepine sedation for surgical procedures. Further experience is being gained in the ICU titration of therapy in pharmacologically paralyzed patients, as well as in monitoring serial changes following TBI that results in brain death.

Pharmacologically Diminished Cerebral Metabolic Rate

Analgesia, anxiolysis, and sedation diminish cerebral metabolism when administered in therapeutic doses. However, the prototypical agent used for decreasing cerebral metabolism and assisting in the control of intracranial hypertension or impaired cerebral oxygenation is sodium pentobarbital.[10] EEG monitoring for the appearance of a burst-suppression pattern correlates well with maximal reductions in CBF and $CMRO_2$.[10] There is poor correlation between serum or CSF levels of barbiturates and reduction in $CMRO_2$, CBF, CBV, and ICP. By reducing the baseline $CMRO_2$ and thus the tightly coupled CBF, barbiturates reduce CBV and therefore ICP. In addition, barbiturates may exhibit neuroprotective effects by scavenging toxic oxygen metabolites and reducing free radical lipid peroxidation of neuronal membranes.[10] Potential deleterious effects of **barbiturate coma** include cardiac depression and hypotension, as well as diminished cellular immune function.[10]

Barbiturate administration for **refractory intracranial hypertension** should employ a systemic loading dose, as well as a continuous infusion that is titrated by continuous EEG monitoring. Patients with refractory intracranial hypertension are estimated to make up approximately 10% of patients with severe TBI. If patients respond to barbiturate administration with a reduction in ICP to levels lower than 20 mm Hg, their mortality rate is reduced (to approximately 10% as compared with approximately 90% with refractory intracranial hypertension).[10] It is also clear that if barbiturate therapy results in hypotension, the beneficial effect of the barbiturate is lost, probably because of the promotion of secondary brain ischemic injury. Pentobarbital use in this setting has been limited by its potent negative inotropic and vasodilating effects. Extensive hemodynamic monitoring with an arterial line and a PAC, in addition to insertion of an ICP monitor, is mandatory when instituting this salvage therapy. Significant inotropic support may be needed to prevent the potentially devastating effects of hypotension and a low-output state on cerebral circulation.

Benzodiazepines are also useful in diminishing the cerebral metabolic rate in a fashion similar to that of barbiturates. The mechanism of action is the potentiation of GABA receptor activity, with subsequent inhibition of the GABA-mediated component of neuronal activity. Propofol (Diprivan) has proved useful in the treatment of status epilepticus; it also results in reduction of the cerebral metabolic rate by approximately 36% from the pretreatment baseline. Propofol has also been demonstrated to help maintain cerebral vasoreactivity to a carbon dioxide challenge without promoting anaerobic metabolism. Finally, etomidate (Amidate) is an imidazole agent that is useful in establishing airway control without respiratory muscle paralysis and has hypnotic effects similar to those of barbiturates. Etomidate is administered as a loading bolus and then followed by a continuous infusion that is titrated to a burst suppression EEG pattern. Significant reductions in ICP may be achieved with etomidate. However, a major detrimental side effect of etomidate therapy is variably reversible adrenocortical suppression, which may require exogenous steroid therapy should it occur. Adrenocortical failure is more common with prolonged etomidate infusion ($\geq$24 hours); thus etomidate is not a common first-line agent for intracranial hypertension management.

Hypothermia Therapy

Hypothermia has been studied over the years with mixed reactions. In humans the depth and duration of induced hypothermia is limited by ventricular dysrhythmias (premature ventricular contractions [PVCs], fibrillation) and disorders of the serine protease coagulation cascade with promotion of coagulopathic-induced intracerebral hemorrhage. Furthermore, myocardial contractility will fall and fibrillation will increase at temperatures below 28° C; increases in stroke volume will compensate for hypothermia-induced bradycardia to 30° C.[38]

The putative mechanism that underlies hypothermic protection is similar to that of pharmacologically induced suppression of the metabolic rate. Reduction in temperature reduces the metabolic activity of living tissue and hence its energy requirements.

In 2000 it was reported that there was an improved neurologic outcome at 6 months following injury in patients with a severe head injury.[30] Using the study's protocol, there was a 62% improvement in independent neurologic function following maintenance of cerebral hypothermia (32° to 33° C, as indicated by tympanic membrane thermography) for up to 7 days. Other important aspects of induced hypothermia were strict maintenance of normoglycemia; DVT prophylaxis with external continuous and sequential compression devices; pressure ulcer prophylaxis with a continuously rotating air pressure bed; aggressive pulmonary toilet with a vibratory/percussion bed, as well as aggressive bronchoscopy for secretion clearance; and full invasive cardiac monitoring with indwelling arterial catheters and PACs. Particular attention was paid to monitoring of coagulation profiles and potassium because of the well-described intracellular shift of potassium with cooling and the prolongation of the clotting profile at lower temperatures.[29]

In a follow-up study, the beneficial effect with regard to the Glasgow Outcome Score was limited to patients with a GCS score of less than 8 and to patients younger than 45 years of age. Further data are needed to define the role of hypothermia more precisely.[30]

Hypertonic Saline

Hypertonic saline (HS), used in small volumes, has been used by some critical care clinicians to enhance blood flow in microvascular beds. HS, which is hyperosmolar, is thought to increase microvascular flows by decreasing viscosity of blood and reducing white cell–vascular wall adherence; this latter property results in decreased white cell diapedesis across vessels in the microcirculation and less lysosomal enzyme release into the perivascular interstitial spaces, resulting in decreased inflammatory reactions. Decreased inflammation results in less edema formation, which may be an important factor in ICP management of brain injury. Numerous animal studies have shown that HS increases cerebral perfusion while limiting brain free water content and ICP. A meta-analysis involving 223 hypotensive patients with TBI showed an improvement in survival with HS when compared with standard crystalloid resuscitation (odds ratio of 2.12, $p = 0.048$).[37] These results should be considered preliminary, and much work is still needed to determine the exact role of HS in the treatment of the brain injury population. When HS is used, hyperosmolarity and hypernatremia may result, which could limit ongoing therapy.

ACUTE CARE

When a neurosurgical patient is to be recovered in the NCCU, the medical director and clinician manager usually receive a request for a postoperative bed during morning rounds. The bed is posted and made available for the expected admission. The assigned NCCU clinician is notified by the OR clinician or member of the surgical team when the patient is ready for transfer and receives the patient report. All equipment and supplies necessary on admission are assembled in the designated room to receive the patient (see Chapters 8 and 18).

On admission the health care team provides the patient report as the NCCU clinician initiates the patient assessment to include the following:

- Patient demographics: name, age, history, premorbid medical condition
- Surgical procedure: intraoperative concerns, length of surgery, intraoperative fluids, blood products, medications, estimated blood loss, intake and output
- Routine admission orders
- Laboratory studies to be completed on admission
- Estimated length of stay (LOS) in the NCCU

Although the details of cerebral debridement and craniectomy are described in Chapter 8, the clinician should be aware of the importance of maintenance of excellent CPP and a normal coagulation profile on the patient's return to the NCCU. An immediate postresection CT scan is useful for evaluating the completeness of resection, as well as the presence of any hemorrhage of the resection bed (the baseline evaluation is used for comparison).[9] If the patient has an open calvarium, particular care needs to be paid to scrupulous aseptic technique in wound care and maintenance of monitoring catheters. Meningitis or an intracranial abscess in this setting is devastating.

Metabolism Management

Techniques to help measure cerebral metabolism include positron emission tomography (PET) scanning and near-infrared spectroscopy (NIS) of cerebral parenchyma.

Two of the most important factors that influence brain activity, temperature and blood glucose, are fortunately some of the most easily controllable. As noted earlier in this chapter, lower brain temperatures reduce cerebral metabolism. Several studies suggest that hyperglycemia for 48 hours following TBI is deleterious to the maintenance of neuronal viability and is thus associated with poorer neurologic outcomes.[2] Therefore stabilization of the critically ill neuroscience patient with metabolic problems includes recognizing and eliminating the precipitating factors as soon as possible. Supportive therapy is provided until clinical and laboratory assessments are completed to evaluate potential causes (see Chapter 5).

The patient history is important, and the patient's current use of prescription medications and drug or alcohol use identifies the need for laboratory and toxicologic screening. Patients with known metabolic disorders may benefit from consultation with their primary health care providers and review of old records from past hospital admissions.

Results of the history, clinical assessment, and laboratory tests allow rapid intervention to eliminate and correct metabolic imbalance or disorders. Disorders of cerebral metabolism require continuous assessment for early detection and treatment to prevent brain damage.

Coagulopathy Management

Disorders of the normal clotting mechanisms may explain inappropriate bleeding in the critically ill neuroscience patient. Coagulopathy in the neurotrauma patient may result from hypothermia or massive fluid administration or blood transfusions during resuscitation. Brain tissue is rich in tissue thromboplastin, and TBI upregulates the synthesis of this important initiator of the coagulation cascade. The result is the induction of a potentially devastating coagulopathy: namely, **disseminated intravascular coagulation (DIC)**.[9,14] DIC will usually be clinically evident as diffuse and possibly severe bleeding from operative sites, venipuncture sites, and uninjured tissue interfaces, such as the gums, nasal passages, tracheobronchial tree, and urinary excretory system. Not all patients develop DIC or have such a dramatic presentation. Laboratory markers of DIC include an elevated PT or APTT, as well as thrombocytopenia (platelet count <100,000), and frequently, elevated fibrin degradation products and decreased fibrinogen levels (<150 mg/dl).

Abnormalities of the coagulation cascade can cause **hypercoagulability** and lead to venous and arterial occlusion and brain infarction. Treatment depends on the underlying cause and may include replacement of blood and blood products on the basis of the patient's coagulation response and analysis of hemoglobin, hematocrit, fibrinogen, platelet count, PT, and APTT.[20]

Infection Management

Infections are the fourth leading cause of death in hospitalized patients. Neurotrauma patients are at high risk for infection because of the mechanism of injury (e.g., automobile collisions with open head wounds and open wound with fractures) (see Chapter 4).

Critically ill patients may have a depressed immune response and develop **nosocomial infections** that can lead to sepsis.[11] Older patients and those with poor nutrition or preexisting medical problems are particularly susceptible. Aggressive assessment and management are needed for early detection of, protection from, and promotion of the patient's resistance to infections, as well as provision of appropriate interventions at the earliest indication. Consultation and follow-up with the infectious disease member of the NCCU team is needed when infections become a concern.

Blood-Brain Barrier Properties and Impact on Antibiotic Usage

The blood-brain barrier is not an actual structure but a term that describes the special permeability of brain capillaries and the choroid plexus. The movement of substances into the brain depends on particle size, lipid solubility, chemical dissociation, and the protein-binding potential of the drug. In general, drugs that are lipid soluble and undissociated at the body's pH will rapidly enter both the brain and the CSF. The CSF is very slow in its uptake of dyes and both organic and inorganic anions and cations (e.g., sodium, potassium, glutamic acid) from the circulating blood. The barrier is highly permeable to water, oxygen, carbon dioxide, other gases, glucose, and lipid-soluble compounds.[19]

Infection in the CNS can arise from the meninges, ventricles, or brain parenchyma, resulting in meningitis, subdural empyema, ventriculitis, or brain abscess. Basilar skull fractures, CSF fistulas, and placement of ICP monitoring devices also pose a risk of infection. The diagnosis of meningitis is based on the analysis of CSF. Ventriculitis is almost always related to a ventriculostomy. The most common organism obtained from ventriculostomy-related infections is either coagulase-negative staphylococci or enteric gram-negative bacteria. Meticulous care of the ventricular catheter is essential both at the time of placement and during subsequent dressings.

A **subdural empyema** is a rare but devastating complication following a skull fracture or an intracranial procedure. This diagnosis should be suspected when the patient's CT scan shows a subdural collection in the presence of fever. Drainage through burr holes or a craniotomy is necessary, and the material should be sent for aerobic and anaerobic cultures. Patients with a subdural empyema should be treated with antibiotics for 4 to 6 weeks.

A **brain abscess** can occasionally be seen secondary to penetrating trauma or as a complication of a neurosurgical procedure. The CT scan shows a characteristic enhancing parenchymal lesion. If the mass is superficial and localized, excision of the abscess may be the best option. Parenteral antibiotics should be continued for 4 weeks or longer. Antibiotic usage comes in three forms:

1. **Prophylactic:** The appropriate antibiotic depends on the anticipated colonizing organisms. Prophylactic antibiotics should be administered such that antibiotic levels are present in the tissues at the time the surgical incision is made. Therapy should proceed for no more than 24 hours.

2. **Empiric:** When agents are selected, their usage should be limited to 72 hours. This practice can be standardized by writing a "72-hour stop" order along with the prescription. This practice mandates a reexamination of therapy and avoids inadvertent continuation of inappropriate antimicrobial agents. Empiric therapy is generally broad spectrum in order to cover multiple organisms and becomes more focused as sensitivity data are returned over the 48 to 72 hours following the culture. Therapy should be based on the likely site of infection, the kinds of organisms likely to be located at that site, and the local hospital antibiogram. For instance, previously healthy patients with an acute infection do not need coverage for nosocomial pathogens. Patients in nursing homes and those who have been hospitalized longer than 7 days (or 72 hours in an ICU) benefit from coverage for nosocomial pathogens. Typical pathogens include methicillin-resistant *Staphylococcus aureus* (MRSA), *Pseudomonas aeruginosa*, *Acinetobacter* species, Enterobacteriaceae, and *Klebsiella* species.

3. **Therapeutic:** The use of therapeutic agents is initiated when the infecting organism becomes identified from an infected site. The choice of agents should ideally be based on sensitivity patterns determined by culture material.

Resistant Pathogens

Coagulase-negative *Staphylococcus aureus* (CNSA) is being recognized as a pathogen in the NCCU patient population. A vigilant watch must occur on a regular basis to identify the presence of extended-spectrum **beta-lactase–producing organisms (ESBLs).** Either these organisms may always make beta-lactase, or the ESBL-producing gene may be induced after a short period of exposure to beta-lactam–containing antimicrobial agents. The typical ESBL-producing microbe is **Klebsiella** species. Klebsielleae are identified by their resistance to ceftazidime by disk diffusion study. Should such an organism be identified, the patient should be placed in strict contact isolation. Antimicrobial selection should be changed from any of the beta-lactam–containing agents to a carbapenem. Fluoroquinolone agents are less effective against ESBL-producing organisms and are not first-line therapy.

When patients are treated with long courses of antibiotics or shorter courses of broad-spectrum agents, normal flora are destroyed and resistant or adapted organisms survive. Two particular types of organisms that are commonly identified in this situation merit mention: **vancomycin-resistant**

enterococci (VRE) and **fungi.** VRE are typically *faceium,* but there are increasingly common vancomycin-resistant *faecalis* species as well. Usually, *faecalis* is sensitive to ampicillin and vancomycin. However, plasmid-mediated transfection can result in vancomycin resistance. It is unclear whether patients die with or because of VRE. Certainly, VRE bacteremia is an infection and merits therapy, but it is not at all clear whether the isolation of VRE from sputum, the urinary tract, or a catheter tip alone merits therapy at all. The most effective current options for VRE eradication are two newer agents: Synercid (bacteriostatic) and linezolid (bactericidal).

The specter of fungal infection is raised when a patient receiving broad-spectrum agents remains persistently febrile. Empiric therapy (72-hour stop) is warranted while specific fungal cultures are being obtained. Initial therapy with an azole agent (e.g., fluconazole 800 mg load, 400 mg/day) is ideal unless there is septic shock, in which case it is our opinion that amphotericin B should be selected as the empiric agent of choice. The reader must bear in mind that only certain **Candida** species are azole sensitive *(Candida albicans);* others *(Candida parapsilosis)* may be sensitive, but there must be confirmatory minimal inhibitory concentrations to document the efficacy of such therapy. *Candida tropicalis* and *Torulopsis glabrata* are not azole sensitive, and amphotericin B therapy is indicated instead. We reserve lipid-formulated amphotericin B for patients with documented central neuraxis infection or patients with abnormal renal function (creatinine >2.0 mg%).

Fungal infection should also prompt consultation with an infectious disease specialist. Fungal infections of the central neuraxis are very difficult to treat. For example, central **Aspergillus** infection carries a virtually 100% mortality rate.

SPECIAL NEUROLOGIC DISORDERS REQUIRING NCCU MANAGEMENT

This section addresses the unique concerns of some types of neuroscience patients who are admitted to NCCUs. Many other neuroscience patient populations also require NCCU management and are discussed in other chapters (e.g., aneurysms and vasospasm [see Chapter 18], tumor resections [see Chapter 7], and seizures and epilepsy [see Chapter 24]).

Myasthenia Gravis

Patients with MG who are developing ventilatory failure but who are not experiencing upper airway problems may at times be managed with **permissive hypercapnia** under close observation in an NCCU. If the upper airway is competent and the patient is not experiencing difficulty handling secretions, intermittent nasal bilevel positive airway pressure (BiPAP) may be a useful temporizing measure. However, the majority of patients who develop hypercapnia in myasthenic crisis require intubation, just the same as those who become fatigued from other processes that increase the work of breathing (WOB). Once a patient is committed to mechanical ventilation, many experts withdraw anticholinesterase treatment for several days (see Chapter 22). If a patient is not weaned within 1 week, the anticholinesterase agent is typically reintroduced at a lower dose.[19]

Guillain-Barré Syndrome

The most immediate threat to life for patients with Guillain-Barré syndrome (GBS) is respiratory failure from intercostal and diaphragmatic muscle paralysis (see Chapter 15). Over a course of several days to weeks, complete muscle paralysis may develop. Patients may often "look good," only to suffer precipitous respiratory arrest because the extent of weakness has not been appreciated. The mainstay of the pulmonary aspect of GBS therapy consists of vigilant monitoring for incipient respiratory failure. ABG monitoring is worthwhile, but hypoxemia and hypercapnia are late findings and indicate that respiratory arrest is imminent. Intubation should not be delayed until there is evidence of deteriorating blood gases. Elective intubation should be performed when the vital capacity approaches 15 ml/kg, or sooner if there is associated pharyngeal paresis and difficulty handling secretions. As the vital capacity drops further, the ability to effectively cough and clear secretions is impaired, resulting in atelectasis and **ventilation-perfusion (V/Q) mismatch,** producing hypoxemia. Hypercapnia usually occurs after the appearance of hypoxemia, when the bellows function of the diaphragm and intercostal muscles is lost. The most common error in caring for patients with GBS is failure to intubate in the presence of marginally compensated ventilatory mechanisms. Failure to intubate early in the course may result in the need for emergency intubation under suboptimal conditions, thereby causing unnecessary risk to the patient.

Autonomic dysfunction is common in GBS and usually responds to the appropriate pharmacologic agents. A **transcutaneous pacemaker** should be readily available. The development of asystole or advanced degrees of heart block may require emergency insertion of a temporary transvenous pacemaker if a transcutaneous pacemaker is not "capturing" or not available. **Neuritic pain** in the limbs and back is common and may respond to quinine or tricyclic antidepressants. Small doses of codeine may occasionally be required to obtain adequate analgesia.

Occasionally, autonomic derangements are of sufficient severity to result in ileus and inability to effectively use the GI tract for feeding; total parenteral nutrition (TPN) should be used while awaiting GI recovery. Depression and psychologic aberration related to the **locked-in** syndrome are common. Patients should be frequently reassured that the outlook for full recovery is good.

Acute Ischemic Stroke

Acute care management of acute ischemic stroke (AIS) has dramatically changed in the past decade (see Chapter 17). The use of lytic therapy has had a major impact in the improved outcome of many patients. Thrombolytic therapy has risks. The management issues concerning postlytic complications are discussed in Chapter 17.

The leading cause of death after stroke is not neurologic but pulmonary, involving pneumonia, usually due to aspira-tion. Since a stroke often causes weakness of pharyngeal muscles and disturbance of the swallowing reflexes, airway protection may be necessary in the first few days after onset (especially in the case of a large hemispheric brain attack/ stroke). Early intubation and mechanical ventilation should be considered in patients with long apneic periods that accompany irregular respirations, and in those with vomiting. The timing of a tracheostomy for clearance of secretions and airway protection varies, depending on the prognosis for neurologic recovery. Many patients recover function within 7 to 10 days, thus avoiding the need for a tracheostomy. Patients should have their oral intake restricted, however, until a **dysphagia consultation** has been done.[13] Stroke protocols in some institutions may require a speech therapist to evaluate a patient diagnosed with AIS in the emergency department (ED) for early identification of patients with dysphagia and strategies to prevent complications.

There is a definite correlation between atherosclerosis in the coronary and cerebral arteries; most stroke patients have underlying coronary artery disease. Some patients will have a concomitant **myocardial infarction (MI)** or will suffer one within a few days of their stroke. The myocardial ischemia is often "silent," or unrecognized, and the patient must be questioned and examined diligently for symptoms that could indicate cardiac ischemia. Because patients are often aphasic, confused, or unresponsive at the time of admission, their ECG (and possibly serum creatine kinase and troponin levels) should be examined so that a possible MI is not overlooked. Preexisting heart disease, combined with the catecholamine release that often accompanies a stroke, accounts for a high incidence of **cardiac dysrhythmias** in these patients. Because these are occasionally serious or even fatal events, each patient must be observed carefully, and treatment individualized.[13]

Seizures

The treatment of seizures and status epilepticus is discussed in other chapters (see Chapter 24). Seizures in NCCU patients, frequently related to noncompliance to anticonvulsant use, have several other causes that must be investigated. Drugs are a major cause of NCCU seizures, especially in patients with diminished renal or hepatic function or when the blood-brain barrier is breached. Drug withdrawal is another frequent offender. Although ethanol withdrawal is common and usually begins on the third day of admission, discontinuing any sedative agent may prompt seizures 1 to 3 days later. In addition, electrolytes and serum osmolarity should be measured for disturbances. Hypoglycemia and nonketotic hyperglycemia can also produce seizures.

GENERAL CARE MANAGEMENT IN THE NCCU

Pulmonary Management

Respiratory compromise and complications are common for neuroscience patients in the NCCU. The clinician should, in addition to completing a thorough neurologic assessment, incorporate into his or her overall patient evaluation a standard respiratory assessment to ascertain if there is respiratory dysfunction that may complicate neurologic recovery. Inadequate oxygenation has significance for all critically ill patients but is particularly challenging for those who fall into the following categories:

- Patients with neuromuscular diseases
- Patients with life-threatening CNS disorders
- Postoperative neurosurgical patients
- Patients with severe neurotrauma, especially with low brain PO$_2$
- Patients with an altered LOC

Work of Breathing

In patients who are difficult to wean from mechanical ventilation, excessive WOB may play a significant role. WOB is the product of the force applied (by the muscles of respiration) to an object (the lung) and the distance the lung is moved (to generate tidal volume) and can be expressed with the following equation:

$$WOB = P \text{ (pressure)} \times V \text{ (volume)}$$

For most patients the WOB is usually negligible (2% to 3% of total energy expenditure by the body). There are patients, however, in whom the WOB does present a problem. These patients include, but are not limited to, those with the following conditions: obesity, atelectasis, pneumonia, pulmonary edema, pulmonary fibrosis, pleural effusion, or pneumothoraces. Included with these patients would be the neuroscience patients who may have prolonged ventilation or require prolonged weaning timetables (e.g., the patient with severe neurologic trauma, MG, or GBS).

Indications and Criteria for Oxygen Therapy

Oxygen therapy is indicated in almost all patients who are in an NCCU. Indications for oxygen include the following:

- Hypoxemia (PaO$_2$ <60 mm Hg; SaO$_2$ <90%)
- Increased myocardial workload (e.g., hypertensive crisis, myocardial infarction, congestive heart failure)
- Decreased cardiac output (e.g., shock or hypoperfusion)
- Increased oxygen demand (e.g., sepsis)
- Decreased oxygen-carrying capacity (e.g., anemia, sickle cell disease, carbon monoxide poisoning)
- Procedures that may cause hypoxemia (e.g., suctioning)
- Decreased LOC

Indications and Criteria for Mechanical Ventilation

Early intubation may prevent exacerbation of intracranial pathologic conditions by avoiding hypercarbia and/or hypoxemia and consequent increases in ICP. (Table 9-2 lists indicators for mechanical ventilation and weaning; Table 9-3 lists modes of mechanical ventilation; and Table 9-4 lists settings of mechanical ventilation.) Indications for intubation and the use of mechanical ventilation include the following:

- Decreased LOC (GCS score <8)
- Inability to protect the airway
- Anticipated deterioration in patient status

- Hemodynamic instability
- Acute respiratory failure with respiratory acidosis
- Hypoxemia refractory to noninvasive therapy
- Apnea
- Hypercarbia with acidemia (pH <7.3)

It is important to mention that any stimulation of the oropharynx, nasopharynx, or trachea may produce a significant rise in ICP. It is advisable that any rise in ICP be avoided if at all possible. Pretreatment of patients undergoing intubation with a short-acting opioid such as fentanyl or a barbiturate such as methohexital may attenuate or prevent this rise in ICP. However, in the patient who is hemodynamically unstable, these agents are not advisable because of the propensity of both agents to depress blood pressure and cardiac output, which will cause a decrease in CPP (Table 9-5).

Intravenous lidocaine (1 mg/kg) is frequently used to blunt the tracheal reactivity and thus the increase in ICP associated with tracheal manipulations.

Indications and Criteria for Tracheostomy

A tracheostomy provides long-term airway access and minimizes the risk of vocal cord damage from an ET tube during long-term airway maintenance. It also decreases dead space and WOB. A tracheostomy should be considered if an artificial airway is required for longer than 2 weeks. The timing of the tracheostomy may depend on the anticipated neurologic and overall outcome of the patient (as early as 3 days or as late as 4 weeks following oral ET intubation). To streamline anesthetic exposures, tracheostomy is commonly performed at the same time as enteral access, most commonly as a percutaneous endoscopic gastrostomy (PEG). In addition, the airway and enteral access make placement in a rehabilitation or long-term care facility easier because of the ability to clear secretions and guarantee that enteral access will not be an impediment to meeting caloric needs.[6,15,16]

Secretion Clearance

Secretion clearance is an essential part of providing ideal pulmonary management. The NCCU patient presents unique challenges with regard to secretion clearance, since the usual secretion clearance maneuvers may induce episodic intracranial hypertension, poorly tolerated hypoxemia, or hypercarbia. Pulmonary secretions, referred to as a mucociliary blanket, are constantly swept toward the proximal trachea by the action of the mucociliary elevator mechanism. The coordinated action of the microvilli moves the mucoid layer proximally, so that a reflexive cough will clear the secretions from the tracheobronchial tree. This process is clearly impeded by dehydration, the use of inhalational anesthetic agents, cold, combustion products (house fire, tobacco), and inhaled poisons (chlorine gas). Also, the clearance mechanism is impeded by an indwelling ET tube (see Table 9-5); just as the secretions may move up into the tube, they can also as easily slide back down into the airway if they are not suctioned completely.

The bedside clinician must exercise care to avoid dehydration of the mucociliary blanket; euvolemia is a minimum. Suctioning of secretions using 100% oxygen and a presuctioning lavage of 0.9% normal saline solution helps avoid

| TABLE 9-2 | Indicators for Mechanical Ventilation and Weaning |

Measurement and Significance		Normal Values*	Mechanical Ventilation Indicated*	Weaning Feasible*
Tests of Ventilatory Reserve or Mechanical Ability				
V_T	Amount of air exchanged during normal breathing at rest	7–9 ml/kg	<5 ml/kg	>5 ml/kg
Respiratory rate per minute		12–20	<10 or >35	12–20
Forced vital capacity (FVC)	Maximal inspiration and then measurement of air during maximal forced expiration; determination of whether patient can sigh deeply enough to avoid atelectasis; best indicator of ventilatory reserve; patient's cooperation necessary	67–75 ml/kg	<10–15 ml/kg	>10–15 ml/kg
Peak inspiratory pressure, negative inspiratory force	Complete occlusion of aneroid manometer attached to airway or mouth for 10–20 sec while negative inspiratory efforts of patient noted; useful index of neuromuscular strength; less patient cooperation necessary	−75 to −100 cm H_2O	>−25 cm H_2O	<−20 cm H_2O
Forced expiratory volume in 1 sec (FEV_1)	Volume of air measured in first second of exhalation of forced vital capacity maneuver; used in patients with COPD to determine degree of obstruction	50–60 ml/kg	<10 ml/kg	>16 ml/kg
Resting minute ventilation	Multiplication of tidal volume by respiratory rate for 1 min, general indication of patient's total ventilation	5–10 L/min	>10 L/min	<10 L/min
V_D/V_T	Estimation from V_T; accurate calculation requiring $PaCO_2$ and partial pressure of CO_2 in mixed expired gas; measurement of portion of each breath that does not participate in gas exchange; indication of lungs' efficiency in removing CO_2	0.25–0.40	>0.6	<0.5–0.6
$PaCO_2$	Indication of lungs' efficiency in removing CO_2 and reflection of body's acid-base status	35–45 mm Hg	>55 mm Hg (acute)	<45 mm Hg
Tests of Oxygenation Capability				
PaO_2/FiO_2	Provision of evidence of lung's ability to oxygenate arterial blood; couples PO_2 with amount of oxygen given	350–400	<200	>300

From Lewis SM, Heitkemper MM, Dirksen SF: *Medical-surgical nursing: assessment and management of clinical problems*, ed 5, St Louis, 2000, Mosby.

*These parameters are only guidelines and must be related to the individual patient's status (e.g., patients with severe COPD may have a normal $PaCO_2$ of 60 mm Hg and values lower than normal for FEV_1, vital capacity, minute ventilation, and maximal voluntary ventilation).

COPD, Chronic obstructive pulmonary disease; *FiO_2,* fraction of inspired oxygen; *PaCO_2,* partial pressure of carbon dioxide in arterial blood; *PaO_2,* partial pressure of oxygen in arterial blood; *PO_2,* partial pressure of oxygen; *V_D,* physiologic dead space in front of tidal volume; *V_T,* tidal volume.

suctioning-induced hypoxemia and aids in clearing secretions that may be thick and viscid (see Table 9-5). Similarly, suctioning should be performed for brief episodes so as to not aspirate the functional residual volume and induce hypercarbia or hypoxemia. Repeated episodes of suctioning for short durations are recommended if there are significant amounts of secretions to clear.

Occasionally secretions become inspissated and may lead to segmental or **lobar collapse.** Immediate progression to bronchoscopic clearance of these inspissated secretions is recommended as opposed to alterations in ventilator management or vigorous attempts at alveolar recruitment with lavage-bagging-suctioning maneuvers.

The issue of suctioning-induced elevated ICP is relevant to the daily care of the NCCU patient. Patients with increased ICP who require suctioning may benefit from the administration of small aliquots of sodium pentothal (50 to 75 mg IV push [IVP]) down the endotracheal tube before tracheal suctioning to control ICP that results from stimulation of the carina, the extracranial site with the greatest density of nerve fiber endings in the body. No randomized trial exists that documents improved outcome with such a strategy, but it is successful in controlling ICP elevations that result from daily care. Etomidate (Amidate) is to be avoided for such a routine strategy because of the risk of inadvertent adrenal suppression. As noted earlier, lidocaine may be helpful here.

Bronchoscopy and Bronchoalveolar Lavage
If secretion mobilization is suboptimal, atelectasis, mucous plugging, and segmental or subsegmental airway obstruction

TABLE 9-3	Modes of Mechanical Ventilation		
Description	Advantages	Disadvantages	Uses
Controlled Mechanical Ventilation (CMV)			
Machine delivers preset number of breaths/min at preset volume. Patient cannot trigger breathing.	Each breath is controlled by the ventilator.	Does not allow patient to initiate breathing or respiratory rate to change with varying patient needs. Airway pressure always positive during inspiration, compromising venous return. Provides limited use of respiratory muscles.	Apnea secondary to brain damage, respiratory muscle paralysis, drug overdose, sedation, intraoperative use during general anesthesia
Assist-Control Ventilation (ACV)			
Delivery of breath is triggered by inspiratory effort of patient after preselected time interval has elapsed. If patient fails to initiate breathing, ventilator cycles as in controlled ventilation.	Patient can initiate own breathing, use respiratory muscles, and alter respiratory rate according to need. Intrathoracic pressure decreases transiently before inspiratory phase.	Problems of overventilation and resultant hypocapnia.	Wide range of situations in which patients are spontaneously breathing but have ventilatory failure or gas exchange inefficiency
Synchronized Intermittent Mandatory Ventilation (SIMV)			
Patient breathes spontaneously at own V_T and rate. Ventilator is synchronized to patient's ventilatory rate. Machine set to give certain number of breaths and is triggered by patient's inspiration.	Ventilator does not compete with patient's breathing.	Allows maintenance of even minor spontaneous excursions. Respiratory muscles remain in use. Ventilator augments patient's own efforts.	Wide range of situations in which patients need ventilatory support; method of weaning

From Lewis SM, Heitkemper MM, Dirksen SF: *Medical-surgical nursing: assessment and management of clinical problems*, ed 5, St Louis, 2000, Mosby.
V_T, Tidal volume.

TABLE 9-4	Settings of Mechanical Ventilation
Parameter	Description
Respiratory rate (f)	Number of breaths the ventilator delivers per minute; usual setting is 4–20 breaths/min
Tidal volume (V_T)	Volume of gas delivered to patient during each ventilator breath; usual volume is 5–15 ml/kg
Oxygen concentration (FiO_2)	Fraction of inspired oxygen delivered to patient; may be set between 21% and 100%; usually adjusted to maintain PaO_2 level greater than 60 mm Hg or SaO_2 level greater than 90%
I/E ratio	Duration of inspiration to duration of expiration; usual setting is 1:2 to 1:1.5 unless IRV is desired
Flow rate	Speed with which the tidal volume is delivered; usual setting is 40–100 L/min
Sensitivity/trigger	Determines the amount of effort the patient must generate to initiate a ventilator breath; it may be set for pressure triggering or flow triggering; usual setting for a pressure trigger is 0.5–1.5 cm H_2O below baseline pressure and for a flow trigger is 1–3 L/min above baseline flow
Pressure limit	Regulates the maximal pressure the ventilator can generate to deliver the tidal volume; when the pressure limit is reached, the ventilator terminates the breath and spills the undelivered volume into the atmosphere; usual setting is 10–20 cm H_2O above peak inspiratory pressure

From Thelan LA: *Critical care nursing: diagnosis and management*, ed 3, St Louis, 1998, Mosby.
I/E, Inspiration/expiration; *IRV*, inverse-ratio ventilation; *PaO_2*, partial pressure of oxygen in arterial blood; *SaO_2*, oxygen saturation of mixed arterial blood.

TABLE 9-5	Complications of Endotracheal Tubes	
Complications	**Causes**	**Prevention/Treatment**
Tube obstruction	Patient biting tube Tube kinking during repositioning Cuff herniation Dried secretions, blood, or lubricant Tissue from tumor Trauma Foreign body	*Prevention:* Place bite block. Sedate patient as required (prn). Suction prn. Humidify inspired gases. *Treatment:* Replace tube.
Tube displacement	Movement of patient's head Movement of tube by patient's tongue Traction on tube from ventilator tubing Self-extubation	*Prevention:* Secure tube to upper lip. Restrain patient's hands. Sedate patient prn. Ensure that only 2 inches of tube extend beyond lip. Support ventilator tubing. *Treatment:* Replace tube.
Sinusitis and nasal injury	Obstruction of paranasal sinus drainage Pressure necrosis of nares	*Prevention:* Avoid nasal intubations. Cushion nares from tube and tape/ties. Ensure proper tube positioning and stabilization. *Treatment:* Remove all tubes from nasal passages. Administer antibiotics.
Tracheoesophageal fistula	Pressure necrosis of posterior tracheal wall resulting from overinflated cuff and rigid nasogastric tube	*Prevention:* Stabilize airway. Inflate cuff with minimal amount of air necessary. Monitor cuff pressures q8h. Use small-bore feeding tube for enteral feeding. *Treatment:* Position cuff of tube distal to fistula. Place gastrostomy tube for enteral feedings. Place esophageal tube for secretion clearance proximal to fistula.
Mucosal lesions	Pressure at tube and mucosal interface	*Prevention:* Inflate cuff with minimal amount of air necessary. Monitor cuff pressures q8h. Use appropriate-size tube. *Treatment:* May resolve spontaneously. Perform surgical intervention.
Laryngeal or tracheal stenosis	Injury to area from end of tube or cuff, resulting in scar tissue formation and narrowing of airway	*Prevention:* Inflate cuff with minimal amount of air necessary to create seal. Monitor cuff pressures q8h. Suction area above cuff frequently. *Treatment:* Perform tracheostomy. Place laryngeal stent. Perform surgical repair.
Cricoid abscess	Mucosal injury with bacterial invasion	*Prevention:* Inflate cuff with minimal amount of air necessary to create seal. Monitor cuff pressures q8h. Suction area above cuff frequently. *Treatment:* Perform incision and drainage of area. Administer antibiotics.

From Thelan LA: *Critical care nursing: diagnosis and management,* ed 3, St Louis, 1998, Mosby.

and collapse may occur. Several initial clinical maneuvers are indicated, which may include the following: chest physiotherapy, postural drainage, and aerosolized bronchodilator therapy. When these initial therapies fail, a more invasive approach is warranted.

The traditional approach to clearance of secretions is **therapeutic bronchoscopy.** The adult **flexible fiberoptic bronchoscope** can easily fit through a size 8.0 or greater ET tube. Unfortunately, airway mucosal irritation is a powerful sympathetic stimulant, and tachycardia, systemic hypertension, and bronchospasm commonly complicate therapeutic bronchoscopy. In the setting of intracranial hypertension, the clinician must take steps to blunt any potential sympathetic stimulation. Mucosal irritation may be minimized by careful bronchoscopic technique that avoids impacting and suctioning the tracheobronchial sidewalls. In addition, topical or systemic lidocaine will also blunt mucosal irritation. Preprocedure blockade with a relatively short-acting agent such as esmolol will blunt the tachycardia and elevated blood pressure that accompanies heightened sympathetic tone. This may diminish the increase in CBF that accompanies sympathetic discharge. Adjuvant therapy with opioid analgesia with a short-acting agent such as fentanyl will enhance sedation and eliminate pain from mucosal injury.[27]

When these measures fail, significant sedation and cerebral protection may be achieved with cautious administration of barbiturates such as sodium pentothal or sedatives such as propofol. These therapies may also be complicated by systemic hypotension. Alternatively, for very short procedures, etomidate is an excellent and powerful hypnotic that has the unique advantage of reducing ICP. Thus excellent IV access for fluid or inotrope administration is mandatory when using barbiturates. A postprocedure chest x-ray study is indicated to assess the results of the bronchoscopy and to look for complications such as a pneumothorax or malposition of the ET tube.

Management of PCO_2, PO_2, and Induced Hypocapnia

Induced hypocapnia has been used for many decades to induce cerebral vasoconstriction and reduce ICP. The mechanism whereby ICP reduction occurs is by restriction of the CBV. A potentially deleterious effect of cerebral vasoconstriction is cerebral ischemia. Therefore the injured brain may be rendered ischemic if the hypocapnia induced to control elevated ICP is severe or prolonged. Normal brain tissue will not become ischemic, since it retains vasoregulatory properties that ensure cerebral perfusion over a wide range of PCO_2 levels, viscosities, and blood pressure readings. There is evidence that after initial constriction in response to hyperventilation, cerebral vessels progressively dilate back to or even beyond their baseline within 24 hours, thus rendering this treatment ineffective. At this stage, attempts to normalize the PCO_2 often produce elevated ICP as the vessels continue to dilate as the PCO_2 rises. Minimal hyperventilation to a PCO_2 of roughly 35 mm Hg is commonly used because this seems to increase cerebrovascular tone slightly and may enhance the cerebral autoregulatory response. In fact, the PCO_2 and CBF are reported to have a linear relationship. Induced cerebral ischemia is clearly and

graphically represented on two-level xenon CT cerebral blood flow (Xe CT CBF) scanning. (See Chapter 3 for further discussion of xenon CT.)

Ventilatory Support in the Neurologically Impaired With Lung Injury

The usual initial manifestation of lung injury, regardless of cause, is impaired oxygenation. As the severity of the lung injury worsens, the "stiffness" of the lung increases, as does the oxygen diffusion barrier. Oxygenation is assessed with arterial PO_2 levels; however, when the PO_2 level is compared to the fractional inspired oxygen needed to achieve that level of oxygenation (PO_2/FiO_2, or P/F ratio), a measure of gas exchange efficiency is obtained. The normal P/F ratio is approximately 600; as lung injury severity increases, the P/F ratio decreases. When the P/F ratio decreases below 300, it requires the clinician to address advanced mechanical ventilation techniques to avoid undesirable hypoxia. The following sections deal with advance ventilatory maneuvers used to treat acute lung injury.

Positive End-Expiratory Pressure and Venous Return

The application of positive end-expiratory pressure (PEEP) is used to increase functional residual capacity and move the zero pressure point of each alveolar unit more proximally in the airway so as to prevent early alveolar collapse. By doing so, the PEEP increases the available number of alveolar units that can participate in gas exchange. The primary effect of PEEP, however, on gas exchange is improvement of oxygenation, not carbon dioxide removal. Carbon dioxide clearance is rather efficient and will be well preserved in situations where oxygenation is not. With the opening of one alveolar unit, the tendency of the adjacent unit is to open as well (i.e., alveolar codependency). There are two primary questions to ask when using PEEP to augment oxygenation: (1) What is the optimal PEEP? and (2) Is the current amount of PEEP compromising the patient's hemodynamics or ICP?[3,31,34]

Optimal PEEP provides an SaO_2 of at least 90% on nontoxic FiO_2 levels (generally <60%) without compromising cardiac output. Tissue oxygen delivery is affected by SaO_2, Hgb, and cardiac output. If SaO_2 is increased but cardiac output is decreased, no true gains in tissue oxygen delivery are achieved.

The intensivist, the neurologist or neurosurgeon, and the clinician all need to work together to determine the effectiveness of all therapies the patient is receiving. An example of multidisciplinary collaboration, with the neuroscience critical care clinician being in the forefront, can be seen with determining optimal PEEP. If one exceeds optimal PEEP and has alveolar overdistention, total intrathoracic pressure may be increased, which results in diminished venous return and hence diminished cardiac output. The decreased venous return may result in cerebral venous hypertension. The team needs to then ask the question, Optimal PEEP for which organ system? Clearly, the optimal PEEP for oxygenation may be the worst PEEP for cerebral venous drainage.

When instituting PEEP therapy in a patient with TBI, one runs the risk of impeding venous return from the cerebral circulation. One would like to be able not only to monitor cerebral venous pressure but also to assess the effects of changes in that pressure on cerebral oxygen metabolism and neuronal homeostasis. At the bedside, only indirect measurements are available for interpretation. Since there are no valves between the cerebral venous beds and the central circulation, central venous pressure (CVP) or jugular bulb venous pressures are reasonable estimates. If PEEP increases either of these measures, cerebral venous drainage may be compromised. If both CVP and ICP rise with PEEP, cerebral dynamics are definitely placed in jeopardy. Another indirect measure is near-infrared spectroscopy (NIS) of cerebral oxygen consumption (see later discussion). In short, if PEEP compromises cerebral metabolism and places neuronal integrity in jeopardy, the measured cerebral "mixed venous" oxygen saturation should theoretically fall. Since this application is still in its infancy, it can only be considered experimental, but it holds great promise as a noninvasive means of assessing cerebral oxygen metabolism.

In practice, most intensivists will initially ventilate a TBI patient with a minimal level of PEEP and assess cerebral dynamics. After obtaining a baseline cerebral profile, PEEP is added as needed to decrease the fraction of inspired oxygen (FiO_2) to 60% or below to avoid pulmonary oxygen toxicity. PEEP is adjusted to achieve the "optimal PEEP" in terms of oxygenation, venous return, and cerebral dynamics.

Pressure-Controlled Ventilation

When oxygenation remains problematic, another strategy to recruit lung function in the setting of low lung compliance, or **"stiff lung,"** is to prolong the inspiratory time to accommodate for the increased impedance to gas flow. The prolonged inspiratory time allows more oxygen-enriched gas to reach the gas-exchanging surfaces of the alveoli where oxygen diffusion into the blood can occur. **Pressure-controlled ventilation (PCV)** is a specialized pressure-limited ventilatory mode that allows gas flow to proceed until a preset pressure limit is reached; this pressure is then maintained for a preset time before passive exhalation. Predetermined assisted ventilation breaths are delivered, and tidal volume (V_T) in this mode is a function of the pressure change for a specified period of time. More uniform gas distribution results from this mode of ventilation, usually at lower peak inspiratory pressures, especially in the setting of low lung compliance. If hypoxia persists despite normal inspiratory/expiratory settings, manipulation of the phase duration of inspiration and expiration may be performed. A normal ratio of inspiration to expiration is 1:3 or 1:4, whereas inverse-ratio ventilation (IRV) uses ratios of 1:1 to 2:1 or greater. As the aspiratory time is increased so that it exceeds the time available for expiration (i.e., IRV), the patient may require sedation or paralysis, or both.[24] In addition, the mean airway pressure increases, as does the impedance to cerebral drainage; therefore elevation of the ICP may result from this ventilatory strategy. It is important to monitor ICP and cerebral oxygen when using PCV in the setting of TBI. Volume expansion is a common solution to decreased venous return but may aggravate cerebral hypertension. When PCV man-

agement compromises cerebral dynamics, more unusual management strategies are required.[34]

Permissive Hypercapnia

The patient's $PaCO_2$ is allowed to increase above normal if normal carbon dioxide clearance cannot be achieved with the ventilation strategy reserved for treating hypoxemia. This type of situation is permitted to occur when the patient has extreme acute respiratory distress syndrome (ARDS). ARDS can occur from numerous causes in the NCCU patient. This ventilator management strategy must be used with extreme caution in patients with a concurrent TBI or the potential for intracranial hypertension. In patients with acute lung injury and TBI, such a management strategy must be accompanied by measures of cerebral perfusion to evaluate for hyperemia and subsequent intracranial hypertension from increased carbon dioxide tension. Data indicating hyperemia may include elevated ICP, increased SjO_2, elevated oxygen concentration on NIS, and increased regional CBF by Xe CT. Permissive hypercapnia is acceptable, provided that hyperemia and intracranial hypertension are not exacerbated, there is no midline shift, and the pH is higher than 7.3.[10]

Airway Pressure Release Ventilation

Airway pressure release ventilation (APRV) is a state-of-the-art technology that is entering the U.S. marketplace after successful trials in Europe. It is essentially a high-level continuous positive airway pressure (CPAP) mode that is interrupted for very brief periods of time. The CPAP level may be as high as 40 cm H_2O. The long period of time during which the high-level CPAP is maintained achieves oxygenation by protracting inspiratory times (creating air trapping and auto-PEEP), and the short release periods achieve carbon dioxide clearance. APRV is fundamentally different from cyclic ventilation. This mode allows the patient to spontaneously breathe during all of the phases of the cycle; this is allowed because of a floating valve that is responsive to the patient's needs regardless of the location within the respiratory cycle. In other words, the patient is allowed to breathe in or out during the high-level CPAP phase, as well as during the release phase. During the high-CPAP phase, a patient may exhale 100 to 200 ml of gas as the lung volume becomes full of gas; this is not a full exhalation, but does give the patient a sense of "control" over the ventilator. Given the spontaneous nature of the mode of ventilation, there should be virtually no need for continuous infusions of neuromuscular blocking agents. The use of APRV may result in a shorter length of ICU stay and a reduced incidence of prolonged neuromuscular blockade syndrome. Furthermore, patients may be ventilated at lower airway pressures than with other ventilatory modes, and there is a reduced need for pressor support of hemodynamics to ensure oxygen delivery. Moreover, there is a reduced need for sedation, since patients are more comfortable with this spontaneous mode than with mandatory ventilation modes.[12,24,25] We have used this type of ventilation at our institution and believe it will change the way ventilated patients are managed.

Of note, when using a PAC in patients receiving APRV, the **pulmonary artery occlusion pressure (PaOP)** must be read at the middle or end of the release phase to maintain the fidelity of the reading. Reading the PaOP at any other point in the cycle will give a significantly different value by comparison with the end-expiratory reading obtained using pressure-controlled ventilation.

Ventilator Weaning Protocol

A well-designed weaning protocol has been demonstrated to be an invaluable aid in reducing the length of stay in the ICU (see Table 9-2). An appropriate protocol will enable the respiratory therapist and the bedside clinician to initiate the weaning process each day before a physician evaluation. Computer order entry may create an ICU admission data set that automatically activates such a protocol once the entry criteria are met (usually that the cause of respiratory failure is improving or has been eliminated, FiO_2 is less than 0.50, PEEP is less than 10 cm H_2O, and there are no pressors other than dopamine at <5 μg/kg/min). A ventilator pathway for charting and modifying the progress of patients on mechanical ventilation is a useful clinical tool. Such a pathway will allow one to engage in a regular review of a patient's progress along what would be considered a usual course for such individuals (Fig. 9-1). Deviation from this course should prompt an investigation into the cause(s) of the deviation. Such a pathway is also an excellent tool to use as a platform for quality assurance and improvement review.

Complications of Ventilatory Support

Pneumothorax. Pneumothorax is an occasional complication of mechanical ventilation in the ICU. It typically occurs following barotrauma or as a complication of an errant placement of a central venous catheter. It is important to recognize that small pneumothoraces that occur in spontaneously breathing patients (i.e., negative pressure ventilation) may be reevaluated with a repeat chest x-ray study in 4 to 6 hours and treated only if expansion occurs. This option is not appropriate for patients receiving any form of positive-pressure ventilation, since a simple pneumothorax may rapidly become a tension pneumothorax with subsequent hypotension and death. Tension pneumothoraces may be recognized by tachycardia, hypotension, elevated peak airway pressures (if mechanically ventilated), jugular venous distention (if not intravascularly depleted), thoracic resonance by percussion on the affected side, diminished or absent breath sounds on the affected side, and tracheal deviation away from the affected side. Clearly, not all signs or symptoms are present in all patients, and treatment is dictated by the patient's clinical condition.[1]

Pneumonia. An indwelling ET tube rapidly increases the risk of nosocomial pneumonia after 3 days. In numerous studies, enteric gram-negative organisms, or **methicillin-resistant *Staphylococcus aureus* (MRSA),** CNSA, and ***Pseudomonas*** species were the predominant organisms recovered from tracheal aspirates and bronchoalveolar lavage (BAL) specimens. Therefore in the clinical context of fever, leukocytosis, infiltrates on chest x-ray, and white blood cells in the sputum, empiric antimicrobial selection should cover this flora and may be guided by the local antibiogram. (An antibiogram outlines an institution's susceptibility pattern to specific microorganisms. It is helpful for the empiric antimicrobial selection process.) If the Gram stain demonstrates gram-negative rods (GNRs), double coverage maybe appropriate and includes the use of a third-generation cephalosporin (antipseudomonal penicillin) or a quinolone in combination with an aminoglycoside. It is important to recall that aminoglycoside dosing should approach the upper end of dosing regimens if a pulmonary infectious process is being treated because aminoglycoside penetration into airway secretions occurs appreciably only with serum levels greater than 6 μg/dl (i.e., 2 mg/kg/dose every 8 hours or 7 mg/kg/day with normal creatinine clearance). Antibiotics should eventually be tailored on the basis of culture results. If the Gram stain reveals only sheets of white cells without organisms, an atypical pneumonia must be considered and cultures should be obtained for unusual organisms such as *Legionella,* acid-fast bacilli, and fungi.

COMPREHENSIVE NEUROSCIENCE PATIENT MANAGEMENT IN THE NCCU

This section addresses six common issues regardless of the proximate cause leading to care in the ICU: (1) nutrition, (2) stress prophylaxis, (3) deep venous thrombosis prophylaxis, (4) pressure ulceration prophylaxis, (5) coagulation issues and disseminated intravascular coagulation, and (6) end-of-life issues.

Nutritional Considerations

The goal of nutritional support in the critically ill patient is not weight gain but support of the hypermetabolic state. Brain-injured patients are assumed to be markedly catabolic, and nutritional support consultation should be considered as soon as the patient arrives in the NCCU. Determining the caloric needs and the amount of protein required is dependent on the patient's body mass index; logistic regression models (i.e., Harris-Benedict equation) relate caloric need directly to gender, height, and weight and inversely to age. A dietitian who is familiar with the needs of the critically ill neuroscience patient population is a valuable asset to the NCCU team.[6,7,16-18]

Feeding of NCCU patients occurs via three modes: oral, enteral catheter, and parenteral (IV). The obvious first choice is by mouth in all patients who can participate in the nutrient intake process. In those patients who have a functional gastrointestinal (GI) tract but are unable to consume nutrients safely, enteral tube feedings is the preferred choice over IV feedings. Advantages of enteral feeding compared with the parenteral route include fewer complications and less expense. When the GI tract is able to maintain its absorptive ability, use of the enteral feeding reduces the incidence of sepsis by preventing the translocation of GI bacteria into the bloodstream or lymphatic system.[6,7,16-18] Gastrointestinal motility and mucosal integrity are the two critical factors in enteral nutrient absorption; in the NCCU population, impaired GI motility—regardless of cause—is the most common limitation to the use of enteral feeding.

	PHASE 1 - DAY 1 (Day of Intubation)	PHASE 1 - DAY 7	PHASE 2 (Day Entry Criteria Met)	PHASE 3 (Active Weaning)	PHASE 3 - DAY 7	PHASE 4 (Extubation)	PHASE 5 (Post Extubation and ICU D/C Plan)
Respiratory Status	• Establish Vent. Settings • Initiate continuous pulse oximetry monitoring • Review chest x-ray for ETT placement, and pathology • **Order ABG and weaning protocols**	• Patient has failed to meet entry criteria for weaning.	• Weaning Protocol entry criteria met. • Consideration given to early T-piece trial in concert with attending physician.	• Weaning Protocol in force by physician's order. • Resp. Therapist Driven	• Patient has failed to be successfully extubated	• Patient meets extubation criteria • Physician's order to extubate	• Step down status and considered for transfer
Consults	• Resp. Therapy Consult • OT/PT consult* • Nutrition consult* • Social Work consult* * = if patient anticipated to be ventilated >48 hr	• As indicated • Confirm OT/PT, nutrition and social service consults	Active follow up from: • Resp. Therapy • OT/PT • Nutrition • SS	• Follow up	• As indicated	• Follow up • Dysphagia consult as indicated	• As indicated
Nutrition/Diet	• IV fluids • Initiate enteral feeding • Fluid balance plan	• Evaluate adequacy	• Enteral nutrition established	• Enteral nutrition		• Gastric tube feedings held for 1 hour prior to extubation.	• Oral feeding or Tube feeding continues
Activity	• Ad lib/As clinically indicated		• OOB when possible • Bedside PT • Good night's sleep			• OOB • PT/OT/Chest PT • Incentive spirometry	
Medications	• Sedation/analgesia anxiolysis PRN • Stress-ulcer prophylaxis • DVT Prophylaxis • Diagnosis-specific meds	• Evaluate for side effects of medications	• Prophylactic agents prescribed • Pharmacologic treatment of primary resp. condition		• As indicated		
Diagnostic Tests	• Baseline ABG • Other ABG per protocol • CXR • Baseline labs	• As indicated • Metabolic cart evaluation • Consider Bicore monitor	• ABG per weaning protocol • Surveillance sputum • Gram stain and C&S		• As indicated • Metabolic cart evaluation • Consider Bicore monitor	• Post extubation ABG	• As indicated
Education/DC Plan	• Introduce patient/family to ventilator, ETT, and other equipment/procedures • Identify patient's decision maker and inquire re: Advance Directives	• Discuss with family the progress and prognosis	• Estimation of weaning success and timing discussed • Patient and family understand goals and participate in process	• Discussion of weaning process with family	• Discuss with family and consultants reasons for protracted weaning	• Discuss communication problems with family and complications of endotracheal intubation	• Transfer orders and note written

Outcomes	**Establish:**
	• **ABG protocol**
	• **Suctioning protocol**
	• **Bronchial hygiene**
	• **Weaning Plan (documented)**
	• Administer sedation/analgesia to ensure patient comfort
	
	Identify patient's decision maker.
	
	Identify and implement appropriate communication methods with patient and family.
		Understanding reason for failure to meet weaning criteria
		• Severity of acute illness
		• New complication
		• New organ failure
		• Complication of procedure or medication
		• Not all consults or treatments are accomplished
		• Excessive respiratory WOB
		• Is the problem ventilation or oxygenation?
			• **Weaning protocol in force**
			• **Primary respiratory condition identified and treated**
			• **PT, nutrition established**
			• Patient and family participate in weaning process
			• Transfer/Discharge planning initiated
				• Reduction in #IMV breaths
				• Reduction of PSV by ≥2 cm H₂O when MV minimal
				• Increased time off ventilator (T-piece, trach collar)
					Establish reason for protracted weaning
					• New complication
					• Fluid overload
					• Bronchospasm
					• Secretion management
					• Muscle weakness
					• Electrolyte abnormality
					• Excessive respiratory
					• WOB
					• Neurological dysfunction
						• Patient successfully extubated
						• No post-extubation laryngospasm
						• Oral feeding begun as feasible
						• OOB during the day
						• PT/OT
						• Consider for step down status
						• Chest PT and incentive spirometry established
						• Bronchial hygiene regimen established.
							• **Patient ready for transfer**
							• Discussed with family, PMD, receiving floor team.
							• Consultants notified for floor follow-up.
							• Social service follow-up for hospital discharge planning
							• No:
							  Fluid overload
							  Electrolyte abnormality
							  Secretion problem
							  Bronchospasm

Acceptable medical practice generally does include a variety of responses to a particular clinical problem.

Peer Review Records: **Confidential pursuant to the Peer Review Protection Act, 63 P.S. 425.1 et. seg. and Health Care Quality Improvement Act, 1986**

TENET   **CLINICAL PATHWAY FOR MECHANICALLY VENTILATED PATIENTS**

Medical College of Pennsylvania Hospital

Patient Name: _____

Medical Record Number: _____

Figure 9-1 Clinical pathway for a mechanically ventilated neuroscience patient.
(Courtesy Medical College of Pennsylvania Hospital, Philadelphia, PA.)

The types and choices of enteral feeding tubes, formulas, and patterns of delivery are many; the reader is advised to consult a nutritional support textbook for more detail. When tube feeding is chosen, it is important for the clinician to always keep the head of the bed elevated if gastric feedings are continuous and for 60 minutes after intermittent feeds. The ET tube or tracheostomy tube cuff should be inflated during feeding, and the clinician should check for residual volume in the stomach every 4 hours. Many NCCU teams prefer nasogastric (NG) or orogastric (OG) feeding catheters since they allow periodic assessment of residual gastric volumes by syringe aspiration. Tube feedings are held if the residual is more than 200 ml (approximately one can of soda). Small-caliber feeding tubes (i.e., Dobhoff-type catheters) do not allow reliable syringe aspiration such that accurate residual assessment can be made or the stomach emptied should the tube feedings not be tolerated.

If **gastric feedings** are not tolerated but the small bowel motility is preserved, a nasojejunal catheter (e.g., Bilboa 8 French duodenal intubation catheter commonly used for enteroclysis studies in radiology) can be placed fluoroscopically. These catheters are long enough to reach the proximal jejunum so that one may feed the patient distal to the pylorus and the ligament of Treitz. Postpyloric feeding may reduce the incidence of pulmonary aspiration.

When a **jejunal catheter** is being used for tube feedings, leaving the NG or OG tube in place has been advocated to keep the stomach empty and to assess for tube feeding reflux. Many NCCUs use liquid charcoal as a marker (enough to color the tube feedings gray) instead of methylene blue or other blue food coloring. Methylene blue is no longer recommended because it is absorbed and then subsequently secreted into gastric secretions and can falsely indicate reflux. In addition, protracted exposure to methylene blue may result in production of clinically significant methemoglobin. Reflux into the NG or OG tube indicates tube feeding intolerance, and the feedings are discontinued. A search should then be undertaken for the proximate cause for the tube feeding intolerance while the GI tract is decompressed.[6,7,16–18]

At the initiation of enteral feeding, caloric goals are calculated as outlined previously. After selection of the most appropriate tube and formula, continuous feeding starts at a low rate of administration (usually between 10 and 25 ml/hr) and then increased by 10 to 25 ml every 8 hours until the estimated goal is achieved. Some studies have shown that patients with severe TBI have a better outcome when receiving full nutritional support via a nasointestinal tube on day 1 than do those who were supported by NG feedings that were increased in a stepwise fashion over a series of days.[6,10,15]

If the patient is unable to tolerate enteral feedings, it is appropriate to initiate **total parenteral nutrition (TPN).**[12] The usual indications for TPN over enteral nutrition include, but are not limited to, the following:[15,17,18]

- High NG (or OG) output (>300 ml/8 hours)
- Shock
- Disordered GI motility
- Abdominal distention
- Acute or chronic pancreatitis

- Proximal small bowel anastomosis
- Hypothermia (core temp <34° C)
- GI bleeding

TPN is commonly constructed using a **"three-in-one" bag formula.** This design allows the lipids to be combined with the protein and carbohydrates in a single bag that will run for 24 hours. The nutritionist or nutritional support team is invaluable in aiding the clinician in selecting the appropriate nutrient and electrolyte composition. If TPN is to be used, the patient requires a central venous catheter with a port that has not been previously accessed.[17,18]

As part of the initial TPN order, a series of biochemical profiles should be done and repeated on a weekly basis (lipid profile, coagulation profile, electrolytes, blood urea nitrogen [BUN], creatinine, glucose, calcium, magnesium, and phosphorus). These profiles may have to be done more frequently if the patient is in a hypermetabolic state. TPN is not a benign therapy, and the reader is encouraged to be thoroughly familiar with the potential complications of its use.[17]

Two such complications that warrant specific mention here are **hyperglycemia** and **refeeding syndrome.** Hyperglycemia in a patient who was previously euglycemic on a stable TPN regimen may herald the onset of sepsis. In this circumstance, in addition to alterations to the TPN formula to reduce the intake of carbohydrates and administration of insulin, a thorough search for a source of infection should be undertaken. The refeeding syndrome occurs in patients who have suffered from severe protein-calorie malnutrition. In this syndrome, cells rapidly consume electrolytes, such as phosphorus and magnesium, and patients become rapidly hypophosphatemic. Seizures may result if the phosphate approaches 0.05 mmol/L. Low phosphate levels may result in low ATP levels, thus making ventilator weaning quite difficult. In extreme cases, spontaneous cardiac and respiratory arrest from inadequate high-energy phosphate levels (PO_4 <1.0 mg/dl) can occur.[6–8,17,18]

Stress Prophylaxis Considerations

Stress Ulcer Prophylaxis

The neuroscience patient is at high risk for gastric or duodenal stress ulceration, or **Cushing's ulcer.** Stress ulceration can be caused by the hypersecretion of acid, but this entity is more related to alterations of mucosal blood flow than to increases in gastric acid output. Blood flow reduction leads to decreased gastric mucus production, which compromises gastric mucosal integrity. This combination allows gastric acid "access" to erode into the submucosa where the vessels reside. Vessel wall erosion will lead to hemorrhage.

There are a variety of methods of stress ulcer prophylaxis, all of which are fairly equivalent in reducing the incidence of hemorrhage and ulceration. These methods are H_2-receptor blockade (i.e., famotidine, ranitidine, cimetidine), proton pump inhibition (omeprazole), oral antacids, and mucosal protectants (sucralfate, luminal feedings).

The NCCU clinician should also be aware that cimetidine may retard the metabolism of drugs such as warfarin, phenytoin, and theophylline, which potentiates their effects. Cimetidine crosses the blood-brain barrier and can produce changes in mental status. Neurologic side effects tend to be more frequent in the population at the extremes of the age spectrum, especially in those with renal or hepatic disease. Physostigmine can reverse cimetidine-induced confusion, but this is recommended only in the presence of life-threatening CNS toxicity.[6,17,18]

Concerns have been raised regarding the promotion of ventilator-associated pneumonia (VAP) with reduction of gastric acid by H_2-receptor or proton pump blockade. Normally, gastric acidity will destroy luminal bacteria. When this protective function is compromised by medications, bacterial growth may occur. Bacterial access to the pulmonary tree may be enhanced by the presence of an OG or NG tube that stents open the lower esophageal sphincter and allows bacteria to "wick" along the tube. Therefore our practice is to use sucralfate as the prophylaxis agent of choice. Patients who are unable to tolerate luminal medications are then treated with an H_2-receptor blocker until their GI tract becomes functional.[17,18]

Glucocorticoids

A special circumstance that commonly affects the neuroscience patient is glucocorticoid administration. Glucocorticoids have been used with great success in reducing edema associated with cerebral neoplasms. There has been no indication for glucocorticoids in patients with TBI. High-dose glucocorticoids have been shown to statistically improve neurologic outcome after blunt spinal cord injury, though the clinical importance of routine steroid use in this setting is being challenged with the new "Guidelines for the Management of Acute Cervical Spine and Spinal Cord Injuries" published in March 2002 in a supplement of *Neurosurgery* (www.neurosurgery-online.com). Unfortunately, steroid use is associated with the relatively rapid development of stress GI ulceration and hemorrhage. Ideally, if the decision to use glucocorticoids is made, the computerized order entry system will link the prescription of glucocorticoids with a stress ulcer prophylaxis regimen of choice.[10]

Deep Vein Thrombosis and Pulmonary Embolus

Neuroscience patients are at increased risk for deep vein thrombosis (DVT) because of immobility, venous stasis, and, commonly, impaired muscular tone and function (see Chapter 10). The greatest risk of DVT is the potential for **pulmonary embolization.** Bedside physical therapy (PT), range-of-motion (ROM) exercises, the use of elastic antiembolic stockings and sequential compression devices (SCDs), and, if medically feasible, pharmacologic DVT prophylaxis (heparinoids) should be included in the NCCU treatment regimen.[29] Heparinoid DVT prophylaxis is frequently contraindicated in neuroscience patients who are at high risk for having CNS bleeding. Since many of the patients demonstrate an abnormal sensorium, accurate reporting of early DVT warning signs, such as calf discomfort, may be impaired. Furthermore, increases in leg circumference may be difficult to interpret if there are orthopedic injuries or if the patient has undergone significant volume expansion during resuscitation from multisystem trauma. Some hospitals screen every NCCU patient on admission and each week thereafter using duplex ultrasonography to detect lower extremity DVT.

Pharmacologic DVT prophylaxis regimens include the following:
- Heparin (unfractionated)
- Low-molecular-weight heparin (fractionated heparin)
- Warfarin

The NCCU patient is frequently at the highest risk stratification for DVT such that combination prophylactic regimens should be undertaken when feasible.[29]

Pressure Ulceration Prophylaxis

Pressure ulceration is a preventable complication. When prolonged pressure is allowed to exist over bony prominences, the overlying skin perfusion is compromised. Pressure ulcers are staged (I to IV) related to the depth of tissue destruction. Increasing depth progresses from any observable pressure-related alteration that may include color, temperature, consistency, or sensation heralding lesion for skin ulceration (stage I); to superficial abrasion, crater, or blister with partial thickness skin loss involving the dermis or epidermis with subcutaneous tissues unaffected (stage II); to full-thickness skin loss with widespread destruction or tissue necrosis with damage extending into subcutaneous tissue with deeper structures unaffected (stage III); to full-thickness skin loss with extensive destruction or tissue necrosis with damage extending to deep structures, including muscle, tendon, and bone, with deep-seeded infections possible (stage IV).[26,36]

Pressure ulcers may be prevented by a variety of interventions. Good nutrition and active mobilization are the best preventive measures for pressure wounds. All NCCU beds should have a well-padded pressure relief mattress. The simplest but most labor-intensive method of preventing pressure ulceration is routine turning and repositioning every 2 hours, with care taken to avoid pressure on bony prominences (e.g., knees, ankles, and the back of the head). It is important to implement all measures to prevent pressure ulcers as the time and expense of healing and recovery are enormous. When patients are discharged from the acute setting with pressure ulcers to the rehabilitation setting, therapies may have to be delayed to allow time for the pressure ulcers to heal. This is critical, for example, with spinal cord injury (SCI), when new modalities such as body weight–supported treadmill training (BWSTT) require the patient to be placed in a supportive harness over a treadmill for ambulation training. A sacral ulcer may delay participation in BWSTT for up to 3 months.

Patients must be positioned in such a way as to avert pressure on nerves that can lead to compression neuropathies, particularly around the ulnar (elbow) and peroneal (lateral knee) nerves. Interventions and measures (e.g., PT) should be initiated early to prevent contractures, footdrop, and muscle atrophy. Neurotrauma patients may be at additional high risk for skin breakdown if they spend many hours on a spine board. Clinicians should check the backboard time to be alert to this problem. In addition, even the use of hard cervical collars can quickly result in skin breakdown to the occipital, submental areas, as well as the clavicular prominences.

Patients with increased ICP may not tolerate the required repositioning, so pressure relief mattresses on continuous lateral rotation frames perform this task in a slow, predictable manner. Many of these specialty beds incorporate percussion therapy as an aid in pulmonary toilet as well. Other beds provide only pressure relief through air bladder mattresses that may be differentially inflated. A change from the standard NCCU bed to a specialty bed with a dynamically inflated pressure relief mattress can be beneficial. A specialty bed is particularly beneficial and cost effective when the patient is able to tolerate turning but is anticipated to be nonambulatory in the NCCU for longer than 48 hours. If the patient does not tolerate turning (e.g., because of increased ICP, decreased MAP, or decreased SaO$_2$), a continuous lateral rotation therapy bed with integrated percussion features (every hour for 10 to 15 minutes) may be used. In addition, if patients are not anticipated to be completely immobilized in bed, a dynamically inflated pressure relief mattress bed is recommended if the patient is nutritionally depleted on admission to the NCCU (i.e., albumin <2.5 g%; involuntary weight loss >15%; temporal wasting). These patients maybe at high risk for ulceration because of the loss of cushioning subcutaneous adipose tissue.[26,36]

Coagulation Issues and Disseminated Intravascular Coagulation

Cerebral parenchyma injury may lead to the release of large amounts of **tissue thromboplastin.** Tissue thromboplastin leads to a pathologic activation of the extrinsic coagulation pathway, which may consume all the coagulation factors. In addition, the fibrinolytic pathway is initiated such that "pathologic" clot lysis occurs to keep the circulation patent. When the factors are depleted, the physiologic clot (clot that is bridging a breach in the circulation) lysis caused by this state results in bleeding from wounds and traumatized membranes. It is imperative that the coagulopathy be corrected as rapidly as possible, especially when the surgical site is in the posterior cranial fossa or the spinal column. These areas are relatively small in size and the structures in these areas are not compressible; increases in volume here result in early pressure increases, thus leading to precipitous herniation or severe and possibly irreversible spinal cord ischemia.[9,20]

When the NCCU team is treating a patient with disseminated intravascular coagulation (DIC), the goal of transfusion therapy should be the establishment of a normal coagulation profile (prothrombin time [PT], activated partial thromboplastin time [APTT], international normalized ratio [INR], platelet count, and fibrinogen). In particular, elevated PT, APTT, fibrin degradation products, prothrombin fragment 1.2, and soluble fibrin monomer levels, as well as depressed fibrinogen and antithrombin (75 units/ml) levels, have been demonstrated to correlate with death from head injury.[20]

Component transfusion therapy is frequently needed to correct DIC along with a thorough search for, and correction

of, the cause of the pathologic clotting process. Fresh frozen plasma (FFP) can be administered in aliquots of 4 units at a time until the PT/APTT and INR are normal. Platelet counts should be kept greater than 100,000/ml. Platelet transfusion (1 unit for every 10,000 increase in platelets desired) should be followed by a 1-hour posttransfusion platelet count to assess whether the thrombocytopenia has been corrected (platelet count increases as predicted), has resulted from ongoing consumption (platelet count is increased but less than predicted), or is due to an antibody-mediated destructive process (no change or decrease in platelet count).[9,20] Fibrinogen should be assayed as well. As a rough guide, levels below 150 mg% should be treated with 1 unit of cryoprecipitate for every 10 kg of body weight. Cryoprecipitate is indicated for the treatment of **hypofibrinogenemia** unless the patient will be receiving 10 or more units of FFP, since those 10 units will be equivalent to 1 unit of cryoprecipitate.

Ionized calcium levels should be measured, since calcium is an integral cofactor for the serine protease system of clotting factors. Since the clotting factor system is enzymatic in nature, the enzymes are also pH dependent with regard to maximal activity. Thus avoidance of significant acidemia (pH <7.25) is essential. Similarly, significant hypothermia (core temperature <32° C) will negatively affect clotting function and is to be avoided.

Blood component therapy carries the well-publicized risks of viral disease transmission, **transfusion-related acute lung injury (TRALI),** hypothermia, acidosis, hypocalcemia, pulmonary edema, alloimmunization, and major and minor transfusion reactions (most commonly a febrile reaction). The clinician must be aware of therapeutic strategies to counter these side effects, as well as the appropriate evaluation of a potential transfusion reaction. In particular, TRALI is among the most difficult adverse reaction to identify. It is not frequently considered as a diagnostic possibility, since it may masquerade as noncardiogenic pulmonary edema and usually responds to similar supportive measures. The routine use of a blood warmer and the monitoring of ionized calcium and base deficit allow early detection and corrective therapy for complications. Unrecognized and untreated hypocalcemia will have significant adverse impact, including reduced cardiac inotropic effects and impairment of the clotting cascade.[9]

Older Adult Considerations

Advanced age in combination with an underlying neurologic illness (e.g., dementia of the Alzheimer's type, alcohol or substance abuse) frequently results in more profound manifestation of disease and longer lengths of stay in the NCCU. Chronic illness, not related to the diagnosis on admission, may complicate recovery.[35] Comorbid factors and multiple medications for underlying conditions (i.e., hypertension, diabetes, and cardiac disease) require careful assessment, as well as evaluation of the potential for drug-drug interactions.

Older adults are often at higher risk for pneumonia and other respiratory complications, become hypoxic and acidotic more quickly than their younger cohort, and experience metabolic and hemodynamic instability more commonly. Electrolyte imbalances, infections, cerebral abnormalities, and immobility may prolong their recovery.

Restlessness, agitation, and sleep deprivation may increase older adults' risk for injury or falls. Patients must be monitored for side effects of therapeutic interventions, including problems such as fluid overload and congestive heart failure. Older patients have an increased risk for delirium in the NCCU that can increase morbidity and is associated with a poor prognosis.

The outcome of the neurologic illness or condition may necessitate a period of rehabilitation and a change in the living status of the older patient. Planned discharge to a rehabilitation facility or long-term care facility instead of return to home may precipitate depression, anxiety, and additional stress. Clinical management should focus on awareness, alleviation, or modification of psychosocial and environmental factors that have negative effects on older patients. Social services providers and other supportive resources should be consulted as needed.

Rehabilitation Considerations

The physiatrist or rehabilitation physician and rehabilitation team members should evaluate patients to determine the timing for acute bedside therapeutic rehabilitation interventions (see Chapter 13). Critical pathways and care maps for stroke, for example, may include physical therapy (PT) with passive range of motion (PROM) or active range of motion (AROM) as early as possible to prevent disuse atrophy and loss of muscle strength and function (see Chapter 13). Occupational therapists (OTs) may provide assistive devices for positioning to prevent contractures, footdrop, dependent edema, and discomfort. Speech and language therapists provide useful consultation for problems with swallowing and speech. Musculoskeletal and other rehabilitation problems (e.g., spasticity) are discussed in Chapter 13. Newer therapeutic rehabilitation concepts (e.g., constraint-induced movement therapy [CIMT]) may be introduced in the critical care setting. For example, the therapist may place a sock on the patient's unaffected hand to encourage the patient to force the affected arm to be used as much as possible to help promote and regain lost function. CIMT therapy can then be continued and reinforced when the patient is transferred to the rehabilitation setting for more intense therapies.

Case Management Considerations

Neuroscience patients present a significant challenge for a hospital case manager, who may be a registered nurse (RN) or in some cases a social worker. Acute head- and spine-injured patients are examples of high-risk catastrophic injuries that require intense hospital-based case management from admission to discharge. Other critically ill neuroscience patients who may require case management include those with a stroke, GBS, MG, or a brain tumor. Patients with significant neurologic impairments, particularly older patients with multiple health problems, may also benefit from active case management involvement. Continuity of case management can be provided when the hospital-based case manager works closely with the community-based or independent case manager to affect the quality of care for patients and their families at the time of discharge to ensure coordination and recovery along the continuum of care.

To be an effective member of the NCCU team, the case manager must be knowledgeable about all aspects of the neurologic illness, the patient's critical pathway, the levels of hospital care for recovery, need for and resources to address aftercare requirements, and the dynamics of the family. The case manager must frequently balance the costs of the health care needs of the patient against the patient's/family's financial resources. Working closely as part of the health care team, the case manager can provide direct input to facilitate discharge, rehabilitation treatment programs, and the patient's return to the community.

Education for the patient and family about specialized long-term needs, durable medical equipment, funding resources, and community nursing and rehabilitation resources facilitates the discharge process. Devices needed for extensive home preparation (e.g., wheelchair ramps, home modifications, special beds, wheelchairs, or environmental control devices) require time to order, receive, and install. Anticipation of these needs, with explanations and discussions with the multidisciplinary team, professionals from other health care disciplines, and the patient and family, assists in a smooth transition from hospital to home. Neuroscience patients with permanent disability, brain damage, or altered states of consciousness often have a life care planner (see Chapter 25), who develops a life care plan (LCP) to project the patient's present and future needs and associated costs.

End-of-Life Considerations

Do not Resuscitate and Do not Intubate

End-of-life issues regarding resuscitation and treatment are common to many patients in an NCCU (see Chapter 25). There should be a formal policy in place to guide patients, their families, and the clinical staff as to the mechanism to enact these therapeutic regimens. During the course of discussions with the patient or family, the clinician should seek out opportunities to explore what the wishes of the patient would be if he or she were in a devastating, medically unsalvageable state. The clinician must help the family to understand that it is the patient's wishes that are the most important and to determine what wishes the patient would express if able to communicate. If the patient is able to engage in this discussion directly, establishment of these goals of therapy are much easier. When the patient cannot participate in these discussions due to lack of capacity for decision making, family members may need significant support to distinguish between what they want for the patient and what the patient would want. It is up to the individual hospital as to whether a form is to be completed or whether progress notes documenting the discussion are sufficient. Our practice is to have the family or patient discussion documented in the physician progress notes by the attending physician. The do-not-resuscitate (DNR) order is written in the order section of the chart. Once a DNR order is written, a DNR label is attached to the front of the patient's chart and a brightly colored DNR band is placed on the patient's wrist to convey the patient's wishes to all health care providers.

Do not Treat and Withdrawal of Therapy

If a patient is unable to reach his or her goals of therapy, or has a nonsurvivable injury, withdrawal of therapy to "allow nature to take its course" is quite appropriate. Most institutions have a process of documentation that precedes activation of the withdrawal of care that is similar to their DNR process: a standardized form or physician progress note is used to document the rationale for withdrawal, and then a separate order is written for each therapy that is to be discontinued. Before therapy is withdrawn, comfort measures are established with the use of a narcotic analgesic and a benzodiazepine sedative. Appropriate visitation for family members should be arranged and individualized provisions made to allow them the option of remaining in the room while therapy is withdrawn. In most circumstances of withdrawal, all support is withdrawn except for one IV line that provides the route for analgesics and sedatives by continuous infusion. These medications are increased as needed for patient comfort. Each withdrawal situation needs to be individualized to be consistent with a patient's advance directive (AD) or the family's prospective of the patient's wishes if a legal AD is not available. Of note, these patients may be eligible for non–heart beating organ donation.

Medical Futility

The issue of medical futility is a complicated and difficult topic to cover. Despite the plethora of literature, there is no single definition that covers all cases. Medically futile care may be defined as delivery of medical services or use of resources that are unable to achieve a patient's stated goals of therapy. Each case is managed individually and may involve the medical ethics committee, the family, and the treating team.

CONCLUSION

Critical care management of the neuroscience patient in the NCCU setting is an expensive, challenging setting where patients are at the greatest risk to develop serious adverse events. All critical care health care professionals should have a comprehensive, in-depth knowledge and understanding of anatomy and physiology and the subtle presentation of pathologic conditions for early detection of potential complications if high quality of care is to be achieved. The NCCU clinician must be part of a multidisciplinary team that has mastered the art of "shared governance"—each team member has the responsibility to exercise his or her expertise in the care of the patient to affect the greatest opportunity for success. Technologic advances and increased understanding of CNS functions provide the NCCU clinician with a rapidly changing environment to apply advanced, specialized skills in patient care, as well as the impetus for lifelong learning.

RESOURCES FOR NEUROSCIENCE CRITICAL CARE MANAGEMENT

Agency for Healthcare Research and Quality, Department of Health and Human Services: www.ahcpr.gov
American Association of Critical Care Nurses: www.aacn.org
American Association of Neurological Surgeons: www.neurosurgery.org/aans
American Association of Neuroscience Nurses: www.aann.org
American Society of Critical Care Anesthesiologists: e-mail: infor@ascca.org
Brain Trauma Foundation: www.braintrauma.org
Guidelines for the Management of Acute Cervical Spine and Spinal Cord Injuries: www.neurosurgery-online.com
Society of Critical Care Medicine: www.neurosurgery-online.com

REFERENCES

1. Alspach JG, editor: *American association of critical care nurses: core curriculum for critical care nursing,* ed 5, Philadelphia, 1998, WB Saunders.
2. Anderson BJ, Marmarou A: Post-traumatic selective stimulation of glycolysis, *Brain Res* 585:184–189, 1992.
3. Ayres SM, Shoemaker WC, Grenvik A, Holbrook PR: *Textbook of critical care,* ed 4, Philadelphia, 2000, WB Saunders.
4. Bader MK, Littlejohns L, March K: Brain tissue oxygen monitoring in severe brain injury, I. Research and usefulness in critical care, *Crit Care Nurs* 23(4):17–25, 2003.
5. Bader MK, Littlejohns L, March K: Brain tissue oxygen monitoring in severe brain injury, II. Implications for critical care teams and case study, *Crit Care Nurs* 23(4):29–48, 40–42, 44, 2003.
6. Beale RJ, Bryg DJ, Bihari DJ: Immunonutrition in the critically ill: a systematic review of clinical outcome, *Crit Care Med* 27:2799–2805, 1999.
7. Bellomo R, Ronco R: How to feed patients with renal dysfunction, *Curr Opin Crit Care* 6:239–246, 2000.
8. Bowling T, Silk DBA: Refeeding remembered, *Nutrition* 11(1):32–34, 1995.
9. Bredbacka S, Blomback M, Wiman B, Pelzer H: DIC in neurosurgical patients: diagnosis by new laboratory methods, *J Neurosurg Anesthesiol* 4(2):128–133, 1992.
10. Bullock R, Chestnut RM, Clifton G, Ghajar J, Marion DW, Narayan RK, et al: *Guidelines for the management of severe head injury,* ed 2, New York, 2000, Brain Trauma Foundation.
11. Cunneen J, Cartwright M: The puzzle of sepsis: fitting the pieces of the inflammatory response with treatment, *Adv Prac Crit Care* 15(1):18–44, 2005.
12. Dart BW IV, Maxwell RA, Richart CM, Brooks DK, Ciraulo DL, Barker DE, Burns RP: Preliminary experience with airway pressure release ventilation in a trauma/surgical intensive care unit, *J Trauma* 59(1):71–76, 2005.
13. Davis M, Barer D: Neuro protection in acute ischemic stroke. II. Clinical potential, *Vasc Med* 4(3):149–163, 1999.
14. Edwards RL, Rickles FR: The role of leukocytes in the activation of blood coagulation, *Semin Hematol* 29:202–212, 1992.
15. Galban C, Montejo JC, Mesejo A, et al: An immune-enhancing enteral diet reduces mortality rate and episodes of bacteremia in septic intensive care unit patients, *Crit Care Med* 28(3):643–648, 2000.

16. Hawker F: How to feed patients with sepsis, *Curr Opin Crit Care* 6:247–252, 2000.

17. Heyland DK: Nutritional support in the critically ill patient: a critical review of the evidence, *Crit Care Clin* 14:423–440, 1998.

18. Heyland D, Dhaliwal R: Immunonutrition in the critically ill: from old approaches to new paradigms, *Intens Care Med* 31(4):501–503, 2005.

19. Hickey JV: *The clinical practice of neurological and neurosurgical nursing,* ed 5, Philadelphia, 2002, Lippincott Williams & Wilkins.

20. Hoots WK: Experience with antithrombin concentrates in neuro trauma patients, *Semin Thromb Hemost* 23(1):3–16, 1997.

21. Hatazawa J, Ito M, Matsuzawa T, et al: Measurement of the ratio for cerebral oxygen consumption to glucose utilization by positron emission tomography: its consistency with the values determined by the Kety-Schmidt method in normal volunteers, *J Cereb Blood Flow Metab* 8(3):426–432, 1988.

22. Jones PA, Andrews PJ, Midgley S, et al: Measuring the burden of secondary insults in head-injured patients during intensive care, *J Neurosurg Anesthesiol* 6(1):4–14, 1994.

23. Kaplan LJ, Bailey H: Bispectral index (BIS) monitoring of patients in continuous infusion of sedatives and paralytics reduces sedative drug utilization and cost, *Crit Care* 4(suppl 1):S110, 2000.

24. Kaplan LJ, Bailey H: A compression of pulmonary artery occlusion pressure (PaOP) measurements using pressure controlled ventilation (PCV) versus airway pressure release ventilation (APRV), *Crit Care* 4(suppl 1):S4, 2000.

25. Kaplan LJ, Bailey H, Formosa V: APRV increases cardiac performance in patients with acute lung injury/adult respiratory distress syndrome, *Crit Care* 3(1):14, 1999. Available at http://ccforum.com.

26. Kaplan LJ, Pameijer C, Blank-Reid C, Granick MS: Decubitus ulceration leading to necrotizing fasciitis, *Adv Wound Care* 11(4):185–189, 1998.

27. Kerwin AJ, Croce MA, Timmons SD, et al: Effects of fiberoptic bronchoscopy on intracranial pressure in patients with brain injury: a prospective clinical study, *J Trauma* 48(5):878–882, 2000.

28. Klessig HT, Geiger HJ, Murray MJ, Coursin DB: A national survey on the practice patterns of anesthesiologist intensivists in the use of muscle relaxants, *Crit Care Med* 20(9):1341–1355, 1992.

29. Knudson MM, Ikossi DG, Khaw L, Morabito D, Speetzen LS: Thromboembolism after trauma: an analysis of 1602 episodes from the American College of Surgeons National Trauma Data Bank, *Ann Surg* 240(3):490–496, 2004.

30. Marion D: Hypothermia in severe head injury, *Eur J Anesthesiol* 17(suppl 18):45–46, 2000.

31. Mason R: *Murray and Nadel's textbook of respiratory medicine,* ed 4, St Louis, 2005, Elsevier.

32. Ostermann ME, Keenan SP, Seiferling RA, Sibbald WJ: Sedation in the intensive care unit, *JAMA* 283(11):1451–1459, 2000.

33. Pavlin JD, Souter KJ, Hong JY, Freund PR, Bowdle TA, Bower JO: Effects of bispectral index monitoring on recovery from surgical anesthesia in 1,580 inpatients from an academic medical center, *Anesthesiology* 102(3):566–573, 2005.

34. Rasanen J, Downs JB: Airway pressure therapy. In Ayers SM, Shoemaker WC, Grenvik A, Holbrook PR, editors: *Textbook of critical care,* ed 3, Philadelphia, 1995, WB Saunders.

35. Santora TA, Kaplan LJ, Trooskin SZ: Care of the injured elder. In Rosenthal RA, Zenilman ME, editors: *Principles and practice of geriatric surgery,* New York, 2000, Springer-Verlag.

36. Schultz A: Predicting and preventing pressure ulcers in surgical patients, *AORN J* 8(5):986–1006, 2005.

37. Wade CE, Grady JJ, Kramer GC, Younes RN, Gehlsen K, Holcroft JW: Individual patient cohort analysis of the efficacy of hypertonic saline/dextran in patients with traumatic brain injury and hypotension, *J Trauma* 42(5S):61–65, 1997.

38. Zurasky JA, Aiyagari V, Zazulia AR, Shackelford A, Diringer MN: Early mortality following spontaneous intracerebral hemorrhage, *Neurology* 64(4):725–727, 2005.

ELLEN BARKER

CHAPTER 10

Intracranial Pressure and Monitoring

Recognition of intracranial hypertension or increased intracranial pressure (ICP) is one of the most important assessments in the management of patients with neurologic disorders. Failure to identify a patient's early and often subtle signs and symptoms of increasing ICP places the patient at great risk. Continued expansion of pressure within the brain can overcome the ability of the cranial structures to compensate, and rapidly increasing ICP can result. The opportunity for timely intervention may disappear if the early warning signals of an escalating pressure go undetected. By the time dilated pupils, vomiting, seizures, and irregular respirations are observed, the patient may have slipped into a state of altered consciousness due to pressure on the brainstem. Herniation can displace nervous system structures so severely that tissue is shifted from one compartment into another. Major complications of unchecked increased ICP can lead to potentially catastrophic consequences (e.g., permanent irreversible brain damage, cardiac or respiratory arrest, and death).[74]

At the time of admission the initial nursing assessment, whether in the emergency department (ED) or intensive care unit (ICU), may indicate that the patient is at risk for increased ICP. Immediate emergency treatment is required. During the course of treatment and recovery, a patient's neurologic status may suddenly change and reflect subtle signs and symptoms of early ICP elevation. It is therefore critical that every nurse clinician be able to recognize the early versus late signs and symptoms of increased ICP and understand the basic anatomic structures and physiologic dynamics involved. An understanding of the etiology of intracranial hypertension, recognition of the signs and symptoms, and appropriate monitoring and timely treatments to prevent herniation and death are fundamental in the management of the neuroscience patient.[8]

Patients with intracranial hypertension present many dilemmas for the clinician, who must prevent elevated ICP while providing critical care. In critical care, monitoring and managing elevated ICP is routine. Clinicians must continually use their assessment skills and recognize when the neurologic status of the patient is compromised.[74] This chapter reviews the key concepts of ICP, assessment guidelines, signs and symptoms of increased ICP, the relationship between ICP and cerebral perfusion pressure (CPP) monitoring, treat-

ment and management of cerebral herniation, herniation syndromes, and barbiturate coma therapy.

DYNAMICS AND CONCEPTS OF INTRACRANIAL PRESSURE

Intracranial pressure (ICP) is a dynamic state that reflects the volume of the contents. ICP is used to describe the pressure of supratentorial cerebrospinal fluid (CSF) in the cranium as exerted by the total volume from the brain tissue, blood, and CSF. All three of these components contain water, which can move between them by bulk flow and osmosis.[49] **Intracranial hypertension** is defined as a sustained resting elevated ICP equal to or greater than 20 mm Hg lasting 5 minutes or longer.[60] Under normal circumstances, the following changes can increase or decrease ICP:[44]

- Arterial pressure
- Venous pressure
- Intraabdominal pressure
- Intrathoracic pressure
- Posture (e.g., position change from supine to standing)
- Temperature, especially hypothermia
- Blood gases, particularly carbon dioxide levels

An increased intracranial volume can raise the ICP to dangerous levels. Increased intracranial volume may result from the following:

- Mass lesion: expanding lesion from a brain tumor
- Vascular congestion: failure of autoregulation
- Head trauma: hyperemia
- Cerebral hemorrhage: hematoma, intracranial, subarachnoid from stroke/brain attack
- Edema: from surgery, mass lesion, infection, hemorrhage
- Central nervous system (CNS) abscess or infection: meningitis, encephalitis
- Hydrocephalus: enlarged ventricles related to communicating, noncommunicating, congenital, or acquired causes, including normal pressure hydrocephalus (NPH)
- Status epilepticus
- Hepatic encephalopathy

As ICP rises from any of these causes, the brain is further compressed against the bony confines of the skull (Fig. 10-1).

CAUSES OF ↑ ICP

SURGICAL

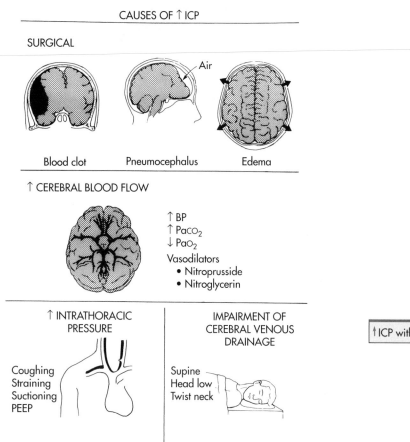

Blood clot   Pneumocephalus   Edema

↑ CEREBRAL BLOOD FLOW

↑ BP
↑ PaCO₂
↓ PaO₂
Vasodilators
• Nitroprusside
• Nitroglycerin

↑ INTRATHORACIC PRESSURE

Coughing
Straining
Suctioning
PEEP

IMPAIRMENT OF CEREBRAL VENOUS DRAINAGE

Supine
Head low
Twist neck

Figure 10-1 Schematic representation of the different causes of increased intracranial pressure.
(*From Frost EAM:* Postanesthesia care unit, *ed 2, St Louis, 1990, Mosby.*)

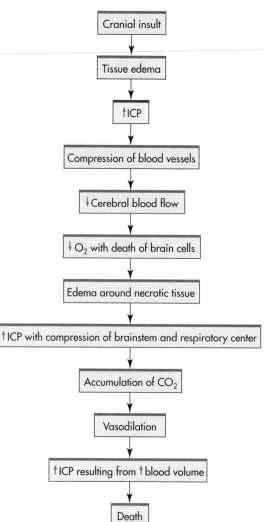

Figure 10-2 Progression of increased intracranial pressure.
(*From Lewis SM, Heitkemper MM, Dirksen RF, editors:* Medical-surgical nursing: assessment and management of clinical problems, *ed 5, St Louis, 2000, Mosby.*)

Progression of **increased ICP** can create a cycle that results in irreversible injury to the CNS, eventually compromising blood flow within the brain and causing death unless treatment is immediate and successful (Fig. 10-2).

The adult cranium is a protective semiclosed, rigid, boxlike, bony structure containing the three components of brain and its structures, blood, and CSF. The intravascular blood from capillaries, arterioles, venules, and large arteries accounts for approximately 12% of the cranium; brain tissue, 78%; and CSF, 12%.[29] The CSF acts internally as a shock absorber to protect the brain. It is theorized that the major parameters that control the resting level and rate of change of ICP are compliance of the CSF space and resistance to the absorption of CSF.

Brain tissue is compressible and can be easily distorted and shifted within the cranial vault. This distortion results in a functional impairment of the brain tissue involved. Factors such as rapidity of increased pressure and degree of distortion are important in determining the effect of a given pressure. It is the location of the increase in volume—not the absolute pressure it produces—that is associated with different alternatives in neurologic status.[57]

Volume adjustment can occur in the normal, uninjured brain because of two properties: compliance and elastance.

ICP is affected not only by the volume of the three intracranial components but also by the elastance of the craniospinal axis.

Intracranial Compliance

Intracranial compliance is the potential expandability of the brain. It is the intracranial content's adaptive capacity. Compliance is the ability of the brain to tolerate stimulation or an increase in intracranial volume without a corresponding increase in pressure. Compliance is affected by volume increases, with smaller increases in volume over longer time accommodated easier than large increases over shorter times. With stimulating bedside activities (e.g., suctioning) that cause a rise in ICP above normal, "B" or "A" waveforms should display a return to baseline within approximately 5 minutes, going back to "C" waveforms when the stimulus has been removed:[70]

$$\text{Compliance} = \frac{\text{Volume}}{\text{Pressure}}$$

Compliance is high when intracranial contents can accommodate a large expanding mass with little change in pressure, and low compliance is seen when high changes in pressure result from small changes in volume.[44]

Intracranial Elastance

Intracranial elastance is defined as a change in pressure as an instantaneous function of change in volume ($E = \Delta P/\Delta V$). The greater the elastance, the less compliant it is to any deforming pressure. Elastance is the inverse of compliance. It is the product of two components: (1) distension (elasticity) of the container of the craniospinal contents (intracranial and spinal dura within the skull and spinal canal), and (2) displacement of blood and CSF. Elastance denotes the tightness of the intracranial compartment—the brain's ability to accommodate changes in volume. A brain with poor compliance is a "tight" brain and has a high elastance; that is, it is stretched to its maximum and has no additional elastic properties:[4]

$$\text{Elastance} = \frac{\text{Pressure}}{\text{Volume}}$$

With high elastance, large increases in pressure occur with small increases in volume.[44]

Intracranial Volume

The total volume of the intracranial contents is estimated at 1700 to 1900 ml and remains virtually unchanged. However, the volume of each of the three components may change. Under normal circumstances (in which intracranial volume remains relatively constant), the balance between these components maintains the ICP. The most significant contributor to this state of elastance is displacement of fluid within the system from inside the intracranial compartment into the spinal compartment. The reason for this is that, unlike the cranial dura, the spinal dura can expand into the epidural space of the spinal canal and can therefore accommodate the displacement of CSF from within the cranium. In addition to this displacement of CSF, there is also bulk absorption of CSF out of the craniospinal axis into the venous circulation.[42] The "A" wave or plateau wave (described later in this chapter) that indicates prolonged rises in ICP of up to 75 mm Hg is pathognomonic of raised ICP and is already at the left-hand edge of the "break point" of a patient's elastance curve.[42]

Modified Monro-Kellie Hypothesis

Two physician researchers, Monro in 1783 and Kellie in 1825, were the first to describe the concept of reciprocal volume. This concept was later modified by others to produce the **modified Monro-Kellie hypothesis.** This hypothesis supports the concept that the three intracranial components are in a state of dynamic equilibrium. An increase in one component must be compensated for by a decrease in the volume of one or more of the other components of the brain (i.e., brain, blood, or CSF) or the pressure will be elevated. This reciprocal volume-pressure relationship maintains a

---

BOX 10-1 Causes of Intracranial Pressure Fluctuations

Increases in Intracranial Pressure
Defecation
Coughing
Airway obstruction
Abdominal breathing
Vomiting
Positive end-expiratory pressure (PEEP)
Suctioning
Muscle exertion or tension
Range-of-motion (ROM) exercises
Isometric exercises
Valsalva maneuver
REM sleep
Position changes (prone, Trendelenburg, extreme hip flexion, neck flexion)
Hypercapnia (PCO_2 greater than 42 mm Hg)
Hypoxia (PO_2 less than 50 mm Hg)
Stress or emotional upsets
Pain and noxious stimuli
Seizure activity
Hyperthermia
Clustering of nursing activities
Discussion of the patient's condition at the bedside
Decreases in Intracranial Pressure
CNS depressant medications
Inspiration

Data from American Association of Neuroscience Nurses: *Core curriculum for neuroscience nursing,* ed 4, St Louis, 2004, Saunders; Barker E: Myths and facts about increased intracranial pressure, *Nursing* 8(12):20, 1988; and Barker E: Avoiding increased intracranial pressure, *Nursing* 20(5):64Q, 1990.
CNS, Central nervous system; *PCO₂,* partial pressure of carbon dioxide; *PO₂,* partial pressure of oxygen; *REM,* rapid eye movement.

---

constant intracranial volume by several compensatory mechanisms, for example, shunting CSF into the spinal subarachnoid space or decreasing the overall production of CSF. By decreasing the volume of one or more of the other components, the total brain volume remains fixed:[4,21]

$$\text{CSF volume} + \text{Blood volume} + \text{Brain volume} = 1700 \text{ to } 1900 \text{ ml}$$

Normal ICP for adults ranges from 0 to 15 mm Hg. In children, the norm is 0 to 10 mm Hg.

Abnormal elevations occur when the ICP is elevated about 20 mm Hg. Fluctuations in ICP occur with coughing, sneezing, straining, or performing a Valsalva maneuver (Box 10-1). Under normal circumstances, changes may cause the ICP to rise momentarily, but the ICP should quickly return to normal. With pathologic conditions, there is an increase in the volume of the cranial contents (e.g., bleeding, tumor, or enlarged ventricles) that causes the displacement of an equal volume of intracranial contents. To compensate, the cerebral blood volume is reduced with no immediate change in ICP. In the early phase of an increase in the volume of cranial contents, ICP remains within normal limits. Patients with cerebral atrophy (e.g., older adults or alcoholics) may have more space for the expanding mass to fill and thus may show delayed signs and symptoms of increased ICP.[9] However, as the small margin of compensation is exhausted, ICP rises:

dCSF s fBrain volume + fBlood volume = 1700 to 1900 ml

Intracranial Volume-Pressure Curve

After the point of compensation has been reached, relatively small increases of 1 to 2 ml lead to a disproportionate increase in ICP. This concept can be explained by the volume-pressure curve, which can be used to represent the four stages of increased ICP[44] (Fig. 10-3). It is important to determine which stage the patient's ICP has reached in providing bedside care and to evaluate the effect *before* the procedure and treatment (e.g., suctioning and repositioning) (Box 10-2).

In the volume-pressure curve, the horizontal axis represents volume and the vertical axis represents pressure. This curve illustrates how the brain accommodates and compensates for changes in the volume of the three components. When the volume increases to the point at which the brain is tight, the addition of a very small volume of 1 to 2 ml causes a precipitous and disproportionate rise in ICP (see Fig. 10-3). The point at which the adaptive mechanisms are exceeded varies according to the following:[79]

- Cranial volume reserve
- Size of the skull
- Size and weight of the brain
- Degree to which the ventricles can shrink or shift to accommodate the added pressure
- Rate of increase in ICP
- Ability of the brain to compensate by redistributing CSF and blood into the extracranial vascular system

Within the cranium, a slowly enlarging lesion is better tolerated than a rapidly expanding mass (e.g., hematoma), which quickly overcomes and depletes the compensatory mechanisms (Fig. 10-4). The compliance phenomenon explains how some patients may tolerate a slowly expanding brain tumor for years with minimal discomfort. A patient with a head injury and intracranial hemorrhage has limited compliance and may decompensate, herniate, and die within a few hours.

Cerebral Blood Flow

Cerebral blood flow (CBF) is affected by respiration and the efficiency of all systems involved in oxygen transport.[75]

BOX 10-2   Stages of Increased Intracranial Pressure

Stage I
There is high compliance and low elastance. The brain is in total compensation with accommodation and autoregulation intact. An increase in volume does not elevate ICP.

Stage II
Compliance is lower and elastance is increasing. An increase in volume places the patient at risk for increased ICP.

Stage III
There is high elastance and low compliance. Any small addition of volume causes a great increase in pressure. There is a loss of autoregulation or a loss of the capacity of the brain to regulate its own cerebral blood flow. There may be symptoms of increased ICP.

Stage IV
ICP rises to terminal levels with little increase in volume. Herniation occurs as the brain tissue shifts from the compartment of greater pressure to the compartment of lesser pressure.

ICP, Intracranial pressure.

STAGES ON THE CURVE

Stage 1: There is a high compliance and low elastance. The brain is in total compensation, with accommodation and autoregulation intact. An increase in volume does not increase ICP.

Stage 2: The compliance is lower and elastance is increasing. An increase in volume places the patient at risk of increased ICP.

Stage 3: There is high elastance and low compliance. Any small addition of volume causes a great increase in pressure. There is a loss of autoregulation, and there may be symptoms indicating increased ICP, such as systolic hypertension with an increasing pulse pressure, bradycardia, and slowing of respiratory rate (Cushing's triad). With the loss of autoregulation and the rise in the systolic blood pressure as a result of the Cushing response, decompensation occurs. The ICP passively mimics the blood pressure.

Stage 4: Finally, when the patient is in stage 4, the ICP rises to terminal levels with little increase in volume. Herniation occurs as the brain tissue shifts from the compartment of greater pressure to the compartment of lesser pressure.

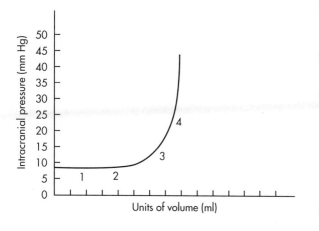

Figure 10-3 Intracranial volume-pressure curve.
(*Modified from Lewis SM, Heitkemper MM, Dirksen RF, editors:* Medical-surgical nursing: assessment and management of clinical problems, *ed 5, St Louis, 2000, Mosby.*)

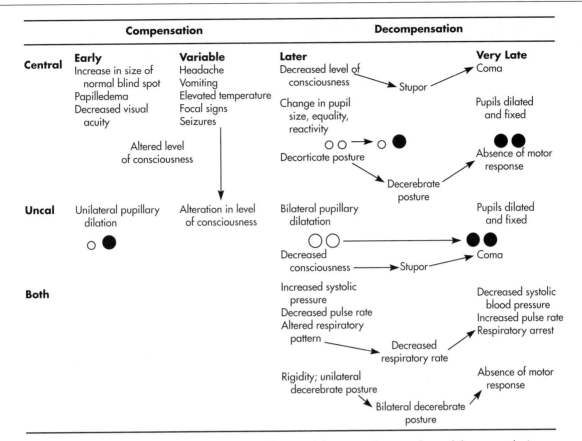

Figure 10-4 Signs and symptoms of supratentorial increased intracranial pressure (compression and decompression). *(From Lewis SM, Heitkemper MM, Dirksen RF, editors:* Medical surgical nursing: assessment and management of clinical problems, *ed 5, St Louis, 2000, Mosby.)*

See Chapter 1 for discussion of CBF. Oxygen tension, carbon dioxide tension, and hydrogen ion concentration affect cerebral vessel tone. If oxygen tension drops, anaerobic metabolism begins, which results in an accumulation of lactic acid. Lactic acidosis causes an increase in vasodilation, an increase in CBF, and an increase in ICP.[44] The threshold of intact spontaneous neuronal electrical activity is approximately 20 ml/100 g/min of CBF. When blood flow falls below this critical value, consciousness is inevitably lost.[42]

CBF remains constant when the oxygen saturation of mixed venous blood (SvO_2) is approximately 70%. Arterial blood saturation (SaO_2) is 96% to 100%. The cerebral arteries dilate when cerebral oxygen tension falls below 50 mm Hg. If oxygenation fails and SvO_2 drops, CBF rises in an attempt to bring additional oxygen to the brain. Blood vessels dilate, more blood enters the brain, and ICP increases.[79] The partial pressure of carbon dioxide in arterial blood ($PaCO_2$) is a potent vasodilator. If the patient retains carbon dioxide, the smooth muscles relax, the cerebral vessels dilate, and CBF increases; this causes the ICP to rise. In this situation, the patient may require intubation with hyperventilation to "blow off" excess carbon dioxide. A low partial pressure of oxygen in arterial blood (PaO_2) in combination with a high hydrogen ion concentration or acidosis is also considered a potent cerebral vasodilator. When available at the bedside, transcutaneous Doppler (TCD) allows for the indirect monitoring of CBF. Results of the TCD measurements of velocity and arterial blood flow can be correlated with ICP measurements.

Carbon dioxide levels increase as ICP increases and ischemia results; this leads to cerebral lactic acidosis. Carbon dioxide is a known **potent vasodilator.** It is estimated that an increase in $PaCO_2$ to 80 mm Hg will double CBF, with the increased blood supply diverted from ischemic tissue. This has been called the "intracerebral steal syndrome."[18] ICP can also affect adequate oxygenation. Cerebral vasodilation occurs when PaO_2 falls below 50 mm Hg, and this further increases CBF.

Cerebral Perfusion Pressure

Cerebral perfusion pressure (CPP) is normally expressed as the difference between mean arterial pressure and intracranial pressure. In other words, it is the difference between the arterial blood entering the brain and the pressure of venous blood exiting. CPP is the pressure needed to perfuse the blood upward to the brain against gravity. For example, following traumatic brain injury (TBI), CPP has two important physiologic roles. First, CPP represents the pressure gradient acting across the cerebrovascular bed and hence is an important factor in the regulation of CBF. Second, CPP contributes to the hydrostatic pressure within the intracerebral vessels and therefore is one of the factors that determine edema formation in the injured brain.[39]

BOX 10-3 | Calculation of Cerebral Perfusion Pressure

$$CPP = MSAP - MICP$$

$$MSAP = DBP + 1/3(SBP - DBP) \text{ or } \frac{SBP + 2(DBP)}{3}$$

Example: Systemic blood pressure = 122/84
MSAP = 97
MICP = 12 mm Hg
CPP = 85 mm Hg

CPP, Cerebral perfusion pressure; *DBP,* diastolic blood pressure; *MICP,* mean intracranial pressure; *MSAP,* mean systemic arterial pressure; *SBP,* systolic blood pressure.

BOX 10-4 | Compensatory Mechanisms for Increased Intracranial Pressure

Initial Compensatory Mechanisms
Increased CSF absorption
Shunting of CSF from the cerebral to the spinal subarachnoid space
Collapse of the cerebral veins and dural sinuses
Later Compensatory Mechanisms
Decreased CSF production
Changes in intracranial blood volume through constriction and dilation
Slight compression of brain tissue
Dispensability of the dura[44]
Increased venous outflow with shunting of venous blood out of the skull[17]

Data from American Association of Neuroscience Nurses: *Core curriculum for neuroscience nursing,* ed 4, St Louis, 2004, Saunders; Hickey JV: *The clinical practice of neurologic and neurosurgical nursing,* ed 3, Philadelphia, 1997, JB Lippincott.
CSF, Cerebrospinal fluid.

CPP is regulated by the diameters of the cerebral blood vessels. Optimal CPP, for example for patients with TBI, ranges from 50 to 70 mm Hg. CPP values over 100 mm Hg represent hyperperfusion. Cerebral hypoperfusion occurs when CPP drops to 40 mm Hg. CPP below 50 mm Hg can be associated with increased levels of extracellular lactate. With decreasing CPP, autoregulation fails. Irreversible ischemia and infarction result when CPP is less than 40 mm Hg. A CPP of 0 to 40 mg signifies brain death.[4] CPP is calculated with the formula shown in Box 10-3.

Mean systemic arterial pressure (MSAP) is a calculated average of blood pressure that can be read from an arterial line monitor or easily calculated by the formula in Box 10-3.

The calculation of CPP is considered an indirect measure of CBF. CPP is always the reciprocal inverse value of ICP. An increase in ICP is associated with a decrease in CPP.

Cerebral Autoregulation

Cerebral autoregulation is an important mechanism that protects the brain against the effects of blood pressure changes so that CBF remains constant (pressure autoregulation) over a wide range of pressure (50 to 150 mm Hg) and the rate of perfusion keeps up with metabolism (CO_2 autoregulation). Autoregulation helps the brain regulate its own CBF to meet the needs of the brain despite variations in systemic arterial pressure. Cerebral autoregulation is accomplished via the automatic changes and alteration in the diameter of the cerebral blood vessels to maintain a constant blood flow for CPP. Vasodilation occurs when pressure is low, in contrast to vasoconstriction when pressure increases and is high. Cerebral vessels have a limit beyond which hypoperfusion or hyperperfusion can occur. Blood vessels dilate and increase blood flow in response to high CO_2 since it is the by-product of high metabolism. CBF is another vital concept in treating elevated ICP. A disruption in autoregulation enables the CBF to surge, which raises cerebral blood volume and ICP. As the neuronal cells become hypoxic from lack of perfusion and autoregulation becomes impaired, the volume of the brain expands and the brain can shift within the cranial vault. When sensitive cells of the reticular activating system (RAS) become hypoxic, the patient's level of consciousness decreases.

Autoregulation protects the brain by three physiologic mechanisms: changes in ICP, cerebral vasodilation, and metabolic factors. Autoregulation is also the process by which the brain maintains its perfusion pressure over a wide range of systemic arterial pressures. The blood pressure limits are 50 to 150 mm Hg. A blood pressure below 50 mm Hg causes CBF to decrease, and autoregulation is lost. Symptoms may include syncope and blurred vision.[44] At this point, CBF becomes pressure dependent.[30] Eventually, autoregulation reaches its physiologic limits and CBF is impaired, causing severe ischemia. When autoregulation fails, CBF follows CPP passively, and the arterioles passively dilate. The veins become compressed, and the blood-brain barrier is disrupted. In the early stages of increased ICP, autoregulation remains intact. Above the upper limits of 150 mm Hg, the cerebral vessels are maximally constricted and ICP increases. For example, an expanding intracranial hemorrhage accompanied by edema places the patient at great risk for herniation. Hyperventilation reduces brain blood flow by reducing CO_2 and causing vasoconstriction—independent of brain metabolism. Autoregulation is frequently impaired with severe TBI, leaving the patient vulnerable to drops in blood pressure. Compensatory mechanisms are described in Box 10-4.

After this protective mechanism has been activated, the normal slack brain appears "tight," with the gyri flattened and smooth when viewed on a computed tomography (CT) scan.

Autoregulation causes a controlled vasodilation in response to reduced CPP. Arterial resistance falls, capillary and venous resistance are unchanged, and CBF is maintained at normal levels. No further vasodilation is possible as the CPP drops to 40 to 50 mm Hg. Bouma and Muizelaar[13] evaluated the relationship between cardiac output (CO) and CBF with and without impaired autoregulation and found that CBF is not related to CO, even when autoregulation is impaired (Box 10-5). Thus the effect of intravascular volume

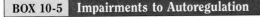

BOX 10-5 Impairments to Autoregulation

- Surgical intervention
- Head trauma
- General anesthesia
- Drug therapy
- Diabetes mellitus, diabetic coma
- Hypertension
- Brain tumor
- Cardiovascular changes (e.g., asystole)

Data from Cummings R: Understanding external ventricular drainage, *J Neurosci Nurs* 24(2):84, 1992.

expansion appears to be mediated by decreased blood viscosity rather than by CO augmentation.[13]

Blood-Brain Barrier

The **blood-brain barrier (BBB)** has been described as an anatomic-physiologic feature of the brain to prevent the passage of large-molecule proteins, toxic chemical compounds, radioactive ions, and disease-causing organisms from the blood into the CNS. The significance of the blood-brain barrier for drug administration is the question of whether a prescribed drug can cross it. The permeability of the blood-brain barrier is altered with brain injury, irradiation, toxic substances, and other causes that allow further insult to interfere with this protective mechanism of the brain.

Conductance of Cerebrospinal Fluid Outflow

Conductance of CSF outflow (C out) is another important parameter to be considered in patients with CSF circulation abnormalities. Research has demonstrated that the mean C out in normal individuals is 0.11 ml/min/mm Hg.[1] The C out value cannot be disregarded because a decrease in C out leads to increased ICP, ventricular enlargement, and hydrocephalus. The determination of C out can be of value and may become another important measurement in evaluating patients with increased ICP, especially those who require shunting.

INCREASED INTRACRANIAL PRESSURE

Etiology and Pathophysiology

Intracranial pressure fluctuates due to the heartbeat, respirations, and neuroregulation. The etiology of increased ICP can be related to TBI, subarachnoid hemorrhage, hydrocephalus, brain tumors, stroke/brain attack, cerebral infectious disorders, Reye's syndrome, hematomas, edema, herniation syndromes, and compressed basal cisterns.[53] As reported in a Dutch journal, a 24-year-old woman with normal blood pressure developed increased ICP after the use of oral tetracycline. She developed reduced visual acuity, papilledema, and concentric impaired visual fields. She recovered after treatment with acetazolamide and recurrent lumbar punctures but suffered disability because she had no improvement in visual acuity and visual fields. The authors concluded that tetracycline should be considered a cause of increased ICP if a patient complains of headache a few days after ingestion and requires urgent referral for treatment.[2]

ALERT: Increased ICP in patients with one or more of the aforementioned conditions or as demonstrated on CT or magnetic resonance imaging (MRI) findings, or with a Glasgow Coma Scale (GCS) score, requires rapid intervention.

The blood vessels in the brain act like a siphon and hold perfusion pressure nearly constant against rather severe degrees of gravitational stress. A drop in transmural pressure that could result in vessel collapse due to negative venous pressure is prevented by a simultaneous fall in CSF pressure. The mechanisms regulating CBF are altered in patients with increased ICP.[61] A thorough understanding of ICP requires an understanding of the anatomy and physiology of ICP. (See Chapter 1 for a review of the neuroanatomy of the brain, ventricles, and production and circulation of CSF.)

After the closure of all sutures and fontanelles in childhood, the brain is well protected but is highly vulnerable to pressure that may build up within the rigid enclosure. The addition of a fourth component to the cranial contents (e.g., a localized tumor or other space-occupying lesion) does not exert a uniform and diffusely distributed ICP but rather a nonuniform or compartmental pressure. Because of this localized effect, the neuraxis within the craniospinal space is displaced, pressure is exerted on other structures, blood supply to and from the brain is interrupted, and the brain is no longer adequately perfused. ICP is governed by the rate of CSF production (0.3 to 0.4 ml/min), resistance of CSF absorption, and the pressure in the superior sagittal sinus as the CSF circulates back to the heart via the jugular veins.

Sustained elevations in ICP, from whatever cause, exert a reciprocal decrease in CPP. Following the intracranial insult, elevated hypertension can cause brain cell ischemia or **oligemia.** Ischemia results in a cascade of events that leads to cell death resulting in cerebral edema, which further increases ICP unless the cycle is interrupted with appropriate medical or surgical interventions.

Major excitatory amino acids, such as glutamate, are found in all parts of the brain and spinal cord. The release of **gamma aminobutyric acid (GABA)** can lead to excessive influx of calcium into the neurons and activate a spectrum of enzymes that alter neuronal function and structure causing injury.[82] Glutamate is released at synapses and taken back up rapidly into presynaptic terminals, exposing glial cells to this amino acid only briefly. More than a brief dose of glutamate is toxic, and prolonged exposure to glutamate triggers a cascade of events that can injure and kill neurons, called **excitotoxicity.** Part of the mechanism of brain damage may involve the release of toxic amounts of glutamate in response to anoxia and some degenerative diseases. Elevated glutamate levels are toxic and may be useful to predict outcomes in disorders such as head trauma, stroke, or Alzheimer's disease.[62] It has been suggested that neuroscience clinicians in the future will measure glutamate levels, with elevated levels signaling poor outcomes. Research for neuroprotective drugs to block toxic levels of glutamate is ongoing.

Cerebral Edema

Cerebral edema is defined as an abnormal accumulation of water or fluid in the intracellular space, extracellular space, or both spaces, and it is associated with an increase in brain tissue volume.[37] The volume of edematous tissue necessary to increase ICP is not known. The edema may be localized to the site of the lesion or diffuse. Three types of edema have been identified, and patients may have one type or a combination of types. The type of edema should be determined for treatment to be effective:

1. **Vasogenic edema** or extracellular edema is the most common type of edema and occurs when autoregulation is lost and the BBB is interrupted. There is an increased permeability of the vessel wall, as changes in the endothelial lining of cerebral capillaries allow the tight epithelial junctions to open and plasma proteins leak from the intravascular space into the extracellular space. Vasogenic edema occurs predominantly in the white matter,[59] from brain tumors, stroke, or hypertensive encephalopathy; it can be visualized surrounding an abscess on a CT scan, and may respond to steroids.

2. **Cytotoxic edema** is an increase of intracellular fluid (predominantly intracellular astroglial cell swelling in the gray matter) from which protein does not escape; this fluid is derived from plasma. Intracellular swelling is related to the inability of the sodium-potassium pump to function normally, and the cells can no longer function because the pump functions to regulate intracellular ion and water balance. As the cell membrane breaks down, an influx of sodium and calcium from the interstitial space moves into the intracellular space, water follows sodium, and the cells swell, lyse, and leak potassium and lactate, contributing to lactic acidosis that can initiate a cyclic affect. This type of edema is commonly seen in cerebral trauma, in stroke patients, or in patients with hypoxia, hypotension, hyponatremia, and syndrome of inappropriate antidiuretic hormone (SIADH).

3. **Interstitial (hydrocephalic) brain edema** occurs primarily in the periventricular white matter, with the periventricular movement of CSF through the ependymal lining with an increase in CSF pressure within the ventricles or hydrocephalus. Shunting relieves ventricular pressure.[58]

Brain Swelling

Brain swelling describes an increase in the bulk weight of the brain caused by a tumor, hyperemia, hydrocephalus, or other factors and can shift and distort the brain (Fig. 10-5). The term **brain edema** is reserved for conditions that are attributed to increased water content of the brain parenchyma. One or both conditions may be present, and the

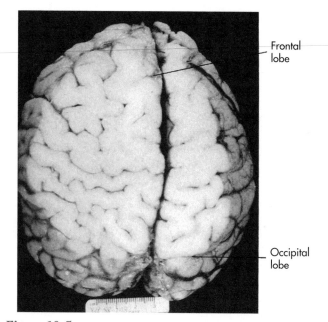

Figure 10-5 Prominent swelling of the left hemisphere with bowing across the midline (horizontal section). *(Courtesy Dr. E. Ross, deceased, Loyola University Medical Center, Chicago, IL.)*

success of treatment is determined by the appropriate interventions.

Brain swelling or edema, singularly or collectively, can contribute to increases in ICP. A sustained increased ICP has a detrimental effect on the delicate structures and functions of the brain. If it continues to increase, CBF is compromised. CBF depends on the blood entering the cranium via the carotid and vertebral arteries, the diameter of the vessels, and the blood viscosity. Each carotid supplies approximately 375 ml/min for a total of 750 ml/min, with the two smaller vertebrals together adding another 250 ml/min for the approximately 1000 ml/min required by the brain. CBF varies the most with significant changes in the CPP and according to the diameter of the vessels. The harmful effects of increased ICP become apparent clinically with any expansion of the cranial contents or with a reduction in blood supply and decreased cerebral venous return.

Benign Intracranial Hypertension

Benign intracranial hypertension (**pseudotumor cerebri**) is a term used for several diverse syndromes characterized by increased ICP, headache, vomiting, and visual dysfunctions with papilledema but without any neurologic signs. Patients may have an occasional sixth cranial nerve palsy, tinnitus, dizziness, or hearing or visual loss. The pathogenesis of pseudotumor cerebri has not been determined, but it has been demonstrated that brain swelling, an increase in cerebral blood volume, and a resistance of CSF outflow may be responsible. Neither an intracranial mass lesion nor a ventricular enlargement is identified on the CT scan. The association of this syndrome with prior exposure to vitamin A, estrogen, or tetracycline indicates that the process may be triggered by extrinsic factors.[58] This syndrome can be treated medically or surgically, and many patients experience spontaneous remissions.

Neurologic Deficits

Intracranial compression can impair the function of the cranial nerves (e.g., III, IV, and VI), with extraocular movements (EOMs) and changes in pupil size and equality. Pressure on the motor tracts causes motor deficits. Brainstem compression at the level of the pons and medulla creates life-threatening cardiac and respiratory complications.

Herniation Syndromes

Herniation is the protrusion of a portion of the brain through an abnormal opening. Increased pressure on one compartment of the cranial vault is not evenly distributed among the other brain compartments (Fig. 10-6). Instead, the brain tissue shifts from the compartment of greater pressure to the compartment of lower pressure.[12] There are two categories of herniation: supratentorial and infratentorial (Fig. 10-7). Herniation can occur without a fixed and dilated pupil.[52]

Supratentorial Herniation There are four supratentorial herniation syndromes: cingulate, central, uncal, and transcalvarial. **Cingulate herniation,** or **subfalcine herniation,** is characteristic of a unilateral hemisphere enlargement or an expansion of the frontal portion of the cerebral hemisphere with a lateral shift, which forces the cingulate gyrus under the falx cerebri (Fig. 10-8). A space-occupying lesion (e.g., tumor, infarct, hemorrhage, and abscess) and the accompanying edema compress blood vessels, primarily the anterior cerebral artery (ACA), and ischemia and necrosis result.[58] A midline shift is seen on CT or MRI with the swollen side forced across the midline or the cingulate gyrus forced under the falx cerebri. The contralateral ventricle may enlarge as CSF outflow is occluded at the foramen of Monro.

Central or **transtentorial herniation** may cause downward pressure from edema or a unilateral mass lesion in the frontal and parietal lobes, where brain tissue from one or both hemispheres is pressed toward the tentorial incisura on either side of the midbrain.[58] The hemispheres, basal ganglia, diencephalon, or midbrain may become displaced downward. Herniated tissue may hemorrhage or become necrotic.

The early signs of central herniation are constricted pupils, decreased EOM, a loss of upward gaze, and small, reactive pupils that may become dilated and fixed. As ICP increases, irregular respirations, temperature changes, motor signs, and posturing (abnormal flexion or abnormal extension) suggest that the patient will likely progress to a comatose state. The patient may exhibit weakness that can progress to paralysis and decreased response to auditory and sensory stimulation. Characteristic **abnormal respiratory patterns** of respiratory changes with compensation, decompensation, and herniation are important signs to alert the clinician of an impending crisis (Fig. 10-9). Later signs may include unequal and unreactive pupils, dysconjugate gaze progressing to eyes fixed, coma state variations in body temperature, unstable vital signs, and the potential for diabetes insipidus (DI).[6]

Uncal or **lateral transtentorial herniation** occurs if one or both cerebral hemispheres expand with the uncus or parahippocampal gyrus of the temporal lobe pressed into the

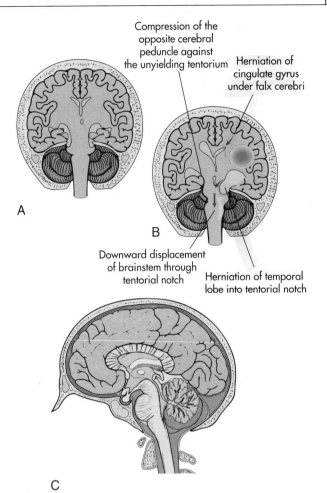

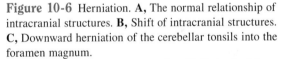

Figure 10-6 Herniation. **A,** The normal relationship of intracranial structures. **B,** Shift of intracranial structures. **C,** Downward herniation of the cerebellar tonsils into the foramen magnum.
(Redrawn from McCance KL, Huether SE: Pathophysiology: the biologic basis for disease in adults and children, ed 3, St Louis, 1998, Mosby; in Lewis SM, Heitkemper MM, Dirksen RF, editors: Concepts of neurologic dysfunction, ed 5, St Louis, 2000, Mosby.)

tentorial incisura or notch (Fig. 10-10). Displacement of the diencephalon or midbrain to the opposite side occurs with contralateral motor signs and unilateral eye signs. Narrowing of the midbrain and compression of the posterior cerebral artery (PCA) with compression or stretching of the third cranial (oculomotor) nerve can produce characteristic symptoms. Early signs and symptoms include third cranial nerve signs with eventual dilation of the ipsilateral pupil, decreased level of consciousness (LOC), contralateral motor changes, and central neurogenic hyperventilation. Prevention of the final stages requires rapid intervention to prevent inevitable progression that leads to herniation with fixed, dilated pupils, coma, and changes in vital signs progressing to cardiopulmonary arrest.

There is one exception to the classic brain lesion that produces contralateral motor/sensory signs and ipsilateral eye signs. **Kernohan's notch** is a paradox in which a unilateral lesion causes the midbrain to be displaced to the oppo-

SUPRATENTORIAL   INFRATENTORIAL

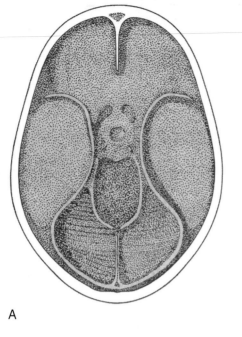

A   B

Figure 10-7 An infolding of the dura mater called the *tentorium* separates the cerebrum from the cerebellum. The compartment above the tentorium is supratentorial (**A**), and the compartment below the tentorium is infratentorial (**B**).

site side (Fig. 10-11). The pressure of the tentorial edge indents the cerebral peduncle (Kernohan's notch) and may produce paradoxic ipsilateral motor signs.[52]

Transcalvarial herniation can occur after cranial trauma or a penetrating head injury with skull fracture and subsequent protrusion of the brain tissue outside the skull (Fig. 10-12). The neurosurgeon can elect not to replace the bone flap after performing a craniotomy in anticipation of severe brain swelling and raised ICP. However, this is not routine procedure.

Infratentorial Herniation   The two types of infratentorial herniation are downward (tonsillar) cerebellar tonsillar herniation and upward transtentorial herniation (see Fig. 10-6).

Tonsillar herniation describes the unique anatomic position of the cerebellar hemispheres as they narrow to rounded points (tonsils) above the foramen magnum and as one or both cerebellar tonsils herniate through the foramen magnum. For example, a mass lesion in the posterior fossa forces the tonsils downward through the foramen magnum; as a result, there is downward displacement of the posteroinferior cerebellar artery (PICA), which produces slow compression of the medulla and upper cervical cord[52] (Fig. 10-13). Nuchal rigidity (stiff neck) is an early sign. Other revealing signs include heart rate and blood pressure changes, small pupils, and ataxic respirations. Coma is a late sign, with eventual cardiac arrest and death caused by compression of the brainstem and medulla.

It is not uncommon for lesions above the tentorium to create downward pressure and herniation. Although rare, pressure can also be generated from below the tentorium with **upward transtentorial herniation** of an expanding lesion of the brainstem and cerebellum. In addition, a patient with an infratentorial mass lesion receiving ventricular drainage from a lateral ventricle site could possibly experience upward herniation. Upward herniation produces cranial nerve deficits, nuchal rigidity, and posturing. The patient may have a loss of upward gaze and a rapid loss of consciousness.[52]

ALERT: Drainage of CSF with a catheter in the lateral ventricle can worsen the upward herniation syndrome.[52]

The **compartmental syndrome** has been recently introduced to explain how ICP varies in each of the three compartments within the brain. When the ICP is measured in each hemisphere with a subarachnoid bolt, elevations in ICP on the same side as the mass lesion often are substantially greater than those on the contralateral side.[58] A lesion within a compartment may raise the pressure of that compartment without affecting the entire intracranial contents and raising the supratentorial pressure.

Assessment

The initial neurologic assessment should determine whether the patient is at risk for increased ICP. Even a subtle change in neurologic status can be very significant in such patients. A high index of suspicion is appropriate for patients who have the conditions listed in Box 10-6.

ALERT: Any changes in level of consciousness (LOC)—one of the most important nursing assessments—should be monitored closely and reported immediately.

The early signs and symptoms of increased ICP are often subtle. The patient may initially appear restless, irritable, and fatigued and may exhibit personality changes or mild confusion. The effects become more noticeable as the reticular activating system (RAS) becomes depressed bilaterally. The patient's speech may be slowed or slurred, voluntary move-

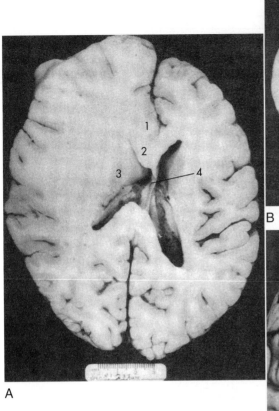

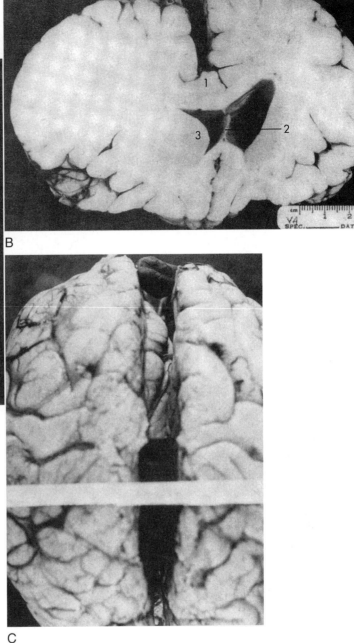

Figure 10-8 A, Swelling of left frontal and parietal lobes with shifting of the cingulate gyrus *(1),* corpus callosum *(2),* caudate nucleus *(3),* and septum pellucidum *(4)* (horizontal section). **B,** Marked swelling of left cerebrum with prominent shifting of the cingulate gyrus *(1),* septum pellucidum *(2),* and caudate nucleus *(3)* (coronal section). **C,** View into the interhemispheric fissure revealing marked shifting of the cingulate gyrus from left to right (frontal lobe section).
(Courtesy Dr. E. Ross, deceased, Loyola University Medical Center, Chicago, IL.)

ments and sensation are diminished, and eye movements are affected. Other symptoms such as headache (especially when supine, early in the morning, and when bending over), coughing, or sneezing may also be reported. Stretching of the pain receptors of the dura around a lesion may lead to dural irritation or head pain. An obstruction of the CSF causes the ventricles to enlarge, resulting in a severe headache.

The patient should also be assessed during sleep for rapid eye movements (REMs), because the decreased respirations that occur during REM sleep cause an accumulation of excess carbon dioxide (a potent vasodilator), and ICP can elevate. If the CT scan shows pressure in or around the medulla (vomiting center), the patient will probably experience nausea and vomiting or projectile vomiting without nausea.

Any patient whose initial assessment indicates a risk for increased ICP should be thoroughly evaluated to diagnose the cause, location, and rate of increasing pressure; to determine the extent of intracranial hypertension; and to plan

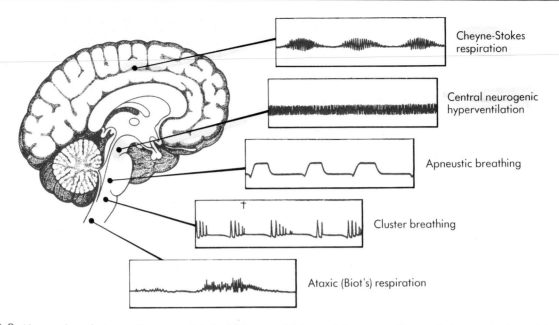

Cheyne-Stokes
respiration

Central neurogenic
hyperventilation

Apneustic breathing

Cluster breathing

Ataxic (Biot's) respiration

Figure 10-9 Abnormal respiratory patterns associated with increased intracranial pressure. Cheyne-Stokes respiration, arising from deep inside the cerebral hemispheres and basal ganglia; central neurogenic hyperventilation, from lower midbrain to middle pons; apneustic breathing, from middle to lower pons and brainstem; cluster breathing, from upper medulla; and ataxic (Biot's) respiration, from the medulla.

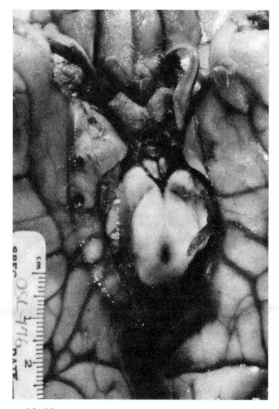

Figure 10-10 Extensive notching of the uncus and parahippocampus with focal hemorrhages.
(Courtesy Dr. E. Ross, deceased, Loyola University Medical Center, Chicago, IL.)

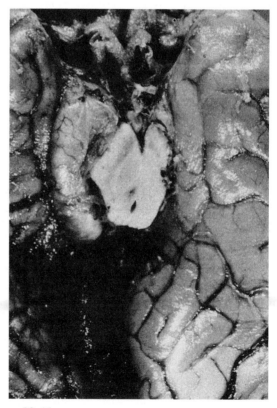

Figure 10-11 Bilateral uncal notching with compression of the left lateral mesencephalon and left cerebral peduncle (Kernohan's notch).
(Courtesy Dr. E. Ross, deceased, Loyola University Medical Center, Chicago, IL.)

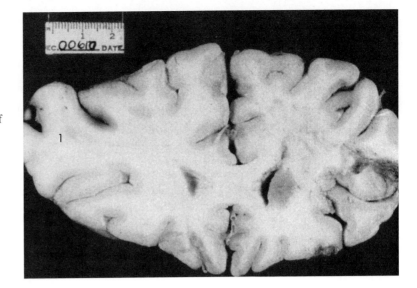

Figure 10-12 Swelling of the left hemisphere out of craniotomy site *(1)*. Note multiple scattered cortical hemorrhagic infarcts (coronal section). *(Courtesy Dr. E. Ross, deceased, Loyola University Medical Center, Chicago, IL.)*

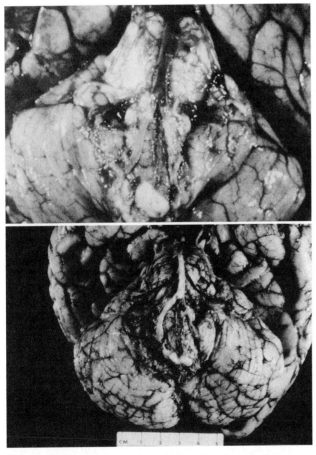

Figure 10-13 Pons, medulla, spinal cord, and cerebellum reveal acute bilateral cerebellar tonsillar herniation and necrosis. *(Courtesy Dr. E. Ross, deceased, Loyola University Medical Center, Chicago, IL.)*

BOX 10-6	Conditions That May Cause Increased Intracranial Pressure

- Brain tumor
- Head injury: contusion, hematoma
- Edema secondary to neurosurgery/neurosurgical procedures, trauma, ruptured aneurysm, or hemorrhage
- Brain attack or ischemic stroke
- Hydrocephalus
- Hypoxic state
- Hypercarbia
- CNS inflammation, infection, or brain abscess
- Colloid cyst of the ventricle
- Metabolic changes (e.g., hyponatremia)
- Reye's syndrome (characterized by encephalopathy with severe edema of the brain)

Data from American Association of Neuroscience Nurses: *Core curriculum for neuroscience nursing,* ed 4, St Louis, 2004, Saunders; Barker E: Myths and facts about increased intracranial pressure, *Nursing* 8(12):20, 1988; and Barker E: Avoiding increased intracranial pressure, *Nursing* 20(5):64Q, 1990.
CNS, Central nervous system.

immediate treatment.[64] The baseline neurologic assessment should be detailed and well documented. Subsequent evaluations are compared with the first assessment to detect changes or trends, particularly in LOC, pupils, vital signs, motor functions, and other parameters (Box 10-7; see also Box 10-1).

Neurodiagnostic and Laboratory Studies

As soon as the patient is stable enough, diagnostic studies will be needed to determine the extent and severity of the underlying cerebral insult (see Chapter 2). The most common tests include the following:

- CT: identifies ventricular size and shape, presence of a shift or collapse of the ventricles, diffuse loss of

BOX 10-7	Early Signs and Symptoms of Increased Intracranial Pressure

- Deterioration in the level of consciousness: restlessness, irritability, personality changes, changes in mental status, mild confusion, agitation, lower Glasgow Coma Scale (GCS) score[42]
- Pupillary dysfunction: ptosis, ovoid pupil, delayed or sluggish reactivity to light, and unilateral change in pupil size or shape as pressure on the oculomotor nerve (cranial nerve [CN] III) causes stretching and then uncal or tentorial herniation
- Vision: blurred vision, diplopia, decreased visual acuity with pressure on the cranial nerves that control eye movement (CNs III, IV, and VI)
- Motor: pronator drift, decreased grasp strength, contralateral hemiparesis
- Sensory: decreased response to touch or pinprick
- Headache: early-morning headache with nausea/vomiting, or headache when straining
- Speech: slow or slurred
- Memory: slightly impaired
- Vital signs: *no change*
- Cranial nerves: may or may not show changes initially
- Seizure activity: may or may not occur depending on cause

Data from American Association of Neuroscience Nurses: *Core curriculum for neuroscience nursing,* ed 4, St Louis, 2004, Saunders; Barker E: Myths and facts about increased intracranial pressure, *Nursing* 8(12):20, 1988; Barker E: Avoiding increased intracranial pressure, *Nursing* 20(5):64Q, 1990; and Hickey JV: *The clinical practice of neurologic and neurosurgical nursing,* ed 3, Philadelphia, 1997, JB Lippincott.

CSF spaces, compression or shift of the ventricles, and presence or absence of cisterns and edema to identify the cause; also identifies acute blood suspicion of mass within the brain and skull fractures; follow-up CT verifies correct placement of intracranial monitoring device

- CT angiogram (CTA): CT for visualization of intracranial vessels or vascular abnormalities
- MRI: may detect changes not apparent on CT; later checks compatibility of ICP monitoring device
- Magnetic resonance angiography (MRA): ability to evaluate cerebral vessels intracranially
- Evoked potentials: for example, brainstem auditory-evoked responses (BAERs); may be used in comatose patients; evaluates extent of CNS injury
- CBF studies: check for compressed cerebral vessels
- Angiograms: may provide additional useful information regarding aneurysms or vascular abnormalities
- Transcranial Doppler (TCD): may also be ordered for a noninvasive test for vasospasm
- Laboratory tests: may include serum osmolarity, electrolytes, platelet count, prothrombin time/partial thromboplastin time (PT/PTT), international normalized ratio (INR), coagulation, and anticonvulsant drug levels[17]

BOX 10-8	Late Signs and Symptoms of Increased Intracranial Pressure

- Deterioration in the level of consciousness progressing: difficult to arouse; requires more stimulus; any decrease in Glasgow Coma Scale (GCS) score; progressing to coma
- Impaired brainstem reflexes: corneal and gag
- Pupillary dysfunction: unilateral enlarging pupil ipsilateral to the lesion that progresses to fixed, dilated "blown pupil"; papilledema; later bilateral dilation and fixation
- Vomiting: usually without nausea
- Motor weakness: progressing to hemiplegia, dense weakness, abnormal flexion progressing to abnormal extension and flaccid muscles
- Sensory deficits: may only posture to painful stimulus
- Headache: worsens with projectile vomiting
- Speech: may only groan/moan to painful stimuli
- Respiratory: irregular respirations; Cheyne-Stokes respirations that progress to central neurogenic hyperventilation, ataxia, and respiratory arrest
- Vital signs: progressive rising systolic blood pressure with widening pulse pressure; after herniation blood pressure may decrease or become hypotensive; bradycardia followed by tachycardia; temperature changes as hypothalamus is compressed; Cushing's triad indicating cerebral dysfunction that may be irreversible; decreased pulse with continued elevation of ICP progressing from irregular to rapid and thready; temperature can increase during decompensatory stage
- Cardiac: Q waves with ST depression, elevated T waves, supraventricular tachycardia, sinus bradycardia, atrioventricular block, PVCs, and an agonal rhythm leading to cardiac arrest
- Cranial nerves: related to supratentorial or infratentorial lesion and edema with brainstem reflexes (corneal, gag)
- Abnormal reflexes: Babinski's sign

PVCs, Premature ventricular contractions.

Continual and Serial Assessment

Patients require continuous neurologic assessment at frequent intervals if they have been determined to be at risk for increased ICP, have a confirmed diagnosis of increased ICP, or display any signs and symptoms of increased ICP. Interventions are focused on preventing late signs and symptoms[25] (Box 10-8).

Patients displaying any late signs and symptoms of increased ICP must be closely monitored and assessed, with any changes reported promptly to the physician. Without the appropriate treatment, the patient's progression to cerebral herniation is imminent.

Cushing's reflex is helpful in explaining the late signs of increased ICP. This response is seen with sudden increases in pressure that result from distortion of a pressure area in the medulla beneath the floor of the fourth ventricle. When the CSF pressure rises to equal arterial pressure, the arteries become compressed and blood supply to the brain is decreased.[22,66] The vasomotor center becomes ischemic and triggers the arterial pressure to rise in compensation for low perfusion. A sympathetically mediated response causes the systolic blood pressure to increase, and there is a widening pulse pressure, slowing of the pulse, and irregular respirations. Patients with Cushing's reflex have recovered after rapid treatment.[22]

Treatment

The goal of therapy is to avoid ICP greater than 20 mm Hg and CPP less than 60 to 70 mm Hg. Otherwise, ischemic may result (see Chapters 9 and 11). Management of the patient with elevated ICP incorporates medical/surgical treatment in collaboration with a physician. The focus is to closely monitor the patient, ensure an adequate airway, maintain adequate ventilation, provide pain control, decrease stimuli, elevate the head of the bed (HOB) (unless contraindicated), and position and turn the patient appropriately. Early treatment may protect the brain and allow time for resolution of the underlying cause and lower the mortality rate. According to the authors of one report in the international literature, the outcomes can be good using the following coordinated aggressive stepwise approach. This protocol focuses on control of increased ICP in the ICU for TBI. Each step is completed until the desired outcome can be achieved without adversely affecting CPP:[78]

- *Step 1:* Slight hyperventilation with a target $PaCO_2$ of 35 mm Hg
- *Step 2:* Insertion of an intraventricular catheter (IVC) for CSF drainage for an ICP greater than 15 to 20 mm Hg
- *Step 3:* Mannitol or hypertonic saline and hyperventilation with a target $PaCO_2$ of 28 to 35 mm Hg
- *Step 4:* Barbiturate coma or decompressive craniectomy

Additional management of this protocol includes seizure prophylaxis, sedation, nutritional support, use of hypothermia, and corticosteroids (except for TBI).[78]

Interventions may include ICP and CPP monitoring with the ability to drain excess CSF fluid, osmotherapy, glucocorticoids, sedation, hyperventilation, normothermia, anticonvulsants, and measures of last resort considered as a final and second-tier treatment. Managing CPP may require the use of pressors to balance the differences between MAP and ICP to maintain CPP greater than 60 to 70 mm Hg, or as ordered. CPP should be assessed individually and continuously, as it may fluctuate over time.

Intracranial Pressure Monitoring

Continuous ICP monitoring of the supratentorial compartment is routine in evaluating intracranial disorders.[58] Monitoring to measure mean ICP (MICP) is useful in detecting early neurologic decompensation in patients suspected of having or presumed to have increased ICP or herniation, in comatose patients, after TBI, when there is CT/MRI evidence of a mass effect, with midline shift, with narrowing or absence of the basal cisterns, or for patients with a Glasgow Coma Scale (GCS) score ≤8 with clinical pathology. ICP monitoring provides an objective measure of the patient's response to interventions used to treat the raised ICP.

Direct therapeutic drainage and ICP monitoring from the posterior fossa have never been accepted in neurosurgical practice because of the risk of CSF leak, cranial nerve palsies, and brainstem irritation. However, one study did determine that posterior fossa monitoring is safe and effective. The study found that posterior fossa pressure was 50% greater than supratentorial pressure in the first 12 postoperative hours. Researchers determined that early detection of and timely intervention for posterior fossa surgery complications can be accomplished with this new method.[67]

Clinical guidelines for ICP monitoring placement include the following:[5]

- *Consent.* Explain/reinforce the purpose, procedure, and risks to the patient or person giving consent and witness his or her signature on hospital form according to policy.
- *Diagnostic studies.* Obtain routine and latest laboratory results, including imaging studies (CT/MRI) and coagulation profile, if indicated.
- *Assessment.* Perform and record a neurologic evaluation.
- *Medication.* Administer sedation or other medications as ordered.
- *Restraint.* Perform according to hospital policy to prevent dislodgment of monitor.

The ICP monitoring device may be placed using sterile technique in the operating room (OR), in the emergency department (ED), or at the bedside in the ICU.

Types of Intracranial Pressure Monitors. There are multiple devices for monitoring ICP, including a subarachnoid bolt; subdural, epidural, or intraparenchymal catheters; or a combination catheter that monitors ICP, CPP, or cerebral temperature. The current method of choice and the "gold standard" is the ventriculostomy using an intraventricular catheter (IVC). Direct access to CSF allows for easy drainage in an effort to assist and maintain the normal compensatory mechanisms of the brain. The types of monitoring devices include fiberoptic, strain gauge, and air pouch. The types of ICP monitors have significance not only in terms of reliability, accuracy, safety, costs, and dependability, but also in terms of clinical applications for compatibility with use in an MRI.

A **subarachnoid screw/bolt** is inserted through a twist drill hole into the subarachnoid space. The bolt can be inserted quickly and connected to an external transducer. A bolt can be used in cases with small or collapsed ventricles and does not penetrate the brain parenchyma. The infection rate is very low, and the cost is minimal. The following are disadvantages: CSF cannot be drained through a bolt, the bolt can become occluded, brain tissue can herniate through the bolt, and the readings may be unreliable a few days after insertion. The bolt requires a closed skull for accurate measurement (Table 10-1).

Parenchymal catheter is an option to monitor ICP into an area of the brain where pressure may be elevated. This serves as a reliable approach when ventricular access is not

TABLE 10-1	**Comparison of Intracranial Pressure Monitors**		
Type	Site	Advantages	Disadvantages
Subarachnoid bolt or screw	Subarachnoid space	Can be used with small or collapsed ventricles; does not penetrate brain parenchyma; low infection rates; low cost; ease and safety of insertion that can be performed quickly	Does not allow CSF drainage or withdrawal; becomes occluded; may have dampened waveform to give unreliable readings after a few days; blood or brain tissue may herniate into bolt; less accurate at higher ICP elevations
Intraventricular catheter (IVC) or ventriculostomy	Ventricles	Ventricular site provides more accuracy; CSF cultures can be collected; allows CSF to be withdrawn to control ICP; contrast materials can be injected for radiologic studies	Risk of hemorrhage due to invasiveness; increased risk of infection; risk of CSF leak at site; artifacts may cause dampening of recordings; more difficult to insert, especially for collapsed, small, or displaced ventricles
Epidural or subdural sensor	Epidural or subdural space	Ease of insertion; least invasive; recommended in case of meningitis and CNS infection; less risk of infection; does not require recalibration	Slower response time; fragile; can become wedged against skull; affected by heat or febrile patient; expensive; diaphragm can rupture; less accurate; unable to sample or drain CSF
Intraparenchymal	Brain parenchyma	Quick insertion, accurate, reliable approach when ventricular access is not an option	Unable to drain CSF, may become clogged

CNS, Central nervous system; *CSF,* cerebrospinal fluid; *ICP,* intracranial pressure.

an option (e.g., collapsed ventricles). Advantages include quick access. A significant disadvantage is the inability to drain CSF, and the catheter may become clogged with brain tissue and need replacing.

The **intraventricular catheter (IVC)** is a popular device because it provides for continuous recordings of pressure and waveform. The measurements are reliable, fluids can be added or withdrawn, and CSF withdrawal can control an elevated ICP. It is usually inserted into the right, nondominant side of the cranium.

Obtaining cultures directly from the ventricles allows frequent sampling. The insertion of a cannula through a burr hole into the nondominant hemisphere requires skill and experience on the part of the neurosurgeon or credentialed practitioner. After connection to a two-way stopcock, the system is ready to hook up to the bedside monitor and the drip chamber with drainage container. It may be unwise to attempt insertion for patients with small or collapsed ventricles or CNS infection. Complications of the IVC procedure include risk of hemorrhage, infection, CSF leakage, and the presence of artifacts (which dampen recordings).

Use of the IVC for supratentorial pressure monitoring is the preferred method because it allows both recording of pressure and drainage of CSF to help lower increased ICP.[58]

An **epidural sensor** is inserted into the epidural space through a burr hole. This device is easy to insert and is the least invasive, but it also tends to be the least accurate because it does not penetrate the dura of the brain. Located between the skull and dura, the epidural monitor is recommended for patients at risk for meningitis or other CNS infections.

Because it does not communicate with CSF, it is not a direct gauge of CSF pressure. The delicate sensor can wedge up against the bone, can be easily damaged, can be affected by heat or febrile patients, and may be expensive. Rupture of the diaphragm with the escape of intracranial air has been reported with this device[33] (Fig. 10-14).

A **fiberoptic catheter** offers the accuracy of *direct* monitoring with several options: intraparenchymal, parenchymal postcraniotomy, subdural, and ventricular placement. The ventriculostomy catheter can be placed in the ventricle as part of a system that includes external drainage and a transducer. This safe, reliable technology offers a closed system for simultaneous monitoring and CSF drainage. According to Crutchfield and colleagues,[19] the fiberoptic device offers certain advantages over conventional monitoring systems, particularly because of its ability to measure the pressure of the brain parenchyma. The study findings suggest that the device be replaced if monitoring is continued for periods longer than 5 days because the device cannot be recalibrated in situ.[19]

The waveform produced by a fiberoptic catheter is sharp and distinct. The system can be disconnected and reconnected by the clinician at any time without interference because the system is calibrated at the time of insertion. Battery operated or adaptable to the bedside monitoring module, the equipment stores and trends the data and is equipped with readout strip capability. The fragile fiberoptic catheters will break if bent and should not be stored near a heat source. The types of transducers vary from external strain gauge, to fiberoptic, air pouch, or combinations.

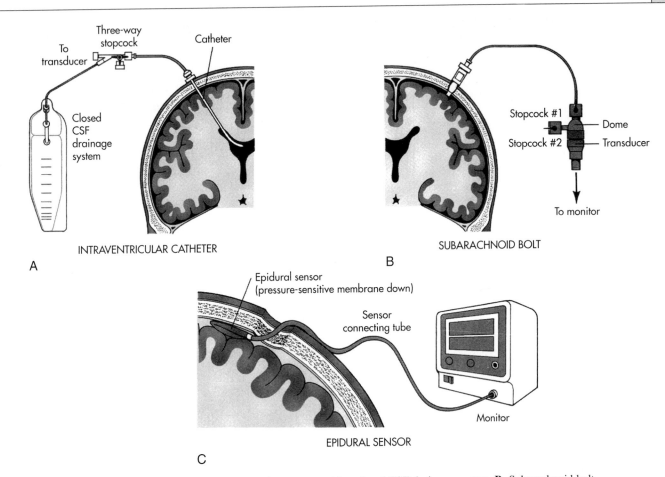

Figure 10-14 A, Intraventricular catheter (IVC) monitoring system with a closed CSF drainage system. **B,** Subarachnoid bolt monitoring system. **C,** Epidural monitoring system.

Waveform Monitoring and Analysis. ICP waveform analysis offers potential as a means of dynamic clinical assessment of intracranial adaptive capacity. The ICP waveform may provide information about intracranial dynamics reflecting compliance or cerebrovascular regulation that will help identify individuals at risk for decreased adaptive capacity (DAC) and adverse responses to nursing care and environmental stimuli.[45]

The level of analysis required is considered when selecting the ICP monitoring device. Examples include IVCs and devices to be inserted into the subdural, epidural, or subarachnoid spaces or into the brain parenchyma. Although all methods produce visually similar waveforms, they may not be adequate for advanced ICP analysis techniques (e.g., spectral analysis). If the transducer needs to be responsive to a frequency bandwidth of at least 20 Hz, fiberoptic transducer-tipped systems are suitable.[31]

Analysis of the ICP waveform begins immediately after catheter insertion and the calibration of all equipment. The goal is to identify risk factors for early identification of individuals with decreased adaptive capacity and to understand the mechanisms. ICP waveforms have three characteristic peaks that correlate with the arterial pulse waveform:[45]

- P_1 (percussion) wave has a sharp peak and a fairly constant amplitude and is thought to be arterial in

origin. Extreme arterial hypotension and hypertension produce changes in the ICP waveform, particularly P_1. With severe arterial hypotension, there is a decrease in mean ICP and ICP waveform amplitude.
- P_2 (tidal wave) is more variable, ends on the dicrotic notch, and is thought to be arterial in origin. As ICP continues to increase, P_2 increases to a greater extent than P_1, and as a result P_1 may become buried. Visual assessment of the P_2 elevation is clinically relevant and provides a rough indicator of decreased adaptive capacity and in predicting the risk for disproportionate increases in ICP.
- P_3 (dicrotic wave) follows the dicrotic notch. It is thought to be venous in origin.

The continuous display reflects a pulsation that corresponds to each heartbeat and a slower wave that corresponds to each respiration, giving the appearance of an upward spike with a systolic (P_1) or percussion wave. This portion has sharp peaks of consistent amplitude that are associated with arterial pulsations. The second wave, the P_2 or tidal wave, is a result of venous pulsations. P_2 varies in amplitude and shape and ends on the dicrotic notch. P_3 follows immediately with a small, superimposed notch (Fig. 10-15).

The P_2 segment may be the most clinically significant. As ICP rises, so does the P_2, which gives the waveform a rounded

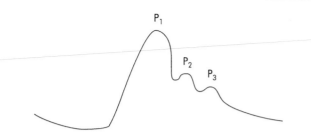

Figure 10-15 Components of the intracranial pulse waveforms.

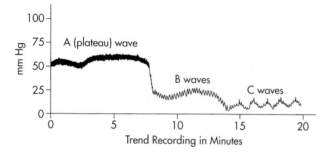

Figure 10-16 Intracranial pressure waves. Composite diagram of *A* (plateau) waves, *B* (sawtooth) waves, and *C* (small, rhythmic) waves.

appearance. The P_2 segment responds to hyperventilation by decreasing in amplitude and is therefore thought to reflect compliance. A decrease in compliance is indicated by an amplitude of P_2 that is greater than that of P_1 or that becomes lost in the tracing.

Each wave and its configuration give additional information regarding the intracranial dynamics. A normal waveform is the rapid rhythmic oscillation of pressure without any relevance and is referred to as the **C wave.** These waves are low-amplitude fluctuations associated with changes in arterial pressures.[58] They occur at 4- to 8-minute intervals and are not as rapid or sharp as B waves. The significance of C waves is not known at this time. They correspond to rhythmic fluctuations of respirations and blood pressure and can rise as high as 20 to 25 mm Hg (Fig. 10-16).

Typical **B wave** oscillations are accompanied by corresponding fluctuations of arterial blood pressure. They also correspond to respiratory fluctuations. These waveforms have a sharp and sawtooth appearance, occur every 30 to 60 seconds, and rise as high as 20 to 50 mm Hg but vary in amplitude. B waves are pathologic and are characterized by less severe elevations in ICP.[58] Patients with an unstable ICP demonstrate this characteristic pattern, and their frequency may increase as compliance decreases. B waves often appear in runs, tend to be associated with a decreased LOC, and indicate a decrease in the brain's normal compensatory mechanism. If B waves do not return to baseline after events such as suctioning or repositioning, they may be forerunners of A waves.

The most dangerous and life-threatening waves are the **A waves** or **plateau waves.** These pathologic waves have diagnostic value and are produced by secondary changes in cerebral blood volume.[58] They occur at varying intervals (often

5 to 20 minutes), are usually superimposed on an already elevated ICP, and are significant because of their elevated value of 50 to 100 mm Hg. A study by Hayashi and colleagues[35] found that patients with a plateau wave phenomenon have a marked impairment of CSF absorption and CSF flow, which suggests that the phenomenon is an important sign that indicates an impairment of CSF absorption capacities. The depressor area of the medullary vasomotor center may also play a role.

CPP may be compromised during plateau waves and produce cerebral hypoxia. Cerebral vasodilation is an important component of a plateau wave. During the waves, a consistent decrease in CPP can be observed and is consistent with a reduced brain compliance, tight brain, or mass lesion. A terminal reduction in CPP causes irreversible ischemia.[23] Herniation may be imminent. Immediate intervention to reduce ICP is necessary (e.g., intermittent manual hyperventilation). Patients are usually comatose, at risk for vomiting (unless a nasogastric tube is in place), display purposeless or no movement, experience a worsening headache, and display irregular forced breathing if not intubated. Vital sign changes may be unreliable during this period.

It is critical during the acute phase of ICP monitoring to evaluate the patient at frequent intervals, check for a loss of or a change in waveform, and closely examine equipment for intact connections or malfunction. The dressing should remain dry and intact and show no evidence of bleeding or CSF leakage. The drainage bag must be secured at the proper height and observed for the color, consistency, and amount of CSF drainage.

Insertion and Removal of Intracranial Pressure Monitoring Devices. There is a movement afoot by organizations other than the American Association of Neurological Surgeons (AANS) and the Congress of Neurological Surgeons (CNS) to sponsor courses that teach non-neurosurgeons the technical aspects of brain monitoring of severely injured patients. These groups wish to instruct physician extenders, intensivists, general surgeons, and others in the techniques of performing brain monitoring. Traditionally, organized neurosurgery held that brain monitoring devices should be placed either by neurosurgeons or under their supervision. Furthermore, the appropriate treatment of complications related to the insertion of ICP monitors often requires skills that are learned only in a neurosurgical residency, as is the ability to perform more extensive neurosurgical interventions that might be needed by these patients.[26]

The neurosurgical physician selects the site and determines the most appropriate type of monitoring device for recording ICP. The right frontal area is usually the first choice because of the important language centers on the left side of the brain. The external ventricular drainage device is commonly used to monitor ICP.

The majority of ventriculostomy insertions are performed under aseptic conditions at the bedside in the neuroscience critical care unit (NCCU); others are placed during surgical procedures in the OR. After obtaining patient consent, explain the procedure and the risks versus benefits to the person who signed for consent, and prepare essential equipment where the procedure will be performed (e.g., the ED,

OR, or ICU). Preoperative medications (e.g., 4 mg midazolam [Versed] and/or 2 to 4 mg morphine sulfate [MS]) or a neuromuscular blockade (e.g., 10 mg vecuronium [Norcuron]) may be ordered. The HOB is elevated 20 to 30 degrees, and the patient is placed supine and appropriately draped. A site anterior to the coronal suture at the level of the midpupillary line is shaved and may be washed with chlorhexidine. The site can then be prepped with Betadine or appropriate solution and draped.

Masks, gowns, and sterile gloves must be worn during the procedure. One percent lidocaine containing epinephrine may be injected at the site, and a number 11 scalpel is commonly used to make a small, 1.5 cm stab incision down to the bone. A small twist drill hole through the outer table is made with a drill from the monitoring kit. A Ghajar guide may be used. A needle or number 18 scalpel is used to penetrate the dura. After saline is used to clean the site, bone bleeding is controlled and the stylet is inserted into the ventricular catheter for placement. No more than three passes should be attempted. The free flow of CSF confirms placement. The stylet is removed, and the transducer is calibrated, inserted, hooked to the pressure monitor, and attached to the bedside monitor. A trocar or another instrument may be used to tunnel under the skin for an exit site away from the burr hole. The incision is closed with sutures, and the exit wound is sutured (Fig. 10-17). The catheter tip is attached to the prepared setup. When the waveform is satisfactory, the system is secured and a sterile dressing is applied. Orders for all abnormal parameters should be established and alarms turned on for continuous monitoring. Neurologic assessments are performed per neuroscience critical care policy (see Chapters 2 and 9).

The initial readings and waveform are recorded. The time, date, location/description of the site, opening pressure, type of monitoring device inserted, and name of the practitioner are documented in the patient's record. The invasive monitoring system will be maintained using strict sterile technique to prevent a CNS infection, particularly when specimens are drawn for cultures. The occlusive dressing should be checked frequently and kept dry and intact.[3]

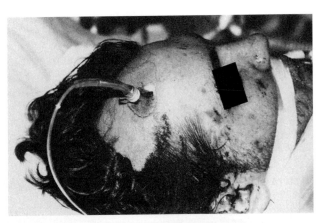

Figure 10-17 Closed head injury; patient following emergent insertion of an ICP bolt.

Leakage around the site should be reported and requires a dressing change. Specimens are obtained per hospital and infection control policies using strict aseptic technique. Collection bags are part of the closed system and are not interrupted unnecessarily or routinely changed until the bag is full. Family teaching includes an explanation of the purpose for ICP monitoring, how to avoid activation of the alarms from stimulation of the patient during visits, and the need to observe the patient's response to visitors and other activities. Request that everyone speak in a soft voice and keep the room as quiet as possible with subdued lighting to promote sleep and rest. Management of patients with multimodality ICP monitoring is described under Acute Care.

The length of time that an ICP catheter or drainage device remains in place depends on the rationale for the drain placement. After several days of treatment—as the patient's condition improves and as the ICP elevations have responded to therapy—the temporary monitoring device is removed. To evaluate the patient's cerebral pressure tolerance, the external drainage system may be clamped for increasingly longer times until the patient's neurologic status remains stable. The patient is placed in the supine position, the dressing removed, and the site checked for any signs of CSF leak or infection and cleaned. The monitoring device is removed, and the catheter or sensor tip may be sent to the laboratory for analysis. The site is stapled or sutured, and a sterile dressing is applied or treated per protocol and the site observed for drainage or signs and symptoms of infection.

Measurement of Brain Temperature and Oxygenation

Advanced cerebral monitoring has become more sophisticated and complex to include methods for multichannel access that include measuring **brain tissue temperature.** A thermistor is a device that measures temperature using a thermal-sensitive resistor. Monitoring the differences in normal brain temperature versus brain temperature following brain injury may help determine factors that influence brain temperature that can be regulated for better outcomes.

Monitoring of cerebral oxygenation is considered to be of great importance in minimizing secondary hypoxic brain damage and detecting ischemic brain damage. **Noninvasive brain oxygenation monitoring** is an option with a device using near-infrared spectroscopy to measure regional oxygen saturation (rSO_2). The sensors are placed on the patient's forehead bilaterally and the infrared light passes through the forehead and skull into the brain. The differences between the arterial O_2 delivered versus arterial O_2 consumed can be measured in number of points or as a percent change. The changes from a patient's normal values guide the treating team in clinical decision making.

Invasive monitoring of cerebral oxygenation with a brain oxygen monitor is capable of detecting harmful events that lead to hypoxic episodes. Using an oxygen-sensitive probe that is inserted into brain tissue for continuous monitoring of partial pressure of brain tissue oxygen (**PbtO₂**) has been found to be accurate, safe, reliable, and sensitive, with good long-term stability. A device, approved by the U.S. Food and Drug Administration in 2000, provides a rapid and potentially more accurate indicator of cerebral oxygenation, thereby allowing for earlier intervention into the prevention of secondary brain injury.[38] Monitoring the partial oxygen pressure of local brain tissue is a safe and reliable method for regulating cerebral oxygenation. Because brain tissue hypoxia occurs often and is significantly related to poor outcome, future efforts should be aimed at the treatment of brain tissue hypoxia.[77]

The brain is highly susceptible to alterations in oxygenation because of its high metabolic energy needs and inability to store oxygen. Multimodal intracranial monitoring may include ICP, CPP, brain temperature, and PbtO$_2$, as well as jugular venous bulb (SjvO$_2$), which monitors global tissue oxygen consumption. The ability to have additional information regarding up-to-date status of brain tissue oxygenation and to indicate the need for early interventions and treatment for local changes versus global changes is weighed against the additional costs, supplies, resources, and expertise of the bedside clinicians (see Chapter 9).

Medical Management

According to the past guidelines published by the joint project of the Brain Trauma Foundation and the American Association of Neurological Surgeons, an absolute and uniformly applicable ICP threshold is unlikely to exist. However, current data support 20 to 25 mm Hg as an upper threshold above which treatment to lower ICP should generally be initiated.[14]

The guidelines for ICP monitoring for head injury are appropriate if patients have the following:

- An abnormal CT scan that reveals hematomas, contusions, edema, or compressed basal cisterns and a GCS score of 3 to 8 after cardiopulmonary resuscitation (CPR)
- A normal CT scan if two or more of the following features are noted on admission: age over 40 years, unilateral or bilateral motor posturing, or systolic blood pressure less than 90 mm Hg

Hyperventilation. **Hyperventilation** is one of the immediate first-line medical interventions for rapid control of ICP. After intubation, the patient can be mechanically ventilated to maintain PaCO$_2$ at 30 to 35 mm Hg for better cerebral tissue perfusion and to constrict the cerebral arteries for decreased CBF. However, hyperventilation is now thought to be effective only briefly for the transient control of ICP. Carbon dioxide reactivity is relatively short lived, and prolonged hyperventilation may be counterproductive or cause a rebound vasodilation effect when discontinued. **Posthyperventilation apnea** may occur if oxygenation is not sufficient to prevent hypoxia or if the PaCO$_2$ level is too low for that individual patient.

Over time, the body's renal mechanism begins to compensate for the prolonged respiratory alkalosis created by hyperventilation and returns CBF to normal. Hyperventilation is also known to elevate the pH up to 7.55. To determine whether hyperventilation is beneficial to the patient, the clinician should allow the PaCO$_2$ to return to normal limits (35 to 45 mm Hg) and should observe for any ICP elevation. Hyperventilation should be gradually discontinued if the ICP remains within normal limits.

Hyperventilation has been used temporarily in certain situations to reduce ICP. Guidelines for severe TBI have recommended that, in the absence of increased ICP, chronic prolonged hyperventilation therapy (PaCO$_2$ $\leq$29 mm Hg) should be avoided, particularly during the first 24 hours after injury, because it can compromise CPP during a time when CBF is reduced. Options include hyperventilation for brief periods when there is acute neurologic deterioration or for longer periods when there is intracranial hypertension refractory to sedation, paralysis, CSF drainage, and osmotic diuretics.[14]

Oxygenation. **Artificial oxygenation** may be required to maintain the PaO$_2$ above 80 to 100 mm Hg to ensure that oxygen delivery to the brain exceeds oxygen consumption. The prevention of hypoxemia is critical. A PaO$_2$ below 60 mm Hg is known to precipitate increases in ICP. Hypoxia and hypercapnia produce synergistic effects and increase CBF more than either factor alone.[61] Measurement of jugular venous bulb oxygen saturation (SjVO$_2$) and cerebral oxygen extraction (CO$_2$E) is becoming part of the monitoring protocols on the NCCU.[20,47,66]

In patients with a head injury, hypoxemia has been associated with significant secondary brain injury. Studies have found that prehospital intubation is associated with enhanced survival for patients with severe TBI, particularly patients with low GCS scores; conversely, a PaO$_2$ below 60 mm Hg is to be avoided.[14]

Osmotherapy. Mannitol has remained a standard therapy to increase intravascular osmotic pressure by drawing water from the interstitial space, thus decreasing brain mass. To exert their maximum effect, these agents require an intact blood-brain barrier. If the blood-brain barrier is disrupted, the osmotic agents may pass into the brain, causing cerebral edema and increased brain size.[63] Osmotic diuretics may lead not only to cerebral edema but also to acute renal failure as serum osmolality increases. Mannitol (20% to 25% solution) is an osmotic agent commonly used because it has a rapid effect on ICP; its peak effect in lowering ICP occurs within 10 to 15 minutes.[52] It reduces blood viscosity and lasts approximately 2 to 6 hours. It is given intravenously in doses ranging from 0.5 to 2.5 g/kg or 0.25 to 1 g/kg with a smaller dose equally effective in some cases and with less effect on serum osmolality. A **serum osmolality** (the osmotic pressure of a solution expressed in mOsm/kg of water) that exceeds 310 to 320 mOsm has been shown to be dangerous and can lead to hyperosmolar coma. Serum osmolality can be measured by the laboratory or estimated via calculation using the following formula:

$$2 \times \text{Serum Na} + (\text{BUN} \div 3) + (\text{Glucose} \div 18)$$
$$= \text{Serum osmolality } (285 - 295 \text{ mOsm/kg H}_2\text{O})$$

The patient receiving osmotic agents should be monitored for hypotension and a urinary output of at least 30 to 50 ml/hr before further administration. After administration, rapid diuresis can be expected. Strict intake and output (I&O) should be measured to record fluid status and monitor for circulatory overload, pulmonary edema, and congestive heart failure (CHF). Side effects from prolonged use of mannitol include hypotension, tachycardia, hemoconcentration, intravascular dehydration, a rebound cerebral edema effect, reduced CBF, and impaired renal function. The rebound effect occurs when water moves from healthy brain tissue, leaving the injured tissue to act as a sponge[63] and pulling fluid into the cell. This action further increases the swelling and as a result increases ICP. Reducing cerebral volume in the injured brain with intracranial bleeding could precipitate a new hemorrhage.

Mannitol has been advocated as a "small-volume resuscitation fluid" to be administered in bolus versus continuous intravenous (IV) infusion. The latest guidelines for treating severe TBI with mannitol before ICP monitoring are signs of tentorial herniation, or progressive neurologic deterioration not attributable to extracranial explanations. The administration of mannitol is common practice in head injury management because it is consistently effective for controlling raised ICP, with the effective dose ranging from 0.25 to 1 g/kg of body weight.[14]

The use of **hypertonic saline (HTS)** as osmotherapy has increased with evidence of its effectiveness as an agent for reducing cerebral edema and in brain resuscitation following brain injury. The advantages may include osmotic mobilization of water across the BBB to reduce cerebral water or augmentation of blood flow and the ability to rapidly achieve and maintain a hypernatremic state as a less expensive and safe continuous infusion. Acceptance in the critical care arena is gaining momentum as clinicians gain experience and understand the hemodynamic profile of HTS therapy and as more data become available (see details below).

Steroids. Controversy continues over the effectiveness of **corticosteroid therapy.** It has been theorized that steroids may be useful in restoring altered vascular permeability in the presence of brain edema. Steroids such as dexamethasone (Decadron) may stabilize cell membranes to reduce leakiness in the BBB, increase CSF resorption, shift the oxygen dissociation curve for easier release of oxygen, and reduce vasogenic edema. The administration of glucocorticoids is common practice in the treatment of edema that accompanies brain tumors. Steroids may therefore increase intracranial compliance. The undesirable side effects of steroids must be weighed against the therapeutic effects. Gastrointestinal (GI) hemorrhage, suppression of the immune system that masks infection, elevated blood pressure, elevated serum glucose levels, and possible hypokalemia are some of the adverse reactions that must be monitored in patients who are receiving steroid therapy.

In the treatment of severe TBI, clinical trials with steroids have revealed no overall beneficial effect on outcome. Therefore the use of steroids is not recommended to reduce ICP in patients with severe head injury.[14] The report from the largest trial ever conducted for TBI, the Corticosteroid Randomisation After Significant Head Injury (CRASH) trial, indicated that the early in-hospital mortality rate after use of corticosteroids was higher than in the control group (23% verus 18% mortality rate).[16]

Diuretics. Diuretics have been shown to be effective in decreasing ICP. Furosemide (Lasix) works by decreasing circulating blood volume and reducing edema. Used before or in conjunction with osmotic agents, it rids the body of water by pulling it from the brain and depositing it in the cardiovascular system. Lasix reaches its maximum effect in about 1 hour. Older patients at risk for pulmonary edema especially benefit from diuretic therapy.

Lasix may also decrease sodium uptake by the brain and reduce the production of CSF.[51] Ethacrynic acid (Edecrin) works in the same manner as Lasix to inhibit the reabsorption of sodium and chloride at the proximal portion of the ascending loop of Henle. Acetazolamide (Diamox) has been administered to reduce CSF formation. The use of diuretics is limited by renal function, electrolyte imbalance, age, and the extent of any renal impairment. The use of concomitant diuretics (e.g., furosemide) along with mannitol boluses in the treatment of severe head injury has not been advocated.[14]

Sedatives and Analgesics. Physician preference guides the selective use of **sedatives** in the patient with increased ICP. Morphine sulfate (MS), either in small IV boluses or by continuous infusion in doses of 2 to 8 mg/hr, permits continuous assessment of the pupils while assisting in blunting the effects of noxious stimuli in the ICU environment. In spite of published reports to the contrary, MS does not mask pupillary dilation if transtentorial herniation occurs.[58]

Fluids. Fluid administration to eliminate excess body water usually calls for an intake of 1000 to 1500 ml per 24 hours. A strict accounting of I&O and central venous pressure (CVP) measurements help in monitoring for potential fluid overload and attaining normovolemia. Colloids are appropriate for fluid replacement in patients with increased ICP. Hypotonic or glucose-containing solutions contain diffusible substances that move passively into the brain to increase brain edema, thus placing the patient at greater risk for increased ICP. For patients who have lost large volumes of blood, rapid restoration of blood is required to promote hemodynamic stability with adequate oxygen-carrying capacity.[58]

Guidelines for severe head injury have included hypertonic saline and mannitol as resuscitation fluids. It is critical to prevent hypotension following severe head injury. Fluid administration should be titrated to maintain a mean arterial blood pressure greater than 90 mm Hg. This is done through the infusion of fluids throughout the patient's course of treatment to maintain a CPP above 70 mm Hg.[41]

Studies using hypertonic saline solution (HSS) indicate that 7.5% saline solution may be a promising approach for the control of elevated ICP in patients with an exhausted response to mannitol and barbiturates. One study found that ICP was reduced by the administration of repeated boluses of HSS to patients with TBI and subarachnoid hemorrhage.[41] Another report found that use of HSS appears to be an inexpensive and reasonably effective treatment for intracranial hypertension. Close monitoring of side effects, including serum sodium, potassium, and serum osmolarity every 4 to 6 hours, is critical, especially adverse side effects of renal failure.[55]

Pharmacologic Agents. The types of pharmacologic agents often prescribed for patients with increased ICP are listed in Box 10-9.

BOX 10-9 | **Pharmacologic Agents Prescribed During Periods of Increased Intracranial Pressure**

- Anticonvulsants to prevent seizure activity
- Muscle relaxants to decrease agitation, posturing, or "bucking" the respirator
- Opioids in small amounts as needed
- Benzodiazepines for amnesia and anxiety
- Sedation as needed
- Antibiotics for infection control
- Antihypertensive drugs to avoid systemic hypertension
- Beta-adrenergic blockers to act against catecholamine release
- High-dose barbiturate therapy to reduce ICP
- Antacids and H_2 blockers to prevent stress ulcers and GI bleed
- Stool softeners and laxatives to allow normal bowel evacuation without straining
- Sedatives as needed to promote periods of uninterrupted sleep and rest

Data from American Association of Neuroscience Nurses: *Core curriculum for neuroscience nursing,* ed 4, St Louis, 2004, Saunders; Barker E: Myths and facts about increased intracranial pressure, *Nursing* 8(12):20, 1988; Boss BJ: Nursing management of adults with common neurological problems. In Beare PG, Myers JL, editors: *Adult health nursing,* ed 3, St Louis, 1998, Mosby; Brain Trauma Foundation and American Association of Neurological Surgeons: *Management and prognosis of severe traumatic brain injury,* New York, 2000, Brain Trauma Foundation; and Hickey JV: *The clinical practice of neurologic and neurosurgical nursing,* ed 5, Philadelphia, 2003, JB Lippincott. *GI,* Gastrointestinal; *ICP,* intracranial pressure.

Other Interventions and Therapy

Hypothermia. **Hypothermia blankets,** cooling devices, and antipyretics (acetaminophen) are used to keep the temperature of the patient with increased ICP within normal limits; low-dose chlorpromazine is used to prevent shivering. Lowering the temperature decreases intracranial metabolism, decreases cerebral blood flow and volume, and decreases ICP. Cerebral metabolic rate is directly proportional to body temperature. Each degree centigrade rise in body temperature raises the metabolic demands of the brain by approximately 10%.[59]

Hypothermia has been tested over the years with mixed reaction. Brain hypothermia is being used as a neuroprotectant to decompress the increased ICP in acute neuropatients. Scientists in Japan have developed a mathematical model for hypothermic decompression for increased ICP resulting from vasogenic brain edema. Their research suggests the possibility of automatic control of increased ICP in brain hypothermia treatment.[32] Regarding the overall incidence or treatment of raised ICP, a prior study conducted by the National Institutes of Health found no significant differences between normal controls and patients who were treated with therapeutic hypothermia. The study found that hypothermia maintained an ICP at lower levels during the cooling phase at 32 to 33 degrees (rectally) within an average of 10 hours after injury and maintained it for 24 hours. However, rewarming with a gradual return of the patient's temperature to 37° C over 12 hours elevated the ICP slightly above or at the same level of the normothermic patients.[73]

Positioning. The head is maintained midline in the neutral position. **Positioning** creates controversy between the traditional concept that elevating the HOB decreases ICP and the latest concept that lowering the head can also compromise CBF to the brain and lower CPP. If the goal is to maintain adequate CPP, CBF must be maintained to perfuse the brain. One recommendation for positioning during elevated ICP is the 30-degree head position for maximum elevation.[61] One study investigated whether patients with raised ICP should be placed in a horizontal position with the potential to increase CPP and improve CBF. It was found that HOB elevation to 30 degrees significantly reduced ICP in the majority of patients without reducing CPP and CBF.[27]

Another study on the effect of head elevation on ICP suggests that patients be positioned by individual prescription based on ICP, systemic arterial blood pressure (SABP), and CPP response.[54] Each patient may respond differently to any one position; therefore each patient should be evaluated to determine the optimal position for adequate CPP and normal ICP.

Barbiturate Therapy. Patients considered for high-dose **barbiturate therapy** typically have the following characteristics:

- Severe head injury with intracranial hypertension refractory to maximum standard medical and surgical ICP-lowering therapy
- Hemodynamically stable
- Are salvageable
- Continue to deteriorate from uncontrolled ICP (e.g., ICP >25 mm Hg for >15 minutes)

The patient with increased ICP should be evaluated for barbiturate therapy if the potential for reversal is present. Thiopental coma to manage ICPs greater than 40 mm Hg in patients with severe head injury was associated with a 37% reduction in lactate, a 59% reduction in glutamate, and a 66% reduction in aspartate in the brain's extracellular space.[14] Barbiturate therapy should be considered only in settings with an available and well-prepared team of specialists, the necessary equipment (mechanical ventilators, arterial line, pulmonary artery catheters, central or Swan-Ganz catheters, and electroencephalographic equipment), and laboratory and respiratory support (see Chapter 9). The risks, potential complications, and requirements of this therapy limit its use.

The goal of barbiturate therapy is to reduce ICP and maintain the pressure between 15 and 20 mm Hg. The mechanism of action in barbiturate therapy is thought to result from a decrease in cortical activity, reduced cerebral metabolism and metabolic demands, constriction in cerebral blood vessels and blood volume, decreased formation of ischemic edema, and reduced (approximately 50%) glucose and oxygen demands.

Research to study the effect of high-dose barbiturate therapy for the treatment of head injury found that barbiturates can produce long-term ICP control when other treatments have failed and that absolute ICP control improves ultimate outcome. Pentobarbital appears to exert its cerebral protection and ICP-lowering effects through the following mechanisms:[14]

- Alterations in vascular tone
- Suppression of metabolism

BOX 10-10	Barbiturate Therapy Guidelines

- CT scan and EEG before therapy; may also be used to identify burst suppression during treatment
- Evoked potentials
- ICP monitoring
- Arteriovenous oxygen saturation
- Jugular venous bulb oxygen saturation
- Pulmonary artery pressure to determine hydration status
- Cardiac monitoring and cardiac output measurements
- Correction of fluid volume (if needed)
- Laboratory tests: serum pentobarbital level, osmolarity, phenytoin (Dilantin) level, PT, PTT, BUN, routine chemistry and electrolytes
- Daily weight

Administer a loading dose of pentobarbital 10 mg/kg over 30 minutes via IV push (pentobarbital is slower to cross the blood-brain barrier; thiopental is shorter acting and crosses the blood-brain barrier faster; phenobarbital has a high degree of anticonvulsant effect). Expect an ICP reduction of 10 mm Hg in 10 minutes. If there is no response, administer second dose of 5 mg/kg every hour for three doses. Continue with a maintenance dose of 1 mg/kg/hr to reach and maintain a barbiturate level of 2.5 to 4.0 mg/dl.

The most reliable form of monitoring is the EEG pattern of "burst suppression." The near-maximum reductions in cerebral blood flow (CBF) and cerebral metabolism occur with the suppression of "burst suppression" EEG.

Modified from Long DL, editor: *Current therapy in neurological surgery*, Philadelphia, 1989, BC Decker.
BUN, Blood urea nitrogen; *CT*, computed tomography; *EEG*, electroencephalogram; *ICP*, intracranial pressure; *IV*, intravenous; *PT*, prothrombin time; *PTT*, partial thromboplastin time.

- Inhibition of free radical–mediated lipid peroxidation
- Coupling of CBF to regional metabolic demands such that the lower the metabolic requirements, the less the CBF and related blood volume, with subsequent beneficial effects on ICP and global cerebral perfusion

Barbiturates have been postulated to act on the CNS as scavengers of free radicals, to prevent membrane damage and destruction, and also to reduce seizure activity. Steroid therapy and mechanical ventilation with hyperventilation can be continued during high-dose barbiturate therapy[34] (Box 10-10). If barbiturate therapy fails to control cerebral metabolism, bursts of activity will be viewed on the electroencephalogram (EEG), which indicates that the level of barbiturate therapy is not adequate to suppress electrical activity.

The side effects of barbiturate therapy include hypotension, hypothermia, lactic acidosis, hyperosmolarity, and decreased cardiac output. It should be noted that drug levels in barbiturate therapy may be unreliable as the drug is stored in fatty tissue. Undesirable side effects should be treated immediately to avoid complications. Maintaining the patient's temperature between 27° and 33° C helps prevent cardiac irritability and arrest. The demonstration of a 30- to 60-second burst-suppression pattern on the EEG has been correlated with effective therapy.

Bispectral index (BIS) monitoring provides an objective way to assess sedation in patients who are on mechanical ventilation, are receiving neuromuscular blockage, or are in a barbiturate coma. When the sensor strip with three EEG electrodes is placed on the patient's forehead, the Bispectral Index calculates the BIS and provides a numerical scale that correlates to sedation endpoints and allows the clinician to adequately assess sedation. Using a sedation protocol, target sedation orders are based on objective numbers. For example, a BIS score of 100 indicates that the patient is awake and alert. Lower numbers (e.g., 30 to 40) indicate that the patient is unresponsive. The bedside monitor displays the BIS value, the trend over time, raw EEG, signal quality, and suppression ratio.

The withdrawal of barbiturate therapy depends on one of the following conditions: resolution of the disease process, management of other forms of therapy, or death of the patient. Barbiturate therapy can be tapered and withdrawn when the ICP is sustained at a level of less than 20 mm Hg.[51] The drug usually clears in 4 to 5 days after discontinuation of the therapy. Seizure activity, agitation, and other mild symptoms that occur after the termination of barbiturate therapy can usually be offset with the appropriate medications.

Surgical Management

When increased ICP is the result of a space-occupying lesion, timely resection of the mass lesion may reduce ICP. Craniectomy with surgical removal of any underlying cause for dural expansion may eliminate the potential for herniation. A bilateral craniectomy alone can lower ventricular pressure to approximately the level of the initial ICP, and dural expansion can further decrease it by 35% in patients with massive brain swelling.[83] Cranial surgery is discussed in Chapter 8.

Hydrocephalus secondary to increased ICP with excessive accumulation of CSF that dilates the ventricles may require surgical intervention. A permanent **shunt** procedure may be required for patients with **hydrocephalus** (see Chapter 8).

There is no clear role for **decompressive craniotomy (DC)** for intracranial hypertension (ICH) treatment in the literature. Actually there is a lack of class I or II published data for DC. It is recommended as a second tier for **refractory intracranial hypertension.** Some neurosurgeons favor the early application of DC for posttraumatic hypertension.

Acute Care

The current goal of acute care for patients with increased ICP is to maximize the potential for recovery, eliminate the cause of the increased ICP (if possible), reduce or prevent increases in ICP or decreases in CPP, provide appropriate interventions and family support, and evaluate the effects of therapy.[56]

An NCCU flow sheet is a suitable tool and guide for assessment and for recording the data described in Box 10-11. The clinician uses the data from the patient's completed admission database, neurologic assessment, and diagnostic studies to develop a management plan that incorporates the concepts of treatment of increased ICP. The expected outcome is that the resting ICP is maintained within the normal limits of 0 to 15 mm Hg.

BOX 10-11   Acute Care Management of Increased Intracranial Pressure

- Patient's level of consciousness (LOC): Glasgow Coma Scale (GCS) score, with documentation and reporting of changes to physician
- Verbal response and subjective complaints (e.g., headache)
- Eye-opening response, diplopia, blurring of vision, change in visual acuity
- Pupillary signs: size, shape (ovoid pupil), equality, and light reaction
- Motor function: strength of all extremities, paresis, flaccid paralysis
- Sensory status: touch and pain, decreased sensory status
- Airway and oxygenation status, ABG studies and pulse oximetry, mechanical ventilation, hyperventilation, suctioning
- Vital signs: widening pulse pressure (systolic pressure minus diastolic pressure equals pulse pressure [S − D = PP]), vital sign changes are late signs of intracranial hypertension
- Temperature: elevated; use of external cooling devices and interventions
- Heart rate and rhythm
- Blood pressure: mean systemic arterial pressure (MSAP), elevated systolic pressure (systolic pressure minus diastolic pressure equals pulse pressure [S − D = PP])

- Respiratory rate and pattern: identify abnormal patterns (e.g., Cheyne-Stokes respiration, Biot's respiration, and other abnormal patterns)
- Pulse rate: bradycardia or tachycardia
- Brainstem response: gag, corneal, oculocephalic, oculovestibular reflexes
- Fluids: administration and use of hypertonic fluids; I&O
- Vomiting without nausea; projectile vomiting
- Seizure activity: description, duration, and interventions
- Cardiac status: dysrhythmias
- Positioning: performed according to orders, with patient's neck in neutral position and an avoidance of hip flexion
- Activity level: bed rest, agitation, restlessness, following of commands, range of motion, REM sleep
- ICP, CPP, brain tissue oxygen pressure ($PbtO_2$) or temperature recordings
- Ventricular drainage: level of collection device, amount, color, consistency, timing of openings to drain CSF to lower ICP
- Medications: hyperosmotics/osmotics, analgesics, antipyretics, anticonvulsants
- Wound: surgical sites with drainage, description, dressing changes

Data from American Association of Neuroscience Nurses: *Core curriculum for neuroscience nursing,* ed 4, St Louis, 2004, Saunders; Barker E: Myths and facts about increased intracranial pressure, *Nursing* 8(12):20, 1988; Boss BJ: Nursing management of adults with common neurological problems. In Beare PG, Myers JL, editors: *Adult health nursing,* ed 3, St Louis, 1998, Mosby; Brain Trauma Foundation and American Association of Neurological Surgeons: *Management and prognosis of severe traumatic brain injury,* New York, 2000, Brain Trauma Foundation; Hickey JV: *The clinical practice of neurologic and neurosurgical nursing,* ed 5, Philadelphia, 2003, JB Lippincott.
ABG, Arterial blood gas; *CPP,* cerebral perfusion pressure; *CSF,* cerebrospinal fluid; *I&O,* intake and output; *ICP,* intracranial pressure; *REM,* rapid eye movement.

For clinicians proficient in direct funduscopic examination, the optic nerve head and adjacent vessels can be examined for **papilledema.** Optic disc swelling resulting from increased ICP can usually be visualized when the patient begins to develop signs of ataxia, altered LOC, headache, nausea and vomiting, and diplopia. If left untreated, elevated ICP leads to vision loss as pressure on the optic nerve causes ischemia and optic nerve atrophy.

Patients with suspected increased ICP need some form of continuous monitoring. Depending on the degree of increased ICP, the patient may require only 24-hour nursing observation with frequent neurologic assessment until the potential for raised ICP has been eliminated, or the patient may require multimodality invasive hemometabolic monitoring. Management incorporates the patient's acuity level, high-risk clinical diagnoses, appropriate treatments to improve outcome, and prevention of complications.[50]

Standard ICU nursing measures and cardiac monitoring are required for patients with increased ICP. In addition, ICP monitoring may be ordered. The goal of continuous ICP monitoring is to provide a standardized method of direct pressure measurement and CSF drainage when clinically indicated. The patient can be expected to have a better neurologic outcome if the CPP can be maintained above 60 to 70 mm Hg and the ICP below 15 to 20 mm Hg. ICP data

provide a valuable prognostic tool in many cases. Advantages of direct monitoring include waveform analysis, a display of mean ICP for rapid assessment and intervention, calculation of CPP, calculation of CSF drainage, and treatment based on actual ICP elevation. With a monitor in place, early treatment can prevent the development of intractable ICP. The effects of treatment can also be evaluated based on results of the ICP waveform pattern and recordings.

Patients in whom ICP can be maintained below 20 mm Hg have an improved neurologic outcome. The measurement and continuous monitoring of ICP and CPP are an accepted invasive modality available in most NCCUs.

Obstruction of jugular veins or an increase in intrathoracic or intraabdominal pressure is to be avoided because this pressure is communicated as increased pressure throughout the open venous system, thereby impeding drainage from the brain and increasing ICP. Trendelenburg, prone, and extreme flexion positions of the hips (for bedpan placement) should be avoided.[74]

A restless patient may require a stiff collar or rolled towels, sandbags, or wrapped IV bags on each side of the neck to ensure that the head is midline for good cerebral arterial blood supply and adequate venous return through the jugular veins. Tight clothing or anything that constricts or compresses the jugular area should be avoided. Activities that might increase ICP should be scheduled at intervals—not in clusters. If the ICP monitor shows significant increases during care and treatment, the patient should be returned to an elevated-head position, the neck should be straightened, and the patient should be returned to rest.[7,11,34] Bruya[15] found that a 10-minute planned rest period between nursing activities was too short to have any noticeable effect on ICP. Talking about the patient's condition at the bedside should be avoided. Stool softeners and measures to eliminate the Valsalva maneuver and straining are also recommended.

Jugular Venous Oxygen Saturation Monitoring. A technique has been proposed to diagnose cerebral ischemia that allows for the continuous monitoring of cerebral oxygenation by fiberoptic catheter oximetry and the simultaneous measurement of arterial and jugular bulb oxyhemoglobin saturation, CPP, and expired carbon dioxide. Jugular bulb oxygen saturation (SjO_2) monitoring is a new method designed to supplement conventional monitoring.[20,47,72] As the blood returns from the brain to the systemic circulation via the jugular vein, a fiberoptic catheter inserted into the jugular vein is used to monitor the oxygen content of the returning blood.

Normal values for SjO_2 are 55% to 70%. If the brain is deficient in oxygen, the brain is oligemic and the SjO_2 remains below 55%. Hyperemia or barbiturates can increase SjO_2. The term **oligemic cerebral hypoxia** defines a state of cerebral hypoxia in which the arterial oxygen content is normal but CBF is critically reduced in relation to cerebral oxygen consumption.[20] Ischemia-infarction episodes and hypoxia may be detected with this new technique if it gains acceptance as an accurate and reliable monitoring device.

Drainage of Cerebrospinal Fluid. The ventricular drainage method has the capability to allow CSF drainage continuously or intermittently as needed. Orders or protocols usually allow the clinician to open the closed system for brief periods when ICP exceeds the set limits. An immediate decrease in ICP can be observed as excess CSF is drained. REM sleep is one example of a situation in which drainage quickly reduces ICP. In situations of bloody CSF, continuous drainage may be ordered to flush blood from the ventricles. Replacement of the system is required for patients with a subarachnoid hemorrhage during which bloody CSF is so thick that it completely occludes the system.

Potential Complications of ICP Monitoring. ICP monitoring is not without adverse effects. After 5 days of monitoring, particularly if the system is opened, complications can occur. Complications to avoid are bacterial colonization with a positive CSF culture that indicates infection (bacterial meningitis),[48] intercerebral hemorrhage, CSF leak, mechanical equipment failure, CSF overdrainage, and hematoma at the site. The main complication is hemorrhage. Improper placement or technical problems occur when the catheter it inserted incorrectly or too deep (e.g., a thalamic hemorrhage).

The patient should be evaluated daily for clinical symptoms and evidence of infection. Frequent CSF cultures, laboratory studies (white blood cell and differential count), and temperature evaluations help identify the first indications of CSF colonization. Written guidelines should be available for all aspects of monitoring from equipment use, to cleaning, to storing, and to dressing changes. Aseptic guidelines must be followed when the clinician changes or manipulates the system. The hospital infection control personnel and neurosurgical team should maintain records to document people involved in patient care during ICP monitoring to track infection rates and to keep the rate at 1% or less. A study relating infection rate to placement of ICP monitoring found that all patients with IVCs who became infected had a diagnosis of hemorrhage; this suggests that the hemorrhage itself possibly raises the risk of infection.[29]

Cerebral bleeding or hematoma may cause bulging at the incision or decreased LOC. The bleeding or oozing may be self-limiting, may reabsorb, or may require emergency neurosurgery. CSF leaks are usually self-limiting but may also require neurosurgical intervention to seal the leak. Close scrutiny of the monitoring equipment and the drainage system is necessary for early detection of mechanical failure. Catheter replacement may be the quickest and safest method to correct mechanical malfunction. To prevent overdrainage from a ventriculostomy, the clinician should maintain the drip chamber at the prescribed position and secure it on an IV pole or other stable device. A drip chamber should never be allowed to fall below the patient's head and overdrain. This could cause the patient to suffer a severe headache, collapse the ventricles, and result in the rupture of bridging veins or in herniation. Drainage ceases when the chamber is positioned too high.

Patient protocols or guidelines during ICP monitoring may include the use of some type of limb restraint to prevent a restless patient from pulling on the equipment, removal of the headboard for easier access to the patient's head, and dates for changing the tubing, head dressing, and drainage bags. Troubleshooting information for dampened waveform, equipment failure, or other problems should be provided to all staff and be readily available in the NCCU. The physician should be notified when the ICP, CPP, or multimodality monitoring parameters are not within the specified orders.

Intracranial pressure up to 15 mm Hg is considered normal. The following are the categories for ICP elevation:

- Normal ICP: 0 to 15 mm Hg
- Mild elevation: 16 to 20 mm Hg
- Moderate elevation: 21 to 30 mm Hg
- Severe elevation: 31 to 40 mm Hg and above
- Very severe elevation: 40 mm Hg and above

Terminal waves, called the "cross of death," indicate the cessation of cerebral pressure as the ICP equals the systemic arterial pressure.

Intracranial compliance, as estimated from a computerized frequency analysis of the ICP waveform, has been studied and in the future may become an indicator that provides an earlier warning of neurologic decompensation than ICP per se. Further research is needed to demonstrate that such early detection would result in an appreciable improvement in clinical outcome.[65]

Multimodality Monitoring. Multimodality monitoring is available at some institutions and may include monitoring of jugular bulb oxygen saturation (SjO_2) as described previously in addition to standard ICP monitoring, especially in head trauma. A study to determine whether there were modifications of management found that intermittent SjO_2 monitoring did not substantially influence the management, and recommendation for its routine use in all patients seems inadvisable.[9] Other clinicians have found that it is complex and difficult to manage the monitoring equipment in addition to multimodality monitoring for critically ill patients with increased ICP.

A cerebral tissue monitoring system is currently available complete with insertion kits and monitor. Through the single probe and with a small sensor, it continuously measures the partial pressure of oxygen (PO_2) in tissue to detect and help reduce cerebral hypoxia, carbon dioxide to detect acidosis and brain tissue metabolic changes, pH to estimate acidosis and early detection of acidemia, and actual core brain temperature to detect hyperthermia and temperature changes.

The Air-Pouch system used in Germany and in selected sites in the United States, particularly in pediatrics, incorporates an air pouch and a standard transducer that can be placed in the ventricles, in the brain parenchyma, or on the dura to monitor cerebral perfusion pressure. It measures intraventricular pressure using an Air-Pouch mounted in the tip of a dual-lumen probe. This system is compatible with other types of ICP transducers for combination ICP and craniospinal compliance monitoring.

A multiparameter monitor has demonstrated that a catheter can be designed to carry a thermistor to measure temperature in addition to measuring ICP and CPP.[40] Options for safe, accurate, user-friendly comprehensive patient multimodality monitoring enhance the management and decision-making abilities of the health care team.[58]

Multisystem Patient Management. The management of patients with increased ICP is challenging and complex. The patient in the acute phase hangs in delicate balance, and the outcome may be to live, permanent disability, coma, persistent vegetative state (PVS), or death. Families require time to understand and adjust, as their emotions fluctuate with every change in the patient's improving or worsening condition. Preventive measures to decrease the risk of an elevated ICP are to be used throughout all phases of treatment.

Neurologic Interventions

Changes in the LOC, CPP, and ICP tracings in conjunction with the neurologic and cranial nerve assessment previously described constitute the focus of clinical management. The prescribed medications listed previously should be administered as ordered. Any seizure activity should be recorded and reported. Anticonvulsant levels must be maintained within the therapeutic range to prevent breakthrough seizures.

Cardiovascular Interventions

In the acute phase during ICP monitoring, systemic arterial blood pressure must be maintained within normal limits, with the CPP high enough to prevent cerebral vasodilation. The cerebral vasodilatory effect preserves CBF until the mean arterial pressure (MAP) drops to about 60 mm Hg. CPP levels must be maintained at 60 to 70 mm Hg for adequate CBF. Irreversible hypoxia occurs at a CPP of less than 30 mm Hg; when ICP equals the MAP, the CPP is zero and CBF ceases. The vascular bed dilates at an exponential rate to decrements in CPP, and the rapid increase in dilation begins as CPP falls below 80 mm Hg. Maintenance of blood

> **BOX 10-12   Measures to Prevent Increased Intracranial Pressure**
>
> - Elevate head of bed 30 degrees (unless contraindicated).
> - Maintain neck in neutral position without pillows; avoid extreme hip flexion; a headache with head rotation may provide a warning of increased ICP.
> - Provide adequate oxygenation.
> - Prevent hypercapnia.
> - Prevent hypertension and hypotension.
> - Strictly control hydration status.
> - Space activities to avoid fatigue and overstimulation.
> - Prevent Valsalva maneuver and straining.
> - Prevent stressors (e.g., sensory overload, emotional stimuli, talking about the patient's condition at the bedside, noxious noise, pain).
> - Prevent electrolyte imbalance.
> - Observe for *early, subtle* changes in the patient's condition and respond appropriately.
> - Prevent hyperthermia.

Modified from Barker E: Avoiding increased intracranial pressure, *Nursing* 20:64Q, 1990.
ICP, Intracranial pressure.

pressure and the control of CPP become the primary goals in the treatment of ICP. Box 10-12 lists measures to prevent increased ICP.

Protocols or written orders for the control of blood pressure, CSF drainage, and hyperventilation or for the administration of medications to lower ICP allow the clinician to use judgment and decision-making skills to protect the patient on a minute-to-minute basis.

Cardiac monitoring can reveal cardiovascular abnormalities or dysrhythmias from either CNS pathology or autonomic nervous system response. Elevated ST segments, prolonged QT intervals, inverted or tall T waves, and other cardiovascular changes usually respond poorly to cardiac medications. Cushing's reflex in response to brainstem compression that elevates the ICP above 45 mm Hg may precipitate cardiovascular decompensation. These systemic effects should resolve when the ICP comes under control.

Pain and fever are common causes of hypertension. The heart rate increases 20 beats/min for each degree of centigrade elevation of temperature. Elimination of the cause could produce the desired return to normal tension.

Pulmonary Interventions

Controlled ventilation is an important adjunct of respiratory support for the patient with elevated ICP. Monitoring oxygen saturation using pulse oximetry and end-tidal carbon dioxide with arterial blood gas (ABG) measurements assists in providing adequate gas exchange. Carbon dioxide pressure can be reduced with ventilatory settings that produce hyperventilation and subsequent vasoconstriction of the cerebral arteries. FiO2 settings increase inspired oxygen concentration. Pulse oximetry can be used to monitor oxygen saturation. The patient often requires ventilator support with the use of positive end-expiratory pressure (PEEP) to maintain adequate tissue oxygenation, yet the addition of PEEP will increase intrathoracic pressure and decrease venous return from the cranium. Avoid high PEEP. A PEEP greater than 5 to 10 cm H_2O can be counterproductive. The use of high-frequency jet ventilation with continuous bursts of air delivered at 80 to 100 breaths/min is useful to avoid the complications of PEEP.[21]

Potential pulmonary complications include **neurogenic pulmonary edema (NPE),** which is believed to be in direct response to increased ICP and hypothalamic dysfunction and stimulates an abnormal sympathetic discharge.[24] An inadequately perfused and hypoxic pulmonary system responds with platelet clumps in the pulmonary capillaries, producing fluid extravasation into the alveoli. The chest x-ray examination depicts a fluffy infiltrate. The patient exhibits shortness of breath, cyanosis, and tachypnea. NPE may progress to congestive atelectasis, respiratory failure, and a syndrome similar to acute respiratory distress syndrome.[24] NPE occurs rapidly, has a high mortality rate, and is resistant to regular treatment. Treatment is aimed at the underlying cause of raised ICP and the pulmonary edema. The patient must be turned frequently, and secretions are suctioned only if necessary and are limited to no more than 10 to 15 seconds with 100% oxygenation before and after suctioning. A plan that includes chest physiotherapy, deep breathing, and coughing is recommended.

Respiratory patterns may be erratic when ICP is elevated and reflect the location, or cerebral compartment, of the increased pressure (see Fig. 10-9). The patient's airway must be assessed for patency, the lungs auscultated for breath sounds, the respirations evaluated for rate and pattern, and the color observed for evidence of cyanosis. Ventilated patients must be turned and the airways suctioned as necessary. Neuromuscular blocking agents may be ordered if the patient fights or "bucks" the ventilator. Sedation with neuromuscular blocking agents is also required.[59] Blood samples for ABG studies should be drawn at frequent intervals to closely assess the adequacy of ventilation, oxygenation, and acid-base status. CVP readings, weight changes, and peripheral or pulmonary edema reflect fluid status and should be used to determine adjustments.

The partial pressure of carbon dioxide and oxygen in arterial blood ($PaCO_2$ and PaO_2) can be affected by endotracheal suctioning (ETS) and are variables of concern in studies evaluating the effects of ETS on ICP. ETS increases ICP and in most cases elevates MAP. For patients with increased ICP, clinicians should be encouraged to include some method of preoxygenation (hyperventilation, hyperinflation, or increased FiO_2 levels) in their ETS procedure.[67] Preoxygenate and suction only when necessary. Limit the number of passes to only two, each lasting only 10 to 15 seconds to prevent hypoxia and hypercarbia. Unless ordered otherwise, the HOB can be elevated 20 to 30 degrees, with nonflexion of the neck. Although raising the HOB lowers the ICP, it could also precipitate a drop in CPP and arterial blood pressure. Codeine sulfate may be ordered for sedation.

To prevent raised ICP associated with ETS, 2% **lidocaine** in the dose range of 1.5 mg/kg, given intravenously 2 minutes before suctioning, has been suggested as an effective drug. If the endotracheal tube route is chosen, 2 ml of 4% lidocaine

can be administered; however, this administration can stimulate the cough reflex, which makes the dose unreliable. The mechanism by which lidocaine works is not known. It does block the cough reflex for about 5 minutes and in this range has minimal effect on hemodynamics and LOC. Other drugs are being tried experimentally or in combination with neuromuscular blocking drugs and topical anesthetics.

Aggressive **chest physiotherapy** supervised by clinicians and in conjunction with respiratory therapy or pulmonary medicine consultation helps prevent atelectasis and pneumonia. The team should review daily or frequent chest x-ray studies to detect respiratory changes. The ICP drainage system can be left open during chest physiotherapy, and all monitor displays should be watched closely. The ventilator alarms should be maintained within appropriate limits and the equipment checked for disconnections, kinks, or water in the tubing.

Renal Interventions

The fluid and electrolyte status of the patient should be maintained with strict I&O measurements and a urinary catheter in place. Observing for polyuria or oliguria and other criteria (see Chapter 5) can prevent diabetes insipidus (DI). The balance between dehydration and overhydration is difficult in patients who are receiving diuretics and hyperosmolar agents for ICP control.[71] To prevent overhydration, the clinician may request the IV pharmacist to mix antibiotics and other medications in smaller volumes of fluid. A strict accountability of feeding, IVs, oral intake, flushing of lines, and total output should be carefully calculated for each shift and every 24 hours to detect trends that signal fluid status complications.

Data concerning IV fluid therapy suggest that certain patients at risk for increased ICP (e.g., those with focal brain injury) may benefit from a slightly hypertonic solution (1.8% saline) versus a hypotonic solution to lower ICP and to improve CBF and oxygen delivery. A study by Shackford, Zhuang, and Achmaker[71] found that hypotonic solutions may contribute to secondary injury.

Gastrointestinal Interventions

Steroids, stress, trauma, brain tumor, and preexisting medical conditions may place the patient at great risk for GI bleeding. H_2 receptor antagonists, proton pump inhibitors, antacids, and tube feeding solutions should be used to keep the gastric pH below 4 to 5. Gastric decompression with a nasogastric tube, head elevation, and the side-lying position are effective interventions to prevent aspiration.

Bowel sounds should be elicited, the abdomen palpated, and a bowel program initiated with stool softeners to prevent constipation with straining and to prevent the Valsalva maneuver.

Musculoskeletal and Skin Interventions

Prolonged steroid use causes delayed wound healing, various skin eruptions, easy bruising, petechiae, and skin that becomes thin and fragile with a shiny appearance. Pressure from immobility and shearing from repositioning are to be avoided. A "lift" or turning sheet is advised with turning every 2 hours unless contraindicated. The patient's head should be supported and the neck maintained in the neutral position as the patient is turned in a "logroll" fashion. Sandbags, IV bags, or, if the patient is very agitated, a soft or rigid collar can be used to extend the neck for adequate venous return. The clinician should avoid using restraints that may cause skin irritation and breakdown when patients work against them. Lamb's wool or appropriate padding can be inserted between the restraint and the patient's skin to reduce friction if restraints cannot be avoided. The clinician should follow hospital policies for patient restraint.

Passive range-of-motion (ROM) exercises every shift with appropriate splinting protect the joints and help prevent foot-drop and contractures. A consultation with the rehabilitation team for evaluation and treatment of these and other problems will prevent complications of immobility.

Pain Interventions

Increased pressure in the patient's head combined with stretching of the dura causes extreme cephalalgia (headache). The clinician should assess for pain in the head and offer appropriate medications for comfort and restlessness. Mild analgesics ranging from acetaminophen to codeine phosphate may provide relief. Opioids should be used cautiously, but small doses of morphine sulfate (MS) and fentanyl have decreased agitation and pain, resulting in a lowering of ICP. Some opioids may not be recommended as a central analgesic for patients with increased ICP because they may affect the CNS, LOC, and pupil reaction and may also lower the threshold for seizures (see Chapter 23).

Postacute and Nonacute Care

Transfer to a postacute unit is appropriate after the patient's elevated ICP has been reduced, the ICP monitoring discontinued, and the patient's condition stabilized. Brain edema from a severe cerebral insult reaches its peak in about 72 hours. Despite aggressive treatment, cerebral edema resolves very slowly, taking weeks or months for CT or MRI scans to document complete resolution. Therefore the role of the clinicians at this level is to continue close evaluation with neurologic checks and vital sign monitoring every 4 hours or according to unit policy and to provide the prescribed medical treatment. The focus is on the prevention of edema or increased ICP. A transfer to a nonacute unit should be considered as the GCS score improves and as the underlying cause of increased ICP responds adequately to treatment, as the patient is able to take fluids and nourishment by mouth, and as the vital signs stabilize (Box 10-13).

With the control of ICP, improvement in the patient's condition, and increased exposure to the patient via extended visiting hours, the family's concerns shift from "Is my loved one going to live or die?" to "What will be the outcome of the illness and what will be the lifelong effect?" If the patient is showing progressive signs of recovery, the clinician can reassure the family while cautioning that edema and recovery from elevated ICP is a slow process.

Families of patients who remain in a PVS (see Chapter 6) or whose condition continues to deteriorate with no hope of complete recovery need the support services of the institution. The clinician should make arrangements for the appropriate consultations. A hospital support group can be very therapeutic at this time.

BOX 10-13 Recovery Following Increased ICP

A patient's recovery from increased ICP and the length of the patient's stay in the NCCU depend on several factors:

- The initial underlying cause of increased ICP (e.g., head injury, brain tumor, subarachnoid hemorrhage, Reye's syndrome)
- Any compounding complications that significantly delay recovery (e.g., complications from the original disease that may continue even after the ICP is controlled)
- Failure of an increased ICP to respond to conventional treatments, even the use of decompressive craniotomy, or barbiturate therapy as a "last ditch" effort
- The inability of the patient to survive despite the best medical treatment and excellent clinical management
- Age—mortality rate is higher in the older population, who do not tolerate extensive therapy as well as younger patients

Centers with extensive experience with large patient populations diagnosed with increased ICP may have better patient outcomes than institutions that lack a specialized team and sophisticated equipment. Researchers worldwide continue to study this complicated disorder and search for better treatments to reduce morbidity and mortality rates.

Anticipatory grieving, depression, fatigue, and exhaustion of the family may be evident. The family, who may not be able to turn to anyone else for understanding, will appreciate extra time and patience by members of the health care team.

Acute and Nonacute Rehabilitation

Rehabilitation needs are directed to the underlying medical condition causing the increased ICP. As soon as the patient is stable, the rehabilitation team provides appropriate support to prevent complications of immobility, such as relieving pressure over bony prominences with assistive devices, preventing dependent edema, and preventing contractures (see Chapter 13). A watchful eye on ICP/CPP monitoring devices will alert physical and occupational therapists when their interventions raise ICP and should be immediately discontinued.

As the patient approaches discharge, neurologic checks and vital signs are required only once per shift or as institution policy dictates. IVs should be discontinued, indwelling catheters removed, and the patient ambulatory (unless he or she is experiencing lingering deficits). Patient and family teaching can concentrate on recognizing signs and symptoms that could signify an elevation in ICP. Written educational material should be reviewed with the patient and family, with instructions to notify the hospital, physician, or health care provider immediately if any symptoms return. Compliance with instructions regarding medications, diet, activities of daily living (ADLs), sleep, and rest must be emphasized, and follow-up visits by home health providers are encouraged. The clinicians should explain and demonstrate hospital equipment or therapeutic devices in the hospital setting, with family members giving a satisfactory return demonstration to verify the correct application.

COMPREHENSIVE PATIENT MANAGEMENT

Nutritional Considerations

Consultation with a dietary specialist during the acute phase is important, because a paralytic ileus often accompanies elevated ICP. For the patient who is hypermetabolic with nitrogen wasting from increased muscle tone, alternatives for nutritional support are gastric, jejunal, and parenteral. Early feeding decisions are individualized between options of IV hyperalimentation or placement of a jejunal or gastric feeding tube and between continuous versus bolus feedings. Caloric expenditure can increase up to 120% to 140%, requiring close calculation of intake versus loss. Jejunal feeding tube or gastrojejunostomy has been placed 3 to 7 days after neurologic injury to replace energy and nitrogen loss requirements and prevent increased mortality risk and improve outcomes. It may take 2 to 3 days to gradually advance feedings for full replacement by day 7. High residuals have been observed in some patients and may be an early warning of increased ICP. Patients with tracheostomy, mechanical ventilation, and feeding tubes should be closely monitored for risk of aspiration and hyperglycemia. All patients should be weighed frequently to monitor weight loss or gain. When recommended, oral feedings are instituted as the patient's condition improves and he or she can swallow without choking and aspiration.

Psychosocial Considerations

The disorder or events that precipitate uncontrolled ICP may happen unexpectedly. The patient and family are unprepared and lack the knowledge to fully understand the seriousness of the diagnosis and the hospital experience. If there is time, the clinician should explain all the procedures to decrease the patient's and family's fear and anxiety. The family should be given permission and encouraged to participate in selected patient care. Families require and deserve regular information, with a mechanism for daily communication and planned sessions for questions and answers with team members to update them on the patient's progress.

A contract can be established with the family and the NCCU nursing staff specifying that one family member or significant other can be selected as the family spokesperson with permission to telephone the NCCU around-the-clock for progress reports from the patient's clinician. The designated person can form a telephone tree with family, friends, and relatives to communicate the patient's status. This communication network prevents the NCCU from receiving numerous phone calls that take the clinicians away from the bedside. It also reassures the family of the clinicians' commitment to establish close communication with the family while stressing patient care priorities.

Therapeutic touch or "soft touch" from a loved one or family member can be viewed as an intervention. Hendrickson's study[36] on ICP changes and family presence found a decrease in ICP when family is present. Walleck's investigation[80,81] reported decreased ICP when family members stroked the patient's cheek. Finally, the results of another small study suggest that the families of head-injured patients with normal ICP can verbally interact with the patients for short periods without significant increases in ICP.[76]

Older Adult Considerations

Initial ICP values are low or normal for approximately 50% of older patients who eventually have abnormal ICP. Older patients with a head injury complicated by conditions such as intracranial hypertension, episodes of apnea or shock, or reoperation for continued mass effect rarely survive with the capacity to care for themselves. A study by Ross and colleagues[68] showed that evaluation of older patients with elevated ICP and other contributing variables at 72 hours is warranted to consider whether aggressive management should be continued.

In general, CBF and metabolism reduce with age. This may be most notable after age 70.[43] MAP and cerebral oxygen consumption rate ($CMRO_2$) also decline. Older adults with increased ICP should be evaluated on an individual basis as cerebrovascular resistance (CVR) shows a reciprocal increase with age.

Health Teaching Considerations

Teaching begins at admission to the NCCU as the patient is determined to be at risk or diagnosed with increased ICP. The clinician explains to the patient and family the reasons for the elevated pressure, the treatment, the procedures involved (e.g., insertion of a monitoring device), and the measures that will be used to reduce the elevation. Important issues are a quiet room with minimal stimuli, avoidance of bedside discussions about the patient's condition, and limits to the number of visitors and the duration of their visits.

Family members need instruction on therapeutic communication and on where and how to touch the patient. When appropriate, families can be taught how to observe the bedside monitors for heart rate to receive feedback on touch and conversation when they interact with their loved one. Monitoring equipment and other devices may shock or frighten the family unless the clinician demonstrates appropriate family interaction. Printed instructional material accompanied by family meetings to answer questions reduces tension and anxiety for the family.

Case Management Considerations

Patients with high-risk neurologic conditions (e.g., severe head injury) often experience increased ICP. The extent and type of case management offered to the patient during the stages of recovery will vary, and more than one case manager may be involved following a catastrophic illness. It is important to provide a coordinated transitional approach until the patient is discharged back home and into the community, where an agency or independent case manager will continue

BOX 10-14	Case Management Considerations

- Is the patient making progress as outlined in the plan of care?
- Has the patient reached his or her maximal functional potential as outlined in the original goals?
- Based on the assessment, is the plan of care appropriate for home care and long-term management?
- What are the skilled or custodial needs that require the attention of the case manager?
- Is the care chronic or custodial? If so, is it covered by the health care payer?
- Have all resources been identified to provide for the total needs of the patient?

Data from Rossi P: *Case management in healthcare: a practical guide,* ed 2, Philadelphia, 2003, WB Saunders.

the treatment plan. Questions to be answered at this time may include those listed in Box 10-14.[69]

After assessment and evaluation of the original plan of care, the necessary changes are made in order to coordinate the skilled care, rehabilitation, equipment and supplies, health teaching, and follow-up care with health care providers to prevent complications and rehospitalization.

CONCLUSION

ICP, CPP, and multimodality monitoring that guides therapeutic interventions are currently employed to guide in the treatment of the injured brain. Direct or indirect monitoring devices measure cerebral oxygenation and perfusion and guide clinicians in providing the appropriate interventions. Analysis of monitoring parameters can be used to implement therapy that can prevent secondary brain injury from cerebral ischemia and edema.

Japanese investigators have shown experimentally that niravoline (RU-51599), a selective kappa-opioid receptor agonist, is effective in reducing ICP and brain water content and in maintaining an adequate CPP, even in the presence of an extradural mass lesion.[10] More research is needed.

As far back as 1925, it was suggested that the pressure of the central retinal vein be recorded to assess ICP. A quick and noninvasive means to determine ICP would have advantages over invasive monitoring. It is now known that the pressure within the optic nerve is exposed to ICP because the optic nerve and nerve sheath have a sleeve of CSF that extends up to the globe. The venous outflow of the entire retina drains through the central vein. With funduscopic examination, the collapse of the central retinal vein can be seen when pressure is increased. Ophthalmodynamometry has been used experimentally in the noninvasive assessment of ICP and has been found relevant for momentary assessment when elevated ICP is suspected.[28]

Continuous long-term measurement of ICP is not yet possible because current sensors are not stable enough to provide accurate measurements for more than a short period of time due to drift and other mechanical problems. A new implantable solid-state sensor that reliably measures ICP for months with minimal drift has been demonstrated. Using animal models, ICP sensors were implanted into the frontal white matter and a fluid-filled catheter was placed in the cisterna magna. The mean ICP and CPP were compared for months and were found to provide accurate and stable data. This method may someday offer hope that the ICP of at-risk patients can be monitored for longer than a few days.[46]

Elevated ICP is one of the biggest challenges in the management of the acutely ill patient with head injury and other neurologic disorders. Expert knowledge, quick decisions, accurate judgment, and a rapid response with appropriate interventions affect the outcome of patients at risk for herniation from increased ICP. With knowledge based on sound scientific principles, managing the care of patients with elevated ICP can be accomplished with competence and confidence.

RESOURCES FOR INTRACRANIAL PRESSURE AND MONITORING

American Association of Neurological Surgeons: 888-566-2267; http://aans.org

American Association of Neuroscience Nurses: 888-557-2266; www.aann.org

Congress of Neurological Surgeons: www.neurosurgeon.org

Brain Trauma Foundation: 523 East 72nd Street, New York, NY 10021; www.braintrauma.org

REFERENCES

1. Albeck MJ, Borgensen SE, Gjerris F, et al: Intracranial pressure and cerebrospinal fluid outflow conductance in healthy subjects, *J Neurosurg* 74(4):597–600, 1991.
2. Altinbas A, Hoogstede HA, Bakker SL: Intracranial hypertension with severe irreversible reduced acuity and impaired visuals fields after oral tetracycline, *Ned Tijdschr Geneeskd* 149(34):1908–1912, 2005.
3. American Association of Neuroscience Nurses: *Clinical guidelines series: intracranial pressure monitoring,* Glenview, IL, 1997, The Association.
4. American Association of Neuroscience Nurses: *Core curriculum for neuroscience nursing,* ed 4, St Louis, 2004, Saunders.
5. American Association of Neuroscience Nurses: *Guidelines: intracranial pressure monitoring,* Chicago, IL, 1997, The Association.
6. Arbour R: Intracranial hypertension: monitoring and nursing assessment, *Crit Care Nurse* 24(5):19–32, 2004.
7. Barker E: Myths and facts about increased intracranial pressure, *Nursing* 8(12):20, 1988.
8. Barker E: Avoiding increased intracranial pressure, *Nursing* 20(5):64Q, 1990.
9. Beindorf AE, Latronico N, Rasulo FA, et al: Limits of intermittent jugular bulb oxygen saturation monitoring in the management of severe head trauma patients, *Neurosurgery* 46(5):1131–1138, 2000.
10. Bemana I, Nagao S, Kuratani H, et al: Niravoline, a selective kappa-opioid receptor agonist, effectively reduces elevated intracranial pressure, *Exp Brain Res* 130(3):338–344, 2000.

11. Boss BJ: Nursing management of adults with common neurological problems. In Beare PG, Myers JL, editors: *Adult health nursing,* ed 3, St Louis, 1998, Mosby.

12. Boss BJ: Concepts of neurologic dysfunction. In McCance KL, Huether SE, editors: *Pathophysiology: the biologic basis for disease in adults and children,* ed 4, St Louis, 2002, Mosby.

13. Bouma GJ, Muizelaar P: Relationship between cardiac output and cerebral blood flow in patients with intact and with impaired autoregulation, *J Neurosurg* 73(3):368, 1990.

14. Brain Trauma Foundation and American Association of Neurological Surgeons: *Management and prognosis of severe traumatic brain injury,* New York, 2000, Brain Trauma Foundation.

15. Bruya MA: Planned periods of rest in the intensive care unit: nursing care activities and intracranial pressure, *J Neurosci Nurs* 13(2):84, 1981.

16. Bullock R, Hesdorffer D: Corticosteroids in TBI: the wider implications of the CRASH trial, *Neurotrauma and Critical Care,* Fall 2005, Rolling Meadows, IL, 2005, American Association of Neurological Surgeons.

17. Cattell E: Neurological system. In Tucker SM, editor: *Patient care standards,* ed 7, St Louis, 2000, Mosby.

18. Cottrell JE, Turndorf H: *Anesthesia and neurosurgery,* St Louis, 1986, Mosby.

19. Crutchfield JS, Narayan RK, Robertson CS, Michael LH: Evaluation of a fiberoptic intracranial pressure monitor, *J Neurosurg* 72(3):482–487, 1990.

20. Cruz J, Miner ME, Allen SI, et al: Continuous monitoring of cerebral oxygenation in acute brain injury: I. Injection of mannitol during hyperventilation, *J Neurosurg* 73(5):725–730, 1990.

21. Cummings R: Understanding external ventricular drainage, *J Neurosci Nurs* 24(2):84, 1992.

22. Cushing H: Some experimental and clinical observations concerning states of increased intracranial tension, *Am J Med Sci* 124:375, 1902.

23. Czosnyka M, Smielewski P, Piechnik S, et al: Hemodynamic characterization of intracranial pressure plateau waves in head-injured patients, *J Neurosurg* 91(1):11–19, 1999.

24. Dettbarn CL, Davidson LJ: Pulmonary complications in the patient with acute head injury: neurogenic pulmonary edema, *Heart Lung* 18(6):583, 1989.

25. Drummond BL: Preventing increased intracranial pressure: nursing care can make the difference, *Focus Crit Care* 17(2):116, 1990.

26. Esposito DP: Who should place and manage ICP monitors?, *Neurotrauma and Critical Care News,* Fall 2005, Rolling Meadows, IL, 2005, American Association of Neurological Surgeons.

27. Feldman Z, Kanter MJ, Robertson CS, et al: Effect of head elevation on intracranial pressure, cerebral perfusion pressure, and cerebral blood flow in head-injured patients, *J Neurosurg* 76(2):207–211, 1992.

28. Firsching R, Schutze M, Motschmann M, Behrens-Baumann W: Venous ophthalmodynamometry: a noninvasive method of assessment of intracranial pressure, *J Neurosurg* 93(1):33–36, 2000.

29. Franges EZ, Beiderman ME: Infections related to intracranial pressure monitoring, *J Neurosci Nurs* 20(2):99, 1988.

30. Frost EAM, editor: *Post anesthesia care unit: current practices,* ed 2, St Louis, 1990, Mosby.

31. Gaab MR, Heissler HE, Erhradt K: Physical characteristics of various methods for measuring ICP. In Hoff JT, Betz AL, editors: *Intracranial pressure VII,* New York, 1989, Springer-Verlag.

32. Gaohua L, Kimura H: A mathematical model of intracranial pressure dynamics for brain hypothermia treatment, *Theoretical Biology* 8(10):463, 2005.

33. Gentleman D, Mendelow AD: Intracranial rupture of a pressure monitoring transducer: technical note, *Neurosurgery* 19(1):91, 1986.

34. Gould KA, consulting editor: *Critical care nursing clinics of North America,* Philadelphia, 1990, WB Saunders.

35. Hayashi M, Handa Y, Kobayashi H, et al: Plateau-wave phenomenon (I). Correlation between the appearance of plateau waves and CSF circulation in patients with intracranial hypertension, *Brain* 114(pt 6):2681–2691, 1991.

36. Hendrickson SL: Intracranial pressure changes and family presence, *J Neurosci Nurs* 19(1):14, 1987.

37. Hickey JV: *The clinical practice of neurologic and neurosurgical nursing,* ed 5, Philadelphia, 2003, JB Lippincott.

38. Hilton G: Cerebral oxygenation in the traumatically brain-injured patient: are ICP and CPP enough? *J Neurosci Nurs* 32(5):278–281, 2000.

39. Hlatky R, Furuva Y, Valadka AB, Robertson CS: Management of cerebral perfusion pressure, *Semin Respir Crit Care Med* 22(1):3–12, 2001.

40. Hoffman WE, Charbel FT, Munoz L, Ausman JI: Comparison of brain tissue metabolic changes during ischemia at 35 degrees and 18 degrees C, *Surg Neurol* 49(1):85–89, 1998.

41. Horn P, Munch E, Vajkoczy P, et al: Hypertonic saline solution for control of elevated intracranial pressure in patients with exhausted response to mannitol and barbiturates, *Neurol Res* 21(8):758–764, 1999.

42. Jellinek DA, Carroll T: Surgical physiology. In Kaye AH, Black PM, editors: *Operative neurosurgery,* London, 2000, Churchill Livingstone.

43. Katzman R, Terry RD: *The neurology of aging,* Philadelphia, 1983, FA Davis.

44. Kerr ME: Nursing management of intracranial problems. In Lewis SM, Heitkemper MM, Dirksen SR, editors: *Medical-surgical nursing: assessment and management of clinical problems,* ed 5, St Louis, 2000, Mosby.

45. Kirkness CJ, Mitchell PH, Burr RL, Newell DW: Intracranial pressure waveform analysis: clinical research implications, *J Neurosci Nurs* 32(5):271–277, 2000.

46. Kroin JS, McCarthy RJ, Stylos L, et al: Long-term testing of an intracranial pressure monitoring device, *J Neurosurg* 93(5):852–858, 2000.

47. Kuluz JW: CNS monitoring in pediatric critical care. Critical Care Pediatrics Conference, March 5, 1992, Lake Buena Vista, FL.

48. Lambert HP: *Infections of the central nervous system,* Philadelphia, 1991, BC Decker.

49. Lee G, editor: *Flight nursing,* St Louis, 1991, Mosby.

50. Littlejohns LR: New technology in critical care, *Surgical Services Management* 3(8):11–13, 1997.

51. Long DL, editor: *Current therapy in neurological surgery,* Philadelphia, 1989, BC Decker.

52. Lyerly HK, editor: *The handbook of surgical intensive care,* Chicago, 1984, Year Book.

53. March K, Wellwood J: Intracranial pressure: concepts and cerebral blood flow. In Bader MK, Littlejohn LR, editors: *Core curriculum for neuroscience nursing,* ed 4, St Louis, 2004, Saunders.

54. March K, Mitchell P, Grady S, Winn R: Effect of backrest position on intracranial and cerebral perfusion pressure, *J Neurosci Nurs* 22(6):375–381, 1990.

55. March P, Bachman T: The use of hypertonic saline solutions in the treatment of intracranial hypertension. Poster presenta-

tion from the Barrow Neurological Institute, St Joseph's Hospital and Medical Center, Phoenix, AZ, AANN Annual Conference, April 2005, Washington, DC.

56. Marik P, Varon J, Fromm R, Sternback GI: Management of increased intracranial pressure: a review for clinicians, *J Emerg Med* 17:711–719, 1999.

57. Marshall LF: Pupillary abnormalities, elevated intracranial pressure and mass lesion location. In Miller JD, editor: *Intracranial pressure VI*, Berlin, 1986, Verlag.

58. Marshall SB, editor: *Neuroscience critical care: pathophysiology and patient management*, Philadelphia, 1990, WB Saunders.

59. Mitchell MS: *Neuroscience nursing: a nursing diagnosis approach,* Baltimore, 1989, Williams & Wilkins.

60. Mitchell PH, editor: *AANN's neuroscience nursing: phenomena and practice,* Norwalk, CT, 1989, Appleton & Lange.

61. Moraine JJ, Berre J, Melot C: Is cerebral perfusion pressure a major determinant of cerebral blood flow during head elevation in comatose patients with severe intracranial lesions? *J Neurosurg* 92(4):606–614, 2000.

62. Nolte J: Synaptic transmission between neurons. In Nolte J: *The human brain,* ed 5, St Louis, 2002, Mosby.

63. Quandt C, de los Reyes R: Pharmacologic management of adult intracranial hypertension, *Drug Intell Clin Pharm* 18:105, 1984.

64. Rauch ME, Mitchell PH, Tyler ML: Validation of risk factors for the nursing diagnosis decreased intracranial adaptive capacity, *J Neurosci Nurs* 22(3):173, 1990.

65. Robertson CS, Narayan RK, Contant CF, et al: Clinical experience with a continuous monitor of intracranial compliance, *J Neurosurg* 71(5):673–680, 1989.

66. Robertson CS, Narayan RK, Gokaslan ZL, et al: Cerebral arteriovenous oxygen difference as an estimate of cerebral blood flow in comatose patients, *J Neurosurg* 70(2):222–230, 1989.

67. Rosenwasser RH, Kleiner LI, Krzeminski JP, Buchheit WA: Intracranial pressure monitoring in the posterior fossa: a preliminary report, *J Neurosurg* 71(4):503–505, 1989.

68. Ross AM, Pitts LH, Kobayashi S: Prognosticators of outcome after major head injury in the elderly, *J Neurosci Nurs* 24(2):88, 1992.

69. Rossi P: *Case management in healthcare: a practical guide,* ed 2, Philadelphia, 2003, WB Saunders.

70. Ruby EB, Stone K, Turner B: The relationship between endotracheal suctioning and changes in intracranial pressure: a review of the literature, *Heart Lung* 15(5):488, 1986.

71. Shackford SR, Zhuang J, Achmaker J: Intravenous fluid tonicity: effect on intracranial pressure, cerebral blood flow, and cerebral oxygen delivery in focal brain injury, *J Neurosurg* 76(1):91, 1992.

72. Sheinberg M, Kanter MJ, Robertson CS, et al: Continuous monitoring of jugular venous oxygen saturation in head-injured patients, *J Neurosurg* 76(2):212–217, 1992.

73. Slade J, Kerr ME, Marion D: Effect of therapeutic hypothermia on the incidence and treatment of intracranial hypertension, *J Neurosci Nurs* 31(5):264–269, 1999.

74. Thelan LA, Davie JK, Urden LD: *Textbook of critical care nursing: diagnosis and management,* St Louis, 1990, Mosby.

75. Thompson JM, McFarland GK: *Mosby's manual of clinical nursing,* ed 2, St Louis, 1989, Mosby.

76. Treloar DM, Nalli BJ, Guin P, Gary R: The effect of familiar and unfamiliar voice treatments on intracranial pressure in head-injured patients, *J Neurosci Nurs* 23(5):295–299, 1991.

77. Van den Brink WA, van Santbrink H, Steyerberg EW, et al: Brain oxygen tension in severe head injury, *Neurosurgery* 46(4):868–878, 2000.

78. Vincent JL, Berre J: Primer on medical management of severe head injury, *Crit Care Med* 33(6):1392–1399, 2005.

79. Vos HR: Making headway with intracranial hypertension, *Am J Nurs* 93(2):28–35, 1993.

80. Walleck CA: Intracranial hypertension: interventions and outcomes, *Crit Care Nurs Q* 10:45, 1987.

81. Walleck CA: The effect of purposeful touch on ICP. Paper presented at the AANN meeting, April 1982, Hawaii.

82. Waxman SG: *Clinical neuroanatomy,* ed 25, New York, 2003, Lange Medical Books/McGraw-Hill.

83. Yoo DS, Kim DS, Cho KS, et al: Ventricular pressure monitoring during bilateral decompression with dural expansion, *J Neurosurg* 91(6):953–959, 1999.

CYNTHIA BLANK-REID,
ROBIN N. MCCLELLAND,
THOMAS A. SANTORA

CHAPTER 11

Neurotrauma:
Traumatic Brain Injury

Traumatic brain injury (TBI), or acquired brain injury, can be defined as a traumatic insult to the brain that is capable of producing physical, intellectual, emotional, social, and vocational changes. Studies indicate that each year approximately 1.5 million Americans sustain a TBI. Of those injured, approximately one-quarter million are hospitalized. It is one of the leading causes of death, with an estimated 50,000 deaths occurring every year in the United States.[14,28] TBI is also one of the leading causes of adult disability. An estimated 5.3 million Americans currently live with disabilities, and each year approximately 80,000 to 90,000 additional individuals become disabled during their most productive years.[55] Approximately 800,000 of those injured receive emergency department or outpatient care, and approximately 270,000 are admitted to the hospital.[14,20,28] TBI has been called a "silent epidemic."

The use of prescription drugs, illegal drugs, and alcohol significantly complicates the assessment and management of a patient with TBI. Early response by highly trained emergency medical service (EMS) personnel with early intubation and rapid transport to the hospital for definitive care has helped reduce prehospital mortality rates. Aggressive resuscitation at trauma centers, early computed tomography (CT) scanning, improved intensive care monitoring, and treatment by a multidisciplinary team have resulted in decreased hospital morbidity and mortality rates.

Despite all these efforts, TBI has a devastating effect on the lives of those injured and on their families. The resulting disability causes a significant loss of productivity and income potential. The cost to society is more than $30 billion annually. Estimates of the average lifetime cost for an individual with severe TBI range from $600,000 to $1,875,000.[14] Survivors of TBI are often left with neuropsychologic impairments that result in disabilities affecting work or their personal life. This will ultimately cause family stress and disruptions; an increased risk for suicide, divorce, and substance abuse; economic hardships; unemployment; and a burden on community, state, and federal agencies.[25,26] Thus TBI is a serious public health problem that mandates continuing efforts in the areas of prevention and treatment.

The reader may refer to Chapter 1 for a review of the anatomic structures and normal physiology of the brain. This chapter focuses on primary versus secondary brain injury; mechanisms of injury; pathophysiology; diagnosis; types of brain injury; medical, surgical, and clinical management; and considerations of comprehensive patient care that relate to patient and family teaching, nutrition, psychosocial concerns, the older adult, rehabilitation and home care, and case management.

INCIDENCE

TBI occurs three times more often in males than in females. The average age of a TBI patient is between 15 and 30 years.[17] TBI crosses all lines of age, gender, race, religion, and socioeconomic status. A majority of patients tend to come from low- to medium-income families and often do not have health insurance. TBI primarily occurs during evenings, nights, and weekends.

ETIOLOGY

Injuries are usually classified by their mechanisms (e.g., blunt or penetrating) and by the type of injury (e.g., focal, diffuse, or fracture). The **mechanism of injury** is the event that caused the injury. Certain mechanisms of injury are associated with specific patterns and may be used to predict the severity of injury. Patients with TBI are injured from either a blunt mechanism, a penetrating mechanism, or a combination of both. Although the most common mechanism of injury associated with TBI is blunt force, neurologic trauma cannot be discussed without mentioning penetrating injuries.[11,40]

Blunt Injuries

Blunt trauma can result from many different causes (Fig. 11-1). The majority of blunt TBI occurs from the following:
- Motor vehicle crashes (e.g., cars, trucks, motorcycles, pedestrians, or bicycle riders)
- Falls
- Acts of violence (e.g., assaults, baseball bats, or other objects)
- Sports-related injuries (e.g., rugby, football, lacrosse, field hockey)
- Other

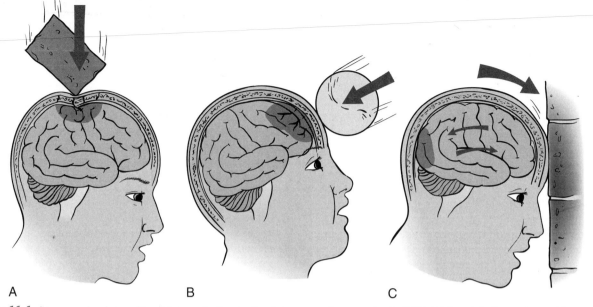

Figure 11-1 Some mechanisms of head injury. **A,** Penetrating injury may fracture the skull. **B,** Diffuse injuries such as a blow to the skull do not result in fractures; they may cause the brain to move enough to tear some of the veins going from the cortical surface to the dura. Note the dark areas of cerebral contusion. **C,** Rebound of the cranial contents may result in an area of injury opposite the point of impact. In addition to the direct damage sustained in the three injuries depicted, additional brain damage may occur. *(From Black JM, Hawks JH: Medical-surgical nursing: clinical management for positive outcomes, ed 7, St Louis, 2005, Elsevier Saunders.)*

The mechanism of injury affects outcome and can result from the following:

- **Deceleration forces:** Injuries result when an individual's head strikes an immovable object, such as the dashboard of a car.
- **Acceleration forces:** Injuries occur when a moving object (e.g., baseball bat) strikes an individual's head.
- **Acceleration-deceleration forces:** Injuries often occur in combination because of the rapid changes in the velocity of the brain within the cranial vault.[47,48]
- **Rotational forces:** These forces refer to the movement of the brain in a side-to-side, twisting manner inside the cranial vault. Rotational injuries often occur in combination with acceleration-deceleration injuries and result in tension and shearing of the brain tissue.
- **Deformation forces:** These injuries are usually the result of direct blows to the head that change the shape of the skull. Such injuries result in a compression of brain tissue. The velocity of the impact determines the extent of deformation and the subsequent injury.[47,48]

Penetrating Injuries

A penetrating TBI can be caused by many things, such as impalement injuries, nail guns, gunshot wounds (GSWs), and stab wounds (SWs). GSWs are the most lethal of all injuries to the brain, and can carry a mortality rate of greater than 90%.[9,11] The pathophysiology of cranial missile injuries is based on three primary events that occur at impact.[9,11]

1. Local parenchymal destruction occurs along the bullet track.
2. A temporary cavity (which may be much larger than the missile's diameter) forms parallel to the primary track and then collapses within milliseconds.
3. A shock and heat wave occurs immediately after the bullet enters the skull and is transmitted throughout the intracranial cavity.

Low-Velocity Injuries

Local parenchymal damage along the bullet path is the most important factor in determining the extent of injury. If the bullet has insufficient energy to exit the skull, it may ricochet off the inner table opposite the entry site or off a dural barrier such as the falx or tentorium, creating a second and occasionally a third track. The course of such a rebounding bullet is highly unpredictable.[11]

High-Velocity Injuries

As the impact energy of a missile increases, temporary cavitation and shock wave effects take on increasing significance in determining the ultimate extent of injury. If the missile crosses vital brainstem structures, the patient usually dies instantly. Even without anatomic disruption of the brain's vital centers, the shock waves themselves can be severe enough to produce transient or permanent medullary failure with cardiopulmonary arrest.[11]

With GSWs to the brain, several secondary phenomena can occur and can lead to death. The pressure wave associated with a bullet that enters the skull can cause distant cerebral injuries such as cerebral contusions and marked increases in intracranial pressure (ICP); such injuries can cause uncal and tonsillar herniation. The mechanism of elevated ICP after a cranial GSW in the absence of hematoma formation is not entirely clear. The blast effect may damage cerebral vessels and may impair autoregulation. The blood-brain barrier (BBB) may be damaged by the shock wave, leading to **vasogenic edema** that occurs in the white matter with loss of autoregulation, increased cell wall permeability, and opening of the tight epithelial junctions that allows plasma protein to leak from the intravascular into the extravascular space. Respiratory arrest may lead to cerebral ischemia, cell death, and **cytotoxic edema** with cellular edema and increase of intracellular fluid of astroglial cell swelling in the gray matter.

Laceration of major cerebral vessels may result in hematoma formation or the development of a traumatic or **pseudoaneurysm.** Local parenchymal damage causes the release of tissue thromboplastin and plasminogen and may result in a **consumptive coagulopathy.** Multiple in-driven bone fragments can create additional areas of brain destruction. Finally, scalp, hair, clothing, and other foreign debris may be pulled in via a vortex effect by the bullet, providing multiple sites for infection.

Stab Wounds

Stab wounds to the head are less common than GSWs in the United States but are more common in countries where guns are not readily accessible. Most stab wounds occur on the left side of the brain because most assailants are right-handed. Neurologic symptoms arise from vessel laceration with hematoma formation, laceration of the brain parenchyma, or cranial nerve injury. Traumatic aneurysm formation, carotid-cavernous fistula, and arteriovenous fistulas occur in approximately half of all SW patients.[11]

PATHOPHYSIOLOGY

TBI can be categorized in several ways, such as intracranial versus extracranial; focal versus diffuse; or mild, moderate, and severe. This chapter categorizes TBI as focal, diffuse, and other.

The mechanisms of injury previously described emphasize the complexity of head injury and the damaging effect that can occur to brain tissue. Besides injury to the cranium, damage may occur to the vascular scalp, the closed bony cranial vault that protects the brain, brain parenchyma, meninges, cranial nerves, cerebral vasculature, and ventricular system.

An understanding of the pathophysiology of TBI has greatly increased during the past two decades. All neurologic damage does not occur at the moment of impact—it is a process. The **primary injury** is defined as the immediate biochemical effects that result from the initial trauma. Primary head injuries include the following:

- Scalp lacerations
- Skull fractures
- Contusions
- Concussions

BOX 11-1 Examples of Secondary Brain Injury

- Cerebral edema
- Hypoxia
- Hypotension
- Hypocapnia
- Hyperthermia
- Sustained increased intracranial pressure (ICP)
- Systemic inflammatory response syndrome (SIRS)
- Anemia
- Electrolyte disturbances
- Vasospasm
- Hydrocephalus
- Seizures
- Infections

- Penetrating injuries
- Hematomas

Although some degree of irreversible damage occurs at the initial or primary injury, TBI is a process in which additional and progressive secondary injury evolves over the minutes, hours, and days following the primary injury. A **secondary brain injury** is anything that worsens the morbidity and mortality risks from the TBI.[12,55] Secondary injuries occur as a complication of the primary injury and are a devastating consequence of the body's physiologic mechanisms. Clinical management is focused on adequately resuscitating the patient and on preventing or minimizing the secondary injuries that accompany the initial injury.[4,5,7,8] As the number, frequency, or severity of secondary injury increases, the prospect of a favorable outcome decreases. Examples of secondary injury are listed in Box 11-1.

To discuss every complication or situation that can cause secondary injury is beyond the scope of this chapter. The publication of the *Guidelines for the Management of Severe Head Injury* by the Brain Trauma Foundation (BTF) and the American Association of Neurological Surgeons (AANS) provides recommendations for practice based on extensive literature reviews.[12] The purpose of this document was to use evidence-based medicine to demonstrate the treatment and prevention of secondary injury.

Focal Brain Injury

Focal injuries account for about half of all head injuries. They are the direct result of trauma to the tissue. In contrast to a diffuse brain injury, a focal brain injury is a localized injury and is limited to a specific, well-defined area. It is the direct result of trauma to the tissue (e.g., contusion, laceration, or intracerebral bleed).

Skull Fractures

The skull has three layers: inner table, diplo, and outer table. The inner and outer table are hard layers of bone, and the diplo consists of cancellous or spongy bone. The skull is very hard and requires a significant amount of force to be fractured. Different types of skull fractures—including linear, basilar, anterior fossa, depressed, and comminuted

BOX 11-2	Types of Skull Fractures

Linear Skull Fracture *Crack; single fx line*

Mechanism of injury: occurs secondary to a force applied over a wide surface area

Percentage of overall skull fractures: accounts for approximately 80%

Location: more than 50% occur in the temporal-parietal area

Extent: may involve either or both of the inner and outer tables of the skull

Outcome: usually benign, except when the fracture crosses a major vascular channel (e.g., middle meningeal artery or dural sinus)

Complications: hemorrhage and epidural hematoma (EDH) may develop

Diagnostic studies: skull x-ray, CT scan

Treatment: generally requires no specific treatment unless it is a basilar skull fracture or involves the base of the skull

Basilar Skull Fracture

Mechanism of injury: usually caused by a direct blow to the base of the skull

Percentage of overall skull fractures: accounts for approximately 20%

Location: commonly arises from an extension of a linear fracture that extends into the anterior, middle, or posterior fossa at the base of the skull

Extent: may traverse air sinuses in the petrous region of the temporal bone

Outcome: depends on the extent of fracture

Complications: dural and brain tissue tears may result because the bones at the base of the skull are sharp and rigid and the brain and its coverings are forced into tight contact with these surfaces; potential for cerebrospinal (CSF) leak with rhinorrhea or otorrhea, hemotympanum, hearing loss, or facial nerve palsy depending on location

Diagnostic studies: CT scan or MRI scans; difficult to diagnose on routine skull radiographs because of the poor visualization of the skull base; therefore patient signs and symptoms are very important

Treatment: goal is to prevent infections with the use of prophylactic antibiotics; CSF leaks may resolve spontaneously within a week; a lumbar drain or surgical repair may be necessary if the CSF leak persists

Anterior Fossa Fracture

Location: usually involves frontal bone, ethmoid, and frontal or paranasal sinuses

Symptoms: characterized by **raccoon eyes** and **rhinorrhea** from bilateral periorbital ecchymosis and free discharge of CSF leak from the nose that occurs in 25% of cases (see Fig. 11-3, *A*); rhinorrhea occurs in 25% of cases and resolves in approximately 2 to 3 days; caution patients against blowing their nose

Middle Fossa Fracture

Location: usually involves fracture of the petrous bone

Symptoms: CSF leak or **otorrhea** with free flow of CSF through the ear (see Fig. 11-3, *B*); 7% of CSF leaks are associated with petrous bone fractures and rupture of the tympanic membrane

Halo sign: yellow ring around bloody drainage on nasal or ear drip pad (see Fig. 11-3, *C*); sample of drainage is sent to the laboratory for accurate testing (rather than using a glucose testing stick)

Hemotympanum: presence of blood in the middle ear; may be associated with hearing loss; packing the ear is avoided; instead a 4 × 4 gauze is placed outside the ear to collect and monitor drainage

Battle's sign: a small hemorrhagic spot behind the ear that may indicate a fracture; develops 12 to 24 hours after the injury (see Fig. 11-3, *B*)

Cranial nerve deficits: CN VII or Bell's palsy (see Chapter 18)

Depressed Skull Fracture

Mechanism of injury: occurs when the bones of the skull are forcefully displaced downward; varies from a slight depression to displacement of the outer table below the level of the inner table

Classification: open **(compound)** or closed **(simple)**

Associated injury: may be accompanied by a concurrent scalp laceration, dural tears, and brain injury directly below the fracture from compression of the tissue below the bony injury and from lacerations produced by the bony fragments

Extent of injury: depends on the amount of brain involved

Treatment: surgical elevation with debridement of fragments, usually within 24 hours

Comminuted Fracture *shattered*

Mechanism of injury: occurs from multiple linear fractures with a depression at the site of impact; originates and radiates toward the site of impact and toward the base of the skull; referred to as **"eggshell fractures"** because the appearance of the skull is similar to that of a cracked eggshell

Treatment: same as for depressed fracture

---

fractures—are described in Box 11-2 and in Figs. 11-2, 11-3, and 11-4.

The assessment of skull fractures is related to the type, extent, location, and signs and symptoms that accompany the fracture. A focused neurologic assessment is needed to determine the impact of the fracture on the underlying brain tissue, whether the fracture was from a blunt or a penetrating force, if the fracture requires surgery or bone replacement with cranioplasty, and if there is evidence of complications (e.g., cerebrospinal fluid [CSF] leak, infection, and brain swelling) associated with the fracture. Treatment is specific to the type of fracture and the need for surgery and patient follow-up.

Contusions

A **cerebral contusion** is when brain tissue has been bruised and damaged in a specific area as a result of a severe **acceleration-deceleration** force or blunt trauma to the head. The Glasgow Coma Scale (GCS) score may range from 9 to 13. Although contusions may occur in any area of the brain, the majority are related to an impact of the brain against the skull and are usually located in the frontal and temporal

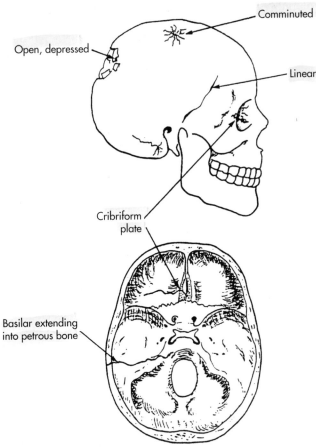

Figure 11-2 Skull fractures. Linear; open, depressed; comminuted fractures; view of base of the skull with fractures.

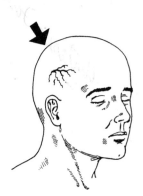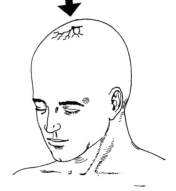

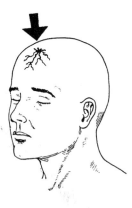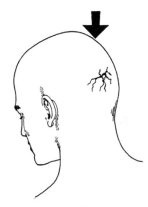

Figure 11-3 Various locations of fractures. Fracture lines originate in the area around the point of impact and radiate toward the base of the skull.

lobes at the poles, around the sylvian fissure, at the orbital areas, and, less commonly, at the parietal and occipital areas (which are more prone to brain lacerations). Other characteristics include the following:

- Tissue alteration and neurologic deficit without hematoma formation
- Significant alteration in consciousness without localizing signs
- Dispersed hemorrhage into the tissue that varies in size from 1 to 3 ml to more than 50 ml[47]
- Cortical and white matter petechial hemorrhages *edema* surrounded by hypodense brain edema

The effects of injury related to contusions (i.e., hemorrhage and edema) peak after about 18 to 36 hours.[9,49] Contusions are characterized as a moderate to severe head injury. They are characterized by loss of consciousness associated with stupor and confusion. Patient outcome depends on the area and severity of the injury.

Temporal lobe contusions carry a greater risk for swelling, rapid deterioration, and brain herniation.[10] These deep contusions are more often associated with hemorrhage and destruction of the reticular activating fibers for arousal.

Coup and Contrecoup Injury

Movement of the brain within the cranial confines causes both contusions and lacerations. These injuries are often

referred to as coup or contrecoup injuries (Fig. 11-5). A coup injury occurs when the damaged area forms directly at the site of impact. A contrecoup injury occurs at the side opposite the injury because of the movement of the brain within the skull. Contrecoup injuries are usually more severe. The size of the area of impact affects the severity of the injury. The smaller the area of impact, the greater is the severity of injury because of the concentration of force in a smaller area.

Hematoma

Three main types of hematomas result from trauma: epidural, subdural, and intracerebral (Fig. 11-6). One third to one half of all TBI patients develop some type of hematoma. One in four patients with skull fractures develops a surgically significant hematoma. The development of a hematoma should be explored if there is any change in level of consciousness (LOC). Mortality rates vary according to the type of hematoma, with a subdural hematoma having the highest mortality rate.[1,19]

Epidural Hematoma. Epidural or **extradural hematomas (EDHs)** account for approximately 1% to 2% of all TBIs and for 20% to 30% of all hematomas.[1,2,19,47] The persons most affected are those in the 20- to 40-year age-group. The

"talk & die"

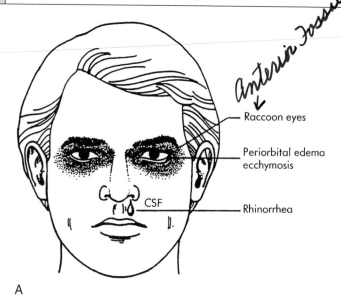

Anterior Fossa fy

- Raccoon eyes
- Periorbital edema ecchymosis
- Rhinorrhea

CSF

A

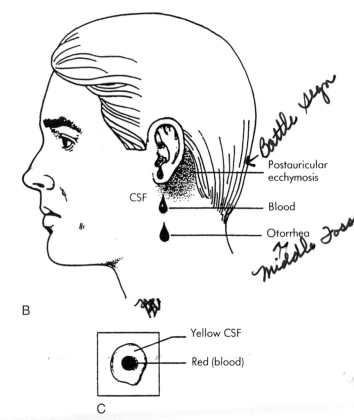

Battle sign

- Postauricular ecchymosis
- Blood
- Otorrhea

CSF

Middle Fossa fy

B

- Yellow CSF
- Red (blood)

C

Figure 11-4 **A,** Raccoon eyes, rhinorrhea. **B,** Battle's sign with otorrhea. **C,** Halo or ring sign.

mortality rate is approximately 8%—the lowest of all hematomas.[47]

EDHs develop from bleeding into the epidural space between the skull and the dura mater. The **middle meningeal artery** runs through a groove in the temporal bone (the thinnest bone of the skull) and is covered by a large muscle mass. A fracture in the temporal bone may cause a tear in the middle meningeal artery, resulting in an EDH.[9,47]

Venous epidural hematomas can occur but are rare and occur from fractures associated with the sagittal or transverse sinuses, which result in venous bleeding. **Posterior fossa epidural hematomas** are associated with fractures across the transverse sinus and constitute approximately 1% to 2% of all EDHs.[9] Because of their positioning, posterior fossa epidural hematomas may cause rapid compression of the brainstem; therefore early operative intervention is necessary to prevent herniation and death.[9]

EDHs are initially characterized by a brief loss of consciousness. This is followed by a lucid interval in which the patient is awake and conversant. The patient then becomes increasingly restless, agitated, and confused; this condition progresses to coma. Herniation is a potential complication of

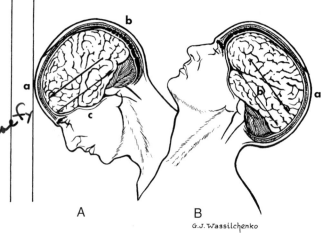

A   B

G.J. Wassilchenko

Figure 11-5 Coup and contrecoup injury. **A,** Coup injury: impact against object. *a,* Site of impact and direct trauma to brain. *b,* Shearing of subdural veins. *c,* Trauma to base of brain. **B,** Contrecoup injury: impact within skull. *a,* Site of impact from brain hitting opposite side of skull. *b,* Shearing forces through brain. These injuries occur in one continuous motion: the head strikes the wall (coup), then rebounds (contrecoup). *(From Rudy EB: Advanced neurological and neurosurgical nursing, St Louis, 1984, Mosby.)*

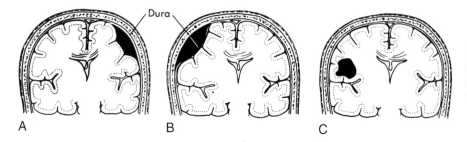

Dura

A   B   C

Figure 11-6 Different types of hematomas. **A,** Subdural (takes on contour of the brain). **B,** Epidural (appears lenticular). **C,** Intracerebral.

EDH; the most common type of herniation syndrome associated with EDH is uncal herniation.[9,47]

With EDHs, an early operative intervention is associated with a more positive outcome.[47] After surgery, 80% of patients have a rapid recovery with little residual neurologic deficit.[9]

Subdural Hematoma. Subdural hematomas (SDHs) are the most common type of hematoma and occur in approximately 10% to 20% of all TBIs. They have the highest mortality rate.[48] SDHs develop from bleeding into the subdural space between the dura mater and the arachnoid, which is usually the result of a rupture of the bridging veins that cross the subdural space.[48] SDHs are most commonly found around the top and sides of the head and are associated with contusions and intracerebral hematomas. They occur bilaterally in 15% to 20% of cases.[47]

There are three types of SDH:

1. **Acute:** An acute SDH occurs within 48 hours after significant impact/injury to the brain. It is nearly always seen with cortical or brainstem injury[9] and represents a mass lesion. An acute SDH results in significant mortality risk because there is injury to the brain tissue, as well as the mass effect caused by the hematoma. The signs and symptoms are those of a rapidly expanding mass lesion or increased ICP, including herniation. Mortality risk decreases when surgical intervention occurs within 4 hours of the injury.

2. **Subacute:** A subacute SDH occurs between 24 and 48 hours to 2 weeks after injury and is associated with moderate TBI. Patients with a subacute SDH show a steady decline in level of response. Bleeding results from ruptured bridging veins, which allows it to occur at a slow rate.[2,3] The hematoma continues to act as a mass lesion; the slower it grows, the better the brain is able to compensate. Surgical removal is required before improvement in the patient's condition is noted.[2,3]

3. **Chronic:** A chronic SDH occurs from 2 weeks to several months after injury. Older adults, chronic alcohol abusers, or those taking the anticoagulant warfarin, Plavix, or aspirin have a higher incidence of this type of injury.[2,3] Patients receiving warfarin need to have their anticoagulation quickly reversed to prevent hematoma growth. There is hope that the use of factor VII will someday assist in the cerebral hematoma damage control process.[33]

A chronic SDH acts as a space-occupying lesion that progressively enlarges. It is often surrounded by a characteristic membrane and may be referred to as a **hygroma.** The mortality rate is 15%.[32,36] A chronic SDH is often bilateral and is usually the result of low-impact injuries such as falling or bumping the head. Patients may have no recall of sustaining an injury or may be unable to relay the event. A chronic SDH is usually treated with burr holes and gradual drainage of the hematoma to prevent recurrence.

Intracerebral Hematoma. Intracerebral hematomas can best be described as large, focal, intraparenchymal hematomas. They are considered mass lesions when they are 25 ml *(frontal & temp region)*

or larger. Approximately 2% to 3% of these hematomas are associated with actual contusions.[2,3,24] They are caused by penetrating injuries (e.g., GSWs, SWs, or lacerations of tissues), deep depressed fractures, and diffuse axonal injuries.[9,11] Intracerebral hematomas develop deep within the hemispheres from contused areas that become confluent and are surrounded by edema.

Summary of Focal Injuries

Lesion size and the patient's overall status dictate treatment. The hematoma must be evacuated if it is large or if the patient's neurologic status is deteriorating.[14] Hematomas act as mass lesions and are often accompanied by progressive edema, producing a steady deterioration in the patient's condition. This deterioration may occur immediately or be delayed for 72 hours to 7 to 10 days.[14] Clot formation and deterioration within a few days after initial insult is called a **delayed traumatic intracerebral hematoma (DTICH).**[20] DTICH occurs in the areas that were injured at the time of impact but appeared normal on the initial CT scan. DTICH is associated with a high incidence of increased ICP and a poor prognosis.[39] There is a higher risk of development of DTICH in patients with disseminated intravascular coagulation (DIC), hypotension, alcohol abuse, and hypoxia.

Diffuse Brain Injury

Diffuse brain injuries are the most common type of head injury. They represent a continuum of brain damage produced by increasing amounts of acceleration-deceleration forces.

Subarachnoid Hemorrhage

A subarachnoid hemorrhage (SAH) is the presence of blood in the subarachnoid space, which lies between the arachnoid and pia meningeal layers. When SAH occurs with trauma, it is often an incidental finding associated with other injuries. The patient's CSF is bloody. If the patient is conscious, he or she may exhibit signs of meningeal irritation such as a headache.[40] Other types of cerebral hemorrhage are discussed in the following sections.

Concussion   *Violent shaking of brain*

A **concussion** is also referred to as **mild traumatic brain injury (MTBI)** or **diffuse injury to the brain.** It may or may not produce a brief loss of consciousness. Early symptoms may appear mild but can lead to retrograde amnesia in the absence of gross cerebral pathology resulting from reticular activating and/or cortical electrophysiologic dysfunction.[47] The mechanism of injury is usually blunt trauma from an acceleration-deceleration force or a direct blow. The GCS score may range from 14 to 15 after 30 minutes. There are two classifications of concussion: **mild** and **classic.** In 2003 the Centers for Disease Control and Prevention issued a report to Congress that defined mild TBI as follows:[37]

- Any period of observed or self-reported
  1. Transient confusion, disorientation, or impaired consciousness
  2. Dysfunction of memory around the time of injury
  3. Loss of consciousness lasting less than 30 minutes

- Observed signs of neurologic or neuropsychologic dysfunction, such as
  1. Seizures acutely following injury to the head
  2. Altered behavior among infants and very young children: irritability, lethargy, or vomiting following head injury
  3. Symptoms among older children and adults such as headache, dizziness, irritability, fatigue, or poor concentration

The latter symptoms, when identified soon after injury, can be used to support the diagnosis of mild TBI, but cannot be used to support the diagnosis in the absence of loss of consciousness or altered consciousness.

Signs and Symptoms of Classic Concussions.

A classic concussion is an injury that results in a loss of consciousness. It is always accompanied by some degree of posttraumatic amnesia, and the length of amnesia is a measure of the severity of the injury. The characteristics of classic concussions may involve the following:

- Loss of consciousness that usually lasts less than 6 hours
- **Posttraumatic amnesia** is the result of the temporary disconnection of the reticular activating system (RAS) from the cortex[20,46]
- No apparent structural sign of injury; may be undetectable by current means of diagnostic study
- Duration of unconsciousness as an indicator of the severity of the concussion (the longer the patient is unconscious, the worse the injury)
- Recovery that may appear complete
- Possible development of rapid, long-term sequelae (**postconcussive syndrome [PCS]**)[29]

Signs and Symptoms of Postconcussive Syndrome.

Symptoms of PCS include headache, dizziness, irritability, emotional lability, fatigue, poor concentration, decreased attention span, memory difficulties, and intellectual dysfunction that may occur from 1 week to 1 year after the initial injury. Patients at high risk for PCS should be identified, and they and their family should be educated about PCS so that all parties involved understand that they are not completely recovered when they leave the hospital. Sequelae may include difficulty at work and at home and may result in interpersonal relationship problems or the loss of employment.[29,38,47]

The field of sports-related concussions is an area of interest associated with PCS that has arisen over the past decade. This topic originally attracted interest because of the injuries sustained by professional ice hockey and football players. After data began to be collected and analyzed, the implications of the findings affected collegiate, high school, and elementary school play and sports as well. At the Second International Conference on Concussion in Sport in 2004, a Sport Concussion Assessment Tool (SCAT) was developed to assist coaches, athletic trainers, and team physicians in deciding when an athlete can play and not play.[34] Patients who have not recovered 6 months after the injury require a referral for further diagnostic workup, treatment, and possibly neuropsychologic testing. Box 11-3 lists the common postconcussion symptoms.

BOX 11-3   Common Postconcussion Symptoms

- Headache: most common complaint possible from nerve fiber damage, abnormal cerebral circulation, or neurochemical changes (some patients develop migraine headaches)
- Dizziness: secondary vestibular changes
- Confusion: may result from electrochemical dissociation
- Nausea/vomiting
- Hearing loss/tinnitus or phonophobia: sensitivity to sound due to impairment of CNs VII and VIII
- Loss of smell/appetite: CN VII involvement
- Visual changes: photophobia, blurred vision, impaired extraocular motor function
- Speech problems: slurred speech from mild brain damage
- Balance and coordination difficulties: dislodging of calcium carbonate crystals of the semicircular canal
- Problems with cognitive function: lack of concentration, short-term memory loss from mild brain damage, axonal fragmentation
- Emotional and behavioral changes: irritability, poor attention span
- Seizures (rare): transient absence or partial seizures with staring spells, memory gaps, and outbursts of temper that improve with anticonvulsants

---

Diffuse Axonal Injury

Diffuse axonal injuries (DAIs), or **axonal shearing,** result from widespread shearing and rotational forces and produce damage throughout the brain. The injured area is diffuse, and there is no identifiable focal lesion.[20,47] DAIs are associated with prolonged traumatic coma, are more serious, and have a poorer prognosis than a focal lesion or ischemia. DAIs may be described as follows:

- Disconnection between the cerebral hemispheres and the RAS that produces widespread white matter injury and degeneration, neuronal dysfunction, and global cerebral edema
- Disconnection due to damage to nerve fibers produced by linear and rotational shear strains related to high-speed deceleration injuries[15]
- Severity that correlates with the amount of shearing force applied

DAIs are commonly located on the corpus callosum and the brainstem.[9] Patients have an immediate loss of consciousness followed by a prolonged coma, abnormal posturing, increased ICP, hypertension, and elevated temperature.[9] The mortality rate is 33%, with another 33% surviving with severe disabilities or remaining in a persistent vegetative state.[9] DAIs create an increase in vasodilation and cerebral blood volume that precipitates increased ICP over time.[30]

DAIs are classified as mild, moderate, and severe:

- Mild: consists of loss of consciousness lasting 6 to 24 hours; occurs in only 8% of all severe head injuries[9]
- Moderate: consists of coma lasting less than 24 hours with incomplete recovery; represents 20% of all severe head injuries and 45% of all DAI injuries; often occurs with basal skull fractures

- **Severe:** occurs in 16% of all severe head injuries; usually involves primary brainstem injury

Other Brain Injuries

Scalp Lacerations and Abrasions

The scalp is composed of five layers of tissue: (1) skin, (2) connective tissue, (3) galea, (4) loose areolar tissue, and (5) the pericranium. The subcutaneous tissue is very vascular and is responsible for the profuse bleeding that usually occurs with scalp injuries. Scalp injuries can be classified as lacerations or abrasions. Important scalp laceration and abrasion considerations are shown in Boxes 11-4 and 11-5.

Cranial Nerve Injuries

The 12 pairs of cranial nerves are often involved in TBI from direct injury, compression from edema, or stretching during periods of increased ICP (see Chapter 16). A careful and thorough assessment of the cranial nerves should be performed at frequent intervals following TBI. Treatment may focus on the primary injury, such as hemorrhage that can irritate or cause cranial nerve compression, edema that compresses the nerves, or trauma that directly injures or destroys the nerves. Treatment focuses on relieving the compression or surgery to reattach or repair the nerves. Careful follow-up cranial nerve assessment is needed to evaluate the patient's response to therapy. Box 11-6 provides a full review of cranial nerve injuries.

Brainstem Injury

Brainstem injuries may be caused by contusions or lacerations and are usually associated with other diffuse cerebral injuries. The prognosis associated with these injuries is poor due to the brainstem's control of vital functions.[32,36] Primary insults to the brainstem produce immediate dysfunction. The dysfunction may also appear in association with other TBIs as a result of secondary injury. Brainstem injuries produce an immediate loss of consciousness, pupillary changes, and posturing, along with cranial nerve deficits and changes in vital functions (e.g., respiratory rate and rhythm).[2,3] Brainstem injuries are also classified under diffuse axonal injuries.

Severe Traumatic Brain Injury

Severe traumatic brain injury (STBI) has a mortality rate of 20% to 35%. Patients usually are admitted comatose with a GCS score of 3 to 8. The patient has a prolonged unconscious state or is comatose, requiring immediate resuscitation and

---

BOX 11-4   Characteristics of Scalp Lacerations

- The most common type of head injury.
- Easily missed if the patient's hair is thick and bleeding is minimal.
- Bleed profusely due to the poor vasoconstrictive ability of the scalp vasculature.
- Rarely the cause of sustained hypotension.
- Scalp lacerations should be inspected cautiously, because the scalp moves on the skull and a fracture may be present in the area of the laceration but not necessarily right below it.
- Consider the possibility of dural tears or brain lacerations.
- Aggressive inspection of the wound may exacerbate the tear and increase the risk of infection.
- After administering a local anesthetic with lidocaine and epinephrine (1:1000) for vasoconstriction, examine the wound with a sterile gloved hand.
- Irrigate the wound thoroughly with normal saline solution after inspection.
- To minimize the risk of infection, debride the wound as soon as possible to remove hair, dirt, glass, and gravel. The venous system of the scalp drains into the venous sinuses of the brain, and a contaminated scalp laceration can lead to a scalp infection, osteomyelitis, necrotizing fasciitis, or an intracranial abscess.
- Suturing may be required to close the wound as soon as possible to prevent the potential for infection and assist in wound healing. The patient is given instructions regarding wound care and suture removal.

BOX 11-5   Characteristics of Scalp Abrasions

- Top layer of the scalp usually associated with minor bleeding
- Occurs when force is applied to the scalp
- Bleeding occurs into subcutaneous layer, with a break in scalp integrity known as "goose eggs"
- Most dramatic in older adults (people in this population most commonly "bump" their heads)
- Usually treated with dressing, ice to the area, and instructions for follow-up if complications occur

---

BOX 11-6   Cranial Nerve Injuries

- There is a potential for unilateral or bilateral cranial nerve (CN) injury.
- The exact site and orientation of the fracture determine the damage.
  CN I: Associated with anterior fossa fracture; results in **anosmia.**
  CN II (rarely injured): Usually causes visual field cuts; associated with orbital fractures.
  CN III: Associated with severe closed head injury. Compression results in increased ICP.
  CNs V, VI, VII, VIII: Usually associated with petrous bone fractures.
  CNs IX, X, XI, XII (rarely injured): May be involved in fractures of the posterior fossa involving the occipital condyle (particularly CN XI).
  CNs VII and VIII: Occurs secondary to fractures when the cervical spine is forced upward and impacts on the base of the skull; fracture may traverse the foramen magnum;[9] can result in peripheral facial palsy and in hearing deficits. CN VII can also be injured with facial fractures.

emergent treatment. The patient with STBI has more complications, has a longer length of stay, and requires extensive rehabilitation.

ASSESSMENT

Initial Assessment

Prehospital providers begin care to the TBI patient in the field by properly immobilizing the patient, securing an airway, and providing oxygen and adequate circulation. They are also valuable sources of information about the patient's status at the trauma scene, the mechanism of injury (e.g., a bull's eye or starring of the automobile's windshield, ejection from the vehicle, or a fall from a balcony), the emergency care provided, and the patient's condition during transport. Advanced trauma life support (ATLS) guidelines and hospital head trauma protocols are immediately implemented. Guidelines from the Brain Trauma Foundation are illustrated in Fig. 11-7. The guidelines demonstrate that hypoxemia and hypotension should be avoided and that there is a need for TBI research to begin in the prehospital arena.

The initial assessment in the emergency department (ED) becomes the baseline against which to compare subsequent serial neurologic examinations to evaluate the patient's condition for deterioration or improvement. Airway (A), breathing (B), and circulation (C) are the immediate priority as the trauma team members quickly complete the initial assessment. Disability (D) of any neurologic function is noted, and total exposure (E) of the patient by removing or cutting away all clothing allows the trauma team to assess the entire body for injuries. Simultaneously, the vital signs are obtained and provide information to the clinician about potential hypoxia, hypotension, or other factors that may influence the patient's neurologic examination. TBI is not usually a cause of hypovolemic shock; therefore other causes of blood loss need to be ruled out before assigning TBI as the cause.

A trauma flow sheet in the ED serves to document the initial and serial assessments. The medical record is a legal document and a communication tool by which members of the team review and observe for trends and changes that require immediate response. Therefore careful, accurate, timely, and legible charting is essential.

Secondary Assessment

The secondary survey follows the initial assessment of the patient. This assessment includes gathering additional information such as a detailed history of how the injury occurred, prehospital care, and any medical history (medications, allergies, surgeries, comorbid conditions) that may affect patient management. A more complete neurologic examination becomes part of the general systems assessment as the patient is provided ventilation and oxygenation and is closely monitored for hypoxia, cardiac dysrhythmias, and adequate perfusion. At this time the patient should have pulse oximetry and an indwelling urinary catheter. Blood samples are

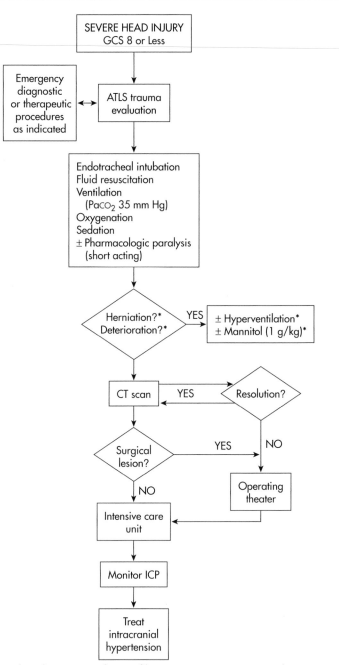

*Only in the presence of signs of herniation or progressive neurologic deterioration not attributable to extracranial factors.

Figure 11-7 Initial resuscitation of the severe head injury patient (treatment option). *ATLS,* Advanced trauma life support. (*From* Management and prognosis of severe traumatic brain injury. I. Guidelines for the management of severe traumatic brain injury: a joint project of the Brain Trauma Foundation and American Association of Neurological Surgeons, *New York, 2000, Brain Trauma Foundation/American Association of Neurological Surgeons.*)

drawn for routine laboratory values and for toxicology and blood alcohol levels (BALs).

Very early after admission to the ED, attention is focused on appropriate management for the prevention of secondary brain damage, such as hypoxia where the patient exhibits apnea or cyanosis and a partial pressure of oxygen in arterial blood (PaO_2) less than 60 mm Hg, hypotension with a systolic blood pressure less than 90 mm Hg, increased ICP with a surgical lesion or edema demonstrated on CT, or metabolic abnormalities.

Level of Consciousness

The most important assessment of the patient with TBI is level of consciousness (LOC), followed by pupillary assessment and assessment of the extremities for lateralized weakness or loss of function. As the trauma team completes the initial assessment, the patient is preliminarily categorized as having mild, moderate, or severe TBI. A mini neurologic examination can be rapidly performed using the AVPU scale to determine if the patient is

A—alert
V—responding to vocal stimuli
P—responding only to painful stimuli
U—unresponsive to all stimuli

The most widely used tool to assess a patient's LOC is the Glasgow Coma Scale (GCS). Since its introduction in 1974, the GCS has become the tool most used to objectively score patient eye opening, motor response, and verbal performance to external stimuli (see Chapter 2). The highest GCS score is 15, which is normal. Any score less than 15 is considered abnormal. A score of 13 to 14 indicates a mild TBI, 9 to 12 a moderate injury, and 8 or less a severe head injury.[1-3,20]

Pupillary Changes

Pupillary changes range from a decrease in reactivity to bilateral fixation and dilation (see Chapter 2). Pupil changes indicate increased ICP resulting in cranial nerve (CN) III compression, as well as injury or ischemia to certain areas of the brain. The pupils are normally round, approximately 3 to 5 cm in diameter, equal in size, and briskly reactive to light. Several factors can influence the size, shape, and reactivity of pupils, such as a history of a previous ocular injury, alcohol ingestion, or the use of certain medications or illicit drugs.[1-3,20]

A pupil that is oval in shape indicates increased ICP and CN III compression and develops into a fixed and dilated pupil if left untreated. This is seen most often in severe closed-head injuries.[3] Bilateral fixed and dilated pupils indicate massive elevations in ICP, which can result in brain death. A metabolically induced coma does not affect pupillary reaction (Fig. 11-8). Changes in pupil size, shape, and reactivity may indicate rising ICP and should be reported to the physician immediately.[1-3,20,30]

Brainstem Reflexes

It is important to assess several reflexes that originate in the brainstem. These reflexes include the cough, gag, corneal, doll's eyes, oculocephalic, cold calorics, and oculovestibular reflexes (see Chapters 1 and 2) and test CN V through CN X. The presence of these reflexes indicates that the integrity of the brainstem has not been disrupted.[3] An absence of these reflexes signifies a poor prognosis.

Vital Signs

Vital sign changes are a late indication of increased ICP. **Cushing's reflex** is seen in approximately 75% of patients

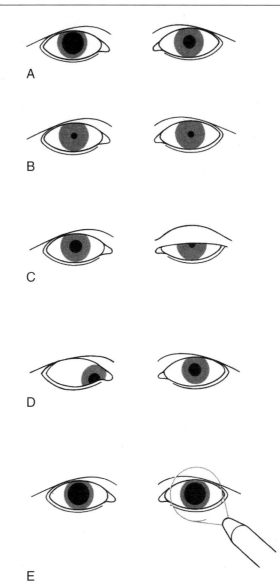

Figure 11-8 Eye signs. **A,** Unilateral fixed dilated pupil: pressure on CN III. **B,** Pinpoint pupils: brainstem hemorrhage. **C,** Unilateral small pupil and ptosis: Horner's syndrome with sympathetic/parasympathetic dysfunction. **D,** Failure of eyes to look downward and inward (left eye is normal eye): CN IV palsy. **E,** Bilateral fixed dilated pupils: herniation.

with increased ICP and is a triad of late symptoms involving vital sign changes that indicate decompensation of the brainstem.[3] These changes include an increase in systolic blood pressure, a widening pulse pressure, and bradycardia. Patients with TBI and increased ICP show a reduced variability in heart rate regardless of activity. The vital signs must be routinely monitored; although the immediate response to TBI is an increase in blood pressure and ICP, these variables should return to normal within 1 to 2 minutes.[30] Blood pressure is decreased with severe injuries and indicates a poor prognosis because of the negative effect on cerebral perfusion pressure (CPP).[30] A decreased blood pressure in the presence of increased ICP results in inadequate CPP, which precipitates further neuronal tissue damage from ischemia and a further increase in ICP. Systemic hypertension can also have deleterious effects on perfusion pressure. Hypertension increases cerebral blood flow, which in turn increases ICP and results in an inadequate CPP. Increased blood pressure may increase cerebral blood flow, but, if autoregulation is not intact, cerebral vasoconstriction will occur to control volume.[30]

Cardiac Changes
Intracranial injuries can produce changes in cardiac rate, rhythm, and conduction, and these changes may be neurogenic in origin.[54] Different intracranial lesions are associated with different cardiac changes. Atrial fibrillation and bundle branch blocks are associated with contusions. A subdural hematoma (SDH) may produce conduction defects, as well as atrial and ventricular ectopy. Junctional escape rhythms, progressive bradycardia, and idioventricular rhythms are seen more often with hemorrhages and increased ICP. ST- and T-wave changes occur with severe TBIs.[50] Neurogenic T waves (inverted T waves of increased amplitude and duration) are seen in a variety of neurologic diagnoses. There are few data to explain the cause of these changes, but they are thought to be related to the catecholamine response that occurs after injury.[50] Because of the nature of these disease processes and their concurrent changes, continuous electrocardiogram (ECG) monitoring is essential in patients with severe TBI.[50]

Respiratory Changes
Respiratory rate and rhythm changes also occur in neurologically impaired patients. **Cheyne-Stokes** respiratory patterns are associated with damage to the bilateral hemispheres and the basal ganglia and often precede cerebral herniation. Cheyne-Stokes breathing is described as rhythmic waxing and waning of the depth of breathing with recurring episodes of apnea.[31] Central neurogenic hyperventilation (CNH) may occur as a compensatory mechanism to increased ICP. Hyperventilation acts by reducing PCO_2 and causing cerebral vasoconstriction and ultimately reduced ICP, but prolonged hyperventilation can produce cerebral ischemia by causing severe cerebral vasoconstriction and impairing cerebral perfusion. CNH is also associated with damage to the midbrain and pons.[9,30] **Apneustic breathing** is characterized by a prolonged inspiration followed by a pause and then a short expiratory phase. This also is associated with pontine injury. **Ataxic or agonal respirations** are associated with medullary damage and may progressively deteriorate to apnea. The clinician should be able to identify changes in a patient's respiratory pattern, because these changes are often indicative of deterioration. Early detection of respiratory pattern changes and immediate, appropriate intervention prevents hypoxia, which contributes to secondary brain damage.[9]

Hypothermia and Hyperthermia
Temperature changes occur rapidly and are common in the TBI patient population. Ongoing monitoring is essential to prevent hyperthermia and hypothermia. Hypothermia has been defined as a core body temperature of less than 35° C (95° F). Hypothermia results when the body can no longer maintain an adequate temperature. With TBI patients, hypothermia needs to be rapidly recognized and treated for life-threatening complications such as apnea, ventricular fibrillation, and acidosis.[23,53,55]

Hypothermia is common with trauma patients as a result of environmental exposures, stress, and the administration of unwarmed IV fluids and blood products to correct massive hypovolemic shock. Age also plays a role in hypothermia, with older adults more at risk because of their high incidence of cardiovascular disease and decreased body fat. In addition, the patient's ability to shiver can be affected by medications (e.g., phenothiazines, neuromuscular blocking agents), an elevated BAL, traumatic injuries, hypovolemic shock, and diseases such as diabetes. Active and passive rewarming are absolutely necessary in order to keep patients from becoming hypothermic.[23,36,45]

Induced hypothermia is a controversial therapy to reduce ICP in TBI patients that has had inconclusive study results. It is an intricate procedure and requires extensive preparation and nursing patient care time. The reader is encouraged to read and refer to the latest literature on hypothermia in the event this therapy is being ordered.[3,45]

Hypothalamic damage and infection often cause temperature increases. Hyperthermia increases the metabolic demands and oxygen consumption in an already overtaxed system. Oxygen consumption increases 10% for every degree of temperature elevation. Increased temperatures cause increased cerebral metabolic activity, increased cerebral blood flow (CBF), and increased carbon dioxide production, all of which increase ICP.[53] Elevations above 38° C should be treated rapidly.[53] Elevated temperatures related to the neurologic injury and not to an infection may be refractory to acetaminophen and aspirin. Other cooling methods such as cool sponge baths or hypothermia blankets may need to be instituted. When using cooling blankets, it is important to prevent shivering, which will also increase metabolic demands. Prevention, early detection, and intervention are essential in minimizing the metabolic demands on the brain. It is important to try to maintain a normothermic temperature with the use of antipyretics, antibiotics, and cooling blankets.[36,53,55]

Neurologic Deficits
Neurologic deficits are evaluated by completing and recording the neurologic assessment, including LOC, motor and sensory evaluations, pupils, and cranial nerves.

Pain
Pain is the **fifth vital sign** and can be evaluated by asking the awake patient if he or she feels pain in any part of the body (see Chapter 23). The extent and severity of pain are determined by using a pain scale or, if the patient is unable to report pain, by observing for facial expressions, body movements, crying, restlessness, and an increased heart rate or blood pressure (see Chapter 23). Sedating the neurologic trauma patient should be avoided until the trauma team leader has cleared the patient to receive analgesics, because pain medications can cause hypotension. It is difficult to determine the extent of pain in patients who are unconscious or pharmacologically paralyzed. The clinician can use a variety of clues to deduce the pain status of an unresponsive

patient. These clues can be determined by assessing the following:

- Vital signs (elevated blood pressure and heart rate)
- Elevated ICP
- Facial grimacing
- Agitation
- Restlessness
- Moaning

Frequently clinical pathways are used to ensure that all aspects of a patient's condition are considered and to bring the standard of care (SOC) to the patient's bedside. The pathway functions as a documentation tool that demonstrates the SOC and functional patient outcome along a time line. The clinical responsibility for each professional discipline is described in clearly measurable outcomes. The advantages of clinical pathways include the following:[55]

- Provide unit-based quality improvement
- Serve as an educational tool for new staff
- Facilitate research
- Ensure continuity of care
- Bring a standard of care to the point of practice

A clinical pathway should be initiated on admission in the ED. If a patient does not have an issue with a category, it is marked as nonapplicable. If a step indicated on the pathway is inappropriate at that time, it is marked as an issue to be readdressed in several days (but no longer than a week). In addition to the pathway, all trauma patients should be discussed weekly during multidisciplinary rounds to review their progress, set short-term goals, and reevaluate long-term goals. Patients who experience complications or fail to recover as predicted are considered a variance and require an explanation (Fig. 11-9).

NEURODIAGNOSTIC AND LABORATORY STUDIES

For a complete description of neurodiagnostic testing, the reader is referred to Chapter 3. The following radiologic tests may be useful:

- Skull radiographs: detect skull or facial fractures, tumors, or foreign bodies.[11]
- CT: best study for rapid diagnosis of type, location, and extent of injury. A CT scan provides a quick comparison with serial scans and detects absent or compressed cisterns. A dual diagnosis of head and spinal injury can be ruled out with both a head and neck CT. CT images are usually repeated every 2 to 3 days after admission or as needed based on the patient's clinical presentation.[48]
- Magnetic resonance imaging (MRI): allows for a better definition of mass lesions, better visualization of the posterior fossa and brainstem, and an increased ability to detect subtle changes in tissue water content. Requires more time than a CT scan and is not usually performed in acute or unstable patients, who are at high risk during scanning. Is used to diagnose DAI but not as an initial diagnostic study; the patient would have had a CT scan first.

- Cerebral angiography: has limited use with trauma unless there are suspicions of cerebrovascular disease, vessel abnormality, or injury.
- Electroencephalogram (EEG): detects abnormal electrical or seizure activity and the absence of electrical potentials as part of the diagnosis for brain death.
- Cerebral blood flow studies (xenon CT, transcranial Doppler): provide noninvasive measurements of CBF velocity, the diameter of cerebral blood vessels, or the presence of vasospasm. These studies can determine whether an increase in ICP is due to an increase in CBF or to cerebral edema. Patients what are brain dead will not have CBF present.
- Evoked potentials (EPs): a noninvasive study that measures the brain's response to auditory, somatosensory, and visual stimuli. It aids in detecting lesions in the cerebral cortex, ascending pathways of the spinal cord, brainstem, and thalamus.
- Near-infrared spectroscopy: noninvasive reflection of tissue oxygenation based on the amount of infrared light that is absorbed by hemoglobin and deoxyhemoglobin.
- Single-photon emission computed tomography (SPECT): provides a qualitative measure of CBF when used as a perfusion study; can also detect areas of increased metabolism, effects of stroke, and several other things.
- Positron emission tomography (PET): evaluates and maps out brain biochemistry and physiology (e.g., oxygen, glucose, blood flow).

TREATMENT

Medical Management

Medical management of the patient with TBI begins in the prehospital setting with the goal of rapid, accurate diagnosis of the primary brain injury and the prevention or management of secondary brain injuries. On-the-scene rescue efforts, rapid transportation, initial resuscitation in trauma-designated hospital EDs, and improved treatment within the "golden hour" are responsible for an increase in the percentage of patients who survive their initial injury.[7] When the patient reaches the ED, resuscitation efforts continue until the patient is stabilized and transferred to the intensive care setting. The ABCDs in the following sections demand evaluation.

Airway

All patients should be evaluated for the ability to protect their airway and oxygenate themselves and for the need for supplemental oxygen. Establishing and maintaining an airway is crucial in patients who are at high risk for hypoxia or aspiration. All patients with TBI who are unconscious should be treated for cervical spine (C-spine) injuries until the diagnosis demonstrates otherwise.[48] Spontaneous, unexpected vomiting is common in these patients 30 to 60 minutes after

CATEGORY/SYSTEM	ADMISSION TO 24 HOURS	24 HOURS TO 48 HOURS	49 HOURS TO 72 HOURS
CARDIOPULMONARY	DVT Prophylaxis (includes TEDS and SCDs) Baseline chest x-ray Pulmonary hygiene for post-op, chest & major abdominal injuries Incentive spirometry, cough & deep breathe, splinting Chest PT, bronchodilators, and pain meds Ventilated PT: Manage per ICU protocol	Assess airway clearance and readjust interventions as needed	→
NEUROLOGICAL	**Evaluation of C-spine completed and findings documented in chart →** Consults: Neuropsychiatric evaluation for head trauma cases	**If patient wearing collar: Skin integrity under collar assessed and skin care initiated** **Refer to skin care protocol** Mobility orders written	Vertebral injury stabilized Pt's cognitive functioning assessed by Neuropsych
GI AND NUTRITION	Feeding route established → Stress ulcer prophylaxis per protocol Admission weight record in chart	Nutrition Orders Initiated: ( ) Tube feeding ( ) Advance Diet As Tolerated ( ) TPN/PPN ( ) NPO	**Nutrition assessed and adjusted:** ( ) TF's tolerated/advanced ( ) TPN modified Consults: ( ) Nutrition consult ( ) Dysphagia/speech consult when extubated, if applicable
INFECTION CONTROL AND PAIN MANAGEMENT	Pain medication ordered: Epidural, PCA, IM, PO Change all lines placed in field or emergency center IV Antibiotics: Specify reason for administration and length of time/number of doses	Pain medication adjustment based on pt. comfort level **Route:** ( ) **Epidural** ( ) **PCA** ( ) **IV/IM** ( ) **PO**	→
MUSCULOSKELETAL AND SKIN INTEGRITY	**Documentation on chart: Injuries, definitive plan for fracture stabilization, plan of care on chart →** Skin assessment evaluation Consult: PM&R, PT & OT per protocol	If patient has not been stabilized: Time frame given for comfort level. **Weight bearing status identified:** Activity level/weight bearing status evaluated and schedule implemented ( ) bedside PROM ( ) OOB/CH ( ) GYM → Wound Care Plan established → **Recommendations and activity plan from PT/OT eval. done**	**PM and R's recommendation for anticipated discharge disposition identified based upon evaluation** Progress activity level →
PSYCHOSOCIAL AND DISCHARGE PLANNING	Patient identified and next of kin notified Current medications documented Consult: Social Work Psychiatry (if situation indicates) Consider pastoral care	Psychosocial needs identified and resources contacted (Substance/Domestic Abuse counseling initiated) Discharge planning initiated with patient and/or family → Verify insurance: If none, full MA application started	**Referrals for appropriate level of care:** ( ) Rehab ( ) SNF ( ) NH ( ) Homecare and DME Education on self-care appropriate to D/C disposition begun.
		EXPECTED OUTCOMES AT 72 HOURS Hemodynamic stability Patent airway and ability to clear secretions Intake that meets metabolic needs to recover	A comprehensive discharge plan that identifies: • Level of care required • Post discharges • Expected time frame for discharge • Education and skills required for self-care and maximum functioning

Patient Name: _____

Medical Record Number: _____

NOTE: This pathway represents guidelines only. Physician practice may vary based upon individual clinical problem. Acceptable medical practice generally does include a variety of responses to a particular clinical problem.
Peer Review Records: Confidential pursuant to the Peer Review Protection Act, 63 P.S. 425.1 et. seg. and Health Care Quality Improvement Act, 1986

Figure 11-9 Trauma pathway.
(Courtesy Medical College of Pennsylvania Hospital, Philadelphia, PA.)

injury, and therefore suctioning equipment must be readily available.[48] Intubation should occur in either the prehospital or ED setting for those patients with a GCS score of 8 or less.[48] Strategies to use in the ED may include a rapid sequence intubation (RSI) protocol, lidocaine, and/or etomidate in recognition that intubation can be a noxious stimulation to the brain and increase ICP.[48]

Breathing

Of those patients with severe TBI, 65% are hypoxic and have PaO_2 levels below 50 mm Hg on admission to the ED. The use of a flow sheet to closely monitor the patient's respiratory pattern and rate provides clues to an expanding lesion. Ventilated patients must be monitored for the need to administer neuromuscular blockade agents (e.g., succinylcholine or rocuronium) and sedatives (e.g., midazolam) to prevent asynchronous ventilation.[35,42,44]

Circulation

The goal is to stabilize and maintain blood pressure and CPP. The systolic blood pressure should not fall below 90 mm Hg,[7] and CPP should not fall below 60 or 70 mm Hg. Hemoglobin and hematocrit should be maintained at normal levels to maximize the oxygen-carrying capacity and oxygen delivery to the brain.[12] Volume expanders and vasopressors (e.g., phenylephrine, epinephrine, or dopamine) allow for the titration of systemic vascular resistance and cardiac output without altering cerebral vascular tone.

Disability

Any apparent neurologic deficits (either cranial or spinal) noted in the primary survey, such as altered LOC, unconsciousness, unequal pupils, cranial nerve abnormalities, and hemiplegia, should be immediately addressed on admission.

Head Injury Guidelines

Patient management is focused on preventing or treating the increased ICP that accompanies the primary injury. Box 11-7 describes the standard therapeutic regimen for the management of head injury.[12] Fig. 11-7 illustrates the algorithm for initial management, and Table 11-1 provides a summary of head injury guidelines from the Brain Trauma Foundation and the American Association of Neurological Surgeons.

Other Variables That Affect Secondary Injury

Seizures

Seizures can increase the cerebral metabolic rate, increase cerebral oxygen demand, and exacerbate ischemic damage (see Chapter 24).[56] Clinicians need to be aware that patients who are pharmacologically paralyzed can still be seizing. A bedside continuous EEG should be used to determine if the patient is seizing. The *Guidelines for the Management of Severe Head Injury* recommend that anticonvulsant therapy be initiated in patients who are at high risk for seizures (e.g., those with a seizure history, or those who have already had a seizure as a result of their injury).[9]

Approximately 5000 new cases of posttraumatic seizures (PTSs) are identified each year in the United States.[18,21] PTSs are classified into two groups:

1. Early: occur within 7 days of the injury or when the patient is still suffering the direct effects of the primary injury. Early PTS may cause increased ICP, hypoxia, and increased metabolic demands that may compromise an already jeopardized brain.[8]
2. Late: occur more than 7 days after the injury.

Tonic-clonic seizures in the acute phase may cause secondary brain injury resulting from increased ICP, compromised oxygen delivery, increased metabolic demands, and excessive neurotransmitter release.[13] Early seizures should be managed with intravenous (IV) lorazepam (Ativan) 0.1 mg/kg up to 10 mg. If seizures persist, lorazepam can be followed with a loading dose of phenytoin or fosphenytoin (Cerebyx). Fosphenytoin is a product of phenytoin sodium equivalents (PSEs). The loading dose for phenytoin is 18 to 20 mg/kg IV at an infusion rate of 50 mg/min; the loading dose for fosphenytoin is 18 to 20 mg/kg PSE IV at 150 mg/min.[8] The goals of the clinician should include patient safety, timely administration of anticonvulsants, first aid for seizures (ABCs), and a thorough documentation of the seizure.

Pulmonary Issues

There is a 20% incidence of acute respiratory failure in the patient with neurologic trauma.[21,22] One type of acute respiratory failure is **neurogenic pulmonary edema (NPE)** (Box 11-8). NPE appears to occur only with massive and often-fatal brain injuries.[15] NPE may develop minutes to hours after the initial insult and usually resolves after 24 to 48 hours.[36] NPE may be caused by a sudden increase in ICP and the subsequent release of catecholamines. The catecholamines cause constriction of the pulmonary vasculature, pulmonary hypoperfusion, and hypoxia. Some experts believe NPE is a form of **acute respiratory distress syndrome (ARDS)**.[20,36]

ARDS may also occur in patients with TBI. Treatment continues to be aimed at minimizing hypoxia. Unfortunately, the treatment of ARDS and NPE conflicts with the

---

BOX 11-7	**Standard Regimen for Clinical Management of Head Injury**

- Intubation with avoidance of mechanical hyperventilation unless ICP becomes acutely elevated and refractory to other therapies
- Maximization of oxygenation to maintain PaO_2 >100 mm Hg
- Osmotic diuresis
- Control of cerebral metabolic rate: sedation, anticonvulsants, antipyretics
- Maintenance of systolic blood pressure >90 mm Hg, avoiding even a single episode of hypotension
- Fluid resuscitation to attain and maintain euvolemia

ICP, Intracranial pressure; *PaO_2*, partial pressure of oxygen in arterial blood.

TABLE 11-1	Summary of Head Injury Guidelines from the Brain Trauma Foundation and American Association of Neurological Surgeons		
Issue	**Standard**	**Guideline**	**Option**
Trauma systems and the neurosurgeon	None	Organized trauma care systems should exist throughout the United States.	Neurosurgeons should be involved in planning, implementing, and evaluating care for patients with neurologic trauma.
Initial resuscitation	None	None	Complete and rapid physiologic resuscitation should occur.
Reduction of blood pressure and oxygenation	None	Hypotension and hypoxia must be avoided and treated.	Maintain MAP >90 mm Hg with a CPP >70 mm Hg.
Indications for ICP monitoring	None	ICP monitoring is indicated in patients with TBI who have an abnormal CT scan and a GCS score between 3 and 8. ICP monitoring may be considered with severe TBI if the patient's CT scan is normal and two of the following apply: age >40 years, posturing, and hypotension (systolic blood pressure <90 mm Hg).	
ICP treatment threshold	None	None	Evaluating the patient's neurologic status and CPP data should coincide with treatment decisions for ICP.
ICP monitoring technology	None	None	None noted, but a recommendation was made: Connecting ventricular catheters to an external strain gauge transducer or a fiberoptic transducer is the most reliable method of monitoring ICP.
Central perfusion pressure	None	None	Maintain CPP >70 mm Hg.
Use of hyperventilation in the acute management of TBI	Chronic hyperventilation ($PaCO_2$ ≤25 mm Hg) should be avoided after TBI if ICP is normal.	Prophylactic hyperventilation ($PaCO_2$ <35 mm Hg) should be avoided for the first 24 hours.	Hyperventilation may be used for short time periods in the event of worsening neurologic situations if all other methods to control ICP have been exhausted. Jugular venous oxygen saturation monitoring (SjO_2) and cerebral blood flow monitoring may help identify the resulting cerebral ischemia from hyperventilation.
Use of mannitol	None	Mannitol can be used for ICP control in small doses of 0.25–1 g/kg. Intermittent boluses may be more effective.	Mannitol can be used before ICP monitoring if the patient exhibits neurologic deterioration or transtentorial herniation; maintain serum osmolarity below 320 mOsm; maintain fluid replacement and euvolemia.
Use of barbiturates	None	Patients with refractory intracranial hypertension in whom all other medical and surgical therapies have failed to lower ICP may receive high-dose barbiturate therapy.	None

TABLE 11-1	Summary of Head Injury Guidelines from the Brain Trauma Foundation and American Association of Neurological Surgeons—cont'd			
Issue	Standard	Guideline	Option
Role of glucocorticoids	Glucocorticoids are not recommended for improving outcomes in severe TBI.	None	None
Critical pathway for the treatment of established intracranial hypertension	None	None	None made, but a comment was noted: a treatment algorithm that describes step-by-step interventions may assist the team in managing patients with TBI.
Nutritional support of patients with TBI	None	Enteral or parental nutrition should be used to replace 140% of resting metabolism expenditure in nonparalyzed patients and 100% of resting metabolism expenditure in paralyzed patients.	Jejunal feeding is preferred related to avoidance of gastric intolerance and ease of use.
Antiseizure prophylaxis	Preventing late posttraumatic seizures using phenytoin, carbamazepine, or phenobarbital is not recommended.	None	May consider use of anticonvulsants for patients at high risk for early posttraumatic seizures.

Data from *Guidelines for the management and prognosis of traumatic brain injury,* a joint project of the Brain Trauma Foundation and American Association of Neurological Surgeons.
CPP, Central perfusion pressure; *CT,* computed tomography; *GCS,* Glasgow Coma Scale; *ICP,* intracranial pressure; *MAP,* mean arterial pressure; *PaCO$_2$,* partial pressure of carbon dioxide in arterial blood; *TBI,* traumatic brain injury.

management of ICP because of the use of **positive end-expiratory pressure (PEEP),** which raises the intrathoracic pressure. This increase in intrathoracic pressure is transmitted through the venous system where, due to the lack of valves in the cerebral veins, venous outflow from the brain is reduced. This reduction in venous outflow causes an increase in cerebral blood volume and therefore increased ICP.[20] The desired level of PEEP is tested by observing for an increase in ICP and a change in the oxygen saturation (see Chapter 11).

Other pulmonary complications may result from the trauma (e.g., pulmonary contusions, hemothorax or pneumothorax, rib fractures, and sternal fractures). The goals are to provide the brain with adequate oxygen between 80 and 100 mm Hg and to keep the PaCO$_2$ at 30 to 35 mm Hg.[35]

Tissue Acidosis
A 40% decrease in CBF results in brain tissue acidosis, and a decrease of 60% results in electrical deterioration.[50] CBF may be normal, increased, or decreased after TBI. Within the first few days after injury, there is a decrease in flow around the injured sites.[5,13] This decrease causes an acidosis, which in turn dilates the vessels and causes hyperemia. This raises the ICP, decreases CPP, and results in decreased blood flow[30,47] (Box 11-9).

TIP: The brain extracts more oxygen from the blood than any other area of the body.

Jugular Bulb Catheterization
Jugular bulb catheterization (SjO$_2$) is an invasive procedure in which the saturation of venous blood is measured as it leaves the supratentorial component in the upper hemisphere. SjO$_2$ monitoring gives the arterial-to-venous oxygen content difference (AVDO$_2$) and lactic acid production.[30,47] This information allows patient treatment to be individualized. SjO$_2$ readings below 55% are referred to as **cerebral oligemia;** readings above 75% are referred to as **cerebral hyperemia.** An increase in AVDO$_2$ that is related to an increase in CBF is better treated with sedation and barbiturates. The ability to monitor CBF and ICP adds new dimensions to the care of the TBI[52] (see Chapter 10).

Brain Tissue Monitoring
A system is now able to monitor brain tissue oxygenation (PbtO$_2$) through a single-lumen or multilumen catheter that is inserted through an ICP monitoring system. It measures PbtO$_2$, brain tissue temperature, and ICP. Since the brain cannot store oxygen, it needs to maintain a constant supply of oxygen[52,58] (see Chapter 10).

Medullary Ischemia
Medullary ischemia appears to be responsible for initiating a massive sympathetic discharge, which releases catecholamines and results in increased systolic pressure, tachycardia, and increased ICP.[55] Catecholamine-blocking agents

Modified from Marshall SB, editor: *Neuroscience critical care: pathophysiology and patient management*, Philadelphia, 1990, WB Saunders.
CO₂, Carbon dioxide; *ICP,* intracranial pressure.

BOX 11-8	Cycle of Neurogenic Pulmonary Edema in Traumatic Brain Injury

Trauma or insult to the brainstem
↓
Increased ICP
↓
Hypothalamic involvement/lesion
↓
Increased sympathetic stimulation from brainstem
↓
Increased vascular resistance and blood pressure
↓
Blood being shunted into lower pressure pulmonary vasculature
↓
Increase in hydrostatic pressure causing fluid leak from lung capillaries
↓
Increased barrier to oxygen and carbon dioxide diffusion
↓
Resulting arterial hypoxemia and hypercapnia
↓
Further increased ICP
↓
Fulminate pulmonary edema with frothy secretions
↓
Massive hypoxemia and CO₂ retention

BOX 11-9	Metabolic Cascade Effects of Brain Injury

Initial brain injury (e.g., head trauma or stroke)
↓
Release of excitatory amino acids (e.g., glutamate)
↓
Opening of the neuron's ion channels (signaled by glutamate)
↓
Massive influx of calcium ions into cells and release of potassium ions
↓
Increased glycolysis for energy to pump ions across the cell membrane
↓
Slowed protein synthesis
↓
Increased cellular lactic acidosis
↓
Acidosis leading to breakdown of cell membrane
↓
Self-destruction of neuronal cells and cellular death

Modified from Barton R et al: The effects of brain injury, *Headlines* 4(1):3, 1993.

may be useful in controlling blood pressure. Agents such as labetalol and esmolol can treat the increase in blood pressure without affecting cerebral vascular reactivity.[15] These agents should not be administered without first checking the CPP. If the blood pressure is increasing secondary to the increased ICP, the first treatment should be aimed at decreasing ICP to preserve and maintain CPP. Catecholamine-blocking drugs may also be helpful in decreasing the myocardial response to the increase in catecholamines and may be helpful in preventing myocardial ischemia.[20] Interventions should done if the blood pressure is greater than 220/130 mm Hg unless there is evidence of other organ dysfunction.[3] Mean blood pressure greater than 130 to 140 mm Hg is the upper limit of autoregulation. Blood pressure that exceeds the upper limits of autoregulation may result in the development of interstitial edema.[3]

Cerebral Edema

Cerebral edema becomes clinically significant when it results in a focal mass effect or when it produces a global elevation in ICP and impairs cerebral perfusion. Two types of cerebral edema can develop after TBI: vasogenic and cytotoxic. Although these two types of cerebral edema are different, both increase brain volume by increasing the water content within the brain. Vasogenic edema is due to a disruption in the integrity of the normal blood-brain barrier. Cytotoxic edema is due to neuronal, glial, or endothelial cell membrane injury. Regardless of the type of cerebral edema, there is an increase in ICP, a decrease in CPP, and a decrease in CBF.

High CBF, called **luxury perfusion syndrome,** is also an indicator of a poor prognosis.[20] Chemical autoregulation is extremely robust and is rarely lost except in cases of severe injury, which usually result in either death or survival in a persistent vegetative state.[20,47]

Studies involving fluid resuscitation of TBI patients with the use of hypertonic saline (HTS) versus standard fluids have shown that while HTS does lower ICP in patients receiving it, there is no impact on outcome.[57] HTS has an osmotic effect on the brain by reducing intracerebral volume and ICP by reducing CSF production and brain water content. Restoration of CBF may occur from local effects on the cerebral microvasculature. HTS maintains extracellular fluid volume and therefore hemodynamic stability is maintained. An example of a protocol for HTS is included in Box 11-10. Further studies are needed to determine the best strength and dose (studies vary from 1.5% to 7.5% HTS), as well as safety and efficacy.[57]

Surgical Management

Patients with an expanding epidural hematoma require emergency surgery for evacuation of the hematoma and cauterization of the bleeding vessel. Trauma patients with a subdural hematoma (SDH) may be managed medically when the clot is small unless the bleeding continues and a craniotomy is needed to locate and stop the bleeding (see Chapter 10). Patients with depressed skull fractures and other serious fractures may also be sent to the operating room for elevation of bone and repair of the dura and brain tissue. Most studies

---

BOX 11-10 **Example of Protocol for Administration of Hypertonic Saline in Severe TBI**

Purpose: 7.5% hypertonic saline (HTS) is used as hyperosmolar therapy to combat the continuation of systemic hypotension and elevated ICP.

Protocal:

- 7.5% HTS has a high potential to cause harm if involved in a medication error. It can lead to myelinolysis (a demyelination syndrome that can cause disorders of central neurons, spastic quadriparesis and pseudobulbar palsy, coma, and death). Always verify the correct indication and the correct patient. To reduce the risk of error, 7.5% HTS is treated as a controlled substance and requires a signature of receipt by the nurse from the pharmacy.
- Use of 7.5% HTS is restricted to use by the neurosurgery service and it is only to be used for the management of traumatic brain injury. The patient must be in the intensive care unit. Use of 7.5% HTS is not allowed in the emergency department or any other hospital location.
- An order is placed either in the chart (written or electronically) for 7.5% HTS 250 ml IV for one (1) dose only. The unit clerk notifies the pharmacy to begin preparation.
- When dispensed from the pharmacy, the IV bag will have the following auxiliary labels attached:
  1. "CAUTION: High Dose Alert"
  2. "For central line administration only"
  3. "For use in traumatic brain injury only"
  4. "Return to pharmacy if not administered within 1 hour of due time"
- The pharmacist delivers the 7.5% HTS infusion to the registered nurse (RN), who signs a narcotic slip with the information "7.5% HTS" written on it. The nurse checks the product and order, and completes the "Hypertonic Saline Checklist" delivered with the IV bag of 7.5% HTS and administers the solution to the patient. The HTS checklist is placed in the chart. The pharmacy follows up and collects the HTS checklist for project review and compliance.
- Administer 7.5% HTS via central line ONLY over 30 minutes. The infusion must begin within 1 hour of receipt from the pharmacy.
- If for any reason the solution is not administered, the nurse returns the 7.5% HTS to the pharmacy immediately and documents the reason for return on the HTS checklist. To prevent medication errors: DO NOT LEAVE THIS 7.5% HTS SOLUTION ON THE UNIT IF NOT ADMINISTERED.
- The pharmacist checks with the nurse 1 hour after delivery of the drug to ensure that it was administered to the patient.
- In some institutions, the trauma service is also able to prescribe and administer 7.5% HTS solution.

---

indicate that the prognosis for recovery from focal TBI is very good with early surgical intervention for mass lesions.

Once it is determined that the injury requires surgical intervention, the neurosurgeon will decide the type of procedure and the timing of surgery. Such decisions are made based on the injury. Surgery may range from burr holes to craniotomy, craniectomy, cranioplasty, or ventriculostomy.

Acute Care

Patients with TBI may be admitted to the neuroscience critical care unit (NCCU) from the ED or after resuscitation, stabilization, or surgical repair of their injuries. Steps must be taken to reduce external stimuli by reducing room lighting, noise levels, and frequent interruptions by the multitude of medical staff to examine the patient. Family can be taught therapeutic touch techniques. The goals of acute care management are to protect the brain from secondary injury and to maintain ICP and CPP within normal limits[22] (see Box 11-7).

Diuresis

Osmotic diuresis is used to manage the excess fluid in brain tissue. Osmotic diuretics must remain in the intravascular compartment to be effective in reducing brain swelling. A hyperosmolar agent such as mannitol is used for osmotic therapy. Mannitol creates an osmotic gradient across the blood-brain barrier. It increases plasma osmolarity and pulls fluid from normal brain tissue to decrease cerebral edema.[4] The usual dose is 0.25 to 1.0 g/kg IV, and when given as a bolus it has a rapid and immediate effect—within 10 to 15 minutes.[15] Mannitol decreases blood viscosity, and its effects last 2 to 6 hours.[7] It is eliminated via the kidneys. Mannitol may leak into the injured brain and pull fluid into these cells, which can result in increased ICP 8 to 12 hours after administration. Mannitol can also have a rebound effect, causing an increase in ICP.

The use of mannitol can cause hypertension. It is important that the patient's vital signs be closely monitored and that mean arterial pressure be maintained at greater than 90 mm Hg. This can be done with the use of albumin, normal saline, packed red blood cells (RBCs), and vasopressors.[1,7]

Lasix is a loop diuretic that is used as an adjunctive therapy in an effort to minimize the negative effects of mannitol. When Lasix and mannitol are used together, Lasix can do the following:

- Enhance the effect of mannitol
- Reduce the incidence of rebound ICP[1,7]
- Decrease blood volume
- Reduce edema by pulling fluid out of the edematous tissue into the vasculature
- Decrease sodium uptake by the brain and reduce CSF production up to 70%[4]

Fluid Replacement and Restriction

Intravenous fluids should be administered as required to resuscitate a patient and to maintain normovolemia. It is very important though that TBI patients not be overloaded with fluids.[7] A patient's serum sodium, potassium, and osmolarity should be monitored to ascertain if the patient is being adequately hydrated despite what clinically appears to be normovolemia.[1,20,36]

Since TBI patients can receive a significant amount of diuresis, the IV replacement formula is based on the amount of diuretic therapy used, the patient's laboratory values, and the patient's clinical condition. Fluid replacement consists of albumin, packed RBCs, and normal saline with potassium chloride (per protocol).

Metabolic Rate

Cerebral metabolic rate can be increased 40% to 100% above normal in patients with TBI.[15] Decreasing the patient's metabolic requirement is a priority, because hypermetabolic states increase the production of carbon dioxide and produce hypercarbia, which further increases ICP.

The following measures are used to lower the patient's cerebral metabolic requirement:

- Keep the patient seizure free.
- Maintain normothermia.
- Maintain a calm, quiet environment, and prevent loud noises and disturbing conversations. This restriction includes having one patient per room and having a door to the room so that the amount of noise and sensory stimulation can be controlled.
- Decrease ICP. Medical interventions that are used in an attempt to lower metabolic needs and decrease ICP include the administration of sedatives, paralytic agents, and anesthetic agents (propofol), as well as the induction of barbiturate coma when increased ICP is refractory to all other forms of therapy.[4,40,53]

Sedation and Analgesia

It is extremely important to obtain a reliable neurologic examination before sedating or administering analgesia to a TBI patient. Sedation reduces restlessness and agitation, and analgesia relieves pain and discomfort. It also decreases the metabolic rate and rate of oxygen consumption. Lorazepam (Ativan) or midazolam (Versed) may be required per the institution's protocol. Opioids (narcotics) have the advantage of being reversed to allow for the completion of an accurate assessment. Morphine can be given in small, frequent doses provided the patient is not hypotensive. Propofol (Diprivan) is lipid based and as such the patient's triglycerides, pH, and liver enzymes should be monitored.[3,36,42]

Intubated patients may have an increase in ICP because the endotracheal tube can act as a noxious stimulus and require fentanyl (small boluses allow for pupil evaluation while decreasing the effect of noxious stimuli). Sedatives should be used very cautiously with nonventilated patients, because a decrease in respiratory rate and respiratory depression may precipitate an increase in ICP.[42]

Paralytic Agents

The objective and guidelines for pharmacologic paralysis include reducing skeletal muscle activity, metabolic rate, and oxygen consumption. Paralytic agents offer no analgesic effect and do not protect the patient from noxious stimuli. However, when used with sedatives, paralytics may help reduce the increase in cerebral metabolic rate related to agi-

tation. The use of neuromuscular blocking agents (i.e., pancuronium [Pavulon], atracurium [Tracrium], vecuronium [Norcuron], and rocuronium [Zemuron]) without sedation should never be allowed as studies suggest that it increases complications and length of stay.

ALERT: Pancuronium can cause tachycardia, which may necessitate the use of a beta blocker.[20]

When paralytic agents are used with ICP monitoring and ventilation, the patient's corneas are protected with artificial tears, and the eyes are taped shut or a moisture chamber is applied. The standard of care requires the use of "train of four" for monitoring the level of paralysis to ensure that the smallest amount of drug is used to achieve the desired level of paralysis. The "train of four" refers to the application of a peripheral nerve stimulator to the ulnar nerve to determine neuromuscular function. The median, posterior tibial, common peroneal, and facial nerves are sometimes used.[7,15,22,42]

Barbiturate Coma

A barbiturate coma is used as therapy for hemodynamically stable patients with severe TBI and intracranial hypertension who are thought to be salvageable but who have been refractory to maximal medical and surgical therapies (see Chapter 10). The diagnosis of a delayed bleed/lesion should be ruled out before the induction of a barbiturate coma.

A barbiturate coma is a pharmacologically induced coma state that lowers cerebral metabolism and CBF. It acts as a neuroprotective therapy and decreases oxygen uptake in the brain, which decreases the cerebral metabolic rate of oxygen consumption ($CMRO_2$) and the CBF by as much as 50%. It may also assist in stabilizing cell membranes, producing a more uniform blood supply, and decreasing the formation of vasogenic edema.[1,3,36]

Pentobarbital is the drug of choice for barbiturate therapy because its half-life is 24 hours. It is a weight-administered drug given as a loading dose of 10 mg/kg over 30 minutes, with a maintenance dosage of 5 mg/kg for 3 hours followed by 1 to 2 mg/kg/hr.[3] Blood pressure and CPP may fall with the loading dose. Vasopressors, inotropes, and volume expanders may be used to help maintain systolic blood pressure and CPP.

Barbiturate infusion levels are regulated by burst suppression pattern appearance on EEG.[20] The barbiturate coma is slowly decreased after the ICP is normal for 24 to 48 hours. This type of therapy requires complex monitoring, nursing care, and medical care. It is instituted only in specially equipped critical care areas.[20,36]

Factor VII

Recombinant coagulation factor VII (rFVIIa) is a new drug that was designed to be used for the treatment of bleeding in patients with hemophilia and inhibitors.[33] It is made by a recombinant DNA technique and is identical in structure to human factor VII. Studies have been conducted in healthy adults, adult and pediatric patients with hemophilia, and adults with cirrhosis and a prolonged prothrombin time (PT).

Factor VII is an effective therapeutic agent for achieving hemostasis in nonhemophilic surgical patients. Studies have been shown that the use of factor VII is effective in reducing the number of blood transfusions needed. There is also improvement in coagulation factors.[33] The use of factor VII has been reported in the literature describing isolated head injury patients who were using blood-thinning agents. The rationale is that it can help correct the prolonged PT. It can be administered by IV bolus and can be given more quickly than fresh frozen plasma (FFP). This will assist with earlier surgical intervention if needed. In various published reports, the dosages have varied, so the optimal dosing of factor VII is not known. There are currently several ongoing clinical trials to determine the effective dose, the timing of the dosage, frequency, and risks. An example of a protocol for factor VII is provided in Box 11-11.

Additional Assessments

A complete neurologic assessment is performed for a baseline evaluation on admission to the NCCU. Subtle changes can be easily detected when subsequent assessments are charted on the neurologic flow sheet to document the patient's changing status. The Rancho Los Amigos scale is a rehabilitative tool that identifies levels of dysfunction and for planning the appropriate nursing interventions (Table 11-2). Some facilities grade a patient on arrival and reevaluate every week to determine progress or what interventions might be helpful at this stage in the patient's care.[46]

In addition to the interventions described previously, acute care for the patient with TBI includes frequent and careful monitoring and documentation to manage the following parameters:

- LOC, GCS score, neurologic status, or 4 SCORE
- Cerebral hemodynamics (ICP: 0 to 15 mm Hg) and blood flow to the brain (CPP: 60 to 100 mm Hg)[30]
- Airway clearance and respiratory rate and rhythm
- Pulmonary capillary wedge pressures, cardiac outputs (should be done based on the patient's overall status)

For patients with a GCS score of 8 or less, ICP monitoring is performed per protocol. For patients with a GCS score of 7 or less, hemodynamic monitoring is performed with a Swan-Ganz catheter and invasive lines. Airway clearance and respiratory rate and rhythm are monitored frequently. The cough, gag, and corneal reflexes are assessed, and the lungs are auscultated every 2 hours to detect adventitious lung sounds that may indicate respiratory failure. Intake and output (I&O) are monitored every shift.

Famotidine (Pepcid) 20 mg IV every 12 hours or Maalox 30 ml orally or via nasogastric tube for a stomach pH less than 5 are administered to prevent stress ulcers.

Patients with TBI are turned every 1 to 2 hours to mobilize secretions and to prevent pressure ulcers. The use of specialty beds, when required, does not negate turning the patients.[1,3] Antiembolic stockings with sequential compression devices are also used as TBI patients are at a very high risk for thromboembolism and pulmonary embolism.[27,32,43]

Suctioning should never be done through the nose, because a basal skull fracture may be present. The patient is suctioned as often as needed but at least every 2 hours. The patient is premedicated with lidocaine 0.5 to 1.5 mg/kg IV or via endotracheal tube to suppress the cough reflex and to prevent ICP elevations;[1,2] the patient is also preoxygenated with 100% oxygen. Suctioning is limited to two passes, and instilling saline down the endotracheal tube is avoided. Secretions are monitored for viscosity, color, and odor (a foul smell may indicate an infection). Humidified air may assist in decreasing secretion viscosity. Chest physiotherapy and postural drainage are performed at least every 2 hours.

Prevention of Complications

Several complications are described in detail in the following sections to emphasize their importance in preventing complications that could cause further neurologic impairment.

Impaired Gas Exchange. Impaired gas exchange is managed by the following:

- Clearing the airway (discussed earlier)
- Auscultating breath sounds every 2 hours to allow for early detection of compromised lung function
- Monitoring arterial blood gas (ABG) results to ensure that the appropriate interventions are provided to maintain adequate oxygenation and perfusion[5,6]

Increased Intracranial Pressure. Nursing activities have been found to contribute to a rise in ICP.[7,19] The clinician should follow the guidelines in Chapter 10 to prevent elevated ICP:[6,7,9]

- Calculate CPP before and after all activities to ensure adequate perfusion to the brain. CPP should be maintained at a minimum of 70 mm Hg.[12] If it cannot be maintained, the activity should be interrupted and the patient allowed to rest.
- Provide a quiet, subdued environment to reduce stimuli and reduce ICP.
- If ICP remains greater than 20 mm Hg, use sedation to decrease agitation.
- For patients with an ICP monitor (Fig. 11-10), evaluate the ICP waveform for an elevated P_2 segment, which indicates decreased compliance.
- For patients with a ventriculostomy, drain CSF by opening the stopcock to release a small amount of CSF, then reevaluate the patient's ICP.

Deficient and Excess Fluid Volume. Deficient or excess fluid volume is managed by the following:

- Judicious monitoring of I&O hourly during the acute phase
- Recording urine specific gravity a minimum of every 2 hours and every hour in the presence of diabetes insipidus (DI)
- Recording daily weights to identify a rapid loss of fluid or fluid retention
- Monitoring electrolytes frequently for DI (e.g., decrease in urine osmolarity, elevated serum sodium, serum osmolarity)[1,3]
- Assessing the oral cavity for dry mucous membranes
- Monitoring for fluid loss ("neurogenic sweats" may cause a loss of 500 to 1000 ml of fluid daily)

Imbalanced Nutrition. Nutrition must be adequate for the injured brain to heal. The following guidelines are recommended:

BOX 11-11	Guidelines for Use of Recombinant Factor VIIa in Warfarin Anticoagulated Patients With Traumatic and Nontraumatic Spontaneous Intracranial Hemorrhage

Statement of Purpose

To define the use of NovoSeven, recombinant factor VIIa (rFVIIa), in the reversal of warfarin anticoagulation in the patient with a traumatic or nontraumatic intracranial hemorrhage.

Definition

NovoSeven: a recombinant human coagulation factor VIIa intended to promote hemostasis by activating the extrinsic pathway of the coagulation cascade; a vitamin K–dependent glycoprotein consisting of 406 amino acid residues (MW 50K Dalton); structurally similar to human plasma–derived factor VIIa.

Mechanism of Action

Recombinant factor VIIa complexed with tissue factor on phospholipid-rich membranes of activated platelets mediates conversion of coagulation factor IX to IXa and factor X to Xa. Subsequently, the prothrombinase complex (factors Xa and Va and phospholipid) produces a procoagulant "burst" that is derived from prothrombin conversion to thrombin. Thrombin then proteolyses fibrinogen to fibrin, which is essential for thrombus formation and cross-linking. Clot stability is further promoted by VIIa-induced activation of thrombin-activated fibrinolytic inhibitor.

Pharmacodynamics

NovoSeven is recombinant factor VIIa and, when complexed with tissue factor, can activate coagulation factor X to factor Xa, as well as coagulation factor IX to factor Ixa, which, in complex with other factors, then converts prothrombin to thrombin, leading to the formation of a hemostatic plug by converting fibrinogen to fibrin and thereby inducing local hemostasis.

Adverse Reactions

Events considered to have at least a possibility of being related to or of unknown relationship to NovoSeven administration include allergic reaction, arthrosis, bradycardia, coagulation disorder, DIC, edema, increased fibrinolysis, headache, hypotension, injection site reaction, pain, pneumonia, decreased prothrombin, pruritus, purpura, rash, abnormal renal function, decreased therapeutic response, and vomiting.

Cautions

Recombinant factor VIIa should not be administered to patients with known hypersensitivity to NovoSeven or any of the components of NovoSeven. NovoSeven is contraindicated in patients with known hypersensitivity to mouse, hamster, or bovine proteins. Caution must be exercised when using rFVIIa in patients with underlying conditions that may predispose them to thrombosis and DIC, including crush injury, septicemia, atherosclerotic diseases, and advanced age. Caution must be exercised in patients with SAH due to evidence showing risk of thrombosis in this patient population.

rFVIIa Protocol

1. **Prescriptive authority:** Trauma attending physicians, neurosurgery attending physicians, emergency department attending physicians.

2. **Target patient population:** Patients who have suffered a traumatic head injury while on warfarin anticoagulation with confirmed intracranial hemorrhage on CT scan (as per the "Anticoagulation Reversal Guideline") or patients on warfarin anticoagulation with confirmed nontraumatic, spontaneous intracranial hemorrhage on CT scan.

3. **Dosing recommendations:** Intracranial hemorrhage in warfarin anticoagulant:
   Patients <100 kg: 1200 µg × 1 dose
   Patients ≥100 kg: 2400 µg × 1 dose (two 1200 µg vials)

4. **Concurrent treatment:** Patients with intracranial hemorrhage on warfarin anticoagulation should also receive FFP and 10 mg vitamin K IV (7th ACCP Chest Guidelines Level of Evidence IC). Vitamin K, 1 to 10 mg per prescriber's recommendation may be repeated every 12 hours if necessary.

5. **Monitoring requirements:**
   • Baseline PT/INR on admission
   • PT/INR drawn 2 hours after rFVIIa infusion to ensure normalization (normalization defined as INR <1.5)
   • PT/INT drawn q4h for the first 12 hours after rFVIIa infusion to ensure normalization. Vitamin K will become active in reversal process within 2 to 4 hours of administration. Vitamin K, 1 to 10 mg per prescriber's recommendation, may be repeated every 12 hours if necessary.

6. **Redosing recommendations:** Redosing is permitted by authorized prescribes only, as indicated by an INR >1.5 (may be a verbal order). FFP based on clinical judgment and patient tolerance of fluid load. Vitamin K, 1 to 10 mg per prescriber's recommendation, may be repeated every 12 hours. Use of rFVIIa after 12 hours of initiation is discouraged.

7. **Procedure:**
   • Send stat order to pharmacy department, including patient weight.
   • Prescriber may request pharmacy to dose.
   • Pharmacy will reconstitute rFVIIa, place dose in syringe, and deliver syringe.

8. **Administration:** Attach suitable injection needle and administer as IV push over 2 to 5 minutes.

CT, Computed tomography; *DIC,* disseminated intravascular coagulation; *FFP,* fresh frozen plasma; *INR,* international normalized ratio; *IV,* intravenous; *PT,* prothrombin time; *SAH,* subarachnoid hemorrhage.

• Nutrition consultation: to establish a feeding route within 24 hours of admission
• Enteral feeding: preferred over parenteral[16,51,54,59,61]
• Gastric residuals: checked every 2 hours, with feedings slowly advanced
• Daily weights

• Calorie counts (when patients are able to take oral nourishment): ensures that high caloric demands are being met

Altered Bowel Elimination. Elimination should be established early after admission. The clinician should keep the following points in mind:[1,3,22]

TABLE 11-2	Rancho Los Amigos Scale of Cognitive Levels and Expected Behavior
Cognitive Level	**Expected Behavior**
Level I No response	Patient is unresponsive to any stimuli.
Level II Generalized response	Patient reacts inconsistently and nonpurposefully to stimuli. Responses may be physiologic changes, gross body movements, or vocalizations. Responses may be delayed.
Level III Localized response	Responses are directly related to the type of stimulus presented but may be inconsistent. Patient may follow simple commands in an inconsistent, delayed manner. Patient may respond to some persons better than others.
Level IV Confused, agitated	Patient is in a heightened state of activity with a severely decreased ability to process information. Behavior is often bizarre and nonpurposeful relative to the environment. Gross attention is often very short, and selective attention is nonexistent.
Level V Confused, inappropriate, nonagitated	Patient appears alert and is able to follow simple commands consistently. Patient is highly distractable and lacks the ability to focus attention on a specific task. Memory is severely impaired with confusion of past and present. It is difficult for the patient to learn new information.
Level VI Confused, appropriate	Patient shows goal-directed behavior. Simple directions are followed consistently. Responses may be inaccurate due to memory problems but are appropriate to the situation. Patient is inconsistently oriented to time and place. Patient is able to carry out functions of activities of daily living.
Level VII Automatic, appropriate	Patient appears appropriate and oriented within familiar settings. Patient is able to complete daily routine but in a robot-like manner. There may be some awareness of condition, but insight is lacking. Patient demonstrates poor judgment and poor problem solving.
Level VIII Purposeful, appropriate	Patient is alert and oriented and able to integrate past and recent events. Patient needs no supervision once activities are learned and is independent in home and community activities. Challenges may be observed in abstract reasoning, tolerance for stress, or judgment in stressful situations.

- Problems of immobility lead to a reduction in gastrointestinal motility.
- Opioids (narcotics) affect the patient's ability for elimination.
- Bowel sounds should be monitored and documented once every shift.
- All bowel movements should be recorded with regard to frequency and type (e.g., soft, hard, small, large, bloody, diarrhea).
- Patients should not go more than 24 to 48 hours without a bowel movement.
- Patients should avoid the Valsalva maneuver, which raises ICP.
- A bowel program (e.g., bowel regimen, stool softeners, laxatives, fiber products) should be established to prevent constipation.
- Adequate hydration and calorie intake are also essential for proper elimination.

Impaired Physical Mobility. Patient immobility affects all body systems. The following guidelines will help prevent complications of immobility:

- Consult with the physiatrist from physical medicine and rehabilitation (PM&R) for a physical therapist and occupational therapist
- Promote optimal level of mobility by following PM&R recommendations for range of motion (ROM)

- Educate the patient and family on how to adapt to the patient's mobility deficits
- Provide interventions such as repositioning, providing stimuli for all senses, and maintaining a safe environment[1,3]
- Ambulation: assessment may indicate appropriate after 24 to 48 hours, bedside physical therapy for passive ROM, out-of-bed to chair usually with assistants

Disturbed Sensory Perception. Sensory alterations are important considerations, and treatment may include the following:

- Repositioning the patient every 2 hours
- Maintaining the bed in a low position with the side rails up and the bed padded for agitated and combative patients
- Strictly following fall prevention assessment and guidelines at all times for patient safety
- Establishing a stimulation/rest routine based on independent patient needs
- Obtaining a physiatrist consultation and physical therapist/occupational therapist consultation to evaluate and intervene as soon as the patient is stabilized for ROM and other exercises, as well as assist in preventing muscle atrophy and contractures

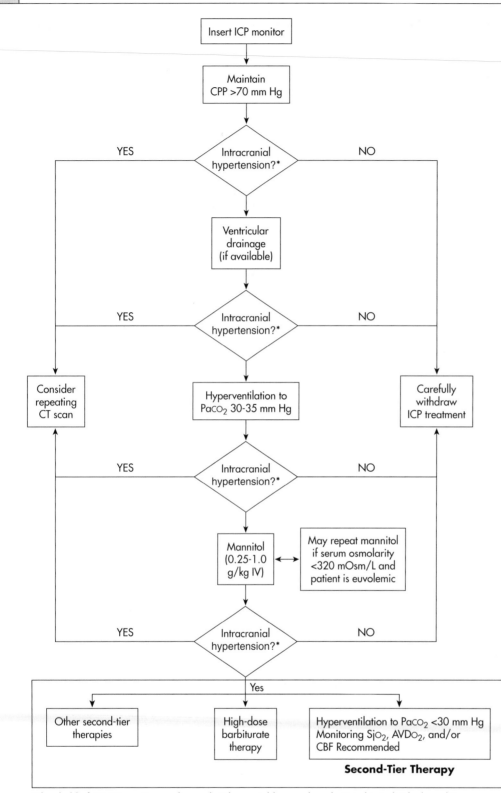

Figure 11-10 Critical pathway for treatment of intracranial hypertension in the severe head injury patient (treatment option). (*From* Management and prognosis of severe traumatic brain injury. I. Guidelines for the management of severe traumatic brain injury: a joint project of the Brain Trauma Foundation and American Association of Neurological Surgeons, *New York, 2000, Brain Trauma Foundation/American Association of Neurological Surgeons.*)

*Threshold of 20-25 mm Hg may be used. Other variables may be substituted in individual conditions.

The occupational therapist may assist with a coma stimulation program, including all types of sensory stimuli (see Chapter 6). Stimulation of the senses may include tactile, gustatory, olfactory, visual, and auditory. The patient should be spoken to in a calm reassuring voice, with all procedures and treatments explained.

Acute Pain. Acute pain may result from injuries sustained from the initial injury, surgery, invasive procedures, or stimulation applied to provoke a response (see Chapter 23). Considerations must be made for the following:

- Pain has an adverse effect on ICP, vital signs, and CPP.

- Pain management is complicated due to the ability of certain agents to interfere with a neurologic assessment.[9,20,42]
- Some agents do not affect pupillary response (codeine and fentanyl allow for continued evaluation of pupils while decreasing noxious stimuli).
- Morphine sulfate (MS) should be avoided because of its effects on the blood pressure and cerebral vasculature.

Neuromuscular blocking agents should not be administered without analgesia because they have no effect on the perception of pain—only on the ability to respond to it.[1,15,20,42]

Ineffective Thermoregulation. Temperature control issues have been discussed previously. All other causes of fever should be evaluated for and eliminated before the cause is attributed to neurologic damage.[53] Tylenol 650 mg per rectum or orally every 4 hours is administered for a temperature over 101.5° F.

Postacute and Nonacute Care

After the patient is physiologically stable and his or her ICP has returned to normal, he or she is transferred to a nonacute unit. The patient is usually more awake and alert, and agitation may increase. There are potential problems for seizure activity, injury from falls, and aspiration as the patient starts oral feedings.

Assessment continues to play a key role. Neurobehavioral testing should be initiated[3,21,29,46,47] to evaluate cognitive, adaptive, and emotional behaviors.[17,39,41,60] These behaviors or responses reflect cortical function. Neuropsychologic testing assists in planning ongoing care, determining rehabilitation potential, and identifying realistic individual goals.[21,46]

The patient may need assistance to regain and build or maintain independent skills (activities of daily living), such as speaking, ambulating, eating, drinking, bathing, and performing personal hygiene to bridge the gap from dependence to independence and rehabilitation.

Level of Consciousness

The higher Rancho Los Amigos Scale (see Chapters 6 and 13) reflects the increased responsiveness that indicates recovery.[21,39] The patient's responsiveness may vary between the following behaviors:

- Confusion
- Agitation
- Emotional lability
- Outbursts of anger, frustration, profanity, and inappropriate behavior

Interventions for this increased responsiveness include a structured environment to reduce overstimulation and distraction and acknowledging behavior calmly while correcting misperceptions and refocusing the patient. The family must be included and educated on how to intercede with the patient; this will help reduce their anxiety and prepare them for the future.[30,46]

Physical or chemical restraints should be used judiciously and only when patients pose a danger to themselves or others.[46] The least restrictive interventions should be used and should include a netted bed and family and/or sitters. Someone should be with the patient at all times during periods of confusion, restlessness, and agitation to prevent the patient from getting out of bed, falling, or self-harm.

Cognitive Functioning

The Rancho Los Amigos Scale of Cognitive Functioning assists in selecting the appropriate actions based on the patient's cognitive status and abilities (see Table 11-2). The following guidelines are useful:

- Take care not to overwhelm or overstimulate a patient who has a low level of response or cognitive function.
- Modulate stimuli such as conversation, music, and environmental noise levels.
- Stimulate the senses by adding only one sensor stimulus at a time; this stimulation may be increased as the patient progresses.
- Provide a structured environment. Give directions in simple language with frequent repetition and reinforcement, and work closely with families and significant others on the type, duration, and methods of stimulation.[3,29] Establish verbal cues and memory aids for the patient.

Self-Care Deficits

The goals of the TBI team are based on some of the following:

- Assist the patient with activities of daily living (ADLs), which may range from teaching patients to dress themselves to performing other self-care activities (e.g., eating, grooming, toileting).
- Teach/educate the patient. Separate activities into small steps, use repetition, and assist only when necessary.[3,29]
- Encourage family involvement. Families can learn how to assist with ADLs and can provide support and encouragement for the patient.

The physical therapist, occupational therapist, speech therapist, and neuropsychologist should evaluate and develop a rehabilitation plan that includes weekly evaluations.

Risk for Injury

The patient with a TBI can be injured as a result of the following:

- *Falls:* To prevent falls, assess for fall precautions, place the patient's bed in the low position, place the patient's call bell within reach (the patient may be ignoring it or may have forgotten how it is used), and remind the patient to call for assistance (he or she will often forget). Use commercial bed alarm systems, or video surveillance, and have a hospital "sitter"/ "patient extender" or family member stay with the patient at all times.
- Unattended or unsupervised activities.
- *Inappropriate behavior:* This includes a reluctance or inability to summon assistance and continuously climbing over the side rails to get out of bed (OOB), most often to use the bathroom.

- Failure to orient the patient to his or her surroundings or not providing adequate lighting or visual aids.
- Failure to provide regularly scheduled toileting that results in patient getting OOB without assistance.

Restraints are used as a last resort to keep the patient from self-harm.[46] Their use should be discussed with family members, and the institution's policy should be followed.

Posttraumatic Epilepsy

Posttraumatic epilepsy occurs after TBI, with both focal and grand mal (tonic-clonic) seizures occurring. Their incidence appears to be greater in those who experience penetrating as opposed to blunt head injuries.[3,11] The onset of posttraumatic epilepsy varies greatly—from 1 month up to 2 years after the original injury. This condition is best controlled with anticonvulsant therapy.[13] It has a propensity to decrease over the years, with some patients becoming seizure free.[13,36]

Situational Low Self-Esteem

Increasing the patient's self-esteem focuses on the following interventions:

- Give the patient as much control as possible and as early as possible.
- Spend time with the patient to enable caregivers to assess the patient's self-concept and direct activities toward his or her abilities, as well as strengthen weaknesses. This will provide a reality base.[3,29]
- Use talk and touch as simple ways of supporting and encouraging the patient.
- Set realistic and patient-directed goals.
- Encourage the family to allow the patient to do as much as possible.
- Help the patient and family locate the nearest TBI support group.

Compromised Family Coping

Like the patient, family members experience a loss of control and feelings of fear and helplessness. Assist the family by using some of the following interventions:

- To reduce their anxiety, identify tasks they can do, and include them in the plan of care.
- Encourage family members to communicate their feelings.
- Answer questions honestly, and provide verbal and written information.
- Mobilize support personnel, such as social services, pastoral care, family liaisons, and case managers.

COMPREHENSIVE PATIENT MANAGEMENT

Health Teaching Considerations

Each day patients and their family experience uncertainty, and with every health care provider they encounter questions and concerns about the injury, treatments, and outcomes. Daily and scheduled family conferences are needed to discuss the injury and the care. Family support is critical in understanding the injury and accepting the goals for each phase of care. Because family members are an important part of the health care team and usually become the caregivers, teaching should begin as soon as they indicate a readiness to learn and participate. Young males are the most likely to sustain brain injuries, with the parents suddenly becoming responsible for caring for and meeting the needs of a son who would normally be leaving home and enjoying the independence of youth.[41] A spouse may become the major caretaker and experience a role reversal, as well as become a major caregiver.[26] A young couple may find that an older parent needs their assistance in recovering from a TBI.

The consequences of caring for a family member with TBI may impede learning until the stress decreases and the reality of the daily routine needs can be explained and demonstrated. Family members should be educated on every aspect of brain injury and rehabilitation (see Resources). A list of treatments and medications can be reviewed with the expectation that family members will be able to recognize what they can do and what follow-up can be expected from other health care providers. Insurance and benefits can be provided by social services. Case managers and life care planners (see Chapter 25) are often consulted for complex cases that require long-term follow-up.

Nutritional Considerations

Swallowing is a complex process that requires a great deal of cognitive function and excellent muscle coordination. Problems with eating and swallowing place the patient with TBI at risk for dysphagia. Interventions include the following:

- *Speech therapy evaluation:* This evaluation determines the type of dysphagia and designs a plan for the patient to ensure adequate nutrition and to prevent aspiration.
- *Speech therapy consultation:* The patient's gag and swallowing reflexes should be tested before introducing any food or fluids.[16]
- *Choking prevention:* If the patient has trouble swallowing (i.e., chokes or gasps), oral feedings should be suspended until a dysphagia consultation can be obtained.
- *Feeding tube maintenance:* A feeding tube remains in place until the team determines that the patient is able to take in enough calories by mouth.[16,51,54,59,61]
- *Oral feeding:* Dysphagia rehabilitation is a slow process but can be done successfully in most instances. Such rehabilitation requires tremendous patience in preventing aspiration and in allowing the patient to consume the adequate amount of food.

Psychosocial Considerations

The psychosocial dysfunction experienced by patients with TBI is perhaps the major obstacle faced after survival. Their lives and the lives of their families are altered forever. Patients and their families must cope with many stressors as they face the fear of unknown and unpredictable outcomes.

Psychosocial support is needed to deal with these concerns, to help reduce stress and anxiety, and to promote adequate coping skills. Patient outcomes range from mild with no residual deficits to a persistent vegetative state, with every condition in between possible. Neurologic deficits may include impairments in language, cognition, personality, mentation, and movement. The patient is evaluated for the need for professional psychologic counseling.

Rehabilitation and education of both the patient and family must start on admission. Families require education and crisis intervention during the initial stages and support throughout hospitalization and often for an extended time after discharge. The Brain Injury Association (BIA) has chapters in every state that can help inform and support families. In the last decade, support groups for patients with TBI and their families have grown in size and number throughout the country. Unfortunately, TBI and its long-term effects (including behavior issues) are not well understood by society, which results in misconceptions about patient behavior and needs and often creates fear and mistreatment for many TBI survivors.

Long-Term Care Considerations

Because of the advances in emergency medical systems during the past 20 years and the current state-of-the-art trauma centers with specialists and new technology, patients who would have died at the scene from a TBI are surviving and living a normal life expectancy. These individuals, however, are not normal. They live each day in communities across the country and struggle with their lifelong disability and cognitive impairments that often lead to early dementia, a shortened work life, the need for early retirement or disability pay, and premature aging with an early onset of medical problems. This population may be at higher risk for Alzheimer's disease and other types of dementia. They are also at a higher risk for sustaining falls and other injuries if their home has not been evaluated and equipped with equipment and safety devices that enable them to live with their special needs. A patient who has lived at home may require early admission to a long-term care facility. The patient's physical limitations and lack of endurance may qualify/classify him or her for disability and the need for expensive equipment (e.g., power wheelchairs, hospital beds) and for the services of physical or occupational therapists. Research on aging and brain injury is needed for patients and their families to successfully prepare them for the final years following a TBI.

Older Adult Considerations

Trauma is the fifth leading cause of death in older adults. The geriatric population (age 65 years and older) has the second highest TBI incidence of all age-groups. The most common causes of TBI in older adults are falls and motor vehicle crashes (MVCs). Older patients are more likely to develop chronic SDHs and experience secondary injury than are their younger counterparts. Indeed, intracranial bleeding in older adults may occur even with minor head trauma because of the cerebral changes associated with aging.

Although TBI is not uncommon in older adults, the diagnosis is often complicated by an atypical presentation. For example, headache is the classic sign of SDH, yet in older adults it is often not a complaint. The presentation of an SDH is delayed weeks or even months, and unfortunately the insidious onset may be attributed to the normal aging process. Chronic SDHs are tolerated better by older adults because of the brain atrophy associated with aging. As the brain decreases in size, the space within the cranial vault increases.[1,3,24] Therefore a hematoma can collect over time without obvious changes in neurologic status until its size is sufficient to produce a mass effect.

The assessment and management of older patients should follow the same algorithm as the care of younger TBI patients. The goals of treatment should focus on returning to the patient's preinjury functional status and future quality of life. It is important to realize that the metabolic, anatomic, and psychosocial changes associated with aging may influence the assessment and care of the older patient with TBI.[18] Injuries that are relatively survivable in younger adults can lead to complications and life-threatening events, including death, in older adults. Thus, in addition to hospital care, nursing interventions should also focus on injury prevention.

Environmental assessments, fall-risk profiles, and appropriate prostheses, assistive devices, and therapies can reduce the older patient's risk for TBI related to falls. A rehabilitation focus that includes an acute-phase prevention of complications should be initiated as soon as the injury is discovered and should be continued throughout the course of recovery.

Rehabilitation and Home Care Considerations

The rehabilitation phase of care for the patient with TBI begins at hospital admission. Admission to the rehabilitation unit is a milestone in a patient's recovery and requires intense work by the patient to complete the daily schedule of therapies. The following are the goals of rehabilitation:

- Maximize the patient's ability to return to his or her highest level of functioning and to his or her home and the community
- Address all concerns before discharge for a smooth transmission to home or rehabilitation
- Promote independence with adaptation to deficits (this becomes a crucial part of care)

The Ranchos Los Amigos Scale of Cognitive Functioning is used as the basis for ongoing assessment of the patient in rehabilitation (see Chapter 13). The patient's neurologic status and GCS score are checked once or twice a day. Cognitive rehabilitation of the patient with a closed head injury requires a dedicated multidisciplinary effort.[3]

The patient should be observed and monitored for postconcussive syndrome (PCS). This condition is most commonly associated with mild TBI but can be seen after any form of TBI. There is no specific treatment for PCS, but it includes neurobehavioral therapy, rehabilitation, and medication.

The symptoms of a TBI may last as long as 6 months postinjury, but it is not unusual for someone in an intellectually demanding role to have significant symptoms for a year before returning to normal (see Chapter 13).

Impaired Physical Mobility

Interventions for the patient with impaired physical mobility include the following:

- Performing ROM exercises on all extremities several times per day
- Splinting weakened extremities and using serial lower extremity casting and upper extremity splinting to treat spasticity and maintain functional position of the extremity, especially during the acute phase of care
- Performing strengthening exercises to prevent atrophy and improve the mobility of the involved extremities (hypertonicity varies from a mild increase in motor tone to rigid states, as seen in flexor and extensor posturing)
- Administering antispasmodic agents such as baclofen, dantrolene (Dantrium), and diazepam
- Performing surgical procedures such as myotomy or muscle/tendon release, peripheral nerve simulator implants, and nerve blocks

Complications of impaired mobility include prolonged spasticity, contractures, and heterotrophic ossification (HO). HO involves the deposition of bone around the major joints and has the potential to cause a frozen joint and a functional loss of the use of the extremity.

Cognitive Functioning

Using the behaviors outlined on the Ranchos Los Amigos Scale of Cognitive Functioning, a care plan can be designed to decrease sensory overload. The plan may include the following:

- A strict and consistent schedule to decrease confusion and increase compliance, because the ability to process information is severely impaired. Short-term memory is also affected in these patients, which means they are unable to understand new information about people, places, and events.
- Sensory stimulation programs are usually started in the NCCU and should be continued in rehabilitation.
- Cognitive retraining improves the patient's executive functioning, judgment, and reasoning.
- Controlled stimulation, order, repetition, and consistency are important in assisting the patient to regain optimal cognitive functioning.
- Cognitive remediation based on an assessment of the deficits and strengths, remedial cuing interventions, and the patient's ability to respond. This program focuses on five core deficit areas: arousal and attention, skill structures, memory, language and thought processes, and emotional activity.

Risk for Injury

Unpredictable and eccentric behavior is often seen in a patient with TBI when arousal occurs. Behaviors include the following:

- Agitation
- Screaming, angry outbursts
- Delusions, disinhibitions

Interventions include controlling the environment by placing the patients in a quiet room, providing consistent caregivers, maintaining a strict schedule, and avoiding loud noises (radio, television), confusion, and too many visitors. Medications include haloperidol (Haldol) and lorazepam (Ativan). Sensory stimuli should be meaningful to the patient and presented in a structured format, because he or she has poor insight and judgment and requires careful monitoring. The use of restraints is discouraged unless no other avenues of preventing harm are successful.

Case Management Considerations

Case managers usually become involved with a TBI case when it becomes clear that the discharge plan will be complex and complicated. The exception is the case manager who becomes involved in the coordination of services and medical care for a patient who has problems from a concussion beyond 6 to 12 months. Almost half of all individuals recovering from a concussion experience symptoms afterward, but fewer than 10% experience disabling symptoms that actually intensify instead of resolving. To help the individual return to work or school, a case manager can facilitate evaluation by a specialist for diagnostic studies, neuropsychologic testing, and treatment. Testing may include the following:

- Evoked potentials, including brainstem auditory evoked responses (BAERs)
- SPECT or MRI imaging
- EEG with a 24-hour Holter monitor or a sleep EEG
- Audiologic evaluation
- Transcranial Doppler (TCD)
- Nocturnal penile tumescence (NPT) monitoring

The goals of cognitive and behavioral rehabilitation after TBI are to enhance the patient's capacity to process and interpret information and to improve his or her ability to function in all aspects of family and community life.[46] Restorative training focuses on improving a specific cognitive function, whereas compensatory training focuses on adapting to the presence of a cognitive deficit. The case manager should be aware that these recommendations include the following:

- Comprehensive, interdisciplinary rehabilitation treatment provided by a diverse team of experienced professionals that contains individualized tailored interventions that are both restorative and compensatory
- Computer-assisted strategies for attention, memory, and executive skills
- Compensatory devices (e.g., memory books and electronic paging systems) to improve cognitive function
- Teaching techniques that use sequenced and repetitive practice
- Psychotherapy to treat depression and the loss of self-esteem and cognitive dysfunction
- Individual and family/significant other psychotherapy for emotional support, self-assessment, reduction of denial, and improvement in interpersonal skills related to family members and the community
- Pharmacologic agents for affective and behavioral disturbances associated with TBI, with additional monitoring provided for detrimental side effects

- Behavior modification for personality and the behavioral effects of TBI
- Short- and long-term vocational rehabilitation and job coaching for individuals who will return to work (a "return to work" is considered prognostic of successful rehabilitation)
- Special education services for students who will return to the classroom
- Structured adult education for nutritional support
- Music and art therapy, therapeutic recreation, acupuncture, and other alternative approaches

The case manager assessment includes a thorough patient assessment and chart review, interviews with family members and members of the health care team, and, in many instances, an evaluation of the patient's home. Placement of the patient following hospitalization and inpatient rehabilitation is the first consideration. If the patient is in a persistent vegetative state or coma, a decision must be made for institutional care versus home care with 24-hour caregivers.

Case managers should be aware of and review the 2000 Medical Rehabilitation Standards for Brain Injury Programs of the Commission on Accreditation of Rehabilitation Facilities (CARF). These standards cover rehabilitation programs, outpatient medical rehabilitation, home and community-based programs, long-term residential services, and vocational services. Through a case management approach, the CARF program addresses the following:[39]

- Ongoing access to information about the services available within a coordinated continuum of care
- Movement through the brain injury continuum of care
- Conservation of funding to meet lifelong needs
- Linkages with the community
- Family and support systems and the community
- Education of the person served, his or her family/support systems, and the community
- Facilitation of opportunities for interaction with individuals with similar activity limitations

The most prevalent impairments subsequent to a brain injury are severe cognitive deficits. With this awareness, a plan of care is developed with the health care team, patient and family members, and approval of the payer. Realistic short- and long-term measurable goals are included. Once approval has been received, the case manager implements the plan in a cost-effective manner to ensure continuity of care, monitors patient compliance, and includes patient and family satisfaction with the plan. The goal is functional restoration, compensatory training, prevention of complications, and avoidance of rehospitalization. The responsibility of the case manager may also include provisions for patient transportation, physician visits, and therapy sessions. Follow-up case management includes arranging for caregivers with appropriate home visits to provide wound care and dressing changes, medications, and nutritional evaluation, with frequent written reports from all members of the home health team.

Issues for the case manager to address include inappropriate patient behavior that may interfere with social relationships and interpersonal relationships and that could cause rejection by the spouse, relatives, friends, and associates.

Sexuality and inappropriate sexual behavior can be another disturbing consequence of TBI. The use and abuse of drugs and alcohol may have contributed to the cause of the head injury and may also be a significant problem after discharge from the hospital or rehabilitation center. The need for a consistent and structured lifestyle may create problems within a family unit. After TBI some individuals experience altered sleep patterns (e.g., napping versus sleeping at night, wandering during the night) that require 24-hour supervision. Quality-of-life issues are some of the more difficult challenges in case management.

The patient and family should be provided with a 24-hour telephone number to call for emergencies following TBI (with the understanding of what constitutes a medical emergency). The consequences of TBI may be lifelong, and the patient may require lifelong services. Preventing a second TBI requires care and injury prevention by all members of the team (and teaching for the family).

CONCLUSION

TBI affects 2 million people per year. The cost is staggering, and the outcome can be devastating. In a time when allocation of limited resources is a growing reality, the care of this population needs to be continually reevaluated, organized, cost-effective, and individualized. Nursing care of the patient with TBI is both challenging and complex. Clinicians must carefully consider how interventions affect patients. Care of the TBI patient is an area in which patient condition and response to care truly dictate the methods of nursing practice. Advanced technologic interventions, new pharmacologic agents, and research have improved the diagnosis and treatment of TBI. This has resulted in an increase in the number of survivors and has helped to reduce disability significantly. As scientists develop modalities for neuronal regeneration and repair, neuroscience clinicians will play a key role in the patient's return to functional independence.

RESOURCES FOR NEUROTRAUMA: TRAUMATIC BRAIN INJURY

American Association for Surgery of Trauma: www.aast.org
American Association of Critical Care Nurses: info@aacn.org; www.aacn.org
American Association of Neurological Surgeons: info@AANS.org; www.aans.org
American Association of Neuroscience Nurses: info@aann.org; www.aann.org
American College of Surgeons Committee on Trauma: www.facs.org
American Trauma Society: 800-556-7890; www.amtrauma.org
Brain Injury Association of America: 8201 Greensboro Drive, Suite 611, McLean, VA 22102; 800-444-6443; www.biausa.org
Brain Trauma Foundation: 708 3rd Street, Suite 1810. New York, NY 10017; 212-772-0608; www.braintrauma.org; copies of publications available:
- *Guidelines for the Management of Severe Head Injury, Third Edition*

- *Guidelines for Prehospital Management of Traumatic Head Injury*
- *Guidelines for the Acute Medical Management of Severe Traumatic Brain Injury in Infants, Children and Adolescents*
- *Guidelines for the Surgical Management of Traumatic Brain Injury* (Bullock MR, Chestnut R, Ghajar J, et al: Guidelines for the surgical management of traumatic brain injury [2006], *Neurosurgery* 58[suppl 3]:S2-1–S2-62, 2006.)

Centers for Disease Control and Prevention: www.cdc.gov
Epilepsy Foundation of America: 800-EFA-1000

REFERENCES

1. Adekoya N, Thurman DJ, White DD, Webb KW: Surveillance for traumatic brain injury deaths—United States, 1989–1998, *MMWR* 51(10):1–14, 2002.
2. Alspach JG, editor: A*merican association of critical care nurses: core curriculum for critical care nursing,* ed 5, Philadelphia, 1998, WB Saunders.
3. Bader MK, Littlejohns LR, editors: *American association of neuroscience nursing: core curriculum,* ed 4, St Louis, 2004, Saunders.
4. Bader MK, Littlejohns L, March K: Brain tissue oxygen monitoring in severe brain injury, I. Research and usefulness in critical care, *Crit Care Nurs* 23(4):17–25; 2003.
5. Bader MK, Littlejohns L, March K: Brain tissue oxygen monitoring in severe brain injury, II. Implications for critical care teams and case study, *Crit Care Nurs* 23(4):29–48, 40–42, 44, 2003.
6. Bader MK, Littlejohns L, Palmer S: Ventriculostomy and intracranial pressure monitoring: in search of a 0% infection rate. *Heart Lung* 24:166–172, 1995.
7. Bader MK, Palmer S: Keeping the brain in the zone: applying the severe head injury guidelines to practice, *Crit Care Nurs Clin North Am* 12(4):413–427, 2000.
8. Bayir H, Clark RS, Kochanek PM: Promising strategies to minimize secondary brain injury after head trauma, *Crit Care Med* 31(1 suppl):S112–S117, 2003.
9. Becker DP et al: Diagnosis and treatment of head injury in adults. In Youmans JF, editor: *Neurological surgery: reference guide to the diagnosis and management of neurosurgical problems,* ed 5, Philadelphia, 2003, WB Saunders.
10. Black KL, Hanks RA, Wood DL, Zafonte RD, Cullen N, Cifu DX, et al: Blunt versus penetrating violent traumatic brain injury: frequency and factors associated with secondary conditions and complications, *J Head Trauma Rehab* 17(6):489–496, 2002.
11. Blank-Reid CA, Reid PC: Penetrating trauma to the head, *Crit Care Nurs Clin North Am* 12(4):477–487, 2000.
12. Bullock R, Chestnut RM, Clifton G, Ghajar J, Marion DW, Narayan RK, et al: *Guidelines for the management of severe head injury,* ed 2, New York, 2000, Brain Trauma Foundation.
13. Callanan M: The prevention and management of posttraumatic seizures, *Clin Nurs Pract Epilep* 1(4):1–6, 2000.
14. Centers for Disease Control and Prevention: Traumatic brain injury: Colorado, Missouri, Oklahoma, and Utah, 1990–1993, *MMWR* 46(1):8–11, 1997.
15. Domino K: Pathophysiology of head injury: secondary systemic effects. In Lam A, editor: *Anesthetic management of acute head injury,* New York, 1995, McGraw-Hill.
16. Donaldson J, Borzatta MA, Matossian D: Nutrition strategies in neurotrauma, *Crit Care Nurs Clin North Am* 12(4):465–475, 2000.
17. Farace E, Alves WM: Do women fare worse: a metaanalysis of gender differences in traumatic brain injury outcome, *J Neurosurg* 93(4):539–545, 2000.
18. Goldstein M: Traumatic brain injury: a silent epidemic, *Ann Neurol* 27(3):327, 1990.
19. Granacher RE: *Traumatic brain injury: methods for clinical and forensic neuropsychiatric assessment,* New York, 2003, CRC Press.
20. Grenvik A, Ayres SM, Holbrook PR, Shoemaker WC, editors: *Textbook of critical care,* ed 4, Philadelphia, 2000, WB Saunders.
21. Henry GK, Gross HS, Herndon CA, Furst CJ: Nonimpact brain injury: neuropsychological and behavioral correlates with consideration of physiological findings, *Appl Neuropsychol* 7(2):65–75, 2000.
22. Hickey JV: *The clinical practice of neurological and neurosurgical nursing,* ed 5, Philadelphia, 2003, JB Lippincott.
23. Jiang J, Yu M, Zhu C: Effect of long-term mild hypothermia therapy in patients with severe traumatic brain injury: 1-year follow-up review of 87 cases, *J Neurosurg* 93(4):546–549, 2000.
24. Jordan KS, editor: *Emergency nursing core curriculum,* ed 5, Philadelphia, 2000, WB Saunders.
25. Jumisko E, Lexell J, Soderberg S: The meaning of living with traumatic brain injury in people with moderate or severe traumatic brain injury, *J Neurosci Nurs* 37(1):42–50, 2005.
26. Katz S, Kravetz S, Grynbaum F: Wives'coping flexibility, time since husbands' injury and the perceived burden of wives of men·with traumatic brain injury, *Brain Injury* 19(1):59–66, 2005.
27. Knudson MM, Ikossi DG, Khaw L, Morabito D, Speetzen LS: Thromboembolism after trauma: an analysis of 1602 episodes from the American College of Surgeons National Trauma Data Bank, *Ann Surg* 240(3):490–496, 2004.
28. Langlois JA, Kegler SR, Butler JA, Gotsch KE, et al: Traumatic brain injury-related hospital discharges. Results from a 14-state surveillance system, 1997, *MMWR* 52(4):1–20, 2003.
29. Lyeth H: Neurocognitive/behavioral outcomes in children and adults. Report of the NIH Consensus Development Conference on the Rehabilitation of Persons with Traumatic Brain Injury, Bethesda, MD, 1999, National Institutes of Health.
30. March K: Intracranial pressure monitoring and assessing intracranial compliance in brain injury, *Crit Care Nurs Clin North Am* 12(4):429–436, 2000.
31. Mason RJ, Broaddus VC, Murray JF, Nadel JA: *Murray and Nadel's textbook of respiratory medicine,* ed 4, St Louis, 2005, Elsevier Saunders.
32. Maull KI, editor: *Complications of trauma and critical care,* St Louis, 1996, Elsevier.
33. Mayer, SA, Brun NC, Begtrup K, et al: Recombinant activated factor VII for acute intracerebral hemorrhage, *N Engl J Med* 352(8):777–785, 2005.
34. McCrory P, Johnston K, Meeuwisse W, Aubry M, Cantu R, et al: Summary and agreement statement of the 2nd International Conference on Concussion in Sport, Prague 2004, *Clin J Sport Med* 15(2):48–57, 2005.
35. Munro N: Pulmonary challenges in neurotrauma, *Crit Care Nurs Clin North Am* 12(4):457–464, 2000.
36. Narayan RK, Gopinath, SP, Robertson CS: Intracranial complications. In Mattox KL, editor: *Complications of trauma,* New York, 1994, Churchill Livingstone.

37. National Center for Injury Prevention and Control: *Report to Congress on mild traumatic brain injury in the United States: steps to prevent a serious public health problem,* Atlanta, GA, 2003, Centers for Disease Control and Prevention.

38. National Institutes of Health: *A report of the task force on trauma research,* Bethesda, MD, 1994, The Institute.

39. Neale PS: CARFs new brain injury programs and spinal cord system of care standards, *J Care Manage* 6(2):40–48, 2000.

40. Newberry L, Sheehy SB, editors: *Sheehy's emergency nursing principles and practice,* ed 4, St Louis, 1998, Mosby.

41. Noppens R, Brambrink AM: Traumatic brain injury in children—clinical implications, *Exp Toxicol Pathol* 56(1–2):113–125, 2004.

42. Ostermann ME, Keenan SP, Seiferling RA, Sibbald WJ: Sedation in the intensive care unit, *JAMA* 283(11):1451–1459, 2000.

43. Page RB, Spott MA, Krishnamurthy S, Taleghani C, Chinchilli VM: Head injury and pulmonary embolism: a retrospective report based on the Pennsylvania Trauma Outcomes study, *Neurosurgery* 54(1):143–148, 2004.

44. Pelosi P, Severgnini P, Chiaranda M: An integrated approach to prevent and treat respiratory failure in brain-injured patients, *Curr Opin Crit Care* 11(1):37–42, 2005.

45. Qiu WS, Liu WG, Shen H, Wang WM, Hang ZL, Zhang Y, et al: Therapeutic effect of mild hypothermia on severe traumatic head injury, *Chin J Trauma* 8(1):27–32, 2005.

46. Rehabilitation of persons with traumatic brain injury, *NIH Consensus Statement* 16(1):1–41, 1998.

47. Shatz DV, Kirton OC, McKenny MG, Civetta JM: *Manual of trauma and emergency surgery,* Philadelphia, 2000, WB Saunders.

48. Sheehy SB, editor: *Manual of clinical trauma care: the first hour,* ed 3, St Louis, 1999, Mosby.

49. Sosin D, Sniezek J, Thurman D: Incidence of mild and moderate brain injury in the United States, *Brain Inj* 10(1):47–54, 1996.

50. Sosin D, Sniezek J, Wazweiler R: Trends in death associated with traumatic brain injury, 1979 through 1992: success and failure, *JAMA* 273:1778–1780, 1995.

51. Spain DA, McClave SA, Sexton LK: Infusion protocol improves delivery of enteral tube feeding in the critical care unit, *J Parenter Enter Nutr* 23(5):288–292, 1999.

52. Stevens WJ: Multimodal monitoring: head injury management using SjvO$_2$ and LICOX, *J Neuro Nurs* 36(6):332–339, 2004.

53. Sund-Levander M, Wahren LK: Assessment and prevention of shivering in patients with severe cerebral injury: a pilot study, *J Clin Nurs* 9(1):55–61, 2000.

54. Taylor SJ, Fettes AB, Jewkes C, Nelson RJ: Prospective, randomized, controlled trial to determine the effect of early enhanced enteral nutrition on clinical outcome in mechanically ventilated patient suffering head injury, *Crit Care Med* 27:2525–2531, 1999.

55. Thurman DJ, Alverson C, Dunn KA, Guerrero J, Sniezek JE: Traumatic brain injury in the United States: a public health perspective, *J Head Trauma Rehab* 14:602–615, 1999.

56. Vespa P, Prins M, Ronne-Engstrom E, et al: Increase in extracellular glutamate caused by reduced cerebral perfusion pressure and seizures after human traumatic brain injury: a microdialysis study, *J Neurosurg* 89(6):971–982, 1998.

57. Vialet R, Albanese J, Thomachot L, Antonini F, Bourgouin A, Alliez B, Martin C: Isovolume hypertonic solutes (sodium chloride or mannitol) in the treatment of refractory posttraumatic intracranial hypertension: 2 ml/kg 7.5% saline is more effective than 2 ml/kg 20% mannitol, *Crit Care Med* 31(6),1683–1687, 2003.

58. Wilensky EM, Bloom S, Leichter D, Verdiramo AM, Ledwith M, Stiefel M, LeRoux S, Grady MS: Brain tissue oxygen practice guidelines using LICOX CMP monitoring system, *J Neuro Nurs* 37(5):278–288, 2005.

59. Wilson RF, Dente C, Tyburski JG: The nutritional support of patients with head injuries, *Neurol Res* 23(2–3):121–128, 2001.

60. Wongavatunyu S, Porter EJ: Mother's experience of helping young adults with traumatic brain injury, *J Nurs Scholarship* 37(1):48–55, 2005.

61. Yanagawa T, Bunn F, Roberts I, Wentz R, Pierro A: Nutritional support for head-injured patients, *Cochrane Database of Systematic Reviews* 3:CD001530, 2002.

CHAPTER 12

KELLY JOHNSON, KELLY MOWREY,
MICHELE J. BERGMAN

Neurotrauma: Spinal Injury

Acute spinal cord injury (ASCI) can be described as one of the most devastating types of injury an individual may experience. Patients with ASCI present neuroscience clinicians with some of the greatest challenges and require an extensive cadre of specialized and experienced health care and community providers to manage an array of complex needs. Clinicians are involved in management of individuals with spinal cord injuries (SCIs) at all levels: prehospital, emergency, critical, and perioperative care; acute and chronic rehabilitation; and home health, case management, and life care planning. Additional support for patients with ASCI may lead to comprehensive services through roles that affect patient advocacy and legislation.

A typical accident leading to an ASCI can occur without warning and often tragically affects the lives of young adults. Momentary inattention coupled with motor vehicles, speed, bad safety practices, and alcohol or substance abuse may play a pivotal role. Emergent and acute care will be managed by a team of experienced SCI clinicians, 24 hours a day, if the individual with an ASCI survives the initial trauma. All too often, such accidents have devastating outcomes that instantly change the life of an individual and his or her family. The consequences of SCI are complex and challenging and have far reaching consequences for everyone involved.

Clinical goals for patients with SCI are to minimize impairment, handicap, and disability. Prevention of secondary complications for these patients is critical and begins with expert trauma and resuscitative care; comprehensive care will extend throughout the individual's lifetime. The ultimate outcomes are to promote maximum health and wellness in this vulnerable population and to assist people with SCI in achieving maximum functional independence, successful community reintegration, and a high quality of life. This chapter covers clinical care of an individual with an acute traumatic spinal injury from the time of injury through a lifetime of follow-up.

NEUROANATOMY OF THE SPINAL CORD

Clinicians must develop an in-depth knowledge of key anatomic features of the spinal structures and spinal cord (see Chapter 1). The value of this knowledge base lies in the fact that the location of injury to the spinal cord affects the pre-sentation of the patient both acutely and long term. Location of injury guides clinical and rehabilitation management.

The spinal column is the bony structure that surrounds and protects the delicate nervous tissue of the spinal cord. The spinal column is formed from vertebrae. There are 7 cervical, 12 thoracic, 5 lumbar, 5 fused sacral, and 3 to 5 fused coccygeal vertebrae. The C1 vertebra is additionally labeled the atlas. The C2 vertebra, also labeled the axis, has a fingerlike projection labeled the odontoid process (dens) that articulates with the anterior arch of the atlas.

The anterior portion of the vertebrae is called the body and the posterior portion is the arch. The arch is formed from two transverse processes and one spinous process and two superior and inferior facets. Two laminae form the roof of the arch and two pedicles attach the arch to the body of the vertebrae. Intervertebral disks are situated between every two vertebral bodies and serve as shock absorbers. The disk is formed from an outer fibrous cartilage ring called **annulus fibrosis** and contains a spongy inner material known as the **nucleus pulposus.** There are two major supporting ligaments, the anterior and posterior longitudinal ligaments. They run from the atlas to the sacrum. There are additionally short, dense ligaments located between the vertebral arches; ligamenta flava run between the laminae; supraspinal and interspinal ligaments run between the spinous processes; and transverse ligaments run between the transverse processes.

As mentioned in Chapter 1, there are 31 pairs of spinal nerves: 8 cervical, 12 thoracic, 5 lumbar, 5 sacral, and 1 coccygeal. Each root has a dorsal (posterior) sensory root that transmits afferent impulses to the cord and a ventral (anterior) motor root that transmits efferent impulses from the cord to target muscles and organs. The C1 nerve roots exit over the top of the body of C1. The C2 nerve root exits between C1 and C2. Other cervical nerve roots exit over the top of the caudal vertebrae until C8, which exits between C7 and T1. All other nerve roots exit under the vertebrae for which they are numbered.

There are several key nerves. C3 to C5 form the phrenic nerve and innervate the diaphragm. C5 innervates the deltoid and biceps muscles. C6 innervates the wrist extensors. C7 innervates the triceps. C8 innervates the finger flexors. T2 to T7 innervate chest muscles. T9 to T12 innervate the abdominal muscles. L1 to L5 innervate the leg muscles. S2 to S5 are significant for innervation of bowel, bladder, and sexual organs. The sensory dermatome figure displays major sensory areas innervated by level (Fig. 12-1).

The nerve tracts are topographically layered within the spinal cord. The central gray matter, the butterfly-shaped core of the spinal cord, contains neuron cell bodies. The posterior or dorsal horn of the gray matter contains sensory cell bodies, and synapse with second-order neurons to send fibers to reflex or higher centers. The anterior or ventral horn of the gray matter contains motor cell bodies that receive input from the brain and synapse with second-order neurons to transmit messages through the anterior root to target muscles and organs. The lateral horns of the gray matter contain autonomic nerve cell bodies.

The white matter contains bundles of neurons that ascend and descend the spinal cord. The ascending tracts contain sensory fibers. The posterior columns are responsible for well-localized touch, pressure, vibration, stereognosis, proprioception, and position sense. These fibers do not cross until the second-order neuron and synapse at the level of the thalamus. The spinothalamic tracts transmit sensations of pain, temperature, and crude touch. These fibers ascend several segments and synapse with a second-order neuron and cross to ascend in the lateral tract. The spinocerebellar tracts transmit joint and position sense, as well as unconscious proprioception, to the cerebellum. The majority of these fibers do not cross. The major descending motor tracts are the corticospinal tracts. These fibers cross at the level of the medulla and travel down the contralateral side of the spinal cord.

The blood supply for the spinal cord arises from descending branches of the vertebral arteries. The **anterior spinal artery** supplies the anterior two thirds of the blood supply to the cord and runs the full length of the cord. The posterior spinal arteries supply the posterior one third of the cord and also run the full length of the cord. Radicular arteries are derived from segmental vessels that supply blood to spinal roots and the outer circumference of the spinal cord.

EPIDEMIOLOGY

The annual incidence of SCI in the United States is estimated to be approximately 11,000 cases per year, not including those who die at the scene. The prevalence is estimated to be approximately 250,000 living in the United States. SCI is primarily an injury of young adult males. The mean age at injury is 37.7, with 19 being the most common age at injury and the range for 50% of those injured being 16 to 30 years of age. Individuals over 60 accounted for 8.4% of injuries, which has steadily risen over the past 25 years. Males make up 79.6% of people living with SCI. Ethnic groups injured include 62.9% Caucasian, 22% African American, 12.6% Hispanic, and 2.5% from other racial or ethnic groups.

Motor vehicle crashes account for 47.5% of reported cases of SCI, with falls (22.9%), violence (primarily gunshot wounds) (13.8%), and recreational sporting activities (8.9%) or other accounting for the majority of the remaining injuries. Incomplete tetraplegia is the largest category of injury (34.5%) followed by complete paraplegia (23.1%), complete tetraplegia (18.4%), and incomplete paraplegia (17.5%). Life expectancy continues to increase for individuals with SCI due to improved medical care but remains slightly lower than the population without SCI. The causes of death that have the greatest impact on reduced life expectancy are pneumonia, pulmonary emboli, and septicemia.[88]

PATHOPHYSIOLOGY

Primary injury to the spinal cord is the damage caused by the initial insult to the spinal cord. It can occur in seconds from biomechanical trauma with hemorrhage and cell death. The primary injury is not reversible. Information about the primary event and mechanism of injury can be provided by paramedics, witnesses at the scene, or the patient and family. The effects of the damage depend on location, severity, and type of nerve damage to the spinal cord[15] and can cause immediate motor, sensory, or autonomic dysfunction. Types of spinal cord injury include contusions (bruising of the spinal cord), compression (pressure on the spinal cord), lacerations, and, less commonly, complete transection. Spinal cord injury can result from vertebral injury, fractures, or injury to the neural elements of the spinal cord without vertebral damage. Damage can also be a result of disruption of the blood supply to the spinal cord.[71]

Types of Vertebral Column Fractures

Mechanism of injury is the force or stress that produced a spinal injury. Blunt injury, the most common mechanism of injury, involves forces, often in combination: forced flexion (anterior) (Fig. 12-2), or flexion with rotation (Fig. 12-3); forced extension (hyperextension) (Fig. 12-4); or vertical compression (axial loading) (Fig. 12-5). Penetrating injuries, such as gunshot or knife wounds, are frequently a result of assault or other violent acts. This mechanism of injury can be attributed to an increasing number of spinal cord injuries. Fractures to the spinal column may or may not result in a spinal cord injury.[26,128] There are numerous types and classifications of vertebral fractures (Box 12-1):

- **Simple fractures:** occur at a spinous or transverse process, facet, or pedicle. Alignment remains intact, and neural compression is usually not present.
- **Wedge fracture:** also called compression fracture. The vertebral body is compressed anteriorly due to a hyperflexion injury; neural compression may or may not be present.
- **Comminuted fracture:** also known as a burst fracture. Results in a shattering of the vertebral body; the bone may be driven into the spinal cord with this type of fracture, which is associated with vertical (axial) loading forces and generally results in serious SCI.
- **Fracture-dislocation injuries:** often combined with ligament injury. Can result in a small fragment of bone breaking off from the anterior edge of the vertebra to lodge in the spinal canal. Neurologic deficits may result if the bone fragment penetrates

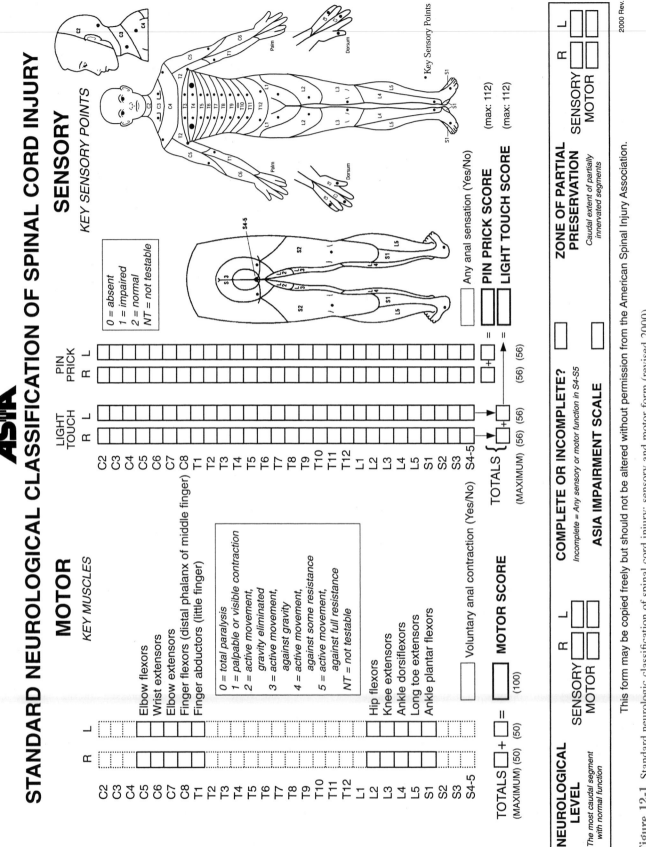

Figure 12-1 Standard neurologic classification of spinal cord injury; sensory and motor form (revised 2000). *(Courtesy American Spinal Injury Association, Atlanta, GA.)*

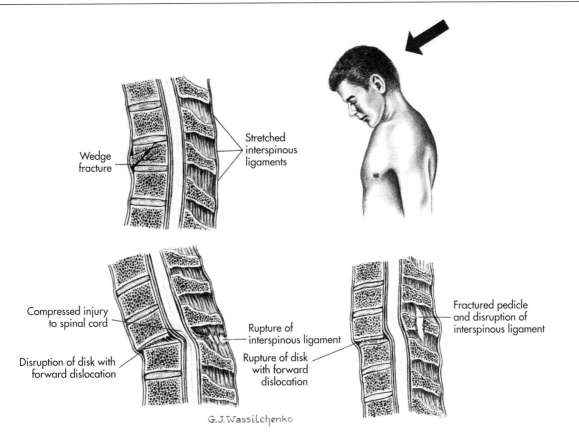

Figure 12-2 Hyperflexion injury of the spine.
(From Thompson JM et al: Mosby's clinical nursing, *ed 3, St Louis, 1993, Mosby.)*

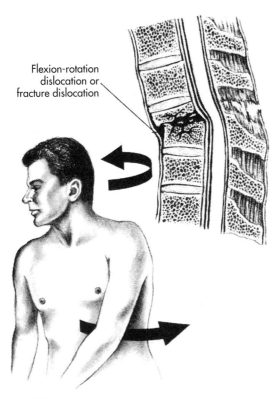

Figure 12-3 Flexion-rotation injuries of the spine.
(From Thompson JM et al: Mosby's clinical nursing, *ed 3, St Louis, 1993, Mosby.)*

BOX 12-1   Vertebral Column Fractures

- Simple fractures
- Wedge or compression fracture
- Comminuted or burst fracture
- Fracture-dislocation
- Dislocation of a vertebra
- Subluxation
- Jefferson fracture
- Atlanto-occipital dislocation
- Odontoid fractures
- Hangman's fracture

---

the spinal cord or if there is severe ligamentous damage.

- **Dislocation of a vertebra:** occurs when one vertebra overrides another and there is unilateral or bilateral facet dislocation. Spinal injury in this case usually results from torn or stretched ligaments that allow excessive movement of the vertebra.
- **Subluxation:** partial or incomplete dislocation of one vertebra over another. Ligamentous injury may also be present after subluxation.
- **Jefferson fracture:** bursting of the ring of C1 as a result of axial loading on C1. The most common complaint is pain in the cervical area. Cervical muscle spasms and a limitation in neck movement also may be present. There is frequently no immediate damage

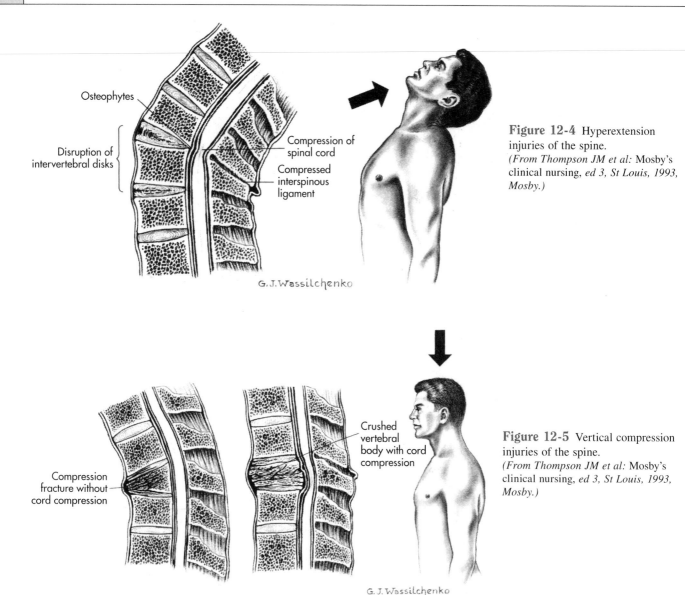

Osteophytes

Disruption of intervertebral disks

Compression of spinal cord

Compressed interspinous ligament

G.J.Wassilchenko

Figure 12-4 Hyperextension injuries of the spine. *(From Thompson JM et al:* Mosby's clinical nursing, *ed 3, St Louis, 1993, Mosby.)*

Compression fracture without cord compression

Crushed vertebral body with cord compression

Figure 12-5 Vertical compression injuries of the spine. *(From Thompson JM et al:* Mosby's clinical nursing, *ed 3, St Louis, 1993, Mosby.)*

G.J.Wassilchenko

to the spinal cord; if the fracture is displaced, the injury may be fatal.

- **Atlanto-occipital dislocation:** produced by an avulsion of the atlas from the occipital bone. Death is usually immediate with this type of injury, but if the patient survives the injury, it is possible to have no neurologic deficit or an incomplete injury.
- **Odontoid fractures:** involve the odontoid process (dens) of vertebra C2. Death or severe neurologic deficits frequently occur if the odontoid process penetrates the spinal cord, but injuries of this type infrequently result in no or minimal neurologic deficit. There are three types of odontoid fractures (Figs. 12-6 and 12-7). Type 1 is an avulsion fracture of the tip of the dens, often involving the alar ligament. This type of fracture is stable and may be associated with atlanto-occipital dislocation.[9] Type 2 is a transverse or oblique fracture through the midsection of the dens. The fracture is unstable. It is often displaced anteriorly

or posteriorly and associated with a high nonunion rate when managed conservatively.[9] Type 3 is a fracture through the base of the dens into the cancellous body of the axis. It may require light traction for initial reduction followed by halo orthosis.[9]

- **Hangman's fracture:** fracture through the arch of the C2 vertebra, often from hyperextension of the neck. The patient may not experience neurologic effects from this injury (Fig. 12-8).

Classification of Stability

Classification of spinal stability can be complex.[5,26] Factors indicative of instability include progressive neurologic deficit, kyphosis of greater than 20 degrees, loss of vertebral height of greater than 50%, and retropulsed bone fragments within the neural canal.[44] There have been several attempts at devising a classification system to assist in determination of spinal stability. The most frequently cited system is the three-

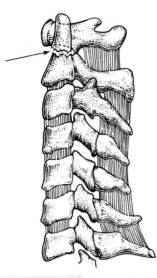

Figure 12-6 Odontoid fractures. Fracture of the odontoid process (the superior projection of the body of C2 that projects into the ring of C1 and orients the two vertebrae) results in instability at this level. Stabilization is required, with the method being determined by the exact type of fracture.

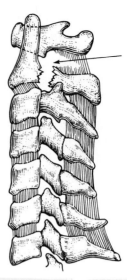

Figure 12-8 Hangman's fracture. A fracture through the pedicles of the second cervical vertebra, separating the posterior neural arch from the body of the axis, resulting in an anterior dislocation with angulation of C1 and the body of C2. These fractures usually will heal spontaneously with prolonged traction or immobilization with a halo brace.

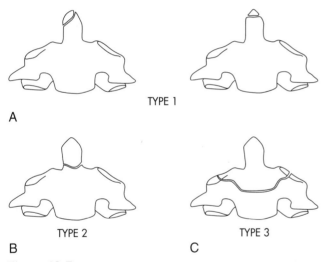

TYPE 1

A

TYPE 2   TYPE 3

B   C

Figure 12-7 Three types of odontoid fractures. **A,** Type I is an oblique fracture through the upper part or tip of the odontoid process. The patient is stable and is usually fitted with a halo-type vest or stiff collar until the fracture heals. **B,** Type II is a fracture at the base of the dens or at the junction of the odontoid process with the vertebral body of C2. Because the blood supply may be impaired, union may be delayed. Depending on the patient, treatment options may include a halo vest for stablization or surgery/halo for stabilization until the fracture heals. **C,** A fracture that actually extends into the body of the C2 vertebrae. With alignment and union of the dens and vertebrae and stabilization with a halo vest, the fracture may heal over a 3-month period.
(From Anderson LD, D'Alonzo RT: Fractures of the odontoid process of the axis, J Bone Joint Surg 56A:1663, 1974.)

column classification of spinal stability. Cervical spinal stability is established using the three-column classification system.[20] The anterior column is formed by the anterior longitudinal ligament, the anterior annulus fibrosus, and the anterior one half of the vertebral body. The middle column is formed by the posterior longitudinal ligament, the posterior one half of the annulus fibrosus, and the vertebral body. The posterior column is composed of the osseous and ligamentous structures posterior to the posterior longitudinal ligament. Spinal stability, in this system, is dependent on at least two intact columns.[42] Gunshot wounds are the exception to the three-column rule, and can be stable even with two- or three-column injury.[20] Even though an injury may be acutely unstable, delayed stability can occur with fracture healing.[128] If severe ligamentous damage has occurred, fractures may remain chronically unstable unless they have been surgically fixated.[6]

Classification of Neurologic Level of Injury

Classification is by neurologic level, clinical syndrome of degree (complete versus incomplete), and mechanism of injury. The American Spinal Injury Association (ASIA) published the most recent edition for classification of SCI in 2000 (see Fig. 12-1). These standards define the neurologic level of injury as the most caudal segment of the spinal cord with normal sensory and motor function on both sides of the body.[5] If the cervical level at C7 is the highest neurologic level of normal function, the neurologic level of injury is documented as C7. It is important to realize that the orthopedic level of injury does not equate to the neurologic level of injury. Neurologic level is more important in functional prediction.

Not all cases of trauma leading to vertebral or ligamentous injury of the spinal column result in SCI, or they may cause varying degrees of neurologic deficit. Neurologic deficit resulting from SCI may occur in the absence of vertebral fracture or ligamentous injury, and may not be detected by radiographic image, either plain films or computed tomography (CT). This occurrence is termed **spinal cord injury without radiographic abnormality (SCIWORA).** SCIWORA is most common in infants and younger children, is occasionally seen in adolescents, and is rarely diagnosed in adults.[23] When trauma to the spinal cord does result in loss of neurologic function, the SCI is classified by level and completeness of injury.

A systematic evaluation of **dermatomes** (sensation) and **myotomes** (motor function) is the basis of determining the cord segments affected by SCI. A thorough examination and documentation of level of injury is critical in determining changes in neurologic status in states of worsening neurologic condition, return of neurologic function, prediction of outcomes, and rehabilitation planning. Cervical dermatomes reflect sensation in the head, neck, shoulders, upper extremities, and chest. Thoracic dermatomes T1 to T12 cover the chest and abdomen. Lumbar dermatomes L1 to L5 reflect the lower extremities, and sacral dermatomes S1 to S5 cover the lower extremities and the perineum.

An injury to the spinal cord in the cervical region may result in **tetraplegia,** defined as an associated loss of muscle strength in all four extremities and the trunk and abdominal region. Injury to the thoracic, lumbar, or sacral regions, including the cauda equina and conus medullaris, may result in **paraplegia** with associated loss of motor and sensory function in the lower extremities and pelvic region.

Complete Versus Incomplete Injury

ASIA has adopted a classification system to determine level of injury and degree of completeness of injury.[5] This classification system consists of five impairment levels, determined by motor-sensory examination. The impairment levels are labeled A through E (Fig. 12-9).

ASIA A, complete SCI, is defined as no sensory or motor function preserved in the sacral segments S4 to S5. **Incomplete SCI** is described by three distinct impairment levels, B, C, and D. **ASIA B** is defined as sensory but not motor function preserved below the neurologic level and includes the sacral segments S4 to S5. At impairment level **ASIA C,** motor function is preserved below the neurologic level, and more than half of key muscles below the neurologic level have a muscle grade less than 3 (grades 0 to 2). At impairment level **ASIA D,** motor function is preserved below the neurologic level, and at least half of key muscles below the neurologic level have a muscle grade greater than or equal to 3. **Normal** sensory and muscle findings on the ASIA impairment assessment are labeled **ASIA E.**

Spinal Cord Syndromes

There are varied clinical presentations by patients who have experienced spinal cord injury with neurologic deficit. Spinal

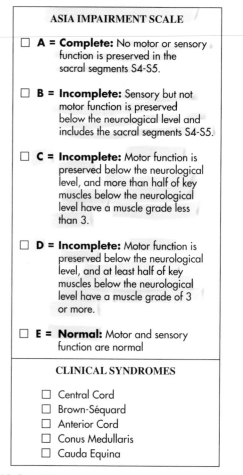

Figure 12-9 ASIA Impairment Scale (revised 2000). *(Courtesy American Spinal Injury Association, Atlanta, GA.)*

cord syndromes are descriptive classifications of incomplete spinal cord injuries (Fig. 12-10).

- **Anterior cord syndrome** affects the anterior two thirds of the cord. It is associated with flexion injury, impaired blood supply or ischemia of the anterior spinal artery, herniated disk, or fracture with bony fragments. There is immediate motor loss and *hypoesthesia,* loss of sensation of pain and temperature below the level of injury. Posterior spinal function is preserved for sensation of light touch, position sense, and vibration. This syndrome results in variable loss of motor function and sensitivity to pain and temperature while preserving proprioception[5] (Figs. 12-11 and 12-12).
- **Central cord syndrome** may follow a hyperextension injury. It is more commonly associated with injuries in older adults and individuals with spondylosis, degenerative changes, spinal disease, or osteoarthritis. It is common in unbelted motor vehicle crashes and particularly after a fall. The lesion occurs almost exclusively in the cervical region. This syndrome is characterized by sacral sensory sparing and greater weakness in the upper extremities than the lower extremities[5] (Fig. 12-13). Microscopic hemorrhage

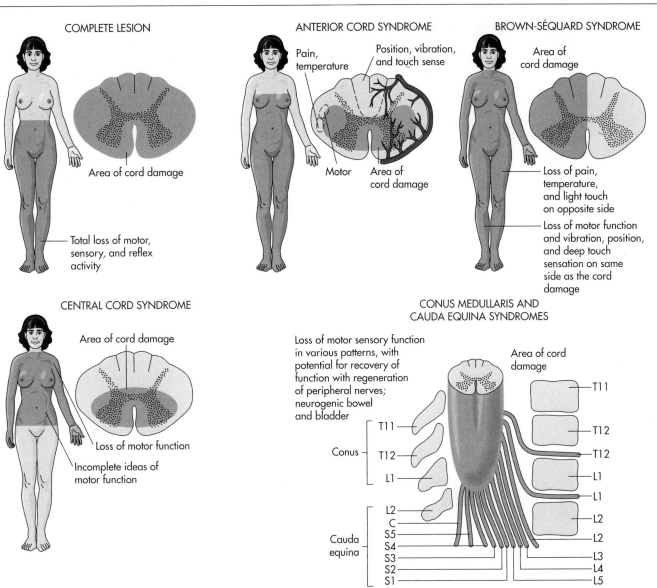

Figure 12-10 Common spinal cord syndromes.
(From Ignatavicius DD, Workman ML: Medical-surgical nursing: critical thinking for collaborative care, *ed 4, St Louis, 2002, WB Saunders.)*

and edema occurs in the central gray matter occurs of the spinal cord.

- **Brown-Séquard syndrome** is a hemisection of the spinal cord most commonly caused by a stab or gunshot wound. It results in greater ipsilateral proprioceptive and motor loss and contralateral loss of sensitivity to pain and temperature[5] (Fig. 12-14). The patient is unable to move the leg (paralysis) but has sensation on the side of injury. Patients have pain, temperature, and light touch sensation on the side opposite the injury.
- **Conus medullaris syndrome** occurs with injury of the conus or sacral spinal cord and lumbar nerve roots. This syndrome usually results in lower motor neuron damage to the bowel, bladder, and lower limbs. Sacral segments may show preserved reflexes such as bulbocavernosus and micturition reflexes.[5]

- **Cauda equina syndrome,** lateral cord syndrome, or root syndrome is an injury or compression to the lumbosacral nerve roots within the neural canal resulting in lower motor neuron damage to the bowel, bladder, and lower limbs.[5] This syndrome should be monitored for following lumbar back surgery when a hematoma or hemorrhage can compress the cord and cause permanent paralysis if not detected early and evacuated for decompression of the nerve roots. Sensation may be lost first, called **saddle hypalgesia.** Patients may develop incontinence and have areflexic bladder and bowel with varying degrees of motor and sensory loss. Because peripheral nerves can regenerate, recovery is often possible.
- **Sacral sparing** is a measure of completeness of SCI and is a significant predictor of neurologic recovery. Patients with sacral sparing are more likely to

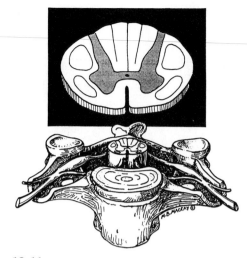

Figure 12-11 Normal spinal cord and column. The relationship between the spinal cord, spinal column, and nerve roots is shown in the midcervical area. The dura has been omitted. The intravertebral disk is depicted. The stippled region demonstrates the gray matter, and the spinothalamic and corticospinal tracts are outlined.
(From Hickey JH, Minton MS, editors: The nursing clinics of North America: neuroscience nursing for a new millennium, Philadelphia, 2000, WB Saunders.)

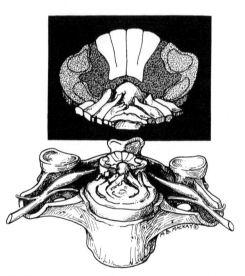

Figure 12-12 Anterior cord syndrome. A large disk herniation is depicted compressing the anterior segment of the cord, which results in damage *(rough stippling)* to the lateral and anterior white matter tracts and to the gray matter. The posterior columns stay intact. This syndrome is known as the anterior spinal artery syndrome. There may be a loss of pain and temperature sensation and motor function below the lesion. Vibration, light touch, and position sensation remain intact.
(From Hickey JH, Minton MS, editors: The nursing clinics of North America: neuroscience nursing for a new millennium, Philadelphia, 2000, WB Saunders.)

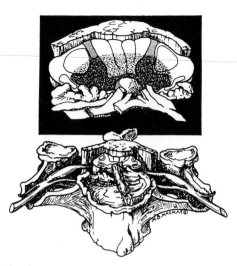

Figure 12-13 Central cord syndrome. This is the most common incomplete spinal cord injury syndrome. It is often seen following acute hyperextension in older patients with preexisting stenosis as a result of anterior spurs. Edema on the central cord exerts pressure on the anterior horn cells. Cervical spondylosis and osteoarthritis of the cervical spine, including anterior and posterior osteophytes, are demonstrated along with hypertrophy of the ligamentum flavum. The spinal cord is compressed anteriorly and posteriorly. The greatest damage *(rough stippling)* occurs in the central portion of the cord. The damaged area includes the medial segment of the corticospinal tracts. There are more motor deficits in the upper extremities.
(From Hickey JH, Minton MS, editors: The nursing clinics of North America: neuroscience nursing for a new millennium, Philadelphia, 2000, WB Saunders.)

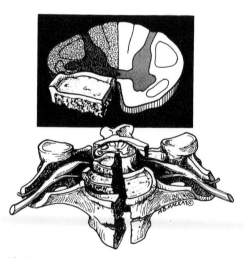

Figure 12-14 Brown-Séquard syndrome. A burst fracture is shown with displacement of the posterior bone fragments and disk. This results in unilateral compression and damage *(rough stippling)* to one half of the spinal cord. This syndrome results in hemisection of the spinal cord, often caused by penetrating trauma. Presentation is ipsilateral paralysis of paresis with an ipsilateral loss of pressure, vibration, and touch and a contralateral loss of temperature and pain sensation.
(From Hickey JH, Minton MS, editors: The nursing clinics of North America: neuroscience nursing for a new millennium, Philadelphia, 2000, WB Saunders.)

experience motor recovery.[75] Sacral sparing is a result of preservation of long tract sacral fibers located at the periphery of the cord.[40] The presence of sacral sensation, including sensation at the anal mucutaneous junction and deep anal sensation, and motor function, including voluntary contraction of the external anal sphincter on digital examination, constitutes sacral sparing.[5] Sacral sparing is determined by stimulation around the anal area to determine if there is any sensation reported by the patient or observation of constriction when a gloved finger is inserted in the rectum.

Autonomic Dysfunction

A primary function of the autonomic nervous system (ANS) is to maintain homeostasis within the body (see Chapter 1). With the presence of trauma to the central nervous system (CNS), the function and stability of the ANS may be impaired. The presence and severity of autonomic dysfunction varies by level and severity of injury. Autonomic dysfunction is more extensive when the level of injury is higher.

Neurogenic shock occurs more commonly in injuries above T6 due to the body's reaction to sudden interruption of the CNS causing the disruption of the sympathetic outflow from T1 to L2 with unopposed vagal tone. Neurogenic shock is manifested as a triad of symptoms: hypotension, bradycardia, and hypothermia. This is caused by the decrease in vascular resistance with associated vascular dilation. Blood pools in the extremities with deceased blood pressure. Neurogenic shock must be differentiated from hypovolemic shock to direct treatment.[40] Bradycardia with hypotension differentiates neurogenic shock from hypovolemic shock.[9]

Spinal shock is a result of the concussive effect of the primary SCI on the nervous system.[9] This concussive effect results in transient depression of all reflexes, including loss of deep tendon reflexes, paralysis, flaccid areflexia, loss of sensation, loss of autonomic function, and loss of bowel and bladder function. The duration of spinal shock is variable and may last days to months.[116] It is not possible to determine completeness of SCI until spinal shock resolves.[9] Resolution of spinal shock is determined with return of the bulbocavernosus reflex, which may return hours or weeks after injury. The onset of spasticity or hyperreflexia is an indication that spinal shock has resolved.

Other early autonomic dysfunctions that may result after SCI are ileus and urinary retention. Later autonomic effects may include autonomic dysreflexia, and hypotension, bradycardia, and poikilothermia that may persist after the spinal shock phase. These later autonomic dysfunctions are more severe with higher levels of injury.

Secondary Injury

Secondary injury is damage to the spinal cord that occurs at the cellular level following the initial trauma. It is important for clinicians to have knowledge of the multiple secondary injuries that can occur and take aggressive measures for early detection and rapid intervention to improve patient outcomes.

There are two ways that cells die in the spinal cord: necrosis and apoptosis. **Necrosis** is a process in which cells swell and burst, leaking toxic substances into surrounding cells. There are several events that contribute to this level of cellular destruction. Immune system reactions are stimulated following trauma. Immune cells are activated and enter the CNS within the first 12 hours after trauma. These cells engulf and eliminate and remove debris, and release a host of powerful regulatory substances. These two functions of the immune cells have beneficial and detrimental effects.[87]

Oxidative damage with oxidizing agents, also known as **free radicals,** are produced by the body's inflammatory cells. Oxidizing agents attack molecules that are essential for cellular function, leading to oxidative damage. Free radicals are a by-product of normal metabolism, and are produced at an increased rate, with increased metabolic processes after trauma. The combination of several of the free radicals can create compounds that are very destructive in the CNS and reduce the antioxidant defenses.[87]

Calcium toxicity and excitotoxicity are phenomena that result from excessive release of neurotransmitters, primarily glutamate, which occurs following trauma to the spinal cord. High levels of calcium enter cells following overactivation of specific glutamate receptors, leading to release of enzymes that are harmful to cells. Calcium additionally contributes to oxidative damage and destruction of cell mitochondria. Glutamate allows entry of ions such as sodium and chloride into cells, which allows water to enter cells leading to cellular swelling, and ultimately cell death.[87]

Apoptosis is thought to be a genetically controlled, **programmed cell death** that has been alternately described as a form of "cell suicide."[87] Cells experiencing apoptosis go through a series of structural changes, including changes in the cell membrane, cell nucleus, and DNA. In the case of traumatic SCI, damaged cells eliminate themselves in order to protect neighboring cells, without releasing chemicals that would be toxic to surrounding cells. Apoptosis has been shown to occur in sites near the impact zone within hours after injury, with more extensive apoptosis occurring days to weeks after injury.[87]

Axonal damage causes motor and sensory changes after spinal cord injury. Neuronal (axon) damage within the spinal cord can be caused at the time of the initial injury with stretching and tearing of the axons. The primary cause of axonal damage, however, is swelling of axons and impaired axonal transport. Axonal transport is a vital function for molecular movement to and from the axon terminals back to the cell body. Disruption in axonal transport has multiple causes. Changes in the cell membrane that allow an abnormal influx of ions, primarily calcium, lead to critical changes in the cytoskeleton. These changes in the cytoskeleton cause interruption of axonal transport. In damaged axons that show no change in membrane permeability, misalignment of neurofilaments is responsible for impairment of transport and swelling of axons. The consequence of axonal damage is cell death. Axons disintegrate after disconnection from the cell body. This process is called wallerian or orthograde degeneration. Retrograde degeneration, whereby the axon degenerates toward the cell body from the site of injury, begins a few weeks after injury and results in severe and permanent effects such as paralysis and loss of sensation. Demyelination of axons also occurs, resulting in cellular degeneration.[87]

Spinal Cord and Brain Injury: Dual Diagnosis

Patients with SCI often have a dual diagnosis, and care becomes an increased challenge for the treatment team. Incidence of concomitant SCI and traumatic brain injury (TBI) is reported between 24% and 59%.[111] A severe TBI may initially mask the presence of an SCI because of the inability to move limbs, or the patient not being able to follow commands. National guidelines should be implemented to manage the TBI; however, review of those guidelines is beyond the scope of this chapter. The main objectives would be to treat the complications of TBI and limit secondary brain damage.[8] Dual diagnosis complicates an already catastrophic injury and presents great challenges to the treating team on admission throughout the acute phase of recovery. Implications for the rehabilitation team involve the potential cognitive deficits and the potential negative impact on patient participation in the rehabilitation program and on the patient's ability to learn management of his or her SCI.

PREHOSPITAL MANAGEMENT

The American Association of Neurological Surgeons and Congress of Neurological Surgeons published a document in 2002 containing 22 evidence-based, best practice recommendations for management of acute cervical spine and spinal cord injuries.[54] The philosophy behind the guidelines is that standardized care will produce better outcomes for this devastating injury. The guidelines address care of cervical spinal cord injury, including the following: prehospital care and transport, neurologic and radiographic assessment, medical management of SCI, closed reduction of cervical fracture dislocations, and specific treatment options, both operative and nonoperative, for each specific cervical injury type known to occur from the occiput through thoracic level one.[54] Although each of the 22 recommendations is not presented here verbatim, most of the 22 recommendations are contained in the following discussion of management of individuals with SCI. The reader is referred to the original document for a complete review of the recommendation. Prehospital emergency medical personnel perform a primary survey of the trauma patient, with the focus being on life-threatening conditions.

Spinal Immobilization and Stabilization

Immediately after an injury, precautions must be taken to immobilize and stabilize the spine. This is usually accomplished by maintaining the spine in a neutral position and avoiding neck flexion. Proper spine immobilization is critical because it is estimated that 3% to 25% of SCIs occur after the initial traumatic injury, such as incorrect management at the scene or during transport.[54] Guidelines for management of acute cervical spine and spinal cord injuries recommend complete spine immobilization, using a rigid cervical collar and sandbags, on a backboard with straps, at the scene and during transport.[54] However, this treatment developed more out of experience in the field than research, and is not without complications.[14] Complications associated with the use of a backboard and rigid collar include lack of lumbar support,[54] airway difficulties, increased cranial pressure, increased risk of aspiration, restricted respirations, dysphagia, and pressure ulcers.[14]

In a study of healthy volunteers who were strapped onto a backboard, a significant reduction in forced vital capacity (FVC) and forced expiratory volume in 1 second (FEV_1) was noted due to chest straps being excessively tight.[14] In the person with SCI with compromised respiratory status, this additional mechanical pulmonary restriction may lead to an otherwise unnecessary intubation. Care must be taken to ensure that chest straps allow adequate respiratory excursion yet maintain spine immobilization.

Methods of moving the patient onto the backboard include the traditional logroll, the HAINES method (acronym for high arm in endangered spine), and the fireman lift.[67] The HAINES method is conducted by placing the patient in the supine position. The upper arm away from the kneeling rescuer is abducted to 180 degrees, the near arm of the patient is placed across the patient's chest, and both lower limbs are flexed. The rescuer's hands stabilize the head and neck and the patient is rolled away onto the board. The fireman lift involves several rescuers on either side of the patient, each of whom slides his or her arms underneath the patient and lifts the patient from one position to another onto the board.[67]

Clinicians must be aware of the potential for the early development of **pressure ulcers** resulting from lengthy immobilization on a backboard. Pressure ulcers can occur during the resuscitation phase because of excessive pressure over bony prominences and lack of weight shifts or padding for prolonged periods. Pressure ulcers present lifelong implications for the people who survive the initial trauma and suffer neurologic deficits. It is not uncommon for people with SCI to acquire early stage III to IV pressure ulcers requiring extended periods of bed rest and surgical intervention. Pressure ulcers not only increase the risk for additional complications such as sepsis, and delay recovery and rehabilitation, but can cost tens of thousands of dollars to manage. Pressure of 35 mm Hg exerted for 2 hours, or 60 mm Hg exerted for 1 hour, is sufficient to cause irreversible tissue damage.[58,74] The tissue pressures on the sacrum of a patient on a backboard may be over 200 mm Hg.[74] Early removal of the backboard after the primary trauma survey and initial resuscitation have been completed is urged to prevent pressure ulcers.[54] Use of padded and vacuum boards has shown some reduction in tissue pressure.[54]

Transportation

Four specific goals for optimal early management of SCI have been identified: resuscitation, immobilization of the patient, extrication from the place of injury, and transport to a hospital or trauma center that has an SCI team.[54] Following initial assessment and stabilization, the patient with SCI requires immediate transportation to a definitive trauma center with the capabilities to manage major multitrauma and neurologic trauma patients.[54] Prolonged medical management at the trauma site can lead to longer hospitalizations and poorer outcomes.[12] The mode of rapid transportation, via ambulance or air, should be determined based on clinical status of the patient, distance to an appropriate facility, and geography.[54] Regardless of the mode of transport, the transport team can elevate the head of the backboard in reverse Trendelenburg position to prevent aspiration and must have access to respiratory support and suction in the event of airway compromise, silent aspiration, or pulmonary dysfunction.[12]

EMERGENCY DEPARTMENT MANAGEMENT AND CARE

Assessment

Initial Assessment and Resuscitation

Initial assessment and evaluation of the patient with ASCI by the trauma team includes primary and secondary surveys using advanced trauma life support (ATLS) and standardized guidelines. Emergency personnel perform a primary survey of the trauma patient, with the focus being on life-threatening conditions. The ABCDEs of the primary survey are as follows:[123]

Airway maintenance with cervical spine control
Breathing and ventilation
Circulation and hemorrhage control
Disability (neurologic status)
Exposure control (completely undressing the patient while preventing hyperthermia or hypothermia)

This assessment is conducted while maintaining a high index of suspicion for SCI based on mechanism of injury, patient report, and pertinent assessment findings.

The secondary survey is a more detailed head-to-toe evaluation, conducted with full spinal immobilization in place. Three providers are required to logroll the trauma patient if warranted to conduct the survey. Evaluation of areas of tenderness on the neck or back by palpation is critical for indication of potential spinal injury. Pertinent assessment findings include neck or back pain (or both) or tenderness with or without palpation; abnormal sensations, including burning, tingling, or numbness; and impaired motor or sensory function (or both). A brief motor examination of grip strength and foot dorsiflexion is conducted, as well as a gross sensory examination. Signs of urinary incontinence and priapism are to be noted. Signs of sympathetic nervous system involvement are assessed, including skin temperature and color.[123] Motor vehicle accidents, falls, and sports injuries have the highest incidence of spinal trauma and potential for SCI. Spine injury should be suspected until ruled out.

Resuscitation techniques recommend the modified jaw-thrust maneuver, and an oral airway may suffice to manage the airway of the trauma patient. Emergent intubation may be required, and careful consideration should be given to maintain the cervical spine in neutral alignment. Intubation should not be delayed if clinically indicated.[106] Suction should be available to remove secretions, foreign bodies, or blood.[123] Aggressive intravenous access and fluid resuscitation are administered by prehospital personnel as warranted by patient condition.[123]

Information and assessment provided by emergency personnel at the scene includes time of injury, mechanism of injury, initial vital signs, and emergency care provided at the scene. Spinal immobilization is maintained with the patient secured appropriately on a backboard. The emergency department's (ED's) routine ABCDE care is initiated, and backboard time is recorded. Intravenous (IV) access with two large-bore IV lines is maintained, and the patient is evaluated and treated for shock. Emergency protocols recommended by the American College of Surgeons for suspected ASCI are initiated on admission. Consultations are called for via a trauma code alert for comprehensive emergent management. In addition to the neurologic assessment, the patient must be assessed for occult injuries, missed injuries, or complications of the original cervical injury, such as airway obstruction, aspiration, or spinal shock. Airway protocols are followed and may include ventilatory support, vital capacity, arterial blood gases (ABGs), and serial pulmonary assessments. A urethral indwelling catheter will be inserted with the initiation of fluid resuscitation for urinary bladder decompression and maintained until spinal shock has resolved. Urine and blood samples are drawn for routine laboratory studies. A pain assessment dictates the management of pain and pain interventions. The patient is reassured and the family is updated on all interventions and the condition of the patient.

NEURODIAGNOSTIC STUDIES

Radiographic imaging may include the following:
- **Lateral C-spine/x-ray examination:** taken and read *immediately* using portable equipment; must be taken with the patient in a neutral position to prevent further SCI. Immobilization of the spinal column is important to prevent additional trauma. All seven cervical vertebrae must be seen to the top of T1 on anteroposterior and lateral films. It may be necessary to depress the shoulders to visualize C7. A **swimmer's view** (one arm up and the other at the side, with the x-ray taken through the axilla) may facilitate visualization. Views of the odontoid process (the dens of C2) may require films taken through the open mouth. Other x-ray studies are performed after first screening has been completed.
- **Thoracic and lumbar x-ray studies:** done if the patient is suspected of having multiple trauma based on the mechanism of injury with the entire spine cleared by x-ray, or if any cervical fracture is found.
- **Computed tomography (CT):** indicated if the spine is not adequately visualized, if the spine appears

abnormal on plain film, or if there is a high index of suspicion of SCI despite normal plain films[54,114] (see Chapter 3).

- **Helical CT:** done commonly for faster time and higher quality and can access several body regions in less time. Magnetic resonance imaging is reserved for complete or incomplete neurologic deficits with x-ray evidence of fracture of subluxation.
- **Magnetic resonance imaging (MRI):** used for complete or incomplete neurologic deficits with x-ray evidence of fracture of subluxation or to determine the extent of SCI. Although MRI may be difficult to perform on some critically ill patients, it is useful for detecting soft tissue involvement (e.g., spinal cord contusion and edema) and intramedullary hemorrhage. MRI can augment the information from the clinical examination and previously mentioned radiographs.
- **Myelogram:** indicated under certain conditions as follow-up; not usually part of the admission diagnostic workup.
- **Angiography or magnetic resonance angiography (MRA):** indicated to rule out other disorders with similar symptoms.

DIAGNOSIS

When a diagnosis of ASCI is suspected, the clinical presentation, diagnostic studies, and ASIA scale are established for the baseline diagnosis and neurologic/functional level. After the initial evaluations, a more thorough neurologic examination should be conducted within 6 hours after injury.[54] The neurologic assessment includes evaluation of motor/sensory function, deep tendon reflexes, level of consciousness, and cranial nerve function.[5] Periodic neurologic assessment should be conducted throughout the critical care phase as comparison to the baseline assessment for early detection of changes that may indicate worsening condition and increasing level of injury or improvement in level of injury and resolution of symptoms. Consistent and reproducible neurologic assessment findings are necessary to define the patient's acute neurologic status and to communicate patient status and changes to care providers.[54] Utilization of valid and reliable tools is necessary for consistent assessments. The ASIA International Standards for Neurological Classification of Spinal Cord Injury is the standard assessment tool recommended for determination of sensory/motor function and to determine the completeness of injury.[5] A comprehensive neurologic examination using the ASIA classification tool is repeated between 3 and 7 days after injury[54] (see Figs. 12-1 and 12-9).

Early Interventions

Cardiopulmonary complications remain the principal cause of death in the critical care phase.[80] The goal of the medical management of the patient in the intensive care unit (ICU) is to prevent life-threatening complications while maximiz-

ing the functioning of all body systems. Assessment of airway and respiratory status includes identifying ineffective breathing patterns and oxygenation status. All patients with cervical injuries, particularly those with cervical spinal cord injury, are likely to have respiratory compromise due to loss or impairment of innervation in the key muscles of respiration, the diaphragm and intercostals. A decrease in FVC of nearly 70% has been noted in patients with acute cervical injuries.[11] In addition, the loss of innervated musculature results in ineffective clearance of secretions and cough. Careful, serial assessments of pulmonary function are performed, including FVC, negative inspiratory force, and ABGs. These data are important to monitor because impaired respiration may initially be compensated for by rapid, shallow breathing.[105] Monitoring by pulse oximetry alone is not sufficient.[105] When signs of fatigue are noted, indicated by declining FVC and oxygenation and increased CO_2, immediate intubation is warranted. Approximately one third of cervical level injuries require intubation.[11] Because of the risk for additional neurologic insult during intubation, it is recommended that intubation be performed by practitioners with extensive experience. Orotracheal intubation with in-line traction has been demonstrated to be safe in this population.[11]

ALERT: Pharmacologic paralysis with succinylcholine should be used with extreme caution in patients with CNS injury because of the risk for rapid and life-threatening hyperkalemia.[57] Other agents such as vecuronium are preferred.

Once the airway is secure and adequate ventilation has been achieved, attention should be shifted to the patient's hemodynamic status. Hypotension, bradycardia, and warm, flushed skin will be present as a result of neurogenic shock. Severe hypotension and cardiac arrhythmias may occur due to hemorrhagic shock.[105] The presence and type of shock must be differentiated to direct treatment. Tachycardia is a classic sign of hemorrhagic shock, whereas bradycardia is a classic sign of neurogenic shock. Because of the potential for these shock states, it is recommended that systolic blood pressure (SBP) be maintained at greater than 90 mm Hg and mean arterial pressure (MAP) at 85 to 90 mm Hg for the first 7 days following ASCI to improve spinal cord perfusion.[54] Initial treatment of hypotension includes administration of IV crystalloid solutions. If the goal of MAP is not achieved with IV crystalloids, the addition of vasopressors with both α- and β-adrenergic actions is recommended (dopamine, dobutamine).[105] Arrhythmias are most common in cervical injuries during the first 14 days.[105] Bradycardia is treated with atropine or temporary transcutaneous pacing.[103] Other arrhythmias are treated per advanced cardiac life support (ACLS) guidelines.

Administration of high-dose steroids or methylprednisolone sodium succinate (MPSS) in the first 24 or 48 hours is controversial. The guidelines describe MPSS as an option in the treatment of patients with SCI that should be "undertaken with the knowledge that the evidence suggesting harmful side effects is more consistent than any suggestion of clinical benefit."[7,54,70,103] The dosing consists of an initial bolus dose of 30 mg/kg over 15 minutes, followed by a 45-minute waiting period. Then a 23-hour infusion at a maintenance dose of 5.4 mg/kg is administered.[52]

Decisions regarding patients initially triaged to a local hospital for treatment and stabilization may be discussed with the patient, family, and treating team for consideration of transfer to a model spinal cord injury system center or a level I or II trauma center.[52] Once initial stabilization has been achieved, it is recommended that "patients with SCI, particularly those with high cervical levels, be transferred to an ICU or a similar monitored setting" because of the level of monitoring required.[54]

ACUTE CARE

Following the diagnosis of ASCI and stabilization in the ED, patients are admitted to the ICU. A comprehensive neurologic assessment is completed and followed by frequent nursing reassessments that include a motor/sensory examination, tests of proprioception, and tests of reflexes.[103] Routine ICU management for ASCI begins immediately following transportation from the ED. The patient should be transferred to an appropriate bed surface for the level of injury, taking into account management of concomitant injuries. A Rotorest-type bed is recommended by the guidelines and may be the best option for the individual with SCI that requires spinal immobilization and easy access for other critical care needs (Fig. 12-15). Methods of cervical spine stabilization include the application of a stiff cervical collar, cervical traction with Gardner-Wells tongs, application of a halo device, and surgical stabilization[103] or orthoses with specific types of bracing. The care of spine stabilization depends on the type of application, with careful attention to the skin. Pin sites should be cleaned and dressed, with immediate reporting of a cerebrospinal fluid (CSF) leak, signs and symptoms of infection, or loosening of any parts of a stabilization device or brace.

The use of a spinal cord assessment or flow sheet is essential to evaluate subtle changes; to evaluate trends in recovery; and to document neurologic checks every 2 hours, intake and output (I&O), and other parameters. Sensory and motor function of the perianal area is a component of the neurologic examination to determine sacral function/sacral sparing and should be tested with each examination.

Hemodynamic stability is maintained with strict blood pressure (BP) parameters greater than 80 mm Hg to prevent hypotension. Respiratory support for patients using a ventilator is needed to keep the lungs clear with the pulse oximetry maintained above 94%. Respiratory assessment and care and meticulous pulmonary hygiene require close monitoring for removal of secretions or effective cough until the patient is able to protect his or her airway.

Ongoing assessment includes assessment for paralytic ileus. Early initiation of a bowel routine is done to prevent constipation. Stress ulcer prevention can be managed with H_2 antagonists or appropriately prescribed medications. A nutritional evaluation is needed to evaluate swallowing and nutritional needs (e.g., a feeding tube). A pneumatic compression device helps prevent deep vein thrombosis (DVT) and pulmonary embolus (PE). Appropriate laboratory studies are collected and results analyzed for abnormal findings that require immediate attention. Marking the skin of the patient with a suitable marker for reference is a strategy to compare findings from each subsequent sensory examination. Meticulous skin assessment and skin care will avoid pressure ulcers, which all patients with ASCI are at high risk for developing. Temperature should be maintained in the normothermic range to avoid extreme temperature changes because patients may be **poikilothermic** and unable to regulate their body heat and will assume the temperature of the environment or setting. Pain is managed to maintain a level of 3 or less on a scale of 1 to 10 with appropriate pain medications (see Chapter 23). Explanations for all interventions are part of the health teaching. Ongoing psychosocial assessment for ineffective coping and the need for additional emotional support

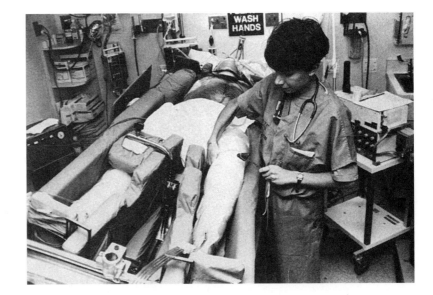

Figure 12-15 Neuroscience nurse performing neurologic assessment on a patient with spine injuries on a Roto-Rest bed.

may indicate the need for psychologic or psychiatric consultations. It is vital for the patient to have a reliable communication system, whether verbal, written, a speech board, or blinks.

The goals of treatment are to preserve neurologic function, decompress the neural elements, reduce pathologic subluxation, restore stability, promote osseous union for long-term stability, and preserve normal motion segments whenever possible. The medical management of the patient with SCI is extremely complex because of the major effects this injury has on many body systems. The goals of patient management in the critical care phase are to prevent **secondary injury,** prevent complications, and prepare for rehabilitation.[52] Many of the interventions initiated in the trauma phase are carried over into the critical care phase.[76] Utilization of a hyperacute SCI protocol or clinical pathway ensures efficient, complete care and helps minimize complications (Fig. 12-16). The spine flow sheet should include the following neurologic assessment parameters:

- **Sensory function:** The sensory assessment is very important in determining the ASIA impairment level. The sensory examination is accomplished by testing all of the sensory dermatomes, bilaterally with pin prick and light touch with a small cotton ball. Sensory examination includes the perianal region (see Chapter 2).
- **Motor function:** All major muscle groups are tested with each examination. To test the major muscle groups, the patient is instructed through the movement of the muscle, beginning with the deltoids and biceps (see Chapter 2). Muscles are assessed by asking the patient to flex, extend, abduct, and adduct each extremity. If the patient is able to move against gravity, resistance is applied by the clinician and the patient is asked to repeat the movement. A five-point motor scoring system is used to grade muscle function (Box 12-2). Absence of a sacral reflex, or "anal wink," and inability to contract the anal sphincter may indicate a complete SCI, spinal shock, or lower motor neuron (LMN) injury (see Chapter 2).
- **Proprioception:** Dorsal column tracts mediate proprioception and vibratory sensation. Proprioception is assessed by asking the patient to close both eyes and identify whether the thumb or great toe is flexed or extended (bent or straight) as it is manipulated through the movements by the examiner.
- **Reflexes:** The biceps (elbow flexion), triceps (elbow extension), knee jerk or patellar (quadriceps—extension of leg), anterior tibialis (ankle dorsiflexion), anocutaneous (pudendal), and bulbocavernous

(pudendal) reflexes are tested. The latter is tested by slightly pulling on the indwelling catheter or by gently pinching the glans penis or clitoris while palpating for anal sphincter contraction (see Chapter 2).

- **Priapism:** This is an abnormal condition of prolonged or constant penile erection following ASCI that can cause vasodilation and vascular engorgement of the external genitalia. It can be painful and may also be indicative of a poor outcome.
- **Respiratory assessment:** The respiratory rate and pattern should be assessed hourly. The respiratory assessment includes measurements of tidal volume, minute ventilation, ABGs, chest radiographs, vital capacity, and continuous pulse oximetry, and will be assessed based on patient need. **Forced vital capacity (FVC)** is often considered the manual muscle test of the diaphragm and is monitored as needed. PaO_2 of at least 80 mm Hg coupled with normalization of the $PaCO_2$ is recommended.[1]
- **Temperature:** The patient may demonstrate poikilothermia. The body temperature may vary according to the temperature of the surrounding environment. Careful monitoring of temperature is important since hypothermia or hyperthermia can result from this loss of thermoregulation. Independent regulation of the patient's room is helpful for precise control to maintain environmental temperature.

Vital Signs, Invasive Lines, and Electrocardiogram Monitoring

Vital signs, invasive monitoring (arterial and pulmonary artery), and electrocardiogram (ECG) monitoring aids in the assessment of the patient with SCI during the phases of neurogenic and spinal shock. In addition to hypotension resulting from decreased systemic vascular resistance (SVR), the cardiac preload is decreased. Cardiac output (CO) drops, and tissue perfusion decreases. The heart rate is closely monitored for bradycardia. Atropine should be available at the bedside in the event the pulse drops below 40 beats/min. Left ventricular function is also depressed from lack of sympathetic outflow. Beta endorphins released as a result of SCI have been implicated in exacerbating poor ventricular performance. Left ventricular dysfunction can lead to cardiac dysrhythmias, including heart block, requiring the use of external, transvenous, or even permanent pacemakers.

Surgical Interventions

Conditions indicating the need for surgical intervention for the patient with SCI include "unstable fractures, a fracture that will not reduce, gross spinal misalignment, evidence of cord compression in the presence of incomplete injury, deteriorating neurological status and persistent instability after conservative management" (pp. 13, 31).[103] The ideal timing of surgical stabilization remains controversial. Early surgical stabilization (less than or equal to 24 hours after injury) is favored by some due to evidence suggesting that systemic complications in patients with SCI may decrease if surgery

BOX 12-2	5/5 Motor Score

5 Active movement, against full resistance
4 Active movement, against some resistance
3 Active movement, against gravity
2 Active movement, gravity eliminated
1 Palpable or visible contraction
0 Total paralysis

UNIT(s)	STABILIZATION PHASE DAY 0-3				
Day		INITIALS			
Date		0	1	2	3
Assessment	Nursing assessment Trauma bath assessment when normothermic Vital signs and Neuro assessment every 1 hour for 24 hours, then every 2 hours Level of injury (motor/sensory) determined by neurosurgeon Respiratory assessment every 2 hours Review laboratory results Skin integrity assessment and risk score Day 0 and 3 Assessment for DVT daily				
Consults	Neurosurgery service Physiatry to coordinate rehabilitation team Nutrition services Social work services Psychiatry liaison services for crisis assessment/intervention plan Substance abuse consult team for positive urine or serum screen Pulmonary service				
Labs	Trauma screen in ED (ABO type & screen, CBC & diff, blood alcohol level, UA, urine drug screen, ABG, HCGF if female age 14-45)				
Tests	In ED, C-spine series, portable CXR, pelvis x-ray Full spine series, CT scan, and/or MRI if not completed in ED				
Meds	Morphine 2-4 mg IVP q 1 hour prn Lorazepam 1-4 IVP q 2-4 hours prn Methylprednisolone ___mg/hr x ___hours Heparin 5000 units SC every 12 hours, begin after 24 hours Famotidine 20 mg IV every 12 hour × 48 hours If vasopressors needed, consider neosynephrine or norepinephrine Docusate sodium daily for bowel training, begin after 48 hours Multivitamin with minerals daily or 1 ampule of MVI daily in IV fluids Vitamin C 500 mg PO daily when taking PO				
IV	D5 1/2 NS with 20 mEq KCl				
Treatments	Pulse oximeter Traction and/or kinetic therapy bed prior to surgical stabilization Pin care every 8 hours wrench attached to halo vest, if applicable Mechanical ventilation if indicated Pulmonary toilet PRN Soft tissue injury repaired Suture line care Replace nasogastric tube with smallest diameter silastic feeding tube after 24 hours of tolerating tube feedings Foley to gravity I&O SCD Consider IVC filter insertion Moisture barrier, PRN if incontinent Rigid cervical collar post-op; check pressure points q shift				
Activity	Bedrest logroll until stabilized Turn and position every 2 hours, if on kinetic therapy bed use 60° continuous rotation Splints per PT/OT on/off every 2 hours				
Nutrition	NPO until surgical stabilization Postop begin feedings, progress to fiber is not used in initial feeding solution				
Teaching	Patient and family updated on tests, procedures, and plan of care SCI expectations Communication techniques Call bell system				
Discharge	Formal multidisciplinary team meeting by Day 3 to establish plan				
Intermediate Outcomes	Hemodynamically stable Injuries identified and treated Neurologically stable Spine stabilized <48 hours Level of functioning identified Pulse Oximeter >92% Nutritional needs met ≤72 hours Patient and family informed of plan of care Multidisciplinary plan established and goals identified Discharged destination options identified <72 hours Pain is optimally managed				
Initials Signature Title					

Figure 12-16 Traumatic spinal cord injury—quadriplegia clinical pathway.
(From Mitcho K, Yanko J: Acute care management of spinal cord injuries, Crit Care Nurs Q 22(2):60–79, 1999. Used with permission. Copyright Allegheny General Hospital.)

is performed within 24 hours of injury.[54,68,103,114] Delayed surgery (more than 200 hours following injury) is preferred by others because it purportedly allows the neurologic status to plateau and the patient to stabilize medically.[52,54,68,103] The goals of treatment are to preserve neurologic function, decompress the neural elements, reduce pathologic subluxation, restore stability, promote osseous union for long-term stability, and preserve normal motion segments whenever possible.

An anterior or a posterior **diskectomy** for decompression of a traumatic herniated disk is performed to remove the herniated tissue or bone fragments (see Chapter 14). Other surgical procedures may be necessary for a burst fracture that would require a **vertebrectomy** to remove damaged vertebral bone and utilize bone grafting or hardware to stabilize the spine and improve function. A **laminectomy** may be performed for decompression, and surgical devices may be used to repair fractures and promote union. Fusion with the use of **pedicle screws** and **spinal instrumentation** has dramatically improved the outcome following spinal fixation.

Nursing management involves routine postoperative management. Close monitoring and neurologic assessment are required with observation of neurologic status, with special emphasis on motor/sensory status, vital signs, respiratory and gastrointestinal (GI) status, wound and skin care, and bowel and bladder care. All immobilization devices or appliances are checked daily. Pain management is important for control of acute pain with appropriate interventions (see Chapter 23). Immediate notification of the attending physician is needed at the earliest signs of complications (e.g., sensory or motor changes, unrelieved pain, or loss of bowel or bladder function that may have resulted from bleeding, infection, or perioperative conditions). Surgery may promotes early ambulation and rehabilitation. Frequent family and patient multidisciplinary meetings to address immediate and long-term needs are scheduled to prepare the patient for early discharge and a lifetime of follow-up to prevent complications and assist the patient and family over the shock of dealing with a catastrophic injury.

Nonacute Care or Acute Rehabilitation

Once stabilized medically, the patient may be transferred to a subacute setting or in many case directly to acute rehabilitation. The clinical management of the patient with SCI is extremely complex because of the major effects this injury has on many body systems. The goals of patient management are to prevent secondary injury and complications and to prepare the patient for reintegration into home and the community. Successful rehabilitation may begin while the patient is in the ICU or nonacute setting, with early implementation of a bowel and bladder management program; prevention of pressure ulcers; maintenance of respiratory, cardiovascular, neurologic, and ANS stability; and early psychosocial support. It is critical that all care providers along the continuum of care for individuals with SCI understand and promote early rehabilitation intervention. Although evaluation by the physiatrist and rehabilitation team may have been initiated in the ICU or subacute care unit, active rehabilitation with full participation by the patient must wait until the patient is physically and psychologically able to participate.

All body systems are affected by SCI. Three body systems—bowel, bladder, and skin—require intense focus by the rehabilitation team, particularly the rehabilitation clinicians, to assist the individual with SCI to a successful rehabilitation and integration to home and the community. Other domains that require nursing management and interventions are the respiratory system, prevention of complications, and the psychosocial effects of SCI. Ineffective management programs or the presence of complications in any of these body systems or domains can be costly and potentially life threatening. They can interfere with the rehabilitation process and later participation in life activities.

Gastrointestinal and Nutrition Concerns

The patient with acute SCI may suffer from gastric dilation and a paralytic ileus during spinal shock. A severe catabolic state occurs during the acute phase.[67] Stress ulcers, particularly if high-dose steroids were administered, can further complicate the GI system and affect nutrition. The nutritional goal is to avoid prolonged catabolism or excessive weight loss greater than 10 pounds throughout the hospitalization. The caloric intake may be as high as 4000 calories per day because of the high rate of catabolism. The patient should be weighed at least once a week to monitor weight loss or gain.[19,30,101] Chronic upper abdominal pain that may be accompanied by diarrhea has been attributed to a rare condition referred to as **superior mesenteric artery syndrome (SMAS).** This condition may be related to visceral ischemia from atrial stenosis or occlusion of branches of the celiac or superior mesenteric artery.

Most patients admitted with acute SCI are previously well nourished, with adequate skeletal muscle (somatic protein) and fat (adipose tissue) stores. Initially, significant muscle atrophy occurs below the site of injury because of loss of nerve innervation and disuse of the affected muscles. Weight loss accompanies this; however, the extent of the loss may be masked by acute expansion of extracellular water. Nitrogen balance is negative for up to 2 months after the injury in spite of adequate caloric and protein intake. Preservation of muscle mass above the level of injury must be the goal. Other nutrients, such as calcium, also reach a negative balance as a result of immobilization.

Caloric needs may closely parallel those of other trauma patients, especially if the patient with spinal cord injury has sustained additional traumatic injuries, such as head injuries (see Chapter 11). In addition, these patients also may have fevers, infections, or sepsis, or they may have received steroids, all of which exaggerate the hypermetabolic response. There is some evidence, however, that even in the acute phase, caloric needs are lower than would be predicted because of decreased metabolic activity of denervated muscle.[67]

The **paralytic ileus** associated with spinal shock generally lasts approximately 3 to 5 days. Oral or tube feedings should begin by this time, if tolerated. Progress is slow until the local gut reflexes become active. Postpyloric tube feedings are generally better tolerated if the adynamic ileus persists. If a patient's total estimated intake via the oral or enteral route does not meet nutrient needs by the fifth to sixth day after injury, parenteral feedings may be required. Decreased gastric motility may also decrease patient tolerance for higher rates and increase the patient's risks for development of increased residual with increased risk of vomiting and aspiration. Prokinetic agents may be indicated.

With impaired bowel function, a bowel program is needed to empty the lower bowel and establish a routine. The plan will depend on the level of injury and is coordinated with dietary and fluid intake.

Neurogenic Bowel

Individuals with SCI experience **neurogenic bowel.** The effects of neurogenic bowel present a different clinical picture based on level and completeness of injury. There are two primary classifications of neurogenic bowel in complete SCI: upper motor neuron (UMN) and lower motor neuron (LMN). The **UMN bowel** occurs in SCI when the damage to the cord is above the conus medullaris and the reflex defecation center remains intact (S2 to S4). SCI above T12 generally results in UMN bowel function that is characterized by presence of rectal tone and intact bulbocavernosus reflex and reflexes of the anal sphincter. The reflexes can be used to stimulate evacuation. The routine bowel program for UMN bowel consists of a chemical stimulant in the form of a rectal suppository, digital stimulation to the anal sphincter while the patient is in an upright or side-lying position, and repeat of the stimulation until bowel evacuation has occurred.[32] A bowel program may be initiated on a daily (or every evening) schedule and may be changed to an every-other-day regimen if results are consistently patterned as such. It is not recommended to increase the time between bowel programs beyond every 2 days.

The **LMN bowel** occurs in SCI of the sacral cord segments in the conus medullaris or the sacral nerve roots in the cauda equina. LMN bowel is characterized by flaccid paralysis and loss of tone in the rectum and loss of anal sphincter contraction. There are more difficulties in management of LMN bowel related to increased frequency of defecation and increased frequency of fecal incontinence.[125] The usual routine for management of an LMN bowel consists of performing the Valsalva maneuver and/or manual evacuation of stool from the rectum until the rectum is free of stool. The LMN bowel requires evacuation once a day and frequently more than once a day after meals.[32]

Assessment of neurogenic bowel is multifaceted and should be conducted at onset of injury and annually throughout the continuum of care.[32] The history includes premorbid or current GI function and medical conditions; current bowel program, including patient satisfaction; current symptoms, including abdominal distention, respiratory compromise, early satiety, nausea, evacuation difficulty, unplanned evacuations, rectal bleeding, diarrhea, constipation, and pain; defecation or bowel care frequency, duration, and characteristics of stool; and medication use and potential effect on the bowel program.[32] The physical examination includes complete abdominal assessment, including palpation along the course of the colon; rectal examination; assessment of anal sphincter tone; elicitation of anocutaneous and bulbocavernosus reflexes to determine if the patient has UMN or LMN bowel; and stool testing for occult blood beginning at age 50.[32] Assessment of function and disability is an additional component of bowel management. Assessment of knowledge, cognition, function, and performance is undertaken to determine the ability of the individual to complete the bowel program or ability to instruct a care provider. This assessment includes ability to learn, ability to direct others, sitting tolerance and angle, sitting balance, upper extremity strength and proprioception, hand and arm function, spasticity, transfer skills, actual and potential risks to skin, anthropometric characteristics, and home accessibility and equipment needs.[32]

A **bowel program** is required to empty the lower bowel and to establish a consistent routine that prevents involuntary stool evacuation and complications such as colorectal distention, hemorrhoids, impaction, diarrhea, and bowel obstruction. This daily routine should be initiated as soon as possible after injury, ideally after the resolution of spinal shock. The bowel program is established taking into account level and completeness of injury, preinjury bowel routine, and anticipated life demands and preferences. The clinician establishes a bowel program, in collaboration with the patient or care providers. To establish a bowel program the clinician will encourage appropriate fluids, diet, and activity; choose an appropriate rectal stimulant; provide rectal stimulation (digital stimulation) initially to trigger defecation daily; select optimal scheduling and positioning; select appropriate assistive techniques; evaluate medications that promote or inhibit bowel function;[125] and provide for balance of fiber, fluid, and requisite medications such as stool softening agents.

A well-managed bowel program without complications is achievable for most individuals with SCI. As individuals with SCI age, the bowel program may develop problems such as increased time for defecation, and may need to be revised. For some individuals with SCI, bowel management is difficult to achieve or maintain. In some cases, individuals with SCI have such severe problems with their bowel program (e.g., frequent bowel incontinence; bowel programs that consume excessive time each day; and complications such as severe bleeding hemorrhoids, constipation, or autonomic dysreflexia with rectal stimulation) that it necessitates consideration of surgical interventions such as colostomy or ileostomy. The decision to undergo surgery for a colostomy or an ileostomy is a complex decision and requires input from the interdisciplinary team, including a surgeon with experience performing surgery in this patient population, and an enterostomal therapist.[32] If the decision is made to perform a colostomy, attention must be paid to placement of the stoma so as not to create seating problems, problems with skin, or difficulty maintaining a colostomy bag. Individuals who pursue colostomy management have reported a significant improvement in quality of life. Benefits of colostomy for bowel management have been reported as reduction in number of hospitalizations for bowel dysfunction; decrease in the time spent each day on bowel management; simplification of bowel routines; increased independence; and improvements in physical health, psychosocial adjustments, and self-efficacy.[102]

Complications that can occur in neurogenic bowel include diarrhea, constipation, and impaction. Hemorrhoids are a common occurrence as well. These complications can be minimized with implementation of a consistent and effective bowel program.

Special consideration is given to the pediatric patient with SCI depending on the child's age. For children injured as infants or toddlers, the bowel program will be initiated at approximately 3 years of age. In children over 3 and in adolescents, the bowel program is initiated as soon after injury as possible.[79]

Neurogenic Bladder

In the past, renal disease was the leading cause of morbidity and mortality in individuals with SCI.[88] With improved treatment of infections and bladder surveillance and management techniques, this is no longer the case. The goals of bladder management are to achieve adequate bladder drainage, low-pressure urine storage, and low-pressure voiding with no urinary leakage or urinary incontinence. This will assist in prevention of urinary tract infection (UTI), bladder wall damage, overdistention of the bladder, vesicoureteral reflux, and stone disease.[94] Similar to effects of SCI on bowel function, bladder function is dependent on level of injury. Bladder dysfunction can be classified into two syndromes: UMN bladder dysfunction and LMN bladder dysfunction. The determination of UMN or LMN bladder dysfunction cannot be made during the phase of spinal shock. Because of the effects of spinal shock and the usual need for aggressive fluid replacement immediately after SCI, patients with acute SCI are best managed with an indwelling catheter. However, it is advised to work toward attainment of a catheter-free status as soon as possible to prevent UTI and other genitourinary complications.[78] Once reflex activity returns, the patient is medically stable, and urine output averges 2 liters in 24 hours, consideration can be given to discontinuing the catheter and starting a bladder management program.[27] A determination of bladder type can be made by physical examination or urodynamic studies. Urodynamic studies may be helpful in determining bladder function and to identify detrusor-sphincter dyssynergia. Once bladder type has been established, bladder management techniques can be determined.

It is critical to include the patient in determination of bladder management technique. If the patient does not have the desire, abilities, or resources to perform and maintain a prescribed bladder management program, the risk for complications is greatly increased.[119,120] Most injuries above T12 will result in UMN bladder function. The UMN bladder will be hyperreflexic or spastic. Additionally there may be dyssynergia or impaired coordination between bladder contractions and relaxation of the bladder neck, and internal and external sphincters during micturition.[27,31] Intermittent catheterization is the management technique of choice in UMN bladder.[27,31,78,94,122] The patient must be willing and able to perform intermittent catheterization at sufficient intervals to maintain low bladder volumes or the therapeutic benefit of this management technique is lost. Clean intermittent catheterization (CIC) may be performed without increased risk of UTI, if performed on a routine schedule with proper technique.[93]

Indwelling catheters, including urethral and suprapubic catheters, are recommended as the management choice of last resort, as they are associated with higher rates of UTI and other complications. Indwelling catheter management may be the most practical and consistent management technique, however, for individuals with higher cervical injuries without the manual dexterity to independently perform CIC or lack of care providers to conduct CIC.[27,120]

Bladder spasticity may lead to problems such as leaking between catheterizations or leaking around indwelling catheters. Anticholinergic agents may be required to prevent leaking. Other bladder management options alone or in conjunction with intermittent catheterization include bladder augmentation; alpha blockers to reduce resistance to outflow; botulinum A toxin injections in the bladder neck to treat dyssynergia; transurethral sphincterotomy or placement of a urethral stent to reduce outlet obstruction; electrical stimulation to stimulate the voiding reflex; and catheterization through a Mitrofanoff channel with or without enterocystoplasty.[27,78,86,96,122] Prevention of urinary complications is of paramount importance. Compliance with the selected bladder management technique is critical to prevent complications such as UTI, deterioration of the upper urinary tract, and urethral trauma.[17,86,120]

Pressure Ulcer Prevention and Treatment

Pressure ulcers may begin within hours or a short period of time following ASCI.[65] Removing the patient as soon as possible from the backboard, checking under the hard cervical collar, and inspecting the skin begin immediately on admission. Development of pressure ulcers in the acute setting can delay rehabilitation and prevent participation in therapeutic activities. Pressure ulcers are of concern to individuals with SCI, all members of the health care system, personal care providers, third-party payers, and those who direct public policy.[37] Pressure ulcers are a complication in approximately 25% of patients with SCI during their initial acute care hospitalization.[29,104] Pressure ulcer prevalence ranges from 8% 1 year following injury to 33% for individuals living in the community with chronic SCI.[37] The most effective approach to addressing this costly complication of SCI is early prevention.

A clinical practice guideline was developed by the Consortium for Spinal Cord Medicine in 2000.[37] The purpose of the clinical practice guideline is to describe effective strategies for identifying risk and reducing the incidence, prevalence, and recurrence of this lifelong complication of SCI.[37] Risk assessment should be conducted on admission and reassessed on a consistent basis. To date there is limited availability of a risk assessment tool that determines heightened risk for patients with SCI. The **Braden scale** is most widely used, but has not been determined to be routinely predictive in this patient population. This is an area in need of further research. Clinical judgment is invaluable in the assessment of risk for pressure ulcer development. All patients with SCI should be considered at high risk for development of pressure ulcers, and appropriate prevention strategies should be employed. The early use of special beds and mattress covers is cost effective. The cost of treatment for pressure ulcers can range from $10,000 to $100,000.

Prevention of pressure ulcers is part of a comprehensive management plan for both acute and long-term SCI. Prevention strategies include avoidance of prolonged positional immobilization; institution of pressure relief as soon as medical condition and stabilization allow; and initiation of intraoperative pressure reduction strategies.[37] Daily skin inspection is a fundamental prevention strategy and includes visual and tactile inspection. Attention is directed to the most vulnerable areas over bony prominences, including, but not limited to, the ischii, sacrum/coccyx, trochanters, and heels.[37] Cervical collars and other immobilization devices are common locations for development of pressure ulcers and require diligent assessment.[37,81]

Turning, padding, and repositioning are conducted every 2 hours in the acute and rehabilitation phases as medical condition allows. Padding with pillows or foam placed above and below all bony prominences, creating a bridging effect, to prevent pressure over bony prominences while the patient is in bed is recommended. Particular attention should be paid to the heels, keeping pressure off, even if the patient is on a pressure reducing mattress or specialty bed. Once the patient is mobilized in a wheelchair, it is critical that the occupational therapist (OT) or physical therapist (PT) be consulted for acquisition of an appropriate wheelchair cushion to place on the seat of the wheelchair. Pillows and foam pads will not suffice as wheelchair cushions. Wheelchairs must be properly fit by OTs or PTs (or both) to prevent pressure from the wheelchair and to allow for a tilt mechanism to facilitate weight shifts if needed.

Other actions to prevent development of pressure ulcers include elimination of stretching and folding of soft tissues, prevention of shearing during repositioning, application of pressure reducing support surfaces, prevention of moisture accumulation and temperature elevation at the support surface–skin interface, and ongoing evaluation of equipment to determine effectiveness of support surfaces.[37] Routine and frequent weight shifts, at no greater interval than every 30 minutes, should be performed while the patient is seated. Timers are an effective way to remind patients and others around them to perform weight shifts.

In the event a patient with SCI does develop a pressure ulcer, assessment must be conducted, findings documented, and frequent reassessment completed. Assessment of a pressure ulcer includes anatomic location and general appearance, size (length, width, depth, and surrounding wound area), stage, exudate/odor, necrosis, undermining, sinus tracts, infection, healing (granulation and epithelialization), and description of wound margins and surrounding tissues.[37] Treatment depends on stage and condition of the pressure ulcer. All wounds should be cleansed at each dressing change. To clean a pressure ulcer use minimum mechanical force, use enough irrigation pressure to enhance cleansing without causing trauma to the wound, use normal saline or commercial wound cleansers, avoid antiseptic agents, and consider hydrotherapy for ulcers containing large amounts of exudates and necrotic tissue.[37] Wounds should be débrided of eschar and devitalized tissue. Only individuals with documented competency should mechanically débride a wound. Commercially available enzymes and other products may be used to débride wounds, but should only be used by competent practitioners. Dressings that will keep the wound bed continuously moist and the surrounding skin dry are recommended. Use a dressing that controls exudates but does not desiccate the ulcer bed or macerate the surrounding tissue. Loosely fill pressure ulcer cavities with dressing material to avoid dead space, but do not overpack the ulcer. Continuously monitor dressings to be sure they remain intact. Perform dressing changes based on needs of the wound or as specified in the manufacturer's directions.[37]

Electrical stimulation may be applied to stage III or IV wounds to promote closure, in combination with standard wound care interventions.[37] The PT or nursing staff generally will provide this modality, but must be competent in the application.

Wounds should be reassessed routinely to monitor healing and adequacy of the treatment plan. The treatment plan should be modified if there is no evidence of healing within 2 to 4 weeks and sooner if the wound worsens.[37]

Individuals with complex stage III or stage IV wounds may require surgical intervention. Surgical protocols routinely require a period of "down time" where the patient is on flat bed rest postoperatively. Progressive mobilization to sitting usually occurs over 4 to 8 weeks postoperatively.[37]

Respiratory Management

Pulmonary complications are the leading cause of morbidity and mortality in acute SCI, and can extend the length of stay of hospitalization.[47,117] Level of SCI will determine the risk and degree of respiratory compromise. The diaphragm, accessory muscles, intercostal muscles, and abdominal muscles are important for ventilation and maintaining a clear airway. The diaphragm is innervated at the C3 to C5 levels. Injuries above C4 will result in total paralysis of the diaphragm and loss of the ability to breathe, which will render these patients ventilator dependent or dependent on other methods of mechanical ventilation. Lesions at the C4 to C5 levels will lead to diaphragmatic dysfunction to a lesser degree with paralysis of accessory, intercostal, and abdominal muscles, leading to lower vital capacity and inability to independently clear secretions. SCI in the low cervical or high thoracic regions produces lack of chest and abdominal movement, resulting in difficulty in deep breathing and clearing secretions,[129] which may result in the need for ventilatory assistance in the early period after injury or with respiratory illness or aging.[69]

Relevant respiratory history includes past medical history, including lung disease, smoking history, current medications, substance abuse, respiratory complaints, and coexisting injuries.[38] Physical assessment includes respiratory effort and vital signs; chest imaging as indicated; continuous pulse oximetry in the early phase of treatment, or with illness; respiratory muscle assessment, including vital capacity (VC) and maximal negative inspiratory pressure; forced expiratory volume in 1 second (FEV_1) or peak cough flow; and neurologic level and extent of impairment.[38] Over the first several days after SCI, end-tidal carbon dioxide (CO_2) is monitored to measure quality of gas exchange.[38] Key medical interventions for respiratory management are aimed at prevention of atelectasis, pneumonia, pulmonary embolism, pleural effusion, and aspiration.[38] Secretion management is critical. If cough is too weak to clear secretions, alternative interventions may be necessary. Suctioning can be performed via nasotracheal, endotracheal, or tracheostomy routes. If suctioning is performed on high-level cervical injuries, the clinician must be alert for a vasovagal response causing severe bradycardia or cardiac arrest. **Manual assisted cough** may be performed in a more stable patient or a patient without artificial airway access. This is accomplished by applying firm pressure, with inward and upward force, over the diaphragm during exhalation. **Chest physical therapy,** intermittent positive pressure breathing, and incentive spirometry are additional interventions for bronchial hygiene.[69]

Aspiration places the patient with SCI at higher risk for pulmonary complications such as atelectasis and pneumonia. The clinician may request a speech therapy evaluation to assess for aspiration. Aspiration may be controlled in the patient with a tracheostomy with tracheostomy cuff inflation. Swallowing and dietary restrictions may additionally be instituted to prevent aspiration.

Communication with the patient who has a tracheostomy and mechanical ventilation can be a challenge. The clinician should ensure that there is an effective means of communicating with the patient, and consult a speech therapist if necessary.

Weaning the patient from the ventilator requires an interdisciplinary team effort.[117] The most common method of weaning the patient with SCI from the ventilator is the **progressive ventilator-free breathing (PVFB) technique.**[38,117] Other methods include **pressure support ventilation (PSV)** and **intermittent mandatory ventilation (IMV).** These techniques are less commonly used in SCI due to fatigue related to neuromuscular involvement of the muscles of respiration.[117]

NONACUTE REHABILITATION

Rehabilitation Program and Team

The patient may be ready for transfer from the acute care hospital in 1 to 2 weeks and move to a rehabilitation facility that can meet the enormous needs of the individual experiencing ASCI. This rehabilitation phase requires involvement of a comprehensive interdisciplinary team. Admission directly to a program in a model spinal cord injury system, of which there are currently 16 in the United States,[88] or a program that has a comprehensive system of care for the patient with SCI and treats sufficient numbers of patients with SCI to have the requisite experience, is the ideal. Spinal cord injury is a complex injury requiring knowledgeable staff and established resources to meet the needs of this patient population. Direct admission to a specialty SCI program from the ICU is preferable. Transfer of the patient with SCI to a program that does not provide services for a significant number of individuals with SCI annually may lead to adverse outcomes for the patient and his or her family.

The interdisciplinary team for rehabilitation of the patient with SCI most commonly includes a physiatrist, a medical specialist in physical medicine and rehabilitation, or a physician who specializes in rehabilitation who functions as the medical team leader. The physician's role is to coordinate all of the medical needs, services, and specialists that the patient with SCI will require. The physician may also provide direct medical rehabilitation services. The team additionally consists of practitioners from the disciplines of rehabilitation nursing; physical therapy; occupational therapy; speech therapy, if there are swallowing or communication needs; recreation therapy; social work or rehabilitation counseling; psychology; chaplaincy; dietary therapy; and respiratory therapy. Other practitioners may join the team based on patient need, such as a tutor for school-age children and integrative therapy practitioners (including massage therapy and acupuncture).

Once the physician and the interdisciplinary team complete the initial comprehensive admission evaluation, a highly individualized, outcome-oriented plan of care is developed (see Chapter 13).

Frequent team and family case conferences are conducted to review the patient's progress in preparation for discharge. Ongoing adjustments are made to the individualized plan of care for the patient based on his or her progress toward discharge goals. The length of stay (LOS) is highly individualized on the basis of the patient's level of injury, complications, and rate of progress. A transition or intensive training period may be planned where the patient's spouse, family, or other care providers stay overnight in a homelike setting and participate in providing care for the patient (e.g., bowel and bladder management, assistance with activities of daily living [ADLs], and management of turns, padding, and positioning). Family members of the ventilator-dependent patient may practice pulmonary hygiene, airway management, and other care in the rehabilitation facility with supervision in preparation for care that will be required at home.

Phases of Rehabilitation

Phases of rehabilitation have been identified for SCI rehabilitation nursing practice.[89-91] Description of these phases is important in assisting the rehabilitation clinician to understand the various roles undertaken by the clinician during the rehabilitation process. The first phase is buffering. *Buffering* is "the nurturing and protective process of helping patients to gather the physical and emotional strength necessary for a strenuous rehabilitation program" (p. 412).[91] The second phase is transcending. *Transcending* is the process of rising above negative and stereotypical beliefs about people with disabilities (p. 216).[90] The third phase is toughening. *Toughening* is "the process of physically and emotionally

preparing the individual for community re-entry" (p. 413).[91] The fourth phase is launching. *Launching* is "the process of exposing the patient with SCI to the real world, exploring the range of options for living in the community, promoting patient autonomy and decision making, and facilitating the discharge of the patient from the rehabilitation program" (p. 414).[91] The patient may move in and out of these phases in response to moving through the trajectory of rehabilitation and community reintegration. It is important for rehabilitation clinicians to understand the variety of important roles they play and to prevent the SCI clinician from taking on the helper role throughout the rehabilitation process, thereby inhibiting progress through rehabilitation for the patient.

Prevention and Management of Potential Complications

Autonomic Dysreflexia

Autonomic dysreflexia (AD) is an acute syndrome of excessive uncontrolled sympathetic output, unique to patients with an injury to the spinal cord. AD does not occur until after the phase of spinal shock when reflexes return. AD occurs in injuries above the major splanchnic outflow at the thoracic 6 (T6) level. AD is a hypertensive emergency that may lead to death if untreated. Intact sensory nerves below the level of injury transmit noxious afferent impulses to the spinal cord. Sympathetic inhibitory impulses that originate above T6 are blocked due to the SCI. Below the injury there is relatively unopposed sympathetic outflow with release of norepinephrine, dopamine-beta-hydroxylase, and dopamine. Symptoms of piloerection, pallor, and severe vasoconstriction in the arterial vasculature leading to sudden elevation of blood pressure are caused by release of these chemicals, which may in turn cause headache. A blood pressure of 20 to 40 mm Hg over baseline may be a sign of AD in this population. Intact carotid and aortic baroreceptors detect hypertension, stimulating vasomotor brainstem reflexes in an attempt to lower the blood pressure. Bradycardia is caused by parasympathetic stimulation of the heart via the vagus nerve. Profuse sweating above the level of injury along with vasodilation and skin flushing occurs above the level of injury. This is the result of a compensatory reflex causing increase in sympathetic inhibitory outflow from vasomotor centers above the SCI.[34]

The most common causes of AD are bladder and bowel problems. Other potential causes of AD include problems of the integumentary system, stimulation from the reproductive system, and other causes such as DVT, excessive alcohol or caffeine intake, fractures or other trauma, functional electrical stimulation, heterotopic ossification, pulmonary emboli, substance abuse, and surgical or invasive procedures.[34]

Treatment of AD should be initiated urgently. Sit the person up if he or she is supine and loosen clothing or restrictive devices. Monitor blood pressure and pulse frequently. Quickly assess the patient for instigating causes and remove the cause. Begin the investigation of cause with an assessment of the genitourinary system. If the patient does not have an indwelling catheter, catheterize the patient immediately. Before inserting the catheter, instill 2% lidocaine jelly into the urethra and wait 2 minutes. If the patient has an indwelling catheter, check the system for kinks or other obstructions and correct the problem immediately. If the catheter is draining, proceed to an evaluation of fecal impaction. If the catheter is not draining, remove and replace the catheter. If the systolic blood pressure is at or above 150 mm Hg, consider pharmacologic management to reduce the systolic blood pressure without causing hypotension. Use an antihypertensive agent with rapid onset and short duration such as nifedipine, nitrates, prazosin, or captopril.[34] Refer to the publication from the Consortium for Spinal Cord Medicine, *Acute Management of Autonomic Dysreflexia*, for a more thorough description of treatment options.[34]

Deep Vein Thrombosis

Deep vein thrombosis (DVT) is a high-incidence complication of SCI, with insidious onset and potentially lethal consequences. Thromboembolic disease is a leading cause of morbidity and mortality in ASCI and in the first year after SCI.[35] Venous stasis, hypercoagulability, and intimal injury are major factors predisposing patients with SCI to thromboembolism.[26,28,35] In spite of this population's high risk for DVT, the incidence is decreasing as a result of improved prevention with pharmacologic agents, standard prophylaxis measures, and increased awareness and surveillance of this complication.[35] Mechanical prophylaxis includes the use of compression hose or sequential compression devices applied to the legs for the first 2 weeks after injury. The compression devices may be knee or thigh length. Compression modalities should be assessed by the clinician every shift for proper placement and functioning. If thromboprophylaxis is delayed more than 72 hours, ultrasound of the extremities is recommended before the initiation of mechanical prophylaxis. **Vena cava filter placement** is indicated for failed anticoagulation prophylaxis or if there is a contraindication to anticoagulation.[35]

Anticoagulant prophylaxis with either low–molecular weight heparin or adjusted-dose unfractionated heparin should be initiated within 72 hours after SCI. Anticoagulants should be continued for 8 weeks for inpatients with uncomplicated complete motor injury and for 12 weeks for those with complete motor injury and other risk factors such as lower limb fractures; history of thrombosis, cancer, or heart disease; obesity; or patients over age 70.[35]

The lower extremity circumference is monitored daily. Increase in size of more than 1.5 cm is promptly reported. Marking the positions on the legs with permanent markers using standard measurement sites is recommended (e.g., at the midcalf and midthigh on each leg). Although there is not strong evidence to support this activity, it is used in some clinical settings. Kinetic treatment beds, used in the acute setting and described previously, rotate the patient for up to 20 hours a day, and also promote circulation in the patient with SCI.[84] Low-grade fever of unknown origin (FUO) and tachycardia are potentially early signs of microemboli.

ALERT: Quad coughing or assisted coughing is contraindicated in patients who have a vena cava filter because of the risk of dislodgement or perforation of the vena cava.

Gastrointestinal Complications

As previously mentioned, delayed gastric emptying and paralytic ileus are common after SCI. Initial treatment includes placement of a nasogastric tube to decompress the stomach and administration of promotility agents. Gastrointestinal (GI) bleeding is a potential complication of SCI from increased gastric acidity and the use of high-dose steroids. Patients require protection from stress ulcers. H_2 blockers are used routinely to neutralize excessive acidity and prevent GI irritation and bleeding.

ALERT: The clinical presentation of acute abdomen (e.g., GI bleed, perforation, obstruction) in patients with SCI above T12 may be muted or absent due to changes in innervation of the gut.[26] Symptoms the patient may report include abdominal fullness and distention, nausea, referred pain, and a general sense of not feeling well. Signs may include temperature elevation, distended or firm abdomen, autonomic dysreflexia, and absent bowel sounds.

Orthostatic Hypotension

Orthostatic hypotension, defined as a drop in blood pressure greater than 20 mm Hg or symptoms of low blood pressure on rising, is common and should not impede efforts to mobilize the patient. Prevention and treatment measures include using an abdominal binder and compression hose, slowly increasing the head of the bed before mobilization, elevating the legs in the wheelchair, and administering pharmacologic agents such as midodrine.

Aspiration, Atelectasis, and Pneumonia

The risk of aspiration in the SCI population is increased because of intubation/tracheostomy, sedation, presence of nasogastric tubes, dysphagia, and supine positioning. Pneumonia, atelectasis, and other respiratory complications occur in 40% to 70% of tetraplegics and are the leading cause of death in this population.[88] Signs and symptoms of these conditions include fever, change in respiratory rate, shortness of breath, tachycardia, anxiety, increased volume or tenacity of secretions, and declining vital capacity. Prevention measures include maintaining the head-of-bed angle at 30 to 45 degrees, use of an endotracheal tube with a dorsal lumen above the endotracheal cuff to allow drainage by continuous suctioning of tracheal secretions, infrequent changes of ventilator circuits, aggressive oral care, monitoring gastric residuals, aggressive turning in bed or kinetic therapy, and administration of promotility agents.

Pain

Pain is a significant and complicated problem in SCI that is reported in ASCI 33% to 94% of the time.[41,110] Severe or disabling chronic pain is reported to range from 18% to 80%.[25,98] Chronic pain is so severe that 30% of individuals with SCI report that the pain interferes with activity and affects quality of life.[25] Management of pain in SCI is a complex process. Usually a single modality is not effective in management of pain in this population.[10] Pain management modalities consist of nonnarcotic and narcotic pharmacologic treatment, physical modalities, ablative procedures, complementary and alternative medicine, and neurocognitive or neurobehavioral interventions (see Chapter 23). Many types of pain are reported by individuals with SCI. It is important to conduct a thorough assessment and determine the type and potential causes of pain before establishing a pain management plan. It is beyond the scope of this text to cover all of the pain syndromes presented by individuals with SCI. General pain categories and treatment options are discussed. Acute pain may be present in the days to weeks following initial injury as a result of the injury to the spinal cord or other injuries suffered in the trauma. These patients may also experience acute postoperative pain if a surgery or procedure is required. Acute pain can be managed by a variety of modalities. Pharmacologic management includes nonsteroidal antiinflammatory drugs (NSAIDs) or opioid analgesics. Physical modalities may be useful and include heat, ice, massage, rest, and immobilization. In addition, cognitive-behavior modalities using relaxation, distraction, and guided imagery may also be helpful.[4]

Musculoskeletal pain is described as dull, aching, and worse with movement or exercise, and appears to arise from musculoskeletal structures.[64] Patients with SCI may experience this type of pain throughout the rehabilitation process and beyond because of therapy interventions, or as a result of the physical effects of completion of ADLs or mobility. Musculoskeletal pain may be acute or chronic. Shoulder pain is a frequent and common form of musculoskeletal pain in SCI.[25] There are numerous modalities that may be effective to manage musculoskeletal pain. Pharmacologic management is the same as for acute pain but additionally may include steroids, benzodiazepines, and muscle relaxants. Topical agents also may be helpful. In severe cases, local steroid injections may be warranted. Physical modalities are similar to those for acute pain management with the addition of chiropractic manipulation and manual therapy or mobilization. Muscle strengthening, stretching, and optimization of posture may also prove helpful. Transcutaneous electrical nerve stimulation (TENS) devices may be effective. Yoga, biofeedback, and acupuncture or acupressure may be effective complementary and alternative medicine interventions.

Neuropathic pain includes radicular pain (arising from nerve root damage, occurring within two levels above or below the level of injury) and central pain (related to segmental spinal cord damage). Pain is described as sharp, shooting, stabbing, electric, or burning in radicular pain syndromes. In neuropathic pain syndromes, the pain is described as tightness, pressure, or burning in thoracic injuries and numbness, tingling, heat, or cold in cervical injuries.[25] This type of pain may be experienced at or just above the level of injury or may be experienced at or below the level of injury.[25,64] Pharmacologic interventions that may be helpful include simple analgesics, tricyclic antidepressants, anticonvulsants, NSAIDs, topical capsaicin, and opioids. TENS, acupuncture, nerve blocks, and surgery, including dorsal root entry zone ablation (DREZ) procedures, may be effective. Relaxation, hypnosis, and cognitive-behavioral techniques may prove beneficial in this pain type.[3,25]

Visceral pain is described as dull or cramping. Visceral pain originates from deep visceral structures and can be identified by location, such as in the abdomen.[64] Pharmacologic interventions identified as useful in this pain type include anticholinergics, H_2 blockers, steroids, and NSAIDs.

Pain can interfere with the rehabilitation process, ability to engage in daily activities, and quality of life and can be a more significant source of disability than the SCI.[77] Pain is underestimated by health care providers in this population[3,64,77] and is undertreated as well (see Chapter 23).

Heterotopic Ossification

Heterotopic ossification (HO) is a condition characterized by formation of mature bone in soft tissues. The specific cause of HO is unclear but is basically the inappropriate differentiation of fibroblasts to bone-forming cells. Early edema of connective tissue proceeds to tissue with central calcification and then maturation of calcification and ossification.[24] HO may be occult, but in symptomatic cases, the earliest sign of HO is decreased joint range of motion (ROM). Other signs and symptoms include swelling, erythema, heat, pain with ROM, and contracture formation. HO can occur anywhere in the body but most commonly forms in the joints or long bones. It always occurs below the level of injury in individuals with SCI.[115] HO must be differentiated from thrombophlebitis, DVT, cellulitis, joint sepsis, hematoma, fracture, and trauma. Routine x-ray and clinical diagnosis are generally sufficient, but bone scan and venogram are necessary to differentiate DVT and early HO (see Chapter 13).[85]

Prevention and treatment of HO includes administration of etidronate disodium (Didronel). This drug seems to have an effect on preventing development of HO or at least minimizing the ossification of bone in the joints.[85] The usual regimen lasts 12 weeks. ROM may be useful in minimizing the effects of bone formation in the joints and in maintaining joint mobility. The only current treatment for severe HO is surgical intervention. Bleeding and postoperative infection, as well as recurrence of HO, is a complication of the surgery.[85]

Spasticity

Spasticity can be useful for transfers, positioning, and mobility in bed if it is not severe. However, severe spasticity can predispose the individual with SCI to complications such as pain, contractures, long bone fractures, joint dislocations, and skin problems.[85] In the event spasticity leads to pain or functional limitations, treatment should be considered. Physical modalities may be useful and include passive ROM exercises; application of ice, heat, or vibration; splinting or bandaging; massage; low-power laser; acupuncture; and electrical stimulation.[85] Pharmacologic agents frequently used to treat spasticity include baclofen, benzodiazepines, dantrolene sodium, clonidine, and soma (see Chapter 13).[85]

Syringomyelia

Syringomyelia is a posttraumatic syndrome that can occur in individuals with SCI caused by development of a fluid-filled cyst in the gray matter of the spinal cord. Symptomatic posttraumatic syringomyelia (PTS) is manifested by neurologic changes and potential functional decline and occurs in 3% to 8% of the SCI population.[72] The signs and symptoms of PTS may include pain at the original site of injury or in the upper limbs and neck. Ascending loss of deep tendon reflexes and pain and temperature sensation, most often unilateral, are early signs of PTS. Worsening weakness and muscle fasciculations and atrophy occur later. Less common signs and symptoms include changes in spasticity, hyperhidrosis, loss of reflex bladder emptying, worsening orthostatic hypotension, scoliosis, central and/or obstructive sleep apnea, new development of Horner's syndrome, reduced respiratory drive, impaired vagal cardiovascular reflexes, and sudden death.[72] Magnetic resonance imaging (MRI) is the definitive diagnostic test. Surgical treatment is warranted if neurologic decline is significant or rapid. Early intervention is encouraged because symptoms may be reversible. The loss of one motor level can make a great deal of difference in independence level or ability to breathe independently in some individuals.

Alterations in Sexual Function

Sexual health care is a vital component of rehabilitation for individuals with SCI.[60] Emotional and psychosocial needs should be addressed as well as physiologic changes after SCI.[66] Sexual health topics related to emotional and psychosocial issues to be addressed for both males and females with SCI include role changes, altered body image and self-esteem, feelings of self-worth, and relationship issues. Physiologic changes vary depending on level and completeness of injury. Sexually transmitted diseases (STDs) are a significant risk in society. Individuals with SCI are not immune to STDs. Sexually active individuals need to take responsibility to practice safe sex to avoid contraction and transmission of STDs. Sadly, individuals with disabilities are at greater risk for physical and sexual abuse.[100] Abuse frequently occurs by caregivers. Individuals with SCI are also vulnerable to perpetrators of abuse that they do not know as well.

Sexual health issues specific to women with SCI revolve primarily around reproductive issues, contraception, and sexual response. Amenorrhea occurs in most women immediately after SCI and lasts up to 6 months after injury. Fertility is relatively unaffected. Birth control should be addressed in sexually active women of childbearing age, particularly if pregnancy is not desired. A woman could become pregnant if engaged in unprotected sexual intercourse before resumption of first menstruation because ovulation may have occurred. Women with SCI should be counseled about resources in the event of physical or sexual abuse as rates of abuse are higher in individuals with disabilities. Vaginal lubrication may be diminished. Water-soluble lubricant should be used during intercourse to prevent trauma to the tissue of the vaginal wall.[60]

Sexual issues specific to men with SCI include reproductive issues, fertility, and sexual response. Fertility in males with SCI is severely compromised. The three primary causes are ejaculatory dysfunction, poor semen quality characterized by low sperm counts and poor sperm motility, and erectile dysfunction. In the event of ejaculatory dysfunction, sperm retrieval can be artificially facilitated by vibrostimulation, electroejaculation, and microaspiration.[60]

Erectile dysfunction is common in SCI. In general, those with UMN injuries experience reflexogenic erections. Those with LMN injuries experience psychogenic erections. Erections may not be firm enough or may not be sustainable for vaginal penetration. There are a variety of options for management of erectile dysfunction. **Vacuum tumescence** devices are one of the least invasive options for management of erectile dysfunction. **Intracavernous injection** of vasoactive drugs is another option, but must be ordered and titrated by a health care provider with prescriptive privileges. Priapism, prolonged or constant, painful penile erection (described earlier), is a potential complication of intracavernous injections and is a medical emergency that, left untreated, may cause permanent damage to the penis. **Intraurethral suppositories** (e.g., MUSE) are another pharmacologic intervention, but one that is not frequently used because of the proliferation of effective oral medications. Oral medications such as sildenafil citrate (Viagra) tablets are effective in individuals with UMN injuries who experience reflex erections. Caution must be used with this medication, which should not be taken within 48 hours of use of nitrate medications. **Penile prostheses** are surgically implanted devices for erection. There are three types: rigid, semirigid, and inflatable. There are a number of potential complications with the use of penile prostheses, including surgical complications and infection, failure of the prosthesis, and extrusion of the rods.

COMPREHENSIVE PATIENT MANAGEMENT

Health Teaching Considerations

Education is foundational to the management of individuals recovering from ASCI. Patients and their families need to learn all they can about SCI to manage and cope during the acute phase and all aspects of life with SCI. Individuals with SCI need to be very knowledgeable on the complete care and be able to instruct others in their care should they need assistance. Prevention of complications requires a thorough understanding of complications that can arise: how to prevent occurrence, recognize signs and symptoms, provide treatment, and seek medical assistance if necessary. After the initial shock and disbelief, the health care team begins the difficult task of preparing the patient and family for a lifetime of living with a permanent neurologic disability. Information about the function of the spinal cord, the effect of the disability according to the level of injury, and strategies for abilities versus disabilities is essential to learning to live successfully with SCI. A plan of care, with appropriate education for each component of the patient's needs and the availability of services to support those needs, provides a sense of security and hope for adjustment and improves the individual's sense of self-worth. The comprehensive plan and teaching must cover medical needs, medications and side effects, safety concerns, and psychosocial adjustments. Education on the significance of continuing rehabilitation and prevention of complications, with an emphasis on the patient

assuming self-control, provides purpose to the patient's new way of life.

Family or other care providers should be encouraged to be involved in all aspects of the rehabilitation program, not only to provide maximal support to the individual with the injury but also to take advantage of every opportunity to learn about management of SCI. Classroom learning, utilization of written materials and other multimedia learning materials, involvement with peers, and hands-on training are teaching methods that can be used with patients and families. A model for assessing learning readiness for self-direction of care, and the role of the clinician within each stage of this model, has been proposed.[92] The model includes five stages of learning readiness with five corresponding nursing roles. The first stage is dependent, and the nursing role is one of authority. The second stage is involvement, and the role of the clinician is guide. The third stage is engagement, and the role of the clinician is motivator. The fourth stage is self-initiation, and the role of the clinician is mentor. The fifth stage is self-direction, and the role of the clinician is consultant. As with the basic rehabilitation program, the patient assumes increasing responsibility for his or her own learning and the clinician moves from an authoritarian role to a supportive, consultative role. A life care plan is another valuable tool to help the individual and family project the short- and long-term needs for the life expectancy of the individual with ASCI.

Nutritional Considerations

Hypermetabolism, accelerated catabolic rate, and extreme nitrogen losses occur with ASCI.[112] This cascade of events results in depletion of energy stores, loss of lean muscle mass, reduced protein synthesis, and ultimately loss of GI mucosal integrity and compromise of immune competence.[112] Risk for prolonged nitrogen losses and advanced malnutrition occurs within 2 weeks of injury, resulting in increased susceptibility to infection, impaired wound healing, and difficulty weaning from mechanical ventilation.[112] Nutritional support for patients with SCI is therefore a priority. The stable patient with SCI in rehabilitation is at increased risk of weight gain after the initial trauma period due to lower than expected resting energy expenditure. Indirect calorimetry is recommended to establish nutritional requirements.[112]

Psychosocial Considerations

The devastating effects of SCI lead to a myriad of emotional reactions and extreme challenges for patients and families as they move toward adaptation to a life with SCI.[46] Stages of adaptation have been proposed but have not been empirically tested. There is limited agreement from experts in the field of SCI that stage theory is applicable in this population. There are, however, a plethora of issues reported related to psychosocial adaptation to SCI. Hospitalization is an **anxiety**-provoking experience under the best of circumstances. The added stress of dealing with a truly life-altering injury may result in excessive anxiety being displayed by patients and families. Patients and families should be given resources and assistance in dealing with anxiety-provoking situations such as financial matters, child care issues, and lifestyle and role changes. **Denial** is a normal coping mechanism employed in the face of overwhelming circumstances. Patients and families may deny the extent or permanency of their situation. Early denial is normal and should not cause extreme concern in health care professionals. If denial begins to hinder the individual's progress in rehabilitation or leads to self-neglect, psychologic intervention may be warranted. Denial may be reframed as hope. Health care professionals need not take hope away from patients and families. An approach may be to encourage the patient to deal with current status and participate in rehabilitation to the extent possible at that time.[83,127]

Anger may surface as a stress reaction or coping mechanism in the patient hospitalized with SCI. Anger may indicate a motivated patient (or family) who is trying to exert control over the situation, or it may arise when the patient and family come to the realization that the SCI is not going away.[83] Anger from patients and families may be directed at staff. Staff should receive education about psychosocial implications of SCI and be given the support and resources to manage potential negative reactions from patients and families. Patents and families should be given outlets to manage their anger such as support from a psychologist and access to support groups.[127] **Depression** is a significant secondary complication of SCI.[43] The prevalence of depression is estimated at up to 25% in men with SCI and 47% in women with SCI.[33] Routine screening should be conducted during the initial rehabilitation phase and with routine health examinations. Once formally diagnosed using established diagnostic criteria, treatment recommendations should be made for specific symptoms.[33]

Community Reintegration Considerations

The ultimate goal of recovery and rehabilitation is reintegration of the individual with SCI back into the community. Reintegration of the individual with SCI into the community can be a challenge.[107] The ability to return to work or school can be complicated by the amount of time the patient takes to perform ADLs. Patients often need specialized equipment to perform simple tasks. In discharge planning, all aspects of the patient's life must be considered, including future goals for reintegration. Members of the rehabilitation team evaluate the individual for all aspects of daily living, including an adapted home that is wheelchair accessible, the need for attendant care, access to resources and ongoing health care, transportation with an adapted vehicle, vocational training, and returning to work or school.

Long-term follow-up for SCI does not occur only with the individual, but affects the entire family. The early phase of rehabilitation and recovery is to help the patient and family focus on potentials and capacities. Since most individuals plateau in neurologic return and functional abilities between 6 and 12 months following SCI, the long-term outpatient rehabilitation process helps the individual adjust to activities and functions for home and community reintegration.

Compensation and remediation is the goal as the individual progresses toward adaptation to a new lifestyle. The team approach to outcome-oriented rehabilitation remains important. Emphasis is on self-care deficits, patient understanding of care, and prevention of long-term complications.[39] Special, caring relationships restore a sense of wholeness and dignity and contribute to the individual's emotional and physical well-being.[73] Comprehensive follow-up and outpatient care includes annual or biannual reevaluations based on the individual's needs, complications, and problems in maintaining a healthy lifestyle. It is recommended for individuals with SCI to receive disability management at a facility with a comprehensive outpatient SCI program. Health care providers with expertise in ongoing medical needs in SCI will best be able to detect early complications and provide necessary health services and rehabilitation.

Primary care includes standard primary care services for health surveillance, health promotion, and disease prevention, as well as management of a variety of short-term (acute) and long-term (chronic) disease states. Individuals with SCI should locate a primary health care provider in their community as soon as they are discharged from acute rehabilitation in case the need arises to use their services. Architectural and attitudinal access of any health care practice, is important to determine.[59]

Recreation, health restoration, and how an individual spends free time are critical components of successful rehabilitation and a happy and successful life. People with SCI are involved in almost every activity of their able-bodied counterparts. The activity may require some adaptation, but most people find several activities they enjoy after their injury. Patients should receive a leisure assessment during their initial rehabilitation program and subsequent evaluations as needed during reevaluations. Recreational resources can be provided for people to explore in their communities. There are a multitude of opportunities for individuals with SCI relative to recreation.

Older Adult Considerations

Age at time of ASCI is increasing.[88] The number of older adults with SCI is increasing in trauma centers and rehabilitation programs. The aging of our patient population creates unique challenges for the rehabilitation treatment team. The first challenge is to determine fit of program for the older individual. Many SCI programs are geared toward younger individuals and may be too strenuous for the older adult. The overall milieu may be geared toward teens and younger adults, and not suitable for some older adults. If an older patient is admitted to a program, the treatment team needs to consider program modifications such as shorter therapy periods, a slower pace, and lighter activities. This does not, however, apply to all older adults, and the program needs to be individualized to specific patient needs. Vocational and leisure programs may require modifications as well. Most individuals with SCI are expected to live into their sixties and seventies.[61,88] This means that for individuals injured in their teens to thirties, they potentially may live several decades with their SCI. These people will face not only the normal changes that occur as we age, but a range of changes attributable to their SCI. Medical, functional, and psychosocial changes can be anticipated.[61,124]

People with SCI appear to experience medical problems sooner than their age-matched peers without SCI. Older people with SCI experience increased rates of metabolic, endocrine, and cardiovascular disorders.[62] Functional changes include potential negative effects on self-care activities, mobility, routine chores, socializing, recreational activities, maintaining family roles, and preserving employment or educational activities. These changes in functional status most commonly are attributed to pain, fatigue, and weakness.[61,62] The psychosocial implications for aging with SCI include the risk for depression and declining perception of quality of life. Depression and a decline in quality of life are both associated with medical problems and changes in functional status.[62] As previously mentioned, the aging individual with SCI is at risk for medical problems and functional decline, which places him or her at greater risk for these psychosocial challenges.

Routine health screening and preventive services are requisite services for the older adult. With SCI as a compounding factor of aging for medical, functional, and psychosocial decline, it is imperative that older adults with SCI have a support system to maintain health, function, and quality of life. This support system consists of access to rehabilitation and specialty medical services. Access to technology, equipment, and personal care assistance will also benefit the older adult with SCI.[62]

Case Management Considerations

With the exception of a handful of catastrophic injury case managers, SCI is not one of the most common disorders found in the case manager's caseload. Long-term case management may be helpful in reintegration of the patient with SCI back to home and community. The initial patient contact requires the expertise of a case manager who is competent to conduct a thorough assessment to determine the patient's potential long-term medical needs and **durable medical equipment (DME)** requirements. Interviews with not only the patient but also members of the interdisciplinary team, family members, and caregivers will assist in the design of a comprehensive plan of care with measurable goals and outcomes. Since costs of services can become extensive, careful research and planning are needed from the onset. A **life care plan (LCP)** can assist the case manager to work with individuals with SCI to manage their resources. A life care plan provides consistency of assessment and services, organization of financial and health resources, and an analysis of the literature to identify services, treatments, and equipment that will enhance long-term health and quality of life and promote functional outcomes and independence.[13,18]

Case management may be required for the lifetime of patients with high-level SCI. After resolution of acute problems, it is important to focus on wellness and preventive care for the highest quality of life while maintaining support from essential health care providers. Measurement of functional improvement, pain relief, avoidance of unnecessary surgery, avoidance of rehospitalization, prevention of and screening for complications, provision of appropriate medical and community resources, and patient compliance and satisfaction are challenging goals for case management of the patient with SCI. The case manager can determine if the individual is eligible for financial benefits and assist the patient and family with the application process to ensure that they receive all the benefits possible.

OUTCOMES FOLLOWING SPINAL CORD INJURY

Motor Recovery

Overall recovery for individuals with SCI has been seen to occur in the early weeks to months after injury, if recovery is going to occur, but slows significantly after that time. For 80% to 90% of patients assessed in the first week of injury as ASIA A complete, injuries will remain complete. Individuals with incomplete injuries experience recovery most often in the first 2 months after injury with some continued but slow recovery for the next 3 to 6 months. Some return of neurologic function may be seen for years after injury, particularly in incomplete injuries. Changes in motor recovery have been documented up to 2 years after injury, and changes in neurologic status may continue beyond 2 years.[36] Return of functional strength in the lower extremities, which would improve the potential for ambulation, occurs in 3% to 6% of individuals who convert to incomplete injuries. Locomotor **body weight–supported treadmill training (BWSTT)** may be appropriate for certain patients who experienced an incomplete traumatic SCI to help recover walking ability (see Chapter 13).

Individuals with sensory incomplete injuries, ASIA B, account for about 10% of new injuries. Approximately 50% of those classified as ASIA B will become community ambulators. Individuals with motor complete injuries who have preserved sacral pinprick sensation have a prognosis for lower extremity recovery similar to the motor incomplete injuries.[36]

Expected Functional Independence Outcomes

A major goal of rehabilitation is to maximize functional independence for individuals with SCI. The Consortium for Spinal Cord Medicine has published a comprehensive document describing expected functional outcomes by level of injury at 1 year after injury.[36] The document includes a table that lists expected outcomes by level of injury in the areas of respiratory, bowel, and bladder function; bed mobility/wheelchair transfers, wheelchair propulsion, and positioning/pressure relief; standing and ambulation; eating, grooming, dressing, and bathing; communication; transportation; homemaking; and assistance required. In each category the equipment is identified that might be required by level of injury to reach maximum independence. An example for an individual with C6 tetraplegia is provided in Table 12-1; functional

TABLE 12-1   Expected Functional Outcomes for an Individual With C6 Tetraplegia

Functionally relevant muscles innervated: clavicular pectoralis supinator; extensor carpi radialis longus and brevis; serratus anterior; latissimus dorsi

Movement possible: scapular protractor; some horizontal adduction, forearm supination, radial wrist extension

Patterns of weakness: absence of wrist flexion, elbow extension, hand movement; total paralysis of trunk and lower extremities

FIM/Assistance Data: Exp = Expected FIM Score, **Med** = NSCISC Median, **IR** = NSCISC Interquartile Range, **NSCISC Sample Size:** FIM = 43, Assist = 35

	Expected Functional Outcomes	Equipment	Exp	Med	IR
Respiratory	Low endurance and vital capacity secondary to paralysis of intercostals; may require assist to clear secretions				
Bowel	Some to total assist	• Padded tub bench with commode cutout or padded shower/commode chair • Other adaptive devices as indicated	1–2	1	1
Bladder	Some to total assist with equipment; may be independent with leg bag emptying	Adaptive devices as indicated	1–2	1	1
Bed mobility	Some assist	• Full electric hospital bed • Side rails • Full to king standard bed may be indicated			
Bed and wheelchair transfers	Level: some assist to independent Uneven: some to total assist	• Transfer board • Mechanical lift	3	1	1–3
Pressure relief and positioning	Independent with equipment or adapted techniques	• Power recline wheelchair • Wheelchair pressure relief cushion • Postural support devices • Pressure relief mattress or overlay may be indicated			
Eating	Independent with or without equipment; except cutting, which is total assist	Adaptive devices as indicated (e.g., U-cuff, tendinosis splint, adapted utensils, plate guard)	5–6	5	4–6
Dressing	Independent upper extremity; some assist to total assist for lower extremity	Adaptive devices as indicated (e.g., button; hook; loops on zippers, pants; socks, Velcro on shoes)	1–3	2	1–5
Grooming	Some assist to independent with equipment	Adaptive devices as indicated (e.g., U-cuff, adapted handles)	3–6	4	2–6
Bathing	Upper body: independent Lower body: some to total assist	• Padded tub transfer bench or shower/commode chair • Adaptive devices as needed • Handheld shower	1–3	1	1–3
Wheelchair propulsion	Power: independent with standard arm drive on all surfaces Manual: independent indoors; some to total assist outdoors	Manual: lightweight rigid or folding frame with modified rims Power: may require power recline or standard upright power wheelchair	6	6	4–6
Standing and ambulation	Standing: total assist Ambulation: not indicated	Hydraulic standing frame			
Communication	Independent with or without equipment	Adaptive devices as indicated (e.g., tendinosis splint; writing splint for keyboard use, button pushing, page turning, object manipulation)			
Transportation	Independent driving from wheelchair	• Modified van with lift • Sensitized hand controls • Tie-downs			
Homemaking	Some assist with light meal preparation; total assist for all other homemaking	Adaptive devices as indicated			
Assist required	• Personal care: 6 hours/day • Homecare: 4 hours/day		10*	17*	8–24*

From Consortium for Spinal Cord Medicine: *Outcomes following traumatic spinal cord injury: clinical practice guidelines for health-care professionals,* Washington, DC, 1999, Paralyzed Veterans of America. Used with permission.
*Hours per day.

independence by level of injury is described in Table 12-2. A newer wheelchair, the iBOT, is available for appropriate individuals that can climb stairs and allow the individual to stand after completing special training and classes (see Chapter 13).

Social Integration

A second major goal of rehabilitation of individuals with SCI is to work toward social integration, including opportunities for societal participation in meaningful roles. Many people with SCI will participate in meaningful social roles beyond those expected for their level of injury.[36]

Quality of Life

A third major goal of rehabilitation is to facilitate opportunities for optimal quality of life. Quality of life is a qualitative measure by people with SCI of their individual perceptions of well-being and satisfaction with life. Individuals with injury report a slightly lower level of quality of life than the average person without SCI, and may not report a significantly different quality of life compared to the preinjury level, although it is contextually driven by their current life condition.[36] Health care professionals underestimate the quality of life of individuals with SCI.[49,50,55] This point must be addressed with providers to assist them to value life with SCI from the perspective of those living it.

Health care providers have the opportunity to enhance quality of life for individuals with SCI, as interventions can be targeted at relationships that affect quality of life, including life and social role barriers; activity limitations; components of social support; social integration; mobility; occupation; family roles; psychologic coping; and pain.[36] Individuals with high-level tetraplegia (above C4) report contributors to quality of life to be autonomy, control over their own life; meaningful use of time, participation in meaningful activities; the need to be busy; the need to have something to wake up for; the ability to explore new opportunities; the need to envision future time engaged in meaningful activities; the need and opportunity to contribute reciprocally to others; meaningful use of time beyond doing, time spent in contemplation and appreciation of things others take for granted; strong relationships with special people; and technologic resources and social policy initiatives that facilitate participation in life and the community.[55] Several complications are associated with quality of life, including neurogenic pain, spasticity, and neurogenic bladder and bowel problems.

CURRENT RESEARCH

It is essential that clinicians working with people with SCI are aware of clinical trials focused on improvement of neurologic outcomes after SCI as patients will assuredly inquire about these options. Although numerous studies are currently underway or in development, few show promise that have withstood the rigorous criticism of experts in the field. It is important to stress that although many studies have given reason for "cautious optimism" in the search for a cure,[70] there are currently only two pharmacologic agents, MPSS and GM-1 (Sygen), that have been investigated in large, multicenter, randomized, placebo-controlled human clinical trials. These agents are currently considered options only in the treatment of ASCI. There remains no cure for SCI, and the best studies to date reveal only mild to moderate improvements in motor and sensory function in a minority of patients.

Of the two pharmaceutical agents considered treatment options, MPSS is the best known and the most controversial. The three landmark trials of this agent include the National Acute Spinal Cord Injury (NASCIS) I, II, and III. These three trials built on one another and led the authors to the following conclusions and recommendations:[22,45] MPSS initiated within 8 hours of injury showed more improvement in motor function than did their counterparts in the placebo group; dosage recommendations include a 30 mg/kg initial bolus followed by a 5.4 mg/kg maintenance infusion for a total of 24 hours.

It is important to note that the interpretation of the NASCIS trials has been called into question by multiple authors, experts, and clinical practice guidelines. Further, there is evidence of severe medical complications associated with its use, including sepsis, pneumonia, respiratory complications, and myopathy.[7,56,70,97] Regardless, MPSS has become a standard of care, for some on the basis of scientific evidence, and for others on the basis of medicolegal risk.[7,56,70]

The second agent, GM-1, studied in the Sygen Multicenter Acute Spinal Cord Injury Study (SMASCIS) a decade ago, initially showed promise in promoting recovery in patients with ASCI.[48] However, by the 6-month follow-up assessment, no significant differences were noted between the control and intervention groups. The drug is not approved by the U.S. Food and Drug Administration (FDA) and is currently only available for use in Europe.[7,70]

In addition to MPSS and GM-1, several other clinical trials are underway. Pharmaceutical agents include minocycline, a semisynthetic analog of the antibiotic tetracycline that is able to diffuse into the central nervous system and has been found to have beneficial effects on inflammation, microglial activation, and apoptotic cell death.[126] Preclinical animal studies comparing minocycline to MPSS have shown superior behavioral recovery.[51,121]

The Rho antagonist Cethrin, a GTPase, has been found to play an important role in neuronal development,[16] including cortical neuron regenerative sprouting leading to rapid recovery of locomotion in animal models.[45] Another agent, Anti-Nogo protein, injected into the injured spinal cords of rats has resulted in significant axon regeneration and regained reflex and locomotor functions.[22] Finally, the nucleoside inosine has reportedly induced new axon growth in rat models.[16]

Studies utilizing clinical interventions in ASCI include the injection of specially prepared macrophages into the spinal cord to attenuate the inflammatory response to injury and scavenge growth inhibitors from the injured tissue

TABLE 12-2 Anticipated Functional Levels in Spinal Cord Injury

	Pulmonary Hygiene	AM Care	Feeding
C3-C4	Totally assisted cough	Total dependence	Unable to feed self; drink with long straw after setup
C5	Assisted cough	Independent with specially adapted devices with setup	Independent with specially adapted equipment for feeding after setup
C6	Some assistance required in supine positions; independent in sitting position	Independent with equipment	Independent with equipment; drink from glass
C7	As above	Independent	Independent
C8-T1	As above	Independent	Independent
T2-T10	T2-6 as above; T6-10 independent	Independent	Independent
T11-L2	Not applicable	Independent	Independent
L3-S3	Not applicable	Independent	Independent

	Pressure Relief	Transfers	Wheelchair Propulsion
C3-C4	Independent in powered recliner wheelchair; dependent in bed or manual wheelchair	Total dependence	Independent in pneumatic or chin-control–driven power wheelchair with powered reclining feature
C5	Most require assistance	Assistance of one person with or without transfer board	Independent in power chair indoors and outdoors; short distances in manual wheelchair with lugs, indoors
C6	Independent	Potentially independent with transfer board	Independent manual wheelchair with plastic rims or lugs indoors; assistance outdoors and with elevators
C7	Independent	Independent with/without transfer board except to/from floor with assistance	Independent manual wheelchair indoors and outdoors except curbs
C8-T1	Independent	Independent, including to/from floor	Independent in manual wheelchair indoors and out
T2-T10	Independent	Independent	Independent
T11-L2	Independent	Independent	Independent
L3-S3	Independent	Independent	Independent

Grooming	Dressing	Bathing	Bowel and Bladder Routine	Bed Mobility
Total dependence	Total dependence	Total dependence	Total dependence	Total dependence
Independent with specially adapted equipment for grooming after setup	Total dependence	Total dependence	Total dependence	Assisted by others and equipment
Independent with equipment	Independent upper dressing; assistance with lower dressing	Independent uppers and lowers with equipment	Independent for bowel routine; assistance with bladder routine	Independent with equipment
Independent with equipment	Potential for independence in upper and lower dressing	Independent with equipment	Independent	Independent
Independent	Independent	Independent	Independent	Independent
Independent	Independent	Independent	Independent	Independent
Independent	Independent	Independent	Independent	Independent
Independent	Independent	Independent	Independent	Independent

Continued

TABLE 12-2 **Anticipated Functional Levels in Spinal Cord Injury—cont'd**

Ambulation	Orthotic Devices	Transportation	Communications
Not applicable	Upper extremity; outside power orthosis; dorsal cockup splint	Dependent on others in accessible van with lift	Read with specially adapted equipment; specially adapted phone; unable to write; type with special adaptations
Not applicable	As above	As above	Same as above
Not applicable	Wrist-driven orthosis	Independent driving in specially adapted van	Independent phone; write with equipment; type with equipment; independent turning pages
Not applicable	None	Independent driving car with hand controls or specially adapted van; independent wheelchair into car placement	Independent with equipment for phone; typing and writing; independent turning pages
Not applicable	None	As above	Independent
Exercise only (not functional) with orthoses	Knee-ankle-foot orthoses with forearm crutches or walker	As above	Independent
Potential for independent functional ambulation indoors with orthoses; some have potential for stairs with railing	Knee-ankle-foot orthoses or ankle-foot orthoses with forearm crutches	As above	Independent
Independent indoors and outdoors with orthoses	Ankle-foot orthoses with forearm crutches or canes	As above	Independent

Developed by the Occupational and Physical Therapy Departments of the Regional Spinal Cord Injury of Delaware Valley, Thomas Jefferson University, Thomas Jefferson University Hospital, and Magee Rehabilitation Hospital, Philadelphia, PA. Data originally compiled by Staas WE et al: Rehabilitation of the spinal cord–injured patient. In Delisa JA: *Rehabilitation medicine: principles and practice,* Philadelphia, 1998, JB Lippincott.

environment, resulting in improved neurologic outcomes.[63,108] Similarly, specially prepared bone marrow injected into the injured cord is thought to activate macrophages and improve neurologic function.[53] One intriguing treatment uses an implanted electrical field over the site of injury, which is thought to facilitate regeneration of sensory and motor fibers.[109]

Clinical trials for chronic SCI aimed at improving neurologic function or sequelae in chronic SCI include pharmaceutical agents such as 4-aminopyridine (Fampridine SR), which improves signal conduction in demyelinated axons and has had mixed results in studies aimed at decreasing spasticity.[2,95] Several studies are underway utilizing various sources of olfactory cells. These cells are of interest because they may participate in the regeneration of olfactory axons and are hoped to stimulate regeneration in the spinal cord. Animal studies have shown positive results.[21] Transplantation of fetal olfactory cells is also being experimented with in China but is surrounded by controversy.[82,118]

Stem cells used for axonal regeneration and remyelination have been and continue to be a popular topic in the lay press. In order to avoid the controversy surrounding the use of human stem cells, researchers are using modified animal cells and autologous bone marrow–derived precursor cells.[99,113] Results of these studies are not published or the studies are underway.

CONCLUSION

Spinal injury continues to be a major consequence of trauma. Although efforts have been increased to prevent traumatic SCI, the number of ASCI survivors each year has remained constant for the past decade. Current prevention efforts need to continue and more aggressive prevention efforts established. Spinal cord injuries are extremely devastating to the patient, the patient's family, the community, and society. Marked changes in lifestyle are required for the survivors of such injuries. Medical, surgical, and rehabilitative advances in the treatment of SCI have been successful in increasing survivability of the initial injury and decreasing the impact of comorbidities. Continued education efforts for health care professionals who manage patients with SCI is a priority. The hope of future scientific developments to provide an improved quality of life may be on the horizon. The future looks bright.

RESOURCES FOR SPINAL INJURY

American Academy of Physical Medicine and Rehabilitation: www.aapmr.org

American Association of Spinal Cord Injury Nurses: 75-20 Astoria Boulevard, Jackson Heights, NY 11370-1177; 718-803-3782; www.aascin.org

American Association of Spinal Cord Psychologists and Social Workers: 75-20 Astoria Boulevard, Jackson Heights, NY 11370-1177; 718-803-3782; www.aascipsw.org

American Paraplegia Society: 75-20 Astoria Boulevard, Jackson Heights, NY 11370-1177; 718-803-3782; www.apssci.org

American Spinal Injury Association: 2020 Peachtree Road, NW, Atlanta, GA 30309-1402; voice: 404-55-9772; fax: 404-355-1826; www.asia-spinalinjury.org

Christopher Reeve Paralysis Foundation: 500 Morris Avenue, Springfield, NJ 07081; 800-225-0292; www.apacure.com

Med Line Plus: www.nlm.nih.gov/medlineplus/spinalcordinjuries.html

Miami Project to Cure Paralysis: www.miamiproject.miami.edu/

National Spinal Cord Injury Association: 8701 Georgia Avenue, Suite 500, Silver Spring, MD 20851; 800-962-9629; www.spinalcord.org

National Spinal Cord Injury Hotline: 2200 Kernan Dr., Baltimore, MD 21207; 410- 448-6623; toll free: 800-526-3456

Nelson A, editor: *Nursing practice related to spinal cord injury and disorders: a core curriculum,* Jackson Heights, NY, 2001, Eastern Paralyzed Veterans of America

Paralyzed Veterans of America: 801 18th Street NW, Washington, DC 20006; 202-872-1300; www.pva.org

Program Development Associates: 5620 Business Avenue, Suite B, Cicero, NY 13039-9576; 800-543-2119; www.pdassoc.com

Spinal Cord Injury Information Network: www.spinalcord.uab.edu

Topics in Spinal Cord Injury Rehabilitation: www.thomasland.com

United Spinal Association: 75-20 Astoria Blvd, Jackson Heights, NY 11370; 718-803-3782; www.unitedspinal.org

REFERENCES

1. Aarabi B, Alibaii E, Taghipur M, Kamgarpur A: Comparative study of functional recovery for surgically explored and conservatively managed spinal cord missile injuries, *Neurosurgery* 39(6):1133–1140, 1996.
2. Acorda Therapeutics: Pipeline: clinical stage. Fampridine-SR: SCI, 2004. Available at www.acorda.com/pipeline_fampridine_sci1.asp (accessed August 1, 2005).
3. Agency for Healthcare Research and Quality: Management of chronic central neuropathic pain following traumatic spinal cord injury: evidence report/technology assessment: 45, 2003. Available at www.ahqr.gov/clinic/epcsums/neurosum.htm (accessed October 16, 2005).
4. AHCPR: Acute pain management abbreviated guidelines. Available at www.medana.unibas.ch/eng/internt/ac_pain.htm (accessed October 16, 2005).
5. American Spinal Injury Association: *International standards for neurological classification of spinal cord injury,* Chicago, 2002, ASIA.
6. Apostolides PJ, Karahalios DG, Sonntag VKH: Surgical treatment of traumatic cervical spine injury. In Kaye AD, Black PM, editors: *Operative neurosurgery,* London, 2000, Churchill Livingstone.
7. Apuzzo MLJ: Pharmacological therapy after acute cervical spinal cord injury, *Neurosurgery* 50(3):S63–S72, 2002.
8. Ayyoub Z, Badawi F, Vasile AT, Arzaga D, Cassedy A, Shaw V: Dual diagnosis: spinal cord injury and brain injury. In Lin VW, editor: *Spinal cord medicine: principles and practice,* New York, 2003, Demos.
9. Bader MK, Littlejohns LR, editors: *AANN core curriculum for neuroscience nursing,* ed 4. St Louis, 2004, Elsevier Saunders.
10. Balazy TE: Management of chronic pain in spinal cord injury, *CNI* 9(1), 1998. Available at www.thecni.org/reviews/09-1-p20-balazy.htm (accessed October 12, 2005).
11. Ball PA: Critical care of spinal cord injury, *Spine* 26:S27, 2001.
12. Barker E, Saulino MF: First-ever guidelines for spinal cord injuries, *RN* 65(10):32–37, 2002.
13. Batten M: Improving quality of life, *Rehab Manag* 12(6):58–64, 1999.
14. Bauer D, Kowalski R: Effect of spinal immobilization devices on pulmonary function in the healthy, nonsmoking man, *Ann Emerg Med* 17(9): 915–918, 1988.
15. Beckley J, Nelson E, Saylor K, Sutheim A: Spinal cord injury: physiological effects and potential treatments, 2005. Available at www.macalester.edu/psychology/whathap/ubnrp/spinalcord05/index.html (accessed October 5, 2005).
16. Benowitz LI, Goldberg DE, Madsen JR, Soni D, Irwin N: Inosine stimulates extensive axon collateral growth in the rat corticospinal tract after injury, *Proc Natl Acad Sci U S A* 96(23):13486–13490, 1999.
17. Berkov S, Sakti D: Urinary tract infection and intermittent catheterization, 2005. Available at www.medscape.com/viewarticle/416648 (accessed October 16, 2005).
18. Blackwell TL, Krause JS, Winkler T, Steins SA: *Spinal cord injury desk reference: guidelines for life care planning and case management,* New York, 2001, Demos.
19. Blissitt PA: Nutrition in acute spinal cord injury, *Crit Care Nurs Clin North Am* 2(3):375–384, 1990.
20. Bono CM, Vives MJ, Kaufmann CP: Cervical injuries: indications and options for surgery. In Lin VW, editor: *Spinal cord medicine: principles and practice,* New York, 2003, Demos.
21. Boyd JG, Doucette R, Kawaja MD: Defining the role of olfactory ensheathing cells in facilitating axon remyelination following damage to the spinal cord, *FASEB J* 19(7):694–703, 2005.
22. Bregman BS, Kunkel-Bagden E, Schnell L, et al: Recovery from spinal cord injury mediated by antibodies to neurite growth inhibitors, *Nature* 378(6556):498–501, 1995.
23. Brockmeyer D: Pediatric spinal cord and spinal column trauma, 2005. Available at www.neurosurgery.org/sections/section.aspx?showprint=true&section=pd&pa (accessed October 12, 2005).
24. Bruno AA: Posttraumatic heterotopic ossification, 2005. Available at www.emedicine.com/pmr/topic112.htm (accessed October 16, 2005).
25. Bryce TN, Ragnarsson KT: Pain management in persons with spinal cord injury. In Lin VW, editor: *Spinal cord medicine: principles and practice,* New York, 2003, Demos.
26. Buckley DA, Guanci MM: Spinal cord trauma, *Nurs Clin North Am* 34(3):661–668, 1999.
27. Burns AS, Rivas DA, Ditunno JF: The management of neurogenic bladder and sexual dysfunction after spinal cord injury, *Spine* 26(24):S129–S136, 2001.

28. Carol MP, Ducker TB: Spinal cord injury and spinal shock syndrome. In Siegel JH, editor: *Trauma emergency surgery and critical care,* New York, 1987, Churchill Livingstone.

29. Chen D, Apple DF, Hudson LM, Bode R: Medical complications during acute rehabilitation following spinal cord injury: current experience of the model systems, *Arch Phys Med Rehabil* 80(11):1397–1401, 1999.

30. Chin DE, Kearns P: Nutrition in the spine-injured patient, *Nutr Clin Pract* 6(1):213–222, 1991.

31. Chua HC, Tow A, Tan ES: The neurogenic bladder in spinal cord injury: pattern and management, *Ann Acad Med Singapore* 25(4):553–557, 2006.

32. Consortium for Spinal Cord Medicine: *Neurogenic bowel management in adults with spinal cord injury,* Washington, DC, 1998, Paralyzed Veterans of America.

33. Consortium for Spinal Cord Medicine: *Depression following spinal cord injury: a clinical practice guideline for primary care physicians,* Washington, DC, 1998, Paralyzed Veterans of America.

34. Consortium for Spinal Cord Medicine: *Clinical practice guideline: acute management of autonomic dysreflexia,* Washington, DC, 1998, Paralyzed Veterans of America.

35. Consortium for Spinal Cord Medicine: *Clinical practice guideline: prevention of thromboembolism in spinal cord injury,* Washington, DC, 1999, Paralyzed Veterans of America.

36. Consortium for Spinal Cord Medicine: *Outcomes following traumatic spinal cord injury: clinical practice guidelines for health care professionals,* Washington, DC, 1999, Paralyzed Veterans of America.

37. Consortium for Spinal Cord Medicine: *Pressure ulcer prevention and treatment following spinal cord injury: a clinical practice guideline for health care professionals,* Washington, DC, 2000, Paralyzed Veterans of America.

38. Consortium for Spinal Cord Medicine: *Clinical practice guideline: respiratory management following spinal cord injury: a clinical practice guideline for health-care professionals,* Washington, DC, 2005, Paralyzed Veterans of America.

39. Davidoff G: Depression and spinal injury: epidemiology, clinical assessment and therapeutic strategies. Presented at the American Spinal Injury Association Conference, 1990, Chicago.

40. Dawodu ST: Spinal cord injury: definition, epidemiology, pathophysiology, 2005. Available at www.emedicine.com/pmr/topic182.htm (accessed October 5, 2005).

41. Demirel G, Yilmaz H, Gencosmanglu B, Kesiktas N: Pain following spinal cord injury, *Spinal Cord* 36:25–28, 1998.

42. Denis F: The three column spine and its significance in the classification of acute thoracolumbar spinal injuries, *Spine* 8(8):817–831, 1983.

43. Elliott TR: Treatment of depression following spinal cord injury: an evidence-based review, *Rehabil Psychol* 49(2):134–139, 2004.

44. Eskenazi MS, Bendo JA, Spivak JM: Thoracolumbar spine trauma: evaluation and management, *Spine* 11(3):176–185, 2000.

45. Fehlings MG, Baptiste DC: Current status of clinical trials for acute spinal cord injury, *Spinal Injury* 36(suppl 2):S113–S122, 2005.

46. Fichtenbaum J, Kirshblum S: Psychological adaptation to spinal cord injury. In Kirshblum S, Campagnolo DI, DeLisa JA, editors: *Spinal cord medicine,* Philadelphia, 2002, Lippincott Williams & Wilkins.

47. Garshick E, Kelley A, Cohen SA, Garrison A, Tun CG, Gagnon D, Brown R: A prospective assessment of mortality in chronic spinal cord injury, *Spinal Cord* 43:408–416, 2005.

48. Geisler FH, Coleman WP, Grieco G, Poonian D: The Sygen multicenter acute spinal cord injury study, *Spine* 26:S87–S98, 2001.

49. Gerhart KA, Koziol-McLain J, Lowenstin SR, et al: Quality of life following spinal cord injury: knowledge and attitudes of emergency care providers, *Ann Emerg Med* 23:807–812, 1994.

50. Gerhart KA, Corbett B: Uninformed consent: biased decision-making following spinal cord injury, *Health Care Ethics Committee Forum* 7:110–121, 1995.

51. Govek EE, Newey SE, Van Aelst L: The role of the Rho GTPases in neuronal development, *Genes Dev* 19(1):1–49, 2005.

52. Gunnarsson T, Fehlings MG: Acute neurosurgical management of traumatic brain injury and spinal cord injury, *Curr Opin Neurol* 16(6):717–723, 2003.

53. Ha Y, Kim YS, Cho JM, Yoon SH, Park SR, Yoon do H, et al: Role of granulocyte-macrophage colony-stimulating factor in preventing apoptosis and improving functional outcome in experimental spinal cord contusion injury, *J Neurosurg Spine* 2(1):55–61, 2005.

54. Hadley MN, Walters BC, Grabb PA, Oyesiku NM, Przybylski JG, Resnick DK, Ryken TC: Guidelines for acute management of acute cervical spine and spinal cord injuries. Written for the Section for Disorders of the Spine and Peripheral Nerves, of the American Association of Neurological Surgeons, of the Congress of Neurological Surgeons, 2002. Available at www.spineuniverse.com/pdf/traumaguide/finished1116.pdf (accessed March 7, 2006).

55. Hammell KW: Quality of life among people with high spinal cord injury living in the community, *Spinal Cord* 42(11):607–620, 2004.

56. Hugenholtz H: Methylprednisolone for acute spinal cord injury: not a standard of care, *CMAJ* 9:168, 2003.

57. Huggins RM, Kennedy WK, Melroy MJ, Tollerton DG: Cardiac arrest from succinylcholine-induced hyperkalemia, *Am J Health Syst Pharm* 60(7):693–697, 2003.

58. Hussain T: An experimental study of some pressure effects on tissue with reference to the bedsore problem, *J Pathol Bacteriol* 66:347–358, 1953.

59. Johnson K, Lammertse DP: Primary care for individuals with spinal cord injury, *CNI Review Spring* 9(1):10–17, 1998.

60. Johnson KMM, Lanig I: Promotion and maintenance of sexual health in individuals with spinal cord injury. In Lanig IS, editor: *A practical guide to health promotion after spinal cord injury,* Gaithersburg, MD, 1996, Aspen.

61. Kemp BJ, Adkins RH, Thompson L: Aging with a spinal cord injury: what recent research shows, *Top Spinal Cord Inj Rehabil* 10(2):175–197, 2004.

62. Kemp B, Thompson L: Aging and spinal cord injury: medical, functional, and psychosocial changes, *SCI Nurs* 19(2):51–60, 2002.

63. Knoller N, Auerbach G, Fulga V, Zelig G, Attias J, Bakimer R, et al: Clinical experience using autologous incubated macrophages as a treatment for complete spinal cord injury—phase I study results, *J Neurosurg—Spine* 3:173–181, 2005.

64. Kogos SC, Richards S, Banos JH, Ness TJ, Charlifue SW, Whiteneck GG, Lammertse DP: Visceral pain and life quality in persons with spinal cord injury: a brief report, *J Spinal Cord Med* 28(4):333–337, 2005.

65. Kosiak M: Prevention and rehabilitation of ischemic ulcers. In Kothe FH, editor: *Krusen's handbook of physical medicine and rehabilitation,* Philadelphia, 1982, WB Saunders.

66. Kroll K, Kline EL: *Enabling romance: a guide to love, sex, and relationships for the disabled (and the people who care about them),* New York, 2002, Harmony.

67. Kwan I, Bunn F, Roberts I: Spinal immobilization for trauma patients, *Cochrane Database Syst Rev* 2:CD002803, 2001.

68. La Rosa G, Conti A, Cardali S, et al: Does early decompression improve neurological outcomes of spinal cord injured patients? Appraisal of the literature using a meta-analytical approach, *Spinal Cord* 42:503–512, 2004.

69. LaFavor KM: Respiratory pulmonary. In Nelson A, editor: *Nursing practice related to spinal cord injury and disorders: a core curriculum,* Jackson Heights, NY, 2001, Eastern Paralyzed Veterans of America.

70. Lammertse DP: Update on pharmaceutical trials in acute spinal cord injury, *J Spinal Cord Med* 27:319–325, 2004.

71. Lindsey L, Klebine P: Understanding spinal cord injury and functional goals and outcomes, 2005. Available at www.spinalcord.uab.edu/show.asp?durki=22409 (accessed October 5, 2005).

72. Little JW: Syringomyelia. In Lin VW, editor: *Spinal cord medicine: principles and practice,* New York, 2003, Demos.

73. Lucke K: Outcome of nurse caring as perceived by individuals with spinal cord injury during rehabilitation, *Rehabil Nurs* 24(6):247–253, 1999.

74. Main PW, Lovell ME: A review of seven support surfaces with emphasis on their protection of the spinally injured, *J Accid Emerg Med* 13:34–37, 1996.

75. Marino RJ, Ditunno JF, Donovan WH, Maynard F: Neurologic recovery after traumatic spinal cord injury: data from the model spinal cord injury systems, *Arch Phys Med Rehabil* 80(11):1391–1396, 1999.

76. McCloskey J, Bulechek GM, editors: *Nursing intervention classifications,* ed 4, St Louis, 2004, Mosby.

77. McDonald H, Fish W: Pain during spinal cord injury rehabilitation: client perspectives and staff attitudes, *SCI Nurs* 19(3):125–131, 2002.

78. Menon EB, Tan ES: Urinary tract infection in acute spinal cord injury, *Singapore Med J* 33(4):3539–3561, 1992.

79. Merenda LA, Hickey K: Key elements of bladder and bowel management for children with spinal cord injuries, *SCI Nurs* 22(1):8–10, 2005.

80. Mitcho K, Yanko JR: Acute care management of spinal cord injuries, *Crit Care Nurs Q* 22(2):60–79, 1999.

81. Molano AE, Murillo PMA, Salobral VMT, Domingues CM, Cuenca SM, Garcia FC: Pressure sores secondary to immobilization with cervical collar: a complication of acute cervical injury, 2005. Available at www.ncbi.nlm.nih.gov/entrez/query.fcgi?cmd=retrieve&db=pubmed&dopt=abstr (accessed October 16, 2005).

82. Mooney P: Fetal cells used to treat ALS, *Scientist* 2004. Available at www.the-scientist.com/news/20040730/02 (accessed August 3, 2005).

83. Moverman RA: Psychosocial factors in spinal cord injury. In Lin VW, editor: *Spinal cord medicine: principles and practice,* New York, 2003, Demos.

84. Murphy M: Traumatic spinal cord injury: an acute care rehabilitation perspective, *Crit Care Nurs Q* 22 (2):51–59, 1999.

85. Nance PW: Management of spasticity. In Lin VW, editor: *Spinal cord medicine: principles and practice,* New York, 2003, Demos.

86. National Institute on Disability and Rehabilitation Research: Consensus statement. The prevention and management of urinary tract infections among people with spinal cord injuries, *SCI Nurs* 10(2):49–61, 1993.

87. National Institute of Neurological Disorders and Strokes, National Institutes of Health: Spinal cord injury: emerging concepts, 1996. Available at www.ninds.nih.gov/news_and_events/proceedings/sci_report.htm (accessed March 6, 2006).

88. National Spinal Cord Injury Statistical Center, Birmingham, Alabama: Spinal cord injury: facts and figures, 2005. Available at www.spinalcord.uab.edu (accessed September, 29, 2005).

89. Nelson A: Patient's perspectives of a spinal cord injury unit, *SCI Nurs* 7(3):44–64, 1990.

90. Nelson A: Developing a therapeutic milieu on a spinal cord injury unit. In Zejdlik CP, editor: *Management of spinal cord injury,* ed 2, Boston, 1992, Jones & Bartlett.

91. Nelson A: Rehabilitation. In Nelson A, editor: *Nursing practice related to spinal cord injury and disorders: a core curriculum,* Jackson Heights, NY, 2001, Eastern Paralyzed Veterans of America.

92. Olinzock BJ: A model for assessing learning readiness for self-directions of care in individuals with spinal cord injuries: a qualitative study, *SCI Nurs* 21(2):69–74, 2005.

93. Perkash I, Giroux, J: Clean intermittent catheterization in spinal cord injury patients: a follow-up study, *J Urol* 5(149): 1068–1071, 1993.

94. Perkash I: Long-term urologic management of the patient with spinal cord injury, *Urol Clin North Am* 20(3):423–433, 1993.

95. Potter PJ, Hayes KC, Segal JL, Hsieh JT, Brunnemann SR, Delaney GA, et al: Randomized double-blind crossover trial of Fampridine-SR (sustained release 4-aminopyridine) in patients with incomplete spinal cord injury, *J Neurotrauma* 15(10): 837–849, 1998.

96. Prabhakaran K, Patankar JZ, Mali V: Meckel's diverticulum: an alternative conduit for the Mitrofanoff procedure, 2005. Available at www.jpgmonline.com/article.asp?issn=0022385 9;year=2003;volume=49;issue=2;s (accessed October 16, 2005).

97. Qian T, Guo X, Levi AD, et al: High-dose methylprednisolone may cause myopathy in acute spinal cord injury patients, *Spinal Cord* 43(4):199–203, 2005.

98. Rariaso AJ: Chronic pain and spinal cord injury, *Clin J Pain* 2:87–92, 1992.

99. Reier PJ: Cellular transplantation strategies for spinal cord injury and translational neurobiology, *NeuroRx* 1(4):424–451, 2004.

100. Rines B, Breen S: *Talking about sexual issues and spinal cord injury: a guide for professionals,* Vancouver, BC, 1989, British Columbia Rehabilitation Society.

101. Rodriguez DJ, Clevenger FW, Osler TM, et al: Obligatory negative nitrogen balance following spinal cord injury, *JPEN J Parenter Enteral Nutr* 15(3):319–322, 1991.

102. Rosito O, Nino-Murcia M, Wolfe VA, Kiratli BJ, Perkash I: The effects of colostomy on the quality of life in patients with spinal cord injury: a retrospective analysis, *J Spinal Cord Med* 25(3):174–183, 2002.

103. Royster R: Critical care in the acute cervical spinal cord injury, *Top Spinal Cord Inj Rehabil* 9(3):11–31, 2004.

104. Salzberg AC, Byrne DW, Cayten CG, VanNieqerburgh P, Murphy JG, Viehbeck M: A new pressure ulcer risk assessment scale for individuals with spinal cord injury, *Am J Phys Med Rehabil* 75(2):96–104, 1996.

105. Sassoon CSH, Baydur A: Respiratory dysfunction in spinal cord disorders. In Lin VW, editor: *Spinal cord medicine: principles and practice,* New York, 2003, Demos.

106. Schreiber D: Spinal cord injuries, 2005. Available at www.emedicine.com/emerg/topic553.htm (accessed October 12, 2005).

107. Schuster R: Enhancing return to work: matching SCI clients with long-term vocational goals, *SCI Nurs* 22(1):26–30, 2005.

108. Schwartz M: Sell Memorial Lecture: helping the body to cure itself: immune modulation by therapeutic vaccination for spinal cord injury, *J Spinal Cord Med* 26(suppl 1):S6–S10, 2003.

109. Shapiro S, Borgens R, Pascuzzi R, Roos K, Groff M, Purvines S, et al: Oscillating field stimulation for complete spinal cord injury in humans: a phase 1 trial, *J Neurosurg Spine* 2(1):3–10, 2005.

110. Siddall PJ, Taylor DA, McClelland JM, Rutkowski SB, Cousins MJ: Pain report and the relationship of pain to physical factors in the first six months following spinal cord injury, *Pain* 81:187–197, 1999.

111. Sommer JL: The therapeutic challenges of dual diagnosis: TBI/SCI, *Brain Injury* 18(12):1297–1308, 2004.

112. Nutritional support after spinal cord injury, *Neurosurgery* 50(suppl 3):S81–S84, 2002.

113. Steeves J, Fawcett J, Tuszynski M: Report of international clinical trials workshop on spinal cord injury: Vancouver, Canada, *Spinal Cord* 42(10):591–597, 2004.

114. Stevens RD, Bhardwaj A, Kirsh JR, Mirski MA: Critical care and perioperative management in traumatic spinal cord injury, *J Neurosurg Anesthesiol* 15(3):215–229, 2003.

115. Stover S: Heterotopic ossification: spinal cord injury, 2005. Available at www.spinalcord.uab.edu/show.asp?durki=21485 (accessed October 16, 2005).

116. Tator CH: Clinical manifestations of acute spinal cord injury. In Tator CH, Benzel EC, editors: *Contemporary management of spinal cord injury: from impact to rehabilitation,* Park Ridge, IL, 2000, American Association of Neurological Surgeons.

117. Wallbom AS, Naran B, Thomas E: Acute ventilator management and leaning in individuals with high tetraplegia, *Top Spinal Cord Inj Rehabil* 10(3), 1–7, 2005.

118. Watts J: Controversy in China, *Lancet* 365(9454):109–110, 2005.

119. Weld KJ, Dmochowski RR: Differences in bladder compliance with time and association of bladder management with compliance in spinal cord injured patients, *J Urol* 163(4):1234–1235, 2000.

120. Weld KJ, Dmochowski RR: Effect of bladder management on urological complications in spinal cord injured patients, *J Urol* 163(3):768–772, 2000.

121. Wells JE, Hurlbert RJ, Fehlings MG, Yong VW: Neuroprotection by minocycline facilitates significant recovery from spinal cord injury in mice, *Brain* 126(7):1628–1637, 2003.

122. Wheeler JS, Walter JW: Acute urologic management of the patient with spinal cord injury: initial hospitalization, *Urol Clin North Am* 20(3):403–411, 1993.

123. Whetstone W: Prehospital management of spinal cord injured patients. In Lin VW, editor: *Spinal cord medicine: principles and practice,* New York, 2003, Demos.

124. Whiteneck GG, Charlifue SW, Gerhart KA, Lammertse DP, Manley S, Menter RR, Seedroff KR: *Aging with spinal cord injury,* New York, 1993, Demos.

125. Yim SY, Yoon IY, Rah EW, Moon HW: A comparison of bowel care patterns in patients with spinal cord injury: upper motor neuron vs lower motor neuron bowel, *Spinal Cord* 39:204–207, 2001.

126. Yong VW, Wells J, Giulliani F, et al: The promise of minocycline in neurology, *Lancet Neurol* 3(12):744–751, 2004.

127. Zejdlik CP: Enhancing feelings of self-worth. In Zejdlik CP, editor: *Management of spinal cord injury,* ed 2, Boston, 1992, Jones & Bartlett.

128. Zejdlik CP: Physiologic consequences and assessment of injury to the spine and spinal cord. In Zejdlik CP, editor: *Management of spinal cord injury,* ed 2, Boston, 1992, Jones & Bartlett.

129. Zejdlik CP: Promoting optimal respiratory function. In Zejdlik CP, editor: *Management of spinal cord injury,* ed 2, Boston, 1992, Jones & Bartlett.

ELLEN BARKER

CHAPTER 13

Neurorehabilitation

An insult to the nervous system can occur at any age. The injury can happen at birth, following an acute illness, or from a traumatic or an ischemic event. Immediately following the event, the goal of rehabilitation for the neuroscience patient is to improve the patient's quality of life and help the individual to "reach the fullest physical, psychologic, social, vocational, and educational potential consistent with his or her physiologic or anatomic impairment, environmental limitations, and desires and life plans."[17]

Rehabilitation is a diverse team approach. It is a dynamic process with an active program to help patients with a neurologic deficit correct their handicaps and maximize their optimal level of functioning as they adapt to the disability. This process begins at the onset of a neurologic insult that results in a disability and may continue indefinitely. Optimal rehabilitation occurs when it begins as soon as the actual or potential disability is identified, which is frequently while an individual is in an acute care setting; rehabilitation may continue with varying levels of intensity throughout the individual's life. Rehabilitation involves a multidisciplinary team approach that includes the patient and family and a variety of health care professionals in all settings from the acute hospital stay to return to the community. Spontaneous recovery, patient motivation, rehabilitation strategies, and a therapeutic environment all affect the individual's ability to reach his or her maximum recovery.

This chapter presents a brief overview of general rehabilitation management principles for promoting functional self-care and health maintenance in patients with neurologic impairment. Specific rehabilitation interventions required by brain-injured and spinal cord–injured patients and stroke patients are discussed. Although many of these principles can be generalized to other neurologic disorders, rehabilitation interventions for patients with other neurologic conditions, as well as suggestions for patient and family teaching, are included in other chapters under "Rehabilitation Considerations." For example, rehabilitation interventions for coma patients including arousal stimulation programs are discussed in Chapter 6. This chapter focuses on principles of rehabilitation, head injury rehabilitation, spinal cord injury rehabilitation, stroke rehabilitation, psychosocial concerns, and the concept of life care planning.

PRINCIPLES OF REHABILITATION

The care of any patient with a neurologic deficit requires basic knowledge of rehabilitation concepts. Rehabilitation interventions begin in the acute phase of care, long before the patient ever reaches a specialized rehabilitation environment. The World Health Organization (WHO) has developed the International Classification of Impairment, Disability, and Handicap that provides a framework for all health care professionals:[52]

- **Impairment:** any loss or abnormality of a psychologic, physiologic, or anatomic structure or function
- **Disability:** any restriction or lack of ability (resulting from an impairment) to perform an activity in the manner or within the range considered normal for a human being
- **Handicap:** a disadvantage for a given individual resulting from impairment or disability that limits or prevents fulfillment of a role that is normal (depending on age, gender, and social and cultural factors) for that individual

The fourth edition of the American Medical Association (AMA) *Guides* provides the following working definitions for the purpose of medical reporting:[52]

- **Impairment:** the loss, loss of use, or derangement of any body part, system, or function
- **Permanent impairment:** impairment that has become static or well stabilized with or without medical treatment, and is not likely to remit despite medical treatment
- **Disability:** a decrease in or the loss or absence of the capacity of an individual to meet personal, social, or occupational demands, or to meet statutory or regulatory requirements
- **Permanent disability:** occurs when the limiting loss or absence of capacity becomes static or well stabilized and is not likely to change in spite of continuing use of medical or rehabilitation measures
- **Handicap:** refers to "obstacles" to accomplishing life's basic activities that may be overcome only by compensation or accommodation

In describing an individual, it is helpful to view his or her ability or inability to perform specific tasks or functions and to describe if this is done independently or with assistance and if there are any barriers that restrict performance.[39] A newer approach and terminology is a systems approach. A systems approach would include the following:

- Pathophysiology
- Impairment
- Functional limitation

- Disability
- Social limitation

Rehabilitation is a patient-centered approach to achieving a maximal level of functioning. It is a goal-oriented process that always emphasizes abilities, including the ability of the patient and family to ultimately assume responsibility for their own self-care. Neuroscience clinicians must promptly recognize the presence of a neurologic impairment and potential disability, as well as assessing the patient's response and potential for rehabilitation. For many patients with a neurologic impairment, rehabilitation is identified as an important component of the overall treatment plan. The patient and family are beginning a journey where they will learn to adjust to the many changes in their lives. Education, adjustment, and change are three critical concepts in rehabilitation.

THE TEAM PROCESS

Rehabilitation is provided within the context of a team.[34] Typical teams include nurse clinicians; physicians who specialize in rehabilitation medicine; physical, occupational, and speech therapists; a psychologist; social workers; and case managers. The rehabilitation team provides care direction via goal setting (both short- and long-term goals). All members of the rehabilitation team collaborate to recommend functional goals for the patient that will facilitate reintegration into the home and community. O'Toole[34] has described the rehabilitation team as being dependent on the collaboration and cooperation of a variety of team members after an accurate assessment to achieve three major functions: (1) establish realistic goals with the patient and family, (2) ensure continuity of care and coordination of resources, and (3) evaluate the progress of the patient and the quality of care.

Rehabilitation teams may function within a variety of models, depending on the setting and the needs of the patient. Three common models for teams are the multidisciplinary, interdisciplinary, and transdisciplinary teams. In a **multidisciplinary team** the efforts of each team member are combined, but there are clear disciplinary boundaries and the goals for the patient are discipline specific. In an **interdisciplinary team** the team members collaborate to develop patient-centered goals as a team. Treatment is still provided by each team member and frequently includes cross-disciplinary problem solving. Interdisciplinary teams are found in structured rehabilitation settings. A **transdisciplinary team** identifies a primary therapist for a patient, depending on the needs of the patient. Input from all relevant disciplines is provided to the primary therapist to establish treatment goals. The majority of therapy is provided by the primary therapist or by a small number of therapists working with the patient. A transdisciplinary team requires cross-training and involves some blurring of disciplinary boundaries. Transdisciplinary teams are most frequently seen in brain injury and behavioral management settings, where minimizing the number of staff interacting with patients can be very beneficial to the treatment process.

Clinicians may be specialized rehabilitation nurses or any nurse clinician who applies rehabilitation concepts in a clinical setting. Nurses are essential members of the rehabilitation team and diagnose and treat the human responses of individuals and groups to actual or potential health problems relative to altered functional ability and an altered lifestyle. The goal is to assist the individual who has a disability or chronic illness in restoring, maintaining, and promoting his or her maximal health.[5]

A **rehabilitation physician** is one who specializes in rehabilitation, or a physiatrist trained in physical medicine and rehabilitation. As a member of the multidisciplinary team who treats neuroscience patients, the rehabilitation physician performs assessments to determine if patients with physical, behavioral, and social problems will benefit from appropriate rehabilitation. The central role of the rehabilitation physician as the rehabilitation medical manager is to provide guidance and leadership in evaluating the patient's potential for rehabilitation, make recommendations to the team, and prescribe appropriate medications, therapeutic modalities, exercise regimens, and assistive devices. After prescribing a comprehensive rehabilitation program, the rehabilitation physician's responsibility includes reassessment of overall functional progress and determination of the length of stay and need for follow-up therapy. The overall goal is to provide appropriate rehabilitation interventions that will lead to optimal care and an optimal outcome for patients with neurologic dysfunction.

Rehabilitation subspecialties have evolved to care for pediatric, adult, and older adult populations. Among the many specialty programs in rehabilitation are those for patients with spinal cord injury (SCI), traumatic brain injury (TBI), brain attack/stroke, or chronic pain. The **speech therapist (ST)** provides an assessment of language and swallowing. The **physical therapist (PT)** evaluates the individual's extremity strength, gait, and fall risks. The **occupational therapist (OT)** helps determine how well activities of daily living (ADLs) can be performed, particularly upper extremity abilities. It is helpful for clinicians, PTs, and OTs to assess an individual as a team to evaluate a patient and develop a plan for safe transfers to and from bed to chair and ambulation to prevent falls. **Neuropsychologic testing** is important to document behavior and impairments related to memory, cognitive and executive functions, visuoperceptual skills, emotional functioning, and any personality changes.

Case management is also frequently used for patients with catastrophic illness or injuries who require placement, treatment, coordination of home therapies, vocational evaluation, or academic programs. The case manager in rehabilitation is frequently involved in the decision making regarding the most appropriate setting for rehabilitation for a given patient. The rehabilitation clinician case manager is responsible for the coordination of care from admission through discharge. Case managers are frequently involved in the initial rehabilitation assessment and identification of patients who are candidates for rehabilitation; they are also involved in planning, in the identification of appropriate resources, and in the coordination of the overall rehabilitation plan.[21] The **social worker (SW)** serves as a valuable resource for

Rehabilitation Team Members

- Patient and family
- Nurse or rehabilitation nurse clinician, advanced practice nurse (APN), nurse practitioner (NP)
- Physicians: neurologist, physiatrist, neurosurgeon, orthopedic surgeon; physician's assistant (PA)
- Occupational therapist
- Physical therapist or recreational specialist
- Psychologist, neuropsychologist
- Speech/language pathologist/dysphagia specialist
- Social worker
- Audiologist
- Case manager
- Chaplain
- Employer
- Home health professionals
- Nutritionist or dietitian
- Orthotist or prosthetist
- Recreational therapist
- Respiratory therapist
- Teacher
- Vocational counselor
- Life coach

financial issues, discharge planning for follow-up care, and community resources. Members of the rehabilitation team vary, depending on the needs of the patient, and usually schedule weekly team meetings working in concert for best outcomes for the individual. Box 13-1 identifies the various professionals who may be a member of a rehabilitation team.

CANDIDATES FOR REHABILITATION

The neuroscience clinician with a background in neuroanatomy and physiology, neurologic assessment, and neurodiagnostics and a through understanding of the neurologic diseases and disorders is a key health care professional for identifying patients who are candidates for rehabilitation. Early identification and referral for rehabilitation is important, regardless of whether the patients are in an acute or outpatient care setting. The notion that "rehabilitation begins at admission" can be applied, beginning in the intensive care unit (ICU). With the universal use of multidisciplinary care plans, the rehabilitation needs can be written in terms of appropriate interventions beginning on day 1. Many rehabilitation interventions can be implemented to prevent secondary complications associated with conditions such as brain attack or stroke, head injury, and SCI. All patients with neurologic impairments that may lead to disability should be assessed for rehabilitation. Any patient with a neurologic injury or disorder and who is in a prolonged immobilized state will benefit from referrals to a physiatrist, a PT, or an OT for positioning recommendations, positioning aids (e.g., splints, wedges, cushions), range-of-motion (ROM) protocols, and activity tolerance assessment.

Therapists, in conjunction with the neuroscience team, can determine which patients are most likely to benefit from rehabilitation. Patients who have permanent lifelong disabilities and have recently experienced an exacerbation of their chronic condition, those who have had a recent onset of a condition that is known to result in a long-term progressive decline in function, and those with a sudden traumatic neurologic injury are prime candidates for rehabilitation.

ASSESSMENT

A complete health history should elicit information regarding the trajectory of a chronic condition or the mechanism of injury, site, and time of injury; any history of loss of consciousness; and a systems review indicating the problems experienced since the injury or illness. Accurate assessment of the individual's functional capacity is also important to determine what the individual can and cannot do following his or her disorder. The international "gold standard" for assessing functional status and for measuring motor, physical, and cognitive elements is the functional independence measure (FIM) (Fig. 13-1). The patient's functional assessment provides the base from which specific rehabilitation management recommendations follow. Functional assessment includes the use of different scales to determine the patient's functional level. The FIM is one tool that is widely used in rehabilitation settings. It is broad based, simple to administer, and well validated (see Fig. 13-1).[47] The FIM is documented as a baseline on admission and to measure changes in functional ability over time. FIM scores may be part of the discharge disposition to determine where to discharge a patient. Higher FIM scores may be seen in patients returning to home and lower scores for discharge to a facility. The FIM has a 126-point scale and 18 individual subscales that measure multiple physical and cognitive functions.

Basic interventions to promote self-care activities should be assessed. Serial assessments provide comparison to follow the patient's progress and highlight the following responses and behaviors that need attention:

- Is the patient progressing from maximal to minimal assistance with self-care?
- Is the patient able to follow simple, repeated one-step instructions?
- Is the patient able to control sensory input, respond to minimal verbal cues, and initiate activities?
- Is the patient consistent in the sequencing of activities?
- Is the patient able to make choices and decisions?
- Is the patient able to respond appropriately to visual cues (e.g., checklist of dressing steps, pictures of staff, and labels on toiletries)?

The assessment aids the clinician to set up a favorable, therapeutic environment; demonstrate new ways to save the patient's energy; and provide assistive devices and adequate utensils to perform the tasks. The assessment helps establish ample or realistic time frames for the patient to complete tasks to maximal independence.

FIM™ Instrument

LEVELS		
	7 Complete Independence (timely, safely) 6 Modified Independence (device)	**NO HELPER**
	Modified Dependence 5 Supervision (subject = 100%) 4 Minimal Assistance (subject = 75%+) 3 Moderate Assistance (subject = 50%+) **Complete Dependence** 2 Maximal Assistance (subject = 25%+) 1 Total Assistance (subject = less than 25%)	**HELPER**

	ADMISSION	DISCHARGE	FOLLOW-UP
Self-Care A. Eating B. Grooming C. Bathing D. Dressing - Upper Body E. Dressing - Lower Body F. Toileting			
Sphincter Control G. Bladder Management H. Bowel Management			
Transfers I. Bed, Chair, Wheelchair J. Toilet K. Tub, Shower			
Locomotion L. Walk/Wheelchair M. Stairs	W Walk C Wheelchair B Both	W Walk C Wheelchair B Both	W Walk C Wheelchair B Both
Motor Subtotal Rating			
Communication N. Comprehension O. Expression	A Auditory V Visual B Both A Auditory V Visual B Both	A Auditory V Visual B Both A Auditory V Visual B Both	A Auditory V Visual B Both A Auditory V Visual B Both
Social Cognition P. Social Interaction Q. Problem Solving R. Memory			
Cognitive Subtotal Rating			
TOTAL FIM™ RATING			

NOTE: Leave no blanks. Enter 1 if patient is not testable due to risk.

Figure 13-1 Functional Independence Measure.
(Copyright 1997 Uniform Data System for Medical Rehabilitation, a division of the UB Foundation Activities, Inc. Reprinted with the permission of UDSMR, University at Buffalo, 232 Parker Hall, 3435 Main Street, Buffalo, NY 14214.)

The FIM is used to examine the degree of dependence in performing 23 items in the following areas: mobility, locomotion, communication, self-care, cognition, social adjustment, and sphincter control.[41] The 18 items include 13 motor and 5 cognitive measures, using a seven-point scale to estimate the severity of the disability and the need for assistance, which ranges from "1" for total assistance to "7" for complete independence. An FIM score of 18 points represent the need for total assistance in all performance areas compared with 126 points representing complete independence. The functional impact of the neurologic deficits is part of the rehabilitation evaluation. The FIM scores are documented at the rehabilitation admission, during hospitalization and at discharge, and at follow-up to determine outcome for individuals undergoing rehabilitation. The patient data collected from rehabilitation subscribers who use the FIM tool is used to prepare special reports that subscribers can use to examine the outcomes of their services and comparisons, both in-house and across clinical sites (e.g., patterns of care, length of stay, charges, and trends and other uses).

Also included is an assessment of the individual's family and the family's role in patient care on discharge. It is important to assess the patient for other health problems; the home situation, including the number of floors and potential barriers for the disabled patient; and the patient's work status, driving status, educational level, and psychosocial status. Physical assessment findings include a neurologic assessment and a rehabilitation assessment to identify specific areas of concern that warrant consideration for rehabilitation, including the following:[2]

- Cognitive dysfunction may be evidenced by impaired orientation, insight, awareness, judgment, arousal, executive function, reasoning, concentration, and memory.
- Communicative deficits may be evidenced by impaired comprehension, confused speech, aphasia, and confabulation.
- Behavioral dysfunction may be evidenced by impulsivity and disinhibition, restlessness, irritability, increased emotional lability, aggression, withdrawal, depression, agitation, and other signs of inappropriate behavior.
- Motor dysfunction may be evidenced by paresis, paralysis, spasticity, ataxia, and pathologic reflexes.
- Impaired respiratory function with reduced airway clearance or an ineffective breathing pattern and impaired cough and respirations that may be altered because of an SCI at C4 and above. Damage at C2 or C3 disrupts breathing signals sent from the brain to the spinal cord. These signals stimulate the diaphragm's respiratory muscles. When muscles become idle, atrophy may result, causing ventilatory dependency.
- Sensory-perceptual deficits may include cortical blindness; impaired position sense; impaired temperature, pain, and touch awareness; apraxia; agnosias; and deficits or loss in the visual field (from damage at the optic chiasm or other sites along the visual pathway).

- Cranial nerve dysfunction may be evidenced by dysphagia, diplopia, dysarthria, impaired taste and smell, and hearing loss.
- Impaired cardiac function may be evidenced by persistent bradycardia, hypotension, primary cardiac arrest, and problems with a past cardiovascular history. Cardiovascular disorders in the acute and chronic stage account for many deaths in individuals with SCI; deep vein thrombosis (DVT), cardiopulmonary arrest, and pulmonary embolism (PE) are major causes of morbidity and mortality in SCI. Orthostatic hypotension can result in light-headedness, dizziness, nausea, loss of consciousness, and seizures.
- Bowel dysfunction is evidenced by an inability to control bowel evacuation. There is loss of control of the nerves that innervate the anal sphincter, causing a loss of anal control. Bowel dysfunction may be related to a situation in which the muscles that control the lower rectal and anal bowel are paralyzed, and the individual is unable to control bowel evacuation.
- Bladder dysfunction is evidenced by an inability to control voiding. There is loss of control of the nerves that innervate the bladder muscles and urinary sphincter. Conscious control of urination is lost. The bladder muscles may become paralyzed in an individual with SCI and the individual is unable to get the urine out of the bladder voluntarily. The risk for urinary tract infection (UTI), calculi, and bladder cancer is increased.

In addition to the routine neurologic assessment, assessments based on the individual's deficits and ability to function are needed (Box 13-2).

NEURODIAGNOSTIC AND LABORATORY STUDIES

Neurodiagnostic studies (see Chapter 3) may not be frequently required in the rehabilitation setting. If needed or when the patient has a change in status or deterioration, diagnostic studies can augment the history and physical assessment findings both in the acute care setting and after discharge from the acute care facility:

- Computed tomography (CT): may be employed to rule out or detect hydrocephalus, brain swelling, and chronic or late-onset intracranial hematomas; can detect pressure on the spinal cord and differentiate between infarction and hemorrhage for patients with brain attack or stroke
- Magnetic resonance imaging (MRI): useful in identifying structural brain changes and/or abnormalities (e.g., central nervous system [CNS] infection)
- Electroencephalogram (EEG): provides extensive information regarding brain damage and possible seizure foci
- Chemosensory evaluation: for assessment of changes in smell and taste

BOX 13-2   Expanded Rehabilitation Assessment

- Chief complaint of the functional loss: described in the individual's own words
- Mobility activities: review of the ability, or inability, to safely perform all mobility needs and the use of any assistive devices related to transfer, sit, stand, ambulate, and stairs
- Activities of daily living (ADLs): eat, groom, dress, bathe, personal hygiene and toilet activities, and the use of any assistive devices
- Household activities: review of activities (e.g., shopping, cooking, cleaning, outdoor home maintenance, and laundry)
- Vocational or academic activities: review of return to work/school requirements and performance; return to work or school
- Smoking and substance abuse: review past and current smoking, drinking, and abuse of prescription or illegal drugs and dependency/addiction
- Home/residence: review issues (may include a home/residence visit by health care provider) as to suitability and livability of home/residence, including need for ramps and retrofitting home in compliance with Americans with Disability Guidelines
- Finances: review with social services loss of income and insurance or coverage for health care needs, especially prescription medications
- Relationships and sexuality: review significant other relationships and need for sexual counseling, medications, and other interventions
- Nutrition: review diet and specific nutritional requirements
- Support and resources: review family and other support systems, use of, and accessibility of local support groups and community resources, and transportation needs
- Medication, durable medical equipment (DME), and supplies: review all prescription, over-the-counter, and alternative therapies and use of DME, including inspection for appropriateness, safety, and state of repair; wheelchair and other equipment evaluations may require evaluations by members of the rehabilitation team (e.g., a "seating evaluation" for wheelchair)

- Gait analysis: informal visual analysis or slow-motion video technology and additional analysis using electromyogram (EMG) and other motion analysis measures
- Polysomnography with median sleep latency test: for assessment of sleep disturbance (see Chapter 6)
- Plain radiography: for assessment to determine deviations from normal, including fractures, dislocations, abnormal bone formation, and infections (osteomyelitis, for example)
- Nocturnal penile tumescence monitoring: for assessment of erectile dysfunction (see Chapter 12)
- Posturographic assessment: for assessment of problems with balance
- Electronystagmography: for assessment of vestibular dysfunction

WELLNESS PROMOTION

The primary goals of rehabilitation management are to help patients improve their quality of life, maximize their level of independence, and promote the ability to attain their personal goals. It is important to teach patients and family how to achieve and maintain a high level of wellness while living with a disability. Wellness, as differentiated from "health" or the passive condition of being free of disease, is best understood as a holistic integration of all facets of the patient's life. Far from being a passive state, wellness requires the patient's full participation and motivation to seek growth-producing challenges, to relate to others in positive and flexible ways, to engage in health-enhancing activities, and to incorporate effective coping strategies to integrate all aspects of the patient's life and achieve a sense of wellness. Similarly, health care professionals must develop attitudes whereby they no longer consider the patient as having an illness, but rather as an individual who must live with functional alterations and integrate them into new life patterns.

Achieving a sense of wellness may be an especially difficult challenge for patients with permanent neurologic deficits, since the social, physical, and psychologic dimensions of their lives are often severely disrupted. Their relationships, goals, careers, and physical abilities may all be altered for the rest of their lives, and these patients may need to acquire entirely new problem-solving, self-care, and psychosocial skills. The neuroscience or rehabilitation clinician plays an integral role in patients' adjustment by assisting them in identifying the ways in which the neurologic impairments have affected various aspects of their lives and in integrating these changed dimensions into their lives to achieve a high level of wellness. The focus on developing a sense of wellness must also consider the patient's cultural, religious, and ethnic background, as well as the patient's ability to change and adapt to his or her new state of health.

DISCHARGE PLANNING AND PROGRAM EVALUATION

Rehabilitation following acute care may occur in various settings; the philosophy in each, however, remains the same. Rehabilitation strives to increase a patient's functional capacity and develop a meaningful lifestyle that adjusts to the neurologic disability. Wellness promotion and patient and family teaching are important for lifelong rehabilitation management.

When choosing a rehabilitation center, evaluating the center's program is essential to patient success. The patient and family must select the most appropriate rehabilitation setting. After the rehabilitation referrals, the family is encouraged to visit the site before making the final decision for transfer. Before a rehabilitation institution is selected,

BOX 13-3	Considerations for Selecting a Rehabilitation Facility

- Geographic location: Is it close enough for family visits?
- Funding and finances: Is there adequate coverage for the duration of the projected stay?
- Transportation: Does it require land, air, or specialized transportation?
- Availability of specialty programs: Is there a dedicated team for spinal cord–injured, head-injured, or stroke patients?
- Family support services: Are there open visiting privileges?
- Vocational therapy: Is vocational retraining available?
- Diagnostic population: Does the program serve a significant population that has the same diagnosis as the transferring patient?
- Patient age: Is there a population of the same age-group in the program?
- Medical care: Is medical care and physician consultation available on site or within the area?
- Length of stay: Can a length of stay be projected before admission?
- Accreditation: Is the rehabilitation program accredited by CARF—The Rehabilitation Accreditation Commission?

BOX 13-4	Common Problems in the Rehabilitation Setting

Adjustment to disability	Behavior
Bladder	Cognition
Bowel	Self-care activities
Skin integrity	Sleep disturbance
Mobility	Potential for injury
Communication	Sexuality
Swallowing	Medical
Level of responsiveness	Vocational
Respiratory	Leisure time activities
Nutrition and fluid balance	Home/Architecture
Pain	Barriers to recovery
Visual or perceptual	Discharge planning

consideration should be given to a variety of concerns (Box 13-3).

The patient's disability and medical history ultimately determine the appropriate rehabilitation program. For example, a patient with TBI who is medically stable but requires cognitive retraining would best be served by a program capable of providing cognitive remediation, life skills training, community reintegration, psychologic counseling, and vocational and academic assessment. Another patient may require a rehabilitation program that specializes in coma management. The patient's financial status and funding sources also must be considered in the selection and design of the rehabilitation program. Catastrophic care, such as that which may be required by those with TBI and SCI, usually involves lifelong management and may cost up to $1 million over a lifetime. Expenditures must be deemed appropriate and cost-effective within the parameters of the funding source policy. The patient's financial limits may also affect the level and intensity of rehabilitation services available. Thus the patient's financial ability to follow care guidelines after discharge, as well as third-party payment options, should be considered when the program is designed. Box 13-4 lists common problems an individual may experience during the rehabilitation period.

Patients who will return to the workplace may respond best to a **work hardening rehabilitation program,** a highly specialized rehabilitation program that bridges the gap between traditional therapeutic modalities and the return to work by simulating the workplace in the rehabilitation environment. These programs bolster the patient's self-confidence and physical condition by using the work routine as the mechanism of rehabilitation. Clinicians can be instrumental

in identifying patients seeking a new alternative to the old problems of delayed recovery from neurologic injury.

The struggle to recover physical functions through a rehabilitation program is only the beginning. The patient with a neurologic impairment and resulting disability who is ready to leave the protective hospital environment must be prepared to face weeks or months of continued physical and cognitive rehabilitation and adjustment to returning to his or her home and community. Beginning with assessment, the rehabilitation interventions are key to the patient's outcome as the clinician continues to monitor the patient's progress and assist with beginning the process of lifelong adjustments.

Measures to minimize disability should be incorporated into every aspect of patient care from the moment of injury or illness through community, home, or long-term care (LTC) placement. Indeed, level I trauma centers require rehabilitation as an integrated part of trauma protocol. Such integrated trauma systems identify problems throughout recovery and seek to match appropriate professionals to the patient's specific needs. This chapter focuses on rehabilitation interventions that can be used by clinicians in acute care settings both in minimizing or sometimes preventing disability and in preparing the patient for rehabilitation. A list of options for patients who require rehabilitation after discharge appears in Box 13-5.

BRAIN INJURY REHABILITATION

Brain injury rehabilitation should begin in the ICU with simple nursing measures (e.g., passive ROM, frequent turning and repositioning to prevent complications of immobility). After stabilization, postacute rehabilitation continues comprehensive treatment for what may be a long course of recovery. **Brain injury rehabilitation** for patients with acute brain injury requires attention to a wide range of changes that includes not just physical recovery. Rehabilitation should not neglect cognitive, social, emotional, and behavioral complications of the injury and their effects on recovery and the family unit (see Chapter 11). Deficits, strengths, and needs are evaluated for an outcome-based plan of care. Of the many

Rehabilitation Options

- Acute hospital (rehabilitation unit)
- Acute rehabilitation hospital
- Independent rehabilitation center
- Comprehensive outpatient rehabilitation facility (CORF)
- Home rehabilitation with visiting therapists
- Extended/step-down rehabilitation
- Work tolerance rehabilitation program
- Transitional program
- Subacute rehabilitation or skilled nursing facility (SNF)
- Group home living
- Supervised living (apartment, community home)
- Respite care
- Behavior program
- Summer camp
- Community center
- School program/intermediate unit
- Vocational facility
- Health club/sports fitness center
- Residential treatment facility

patients who survive TBI each year, many experience moderate to severe neurobehavioral and physical sequelae, although the long-term responses to injury are highly individualized and often difficult to anticipate exactly. It is estimated that 20% of people who experience a brain injury incur long-term disability[26] and that there are 5.3 million Americans living with TBI-related disability.[46]

The recovery of brain-injured patients is influenced by many disparate factors, including the site of injury, extent of neurologic damage, complications and associated or secondary injuries, patient age, premorbid level of function and physical ability, and medical risk factors. Musculoskeletal problems occur from immobility and disuse atrophy (Table 13-1).

Acute and Postacute Care

Assessment

A neurologic assessment (see Chapter 2) and other evaluation tools may be included in the rehabilitation assessment

TABLE 13-1 | **Problems Associated With Injury of the Musculoskeletal System**

Problem	Description	Clinical Considerations
Muscle atrophy	Decreased muscle mass normally occurs as a result of disuse following prolonged immobilization.	An isometric muscle-strengthening exercise regimen within the confines of the immobilization device assists in reducing the amount of atrophy. Muscle atrophy interferes with and prolongs the rehabilitation process.
Contracture	Abnormal condition of joint characterized by flexion and fixation. Caused by atrophy and shortening of muscle fibers or by loss of normal elasticity of skin over a joint. Related to improper support and positioning of a joint.	This condition can be prevented by frequent position change, correct body alignment, and active-passive range-of-motion exercises several times a day. Contracture of a joint immobilized for a long time with a cast is common. Intervention requires gradual and progressive stretching of the muscles or ligaments in the region of the joint.
Footdrop	Plantar-flexed position of the foot (footdrop) occurs when the Achilles tendon in the ankle shortens because it has been allowed to assume an unsupported position. This may signify damage to the peroneal nerve.	Nursing management of the patient with long-term injuries must include preventive measures by supporting the foot in a neutral position. Once footdrop has developed, ambulation and gait training may be significantly hindered.
Pain	Frequently associated with fractures, edema, and muscle spasm; pain varies in intensity from mild to severe and is usually described as aching, dull, burning, throbbing, sharp, or deep. Acute versus chronic pain should be assessed.	Important causal factors of pain include incorrect positioning and alignment of the extremity, incorrect support of the extremity, sudden movement of the extremity, an immobilization device that is applied too tightly or in an incorrect position, constrictive dressings, motion occurring at the fracture site, and psychosocial factors. Pain is a valuable assessment parameter, and the underlying causes should be determined so that corrective nursing action can be taken before analgesics are administered.
Muscle spasms	Caused by involuntary muscle contraction after fracture, but not limited to fracture, and may last as long as several weeks. Pain associated with muscle spasms is often intense. The duration varies from several seconds to several minutes.	Nursing measures to reduce the intensity of the muscle spasms are similar to the corrective actions for pain control. The area involved in muscle spasms should not be massaged. Thermotherapy, especially heat, may reduce muscle spasm.

From Lewis SM, Heitkemper MM, Dirksen SF: *Medical-surgical nursing: assessment and management of clinical problems*, ed 5, St Louis, 2000, Mosby.

(e.g., the Glasgow Coma Scale, the Glasgow Outcome Score, and the Rancho Los Amigos Scale, or FOUR score). The Glasgow Coma Scale (GCS) (see Chapter 2) is performed for a quick numerical assessment of the degree of conscious impairment for patients with head injury. It measures eye opening, verbal response, and motor response, and the score ranges from 3 to 15. A GCS score of 3 is considered comatose and may be compatible with brain death. A GCS score of 15 is awake and fully alert with no impairment. The GCS has some prediction for duration or outcome of coma. In the face of a sudden decline in the GCS or FOUR score (see Chapter 6), the scores can be used as an indicator for diagnostic test (e.g., an emergency CT scan), the need for intubation and mechanical ventilation, or the need for intracranial pressure monitoring.

The Glasgow Outcome Score (GOS) is commonly used as a functional assessment inventory to measure outcome from head injury. It has five global categories: (1) death; (2) persistent vegetative state with absence of cortical function; (3) severe disability, conscious but disabled; (4) moderate disability, disabled but independent; and (5) good recovery with resumption of "normal life." Many studies group the various levels into poor outcome (GOS 1 to 3) or good outcome (GOS 4 to 5).[1]

The Rancho Los Amigos Scale is a scale of cognitive functioning (see Chapter 6) developed as a behavioral rating scale used in the assessment and treatment of patients with head injury. A scale ranges from I (no response) to VIII (purposeful/appropriate) up to X (postacute, stable, and can handle multiple tasks). In the acute phase, the Rancho scale is used on admission to categorize a patient's status as a benchmark and for comparison during admission to measure cognitive improvement. At the time of discharge, the patient's Rancho level may determine placement and the level of care required. Patients admitted for rehabilitation may have a Rancho as low as II to III. To begin rehabilitation, a patient with a Rancho of I should demonstrate some level of arousal and awareness to begin the rehabilitation process.

In addition to these assessments tools, it is generally accepted that preinjury conditions, age, gender, the severity of the brain injury, secondary complications, and other influences during the acute phases of recovery will influence the rehabilitative treatment and recovery. The clinical assessment includes the following:
- Past medical and surgical history, family history, social history
- Functional history
- Vital signs
- Review of systems: cardiovascular, neurosensory, gastrointestinal (GI), genitourinary (GU), musculoskeletal, endocrine, pulmonary, hematologic, psychiatric, ears/nose/throat/mouth
- Cognitive level: orientation, memory judgment, impulsiveness
- Motor evaluation: upper and lower strength, balance, and gait
- Functional mobility
- Activity level, transfers, ambulation
- Pain flow sheet with pain score, location, duration

- Complete the FIM flow sheet
- Medications
- Allergies
- Bladder: continent, incontinent, incontinent device in place (catheter)
- Bowel: continent, incontinent, suppositories, enema, frequency of accidents
- Self-care evaluation and training
- Strength and energy conservation
- Adaptive equipment, assistive devices, orthotics
- Dietary, nutrition, and fluids
- Safety and mobility issues, need for restraints
- Fall risk
- Skin inspection, wound inspection: location and description to include diameter and depth, drainage, odor, Pressure Ulcer Stage
- Community living skills
- Laboratory and other diagnostic study results
- Social interactions
- Patient and family education

After completing the admission baseline assessment, patient goals are discussed to establish an individualized plan of care. Current medications are reviewed. The patient is further evaluated as to the need for physical restraints, more vigilant observation, 1:1 care, or family members staying with the patient secondary to poor insight, safety awareness, and lack of judgment for safety and risk of injury. The patient's functional status is recorded, the need for counseling evaluated, wound care determined, and a bowel and bladder program initiated as needed. The nursing assessment is integrated into the multidisciplinary team's comprehensive care plan and implemented with regular communications verbally or through progress notes in the patient's medical record.

Complications Associated With Brain Injury

The following areas of functioning can be impaired after brain injury and should be closely monitored:
- Motor and sensory
- Language and communication
- Visual-perceptual
- Attention
- Memory
- Executive functions
- Personality and emotions

Hydrocephalus is a pathologic condition marked by dilation of the cerebral ventricles, most often occurring secondary to obstruction of the cerebrospinal fluid (CSF) pathways inside or outside the brain and accompanied by an abnormal accumulation of CSF within the ventricles or subarachnoid spaces of the brain—the fluid often being under increased pressure. Hydrocephalus appears to affect the long-term neuromedical status of individuals with TBI.[50] Hydrocephalus is one of the most common treatable complications during rehabilitation of patients with TBI. Symptoms may include lethargy, incontinence, changes in behavior, or ataxia. **Obstructive (noncommunicating) hydrocephalus** occurs when the flow of CSF is blocked within the brain along one of the internal pathways between the ventricles, or at the exits from the brain. **Communicating hydrocephalus** occurs when the external CSF pathways are blocked or, more commonly, when there is failure of CSF absorption that results in enlargement of the ventricles. Hydrocephalus can be surgically managed with an external shunt or shunt placement (see Chapter 8).

Normal pressure hydrocephalus (NPH) is classified as an acquired communicating hydrocephalus. In its most common form, or **idiopathic normal pressure hydrocephalus (iNPH),** it is seen among older adults and is thought to be related to a failure of CSF to be properly absorbed.[24] Whether or not intracranial pressure (ICP) is truly normal remains controversial. The assessment begins with a history, date, and description of the precipitating event: subarachnoid hemorrhage (SAH), TBI, CNS infection, or a brain tumor. Box 13-6 lists NPH assessment guidelines.

The classic triad of symptoms is as follows: (1) gait disturbance may occur first that may be wide based, short stepped, slow, or shuffling; (2) dementia typically includes short-term memory loss; and (3) urinary incontinence may include nocturia, urgency, or frequency. In its idiopathic form, NPH is typically a chronic, progressive disorder in adults older than age 60 and is characterized by a general slowing of the thought process, as well as mobility. A copy of the seven-page *NPH Questionnaire* developed by

---

BOX 13-6	**Assessment for Normal Pressure Hydrocephalus (NPH)**

- History of precipitating event: SAH, TBI, CNS infection
- Ambulation: problems with gait (early sign), imbalance; ambulation: wide-based gait, difficulty turning, short length of stride; "magnetic gait" or forgetting how to take a step or even stand; ask the patient to walk in a straight line (count steps), turn, and walk back; may repeat for three trials for comparison
- Urinary: incontinence (late sign), urgency, not making it to the bathroom in time, soiling themselves without notice (much later sign), UTIs
- Memory: trouble remembering, problems with recent memory, long-term memory, mini mental status examination
- Cognition: trouble thinking normally, decline in problem-solving skills, difficulty with word-finding
- Attention: problems with attention, understanding, loss of interest in activities
- Personality changes
- Changes in eating habits, reduced oral intake
- Inability to perform or unsafe in performing mechanical activities
- Loss of driving privileges or recent changes in driving
- Medications
- Neuropsychologist consultation: neuropsychologic testing if needed
- Urology consultation: referral for urodynamic studies if needed

See Resources for the author's *NPH Questionnaire.*
CNS, Central nervous system; *SAH,* subarachnoid hemorrhage; *TBI,* traumatic brain injury; *UTI,* urinary tract infection.

---

the author can be accessed at www.aesculapusa.com (see Resources).

NPH may result over weeks or months from scarring of the basal cistern following TBI with ventricular enlargement and brain compression with normal or abnormal CSF pressure. A lack of clinical indicators may include headache or papilledema. Even though there may be an enlargement of ventricles, a normal opening pressure after a lumber puncture (LP) is possible. A tap test may be performed in which 50 to 200 ml of CSF is drained to evaluate the clinical response. Other diagnostic studies may be needed to confirm NPH. Early diagnosis includes assessment of the triad of symptoms, comprehensive neurologic assessment, and a documented mini mental status examination. In addition, other studies (e.g., functional brain imaging, CT/MRI imaging, neurologic testing, urodynamic studies, or EEG) will exclude other disorders. Early treatment will improve outcome. A 45- to 60-minute ventricular shunting under general anesthesia is the accepted intervention in most cases. A variety of programmable and nonprogrammable valves have been developed to specifically address the needs of NPH patients and to minimize the risk of overdrainage, including catheters impregnated with antibiotics to reduce shunt infection (Fig. 13-2). The gravity-assisted valve (GAV) allows for prompt switching function as soon as the individual changes position from lying down to sitting. Following surgery, patients may be discharged in 1 to 2 days and mobilized with a short stay in a rehabilitation facility to prepare for home and an improved quality of life.

Chiari malformations (CMs) include a complex group of disorders that are characterized by herniation of the cerebellum through the foramen magnum into the spinal canal. The herniated tissue blocks the circulation of CSF in the brain and can lead to a formation of a syrinx or cavity within the spinal cord. CM is classified into three types, according to severity, with CM I being the most prevalent form when the cerebellar tonsils prolapse into the spinal canal without elongation of the brainstem. Hydrocephalus and syringomyelia are Chiari-related disorders related to CSF disturbances.[28] A **syringomyelia** is a tubular cavity called a syrinx that develops within the spinal cord, caused by obstruction of the CSF circulatory pathways. Approximately 80% of cases are a result of a Chiari malformation. There may be a genetic component. The American Syringomyelia Alliance Project (ASAP) has developed a questionnaire to elicit information regarding the familial incidence of CM I (see ASAP Web site under Resources). TBI from a whiplash, or a direct blow to the head, may be the precipitating event that is followed by a marginally compensated CSF flow that causes destabilization in individuals with a congenital CM I.[28]

The patient may give a positive family history that suggests a genetic component for transmission of CM. The past medical history may include Chiari-related headaches, ocular symptoms, dizziness, vestibular dysfunction, hearing loss, and other symptoms that were previously explained as psychogenic. A comprehensive neurologic evaluation and imaging of the brain with MRI, CINE-MRI, and other diagnostic studies will determine treatment options. On the basis of the diagnostic findings, an operative technique for CMI

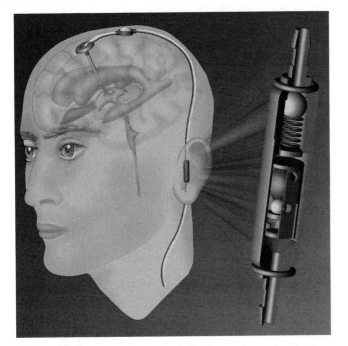

Figure 13-2 The new Aesculap Miethke gravity-assisted valve (GAV) is a combination of a ball-cone valve and a gravitational valve. The ball-cone valve, set to a low opening pressure, keeps the individual's intraventricular pressure (IVP) within physiologic limits, always keeping the gravitational valve open in the horizontal position. When the individual rises, the gravitational valve is activated automatically, because both balls in the valve drop as soon as the posture of the patient departs by more than 30 to 40 degrees from the horizontal position. Because of the prompt switching function as soon as the individual changes his or her position from lying down to standing up, the GAV may be suitable for NPH.
(Used with permission from Hydrocephalus Management Systems, Center Valley, PA.)

for posterior fossa decompression to reestablish optimal CSF is tailored to patient-specific variables.[28]

Seizures are a hyperexcitation of neurons in the brain leading to a sudden involuntary series of contractions of a group of muscles (see Chapter 24). They are classified by whether they appear to start from a localized cortical region or from the entire brain at once. Following brain injury, seizures should be considered when episodes of discrete and stereotypic behaviors occur with altered or lost consciousness. Approximately 5% of patients with TBI eventually experience a **late-onset seizure disorder** up to 4 years after injury, and another 5% experience **posttraumatic epilepsy** during the acute phase after injury.[49] After a thorough assessment and diagnostic evaluation, the treatment modality of choice for most TBI patients with seizure activity is pharmacologic management (see Chapter 24). Status epilepticus is a rare but significant complication that may accompany seizure activity in individuals with TBI. Status epilepticus increases the morbidity and mortality rates associated with TBI. The severity of the brain injury best predicts whether posttraumatic epilepsy will occur. Other risk factors include genetic susceptibility to epilepsy, duration of coma, and age,

with older patients at higher risk.[21] An EEG is a useful diagnostic tool, but a normal EEG does not exclude the possibility of epilepsy. Initiation of antiepileptic drug (AED) therapy should begin only after careful evaluation of the patient and seizures have been clearly identified. Almost all clinicians will begin therapy once two seizures have occurred, but there is debate on whether therapy should be initiated after the first seizure. In general, after head injury, all AEDs should be introduced slowly to avoid problems with neurotoxicity, including somnolence and altered mental status.[21]

Heterotopic ossification (HO) is a frequent musculoskeletal condition that has been associated as a complication of TBI and other neurologic conditions, including SCI and stroke. HO involves osteoblastic activity and an abnormal deposition of new bone formation in soft tissues at abnormal sites of paralyzed limbs, such as large joints. The osteoporotic changes of HO are a common complication in brain-injured patients with decrease in bone density that may result from the initial injury, prolonged immobilization, and comatose states. HO has been described as true osseous tissue rather than calcified soft tissue. Several months after TBI, patients may initially experience limited joint motion and pain. Other symptoms follow (e.g., joint swelling, decreasing ROM, pain associated with ROM, heat, and an increase in spasticity) and increasing pain in joints (e.g., shoulders, elbows, hips, and knees).

> **ALERT:** An increase in pain, spasticity, or muscle guarding should alert the examiner to the impending onset of HO.[20]

Patients older than 30 years of age and who have spasticity may be at higher risk. Confirmation is by erythrocyte sedimentation rate (ESR), elevated levels of serum alkaline phosphatase (SAP), radionuclide bore imaging (RNBI), or the "three phase" bone scan. It may be necessary to rule out other problems (e.g., thrombophlebitis, septic arthritis, trauma, hematoma, or even a fracture) before initiating treatment. A patient with minimal HO may not require therapy. Others may require physical therapy, medications, manipulation, or in severe cases surgical excision. Preventive treatment to decrease new bone development has been recommended in some cases and consists of etidronate (Didronel) 20 mg/kg taken orally each day for 2 weeks, followed by 10 mg/kg per day for 10 weeks for a total of up to 6 months.

> **ALERT:** Etidronate should not be given for more than 6 months because prolonged treatment at this dosage can cause osteoporosis and fractures may occur.[20]

In addition to etidronate, medical treatment may include nonsteroidal antiinflammatory drugs (NSAIDs) such as indomethacin (Indocin), physical modalities (e.g., ROM), and in severe cases surgery or radiation to arrest further HO. Selected TBI patients with spasticity have reported benefits from forceful manipulation under anesthesia to maintain or increase motion.

Nutritional deficits may result from decreased intake and swallowing disorders. The metabolic response to head injury is characterized by increased metabolism and catabolism. It has been estimated that resting energy expenditure following brain injury can increase up to 40%. After admission for rehabilitation, most patients will benefit from aggressive nutritional management. Inadequate nutrition creates problems of malnutrition, muscle weakness, skin problems, fatigue, and other problems in patients with TBI. Patients may have special nutritional needs if the injury produced severe increases in basal metabolism, resulting in weight loss, low serum albumin levels, and a negative nitrogen balance. A deficit in olfaction is not uncommon following brain injury and affects appetite. Weight should be closely monitored and skin thickness (anthropometry) measured. Routine laboratory studies to evaluate nutritional status may include serum albumin, total protein, total lymphocyte count, transferrin, and thyroxin-binding prealbumin.

Brain damage with impaired cognition and the impaired swallowing process may result in **dysphagia** (a swallowing disorder that interferes with oral feeding). The incidence of dysphagia in patients with TBI at the time of transfer to rehabilitation is about 27%.[13] Individuals with a right-hemispheric lesion may be more likely to have a deficit in the pharyngeal phase of swallowing. A swallowing evaluation by a speech pathologist or dysphagia specialist helps determine a plan of care to address the potential for aspiration, and the need for a safe nutritional program to ensure adequate protein and caloric intake to reach nutrition goals. **Videofluoroscopy** is the standard test for evaluation to determine the exact swallowing dysfunction. The use of a jejunostomy for continuous nutritional tube feedings in the acute setting may be switched to gastrostomy on admission to rehabilitation for bolus feedings depending on the patient's aspiration risk.

Impaired Physical Mobility

Orthopedic and related injuries (e.g., long-bone fractures, joint dislocations, fractures to the pelvic girdle, soft tissue injuries, and vertebral fractures) are prevalent with acute brain injury. Interventions include limited periods of traction, external fixation devices, open reduction with internal fixation (ORIF), serial casting (Fig. 13-3), splints, and various orthotics. It is critical to identify orthopedic impairments and provide appropriate intervention.

To prevent **pressure ulcers,** the clinician should assess the patient's response to ROM and observe the skin for redness, edema, and physiologic responses (temperature elevation, diaphoresis as a response to pain, or autonomic dysfunction). Frequent repositioning and avoidance of positions that increase tone are important interventions. Immobility, dehydration, incontinence, advanced age, spasticity, and poor nutrition are risk factors for pressure ulcers. Interventions for prevention include a prescribed and documented turning schedule, assessment using the Braden Scale (www.bradenscale.com), or other tools and consultation with therapists for assistive and protective devices. At the earliest sign of breakdown, consultation with a wound specialist and aggressive treatment for wound closure are needed. Treatment may include pressure-relieving mattress covers, special beds, and dressings. If those interventions are not effective, enzymatic, mechanical, and surgical debridement in combination with good medical and clinical care optimize recovery. Surgical repair with skin grafts or musculocutaneous flaps is needed to promote deep soft tissue healing.

Pain management is essential and is covered in Chapter 23.

Spasticity or spastic hypertonia is a motor disorder characterized by a velocity-dependent increase in muscle tone with exaggerated tendon jerks resulting in hyperexcitability of stretch reflex. This is often referred to as part of an upper motor neuron syndrome seen in brain injury. Spasticity leads to an involuntary rhythmic contraction of the part in response to a relatively quick movement.[51] Spasticity following brain injury is similar to spasticity with stroke but often very different from that of SCI. Cerebral origin spasticity characteristically causes greater extensor tone in the

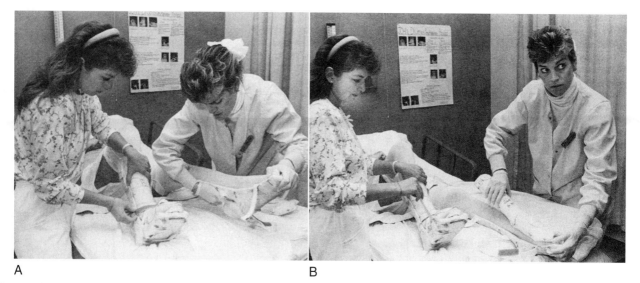

A   B

Figure 13-3 Application of serial casts for contractures. *(Courtesy Bryn Mawr Rehabilitation Hospital, Malvern, PA.)*

BOX 13-7	Assessment for Spasticity

- Pain, or painful muscle spasms
- Passive ROM may reveal increased muscle tone with increased resistance to stretching
- Abnormal posturing patterns with severe extension or flexion, deformities, or contractures
- Swelling or tenderness of involved extremities
- Grading of reflexes demonstrates hyperexcitable reflexes or clonus
- Interferes with functional limb control
- Interferes with or prevents ambulation, transferring in and out of bed, sitting in a wheelchair
- Interferes with performance of ADLs
- Monitor for noxious stimuli that trigger spasticity (e.g., UTI, pressure ulcers)
- Interferes with caregiving, positioning, or bathing, or close approximation of thighs prevents personal care
- Babinski response with up-going toes
- Recent slips, trips, falls, or fractures related to spasticity
- Increased caregiver time for bathing, dressing, transferring in and out of bed
- Totally confined to bed related to spasticity
- Record the progression and level of spasticity based on tools, such as the modified Ashworth, or other scales

ADLs, Activities of daily living; *ROM,* range of motion; *UTI,* urinary tract infection.

BOX 13-8	Modified Ashworth Scale

0	No increase in muscle tone
1	Slight increase in tone (catch and release at end of the ROM)
1+	Slight increase in tone, manifested by a catch, followed by minimal resistance throughout remainder (less than half of the ROM)
2	More marked increase in muscle tone through most of ROM, but affected part(s) easily moved
3	Considerable increase in tone; passive movement difficult
4	Affected part(s) fixed in flexion and extension

From Bohannon RW, Smith MB: Interrater reliability of a modified Ashworth scale of muscle spasticity, *Phys Ther* 76:206–207, 1987. *ROM,* Range of motion.

lower extremities and a lesser tendency to "spasms."[13] Spasticity may include an upper motor neuron (UMN) lesion. The neurologic evaluation, spasticity assessment (Box 13-7), gait analysis, balance, and modified Ashworth scores (Box 13-8) may identify loss of limb control with specific muscles affected that results in motor dysfunction, muscle stiffness, contractures, and spasticity. See Appendix D: Spasticity Questionnaire for a comprehensive evaluation for long-term management for individuals with spasticity.

Spasticity has positive and negative qualities. Patients may use the increased muscle tone of spasticity to assist with weight bearing, for transfers or taking a few steps. The increased muscle tone may improve muscle bulk or may help prevent DVTs by increasing venous return. Spasticity with excessive tone may increase muscle fatigue, reduce dexterity, interfere with sleep, or interfere with ambulation by producing a plantar-flexed foot that makes ambulation impossible. The goal is to achieve an adequate balance. Treatment should begin when the spasticity has progressed to a level that it is beginning to interfere with the individual's function with negative consequences: creating safety risk, causing pain/discomfort, or increasing caregiver burden.[9]

Assessment may reveal the progression of spasticity and determine the current level. Review diagnostic studies (e.g., EMG, dynamic EMG, or x-ray findings) to rule out missed fractures or HO. EMG results may indicate the need for nerve blocks or other treatments.

Treatment should begin when the spasticity has progressed to the level where it is beginning to interfere with the individual's function with negative consequences, creates a safety risk, causes pain/discomfort, interferes with sleep, and increases caregiver burden. Working as a team, the rehabilitation physician will prescribe a program of spasticity-preventing measures with realistic functional goals to decrease spasticity, improve strength, and improve mobility and ambulation. Cosmetic goals for management include better alignment and positioning, or decreasing or preventing contractures. Caregiver goals may include helping to improve self-hygiene or decrease caregiver time, improve sleep, and decrease complications.

Early treatment with conservative management is often a combination of many therapies and may begin with therapeutic exercises or massage, ROM, a muscle stretching program once or twice a day, cold/heat application, aquatic therapy, continence management, appropriate positioning, frequent turning, and consultation with physical and occupational therapy to evaluate for orthotics, splinting, bracing, a **transcutaneous electrical nerve stimulation (TENS) unit,** or casts with serial casting. **Serial casting** (using progressive bivalved casts to gradually increase extension or flexion of an extremity by inhibiting spasticity) may also be effective. A patient could have serial casts on all four extremities. Clinicians must monitor for weight changes or skin conditions that would influence the comfort and fitting of the cast (e.g., impaired sensation and circulation, and skin irritation). Temperature elevation, pulse changes, diaphoresis, pain, and agitation are frequent patient symptoms as a result of casting. On-off cast application schedules must be followed for therapeutic effectiveness (see Fig. 13-3).

Potential modalities to consider include effective pain management and antispasticity medications (e.g., baclofen) (Table 13-2). A 24-hour schedule should be implemented that balances rest therapy with active physical exercise. When the patient establishes and reaches rehabilitation goals, it is rewarding not only for the patient but also for the caregivers. Positive reinforcement with praise and encouragement for each goal achieved can be extremely motivating for the patient.

With severe spasticity that interferes with function and ADLs or caregiver health care, or if there are intolerable side effects from oral therapy, other options are available.

TABLE 13-2	Pharmacologic Options for Spasticity Management	
Drug	**Daily Dosage Range**	**Side Effects**
Baclofen*	5–80 mg/day but individual patients have required larger doses without adverse side effects	Sedation Withdrawal effect
Tizanidine	2–36 mg	Fatigue Dry mouth Sedation Elevated LFTs
Dantrium	25–400 mg	Elevated LFTs Weakness
Diazepam	5–40 mg	Sedation Tolerance Cognitive dysfunction
Gabapentin	100–4000 mg	Sedation Fatigue Ataxia Dizziness
Clonidine	0.1–0.6 mg	Orthostatic hypotension

*Intrathecal form available.
LFTs, Liver function tests.

Botulinum toxin A (Botox) injections that selectively target only specific limbs or muscle groups can be injected without anesthesia. Although Botox is lethal when ingested orally, it is safe to use as an injection into the selected muscles to block the release of acetylcholine, the substance necessary for muscular contraction. This chemical denervation lasts about 3 to 4 months. Botox injections often work best when combined with other therapeutic treatments because the patient will discover uncovered muscle weakness when the spasticity has been removed. Botox can produce neutralizing antibodies and become ineffective over time.

When other therapeutic interventions fail and the individual becomes intolerant of oral therapies, intrathecal (IT) drug delivery with baclofen with an implantable programmable pump surgically placed may be recommended for severe spasticity. **Baclofen** is a skeletal muscle relaxant that inhibits transmission of reflexes at the spinal cord level. **Intrathecal baclofen (ITB) therapy** is a muscle relaxant and antispastic in a sterile isotonic-free solution. ITB therapy delivers a precise dose of preservative-free baclofen into the CSF around the spinal cord. The pump can be programmed to provide various bolus doses or a constant infusion rate during the 24-hour period. The precise mechanism of action is not fully understood. The intrathecal or subarachnoid space contains CSF. Intrathecal baclofen is delivered via the pump and catheter directly to the CSF surrounding the spinal cord for effective CSF concentrations, with plasma concentrations dramatically less than those occurring with oral administration. The much smaller dose minimizes potential side effects versus large oral amounts of baclofen. ITB therapy delivers a continuous and precise dosage with a flexibility rate that can be programmed to the lifestyle of the individual. For example,

a 20% increase of baclofen can be delivered 2 hours before bedtime to ensure restful sleep and programmed to deliver the daytime dose 2 hours before waking.

Indications for ITB therapy are individuals with severe spasticity of spinal origin who are unresponsive to oral baclofen, who experience unacceptable side effects at effective doses of oral baclofen, who experience spasticity or contractures that affect quality of life (e.g., decreased ambulation or immobility), or increased caregiver burden that interferes with providing personal hygiene and ease of care. Assessment includes a history and review of oral medications; an examination that includes the patient's spasticity, clonus, muscle strength, pain level, and seizure activity; psychosocial considerations; family support system; and patient motivation to comply with long-term ITB therapy. The OT and the PT may assist in evaluating orthotics and equipment such as a walker or wheelchair, functional status, and overall goals of therapy.

Patients are admitted as outpatients or short-stay inpatients to the hospital for a standard screening test via an LP administered to selected patients to determine eligibility for long-term ITB therapy. Following administration of the bolus test dose, the patient is closely monitored for one-half hour, 4 hours, and 4 to 8 hours after the bolus for strength and muscle tone and a reduction in spasticity to see if ITB therapy may be beneficial. ROM, the modified Ashworth scale (see Box 13-8), the spasm scale, the Tardieu scale, video taping, or other screening tools may be used by therapists to distinguish spasticity and tone from strength because spasticity can mask muscle weakness. A positive test response consists of a significant decrease in muscle tone or frequency or severity of spasms, and the patient is scheduled for surgical pump implantation.

Patients are admitted for the 1- to 3-hour procedure performed by neurosurgery under general anesthesia. The pump and catheter are surgically placed with the pump placed under the skin, usually on the patient's lower abdomen. A needle is inserted into the intrathecal space below the spinal cord, usually L2 or L3, and the catheter is advanced to about the T10 or T11 level and then connected to the programmable pump. Initially the patient may appear weaker because the spasticity is significantly reduced. After a brief hospital stay the patient may be admitted to rehabilitation for several days of occupational therapy, speech therapy, and physical therapy for therapeutic exercise, strengthening, functional electrical stimulation, mobility and ambulatory gait training, and functional training in ADLs, to prevent falls and improve balance and posture to increase independence. Reassessment for adaptive equipment may show that a wheelchair is no longer needed or that a walker is more appropriate.

ITB therapy provides effective long-term treatment of spasticity of cerebral origin, and its effects do not appear to diminish with time. The therapy is frequently associated with adverse side effects that usually can be alleviated by adjustments in dosage.[3,33] The goal of long-term ITB therapy is to maintain muscle tone as close as possible to normal and to decrease the frequency and severity of spasms and to alleviate without inducing intolerable side effects. Long-term follow-up with a health care provider for dose titration and scheduled baclofen pump refills helps achieve the minimal dose to relieve spasticity and allow the best quality of life. ITB therapy has safeguards with alarms signaling when to refill and for battery replacement. Patient and family teaching emphasizes dosing schedule, pump replacement, and potential complications.

Self-Care Deficit

Patients with posttraumatic brain injury (PTBI) exhibit impairment in self-care activities because of cognitive, motor, and behavioral impairments interfering with their ability to perform ADLs. Very basic activities may require numerous rehabilitation team referrals to address appropriate skills and provide the necessary assistive devices. A structured environment adapted to the patient, both physically and cognitively, helps the patient successfully perform most self-care activities. The patient's specific areas of cognitive impairment necessitate an individualized nursing care plan for ADLs.

Risk for Injury

To prevent injury from behavioral impairments that commonly occur after brain injury, the clinician must be prepared for agitated behavior by the patient. The Rancho Los Amigos Scale of Cognitive Functioning is used to evaluate the patient with TBI (see Chapter 6). This tool is commonly used during inpatient and outpatient rehabilitation and is used to evaluate neurobehavioral functioning for individuals with brain injury at any stage of recovery. The patient's level is documented to record the sequence of recovery and provide the rationale for interventions for each stage of recovery, as well as evaluation of the treatment modalities and plan of care.

Agitation is a behavioral change or state of heightened activity, restlessness, or increased psychomotor activity that can be sudden and unpredictable. Patients at level IV on the Rancho Los Amigos Scale are typical of the patient who displays a heightened state of activity. The clinician, nonetheless, must ensure the safety of the patient, other patients, personnel, family members, and other visitors (see Chapter 6). It is important to identify and remove noxious stimuli and rule out seizure activity, withdrawal from substance abuse, or other potential causes.

The interdisciplinary rehabilitation team chooses the appropriate interventions. The patient's clinical status must first be assessed, and then management focuses on controlling the head-injured patient's environment. Specific interventions include removing the source of agitation, if possible, and performing various tests before making the diagnosis of agitation (Box 13-9). Treatment may include medications, behavioral strategies, and environmental management.[13] The most frequently prescribed medications include pain medications, if pain is the source of agitation, and the following: carbamazepine (Tegretol), tricyclic antidepressants (nortriptyline [Pamelor]), trazodone (Desyrel), amantadine (Symmetrel), and beta-blockers (propranolol [Inderal]).[13]

A protective environment with padding on the floor and walls using the Craig bed allows the patient freedom of movement. Seat restraints are added to wheelchairs as appropriate. A unit or room, also padded, where the patient can stay during an episode of agitation, is secured. (This should

BOX 13-9	Suggested Tests for the Evaluation of the Confused and Agitated Patient

- Serum electrolytes
- Blood urea nitrogen (BUN), serum creatinine
- Glucose, calcium, magnesium, and liver enzymes
- Thyroid function
- Complete blood count (CBC) with differential
- Urinalysis
- Serum B_{12} and folate levels
- Drug and alcohol screen
- Brain CT or MRI
- EEG
- Plain radiograph (to evaluate for occult fractures or heterotopic ossification causing pain)

From Boake C, Francises GE, Ivanhoe CB, Kathani S: Brain injury rehabilitation. In Braddom RL, editor: *Physical medicine and rehabilitation*, ed 2, Philadelphia, 2000, WB Saunders. *CT*, Computed tomography; *EEG*, electroencephalogram; *MRI*, magnetic resonance imaging.

be separate from the patient's room so that the two rooms are not associated.) A Craig bed allows the patient to move in bed and sit up and prevents falling or getting out of bed (Fig. 13-4). Physical restraints are used with caution and with the least amount of restriction required for the patient's safety (e.g., mitted gloves are preferable to securing the patient's arms to the bed). Because restraints may pose a physical risk to the patient, minimal-restraint or restraint-free environments are advocated. Having a family member or sitter stay with the patient has a calming effect. Medication is used only as necessary, and those agents that have associated side effects that suppress cognitive function are avoided. The clinical staff should also formulate a plan of action that will minimize stimuli in anticipation of an episode of agitation, such as performing in-room or in-unit therapy to avoid moving the patient when possible. Therapeutic touch, massage, or music therapy may reduce agitation. Some patients respond better to a Geri chair, Q Foam International Chair, or Planet Chairs (shaped like a disk, hard to get out of, and therefore good for an impulsive patient). Other options include moving the individual near the nursing station for closer observation, and in some cases consultation with psychiatry for assistance with management of medications.

An individualized assessment is needed to determine the most effective and safest method to reduce agitation. Daily documentation is essential and required by the Joint Commission on Accreditation of Healthcare Organizations (JCAHO).

At discharge, the GOS is used as an indicator of outcome in TBI. One study found that the baseline GOS was a reliable predictor of outcome in patients with an initial score of 5 (no disability) or 4 (mild disability), but not in patients with an initial score of 3 (severe disability). Patients who remained unconscious for more than 24 hours did not have significantly lower outcomes than those who experienced loss of consciousness for less than 24 hours at 15 months after injury. The authors concluded that the duration of unconsciousness did not affect the likelihood of an improved score

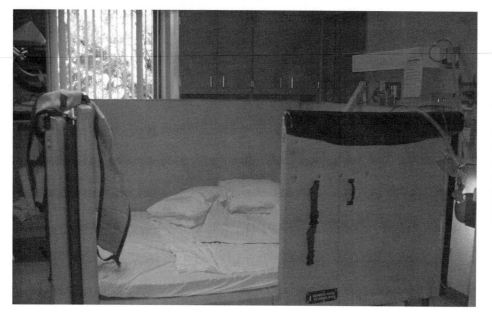

Figure 13-4 Craig bed. Agitated or nonambulatory patients may often benefit from the use of a bed on the floor (or slightly elevated) that eliminates the need for restraints. A panel opens to allow the clinician to provide case. *(Courtesy Craig Hospital, Englewood, CO.)*

during the study period in patients with a baseline GOS of 3 to 4.[29]

Advancing age is known to be a determinant of outcome in brain injury. As the brain ages, it is thought to undergo a variety of changes. Outcomes in older adults include a higher percentage of death, vegetative state, and moderate or severe disability, or no recovery.[48] Recovery from brain injury was studied in an outpatient rehabilitation program; the study found that older patients who survive have a greater likelihood of becoming physically and financially dependent on others. The authors recommend that rehabilitation should focus on maximizing levels of independence to limit financial and emotional costs to patients and their families.[45]

To establish long-term mortality rates for individuals after TBI, researchers analyzed records of patients from one large rehabilitation hospital. Their data constituted evidence for premature death in the postacute TBI population following a moderate to severe head injury.[37]

In addition to the modalities described, rehabilitation facilities may offer vocational and educational services, community reentry programs, recreational activities, and ongoing support groups. It is beyond the scope of this chapter to review these programs, and the reader is referred to other texts for details. The brain may lose up to 5% to 10% of its weight beginning during an individual's twenties. Lifestyle factors may affect the brain's rate of aging (e.g., regular exercise, a cognitively challenging environment with social contacts, reading, playing card games, and lowering blood glucose levels with a healthy diet).

SPINAL CORD INJURY REHABILITATION

Following SCI, the patient's resulting condition may range from temporary neurologic deficits to permanent, total paralysis (see Chapter 12). Similarly to brain injury rehabilitation, successful SCI rehabilitation should begin in the ICU. Some

aspects of early rehabilitation include protection of joints, passive ROM exercises three to four times per day depending on the degree of muscle tone present in the extremities, application of wrist and ankle protective splints, and very careful monitoring of skin to prevent pressure ulcers.[19] After stabilization and transfer to a rehabilitation hospital, the entire rehabilitation team must work with the goal to maximize the patient's projected functional abilities, minimize the complications, and encourage the psychosocial adjustment of patients who have sustained SCIs. Table 13-3 outlines rehabilitation potential based on the functional level of spinal cord disruption. Therapeutic modalities and training by the multidisciplinary team to restore functions lost to paralysis are augmented by adaptive equipment, orthotic devices, wheelchair training, and psychosocial support.

SCI necessitates the patient's participation in the management of his or her health care needs and the progress toward independence from the medical system. Even a patient with a C4 injury on mechanical ventilation can and should direct his or her own care, regardless of the 24-hour nursing care. The health care providers should consciously promote self-reliance and not foster dependence.

Acute and Postacute Care

Paralysis can affect every body system and presents the patient with many medical challenges and potential for complications (see Chapter 12). Shorter length of stay (LOS) in rehabilitation with less time to make functional gains before discharge can be overwhelming for an individual with SCI. The patient may be unable to quickly adapt to the physical and emotional demands of an intense program while coping with some of the following medical conditions.

Assessment

The comprehensive assessment for SCI can be reviewed with the neurologic classification and American Spinal Injury

TABLE 13-3	Functional Level of Spinal Cord Disruption and Rehabilitation Potential	
Level of Injury	**Movement Remaining**	**Rehabilitation Potential**
Quadriplegia		
C1-C3		
Usually fatal injury, vagus nerve domination of heart, respiration, blood vessels, and all organs below injury	Movement in neck and above, loss of innervation to diaphragm, absence of independent respiratory function	Ability to drive electric wheelchair equipped with portable respirator by using chin control or mouth stick, headpiece to stabilize head, lack of bowel and bladder control
C4		
Vagus nerve domination of heart, respirations, and all vessels and organs below injury	Sensation and movement above neck	Ability to drive electric wheelchair by using chin control or mouth stick, lack of bowel and bladder control
C5		
Vagus nerve domination of heart, respirations, and all vessels and organs below injury	Full neck, partial shoulder, back, biceps; gross elbow, inability to roll over or use hands; decreased respiratory reserve	Ability to drive electric wheelchair with mobile hand supports, ability to use power hand splints (in some patients), lack of bowel and bladder control, feed self with setup and adaptive equipment
C6		
Vagus nerve domination of heart, respirations, and all vessels and organs below injury	Shoulder and upper back abduction and rotation at shoulder, full biceps to elbow flexion, wrist extension, weak grasp of thumb, decreased respiratory reserve	Ability to assist with transfer and perform some self-care, feed self with hand devices, push wheelchair on smooth, flat surface; lack of bowel and bladder control
C7-C8		
Vagus nerve domination of heart, respirations, and all vessels and organs below injury	All triceps to elbow extension, finger extensors and flexors, good grasp with some decreased strength, decreased respiratory reserve	Ability to transfer self to wheelchair, roll over and sit up in bed, push self on most surfaces, perform most self-care; independent use of wheelchair; ability to drive car with power hand controls (in some patients); lack of bowel and bladder control
Paraplegia		
T1-T6		
Sympathetic innervation to heart, vagus nerve domination of all vessels and organs below injury	Full innervation of upper extremities, back, essential intrinsic muscles of hand; full strength and dexterity of grasp; decreased trunk stability, decreased respiratory reserve	Full independence in self-care and in wheelchair, ability to drive car with hand controls (in most patients), ability to use full body brace for exercise but not for functional ambulation, lack of bowel and bladder control
T6-T12		
Vagus nerve domination only of leg vessels, GI, and genitourinary organs	Full, stable thoracic muscles and upper back; functional intercostals, resulting in increased respiratory reserve	Full independent use of wheelchair; ability to stand erect with full body brace, ambulate on crutches with swing (although gait difficult); inability to climb stairs; lack of bowel and bladder control
L1-L2		
Vagus nerve domination of leg vessels	Varying control of legs and pelvis, instability of lower back	Good sitting balance, full use of wheelchair
L3-L4		
Partial vagus nerve domination of leg vessels, GI, and genitourinary organs	Quadriceps and hip flexors, absence of hamstring function, flail ankles	Completely independent ambulation with short leg braces and canes, inability to stand for long periods, bladder and bowel continence

From Lewis SM, Heitkemper MM, Dirksen SF: *Medical-surgical nursing: assessment and management of clinical problems,* ed 5, St Louis, 2000, Mosby

GI, Gastrointestinal.

Association (ASIA) score. Care plans for specific interventions are based on injury impairments.

Complications Associated With SCI

Pulmonary: Ineffective Breathing Pattern. Respiratory complications have been acknowledged as one of the leading causes of death for individuals with tetraplegia. Mechanical ventilation may be required. Respiratory fatigue (including absent or weak cough ability or inability to clear secretions), obesity, smoking, atelectasis, respiratory infections or pneumonia, pulmonary edema, and age affect respiratory function. Respiratory impairment for SCI, especially high-level injury (C1 to C4), may require tracheostomy, quad coughing (assisted coughing), intermittent ventilation or long-term ventilator support, secretion management with suctioning, and oxygen supplementation. Incentive spirometry and intermittent positive-pressure breathing (IPPB) or nebulizer treatments may be necessary.

Although long-term tracheostomy care and mechanical ventilation do not prevent the patient from participating in vocational, academic, or community activities, patients with respiratory impairment do require ongoing, close assessment. Prevention of respiratory infection is a central goal of management. Moreover, a speech pathologist may be needed on the interdisciplinary care team if augmentive communication devices or recommendations regarding pacing and breath support are warranted. The Passy-Muir valve has been used in some cases instead of a tracheostomy. A noninvasive diaphragmatic phrenic nerve pacemaker (DPNP) implantation is an option for appropriate candidates. Surgical implantation of electrodes that electrically stimulate muscles of the phrenic nerve causes the muscles to contract and air to enter the lungs.

Extensive patient education and review of equipment for long-term use helps in the adjustment of impaired breathing and decreases patient and family anxiety. Good pulmonary toilet with a routine 'for coughing, breathing, exercises, mobility, adequate fluid intake, moisture, chest physiotherapy (CPT), and positioning, as well as using an abdominal binder, may be useful to improve elastic recoil of the diaphragm.

Pressure Ulcers: Impaired Skin Integrity. Prevention of pressure ulcers is the primary goal of clinical management. Devices such as gel cushions, water mattresses, positioning aids, and seating systems are often recommended to decrease skin breakdown, but weight shifts and routine skin inspections are the keystones of management. Patients should be taught techniques to relieve pressure over bony prominences every 20 minutes and how to inspect their own skin, including using a mirror to help check unexposed areas (Box 13-10). Prevention techniques include avoidance of shearing during transfers or when moving the patient in bed, meticulous skin care, frequent repositioning, good nutrition and hydration, avoidance of incontinence, and prevention of dependent edema through elevation of limbs.

It is hoped that death from infection caused by pressure ulcers and septicemia is a complication of the past. Pressure sore management protocols must be instituted immediately for any skin breakdown. Patients with a halo vest need special

---

| BOX 13-10 | **Skin Care for Patients With Spinal Cord Injury** |

Skin breakdown is a potential problem following spinal cord injury. The following measures are used to decrease this possibility:

Change Position Frequently

If in a wheelchair, lift self up and shift weight every 15 to 30 minutes.

If in bed, a regular turning schedule (at least every 2 hours) that includes sides, back, and abdomen is encouraged to change position.

Use special mattresses and wheelchair cushions.

Use pillows to protect bony prominences when in bed.

Monitor Skin Condition

Inspect skin frequently for areas of redness, swelling, and breakdown.

Keep fingernails trimmed to avoid scratches and abrasions.

If a wound develops, follow standard wound care management, which includes keeping wound open to air and applying treatments as prescribed. Assess nutrition status.

From *Mosby's patient teaching guides,* St Louis, 1996, Mosby.

---

teaching for home care and especially to prevent infection (Box 13-11). Treatments for pressure ulcers vary widely based on the location, stage, and extent; pressure ulcers can be effectively managed if treated early and in consultation with a wound care specialist. Frequent inspection to remove pressure and good nutrition help prevent skin breakdown, but when preventive measures fail, surgery may be needed for stage IV ulcers with myocutaneous skin flaps or artificial skin.

Genitourinary: Impaired Urinary Elimination and Sexual Dysfunction. A **neurogenic bladder** is a neurologic condition with disruption at the level of the cerebral cortex in which the bladder muscles are paralyzed and the individual is unable to get urine out of the bladder voluntarily (Table 13-4). The overall goal for bladder management is to reduce or eliminate factors leading to incontinence, maintain adequate hydration, prevent overdistention of the bladder, and teach the patient management of an effective bladder program. Patients with incontinence may increase their disposition to a long-term care facility versus home, making teaching the patient meticulous bladder self-management important. Patient education has also led to a significant decrease in renal failure in patients with SCI.

The bladder often has bacterial colonization. Bacteria are commonly forced into the bladder without necessarily resulting in infection. The occasional presence of bacteria in the urine does not necessarily indicate a UTI and does not require aggressive pharmacologic interventions. The determinant of bacterial cystitis, for example, depends on the virulence and inoculum size of the invasive bacteria and the adequacy of the host's defense mechanism. Regular voiding or emptying of the bladder flushes bacteria that would ultimately colonize the urine if residual urine is allowed to remain and pool within the bladder. Clinically significant

BOX 13-11	Halo Vest Care for Patient and Family Home Care

The following are teaching guidelines for a patient with a halo vest:

- Inspect the pins on the halo traction ring. Report to the health care provider if pins are loose or if there are signs of infection, including redness, tenderness, swelling, or drainage at the insertion sites.
- Clean around pin sites carefully with hydrogen peroxide on a cotton swab. Repeat the procedure using water.
- Use alcohol swabs to cleanse pin sites of any drainage.
- Apply antibiotic ointment as prescribed.
- To provide skin care, have the patient lie down on a bed with his or her head resting on a pillow to reduce pressure on the brace. Loosen one side of the vest.
- Gently wash the skin under the vest with soap and water, rinse it, and then dry it thoroughly. At the same time, check the skin for pressure points, redness, swelling, bruising, or chafing. Close the open side and repeat the procedure on the opposite side.
- If the vest becomes wet or damp, it can be carefully dried with a blow dryer.
- An assistive device (e.g., cane or walker) may be used to provide greater balance. Flat shoes should be worn.
- Turn the entire body, not just the head and neck, when trying to view sideways.
- In case of an emergency, keep a set of wrenches close to the halo vest at all times. A flat wrench can be Velcroed onto the vest.
- Mark the vest strap such that consistent buckling and fit can be maintained.

Modified from *Mosby's patient teaching guides*, St Louis, 1996, Mosby.

bacteriuria may be indicated by bacterial colonies greater than 100,000/ml in a culture. One of the most common complications of SCI, however, is UTI, and the resistant strains of bacteria make UTI more difficult to treat. Other GU complications include the following:[11]

- Bladder cancer
- Calculi
- Urethral tears
- Hydronephrosis
- Bladder dilation
- Bladder trabeculations
- Chronic cystitis
- Prostatitis
- Epididymo-orchitis

Because the predisposition for UTI continues for life, the patient should be taught the signs and symptoms of UTI to enable early detection and treatment. Renal calculi formation is another complication seen with SCI. A fluid intake of 2000 to 4000 ml/day is encouraged, along with mobilization, to decrease the risks of both UTI and calculi formation; however, the plan must be individualized and must reflect the patient's overall medical status. For example, a patient with a cardiac history might have fluid restrictions.

Various types of catheters (urethral and suprapubic), external collection devices (e.g., condom/Texas catheter), and drainage systems (e.g., leg bag, indwelling catheter, and bladder incontinence pads) are available for neurogenic bladder management. Frequently, the patient's lifestyle or an infection may necessitate a combination of devices. The appropriate mode of urinary elimination management considers the patient's history, lifestyle, environment,

TABLE 13-4	Types of Neurogenic Bladder		
Type	**Characteristics**	**Cause**	**Clinical Manifestations**
Uninhibited	No inhibitions influence time and place of voiding	Corticospinal tract lesion; observed in CVA, multiple sclerosis, brain tumor, brain trauma	Incontinence, increased frequency, urgency
Reflex	Bladder behaves as part of spinal reflex arc with no connection to brain	Lesion of motor and sensory fibers; occasionally seen in multiple sclerosis, pernicious anemia	Incontinence, urinary frequency, lack of sensation of bladder filling
Autonomous	Bladder behaves autonomously, as if it were cut off from brain and spinal cord	Lesions of cauda equina, pelvic nerves, spina bifida	Incontinence, difficulty initiating micturition
Motor paralysis	Bladder acts as if there were paralysis of all motor functions	Lower motor neuron lesion caused by trauma involving S2-S4	If sensory function intact, feels bladder distention and hesitancy; no control of micturition, resulting in overdistention of bladder and overflow incontinence
Sensory paralysis	Bladder acts as if there were paralysis of all sensory modalities	Damage to sensory limb of bladder spinal reflex arc; seen in multiple sclerosis, diabetes mellitus, pernicious anemia	Poor bladder sensation, infrequent voiding, large residual volume

From Lewis SM, Heitkemper MM, Dirksen SF: *Medical-surgical nursing: assessment and management of clinical problems*, ed 5, St Louis, 2000, Mosby.
CVA, Cerebrovascular accident.

compliance, and financial resources. Research can be found that supports or criticizes any procedure, but in all cases the overall goals of bladder management are the prevention of long-term complications (i.e., reflux or chronic infection resulting in urinary diversion surgery) and the assimilation of bladder control into the patient's lifestyle. Systems for urinary elimination include the following:[12]

- Voluntary voiding at scheduled intervals, sensory signaled voiding, reflex-triggered voiding, and Valsalva voiding are the least invasive methods.
- Condom catheter drainage with a collecting device is an effective method, although the adhesive material may cause skin irritation and may be difficult for some individuals with SCI to use.
- Intermittent catheterization is an effective invasive method, and with good technique and timing, the patient can have scheduled emptying and remain catheter free in between.
- Indwelling urinary catheter with a drainage container via the urethral or suprapubic route is the method of choice for many patients but requires daily cleaning of the bag and changing monthly and creates a higher risk of UTI and calculi.

Periodic testing (e.g., routine urinalysis) and yearly urodynamic evaluation help reduce morbidity and mortality rates from GU complications. Ultrasound, 24-hour urine studies, renal radionucleotide scans, intravenous (IV) pyelograms, and cystoscopy are performed for specific complications. Management of neurogenic bladder, including drug therapy, is described in Box 13-12.

Changes in sexuality are based on the level of injury and whether the SCI was complete or incomplete. Women with SCI may maintain their capacity for orgasm with the potential for a satisfactory sexual relationship with their partners.

Selection of appropriate birth control must weigh the benefits and risks of each method in consultation with the SCI physician, the patient's gynecologist, and other specialists. After the acute phase of SCI, women usually resume their normal menstrual cycles in approximately 6 to 12 months. Women who plan to have a family and become pregnant usually deliver a normal, healthy infant. Careful planning with a team of experts is needed to manage potential problems during pregnancy that are associated with SCI (e.g., autonomic dysreflexia, spasticity, ITB, and respiratory problems).

Gastrointestinal: Bowel Incontinence. The **neurogenic bowel** results in paralysis of the lower rectal and anal muscles and the individual is unable to control bowel evacuation. A neurogenic bowel program may include medical management, dietary limits, hydration requirements, scheduled intervals between evacuations, and stimulation techniques for evacuation (Box 13-13). Often the patient needs to schedule the

---

BOX 13-12	**Management of Neurogenic Bladder**

Diagnostic
Neurologic examination
Cystourethrogram
IV pyelogram
Urine culture
Drug Therapy
Increasing detrusor muscle strength (bethanechol [Urecholine])
Acidification of urine (ascorbic acid [vitamin C])
Relaxation of urethral sphincter
Nutrition
Low-calcium diet (<1 g/day)
Fluid intake at 1800 to 2000 ml/day
Urine Drainage
Reflex training
Intermittent catheterization
Indwelling catheter
Urinary diversion surgery

From Lewis SM, Heitkemper MM, Dirksen SF: *Medical-surgical nursing: assessment and management of clinical problems,* ed 5, St Louis, 2000, Mosby.
IV, Intravenous.

BOX 13-13	**Bowel Management After Spinal Cord Injury**

The following are teaching guidelines for a patient with a spinal cord injury:
- Optimal nutritional intake includes the following:
  - 3 well-balanced meals each day
  - 2 servings from the milk group
  - 2 or more servings from the meat group, including beef, pork, poultry, eggs, fish
  - 4 or more servings from the vegetable and fruit group
  - 4 or more servings from the bread and cereal group
- Fiber intake should be approximately 20 to 30 g per day. Gradually increase amount of fiber eaten over 1 to 2 weeks.
- Three quarts of fluid per day should be consumed unless contraindicated. Water or fruit juices should be used, and caffeinated beverages such as coffee, tea, and cola should be avoided. Fluid softens hard stools; caffeine stimulates fluid loss through urination.
- Foods that produce gas (e.g., beans) or upper GI upset (spicy foods) should be avoided.
- Timing: A regular schedule for bowel evacuation should be established. A good time is 30 minutes after the first meal of the day.
- Position: If possible, an upright position with feet flat on the floor or a step stool enhances bowel evacuation. Staying on the toilet, commode, or bedpan for longer than 20 to 30 minutes causes skin breakdown. Based on stability, someone may need to stay with the patient.
- Activity: Exercise is important for bowel function. In addition to improving muscle tone, it also increases GI transit time and increases appetite. Muscles should be exercised. This includes stretching, range of motion, and position changing.
- Drug treatment: Laxatives, including suppositories, may be necessary to stimulate a bowel movement. However, these drugs can be habit forming and thus should only be taken when necessary. Manual stimulation of the rectum may also be helpful in initiating defecation.

From *Mosby's patient teaching guides,* St Louis, 1996, Mosby.
GI, Gastrointestinal.

bowel program around daily activities; it is critical that the patient's normal routine not be structured around the bowel program or the caregiver's requests. It is also important that the regimen remain constant and not change more than every 3 to 5 days. Although the patient may take several weeks to arrive at a consistent schedule, diligent bowel training usually prevents embarrassing accidents, promotes independence, and prevents bowel impaction and obstruction. The choice of regimen depends on the level of injury, amount of assistance required, and individual preference. A bowel movement every 1 to 3 days is a traditional pattern for evacuation. Possible bowel programs include the following:

- Stool softeners: docusate
- Digital stimulation for reflex neurogenic bowel
- Regular addition of fiber to the diet
- Diet limitations
- Small-volume enema/suppository
- Special positioning
- Detailed bowel program

It may take weeks to months, and careful management, to establish a successful bowel program. The goals of an effective bowel program are as follows:[16]

- Minimize or prevent incontinence
- Evacuate stool at a regular and predictable time
- Minimize the secondary complications of colonic overdistention, fecal impaction, and diverticula

A large majority of patients with SCI report problems with constipation that may cause gastric pain. The embarrassment of bowel accidents may prevent patients from traveling or leaving home when they are unable to maintain a satisfactory bowel program. Hemorrhoids are also problematic. One study from the model spinal cord injury systems revealed that 30.4% of patients with either complete or incomplete SCI required assistance with bowel management. The level of assistance varied according to the severity of injury, ranging from 78% for individuals with complete tetraplegia who required complete assistance to 11.8% for individuals with complete paraplegia who required complete assistance. Of the individuals with complete paraplegia, 53.3% managed their bowel care with modified assistance. In general, patients with SCI at or above the C5 level will be dependent and require total assistance for all aspects of bowel care.[14] Medications must be evaluated for side effects of diarrhea or constipation, which make it difficult at times to treat spasticity, neurogenic bladder, infections, pain, and depression.

Factors that should be considered in designing a bowel program include the availability of caretakers for assistance (if needed), daily life schedules, and the availability of adaptive equipment.[42] The following may be part of the bowel program management:

- Patient's normal pattern of bowel elimination
- Dietary modulation of stool consistency with fiber and liquid intake
- Increased physical activity
- Regular scheduling of bowel care time and frequency
- Adaptive equipment (e.g., commode chair, digital stimulation devices) based on the individual's

functional status and home/community environmental needs
- Oral medications (that either promote or inhibit bowel function)
- Rectal medications (suppositories)

Impaired Physical Mobility. Acute assessment of mobility status is required after SCI to identify positioning and equipment needs. A wide array of assistive devices is available, including wheelchairs and accessible modified vans that allow even patients with quadriplegic levels of injury to continue driving.

Bed mobility must be assessed to determine the patient's level of independence in performing ADLs. Splints and braces (e.g., **molded ankle-foot orthoses [MAFOs]** and **ankle-foot orthoses [AFOs]**) may be appropriate to assist the patient with mobility and self-care activities. These devices also support appropriate positioning for body alignment and at times inhibit spasticity.

Functional electrical stimulation (FES) is a growing area of research in SCI. FES stimulates specific muscle groups to create the contraction and relaxation necessary for assisted ambulation. Bioengineering has been instrumental in the development of FES, which has enabled some patients to stand and actually take steps with a walker. FES candidates are vigorously evaluated by the rehabilitation team and undergo prolonged cardiovascular conditioning. These patients must continue with a home exercise program designed to maintain functional ability.

The U.S. Food and Drug Administration (FDA) approved the **iBOT,** an innovative high-technology power mobility system, in August 2003. It has been described as potentially revolutionary. The iBOT requires the patient to have the use of one arm to operate the iBOT. The system has four wheels and uses sensors and gyroscopes to navigate stairs while balancing on two wheels. A physician's prescription is required, and the user must undergo special training at a designated center to learn safe operation of the device (Fig. 13-5).

Autonomic dysreflexia can result if bladder, bowel, and skin management are not appropriately implemented in SCI patients with injury at T6 or above (see Chapter 12). Precipitating factors include kinked or obstructed catheters, overdistention, UTI, calculi, constipation, and pressure ulcers or other noxious stimuli. Ongoing assessment is necessary to prevent such complications and to reevaluate the effectiveness of interventions in these areas.

Osteoporosis is a long-term complication for many patients with SCI. Exercise, medications, and the use of weights placed on the lower extremities help prevent osteoporosis and bone fractures.

Heterotopic ossification (HO) is present in approximately 16% to 53% of the SCI population.[15] As described earlier in the section on head injury rehabilitation, HO is an accumulation of uncharacteristic bone that is usually deposited between layers of connective tissue. It is called myositis ossificans when the bone forms between muscles. The exact cause is unknown, but HO is found in patients who have experienced trauma. As rehabilitation progresses, the patient with SCI may experience severe limitations of mobility,

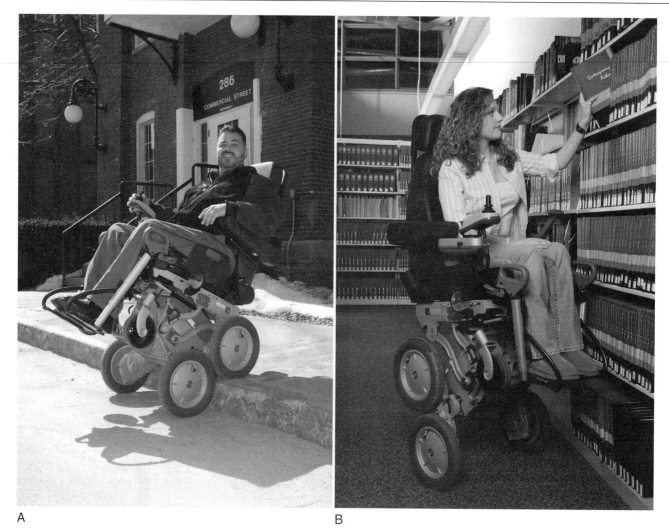

A   B

Figure 13-5 A, iBOT wheelchair climbing over a curb. **B,** Elevated iBOT wheelchair for upright positioning. *(Courtesy Independence Technology, Endicott, NY.)*

including impairment of motion to joints or impairment of functional use of extremities.

Prevention of HO has not been clearly documented in the literature; however, it is an area of extensive investigation, particularly in the area of medical management, including the use of prophylactic medication such as etidronate (Didronel). Aggressive ROM and other exercises recommended by the PT to prevent contractures may also be effective in reducing the incidence of HO. As in patients with TBI, severe cases of HO may require surgery or radiation therapy.

Psychosocial Implications

The overall incidence of a major depressive episode associated with acute SCI has been estimated at 10% to 50%. The etiology of the depression (i.e., whether it is a natural part of recovery after SCI or caused by the psychosocial ramifications and reactions of catastrophic injury) is controversial. Clinicians may be confronted by various behaviors after SCI that can be misinterpreted as anger directed toward caretakers, rather than as behaviors resulting from catastrophic trauma. Clinicians who care for the patient with SCI, regard-

less of the care setting, must be familiar with all possible behaviors, which may range from withdrawal, extreme anger, and verbal abuse to demonstrations of frustration. These behaviors are a result of the injury and the attempts of the injured patient to cope with a devastating and life-altering condition.

It is critical to assess the level of the patient's support, including friends, significant others, and vocational/academic peer groups, as well as the patient's own capacity to participate in counseling. Often support groups, patient advocacy groups, and peer groups with a specific focus (e.g., sports or a political issue) benefit both the patient and the family. A support network may enable the patient to direct his or her reactions and responses to catastrophic injury in a productive, positive manner. Health care providers, particularly clinicians who interact with the patient in postacute or home settings, are responsible for making appropriate referrals for psychologic counseling for both the patient with SCI and the immediate family as indicated. The entire family should understand the patient's behavior and the appropriate interventions as much as possible.

Pain Implications

Spinal pain has been described by many patients as a burning, hot poker, throbbing type of sensation that never completely leaves. When present, spinal pain is within the zone of injury or below the level of injury, and it may be exacerbated by spasticity. Biofeedback and diversion therapy have been partially effective, but chronic pain programs are recommended for patients with long-term chronic pain symptoms (i.e., pain persisting longer than 6 months) (see Chapter 23).

Pain rehabilitation programs may consist of medication, behavior modification, creative imagery, aquatic therapy (hydrotherapy), leisure counseling, and psychologic counseling. Total pain alleviation may not be a realistic goal; pain management, which encourages a lifestyle that is not pain oriented, is the overall goal.

Spasticity

The evaluation and treatment of spasticity in SCI are comparable to that done in individuals with other types of upper motor neuron (UMN) neurologic diseases. Spasticity is usually not painful but in some cases can be so powerful as to make wheelchair use and transfers dangerous.[19]

As spinal shock wears off and the patient's limbs are no longer flaccid, **spasticity** may develop. As described under brain injury, this is a form of **muscular hypertonicity** with increased resistance to stretch. In some situations, limited spasticity may actually assist the patient. For example, a patient with spasticity in the lower extremities may have greater standing tolerance or transfer ability. In most instances, however, spasticity remains burdensome, interfering with ADLs and general functioning.

Treatment is initiated when spasticity interferes with functions and causes complications. An unexplained worsening of spasticity can signal the development of secondary complications, such as spinal instability or syringomyelia. Eliminating contributing factors or noxious stimuli is the first step in comprehensive management. Spasticity is probably more severe in individuals with incomplete SCI. A stepwise approach to eliminate or reduce spasticity begins with muscle stretching as described in the section on brain injury, and then progresses to nonpharmacologic interventions and then medications. Four medications have been the mainstay for therapy:

1. Baclofen (Lioresal) is often the first-line agent. It acts on the spinal cord level. The manufacturer's maximum recommended dose of 40 to 80 mg/day is often prescribed at higher doses and is well tolerated by some patients.
2. Diazepam (Valium) acts on the spinal cord level and is recommended in doses that can be slowly increased up to a maximum of 40 mg/day.
3. Tizadine (Zanaflex) acts on the spinal cord level and is given at low doses but can be increased up to 12 to 36 mg/day.
4. Dantrolene (Dantrium) acts on peripheral muscles at the neuromuscular junction. Weakness can be a major limitation to the use of this agent. The initial dose usually starts with 25 mg/day and can be increased slowly up to a maximum of 400 mg/day.[32]

When the magnitude of the spasticity becomes intolerable, ITB therapy, with lifetime refills and pump replacement, offers improved function and follows the same test dose and surgical implantation as described in the section on brain injury. ITB therapy has evolved into a standard treatment for spasticity.[38] Surgical management may include rhizotomy (cutting of the roots of the spinal nerves) or tenotomy (cutting of a tendon to release contracture).

Body Weight–Supported Treadmill Training

As patients recover from the shock and disbelief of an acute SCI, they ask when they will walk again at every phase of their recovery. Body weight–supported treadmill training (BWSTT) is a new therapy that has combined the efforts of experts in medicine, bioengineering, and computer science to develop a new kind of therapy aimed at restoring lost function.[10] BWSTT has shown promise as a means of enhancing walking/gait recovery. A harness is worn to "unweight" the individual to allow for easier lower extremity movement. Patients are then capable of learning how to control their pelvic movement and weight-shift during assistance from therapists with breakdown of the walking components. The harness is attached to an overhead support suspended above a treadmill, and is worn by the individual to provide support and stability. The individual is carefully positioned on the treadmill by therapists in front of a mirror for feedback. A bar in front allows the individual to hold on as the treadmill is activated at a very slow speed. Four therapists remain stationed around the individual—one in front to monitor the patient and the controls, one on each side of the treadmill to physically lift the individual's legs up and down in a walking action on the moving treadmill, and the fourth straddling the treadmill to support the individual's hips and trunk for proper alignment and in concert with the movement (Fig. 13-6, A). Sessions may last 30 to 60 minutes for the prescribed number of days and weeks of therapy.

One theory behind BWSTT is based on the belief that the spinal cord can generate steplike electrical patterns when exposed to the sensation of walking. When a paralyzed individual has intense and repetitive retraining to walk, it stimulates the spinal cord to respond.[40] This type of therapy may enhance locomotor activity. Another concept is the so-called plasticity of the brain to adapt and reorganize. Once the legs are paralyzed, the individual experiences behaviorally based "learned nonuse" of the muscles. Traditional rehabilitation offers compensatory methods of functioning, provides a wheelchair for mobility, and offers therapeutic exercises for strength and muscle building.

Work with experimental animals, paralyzed from a transected spinal cord, demonstrated the ability to walk when placed on a moving treadmill. These early animal studies led to the theory of central pattern generators (CPGs).[4] CPGs are neural circuits that produce self-sustaining patterns of behavior with localizations outside the brain. Since walking is a cyclic behavior, it is believed that walking is controlled in the spinal cord by CPGs.[6] In addition to therapist-assisted BWSTT, robotic-assisted BWSTT therapy is available. A computer controls the AutoAmbulator robotic devices attached to the patient's legs and simulates walking while

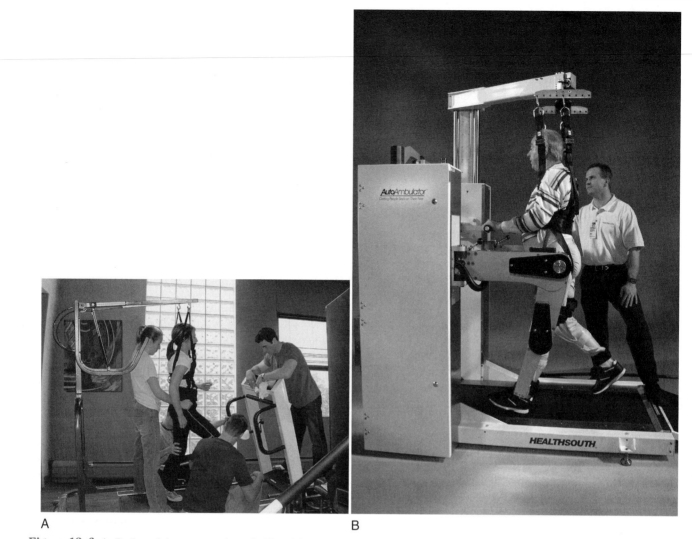

Figure 13-6 A, Body weight–supported treadmill training (BWSTT) session with four physical therapists. Two therapists manually move the patient's legs over a treadmill with a harness supporting the patient's weight. **B,** The FDA-approved AutoAmbulator, developed by HealthSouth and used in 86 HealthSouth centers in the United States, is a sophisticated treadmill device to simulate walking while robotic braces move the patient's legs across the treadmill using integrated computer system controls.
(A, Courtesy Darcy Reisman, PhD, PT, with permission from the University of Delaware's Neurologic Physical Therapy Clinic, Newark, DE.
B, Courtesy HealthSouth, Birmingham, AL.)

measuring the body's response to movement (Fig. 13-6, *B*). Only one therapist is needed to monitor the individual and operate this equipment.[30] Research continues on the application of BWSTT, selection of candidates, the timing after SCI, development of standardized protocols, and reimbursement issues.

For additional clinical practice guidelines in spinal cord medicine, the reader is encouraged to obtain copies of the complete series published by the Consortium for Spinal Cord Medicine sponsored by the Paralyzed Veterans of America.

Dual Diagnosis: Brain and Spinal Cord Injury

An incidence of 24% to 59% of patients with concomitant brain and spinal cord injury is challenging to therapeutic rehabilitation providers. The dilemma often begins at admission with the decision of assigning the patient to the most appropriate nursing unit. Severity of each injury, overall admission status, and level of care needed for each diagnosis go into the decision-making criteria. The cognitive impairments from the brain injury may initially be overlooked with a suspected SCI. The implications of dual diagnosis encountered during rehabilitation to recover from the cognitive impairments of brain injury and motor deficits of SCI require extensive management strategies and a higher vigilance for prevention of complications.

STROKE REHABILITATION

Although stroke is recognized as the leading cause of long-term disability, an estimated 1 in 10 stroke victims recover almost completely. Nearly half may experience moderate to severe impairments that could require special care. Rehabilitation of the stroke patient helps stroke patients reclaim function and mobility. A comprehensive stroke rehabilitation plan sets goals that may help lessen physical and cognitive impairments, increase functional independence, lessen the burden of care provided by significant others, reintegrate the patient into the family and community, and restore the patient's health-related quality of life. Such plans include long-term interventions that may prevent complications of immobility, reduce impairments and disability, and improve quality of life[18] (see Chapter 17).

Approximately half of individuals who survive a stroke have some type of residual physical or social disability.[25] Rehabilitation for individuals who have experienced a stroke begins immediately in the acute care setting as soon as the patient is stable, usually after 24 hours. Depending on the severity of neurologic impairment following a stroke, individuals may continue their rehabilitation in rehabilitation settings, long-term care centers, home, or outpatient settings. Most stroke patients returning to the home setting require ongoing rehabilitation and recovery. The rehabilitation goals are the maintenance of functioning and the promotion of additional recovery. Outpatient therapy often includes physical therapy, occupational therapy, speech therapy, and psychology. Case management is also necessary to coordinate the physician's recommendations for care, equipment rental, transportation services, and day care center enrollment.

Acute and Postacute Care

Assessment

A comprehensive neurologic assessment is performed as a baseline on admission (see Chapter 2). Multiple assessment scales and tools may be of use and available to evaluate the patient during rehabilitation (e.g., the FIM, described earlier, and the Barthel Index [BI] to evaluate the level of independence in ADLs). At admission the majority of patients have a moderate level of disability or a total FIM score of 40 to 80.[18] The National Institutes of Health Stroke Scales (NIHSS) (see Chapter 17) is routinely performed on admission in the acute care setting and repeated daily. Research has shown that the NIHSS performed 7 days after a stroke forecasts good recovery on severe disability at 3 months.[1]

Today, with the modest amount of formal inpatient and outpatient stroke rehabilitation from an interdisciplinary team, the family and home health providers are assuming early and increasingly greater responsibility. Patient and family education becomes extremely important in teaching how to provide or supervise continuing therapy after discharge. During inpatient rehabilitation, about one third of patients have a UTI, urinary retention, musculoskeletal pain, or depression. It has been estimated that up to 20% of patients fall, experience a rash, or need continuous management of blood pressure, hydration, nutrition, or glucose levels. Another 10% of patients may have a transient toxic-metabolic encephalopathy, pneumonia, cardiac arrhythmias, pressure ulcers, or thrombophlebitis. A smaller percentage of patients (up to 5%) may have a pulmonary embolus, seizures, GI bleed, heart failure, or other medical complications. Many of these conditions are discussed in Chapter 17; this chapter reviews the four most common medical disorders.

Impaired Physical Mobility

Recovery of ambulation correlates directly with residual leg strength. In general, patients who can flex the hip and extend the hemiparetic knee against gravity after stroke will be able to ambulate without assistance.[18] The overall goals for a patient with impaired physical mobility resulting from a stroke include maintenance of normal alignment; prevention of edema, which can further decrease movement; reduction of spasticity; and prevention of the complications associated with immobility. Therapeutic exercises and muscle strengthening, compensatory training, and task-oriented retraining are provided by the members of the rehabilitation team at the bedside and in the therapy area or gymnasium. Depending on the level of disability, a patient with a stroke may require a home evaluation to determine whether home modifications are necessary. Recommendations may include nonskid floor surfaces, handrails in living areas, short-pile carpeting, safety bars in bathrooms, and double stair rails. If the patient is dependent on a wheelchair, modifications might include entrance/exit ramps, a safety intercom system, a roll-in shower stall, a shower chair, and a transfer bench or sliding transfer board. Above all, concern for the patient's safety determines which home modifications are necessary. The patient with severe impairments must rely on caregivers for ADLs, positioning, turning, joint mobility, and safety.

Since 1986, a new therapeutic approach to rehabilitation of movement after stroke, termed **constraint-induced movement therapy (CIMT),** has been developed. Years of basic animal and human neuroscience research began with monkeys given somatosensory deafferentation. Edward Taub, the pioneer of this neurorehabilitation technique, experimented with constraint of the affected arm and "forced use" by the individual to actively use the limb disabled by the stroke.[44] CIMT is an innovative, research-supported intervention that assists individuals in increasing the functional use of their weakened arm following a stroke as compared with traditional therapy for the affected arm that may have only a negligible impact. Restitution of function in the affected arm improves skills for acute, subacute, and chronic stroke patients and has been shown to actually cause the brain to rewire. The CNS of adults was thought to be minimally responsive to environmental demands, or "hardwired." Areas surrounding the damaged motor area appear to respond to repetitive tasks that have a functional purpose (e.g., shaping techniques with progressively more difficult tasks using the affected arm with a goal of eating independently).

As in BWSTT, "learned nonuse" occurs when individuals recovering from a stroke realize their deficit and adapt to their hemiparetic arm by becoming increasingly or totally dependent on the nonaffected arm. CIMT involves constraining the functioning arm to induce stroke patients to greatly increase the use of the affected upper extremity for many hours a day over a consecutive period of 1 to 14 days.[7] The theory is based on intense and repetitive activity, the plasticity of the brain, and its ability to rewire itself and to make new neural connections. The individual may attend a 6-hour therapy session 5 days per week for 2 to 3 weeks. The repetitive tasks are performed for 15 to 20 minutes as part of the behavioral technique called "reshaping" with tasks broken

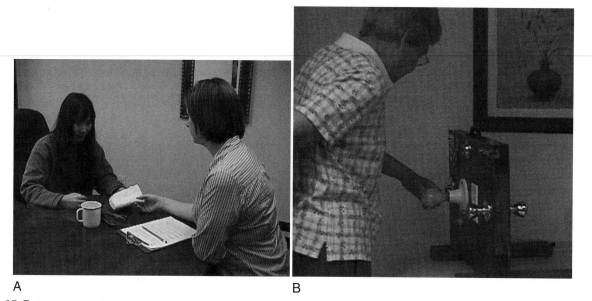

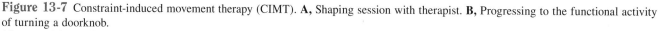

Figure 13-7 Constraint-induced movement therapy (CIMT). **A,** Shaping session with therapist. **B,** Progressing to the functional activity of turning a doorknob.
(Courtesy Advanced Recovery Rehabilitation Center in Sherman Oaks, CA.)

down into small steps (Fig. 13-7). The therapist may record or videotape the steps and encourage the individual to wear a mitt or even a sock on the unaffected arm at home for follow-up.

CIMT has significantly improved quality of movement and substantially increased the amount of use of the affected extremity in ADLs. CIMT therapy has potential benefits for patients with chronic stroke who meet specific inclusion criteria for upper extremity motor function[31] (see Chapter 17). Trials are underway to determine cost-effective ways to offer CIMT:

- Group sessions for 2 weeks versus one-on-one therapy
- One hour per day of outpatient CIMT with 5 hours of home therapy for 2 weeks with a family member or caregiver supervising a structured home protocol
- Modified CIMT (mCIMT) over a 10-week period of only 5 hours per day of repetitive exercise therapy and wearing the constraining mitt on the unaffected arm
- Totally home-based computer-assisted CIMT with a computer camera connected to the rehabilitation facility with live interaction between the patient and therapist
- Surface electromyography-triggered neuromuscular stimulation (ETNS) with biofeedback for patients with no active movement in their affected wrists/fingers who participate in ETNS and regain some active function and progress to mCIMT[35]

Preliminary evidence suggests that BWSTT, discussed previously as an intervention for spinal cord–injured patients, may be an effective treatment to increase walking speed in individuals after stroke.[43] As illustrated in Fig. 13-6, *A,* a harness attached to an overhead support suspended above a treadmill is worn by the individual to provide support and

stability. Typically the application of this intervention in individuals after stroke requires the assistance of two therapists; one therapist provides input to the patient's hips and trunk to encourage proper alignment and stability and a second therapist assists the patient or provides cues for the advancement of the hemiparetic leg. As the patient's skill advances, the amount of BWSTT is decreased, as is the assistance of the therapists. This intervention has been shown to be particularly promising in patients with a lower level of baseline walking function.[6]

Impaired Swallowing

Described previously under head injury, a **dysphagia program** is usually initiated in the acute care setting and continued with the help of a rehabilitation dysphagia specialist, a speech/language pathologist, or an occupational therapist. Aspiration occurs in the majority of individuals recovering from a stroke, particularly with a right-hemispheric stroke with deficits in the pharyngeal phase. Swallowing should be continually evaluated to minimize malnutrition, dehydration, and aspiration pneumonia. Ongoing assessment of the patient's ability to chew, drink, and swallow is needed to ensure that a correct diet with an appropriate consistency has been ordered. Attention must be paid to the caloric and fluid intake that a patient is consuming to avoid dehydration and ensure adequate caloric intake.

After a bedside swallowing assessment, further studies may be required, such as the **videofluoroscopic modified barium swallow (MBS).** The radiologist and dysphagia specialist or speech therapist (or both) may perform the evaluation. The MBS allows the team to observe the different aspects of swallowing, signs of aspiration, and compensatory strategies used by the patient. Ultrasound may be performed for patients who need only an assessment of oral function.

Fiberoptic endoscopic evaluation of swallowing (FEES) is used to evaluate laryngeal/pharyngeal function and risks of aspiration. An endoscope is passed transnasally during the evaluation. With results of the bedside assessment and diagnostic test results, the team makes the decision regarding the type of nutritional support needed by the patient.

Enteral feedings include short-term tube feedings (i.e., passing a nasogastric [NG] tube with selected commercial supplements using the GI route). If this method is not appropriate and a longer period of alternative nutrition is needed, invasive methods may be needed (e.g., a percutaneous endoscopic gastrostomy [PEG] tube may be placed surgically with the feeding passing directly into the stomach or a transpyloric or gastrojejunostomy feeding may prevent aspiration and gastric intolerance).[22]

If enteral feedings are being tapered, with oral feedings increasing, a dietitian should be consulted to ensure adequate caloric intake and hydration. When oral feedings are begun, the patient must be positioned to facilitate the swallowing process and minimize the risk for aspiration. The patient should be sitting upright with the head and neck positioned slightly forward and flexed. Soft or semisoft foods and fluids are preferred. Thickening powders are available to add to foods and fluids to increase the consistency to the appropriate thickness. Some individuals may have a tendency to pocket food on the side of the mouth where there is decreased sensation, which can pose a risk for choking. These patients should be taught to use their tongue to sweep the inside of their cheek for food. These patients should be supervised throughout the meal. They may become compulsive and "shovel" food, thereby overfilling the oral cavity, which may result in choking or aspiration.

Some patients who have experienced a stroke have no difficulty with swallowing but may be easily distracted and impulsive, which can also lead to an increased risk for aspiration. Individuals exhibiting these behaviors should eat their meals in a quiet environment with minimal distractions.

Psychosocial Implications

Depression following stroke is common and may be correlated with premorbid depression and the area of the brain affected by the stroke. The stroke patient may demonstrate significant cognitive impairments that require counseling, cognitive retraining with professional assistance, and treatment with tricyclic or selective serotonin reuptake inhibitor (SSRI) antidepressants. If depression and apathy limit the individual's participation during inpatient rehabilitation, methylphenidate (Ritalin) may be ordered at a dosage of 10 mg after breakfast with a buildup to 20 mg twice per day. Fluoxetine (Prozac) 10 mg or sertraline (Zoloft) 25 to 50 mg may be started several days later, and then increased as needed.[18] It is important the family be taught that the patient may show some of the signs of cognitive impairment listed in Box 13-14.

The clinician can assist the patient in developing coping skills to compensate for these cognitive deficits. The patient must understand that these cognitive deficits are the result of brain damage after a stroke. Effective teaching strategies include the following:

| BOX 13-14 | **Signs of Cognitive Impairment Following Stroke** |

- Decreased ability to understand new ideas, conceptualize, or make decisions
- Abnormal interpretations of environment
- Distraction or impatience
- Inappropriate social behavior
- Altered sleep patterns
- Hallucinations or delusions
- Disorientation
- Temperamental outbursts

- Reduce distractions and nonessential information
- Associate new skills with old skills
- Encourage the patient to structure relationships between particular facts, wider principles, and generalizations
- Use memory aids as needed
- Maintain consistency in the structure, scheduling, and duration of teaching sessions

Impaired Verbal Communication

Strategies used for rehabilitation in the area of impaired verbal communication depend on the type of aphasia present: receptive, expressive, or mixed (see Chapter 2). In all cases the goal is to establish an effective mechanism for communication. A speech and language pathologist should be involved in the assessment of the type and degree of aphasia and in the development of effective, alternative communication strategies, such as picture boards. Individuals with receptive aphasia will require that directions be provided in a simple, step-by-step, and repetitive manner. Communication with the patient should be slow, and simple sentences and phrases should be used with sufficient time allowed for the patient to understand and process the information. Staff and family members should take opportunities to repeat the names of common objects throughout the day. Individuals with expressive aphasia are frequently aware of their difficulties with communication and become very frustrated with their inability to express themselves. Constraint-induced aphasia therapy (CIAT), based on restraining the use of writing, gesturing, and any other nonverbal form of communication with selected patients who are limited to one or two words, is available. Reshaping techniques, forcing speech with intense repetition and intensity based on the same models for CIMT, have resulted in success in speaking sentences after 2 to 3 weeks of therapy in some cases.

COMPREHENSIVE PATIENT MANAGEMENT

Health Teaching Considerations

Patient and family health teaching is the key to helping the patient reach and maintains a high level of wellness. A multidimensional education program should begin as early as possible in the patient's care and should include the patient's family or significant others. Teaching addresses the psychosocial and physiologic aspects of the patient's life and offers opportunities for the patient to develop new skills, coping mechanisms, and behaviors to adjust to aspects of a temporary or permanent neurologic impairment.

Several factors may influence the patient's ability to learn, including his or her neurologic status (i.e., cognitive and sensory deficits, impaired memory, and pain) and developmental level. With time, however, the patient can be taught the skills necessary to begin a lifelong course toward the highest possible level of wellness within the context of his or her disability.

Patient and family education is essential to a successful rehabilitation experience. This education most appropriately begins in the acute care setting. The current health care delivery system results in patients and families being moved quickly along the continuum of care. The rehabilitation process is enhanced when patients and families have been provided with accurate information conveyed in a manner that is simple and straightforward about the care that is being provided in the acute care phase. Patient education requires a high level of skill on the part of the clinician to determine the amount of information to provide and how to deliver the information to patients and families. An individual, for example, with SCI is likely to have an alteration in bowel function that will require extensive learning before discharge home. In-depth detailed teaching and establishment of a new bowel elimination program will most likely occur in the rehabilitation phase of care. Early simple and factual information about what is being done to avoid constipation and bowel obstructions, beginning in the acute care phase, will serve to familiarize the patient and family with the terms and importance of this area of care when detailed teaching is done in the rehabilitation phase.

Patient education is closely related to the concepts of adjustment and change. For many patients and families with neurologic impairments leading to disability, the magnitude of changes that occur is enormous. Rehabilitation may require months of relearning the most basic ADLs, including mobility, bathing, dressing, toileting, grooming, and feeding. In addition, brain injury requires cognitive intervention for the patient and family to adapt to the onset of a major neurologic event—patients and families require considerable support to develop successful strategies to adjust to the changes. Clinicians along the continuum of care need to recognize the importance of repetition and reinforcement of information in ways that are meaningful and accessible to patients and families. Paterson, Kieloch, and Gmiterek[36] report that families of survivors of TBI did not remember being taught what to expect after discharge or what resources were available to them, despite health care professionals reporting that extensive discharge planning and teaching had occurred. These findings point out how critical it is that clinicians and caregivers along the continuum understand the stress that patients and families encounter. There is also a need to develop strategies that regularly assess the patient's and family's understanding of the individual's condition and the care that will be needed.

Psychosocial Considerations

Sexuality

Preliminary teaching for altered sexual functioning may begin in acute care when the patient voices a readiness to deal with the topic (see Chapter 14). Cognitively impaired patients may express sexual inappropriateness (e.g., male patients making advances toward female health care providers or using sexually explicit language). Firm responses that let the patient know that the behavior is unacceptable will extinguish the inappropriate behavior over time. Initially, health care professionals are responsible for preparing the patient to discuss sexual relations, focusing on bowel and bladder management, spasticity, and problems with performing ADLs that may affect sexual activity. Sexual concerns should be integrated into the rehabilitation treatment program, which includes counseling, educational tapes, books, and discussion groups. Sexual therapists often counsel both the patient and his or her partner to discuss expectations and changes in their sexual relationship. The clinician can help patients maintain their sexual identity by minimizing embarrassing situations, supporting patients' attempts to maintain their physical appearance, providing uninterrupted, private time for patients and their partners, and encouraging the patient to explore sexual feelings and alternative modes of sexual expression.

Fertility and sexual performance are frequent concerns, particularly in patients with SCI. Sildenafil (Viagra) is an effective, well-tolerated treatment for erectile dysfunction (ED) that is taken orally before sexual activity. Viagra is currently under investigation for neurologically impaired women. For the male patient, erection assistive devices are available, such as vacuum suction pumps, prostaglandin penile injections, and penile prosthetics or implants. Electroejaculation, vibratory stimulation, and pharmacologic intervention may be useful for ejaculation and producing sperm. For female patients, issues of bowel and bladder management and childbirth are continuous. These patients have special needs for accessible gynecologic and obstetric care during childbirth.

The Patient's Self-Perception

The neurologic patient experiences periods of frustration and depression intermittently throughout the recovery process or as a new phase in the trajectory of a chronic illness is experienced. Confronting the aging process and its effect on residual neurologic deficits may prove especially difficult. People in America have expressed that they are more fearful of being disabled by stroke than of death itself. When individuals are diagnosed with a stroke, they may develop a negative body image reinforced by memories of a friend or relative who was disabled by a stroke and left helpless, physically impaired, and unable to speak, move, or control his or her bowels or bladder. Referrals for psychologic counseling, support groups, patient advocacy groups, and community organizations are often helpful, especially if the patient will be discharged to the community from the acute care setting and will be receiving rehabilitation services on an outpatient basis or at home.

Adjustment to and coping with SCI may result in emotions that range from sadness to varying stages of depression during the initial recovery phase. Long-term psychologic adjustment for individuals with SCI may be enhanced with rehabilitation counseling, support groups, and a supportive family. Individuals unable to successfully cope may benefit from professional psychologic evaluation and antidepressant medications.

Depending on the extent of neurologic deficit, the patient may be able to live a completely independent life. Unfortunately, this is often not possible, and appropriate caregiver services must be secured. If the patient hires caregivers independently, the patient may become the employer of several attendants, nurses, or therapists. This, along with the duties of health maintenance, may be overwhelming. In such instances the patient may need medical services or therapy to be reinitiated. Nonetheless, independence in directing his or her own care and maintaining his or her functional status is critical to the patient's self-concept. Health care professionals should encourage independence rather than foster dependence on health care systems.

The clinician can help improve the patient's self-esteem by assisting with the identification of realistic goals that capitalize on the patient's strengths and resources. The rehabilitation patient needs to verbalize a clear understanding of the rehabilitation process and the nature of the injury or illness to the extent possible. This helps the patient feel in control. A supportive environment should also be provided so that the patient can be encouraged to explore new feelings and activities without fear of failure or criticism.

Family Support

By the time the patient with TBI, SCI, or a brain attack or stroke is in rehabilitation, the family or significant others often have become very knowledgeable in many aspects of the care. Nevertheless, the rehabilitation phase may prove to be the most challenging for the family. Teaching the patient and family to function without health care providers or hospital resources may invoke stress and anxiety. Teaching the patient to take control of his or her care may meet with some resistance, and teaching the family to allow the patient to take control may also be difficult. Finding an appropriate **support group** for the patient or family is usually very therapeutic.

Stress

Stress has been described as a prevalent health problem in America. Stress can increase during recovery and rehabilitation and actually become a barrier to improvement by tightening muscles and causing discomfort. Stress reduction is helpful in boosting the immune system, relaxing muscles, and promoting a sense of well-being. Stress reduction classes or individual sessions with a therapist can be recommended to determine the most appropriate therapeutic relaxation procedures. Choices may include biofeedback, Herbert Benson's "Relaxation Response," deep breathing, guided imagery, therapeutic touch, music therapy, or meditation. Aquatic therapy, or hydrotherapy, is another therapeutic modality whereby patients can use flotation devices in the deep end of the pool and relax to music or close their eyes for fantasy exercises (e.g., a trip to Hawaii). Once patients learn to recognize when tension is developing, they can learn how to avoid tension buildup and use their progressive relaxation techniques.

Suicide

Patients who are unable to cope with their disability, who suffer from severe depression, who become reclusive following their neurologic injury, and who feel helpless and hopeless in their rehabilitation efforts should be assessed for the potential for suicide. Early counseling and psychologic support, in addition to rehabilitation, is often needed for individuals with chronic or catastrophic neurologic outcomes. Older adults may not exhibit the typical signs of suicide and are often successful using lethal means. Risk assessment with early referral to a mental health professional is important for patients who have severe depression and are at risk for suicide.

Rehabilitation is physically taxing and requires a highly motivated patient and a strong support system to be successful. The rehabilitation process may be particularly stressful for the families of patients with TBI, and to intervene effectively, neuroscience clinicians should act on three main premises:

1. Crisis theory is applicable to the family situation.
2. Clinical interventions must be based on the behavioral response of the family.
3. Family dynamics directly correlate with the recovery status of the patient.

Living in a constant crisis state reduces the family's ability to mobilize and use all available resources. The key clinical goal is to assist the family in identifying and using all coping resources.

Older Adult Considerations

With about 15% of the population now over 65 years of age and older adults making up the majority of the rehabilitation population, the Association of Rehabilitation Nurses in 1994 described the subspecialty of rehabilitation for older adults as follows:

> Gerontologic rehabilitation nursing practice provides care and expertise to promote health, maintain and restore function, and provides education and counseling to older clients and their families. Gerontologic rehabilitation clinicians combine rehabilitation knowledge and skills with gerontologic principles to focus on individuals who are 65 years of age and older.[5]

With the aging of the 78 million baby boomers, by 2010, 50% of the population will be 50 years of age or older. Gerontologic rehabilitation is a specialty that will require a large body of health care providers to focus on the unique needs of the older population with neurologic deficits. The older patient, as a result of the normal aging process, may have physical and cognitive limitations, visual and hearing deficits, increased fatigability from poor nutrition and weight loss, delayed healing, decreased muscle mass, and frail,

TABLE 13-5	Older Adult Differences in Assessment of the Musculoskeletal System
Changes	**Differences in Assessment Findings**
Muscle	
Decreased number and diameter of muscle cells, replacement of muscle cells by fibrous connective tissue	Decreased muscle strength and bulk, abdominal protrusion, muscle flabbiness
Loss of elasticity in ligaments and cartilage	Decreased fine motor activity, decreased agility
Reduced ability to store glycogen; decreased ability to release glycogen as quick energy in times of stress	Slowed reaction times, slowing of most muscle neuronal reflexes, slowing of impulse conduction along motor units, easy fatigability
Joints	
Erosion of articular cartilage, possible direct contact between bone ends	Manifestations of osteoarthritis, joint stiffness, possible crepitation on movement of joints, pain with range-of-motion movements
Overgrowth of bone around joint margins (osteophytes)	Heberden's nodes in fingers (especially in women), limited mobility in affected joints
Loss of water from disks between vertebrae, narrowing of joint vertebral spaces	Loss of height, back pain, joint subluxation
Bone	
Decrease in bone mass	Dowager's hump (kyphosis) caused by compression of vertebral bodies
	Decreased height

From Lewis SM, Heitkemper MM, Dirksen SF: *Medical-surgical nursing: assessment and management of clinical problems,* ed 5, St Louis, 2000, Mosby.

thinner skin that rapidly breaks down (Table 13-5). These normal aging processes, in combination with a major neurologic injury, make rehabilitation a challenge that requires additional time and resources to help the patient adapt and recover from a neurologic disability.

Gerontologic specialists are available in most acute care hospitals and rehabilitation facilities to deal with the special needs of older adults. After discharge, however, the older patient who returns home may require a home assessment with potential home alterations, someone to adapt the home environment for the older patient with a disability, a hospital bed, and other special equipment to continue the rehabilitation. The spouse, who may also be older, may be anxious and frustrated if he or she is the only caregiver 24 hours per day. Attendant care is therefore essential in these cases to supervise and provide relief for the spouse, who often claims to have become a prisoner in his or her own home.

A personal attendant can provide ROM, ambulation, and good nutrition, as well as teach safety and how to prevent falls and injury. Patients who display poor judgment, impulsiveness, and unwillingness to accept help can benefit from an attendant using behavior modification and positive reinforcement until the older patient adapts and learns to cope with the disability.

In addition to physical therapy and occupational therapy, rehabilitation centers and community fitness clubs now offer therapeutic recreation. Included are exercise and fitness programs for rehabilitation of the older adult that include land (tai chi) and water therapy. Aquatic classes for aquatic motion and strength training, gait therapy, muscle lengthening, and stress release improve gait with less energy expended, improve balance, provide relief of back pain, and increase

muscle flexibility. Many programs offer wheelchair accessibility and maintain the ideal temperature for older patients. Socializing with other older adults with disabilities is an added benefit. Pet therapy and a canine companion have proven therapeutic benefits, especially for older patients who have fond memories of pets they have owned (see Chapter 14).

The potential for **elder abuse** should be considered when the stress and strain appear to overtax the spouse or family members. Abuse is suspected when there is evidence of neglect, unexplained wounds, dehydration, malnutrition, an unkempt home appearance, the patient's being left alone for long periods of time, poor personal hygiene of the older patient (including soiled bed linen), and no evidence of shopping for food or cooking. Older patients may be reluctant to report family violence or abuse for fear of abandonment or being moved from the home to long-term care. Frequent checks or unannounced follow-up visits by home health personnel can dispel the suspicion or give evidence for contacting protective services to get involved. Patients in imminent danger should be removed immediately.

Adequate support and rehabilitation are rewarding when older adults regain their independence and function. With community services and family support, older patients can recover from neurologic disorders to live long and productive lives. Financial concerns should be discussed with a social worker, and referral to local community services for older adults is helpful. There are family situations where long-term care is sometimes necessary due to caregiver issues (e.g., the advancing age of the caregiver), or the level of caregiver burden requires a facility that is able to provide full services for inpatient health care.

Case Management Considerations

Case management goals may include interventions listed in Box 13-15. Effective care coordination is the responsibility of the case manager, who will continue the patient's prescribed rehabilitation plan in the home setting.[23] After the patient evaluation, the case manager will meet with the health care team of rehabilitation professionals and family to carefully develop a plan designed to restore the individual to his or her highest level of functioning and increase his or her mobility and capacity for independence. Once the cost-effective plan has been approved by the third-party payers to cover the needed funding for services and equipment, the goal is to help the patient complete the rehabilitation process, prevent complications, and avoid rehospitalization.

Familiarity with not only the patient's neurologic condition and concepts of rehabilitation, but also safety and equipment, is essential. Patients and families also require health teaching regarding medications, including their side effects or adverse reactions; the use of special equipment for transfers and ambulation; and transportation using automobiles and vans, properly fitted wheelchairs, and devices to assist caregivers (e.g., lifts).

Steps and bathrooms, for example, can pose serious problems as patients return to their homes with walkers, braces, power wheelchairs, and physical disabilities that are new and frightening. Case managers can assess how the patient functions in the home setting and can offer appropriate recommendations. For those patients with a lifelong catastrophic neurologic injury (e.g., SCI, TBI, or stroke), the challenge of case management includes advocating for funds and resources to cover the rehabilitation services long enough to help achieve the individual's goals of independence and a satisfactory quality of life.

Life Care Planning Considerations

Life care planning (LCP) is the process of identifying a patient's current health status, future health care needs, and appropriate resources and associated costs to address life-long disability/illness management.[8] Many neurologic disorders may require LCP—especially TBI, SCI, stroke, and brain tumors. When the clinician prepares a life care plan, the nursing process functions as the conceptual framework and nursing and medical diagnoses serve as the rationale for the recommendation of future care and related expense. LCP is reviewed in Chapter 25.

Clinical trials are underway for exciting new research that holds hope for future technologic advances. One example is the pioneering research by Todd Kuiken at the Neural Engineering Center for Artificial Limbs at the Rehabilitation Institute of Chicago. Dr. Kuiken has developed a procedure that connects an amputee's own nerves to healthy muscle, allowing the user to move a prosthetic limb in the same manner as a real limb.[27] The development of the first bionic arm, or myoelectric arm, works using electrical signals from the amputee's chest muscles activated by the user's thought processes. This breakthrough was publicized with the 2005 announcement of Jesse Sullivan as the world's first "bionic man" (see Resources).

CONCLUSION

Rehabilitation of the patient with a neurologic illness is a specialty that has made significant contributions to patients' quality of life. This chapter has provided the reader with an overview of common rehabilitation interventions. Rehabilitation encompasses a vast range of treatment methods of various disciplines to accomplish the patient's goals. It does not stop with the rehabilitation team's final session. Coping with disability, maintaining a state of wellness, exercises, and individual therapy can be continued for a lifetime.

Acknowledgments

Peter Rossi, MD, FAAN, President of the American Society of Neurorehabilitation; Fellow, American Academy of Neurology and Fellow, American Academy of Disability Evaluating Physicians and Medical Director, Neurorehabilitation Services, Rehabilitation Hospital of the Pacific, Honolulu, Hawaii, was a chapter consultant.

RESOURCES FOR REHABILITATION

American Academy of Orthopaedic Surgeons: www.aaos.org
American Academy of Physical Medicine and Rehabilitation: www.aapmr.org
American Association of SCI Nurses: www.aascin.org
American Paraplegia Society: www.apssci.org
American Syringomyelia Alliance Project, Inc.: www.ASAP.org
Association of Rehabilitation Nurses: 800-229-7530; www.rehabnurse.org
CARF—The Rehabilitation Accreditation Commission: www.carf.org

---

BOX 13-15	Case Management Goals Checklist

The following case management goals may be appropriate following discharge:
- Home health referral
- Prescribed medications available at time of discharge
- Support and education with verbal and written information
- Equipment procurement delivered and ready for use in the home
- Financial referral completed
- Transportation home arranged to coincide with date/time of discharge
  - Home assessment completed and appropriate recommendations completed
  - Home attendant care agency referral completed and available at prescribed level/date
  - Vocational and educational services arranged
  - Substance abuse with drug/alcohol counseling referral
  - Sexuality needs addressed or referral completed
- Institutional placement arranged
  - Transportation available for future follow-up return medical/therapy appointments

Chiari Institute, North Shore–Long Island Jewish Health System: www.chiariinstitute.com

disAbility Resources: www.disabilityresources.org

Hydrocephalus Association: www.hydroassoc.org

Model Spinal Cord Injury Systems: www.ncddr.org/rpp/hf/hfdw/mscis

National Center for the Dissemination of Disability Research: www.ncddr.org

National Rehabilitation Information Center: www.naric.com

New Mobility: www.newmobility.com

Normal Pressure Hydrocephalus (NPH) Questionnaire: Download free copy by Ellen Barker at www.aesculapusa.com and go to Products, scroll down to Neurosurgery and access the NPH Questionnaire PDF file

Rehabilitation Institute of Chicago: 345 East Superior Street, Chicago, IL 60611-4496; Bionic Arm Info at www.ric.org/bionic

Senelick RC, Dougherty K: *Living with brain injury: a guide for families,* ed 2, Clifton Park, New York, 2001, Thomson Delmar Learning.

Senelick RC, Rossi PW, Dougherty K: *Living with stroke: a guide for families,* New York, 1991, McGraw-Hill.

Senelick RC, Ryan CE: *Living with head injury: a guide for families,* 1991, Rehab Hospital Services Corp.

Spinal Cord Resources: www.makoa.org/sci.htm

U.S. Department of Education, National Institute on Disability and Rehabilitation Research: www.ed.gov/offices/OSERS/NIDRR

REFERENCES

1. Adams H, Davis P, Leira E, et al: Baseline NIH stroke scale score strongly predicts outcome after stroke, *Neurology* 53(1):126–131, 1999.
2. Agency for Health Care Policy and Research (AHCPR): Pub no 99-E006, prepared by Oregon Health Sciences, Portland, OR, February 1999.
3. Albright AL, Gilmartin R, Swift D, Krach LE, Ivanhoe CB, McLaughlin JF: Long-term intrathecal baclofen therapy for severe spasticity of cerebral origin, *J Neurosurg* 98(2):291–295, 2003.
4. Alford S, Schwartz E, DiPresco GV: The pharmacology of vertebrae spinal central pattern generators, 2003. Available at http://nro.sagepub.com/cgi/content/abstract/9/3/217 (accessed April 22, 2005).
5. Association of Rehabilitation Nurses: *Standards and scope of rehabilitation nursing practice,* Glenview, IL, 2000, The Association.
6. Barbeau H, Visintin M: Optimal outcomes obtained with body-weight support combined with treadmill training in stroke patients, *Arch Phys Med Rehabil* 84:1458–1460, 2003.
7. Barker E: New hope for stroke patients, *RN* 68(2):38–42, 2005.
8. Barker E: Life care planning, *RN* 52(3):58–61, 1999.
9. Barker E, Saulino M: Life care planning for the client with severe spasticity: intrathecal baclofen therapy, *J Life Care Planning* 3(11):3–15, 2004.
10. Barker E: SCI patients take a big step forward, *RN* 68(7):30–34, 2005.
11. Bickel A, Culkin DJ, Wheeler JS Jr: Bladder cancer in spinal cord injury patients, *J Urol* 146(5):1240–1242, 1991.
12. Blackwell RL, Krause JD, Winkler T, Stiens AS: *Spinal cord injury desk reference: guidelines for life care planning management,* New York, 2001, Demos Medical Publishing.
13. Boake C, Francisco GE, Ivanhoe CB, Kothari S: Brain injury rehabilitation. In Ashley MJ, editor: *Traumatic brain injury: rehabilitative treatment and case management,* ed 2, Boca Raton, FL, 2004, CRC Press.
14. Cardenas DD, Hooton TM: Urinary tract and bowel management in the rehabilitation setting. In Braddom RL, editor: *Physical medicine rehabilitation,* Philadelphia, 1996, WB Saunders.
15. Colachis S, Clinchot D, Venesy D: Neurovascular complications of heterotopic ossification following spinal cord injury, *Paraplegia* 31:51–57, 1993.
16. Consortium for Spinal Cord Medicine: *Clinical practice guidelines: neurogenic bowel management in adults with spinal cord injury,* Washington, DC, 1998, Paralyzed Veterans of America.
17. DeLisa JA, Currie DM, Martin GM: Rehabilitation medicine: past, present, and future. In DeLisa JA, Gans BM, editors: *Rehabilitation medicine: principles and practice,* Philadelphia, 1998, Lippincott-Raven.
18. Dobkin BH: Rehabilitation and recovery of the patient with stroke. In Mohr JP, Choi DW, Grotta JC, Weir B, Wolf PH, editors: *Stroke: pathophysiology, diagnosis, and management,* ed 4, Philadelphia, 2004, Churchill Livingstone.
19. Frost FS: Spinal cord injury medicine. In Braddom RL: *Physical medicine and rehabilitation,* Philadelphia, 2000, WB Saunders.
20. Garland DE, Varpetian A: Heterotopic ossification in traumatic brain injury. In Ashley MJ, editor: *Traumatic brain injury: rehabilitative treatment and case management,* ed 2, Boca Raton, FL, 2004, CRC Press.
21. Hernandez TD, Levisohn PM, Naritoku DK: Posttraumatic epilepsy and neurorehabilitation. In Ashley MJ: *Traumatic brain injury: rehabilitative treatment and case management,* ed 2, Boca Raton, 2004, CRC Press.
22. Heyland DK, Drover JW, MacDonald S, Novak F, Lam M: Effect of post-pyloric feeding on gastro-esophageal regurgitation and pulmonary micro aspiration: results of randomized controlled trial, *Crit Care Med* 29:1495–1501, 2001.
23. Hines JA: Case management: a client-focused service. In Derstine JB, Hargrove SD, editors: *Comprehensive rehabilitation nursing,* Philadelphia, 2001, WB Saunders.
24. Hydrocephalus Association: *About normal pressure hydrocephalus: a book for adults and their families,* San Francisco, 2002, The Association.
25. Kong KH, Chua KSG, Tow A: Clinical characteristics and functional outcome of stroke patients 75 years old and older, *Arch Phys Med Rehabil* 79:1535–1539, 1998.
26. Kraus JF, McArthur DL: Epidemiology of brain injury. In Evans RW, editor: *Neurology and trauma,* Philadelphia, 1996, WB Saunders.
27. Kuiken T: Targeted reinnervation for improved prosthetic function, *Phys Med Rehabil Clin North Am* 17(1):1–13, 2006.
28. Milhorat TH: Personal communications, Feb 10, 2006, Chiari Institute, North Shore–Long Island Jewish Health System, Great Neck, NY.
29. Miller KJ, Schwab KA, Warden DL: Predictive value of an early Glasgow Outcome Scale score: 15-month score changes, *J Neurosurg* 103(2):239–245, 2005.
30. Mobility Research: Partial weight bearing gait training protocol using LiteGait, 2005. Available at www.litegait.com/products,htm (accessed April 25, 2005).
31. Morris DM, Crago JE, DeLuca SC, et al: Constraint-induced movement therapy for motor recovery after stroke, *Neurorehabilitation* 9(1):29–43, 1997.

32. *Mosby's 2005 drug consult for nurses,* St Louis, 2005, Elsevier Mosby.

33. Ordia JI, Fischer E, Adamski E, Chagnon KG, Spatz EL: Continuous intrathecal baclofen infusion by a programmable pump in 131 consecutive patients with severe spasticity of spinal origin, *Neuromodulation* 5(1):16–24, 2002.

34. O'Toole M: The rehabilitation team. In Derstine JB, Hargrove SD, editors: *Comprehensive rehabilitation nursing,* Philadelphia, 2001, WB Saunders.

35. Page SJ: Modified constraint-induced therapy ties patients down to bring them up, *BioMechanics* X111(2):22–29, 2006.

36. Paterson B, Kieloch B, Gmiterek J: "They never told us anything": postdischarge instruction for families of persons with brain injuries, *Rehabil Nurs* 26:48–53, 2001.

37. Ratcliff G, Colantonia A, Escobar M, Chase S, Vernich L: Long-term survival following traumatic brain injury, *Disabil Rehabil* 27(6):305–314, 2005.

38. Rawlins PK: Intrathecal baclofen therapy over 10 years, *J Neurosci Nurs* 36(6):322–327, 2004.

39. Rondinelli RD: Practical aspects of impairment rating and disability determination. In Braddom RL, editor: *Physical medicine and rehabilitation,* ed 2, Philadelphia, 2000, WB Saunders.

40. Rossignol S: Locomotion and its recovery after spinal injury, *Curr Opin Neurobiol* 10(6):708, 2000.

41. Rothstein JM, Roy SH, Wolf SL, Scalzitti DA: *The rehabilitation specialist's handbook,* Philadelphia, 2005, FA Davis.

42. Steins SA: Gastrointestinal system. In Hammond MC, editor: *Medical care of persons with spinal cord injury,* Washington, DC, 1998, US Department of Veterans Affairs.

43. Sullivan KJ, Knowlton BJ, Dobkin BH: Step training with body-weight support: effect of treadmill speed and practice paradigms on poststroke locomotor recovery, *Arch Phys Med Rehabil* 83:683–691, 2002.

44. Taub E, Miller NE, Novack TA, et al: The goal is to maximize or restore its motor function: techniques to improve chronic motor deficit after stroke, *Arch Phys Med Rehabil* 74(4):347–354, 1993.

45. Testa JA, Malec JF, Moessner AM, Brown AW: Outcome after traumatic brain injury: effects of aging on recovery, *Arch Phys Med Rehabil* 86(9):1815–1823, 2005.

46. Thurman DJ, Alverson C, Dunn KA, et al: Traumatic brain injury in the United States: a public health perspective, *J Head Trauma* 14:602–615, 1999.

47. Uniform Data System for Medical Rehabilitation: *Guide for the uniform data set for medical rehabilitation,* Buffalo, NY, 1996, State University of New York, Buffalo.

48. Ushewokunze S, Nappapaneni R, Gregson BA, Stobbart L, Chambers IR, Mendelow AD: Elderly patients with severe head injury in coma from the outset—has anything changed? *Br J Neurosurg* 18(6):604–607, 2004.

49. Vollmer DJ, Dacey RG, Jane JA: Cranio-cerebral trauma. In Joynt RJ, editor: *Clinical neurology,* vol 3, Philadelphia, 1992, JB Lippincott.

50. Weintraub A, Ashley MJ: Traumatic brain injury: aging and related neuromedical issues. In Ashley MJ: *Traumatic brain injury: rehabilitative treatment and case management,* ed 2, Boca Raton, FL, 2004, CRC Press.

51. Winkler T: Pathophysiology of spasticity and hypertonicity, *J Life Care Planning* 2(4):191–194, 2003.

52. World Health Organization: *International classification of impairments, disabilities, and handicaps,* Geneva, 1980, The Association.

CHAPTER 14

ANNE G. MIERS

Nontraumatic Disorders of the Spine

The spinal cord and peripheral nervous system function to sense changes in the external and internal environment, carry information about changes to the central nervous system and brain, and carry commands to tissues required to perform a response. The **spinal cord** is an elongated, cylindric continuation of the medulla oblongata that extends from the cranial border of the atlas and terminates at the level of the first lumbar vertebra (L1). Spinal nerves enter and exit the cord. Lumbar and sacral nerves form the cauda equina and remain in the vertebral foramen until they exit at the appropriate level of the spinal column. The spinal cord is protected by meninges and surrounded by adipose tissue and blood vessels. Clinicians must be familiar with the anatomy and physiology of the spine, spinal cord, and supporting structures to understand nontraumatic spinal cord disorders. (See Chapter 1 for a comprehensive review of the anatomy and physiology of the spinal cord.)

This chapter focuses on the management of patients with nontraumatic disorders of the spine, including tumors, infections, arteriovenous malformations (AVMs) of the spinal cord, degenerative disk disease, compression fractures, syrinxes (both syringomyelia and syringobulbia), and spinal cord infarction. **Nontraumatic disorders of the spine** are those caused by forces occurring within the spinal canal as opposed to sudden external physical forces. Although they often occur less acutely, they may have an outcome similar to a traumatic cord injury—even if diagnosed and treated in a timely manner. Newer treatments of some disorders have led to more favorable outcomes.

ETIOLOGY

Because of the fixed size of the spinal canal, growth, edema, and inflammation from spinal cord disorders may quickly cause symptoms or the disorder may occur over time (e.g., in spondylosis). The major causes of nontraumatic disorders of the spine include the following:

- Tumors: can be primary or metastatic affecting the cord or the spinal column
- Infections: can be primary or secondary (i.e., from another place in the body)

- **Arteriovenous malformations (AVMs):** a tangle of blood vessels in which there is an abnormal direct connection between an artery and vein without a capillary bed (local dilation of the vessels, ischemia of distal areas, and pressure effects of the AVM cause the pathologic condition)
- Disk disease: caused by degenerative problems and compression from conditions such as disk herniations; may result in failed-back syndrome
- Nontraumatic vertebral compression fractures: most often result from osteoporosis but can occur from neoplasms of the vertebral body such as metastasis or myeloma
- **Syrinx:** an abnormal cavity that forms in the central portion of the spinal cord and can be caused by previous trauma, neoplasms, and congenital malformations
- Infarctions: in general, are caused by a disruption of blood supply to the spinal cord

PATHOPHYSIOLOGY

The pathophysiology of nontraumatic disorders of the spine is attributed more to changes caused by compression and ischemia than to external invasion or destruction of the spinal cord. Common pathophysiologic changes include the following:

- Compression, irritation, and traction on the spinal cord, spinal nerve roots, or blood supply
- Mechanical displacement of the spinal cord from forces other than direct trauma
- Ischemia caused by interference with the spinal cord blood supply
- Obstruction of cerebrospinal fluid circulation
- Invasion and destruction of spinal cord tracts

The pathophysiology often depends on anatomic location. Various terms are used to describe a disorder and its relationship with the spinal cord. A cross section of the spinal cord showing lesion types is presented in Fig. 14-1.

The following terms are used to describe the location of nontraumatic disorders of the spine:

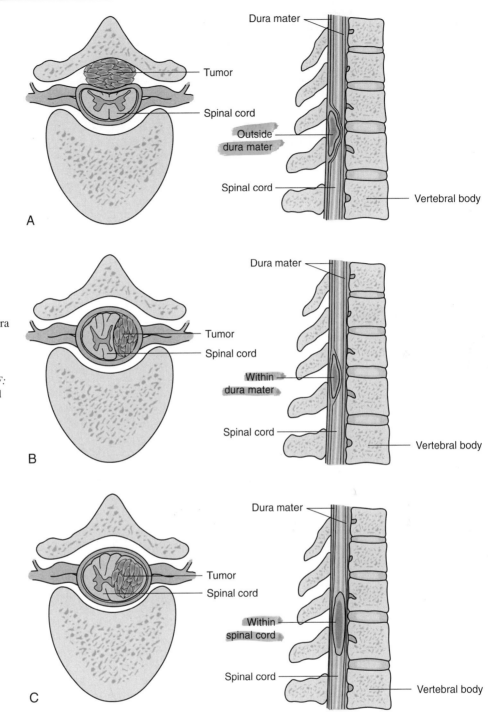

Figure 14-1 Spinal tumors. **A,** Extradural tumors (outside the dura mater). **B,** Subdural tumors (within the dura mater). **C,** Intramedullary tumors (within the spinal cord). *(From Phipps WJ, Sands JK, Marek JF: Medical surgical nursing: concepts and clinical practice, ed 6, St Louis, 1999, Mosby.)*

- **Extradural:** lesions located outside the dura mater in either the epidural space or the bones of the spinal column or paraspinal tissue
- **Intradural:** lesions located within or under the dura mater of the meninges
- **Intramedullary:** intradural lesions arising within the substance of the spinal cord, within the tracts and central gray matter
- **Extramedullary:** lesions arising outside of the spinal cord in the meninges, nerve roots, or vertebral bodies

Spinal Cord Tumors

Spinal cord tumors are one source of nontraumatic disorders of the spine. They can be **primary** or **metastatic,** but many are benign. Spinal cord tumors are rare in terms of overall central nervous system (CNS) tumors, and the pathologic condition depends on their location, as well as histologic cell type. Metastatic extradural tumors causing epidural spinal cord compression are most commonly a result of lung tumors in men and breast tumors in women. Table 14-1 shows the most common tumor types, characteristics, and treatment.

TABLE 14-1	Common Tumor Types		
Tumor Type	**Incidence**	**Most Common Site**	**Treatment**
Extradural			
Metastatic tumors	Most common extradural	Thoracic spine	Steroids + radiation therapy (RT) +/– surgery
• Multiple myeloma	Most common malignant		
• Lung			
• Breast			
• Lymphoma			
• Renal cell			
• Plasmacytoma	Rare		
Hemangioma	Most common spinal tumor	Thoracic spine	Surgery and RT
Chordoma	Rare	Sacrococcygeal	
Osteoid osteoma	Common	Lumbar spine	
Aneurysmal bone cyst	Rare	Lumbar-sacral spine	
Giant cell tumor	Rare	Sacral spine	
Eosinophilic granuloma	Rare	Thoracic spine	
Intradural—Extramedullary (EM) Tumors			
Schwannomas	Benign tumor arising from Schwann cells from the dorsal (sensory) root of spinal or cranial nerves	Lumbar spine	Surgery or stereotactic RT
Neurofibromas—nerve sheath tumors	Most common benign EM tumor; may be multiple in von Recklinghausen's neurofibromatosis	Thoracic spine	Surgery or stereotactic RT
Paraganglioma	Rare	Conus	Surgery +/– RT
Meningioma	Second most frequent benign tumor; arises from arachnoid villi of the dura	Upper cervical spine/foramen magnum/thoracic spine	Surgery +/– RT if subtotally resected
Intradural—Intramedullary (IM) Tumors			
Ependymoma	Most common IM—arises from ependymal cells	Cervical spine or conus	Surgery +/– RT +/– chemotherapy
Astryocytoma	Second most common IM—arises from astrocytes; most are low grade	Thoracic spine or cervico-medullary area in the young	Surgery +/– RT +/– chemotherapy for unresectable, progressive, or malignant tumors
Hemangioblastoma	Rare; benign; some may be EM; 25% are associated with von Hippel-Lindau syndrome; some cause subarachnoid hemorrhage	Thoracic spine	Surgery +/– RT for unresectable or recurrent tumors
Metastases	Cause pain, weakness, paresthesias, and sphincter dysfunction	Up to 70% involve thoracic spine; 20%–30% involve cervical and lumbar spine	Steroids +/– RT +/– chemotherapy
• Lung			
• Breast			
• Colorectal			
• Melanoma			
• Lymphoma			

Data from Maher De Leon ME, Schnell S, Rozental JM: Tumors of the spine and spinal cord, *Semin Oncol Nurs* 14(1):43–52, 1998; Van Goethem JW, van den Hauwe L, Ozsarlak O, et al: Spinal tumors, *Eur J Radiol* 50(2):159–176, 2004.

Extradural tumors account for approximately 60% of all spinal tumors, are usually malignant, and produce a rapid onset of symptoms.[50,54] Pain at the tumor site is common and occurs before the symptoms of spinal cord dysfunction.[97] Early symptoms include weakness and a loss of vibration sense; later symptoms are a loss of bowel and bladder control. In fast-growing tumors, symptoms can progress rapidly to paralysis. Early recognition and prompt treatment (while the patient still has motor function) are the most important factors in preventing permanent and debilitating neurologic dysfunction.

Intradural tumors account for 20% to 25% of spinal tumors, with one third of them being **intramedullary** (within the cord substance) and two thirds of them being **extramedullary**.[91] The signs and symptoms of intramedullary tumors usually develop slowly and progressively as the spinal cord is compressed.[91] Pain is a common symptom at the time of diagnosis. Local, **radicular pain** (i.e., following a nerve root) is often an early sign of extramedullary tumors, with neurologic dysfunction a later sign.[9] Clues to the exact location of the lesion may be obtained from a careful history. For example, lesions occurring in the posterior aspect of the spinal cord will produce posterior column dysfunctions, such as joint position and vibratory sensation loss.[9]

The pathophysiology of a spinal cord tumor also depends on the cell type. The histologic types of intradural spinal cord tumors are neurilemomas (schwannomas, neurofibromas), meningiomas, astrocytomas, and ependymomas.[9] Each of these tumor types is described in more detail in the following paragraphs.

Neurilemomas are the most common intradural primary tumors of the spinal cord and are classified as schwannomas or neurofibromas.[54] These tumors arise from the nerve root sheaths and therefore are found in the spinal, cranial, and peripheral nerve systems. Most commonly they are extramedullary. The majority of nerve sheath tumors arise from the dorsal sensory nerve root and are benign.[54] They tend to involve both the spinal and cranial nerves. The tumors of neurofibromatosis, or von Recklinghausen's disease, are of the neurilemoma type.

Meningiomas are well-circumscribed intradural or extramedullary primary tumors that arise from the arachnoid cells.[54] Most commonly found in the thoracic area, they are more prevalent in women than in men.[22,54] They are usually loosely attached to the dura, which permits easy surgical removal. They may also erode into bony structures.

Astrocytomas are most often intradural and intramedullary. They are the most common type of intramedullary spinal cord tumor in adults and children in the cervical and thoracic spine region.[54,80] In adults they occur most often in the third through fifth decades of life.[80] Similar to the classification of brain tumors, astrocytomas occur along a continuum of grades I to IV (see Chapter 7). The majority of spinal cord astrocytomas are grade I, with 75% being low-grade gliomas.[54] Grade II tumors contain a number of anaplastic cells, and grade III and IV tumors are considered malignant. A malignant astrocytoma may lead to rapid neurologic deterioration and death. Radiation is indicated only in patients with anaplastic cells; however, the benefit of this may be limited.[56]

Ependymomas can be found throughout the spinal cord and tend to be intradural and intramedullary. More than half occur in the fourth and fifth decades of life, and approximately one third of them involve an increased number of anaplastic cells.[54] Unlike astrocytomas, ependymomas tend not to invade normal tissue.[91] They can therefore be debulked with minimal morbidity. The 10-year survival rate is greater than 75% without further treatment.[56] Disease-free survival following recurrence is unusual (15% at 5 years) and suggests that intensification of initial adjuvant treatment may best prevent relapse.[17]

Other types of tumors include epidermoids, dermoids, teratomas, lipomas, and hemangioblastomas.[54] These make up about 10% of the total number of intradural spinal cord tumors, with each type accounting for less than 2% of such tumors.[9] **Hemangioblastomas** are the most vascular intramedullary tumors, although their vascularity varies.[56] They are benign, discrete, and well circumscribed and generally can be surgically removed.

Tumors that metastasize to the bones of the spinal column can cause fractures of the bones or pressure on the cord. The most common types of bony metastases are from primary breast, prostate, kidney, lung, and thyroid cancers.

Infections

Infections in the spine are rare and manifest in a variety of ways; therefore they are relatively difficult to diagnose. The neurologic deficits that accompany an infection range from minor weakness and pain to nuchal rigidity and the loss of bowel and bladder function. Signs and symptoms depend on whether the infection is extradural, subdural, or intramedullary. Infectious sources include pyogenic infections (primarily abscesses and osteomyelitis), fungal infections, parasitic infections, and spinal tuberculosis. Human immunodeficiency virus (HIV) can cause severe neurologic problems, including perivenular demyelination of the spinal cord.[27] Vacuolar myelopathy is the cause of gait difficulties in HIV-infected patients and it is only seen in this population.[27] Fungal and parasitic infections are rare and therefore are not discussed here.

Pyogenic Infection

Pyogenic infections of the spine include osteomyelitis and epidural, subdural, or intradural abscesses. All of these infections are usually caused by the organism *Staphylococcus aureus,* which spreads by direct invasion or hematogenously to the vertebral bodies or spinal cord.[79,95]

The most common pyogenic infection of the spine is vertebral osteomyelitis. **Osteomyelitis** is a bone infection and is commonly associated with a primary bacterial (staphylococcal) infection elsewhere in the body. Typically the thoracic and lumbar vertebrae are affected. There may be little or no fever or malaise, but the patient's erythrocyte sedimentation rate (ESR) is usually elevated. Osteomyelitis of the thoracic region can occur after insertion of a chest tube, especially when sterile conditions are less than optimal, such as with a traumatic injury. The patient can develop osteomyelitis months after a chest tube has been placed. Patients usually complain of back pain and have an elevated ESR.

Other organisms can cause osteomyelitis. Cryptococcal spondylitis can mimic spinal tuberculosis, and therefore tissue samples are often sought to confirm the diagnosis.

Abscess

A **spinal abscess** is a localized collection of pus. Abscesses of the spine occur in epidural, subdural, and intramedullary areas. They can be classified as primary versus secondary, single versus multiple, and acute, subacute, or chronic. Epidural abscesses of the spine are localized bacterial infections above the dural layer of the spinal meninges. Figure 14-2 illustrates the layers of spinal meninges. These spinal epidural abscesses were once considered rare or unusual; however, because of the increased incidence, this is no longer the case.[58] The increase in these abscesses may be due to an aging population, an increase in intravenous (IV) drug abuse, diabetes mellitus, alcoholism, resistant organisms, an increase in the use of spinal instrumentation, or epidural anesthesia.[58] Patients can have either acute, subacute, or chronic forms depending on whether the clinical course has evolved over a few days or several weeks.

Subdural spinal abscesses and intramedullary spinal cord abscesses are rare. The thoracic section is the most common site of intramedullary abscesses.[74]

Abscesses can cause a wide variety of signs and symptoms in patients, but the usual complaints include progressive weakness, sensory loss, back pain, nuchal rigidity associated with movement, and incontinence.[23] The ESR is a more sensitive and specific test than the white blood cell count as a screen for spinal cord abscesses.[24] Patients with localized back/neck pain and raised inflammatory markers need urgent magnetic resonance imaging (MRI).[39] Neurologic recovery

is excellent if spinal cord damage is minimal at the time of presentation and decompression, but is very poor if paraparesis or paralysis has been present longer than 48 hours.[74]

Tuberculosis

Tuberculosis (TB) is an infectious disease affecting primarily the lungs, but it can involve any body organ. Although many persons mistakenly believe that TB is no longer a health threat, the incidence of TB has risen dramatically in the United States during the last decade.[15] The World Health Organization estimates that between 19% and 43% of the world's population is infected with TB, with approximately 15 million Americans infected with the bacterium.[65] With greater world travel and increased immigration, health care workers must be vigilant to include TB in differential diagnoses.[2] Extrapulmonary TB, including tuberculous meningitis and TB of the joints and bone, is most often seen in older adults as a result of reactivation of a dormant focal infection in the CNS.[99] Although rare in younger adults, the relative rate of new cases of active TB in the United States is highest among older adults, and deaths caused by TB are highest in those over age 65.[99] The most serious aspect of this problem is an increase in multidrug-resistant TB.

TB can occur as a localized form that involves the vertebral body, epidural space, dura, arachnoid, or spinal cord, but often it is confined to one anatomic area. A tuberculous spinal infection involving the vertebral body is known as **Pott's disease** (or **Pott's paraplegia** if paralysis occurs). Pott's disease develops when the hematogenic spread of tubercle bacilli to the spine causes vertebral osteomyelitis, adjacent joint space infection, and subsequent paravertebral abscess.[75] Signs of spinal tuberculosis include fever, pain, and weakness according to location in the spine.

Skeletal TB can involve the cervical, thoracic, or lumbar spine areas; however, it is most common in the midthoracic area.[93] Insidious pain over the involved vertebrae may be the initial symptom of TB infection in the older adult. Other signs and symptoms include fever, fatigue, weight loss, and anorexia. Older adults are also at risk for tuberculous arthritis. Because older persons often experience a variety of joint diseases, tuberculous arthritis may be undetected or overlooked when pain and swelling of hips, knees, ankles, wrists, and hands occurs.

Arteriovenous Malformations

Spinal cord arteriovenous malformations (AVMs) can be either dural or intradural according to whether they are located inside or outside the dural meningeal layer of the spinal cord. They consist of either one or multiple abnormal arteriovenous channels or **fistulae.** This disorder results in ischemic necrosis of affected areas of the spinal cord caused by shunting of the blood or by direct compression from dilated vessels. These lesions can lead to epidural or intramedullary hemorrhage and can have devastating neurologic consequences. The signs and symptoms of AVMs include the following:[71]

- Spastic paresis of the lower extremities
- Loss of pain and temperature sensation

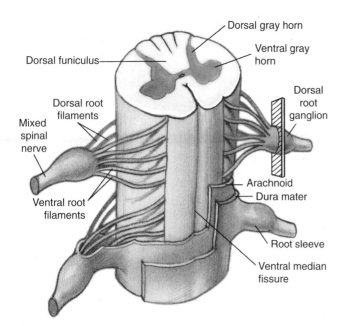

Figure 14-2 Meningeal layers of the spinal cord. *(From Mayo Clinic Foundation, Rochester, MN.)*

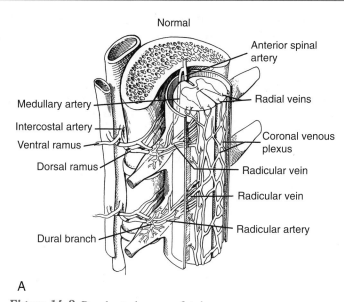

Normal

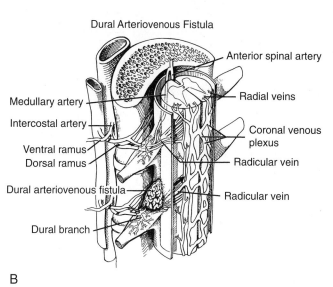

Dural Arteriovenous Fistula

A

B

Figure 14-3 Dural arteriovenous fistula.
(From Mayo Clinic Foundation, Rochester, MN.)

- Bladder dysfunction
- Impotence
- Nerve root pain
- Back pain aggravated by physical activity

Dural AVMs of the spinal cord are the most common type of AVM. These are lesions in which an abnormal arteriovenous shunt is embedded in the dura covering the proximal nerve root and the adjacent spinal dura[33] (Fig. 14-3). Males are affected four times as often as females.[72] The most common age of onset is in the fifth and sixth decades.[41] Intradural AVMs are lesions in which the abnormal shunt is internal to the dura and involves the spinal cord. The age of clinical presentation of these lesions is between 20 and 40 years.[41]

Disk Disease

The incidence of low back pain in the United States is very high; some authors estimate that 50% of working adults will experience back pain in any given year.[96] Low back pain (LBP) is responsible for the loss of millions of hours of work per year, with the economic impact of billions of dollars per year. The greatest risk factor for a back injury is a previous back injury. New technology is providing better insight as to the different causes of LBP and is leading to refined ability to treat a variety of back conditions.[18]

Degenerative Disorders

Degenerative disorders of the spine have risen dramatically along with the national increase in life expectancy. They are the result of the normal aging process—after 20 years of age the disk and the annulus tend to lose their hydrostatic and elastic properties. As the disk becomes more inflexible, movement between the adjacent vertebral segments becomes uneven, excessive, and irregular. The degenerative process varies among individuals and can be accelerated by trauma or constant strain to the back. Degenerative disk disease is thought to have some correlation with certain strenuous occupations such as nursing, but other factors (e.g., genetics) may be involved.

Most individuals with intervertebral disk disorders are between 30 and 60 years of age, although it is seen in people of all ages. The pathology of degenerative disk disease can lead to stenosis, spondylosis, subluxation, and ruptured intervertebral disk. **Stenosis** is narrowing of the spinal canal caused by soft tissue, bone, or subluxation. **Spondylosis** is the formation of vertebral osteophytes secondary to degenerative disk disease.

Ruptured intervertebral disks most commonly cause compression on the cervical or lumbosacral nerve roots.[16] "Myelo" pertains to the spinal cord whereas "radiculo" pertains to an individual spinal nerve. The term **radiculopathy** is a disease of a spinal nerve root or disk herniation. Symptoms can cause pain, motor changes, or sensory changes that result from neural compression. Figure 14-4 illustrates a ruptured intervertebral disk. The cervical and lumbar areas of the vertebral column are the most flexible, and therefore disk disease tends to be found most often in these areas. The lumbar spine has the highest incidence of disk disease, especially between L4 and L5 and between L5 and S1.[31] Herniations occur approximately equally among men and women; stenosis is more common among women than men.[31]

The clinical criteria for the diagnosis of lumbar disk rupture associated with severe **sciatica** include the following:[16,96]

- Leg pain (including buttock pain and pain radiating below the knee) is present.
- Pain should follow a radicular distribution and should be the dominant complaint when compared with back pain.
- Straight-leg raising (SLR) must be significantly reduced.

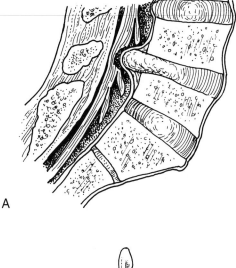

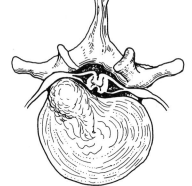

Figure 14-4 Ruptured invertebral disk. Diagram shows herniation of the nucleus pulposus. **A,** Herniation presses on the structures of the spinal cord. **B,** Herniation may press on the exit of the spinal nerve and produce pain and other symptoms.

- Neurologic symptoms (paresthesias or weakness) should be present in a radicular distribution.
- Neurologic signs (motor, sensory, reflex changes, muscle wasting) should be present in a radicular distribution.

Cervical disk syndromes occur most often at C5-6 and C6-7 where great forces are exerted on the disks.[31] The cervical disk is considerably smaller than the lumbar disk and almost invariably does not contain enough nucleus for more than one herniation.[86] It is extremely rare to encounter cervical disk herniation at more than one level.[86] Because of the relative immobility of the thoracic spine, disk problems in this area are relatively rare.

Failed Back Surgery Syndrome

Failed back surgery syndrome (FBSS) has been defined as the failure of medical or surgical treatment interventions to relieve pain after 6 months of treatment and the continued incapacitation from low back or leg pain secondary to disease of the lumbar spinal region. Naming this a syndrome may be a misnomer in that it does not follow a consistent pattern. There may be multiple reasons for this condition, including recurrent or retained disk fragments, unrecognized lateral recess or foraminal stenosis, spinal canal stenosis, nerve root injury, and multiple other possibilities.[57] There is evidence that scar tissue may form around the nerve roots and cause pain and spasm with movement of the spine or legs.[85] There is evidence that segmental instability after lumbar microdiskectomy may cause or contribute to FBBS.[77] Accurate diagnosis and patient selection for surgery are needed to reduce the number of inappropriate lumbar surgeries and resultant rate of FBSS.[85] This major health problem often involves a complex interplay of organic, psychologic, and socioeconomic factors that further complicate the syndrome.

Compression Fractures

In 2000, osteoporosis was estimated to affect 10 million people in the United States, 80% of them women.[89] Of the 1.5 million fractures attributed to osteoporosis, 700,000 are benign osteoporotic vertebral compression fractures.[89] Vertebral compression fractures also occur due to vertebral metastasis and to individuals as the result of chronic steroid use (e.g., transplant recipients). These fractures can result in significant morbidity and mortality rates.

Syrinxes

A syrinx is the formation of a cavitation in the central cord canal. Two types of syrinx formations occur in the spine: syringomyelia and syringobulbia. **Syringomyelia** is a central cavitation of the spinal cord. Depending on the degree of cavitation, it may be asymptomatic or result in sensory changes, weakness, and muscle wasting.[75] Syringomyelia may mimic a spinal tumor or an abscess because of its similar symptom manifestations, but syringomyelia develops more gradually. **Syringobulbia** is a cavitation of the medulla, a very serious condition that can result in respiratory compromise and death.[6] Syringomyelia and syringobulbia can lead to involuntary limb movements due to increased excitability of the spinal motor neurons.[75] Syringomyelia and syringobulbia are commonly found in association with Chiari malformations, neoplasms, and conditions subsequent to spinal cord trauma.[35,37] **Chiari malformations** I and II are congenital malformations in which the cerebellar tonsils protrude through the foramen magnum.[14]

Infarction

Vascular disease of the brain can cause strokes. Vascular disease of the spinal cord, although rare, can result in infarction. An **infarction** is a lesion caused by inadequate blood supply to an area of the spinal cord. There are many causes of infarction; a few of the more common causes are trauma, clamping of the aorta in surgery, stenosis, infections, emboli, and hypotension. Similar to vascular disease in the brain, the onset of vascular disease in the spinal cord is often abrupt, dramatic in scope, and disabling.

Anterior spinal artery (ASA) occlusion is the classic syndrome described in infarction. The anterior spinal artery supplies two thirds of the blood supply to the ventral spinal cord. A review of the blood supply to the spinal cord is neces-

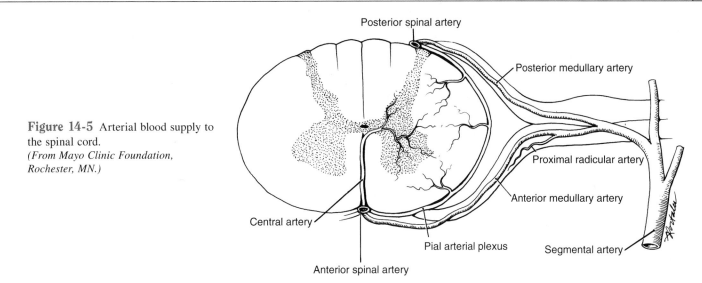

Figure 14-5 Arterial blood supply to the spinal cord. *(From Mayo Clinic Foundation, Rochester, MN.)*

sary for a thorough understanding of this condition. Figure 14-5 illustrates the arteries of the spinal cord. The ASA is formed at the level of the foramen magnum by two branches of the intracranial vertebral arteries, and it perfuses the anterior two thirds of the cervical spinal cord. Interruption in this blood supply from emboli, trauma, or stenosis gives rise to the neurologic deficits associated with infarction. The clinical picture of ASA occlusion is that of initial flaccid paralysis and diminished or absent reflexes. With time, the reflexes become hyperactive, and symptoms usually include weakness, muscle atrophy, numbness, aching, tingling, cramping, loss of bowel and bladder function, and pain.

ASSESSMENT

When a patient is admitted, it is important to complete a thorough assessment to obtain a baseline evaluation (see Chapter 12 for a full review of spinal cord assessment). When assessing the patient with a nontraumatic disorder of the spine, the clinician must assess functional status and ascertain the level of the lesion. The functional assessment encompasses the areas of pain, sensory impairment, motor impairment, and sphincter control.

Pain

Many nontraumatic disorders of the spine manifest with pain as the initial symptom. The pain is thought to be caused by compression, invasion of the spinal tracts, tension on the nerve roots, or attachment to the dura.

Extradural and extramedullary spinal tumors can cause severe local pain and tenderness. Intramedullary tumors also cause pain, but it is generally less severe. **Radicular pain** runs through the distribution of a sensory nerve root and is caused by irritation, tension, or pressure on the nerve root.[56] Patients often describe radicular pain as knifelike or as a dull ache with accompanying bouts of sharp, piercing pain. Performing the Valsalva maneuver (movements such as gagging, coughing, and straining to have a bowel movement) intensi-

fies radicular pain and causes radiation to the dermatomes supplied by the affected nerve root.[56]

The pain caused by a spinal cord tumor is aggravated by bed rest and is therefore worse at night; conversely, the pain of a herniated disk is relieved by bed rest.[56] The nocturnal pattern of pain with spinal cord tumor is thought to occur secondary to venous congestion in the recumbent position and distention of the spinal cord.[91] The pain in cervical disks will vary according to the type of herniation, with some people having no pain. Pain with cervical disks can be just in the neck or radiate to one or both arms.

Back pain associated with vertebral collapse occurs most commonly in older women with osteoporosis and is characterized by intense muscle spasm and girdle-like radiculopathy. Pain associated with vertebral compression often resolves in 4 to 6 weeks; in a subset of people this pain is prolonged and debilitating.[52] Vertebral compression fractures typically cause severe axial spine pain that is referable to the compressed vertebral body.[89] In addition, because of kyphosis or neural foraminal compromise, these patients often have paraspinal or radicular pain secondary to muscle or ligamentous strain[89] (see Chapter 23).

Back pain is present in approximately two thirds of the cases of patients who have **vertebral osteomyelitis.** The cervical or lumbar areas can both be affected by vertebral osteomyelitis. Point tenderness is usually present on palpation of the involved site.[42]

The lumbar pain experienced by the patient with FBSS may have originally resulted from muscle strain, rheumatoid arthritis, osteoarthritis, a herniated intravertebral disk, or multiple other etiologies. **Sciatica,** or radicular leg pain, may also contribute to this syndrome, with inflammation of the sciatic nerve usually marked by pain and tenderness of the sciatic notch in the buttocks and along the course of the nerve through the thigh and leg.

A multitude of pain scales may be used to assess and document pain levels. Initially, the key factors that are essential for the clinician to assess and document are the location, duration, and level of pain. Level of pain is usually described on a scale of 0 to 10, with 0 being no pain and 10 being the worst pain. Pain is considered the "fifth vital sign" and should be assessed with great vigilance (see Chapter 23).

Sensory Impairment

Regardless of the etiology of the nontraumatic disorder of the spine, sensory disturbances depend on the degree to which ascending fibers are affected. Affected dorsal columns produce impairments of light touch, joint and position sense, vibration, two-point discrimination, and stereognosis (see Figs. 2-12 and 12-1 for dermatomes). Impairments of pain and temperature discrimination result when fibers of the anterolateral columns are affected. At first the lesions may affect only peripheral fibers, leading to sensory loss in a level below the spinal segment of the lesion. Sensory loss will ascend as lesions increase in size.

The clinician concisely documents the initial sensory assessment by noting the areas of sensory deficit on an outline of the human body. A narrative description is also useful.

Motor Impairment

In general, motor weakness is a late symptom in spinal disorders of nontraumatic origin. Weakness is due to the involvement of the pyramidal or corticospinal tract or to involvement of a spinal nerve. The degree of motor impairment may range from clumsiness of one extremity to complete quadriplegia.

Spinal cord tumors usually cause motor weakness of the upper motor lesion type, especially if the pyramidal tracts are involved. The following symptoms are then manifested:[9]
- Paresis
- Spasticity
- Hyperactive reflexes
- Babinski's sign (typically present)

Brown-Séquard syndrome may be found with spinal cord tumors of the lateral aspect of the spine, with severe central cervical disk herniation or from a traumatic penetrating stab or bullet wound.[20] This is characterized by ipsilateral (same side) motor loss and by contralateral (opposite side) loss of pain and temperature sensations (see Figs. 12-10 and 12-14). The patient may not be able to move the leg on the side of the tumor but has sensation on that side with loss of pain and temperature on the opposite side because of the spinothalamic tract involvement.

Many motor findings are specific to patients with a syrinx; they can be unilateral or bilateral and can develop slowly—usually over years. In assessing the motor system in these patients, the clinician must assess reflexes, motor strength, and size in all extremities.

Figure 14-6 provides an easy guide to muscle testing that will assist the clinician.[26] Explanations for levels C3 to S1 include the specific muscle being tested, the function of that muscle, how to provide resistance, and a figure illustrating the muscle action.

Sphincter Control

Disturbances of sphincter control, with loss of bladder and bowel control, can occur as a late symptom of a spinal tumor.[91] When a nontraumatic disorder of the spine causes compression of the second or third sacral segments or nerve roots, micturition is affected and there is paralysis of bladder contractions, bladder distention, and retention of urine with overflow incontinence. Urinary incontinence is often associated with a syrinx when the lesion causes disruption of the sacral pathways (see Chapter 12).

Sexual dysfunction may also occur when there are problems with sphincter control. This occurs because the spinal nerves for all of these functions are located in the same lumbosacral area of the spine. Males may experience difficulty with erection and impotence. Sexual dysfunction in females may be more difficult to identify; therefore women should be asked about diminished response to sexual stimulation.

Lesion Levels

Along with a baseline assessment of pain, sensory impairment, motor impairment, and sphincter control, the clinician must ascertain whether the lesion is at the cervical, thoracic, or lumbar level of the spinal cord. Table 14-2 provides an overview of symptoms based on tumor location.

Cervical Lesions

Lesions at the level of the foramen magnum (the upper cervical segments) can be complicated. The clinician should be alert to the tendency of patients with lesions at this level to hold their head stiffly and experience difficulty with shoulder elevation.

Lesions at the C4 level can be particularly dangerous because of the involvement of the phrenic nerve, which affects respiration. With lesions involving the unilateral cord, the patient may experience respiratory difficulty and bilateral respiratory failure. High cervical lesions also produce the following symptoms: quadriparesis, occipital headache, stiff neck, and downbeat nystagmus.

Lesions below the C4 level are less life threatening because the phrenic nerve (and therefore the diaphragm) is not involved. Pain and muscle weakness follow patterns according to root distribution. For example, if sensation is not impaired, the patient with a C5-6 lesion will experience pain in the medial aspect of the arm.

Horner's syndrome may occur with lesions at the cervicothoracic junction (C8) as a result of autonomic nervous system dysfunction. **Horner's syndrome** includes **ptosis** of the eyelid with pupillary constriction or **miosis** and **anhydrosis** on the affected side. This can occur unilaterally or bilaterally (see Fig. 16-4).

Thoracic Lesions

Metastatic lesions from the lung tend to spread to the thoracic area. Whether metastatic or primary, lesions of the thoracic region are more difficult to localize than are cervical or lumbar lesions. Pain and sensory changes usually precede muscle weakness. Sensory changes are relatively easy to identify because of the regular bandlike distribution of the dermatomes at this level.

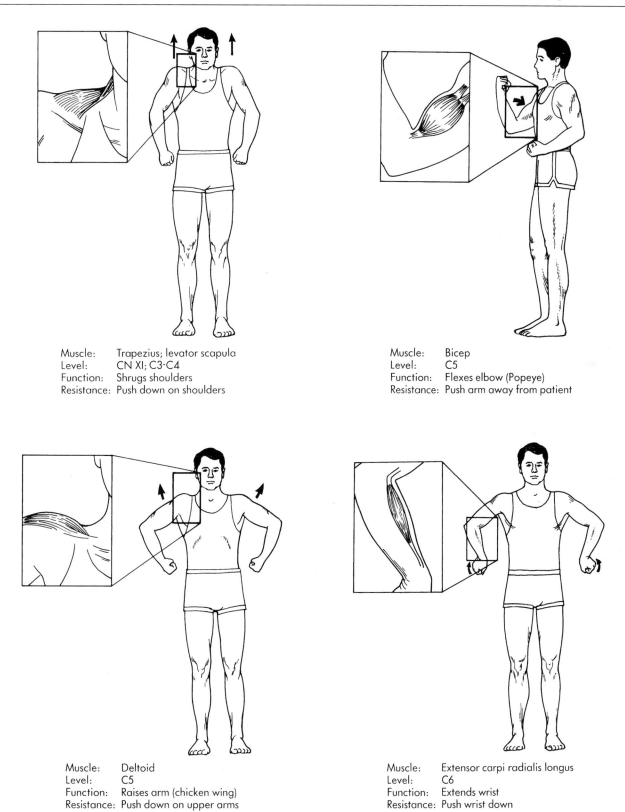

Muscle: Trapezius; levator scapula
Level: CN XI; C3-C4
Function: Shrugs shoulders
Resistance: Push down on shoulders

Muscle: Bicep
Level: C5
Function: Flexes elbow (Popeye)
Resistance: Push arm away from patient

Muscle: Deltoid
Level: C5
Function: Raises arm (chicken wing)
Resistance: Push down on upper arms

Muscle: Extensor carpi radialis longus
Level: C6
Function: Extends wrist
Resistance: Push wrist down

Figure 14-6 An easy guide to muscle testing of upper and lower extremities (C3 to S1). In general, if you ask the patient to move the limb in a vertical position, you are adding gravity. If you ask the patient to move the limb in a horizontal field, you are taking away gravity.

Continued

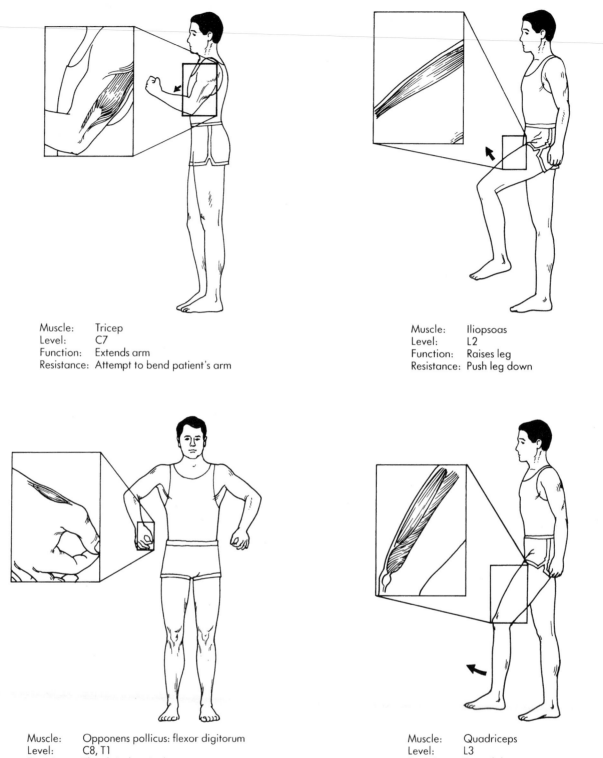

Muscle: Tricep
Level: C7
Function: Extends arm
Resistance: Attempt to bend patient's arm

Muscle: Iliopsoas
Level: L2
Function: Raises leg
Resistance: Push leg down

Muscle: Opponens pollicus: flexor digitorum
Level: C8, T1
Function: Thumb-index pinch
Resistance: Try to pull fingers apart

Muscle: Quadriceps
Level: L3
Function: Extends knee
Resistance: Try to bend leg

Figure 14-6, cont'd

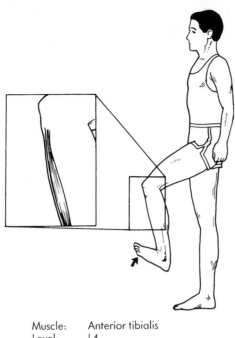

Muscle: Anterior tibialis
Level: L4
Function: Pulls foot up (dorsiflexion)
Resistance: Attempt to pull foot down

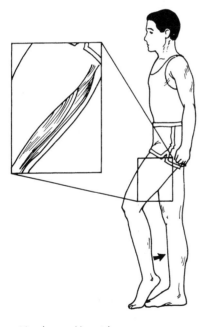

Muscle: Hamstrings
Level: L5, S1
Function: Flexes the knee
Resistance: Try to straighten the knee

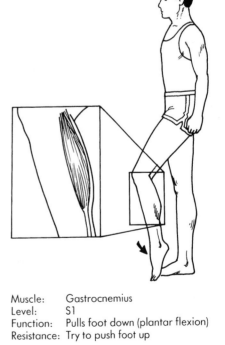

Muscle: Gastrocnemius
Level: S1
Function: Pulls foot down (plantar flexion)
Resistance: Try to push foot up

Figure 14-6, cont'd

TABLE 14-2	Symptoms Based on Tumor Location			
Location	Pain	Motor Impairment	Sensory Impairment	Sphincter Involvement
Cervical				
C4 and above	Occipital headache Stiff neck	Quadriparesis Diaphragm involved Respiratory failure when bilateral Respiratory difficulty with loss of intercostal and abdominal muscles if loss is unilateral Downbeat nystagmus Atrophy of shoulder and neck muscles Dysphagia Dysarthria	Vertigo Sensory loss within area of weakness	May have sacral sparing
C4 and below	Arms and shoulders	Atrophy of shoulder, arm, and hand with muscle fasciculations	Paresthesias without pain	
C5-C6	Medial aspect of arm			
C7-C8	Lateral forearm and hand	Horner's syndrome with C8 involvement		
Thoracic				
	Percussion tenderness over tumor location			
	Dermatomal pain	Beevor's sign* Spastic paresis in lower extremities Positive Babinski's sign	Band of hyperesthesia at dermatome of tumor site	Impaired bladder and bowel control
Lumbar/Cauda Equina				
	Lower extremities Low back One leg longer than other	Paresis of lower extremities Atrophy of lower extremity muscles Selected muscle groups involved in each patient Achilles and plantar reflexes absent or diminished	Paresthesias Loss in legs and saddle area	Early loss of bladder control

From Raney D: *J Neurosci Nurs* 23(1):44–49, 1991.
*Beevor's sign: when sitting up or raising head from the recumbent position, the umbilicus appears to displace toward the head because of paralysis of the internal portion of the rectus abdominal muscle.

Beevor's sign may be present with a lesion at the T10 level. When a patient sits up or raises the head from a recumbent position, the umbilicus is displaced toward the head. This is a late sign that occurs secondary to paralysis of the interior portion of the rectus abdominal muscle.

Lumbar Lesions
Patients with cancer of the lung, breast, prostate, and kidney may have metastases to the lumbar or cauda equina region.[78] Whether metastatic or primary, lesions of the lumbar and cauda equina region are characterized by pain, paresis, and a loss of strength in the lower extremity muscles. The pain can be very severe, and early loss of sphincter control is not uncommon.

Ongoing Assessment

The findings of the initial assessment determine the pain, sensory, and motor parameters pertinent to ongoing assessment for the individual patient. The use of a spinal cord flow sheet is recommended for continued assessment. The results of the initial neurodiagnostic studies will indicate follow-up studies that are pertinent to the ongoing care and treatment of the patient with a nontraumatic spinal cord disorder.

NEURODIAGNOSTIC AND LABORATORY STUDIES

Many neurodiagnostic studies are used in the initial evaluation of nontraumatic disorders of the spine. Clinicians should have some knowledge about these studies because of their role in preparing the patient for and educating the patient about these procedures, as well as providing postprocedure care (see Chapter 3). In a time of increasing awareness of costs, the choice of studies should be based on availability, perceived accuracy of the test, patient tolerance, and physician familiarity and comfort with the study.
- Myelography: useful in obtaining information about the characteristics, location, and spatial relationships among

spinal structures; can demonstrate the level of an abscess, widening of the cord, and blockage of cerebrospinal fluid (CSF) flow around the cord. Myelography was used in the past to differentiate spinal AVMs from other pathologies but is now performed most often when computed tomography (CT) and MRI are not feasible or available or in combination with CT and MRI.[33,64]

- Spinal angiography: gold standard for making a conclusive diagnosis of spinal AVM and for localizing the source of hemorrhages;[3,73] sometimes used intraoperatively to assess for residual filling of spinal AVMs;[7] contrast-enhanced, time-resolved MRA is being shown to be a diagnostic tool for safe, accurate diagnosis of spinal AVMs.[68]
- CT: beneficial in diagnosing osteomyelitis, spinal tuberculosis, disk disease, compression fractures, and other conditions that affect the vertebral column; useful in evaluating back pain, including FBSS. As many as 60% of cases of FBSS have been attributed to bony abnormalities, which a CT scan will readily demonstrate.[57]
- MRI: provides more detail of the pathologic condition of the spinal cord and surrounding soft tissue than either a CT scan or myelography; valuable in the diagnosis of spinal cord infarcts and fistulae;[3,46] an excellent technique for delineating a syrinx.[54,66] A gadolinium-enhanced MRI scan is useful in differentiating scar tissue from recurrent intervertebral disk herniation, as well as in delineating tumors.[11] It is useful in differentiating spinal cord infections from other intramedullary lesions.[61,75]
- Radionuclide scanning: can be performed with technetium, indium, and gallium; technetium labeling is useful for evaluating primary and metastatic neoplasms involving bone, stress fractures, osteomyelitis, and tuberculosis.[60]
- Single-photon emission computed tomography (SPECT): useful for localizing metastatic lesions. Where available, it is replacing general radionuclide scanning for localizing metastatic lesions.[82] It can define the site of the lesion within a given vertebra (i.e., pedicle versus facet), which cannot be done well with planar images.
- Electrodiagnostic studies: include electromyography (EMG), nerve conduction studies, somatosensory-evoked potentials (SSEPs), and motor-evoked potentials (MEPs). These studies help differentiate between motor neuron diseases, peripheral neuropathies, peripheral nerve entrapments, radiculopathies, and CNS disorders by supplying more detailed information about the muscles and the nerves innervating them. If available, they are more helpful when compared with previous studies and are most useful in the setting of new neuropathic complaints and symptoms.
  - MEPs: Used during embolization of an arteriovenous fistula to detect functional changes.[76]
  - SSEPs: Have become a valuable tool in the diagnosis of acquired immunodeficiency syndrome (AIDS)–associated myelopathy, particularly when myelopathy

and peripheral neuropathy coexist.[84] SSEPs are being tested in the evaluation of lumbosacral spinal stenosis and for intraoperative monitoring of spinal surgery.[49]
- Plain spinal films of the vertebral column: often helpful in identifying spinal tumors, but they do not image the spinal cord.

TREATMENT

Medical Management

The medical management of nontraumatic disorders of the spine varies according to their cause.

Tumors

The medical management of spinal cord tumors includes preoperative control of cord edema, as well as radiation and chemotherapy after surgical resection. The exact course of medical therapy depends on the pathology of the tumor.

Edema caused by a tumor is most commonly controlled with the corticosteroid dexamethasone (Decadron). Decadron is administered in an IV form using a large loading dose and then tapering the amount over the next few days. The patient's neurologic deficits should stabilize or improve as spinal cord edema decreases. Emergent surgical decompression is indicated if the patient's neurologic condition deteriorates.

Infections

IV antibiotics are begun as soon as any infection of the spine is suspected. As stated previously, the most common causative organism in spinal abscesses is *S. aureus*. The patient is thus started on an antibiotic appropriate to this organism until culture and sensitivity results prove the causative organism to be otherwise.[81]

Vertebral TB lesions and tuberculous meningitis are treated with immobility and appropriate drug therapy. The drug regimen of choice for TB is a combination of isoniazid, rifampin, and pyrazinamide for 2 months followed by a 4-month (or longer) course of isoniazid and rifampin.[93] Careful consideration goes into choosing a drug regimen for the individual with multidrug-resistant tuberculosis. Multidrug treatment may be instituted in geographic areas where drug-resistant disease and HIV infection are common. Treatment may begin with five to seven drugs until drug susceptibility results are known.[93]

Arteriovenous Malformations

Although open surgical procedures are still used for treatment, certain dural arteriovenous malformations (AVMs) can be treated with **embolization**.[33] This treatment was introduced in the 1970s but is not performed at all hospitals.[19] This procedure is most commonly performed in the angiography suite. To embolize an AVM, a catheter is introduced and placed as distal to the feeding artery as possible; an occluding substance is then introduced.[33] Embolization is sometimes performed as an isolated treatment. It is often performed in conjunction with surgery, whereby a portion of the AVM is embolized and a portion surgically removed. The complications of embolization include hematoma at the catheter insertion site, occlusion of the wrong artery, an inability to introduce the catheter into the intended artery, and emboli resulting from occlusive material. Arteriovenous fistulae are often embolized. Detachable coils, originally used for occlusion of cerebral aneurysms, are now being used in some centers for the treatment of these fistulae.[8] Radiosurgical treatment of spinal AVMs is becoming a practical therapeutic option as methodology is improving.[34]

Degenerative Disk Disease

Medical management may be used before or instead of surgical management to treat degenerative disk disease. Most cases of LBP and sciatica may improve with conservative treatment consisting of 1 to 2 days of bed rest, nonsteroidal antiinflammatory medications, exercise regimens, epidural steroids, and patient education.[18] A cervical collar may be ordered for cervical disorders to assist in pain relief. For those receiving conservative therapy, efforts should be made to strengthen back muscles, because fitness and strength are postulated to protect an individual from disk rupture.[40] Samples of appropriate exercises are found in Fig. 14-7.

Long-term follow-up (4 to 10 years) of patients undergoing conservative treatment has showed no difference in outcome from those treated with surgery. There was approximately 60% improvement in both groups. However, there were indications that patients who did not receive surgery experienced more episodes of LBP and sciatica and lost more time from work. Studies done more recently indicate that patients with mild symptoms on presentation show no significant advantage with surgery.[96] Approximately 90% of patients will experience resolution of symptoms within 1 month without surgical treatment.[96] However, patients who had surgery for severe or moderate symptoms showed significantly greater improvement in leg and back pain at the 1-year follow-up.[69]

FBSS is best treated on an outpatient basis through a comprehensive team approach. Newer diagnostic studies have made it possible to identify the pathology of previously unrecognized FBSS. A referral to a pain clinic is often the most appropriate course of action, because an interdisciplinary team is generally available in these clinics. Many new treatments or improvements on historically used treatments are being used to help patients cope with the continuing pain associated with this syndrome. Some of these methods include intraspinal opioids delivered via implanted pumps, intrathecal medications, and spinal cord stimulators.[57]

Medical treatment may first include a thorough evaluation of medications to ensure the proper use of narcotics and muscle relaxants. In general, a program of education, physical reconditioning, behavior management, and vocational counseling is used. Team members focus on educating the patient, significant others, and other family members on the following:

- Physiology and psychology of chronic pain
- Structure and function of the human back
- Behavioral principles for managing symptoms and lifestyle

- Body mechanics and back care
- Pharmacology of pain medications
- Appropriate use of the medical system

Compression Fractures

The treatment of benign osteoporotic compression fractures includes bed rest, analgesics, external bracing, and medical management of the osteoporosis in an attempt to prevent future fractures.[52] Surgical procedures are occasionally offered to patients suffering from compressions resulting from metastases, myeloma, or hemangioma.[12]

Surgical Management

Surgery is usually indicated if the nontraumatic disorder is causing compression on the spinal cord or for patients with radiculopathy that fails conservative treatment. Progressive neurologic deterioration constitutes a surgical emergency except in the case of overwhelming metastatic invasion. Rapid decompression may lead to a successful return of full function. Surgery may be scheduled electively if rapid neurologic deterioration is not present. Clinicians must be familiar with the parts of a vertebral body to understand the surgical procedures used to treat these disorders. A cross section of the L5 vertebral body and its parts is shown in Fig. 14-8.

Surgical techniques for nontraumatic disorders are rapidly changing and improving. The most common procedure is the decompression laminectomy. A **laminectomy** is the removal of the lamina portion of the vertebrae to gain access to the spinal cord. A posterior approach is the most common method, but anterior approaches are becoming more common. Clinicians should understand several other terms used in surgical discussions:

- **Hemilaminectomy:** a procedure in which only a portion of the lamina is excised.
- **Foraminotomy:** the enlargement of the intravertebral foramen to remove tension on the nerve root. This procedure is very effective when one nerve root is affected and radicular symptoms are present.
- **Vertebrectomy/corpectomy:** the removal of the body of the vertebra.
- **Fusion:** involves the use of a bone graft across the vertebral space to prevent active motion across that space. Autologous grafts are most commonly obtained from the lateral aspect of the ilium. Freeze-dried or irradiated bone bank graft material can be used.[29] Interbody **titanium cages** have been introduced as a method of providing structural support and encouraging fusion (Fig. 14-9).[67] These devices provide immediate stabilization, reduce or eliminate pain, promote bone fusion between the vertebrae adjacent to the cage by allowing bone growth through the cage, reestablish and maintain the intervertebral space, reduce the average hospitalization time, and allow a quicker return to work.[67]
- **Instrumentation:** the use of rods, screws, plates, wires, or other devices with laminectomy to provide stability to the spine (Fig. 14-10).

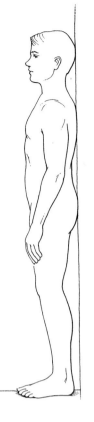

A

STANDING POSTURE

Components of standing with a neutral spine **(A)**:

- Head held with chin tucked in
- Chest held high with shoulders and arms relaxed
- Stomach muscles held firm
- Knees straight but not locked
- Feet parallel

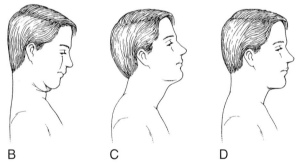

B   C   D

Exercises to help find neutral spine position and maintain a healthy standing posture:

1. Head and neck neutral spine
   - While standing, tuck chin down slightly and pull head back and up as if to flatten neck against a wall **(B)**.
   - Looking straight ahead, jut chin forward as if moving neck away from the wall **(C)**.
   - Slowly repeat these movements five times to learn the range of comfortable movement of neck.
   - After the last repetition, allow head to find a comfortable position between the two movements **(D)**.
   - This is the healthy posture position for head and neck.

Figure 14-7 Sample exercises to strengthen back muscles. (*From* Care of the Back, *Mayo Clinic, Rochester, MN.*)

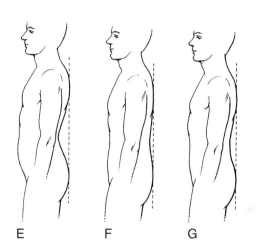

E   F   G

2. Lower back neutral spine
   - While standing, arch lower back **(E)**.
   - Tighten abdominal muscles as if to flatten lower back against a wall **(F)**.
   - Slowly repeat these movements five times to learn the range of comfortable motion of lower spine.
   - On the last repetition, instead of flattening lower back, slowly move from the arched position to find a relaxed, balanced, comfortable position for spine **(G)**.
   - This is the healthy posture position for lower back.

Maintain a healthy posture for head, neck, and lower back when moving about by making slight adjustments of neck or abdominal muscles. Help prevent or manage back pain by maintaining a neutral spine position.

Practice finding healthy posture positions during daily activities.

3. The wall test
After finding neutral spine position, use the wall test to help develop and maintain a healthy posture while standing:

- Stand against a wall with heels approximately 2 to 4 inches away from the wall.
- Stand with head, shoulder blades, and buttocks against the wall.
- Reach back with hand and place palm flat against the wall.
- Slide your hand behind the small of back.
- There is typically one hand's thickness of space between the small of back and the wall.
- If there is more than one hand's thickness of space between the small of back and the wall, tighten abdominal muscles and gently push back against your hand.
- If there is too little space, arch back just enough so hand fits comfortably behind back.

Continued

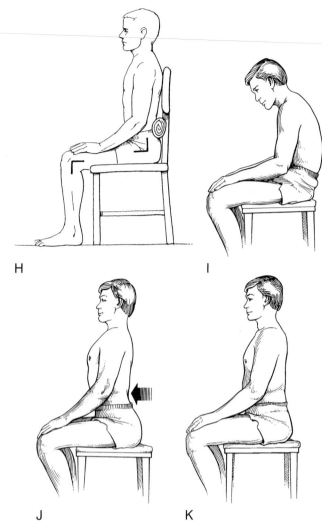

H   I

J   K

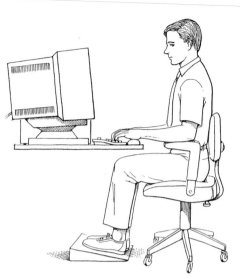

L

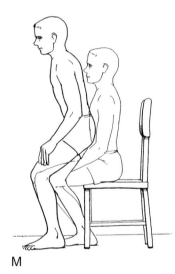

M

SITTING POSTURE

When sitting with a neutral spine (**H**), feet are flat on the floor, knees and hips are bent at a right angle (the rule of "90s"), and low back curve is supported by the chair or by a lumbar support such as a rolled towel or cushion.

- For most people, the height of the chair should allow both feet to rest flat on the floor, while the knees are at the same level as the pelvis.
- If position is not comfortable, adjust the height of chair or place a foot support under feet to find the best position.
- Choose a sitting surface that provides support of lower back (lumbar region).
- Ideally, chair should have a back rest located to fit in the small of back. If one is not available, a rolled towel can be used.

Develop and maintain a healthy posture while sitting by finding neutral spine position. To find this position, practice the following exercise:

- Slouch while sitting in chair by allowing head to come forward and rounding out upper back (**I**).
- Sit up straight, arching the small of back (**J**).
- Repeat these movements 5 times.
- After the last repetition, instead of slouching, slowly move from the arched position to find a relaxed, balanced, comfortable position for spine (**K**).

Figure 14-7, cont'd

- This position is a neutral spine or healthy posture while sitting.
- Practice maintaining healthy posture during daily activities.

Maintaining proper sitting posture at a computer or desk

When working at a computer or desk (**L**), it is important to sit with balanced posture, maintaining the same spinal curves as when sitting in a neutral spine position (**M**).

To develop a balanced sitting posture, practice the following:

- Stretch the top of head toward the ceiling.
- Tuck chin in slightly.
- Keep upper back and neck comfortably straight.
- Keep shoulders relaxed, not elevated, rounded, or pulled backward.
- Maintain low back curve (adjust chair's lumbar support).
- Adjust seat so that it does not press into the backs of knees (allow 2 to 3 finger widths between chair and back of knees).

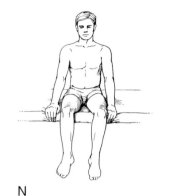

N

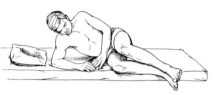

O

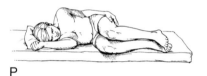

P

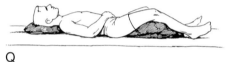

Q

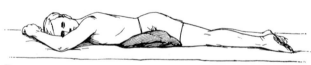

R

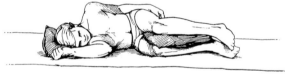

S

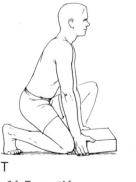
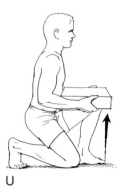

T   U

Figure 14-7, cont'd

- Rest feet comfortably on the floor or on a foot rest.
- Distribute weight evenly over back of thighs.
- Keep knees about level with hips.

The purpose of a balanced posture while sitting at a desk is to keep neck, shoulders, and upper back muscles relaxed. Developing a healthy posture requires practice. The basic skills can be learned quickly, but need regular practice and use over months or even years for posture to become balanced, relaxed, and automatic.

LYING DOWN

When lying down from a sitting position, be sure to maintain a healthy posture.

- Start by sitting on the bed so that head will *hit the pillow* when lying down **(N).**
- Using arms for support, slowly lower onto the bed while bringing legs up to a side-lying position **(O, P).** This allows maintenance of neutral spine while changing positions.
- When sitting up from a lying position, first roll to side with your knees bent. Then slide feet over the edge of the bed while using arms to push body up to a sitting position.

Maintain position of healthy posture while lying down.

- When lying flat on back, place a small pillow under knees or thighs to help maintain the normal curve of lower back **(Q).**
- A small rolled towel may be placed under the small of back for additional support.
- When lying on abdomen, place a pillow under pelvis and lower abdomen **(R).**
- When lying on side, bend knees and place a pillow between them **(S).** A small rolled towel may be placed under waist to help maintain normal spinal curves.

REACHING

When reaching for objects, be certain to get as close to the object as possible to avoid overextending arms and trunk. Use positions that prevent arching and twisting of back.

KNEELING METHOD

- Stand as close as possible to the object to be lifted **(T).**
- Find a neutral spine position, and maintain it during the activity.
- Keep feet 8 to 12 inches apart.
- Place one foot forward.
- Keep weight on the balls of your feet.
- Lower body down to one knee by bending at the hips and knees.
- Lift the object from between the legs and hold it close to body.
- If the object is heavy, first lift it to rest it on bent knee **(U).**

Continued

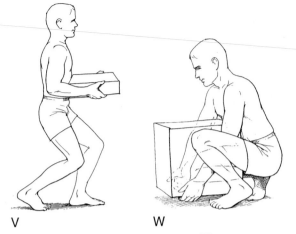

V   W

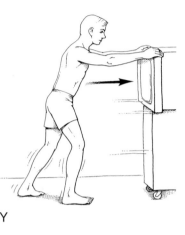

Y

- Use leg muscles to rise from the floor (**V**).
- **Do NOT twist** body while lifting or carrying the object—turn by pivoting on feet.
- Use this method for lifting and carrying small children.

SQUATTING METHOD

Following the same procedure as with kneeling but squat rather than kneel (**W**). Lift the object from between legs, holding it close to body.

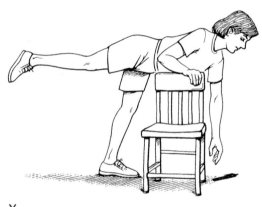

X

GOLFER'S LIFT

Use the golfer's lift when picking up light objects. Stand on one leg. Bend forward at the waist, maintaining neutral spine position, and extend other leg out behind for balance. Reach down with the arm opposite extended leg to pick up the object (**X**). Hold on to the back of a chair or other support for added balance.

When returning to a standing position, bring extended leg down while maintaining neutral spine position.

PUSHING

When pushing an object, bend knees so arms are level with the object. Keep elbows slightly bent. Lean toward the object while maintaining a neutral spine position. Push the object forward using leg muscles (**Y**).

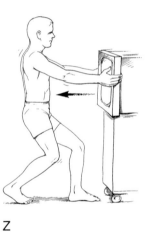

Z

PULLING

When pulling an object, bend knees so arms are level with the object. Keep elbows slightly bent. Lean away from the object while maintaining neutral spine position. Pull the object by using body weight and leg muscles (**Z**).

Reminders about pushing or pulling objects:
- If possible, push rather than pull.
- Place heavy objects on casters.
- If the object is too large or heavy, seek help.

Figure 14-7, cont'd

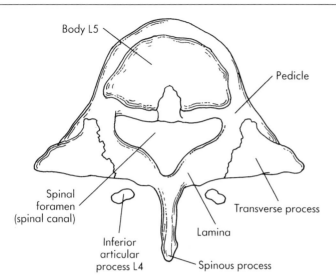

Figure 14-8 Cross section of vertebra.

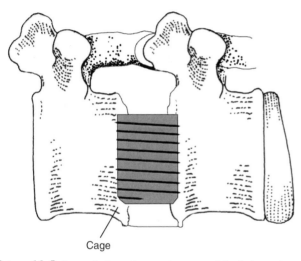

Figure 14-9 Lateral view of cage placement *(shaded area)*. *(From Kaye AH, Black P, editors:* Operative neurosurgery, *New York, 2000, Churchill Livingstone.)*

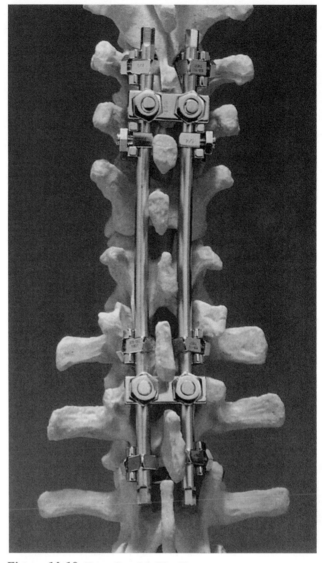

Figure 14-10 Texas Scottish Rite System. *(Courtesy Medtronic Sofamor Danek, Memphis, TN.)*

Tumors

The surgical management of the patient with a spinal cord tumor depends on the tumor type and neurologic status of the patient. The most common procedure is the decompression laminectomy. The use of a laminectomy in these cases generally involves decompression, stabilization, and fusion.[12,48] Radiation and IV chemotherapy are commonly used after the tumor has been debulked surgically. The prognosis for benign spinal cord tumors that have been resected and irradiated is excellent.[98] Radiation, if given, is started 3 to 4 weeks after surgery. This allows the incision time to heal.

Malignant spinal cord tumors have a dismal prognosis after resection and radiation; therefore radiation is used as a palliative treatment in many patients with malignant tumors. Procedures such as endoscopy, vertebroplasty, kyphoplasty, and stereotactic radiosurgery are also being offered to patients with metastatic disease.[1,12,43]

Infections

The surgical management of infections corresponds to the location and degree of spinal cord compression.[25] An abscess can be easily removed if it is encapsulated or has a wall surrounding it. If the abscess is localized with no wall, it can usually be aspirated.[79] Hemilaminectomy at one or more levels can be sufficient to drain an abscess posterior to the dura.[58] More extensive infections may include the vertebra, and a vertebrectomy may be warranted.[58] Fusion or instrumentation is generally included in these surgeries to provide stabilization.[48] Devices such as the halo vest can be used with cervical spine (C-spine) surgeries to provide postoperative stability and allow bone to heal. Organism-specific antibiotics with surgery remains the treatment of choice.[62]

Arteriovenous Malformations

Laminectomy is the surgery of choice for AVMs of the spine to expose the lesion. In dural lesions, the abnormal arterialized draining vein is clipped and excised.[33] A microsurgical technique is usually used for intradural lesions. The arachnoid is opened, and the largest vessels are clipped and cauterized. The lesion is gradually pulled away from the spinal cord, and any additional arterial feeders are coagulated and divided.[33]

Disk Disease

Surgical treatment of disk disease uses a variety of procedures depending on the pathologic condition and location. An anterior diskectomy and fusion is used for single-level or multilevel cervical disease. Posterior cervical fusion often includes wiring and screw fixations. As with spinal cord tumors and infections, laminectomy is the most common surgical procedure used for a degenerated or herniated lumbar disk.

A laminectomy is performed on the thoracic or lumbar spine. During the procedure, the affected vertebrae are exposed by dissecting the muscles of the spine. After the lamina of the vertebrae is removed, the ligament is incised to expose the underlying dura mater and nerve root, and the degenerated disk is removed.[64] The purpose is to relieve pressure exerted on the exiting nerve root by the disk, which is producing neurologic findings or pain.[64] Figure 14-11 illustrates the laminectomy procedure for the removal of a protruding disk.

Indications for a lumbar laminectomy in disk disease include the following:[69]

- Progressive neurologic deficits
- Loss of bladder and bowel control
- Significant neurologic deficit with reduced ability for straight-leg raising
- Radiographic evidence of an extruded disk within the spinal canal
- Recurrent episodes of sciatica
- Failure of conservative medical treatment

The operating microscope has allowed surgeons to use a smaller incision for disk removal. The microscope provides excellent illumination and magnification of the surgical field, thereby facilitating a less traumatic surgical technique.[69] Proponents of this technique believe that patients experience less morbidity and improved surgical outcomes.[69] Patients who

have been found to be good candidates for the microscopic approach include those with the following conditions:[69]

- Foraminal disk herniation
- Disk rupture in the setting of a stenotic canal
- Axillary disk herniation (most common at L5-S1)
- Reoperation for recurrent disk rupture

Artificial Disk Replacement. Technologic developments are improving such that some proponents believe that total disk replacement may have the potential to replace fusion as the gold standard surgical treatment for degenerative disk disease. Devices are coming into the market that fall into two main categories: disk nucleus replacement devices and total disk replacement devices.[90] The aim of this technology is to develop a prosthesis that would restore disk space height and lordosis, restore segmental motion, generate physiologic kinetics at the spinal triple joint complex, and serve as a shock absorber. It would also be biocompatible and durable for greater than 40 years.[90] Success has been reported by some surgeons with these devices;[90] however, only short-term and midterm results have been reported in the literature.[90,92] Complications from the surgery have also been reported, which are related to technical difficulties that need to be solved.[92]

Minimally Invasive Disk Decompression. Several percutaneous intradiscal therapies have been developed over the past 40 years. These are aimed at relieving chronic discogenic back pain or radicular leg pain without the risks of open disk surgery. They include chemonucleolysis, percutaneous nucleotomy, percutaneous diskectomy, intradiscal laser treatments, intradiscal radiofrequency ablation, intradiscal electrothermal annuloplasty, and nucleoplasty.[18] All of these techniques are designed to partially remove the nucleus pulposus and reduce intradiscal pressure.

Chemonucleolysis was the first percutaneous intradiscal therapy introduced approximately 40 years ago. The enzyme chymopapain was used to dissolve the nucleus pulposus. This procedure was studied extensively, and although it did provide relief to carefully selected patients, it had anaphylactic immunologic reactions thought to be induced by antigens of the chymopapain protein.[18] This led to neurotoxic side effects of the procedure. The production of chymopapain was

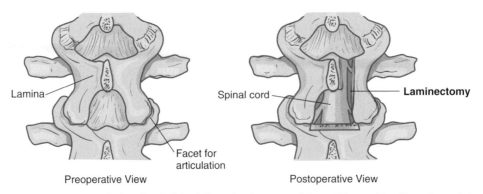

Lamina

Facet for articulation

Preoperative View

Spinal cord

Laminectomy

Postoperative View

Figure 14-11 Laminotomy exposure of a herniated disk. A 2 cm laminotomy of the trailing and leading edges of the opposing laminae followed by excision of the ligamentum flavum exposes the epidural space. Retraction over the shoulder of the nerve root should expose a ventral, medial, or lateral disk herniation. The integrity of the facets and facet joint is preserved.
(From Black JM, Hawks JH: Medical-surgical nursing: clinical management for positive outcomes, ed 7, Philadelphia, 2005, WB Saunders.)

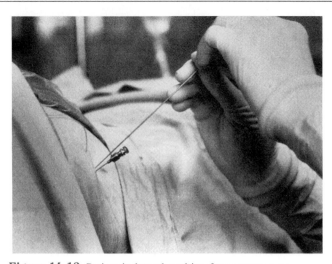

Figure 14-12 Patient in lateral position for percutaneous lumbar surgery.

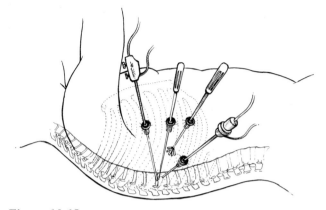

Figure 14-13 Endoscopic thoracic diskectomy. The instruments are inserted under direct vision and centered around the affected disk space.
(From Kaye AH, Black P, editors: Operative neurosurgery, *New York, 2000, Churchill Livingstone.)*

stopped in the United States in 1999.[18] It is mentioned in this chapter because clinicians may encounter patients who had chemonucleolysis in the past and are returning with follow-up issues or problems.

Percutaneous Lumbar Diskectomy. Since the introduction of arthroscopic techniques for percutaneous disk removal in the 1990s, numerous endoscopic procedures have been developed. Endoscopic procedures have been used in lumbar and thoracic disk removals and may soon be used for cervical procedures.[32] With the patient in a prone position, percutaneous arthroscopic microdiskectomy allows direct visualization of the annulus, periannular structures, and disk space in the lumbar region[32] (Fig. 14-12). It facilitates debulking of the nucleus pulposus with decompression of the posterior portion of the intervertebral disk and extraction of the posterior nuclear fragments.[32] Use of the technique has expanded for treatment of far-lateral disk herniations.[18]

Endoscopic Thoracic Diskectomy. Endoscopic thoracic diskectomy is another relatively new procedure. Less than 1% of disk-related hospital admissions are for thoracic disk herniations. However, a classic laminectomy for thoracic disks is associated with high rates of morbidity and mortality because of the need for excessive cord manipulation.[32] The technique of microsurgical endoscopy allows for the exposure of T2 to T12-L1 disk spaces.[32] Patients are placed in a lateral decubitus position with the affected side up.[32] Figure 14-13 shows the introduction of the endoscope.

Laparoscopic Diskectomy. Laparoscopic diskectomy has been used in some centers since the 1990s.[87] Retroperitoneal laparoscopic procedures have been tried for lateral disk lesions, with successful cases reported.[87] Laparoscopic spinal fusions are also reported.[44] A **laser-assisted laparoscopic lumbar diskectomy** excises the disk with the aid of a laser and standard disk instruments that have been modified to fit through the laparoscopic cannulae.

During laparoscopic lumbar procedure, the patient is placed in a steep Trendelenburg position before the abdomen is prepared for surgery. A laparoscopic trocar is inserted periumbilically, the abdomen is inflated with carbon dioxide,

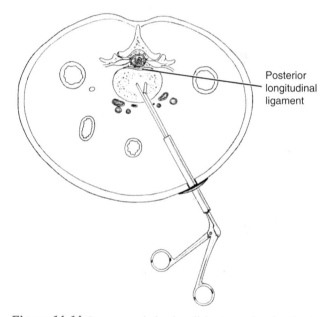

Figure 14-14 Laparoscopic lumbar diskectomy showing the insertion of a laparoscopic trocar at the L5-S1 interspace.
(Courtesy Dr. S. C. Stein, MD, Cooper Medical Center, Camden, NJ.)

and additional trocars are placed above the pelvic brim. After the large and small bowels are retracted and the iliac bifurcation has been identified and confirmed by Doppler ultrasound, the posterior peritoneum is sharply opened and retracted. After the disk is located by direct inspection and its margins are confirmed by x-ray examination, the annulus of the disk is opened and removed[87] (Fig. 14-14). New developments in lasers and endoscopy that improve the view may facilitate the use of this technique and permit treatment for more severe herniated disks.[18]

Intradiscal Radiofrequency Ablation. Intradiscal radiofrequency ablation is another technique being studied for treatment of chronic LBP. This technique uses a high-frequency alternating current through the intradiscal needle electrode to produce a lesion in the nucleus pulposus, reducing nociceptive input from a painful intervertebral disk.[18] Needle position and heating parameters are undergoing research at this time.

Intradiscal Electrothermal Annuloplasty. Intradiscal electrothermal annuloplasty is another minimally invasive procedure receiving study.[18] This procedure is believed to relieve pain by way of thermal ablation of nerve endings and not by decreasing intradiscal pressure. It has shown promising results in carefully selected patients.

Nucleoplasty. Nucleoplasty was approved for use by the U.S. Food and Drug Administration (FDA) in 2001 as a treatment for contained herniated disks. It is a non–heat-driven process that uses Coblation technology, based on bipolar radiofrequency technology applied to a conductive medium (e.g., saline) to achieve tissue removal with minimal thermal damage to collateral tissues.[18] Many physicians find this procedure easier to perform than nucleotomy.[18] Nucleoplasty does not replace microdiskectomy or fusion, but helps fill the gap between conservative treatments and open spinal procedures.

Compression Fractures

Patients with vertebral compression fractures who have prolonged and debilitating pain may be offered a procedure called **vertebroplasty.** This procedure was developed in France in the 1980s and became popular in the United States in the 1990s. Before the procedure, the patient's x-ray films, MRI scans, CT scans, or bone scans are reviewed by the radiologist to determine the fracture(s) causing the pain. The patient is seen for an initial consultation with a radiologist who reviews the patient's history. A physical examination of the back is performed under fluoroscopic observation in order to localize the patient's pain and thus identify if the patient could potentially benefit from vertebroplasty.

To be considered for the procedure, the patient's pain must be reproducible with manual palpation directly over the posterior aspect of the compressed vertebra.[52] Currently only one out of seven patients who undergo initial fluoroscopic screening is identified as an appropriate candidate for vertebroplasty.[89] Relative contraindications include patients with uncorrectable coagulopathies and patients with coexisting medical conditions that prohibit lying prone for the expected 1 to 2 hours of the procedure.[4] Patients with metastatic lesions and a loss of integrity of the posterior cortex of the vertebral body are considered to have a relative contraindication and are approached on a case-by-case basis.

Vertebroplasty is performed by a radiologist in an angiography suite using fluoroscopic x-ray guidance to place a large-bore hollow needle into the compressed vertebral body. The patient is placed under conscious sedation. Once the needle is positioned, polymethylmethacrylate bone cement is injected into the vertebral body under direct fluoroscopic observation[4] (Fig. 14-15). The cement stabilizes the fracture and, for approximately 80% of patients, relieves the pain.[4] The patient remains on bed rest for 1 hour to allow the cement to harden and the patient's conscious sedation to wear off.[4] Depending on their preexisting health status, patients may stay overnight or be discharged later the same day of

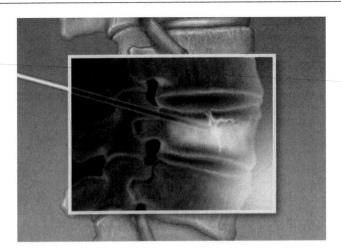

Figure 14-15 Percutaneous vertebroplasty. In the vertebroplasty procedure, a needle is inserted into the compressed vertebral body by a percutaneous transpedicular approach, and the compressed vertebral body is filled with bone cement.
(From Mayo Clinic, Mayo Clinical Update *15[3], 1999, Rochester, MN.)*

the procedure. The patient may resume normal activity and should experience a significant reduction in pain within a few days. Patients may report muscle spasms or tenderness at the puncture sites for a few days following the procedure.

Complications related to vertebroplasty are rare but include "cement" pulmonary embolism, infection, neurologic injury, and rib fracture.[4] Because of increased activity by the patients as the result of less pain, some develop additional new compression fractures of other vertebral bodies.

Kyphoplasty is another technique with the goal to stop pain caused by bone fracture and to stabilize the bone; however, this procedure also restores some or all of the lost vertebral body height due to the compression fracture. The procedure is similar to vertebroplasty in terms of positioning and technique. The difference is that special balloons are inserted into the vertebrae and inflated. The balloon inflation elevates the fracture and compacts the soft inner bone to create a cavity inside the vertebrae. The balloon is removed and polymethylmethacrylate is injected into the cavity under low pressure, decreasing the risk of cement leakage.[10,51] Additional research on this technique is occurring worldwide.

Syringomyelia and Syringobulbia

The goal in the treatment of syringomyelia and syringobulbia is to halt destruction of the nervous system by compression. Surgery is most commonly undertaken to drain and decompress the syrinx cavity. A laminectomy or hemilaminectomy is used to expose the spinal canal, and a shunt or a small tube is inserted to divert the fluid.[88] This fluid is usually diverted to the subarachnoid space or peritoneal cavity.[45] Posterior fossa decompression utilizing suboccipital craniectomy and duraplasty remains the standard surgical treatment for Chiari-associated syringomyelia.[21] A syringosubarachnoid shunt can be used for syringomyelia associated with **Chiari malformation.**[36] A lumboperitoneal shunt combined with myelotomy of the caudal spinal cord may also be used for surgical treatment of a syrinx.[88]

Acute and Preoperative Care

Management of the patient with a nontraumatic disorder of the spine presents a challenge because of the diverse variables involved. If spinal instability is present, care is similar to that of a patient with a spinal cord injury (see Chapter 12). Specific care depends on the findings of the initial assessment concerning functional status, the level of the disorder, and the associated neurologic signs, symptoms, and deficits.

Acute care management of the patient with a nontraumatic disorder of the spine is directed toward stabilizing the patient's condition and preparing him or her for therapy. The primary goal during this period is preventing neurologic deterioration through early detection of changes and appropriate interventions. The problem of spinal instability is less prevalent in these patients than in patients with a traumatic disorder. Nevertheless, instability must be considered in cases in which a tumor or infection invades the vertebral column.

Assessment

Assessment begins on admission and should provide baseline data about functional status, level of the lesion, and associated problems.

If the surgery is elective, the patient should be questioned about the availability of donating autologous blood for surgery. If autologous blood is not available, family members can be encouraged to donate for the patient. The clinician must check with the local blood bank for requirements, because procedures do vary, and a physician prescription is sometimes required for patient-directed donations. Patients should be assessed for smoking habits. Smokers are both more likely to have degenerative disk disease and spondylosis and more likely to experience fusion failure.[13] Patients who smoke have been shown to experience a decrease in bone mineral density that is believed to interfere with healing and increase the risk of fracture.[13]

Expected Outcomes

Expected outcomes for the patient during the preoperative phase include the following:[53]
- Safety behavior and fall prevention
- Knowledge of the disease process and treatment regimen
- Fear control

Interventions

Interventions to prevent further injury need to be individualized according to the level of neurologic dysfunction. Regardless of the level of neurologic injury, each patient needs ongoing assessment and documentation of signs and symptoms, with attention given to the area of deficit. Any significant worsening of deficits (e.g., progressive weakness) needs to be reported to the physician for immediate attention. In addition to the ongoing assessment, the clinician must use interventions to protect the patient from injuries that

---

BOX 14-1	**Interventions for Patients With Sacral and Lumbar Lesions Causing Neurologic Dysfunction**

- Provide range of motion to affected extremities at least once a shift.
- Turn patient every 2 hours if he or she is unable to do so voluntarily.
- Establish a bowel program with increased dietary fiber, increased fluids, stool softeners, and stimulants as needed.
- Use a urinary catheter or intermittent catheterization program for bladder management.
- Use heparinization or a sequential compression device (SCD) to prevent deep vein thrombosis (DVT) and pulmonary embolism (PE).

---

result from respiratory complications or complications of immobility.

A patient with a complete lesion at the C4 level and above will be intubated and mechanically ventilated. The patient with a lesion below the C4 level may need temporary ventilatory support. Any patient with a cervical lesion may need assistance with secretion management, including suctioning at least every 2 hours. A multidisciplinary approach is needed, with the goal being to wean the patient from the ventilator as early as possible (see Chapter 12).

Patients with a C4 to T1 lesion experience a loss of intercostal muscle innervation, which results in total reliance on the diaphragm for breathing. These patients also need respiratory support, including possible assisted coughing at least every 4 hours because they have difficulty bringing up secretions and maintaining a patent airway (see Chapter 12).

Patients with sacral and lumbar disorders may have lower extremity weakness and altered bowel and bladder function, and appropriate nursing interventions are needed (Box 14-1).

The coordination of preoperative responsibilities is an important nursing function in preparing the patient for surgery. In addition to following the institution-specific checklist, the clinician must make sure that all needed equipment accompanies the patient to the operating room (OR). If the patient is scheduled for cervical surgery, a collar is often ordered and stays with the patient for immediate postoperative application. Depending on the length of the surgical procedure or the patient's medical history, thigh-high compression stockings with an alternating sequential compression device (SCD) may need to be applied before surgery. These may be ordered for delivery to the OR, or may accompany the patient. IV antibiotics also sometimes accompany the patient to the OR. The necessary equipment varies according to the individual institution and physician protocols.

Health Teaching. Family and patient teaching is the most important intervention in alleviating knowledge deficits and fear. There is little time for preparation and teaching of the patient and the family if the patient is admitted through the emergency department. Patient and family teaching should focus on information about the diagnosis and surgical procedure, especially if the patient has never undergone surgery. The patient and family should be prepared for the postoperative experience, and printed material should be provided during the admission workup. This material varies according to institution, but general topics to be addressed are outlined in Boxes 14-2 and 14-3.

Nutritional Care. Optimal nutritional status is important for the surgical candidate to facilitate wound healing. In the absence of progressive neurologic deterioration, the physician may require the obese patient to lose a specified amount of weight before surgery. The malnourished patient may need nutritional supplements during the preoperative and postoperative periods. Providing good nutritional support is always a collaborative venture among the patient, physician, nurse, nutritionist, and family.

Attention should also be directed toward addressing nutritional and patient/caregiver/family teaching. Preoperative assessment of mental and functional status in the older patient can be a useful guide when planning postoperative goals and can provide early identification of those patients who may be at highest risk for perioperative complications.

Recovery Pathways

Patients with nontraumatic disorders of the spine are admitted to the neuroscience unit in one of three ways: (1) through the emergency department, (2) preoperatively (occasionally) as a scheduled elective admission, or (3) postoperatively from a same-day surgical unit. The pathways for recovery for each of these types of admissions will differ.

Patients admitted through the emergency department are emergencies and are experiencing acute neurologic deterioration. These patients undergo diagnostic testing, emergency surgery, and treatment as indicated by their condition. The pathway for recovery for these patients is affected by many variables, including level of injury, number of diagnostic tests used, extensiveness of surgery, and family support.

Patients with a scheduled elective admission may undergo diagnostic studies one day and surgery the next day. Some admitted patients have had their diagnostic workup completed on an outpatient basis and have surgery on the day of admission. The office nurse, the nurse admitting the patient in the same-day surgery area, or the admitting nurse practitioner will prepare and teach patients who are admitted electively.

Patients who arrive on the neuroscience unit postoperatively have the shortest pathway for recovery. The variables affecting recovery in these patients include age, preoperative condition, and postoperative complications. Postoperative complications for this patient group are discussed later in this chapter.

BOX 14-2	Laminectomy: Topics for Discussion

Lumbar Laminectomy

Expect pain or spasms in the low back, abdominal, or thigh regions.

Efforts will be made to manage postoperative pain.

Preoperative pain may not be relieved immediately after the operation; some patients do not experience pain relief until after discharge from the hospital.

A brace may be ordered postoperatively depending on physician preference.

Cervical Laminectomy/Fusion

Pain or spasms are present in the upper back, shoulder, neck, or arm region.

A cervical collar is sometimes required postoperatively.

A sore throat should be expected for an anterior approach.

BOX 14-3	General Preoperative Teaching Guidelines

Preoperative Procedure

Nothing by mouth (NPO status) after midnight the day of surgery

Special skin scrub, shave (not all physicians order a shave), or shower IV started (when, by whom)

Preoperative medication (when, route)

Precautions after medications (two side rails up after narcotics)

Safekeeping of jewelry, dentures, personal belongings, valuables

Gown only to operating suite

Other procedures that might occur

Postoperative Procedure

Waking up in the postanesthesia care unit (PACU)

Pain control (patient-controlled analgesia [PCA] or IM/IV injections)

Use of a pain scale for communicating pain intensity

Use of incentive spirometer and coughing

Sequential compression device (SCD) (if not able to walk within hours of surgery)

Mobility expectations

Frequency of isometric exercises

Rate of diet advancement

IM, Intramuscular; *IV,* intravenous.

Postoperative Management

The goals of postoperative care following a laminectomy are to prevent injury and manage acute pain.

Assessment

There are many areas to assess in the patient following a laminectomy. The clinician conducts a comprehensive assessment, and a postoperative flow sheet assists in concise documentation of the following:

- Review of systems: with attention given to any problem areas identified in the preoperative assessment
- Vital signs: every 15 minutes for the first hour, every 30 minutes for the next hour, every hour for the next 2 hours, and then every 4 hours until the patient is assessed to be stable
- Level of consciousness: should be assessed each time vital signs are monitored

- Extremities: evaluation for movement of all four extremities
- Output: urinary output
- IV: site and dressing
- Skin: redness, intact skin

The clinician needs to know the position in which the patient's surgery was performed (e.g., prone, supine, knee-chest, sitting, lateral position). Figures 14-16 to 14-19 show intraoperative positioning. Special attention is given to padding dependent areas in the OR, but it is essential to assess and document any skin breakdown postoperatively. Patients who are immobile should be turned every 2 hours around-the-clock to prevent skin breakdown (or more frequently based on skin assessment).

Much of the focus of the postoperative assessment is on detecting the signs and symptoms of surgical complications. For example, a decrease in blood pressure, an increase in heart rate, a change in level of consciousness, a decrease in movement or sensation, and saturation of surgical dressing may indicate hemorrhage, and the physician should be notified immediately.

Expected Outcomes

Expected outcomes for the patient in the postoperative phase of care include the following:

- Risk control[53]
- Mobility level
- Pain control

Potential Complications

The patient is at high risk for injury following a laminectomy related to postoperative surgical complications. The main goal is early detection of complications to prevent permanent injury. Complications can result from the following:

- Hematoma formation
- Cord edema
- Surgical trauma
- Cerebrospinal fluid leak
- Infection (symptoms develop later)
- Diskitis (symptoms develop later)

Hematoma formation is a rare but a serious complication following a laminectomy.[28,47] **Cauda equina syndrome (CES)** is an injury or compression of any of the lumbosacral nerve roots within the neural canal below the lumber vertebra (L1). Considered a lower motor neuron (LMN) injury, the patient may initially complain of loss of sensation in the

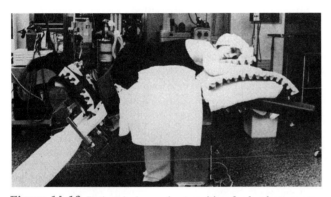

Figure 14-16 Patient in knee-chest position for lumbar surgery. Blanket chest rolls are used, with the arms padded, placed on armboards, and flexed less than 90 degrees. Upper and lower legs are padded, flexed, and supported in table knee supports. The head is turned to the side.

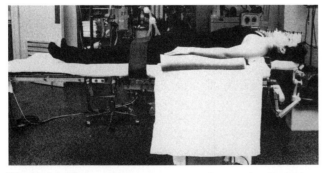

Figure 14-17 Patient in supine position for anterior cervical surgery, with head resting on Mayfield head holder–horseshoe adapter and arms at side with padding. Shoulder roll is under shoulders, and head is in neutral position and can be hyperextended.

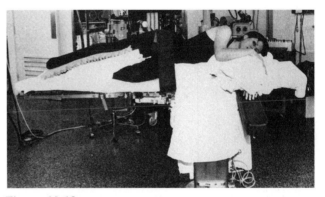

Figure 14-18 Patient in lateral position for lumbar spine surgery with bottom leg flexed, top leg straight, auxiliary roll to left axilla, upper arm supported with blanket roll, and padding between legs. Patient secured with tape and table strap.

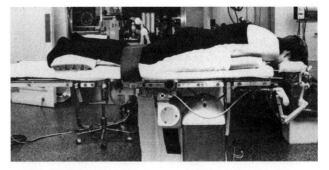

Figure 14-19 Patient prone in horseshoe head holder for posterior cervical or posterior fossa surgery. Arms are at side and padded, lower legs are flexed, ankles and feet are padded, and toes are hanging free.

buttocks area—**saddle hypalgesia.** The patient may exhibit incontinence with areflexic bladder and bowel with varying degrees of motor or sensory loss. The lower extremities may become paretic and later paralyzed. If the hematoma is detected early, recovery is often possible because peripheral nerves may regenerate. If reported at the first signs and symptoms, the hematoma can be evacuated immediately with operative decompression. If the hematoma is not detected early, recovery is often not possible and injury may be permanent.

Patients who require multilevel procedures or have preoperative coagulopathy are at significantly higher risk for developing a postoperative epidural hematoma.[47] Laceration of a major vessel during surgery results in acute hemorrhagic shock. A partial laceration of a major vessel results in a delayed hematoma formation. The clinician should listen for complaints of severe, localized incisional pain that is often described as throbbing. The combination of severe incisional pain and decreased motor and sensory function suggests a hematoma.[83] The physician should be notified immediately.

Signs and symptoms of a retroperitoneal hematoma include flank pain and nausea; these are nonspecific and may accompany an uncomplicated case. The clinician must watch for hypotension and tachycardia. Another complication is the formation of a traumatic AVM or a fistula between an artery and vein as a result of surgical manipulation. Patients exhibit signs and symptoms of high-output cardiac failure, and a bruit can be auscultated over the abdomen when an AVM has developed.

Interventions

Interventions must be instituted to detect and prevent general surgical complications. The patient who is not mobilizing quickly must be assisted in using the incentive spirometer and to turn, cough, and deep breathe every 2 hours to prevent respiratory complications and skin breakdown. Patients who are discharged within 24 hours of surgery should be instructed to continue respiratory care. Patients are encouraged to participate in their care to the fullest extent possible to decrease feelings of dependence. Patients commonly return from the OR with SCDs, which are maintained until they are fully ambulatory. If the patient has been prescribed prolonged bed rest, compression stockings and low-dose heparin (5000 U every 12 hours subcutaneously) or a low-molecular-weight heparin may be initiated for antithrombotic treatment. The patient should also be assessed for the return of bowel sounds. When bowel sounds return, the patient can begin a clear liquid diet and advance to a regular diet as tolerated. Patients can have their IV lines discontinued or heparin locked as soon as they have a good liquid intake. If a urinary catheter was needed, it should be discontinued on the first postoperative day, and interventions should be used to encourage the patient to void. The use of a bedside bladder scanner is helpful in assessing the amount of urine in the bladder. If the patient is unable to void, intermittent catheterization may be necessary until bladder function returns.

Impaired physical mobility is a concern for patients following a laminectomy for several reasons. They may be reluctant to move after surgery, may have neuromuscular or musculoskeletal impairment, or may have restrictions imposed by their physicians. Patients should be mobilized as soon as possible after surgery, taking into account preexisting deficits and activity restrictions.

Patients who were able to ambulate before surgery should be assisted to do so as soon as possible after surgery. If the physician imposes no restrictions, patients should be assisted out of bed the evening of the surgery or first thing the next morning. Some physicians want patients who have undergone a simple laminectomy to stand at the bedside 1 hour after returning from the recovery room and to do slow knee raising (marching in place). These patients are not encouraged to sit for long periods of time but should ambulate progressively. The following is a sample progression:

- Out of bed, standing at bedside
- Ambulate to bathroom or across room
- Ambulate in hallway 50 feet
- Ambulate in hallway 100 feet

Many patients who undergo a laminectomy for uncomplicated disk removal leave the hospital the day of the procedure or 1 to 2 days after surgery depending on the individual patient. These patients require teaching regarding their need to progressively increase ambulation.

The clinician should continue to increase the distance of ambulation until the patient is able to walk with minimal assistance on the day of discharge. The number of days a patient takes to accomplish this progression depends on age, preoperative condition, surgical procedure, and physician restriction. The patient should be cautioned not to attempt too much in one day and become overly fatigued. The clinician should administer pain medication before assisting the patient to get out of bed or to ambulate.

If the patient is unable to get out of bed because of neurologic deficits or physician restriction, nursing interventions must be used to prevent complications of immobility. A physical therapy consultation may give the patient added support and resources for preventing complications. The clinician should work with the physical therapist to ensure that range-of-motion exercises are performed on all extremities at least once every shift and should also teach the patient and family correct range-of-motion exercises. The patient should be taught and encouraged to use isometric exercises (e.g., quadriceps-setting exercises). The patient should continue to wear an SCD device until he or she is fully ambulatory. Some physicians maintain the patient on bed rest until he or she has been measured and fitted for a back brace. Many types of braces are designed to provide support or immobilization. The patient and family need to learn about the type of brace, how to put it on and take it off, and any other pertinent care. The various companies that manufacture braces can provide information about their products.

Pain Management. Pain related to the surgical incision is almost always present postoperatively; therefore pain management is a concern for all patients. The drugs chosen for pain management depend on patient history, the procedure, and the expected length of stay.

Patient-controlled analgesia (PCA) is used in many institutions and provides the patient with pain relief immediately after the operation. The patient is given narcotic IV medication for the first few hours or days via a PCA pump. Intramuscular (IM) injections are ordered as needed, and the patient is gradually switched to an oral medication before discharge (see Chapter 23). The clinician should be alert for side effects such as nausea and vomiting, which are common with narcotics. Problems with pain management are best handled by using a multidisciplinary approach and a pain team, if one is available in the institution.

If a bone graft is obtained from the iliac crest for fusion, patients may experience more postoperative discomfort at the donor site than at the operative site. Some patients may benefit from the use of a walker. A heating pad on the low setting and applied at intervals helps relieve pain for some patients, whereas ice packs are more helpful for other patients.

Patients who have undergone an anterior cervical procedure usually experience fewer muscle spasms because the large muscles of the posterior neck have not been cut. Many patients who have undergone posterior procedures experience muscle spasms resulting from edema caused by nerve root and muscle irritation secondary to surgical manipulation. The pain may be greater postoperatively than preoperatively because of spasms, and this may be very discouraging to the patient. Spasms should subside as the edema decreases. The neuroscience clinician can reassure the patient that this is a normal occurrence. Nonsteroidal antiinflammatory drugs (NSAIDs) and muscle relaxants may help control spasms. The appropriateness of NSAIDs should be checked for patients with fusion (see Chapter 23).

The following interventions may assist in decreasing pain following surgery in the cervical area:

- Provide a soft diet and throat lozenges for the first 48 to 72 hours to alleviate a sore throat
- Maintain a cervical collar to prevent flexion of neck (per physician preference)
- Place a small cervical pillow under the patient's head for comfort
- Provide diversional activities

Health Teaching. The goal of patient and family teaching in the postoperative period is preparation for discharge. General discharge teaching should address diet, medications, activity, when to call the doctor, precautions, and other pertinent information. General discharge instructions for laminectomy patients are listed in Box 14-4.

Patients who have undergone cervical surgery and have a cervical collar for immobilization and support need preparation before discharge. There are many types of cervical collars. Box 14-5 contains instructions for the patient being discharged with a cervical collar. The clinician needs to review the purpose of the collar, how to care for it, and the amount of time the patient must wear it. The clinician also needs to address any other patient concerns.

The patient with acute low back pain needs instruction about maintaining optimal weight, avoiding periods of excessive physical activity, and using proper back care and body mechanics. Nursing and physical therapy can collaborate in teaching the proper methods of lifting, carrying, reaching, pushing, pulling, and proper posture while sitting or driving (Box 14-6).

BOX 14-4	General Discharge Instructions: Laminectomy

After discharge from hospital, your activities should be restricted in the following manner:

- **First week:** Get adequate sleep; rest in the afternoon; go to bed early. You may be driven in a car, but do not drive yourself. Do not do any lifting. You may take a shower or a tub bath.
- **Second week:** Increase activities within the limits set by fatigue (light housework). Go to bed early. You may drive your own car.
- **Third week:** You may return to light work.
- **Fourth week:** Normal activities except those that involve repetitive bending, rotation under stress, or lifting more than 50 pounds as a straight lift or 20 pounds with the weight held at arm's length.
- **Eighth week:** No restrictions.

It is common to get occasional twinges of pain in one or both legs, and it is also common to have cramps in the calf, particularly at night. These are not significant and will diminish by themselves.

If you had any numbness or weakness before the operation, it may take several weeks to recover and return to a normal state.

When activities are increased, you are bound to get some aching in the back (if there was scar tissue) that is stretched. This need not cause any alarm and need not indicate any curtailment of activities. A backache of this type may last for 1 or 2 months.

Modified from Rudy E: *Advanced neurological and neurosurgical nursing*, St Louis, 1984, Mosby.

Recovery Pathway

The use of critical pathways is becoming more common in this age of managed care, and several pathways exist for lumbar laminectomy. Standardized pathways for laminectomy patients vary considerably because of the variety of operative procedures now being performed. The pathway in Table 14-3 follows a 4-day stay.[63] Although many patients return home from some institutions within 1 to 2 days, this pathway provides helpful information to consider when caring for patients with an extended length of stay.

Management of the Patient With an Inoperable Lesion

Patients with inoperable lesions of the spinal cord include those with malignant spinal cord tumors. As noted previously, compression of the spinal cord most commonly causes severe back pain, disturbed sensation, loss of sphincter function, and paraplegia. The prognosis is poor, and the course of the disease is swift. The major objectives are to keep the patient as comfortable and functional as possible.

Assessment

The baseline assessment of the patient with an inoperable lesion of the spinal cord is best divided into motor assessment, sensory assessment, reflexes, and sphincter function.

This information will help in your recovery after neck surgery. Please read this information carefully. Feel free to ask the doctors and nurses any questions you may have. You will receive further instructions at your next doctor's visit. Instructions are as follows:

- Wear your collar at all times or as directed by your physician or health care provider.
- Wash your neck under the collar twice a day. If you have an incision, clean the incision with a mild soap and dry.
- To clean under your collar, have someone follow these steps when assisting you:*
  1. Lie flat on your back.
  2. Open the Velcro tabs on each side of the collar and remove the front part of the collar.
  3. Keep your head still while the collar is open!
  4. Gently wash and dry your neck.
  5. Replace the front part of the collar and fasten the Velcro tabs.
  6. Turn to one side with a thin pillow under your head and open one Velcro tab.
  7. Gently wash the back of the neck, and dry it well.
  8. Fasten the Velcro tab.
  9. Turn to the other side and repeat.
- Men should shave *only with help* and while lying flat in bed.* To do this, remove only the front part of the collar. Keep your head and neck still while shaving.
- For comfort, you may find it helpful to place a silk scarf under the collar or to use the silk cover that comes with some collars. Be sure there are no wrinkles.
- If your doctor allows, you may ride in a car, but you cannot drive.

*Depending on stability of the neck, the patient may be able to perform care in front of a mirror.

Ongoing assessment focuses on areas of deficit identified in the initial assessment. Findings from the assessment of the patient with an inoperable spinal lesion will guide the appropriate planning of nursing interventions.

The signs and symptoms exhibited by the patient depend on the level of the lesion in the spinal cord. Degree of pain, motor impairment, sensory impairment, and sphincter involvement are assessed at each level. The location and intensity of pain are assessed and documented. The motor system is assessed and findings are documented in terms of gait, muscle size, tone, and strength. Sensory assessment includes superficial sensations and deep sensations. The right and left sides of the body are compared in the motor, sensory, and reflex assessment. Reflexes that are assessed include the deep tendon, superficial, and pathologic reflexes. Bowel and bladder function are assessed for sphincter function.

Careful assessment of the neurologic deficits determines the nursing care of the patient with a malignant spinal cord tumor. Motor deficits, activity intolerance, or a lack of physical mobility are of concern to the clinician. Safety of skin integrity may be important for patients with sensory deficits.

Inspection of wound for signs and symptoms of infection. Notify your physician of a temperature of 101.5° F or more, redness of the incision, drainage, increased swelling or warmth at incision site, or increased pain.

Care of incision. Keep the wound clean and dry.

Lifting restrictions. Avoid lifting, pushing, pulling heavy objects (5 to 10 pounds) for 6 weeks, then progress as tolerated.

Bending. Avoid excessive bending; use your legs to squat down.

Driving. Do not drive for 2 weeks following surgery or until safe (patients who have undergone cervical surgery may not be able to turn their head enough to drive safely).

Sexual activity. As tolerated; use comfort and common sense.

Return to work. Discuss with physician.

It is common to get occasional twinges of pain in one or both legs, and it is also common to have cramps in the calf, particularly at night. These are not significant and will go away by themselves.

If you were experiencing any numbness or weakness before the operation, it may take several weeks to recover and return to a normal state.

When activities are increased, you are bound to experience some aching in the back if the scar tissue is stretched. This need not cause any alarm and need not indicate any curtailment of activities. A backache of this type may last for 1 or 2 months.

Clinical management often involves keeping the patient as comfortable and as free of complications as possible until death. A multidisciplinary approach will best meet the needs of the patient and family. This approach is most effective in assisting the patient to maintain as optimal a level of functioning as possible.

Expected Outcomes

Expected outcomes for the patient with a malignant spinal cord tumor include the following:

- Maintenance of endurance[53]
- Pain control
- Bowel continence/elimination
- Urinary elimination
- Spiritual well-being
- Hope
- Grief resolution
- Dignified dying
- Anticipatory grieving related to terminal illness

Health Teaching

Patient and family teaching for the patient with a malignant tumor of the spinal cord focuses on the disease process, diet, medications, and physical care. Many patients prefer to die

TABLE 14-3 Clinical Pathway: Lumbar Laminectomy

	Inpatient Care			
Preadmit Phase	**Day 1 (or Schedule Readmission Screening)**	**Day 2**	**Day 3**	**Day 4**
Diagnostic Tests				
Complete blood count (CBC)	Hemoglobin	Pulse oximetry	CBC	Same as previous day
Serum electrolytes (lytes)	Hematocrit		Lytes if indicated	
Prothrombin time/international normalized ratio	Pulse oximetry			
Activated partial thromboplastin time				
Type and screen				
Urinalysis				
Chest x-ray				
Myelogram				
Computed tomography scan				
Magnetic resonance imaging				
Electrocardiogram				
Medications				
Take medication history	Analgesics as ordered (patient-controlled analgesia/IM)	Analgesics as ordered (wean to PO)	Analgesics as ordered	Analgesics as ordered
Discontinue (D/C) aspirin (ASA) and nonsteroidal antiinflammatory drugs 24 hours before surgery and warfarin (Coumadin) 5 to 7 days before surgery	IV antibiotics	IV antibiotics	IV antibiotics	D/C IV
	IV fluids if not tolerating fluids by mouth (PO)	Heparin or saline lock IV device	Stool softener	Stool softener
	Stool softener	Stool softener		
	Antiemetic for postoperative nausea and vomiting	Laxative if no bowel movement (BM) in 3 days	Laxative if no BM in 3 days	Laxative if no BM in 3 days
Procedures				
Apply thigh-high antiembolism (TED) stockings or intermittent sequential compression device (ISCD)	Check VS and perform neurovascular and wound assessment every 15 minutes for 4 hours, every 30 minutes for 4 hours, every hour for 4 hours, and then q4h and as needed	Check VS and perform neurovascular and wound assessment q4h and as needed	Check vital signs q4h and as needed	Check VS q4h
			Assess neurologic, respiratory, urinary, musculoskeletal, and GI status q4–8h	Assess neurologic, respiratory, urinary, musculoskeletal, and GI status every shift
Take baseline vital signs (VS)		Assess neurologic, respiratory, urinary, musculoskeletal, and GI status q4–8h	Assess wound drainage q4h	Assess wound drainage q4h
Discuss need for early ambulation	Assess neurologic, respiratory, urinary, musculoskeletal, and GI status q4–8h	Assess wound drainage q2–4h	Have patient use IS until fully ambulatory	Have patient use IS until fully ambulatory

Continued

| TABLE 14-3 | Clinical Pathway: Lumbar Laminectomy—cont'd |

Inpatient Care

Preadmit Phase	Day 1 (or Schedule Readmission Screening)	Day 2	Day 3	Day 4
	Assess wound drainage q2–4h	Provide incentive spirometry q2h	Remove and replace TED stockings or compression boots every shift	Remove and replace TED stockings or compression boots every shift
	Have patient perform inflatable sequential (IS) q2h	Remove and replace TED stockings or ISCD every shift	Remove Hemovac or Jackson-Pratt drain	Change dressing bid
	Remove and replace TED stockings or ISCD every shift	Assess straight catheter q8h and as needed	Change dressing bid	Provide wound care
		Change dressing bid; first change by doctor, subsequent changes by RN	Provide wound care	
		Provide wound care		
Diet				
Assess nutritional status	Keep nothing by mouth for 4 hours	Give diet as tolerated (DAT)	Give DAT	Give DAT
	Progress to ice chips, then clear liquid, and advance as tolerated			
Activity				
Assess limitations	Encourage bed rest	Have patient TCDB q2h and as needed (logroll)	Have patient walk qid with assistance	Have patient walk ad lib
Assess ability to perform activities of daily living (ADLs)	Have patient get out of bed (OOB) to chair in afternoon with assistance		Increase walking distance each time	Encourage participation in ADLs as tolerated
	Have male patient stand to void	Have patient walk with assistance in room qid	Encourage participation in ADLs as tolerated	
	Have patient turn, cough, and deep breathe (TCDB) q2h and as needed (logroll)	Encourage participation in ADLs as tolerated		
	Place "Logroll Only" sign at bedside			
	Have patient perform passive and active range of motion to all extremities three to four times daily			

From Poirrier GP, Oberleitner MG: *Clinical pathways in nursing,* Philadelphia, 1999, Springhouse.

at home with their family as caregivers. Family members must be instructed in the physical care of the patient and how to prevent complications. This is best accomplished by having the family participate in the patient's care, treatments, and administration of medication before discharge from the hospital. The clinician should explore hospice and the availability of a parish nurse and respite care in the community for these families.

Recovery Pathway

The time until the death of the patient depends on the pathology of the lesion, the level of the lesion, and the complications. For example, patients with a malignant astrocytoma of the spinal cord have a median survival period of 6 months.[55]

Because of the high cost of care, patients with inoperable lesions tend not to stay in the hospital but are discharged to their homes or to a nursing home. If the patient has a life expectancy of 6 months or less, residential or home hospice care may be an option.

Rehabilitation and Home Care

The patient with a nontraumatic disorder of the spine is likely to be in a deconditioned state as a result of a slow, progressive preoperative course. These patients may need rehabilitation or home care services.

Assessment

As mentioned in the preceding assessment sections, the clinician must assess the degree of neurologic deficit of the patient. The areas of pain, motor assessment, sensory assessment, and sphincter control are all important. Functional status and degree of disability are also important factors to assess in preparing for rehabilitation or home care of the patient with a nontraumatic disorder of the spine.

The **Functional Independence Measure (FIM)** is a useful tool in assessing functional ability (see Fig. 13-1). This scale measures six domains: self-care, sphincter control, mobility, locomotion, communication, and social cognition (see Chapter 13). Box 14-7 lists the components included under each of the six categories. These components are scored on a seven-point scale that ranges from complete dependence (1) to complete independence (7). This scale has demonstrated acceptable reliability across a wide variety of settings, raters, and patients.[59]

BOX 14-7	Categories Used for the Functional Independence Measure

Self-Care
1. Eating
2. Grooming
3. Bathing
4. Dressing (upper body)
5. Dressing (lower body)
6. Toileting

Sphincter Control
7. Bladder management
8. Bowel management

Mobility
9. Transfer
10. Bed, chair, wheelchair
11. Toilet
12. Tub, shower

Locomotion
13. Walk/wheelchair
14. Stairs

Communication
15. Comprehension
16. Expression

Social Cognition
17. Social interaction
18. Problem solving
19. Memory

The identified areas of deficit can guide the planning of appropriate nursing interventions to assist the patient in returning to as functional a life as possible.

Expected Outcomes

Expected outcomes include the following:
- Self-care (bathing)[53]
- Self-care (dressing)
- Coping
- Decision making
- Symptom control behavior
- Safety behavior (home physical environment)
- Social support

COMPREHENSIVE PATIENT MANAGEMENT

Management of the rehabilitation patient with a nontraumatic disorder of the spine involves assisting him or her in attaining the highest level of self-care possible given his or her residual deficits. Many of the specific interventions and expected outcomes for these patients are similar to those for patients with traumatic spinal cord disorders (see Chapter 12). For example, the patient with residual weakness needs a program of gradual strengthening and endurance building. Patients also need to learn to compensate for permanent deficits by undertaking regimens such as bladder and bowel programs. Patients and their families must be prepared to manage the altered health state for the remainder of the patient's natural life.

Special rehabilitation programs can assist the patient with disk disease in returning to work. Physical therapy is commonly prescribed for patients with low back pain. Other modalities include heat, cold, and electric stimulation. Exercise programs are prescribed as tolerated. A multidisciplinary program is often needed for a comprehensive plan of care.

With early discharges and more acutely ill patients going home, home nursing care may be necessary for many patients with nontraumatic disorders of the spine. Before discharge, the goal is for the patient or family to be able to verbalize an understanding of the overall plan of care in the home. Clinicians and discharge planners should work with the family to assess insurance or third-party reimbursement for home care needs. Interventions in the home include assessment for complications, physical care, and treatments. Care is individualized according to the needs of the patient and family. The home health care teams teach the patient and family how to perform interventions as they are being carried out. The ultimate goal is for the patient or family to manage home care on their own and successfully.

Health Teaching Considerations

In addition to physical care and treatments, the rehabilitation and home care nurse must teach the patient and family about the many complications for which these patients are at risk. Complications include contractures, thrombophlebitis, orthostatic hypotension, skin breakdown, autonomic dysreflexia (for those with complete spinal lesions above T6), infections, unsuccessful bowel or bladder programs, and decreased range of motion. The patient and family should be able to verbalize the symptoms of complications, understand how to prevent them, and take the appropriate course of action when they occur.

Psychosocial Considerations

Patients with nontraumatic spinal cord disorders may be faced with many issues because of the possible chronic nature of their condition. Neurologic impairments may lead to temporary or permanent job changes. Chronic pain can cause psychologic distress. Family role changes may be experienced. All clinicians must be sensitive to these possibilities.

Older Adult Considerations

A variety of care concerns affect management of the older adult patient. Older patients who receive drug therapy for TB should be carefully monitored for side effects and toxicities. For example, isoniazid treatment increases the risk of hepatitis. Older adults should receive baseline liver function tests before the initiation of drug therapy, as well as periodic measurements of serum glutamic oxaloacetic transaminase (SGOT) at 1, 3, and 6 months after beginning the drug regimen.[65] Rifampin may also cause hepatitis. Ethambutol may cause a loss of color discrimination and visual acuity; therefore older adults should be tested for color discrimination and visual acuity.[65] One of the most devastating adverse effects of streptomycin is irreversible hearing loss. Clinicians must consider alterations in pharmacokinetics, especially renal impairment, when adjusting the dosage of streptomycin in older patients.

Elective lumbar spinal decompression surgery in older adults is becoming as common as total hip arthroplasty, and recent studies have shown it to be as safe in this population as hip surgery.[5,70] Older adults, however, are likely to suffer minor perioperative complications warranting increased vigilance and careful monitoring.[5]

Care of the older surgical candidate includes a preoperative assessment of medical, psychosocial, medication, and functional status history. Alterations in any of these areas can influence the perioperative course. Clinical goals should be directed toward maintaining function and preventing iatrogenic complications.

With age, physiologic changes in the pulmonary system may influence the operative course, especially if the patient requires intubation. These changes include an increase in residual volume and functional residual capacity, a decrease in vital capacity and maximum oxygen consumption, and a decreased cough reflex. Clinical actions should include increased surveillance of ventilator weaning and the prevention of pneumonia, especially aspiration and atelectasis.

Case Management Considerations

Because nontraumatic disorders of the spine can lead to chronic problems, case management is often necessary. Following a medical or surgical intervention, the majority of patients are expected to experience symptom relief and resume their previous lifestyle. Other patients are referred for evaluation for case management services. After conducting the initial patient interview and evaluation and meeting with members of the health care team, the case manager develops an individualized plan of care with measurable outcomes and seeks approval for reimbursement of recommended services. Points to remember with patients in this population include the following:

- Low back pain related to disk disease is usually a self-limiting problem, with 51% of patients better within a month and 95% better within 3 months.[30]
- The patient's diagnostic studies must be carefully assessed to ensure that the proper tests were used.
- Predictive factors for return to work following lumbar disk herniation include the following:[94]
  - No preoperative comorbidity
  - Duration of sciatica less than 7 months
  - Education or vocational training in addition to compulsory school
  - Age younger than 41 years
  - Male gender
  - No previous nonspinal surgery

The 5% of patients who have not recovered within 3 months of treatment are at a high risk for falling into a life pattern marred by chronic pain and disability.[30] Patients out of work at 6 months have only a 40% chance of returning to work. This chance drops to 20% for patients disabled for 1 year and close to zero if disabled for 2 years.[30]

Eighty-five percent of the total cost of caring for patients with low back pain is spent on the 5% of patients who have pain that persists for more than 3 months.[30] A postoperative positive straight-leg raising test sometimes correlates with an unfavorable surgical outcome.[38] The clinician should ensure that patients with failed back surgery syndrome receive a coordinated management of pain even though surgical options may not be available.

Close patient follow-up by phone or home visits is needed to validate the patient's and family's satisfaction with the plan of care, patient compliance with the therapy, patient progress toward the expected outcomes, and prevention of complications and rehospitalization. It is the responsibility of the case manager to ensure that all services, medications, and rehabilitation have been provided as prescribed. For example, follow-up physician appointments may also include the need to provide handicap transportation.

The patient, family, and caregivers must be instructed on how to detect and immediately report any medical emergency, neurologic changes, medication side effects, or injuries (e.g., falls). In some cases in which reimbursements for care are exhausted and the patient's health care team wants to continue therapy, the case manager must be very resourceful, creative, and knowledgeable about all available community resources.

CONCLUSION

Caring for the patient with a nontraumatic disorder of the spine is a challenge because of the diversity of this population's needs and because of the ever-changing health care environment. A well-prepared plan of care with input from the patient and family is essential. Ongoing evaluation with attention to comprehensiveness and individual patient needs is important. The patient's hospital course may be long and difficult with many revisions of the plan of care, or it may be a short stay with a straightforward plan of care. The challenge is to keep up with individual patients and to keep abreast of new medical and surgical developments in the ever-changing area of nontraumatic disorders of the spine.

Acknowledgments

The author acknowledges and thanks Dennis Nath, RN, and Alicia Pfeilsticker, RN, for their suggestions to revisions of this chapter.

RESOURCES FOR PATIENTS AND CAREGIVERS

Krames Communications: Division of Staywell Company, 1100 Grundy Lane, San Bruno, CA 94066-3030; 800-333-3032; https://shop.krames.com/OA_HTML/default.jsp; info@krames.com

REFERENCES

1. Aebi M: Spinal metastasis in the elderly, *Eur Spine J* 12(S2): S202–S213, 2003.
2. Almeida A: Tuberculosis of the spine and spinal cord, *Eur J Radiol* 55(2):193–201, 2005.
3. Andersson T, Van Dijk JM, Willinsky RA: Venous manifestations of spinal arteriovenous fistulas, *Neuroimaging Clin North Am* 13(1):73–93, 2003.
4. Andreula C, Muto M, Leonardi M: Interventional spinal procedures, *Eur J Radiol* 50(2):112–119, 2004.
5. Arinzon ZH, Fredman B, Zohar E, et al: Surgical management of spinal stenosis: a comparison of immediate and long term outcome in two geriatric patient populations, *Arch Gerontol Geriatr* 36(3):273–279, 2003.
6. Aryan HE, Yanni DS, Nakaji P, et al: Syringocephaly, *J Clin Neurosci* 11(4):421–423, 2004.
7. Benes L, Wakat JP, Sure U, et al: Intraoperative spinal digital subtraction angiography: technique and results, *Neurosurgery* 52(3):603–609, 2003.
8. Briganti F, Tortora F, Elefante A, et al: An unusual case of vertebral arteriovenous fistula treated with electrodetachable coil embolization, *Minimally Invasive Neurosurg* 47(6):386–388, 2004.
9. Brotchi J: Spinal intradural extramedullary tumors. In Rengachary SS, Ellenbogen RG, editors: *Principles of neurosurgery,* St Louis, 2005, Elsevier Mosby.
10. Brown CW, Wong DC: Spine-health.com, July 7, 2000. Available at www.spine-health.com/research/kyph/khph02.html (accessed August 31, 2005).
11. Burns AS, Dillingham TR: Importance of gadolinium enhancement when using MRI to evaluate spinal cord pathology, *Am J Phys Med Rehabil* 79(4):399–403, 2000.
12. Byrne TN: Metastatic epidural cord compression, *Curr Neurol Neurosci Rep* 4:191–195, 2004.
13. Cahill DW, Vale F, Hajjar MV: Lumbosacral pseudoarthrosis and instrumentation failure. In Batjer HH, Loftus CM, editors: *Textbook of neurological surgery,* Philadelphia, 2003, Lippincott Williams & Wilkins.
14. Caldarelli M, Di Rocco C: Diagnosis of Chiari I malformation and related syringomyelia: radiological and neurophysiological studies, *Childs Nervous System* 20(5):332–335, 2004.
15. Centers for Disease Control and Prevention: Division of tuberculosis elimination. Available at www.cdc.gov/nchstp/tb/surv/surv2003/default.htm (accessed September 13, 2005).
16. Chad DA: Disorders of nerve roots and plexuses. In Bradley WG, editor: *Neurology in clinical practice,* Philadelphia, 2004, Butterworth Heineman.
17. Chamberlain MC: Ependymomas, *Curr Neurol Neurosci Rep* 3:193–199, 2003.
18. Chen Y, Derby R, Lee S: Percutaneous disc decompression in the management of chronic low back pain, *Orthop Clin North Am* 35(1):17–23, 2004.
19. Choi IS, Tantivatana J: Neuroendovascular management of intracranial and spinal tumors, *Neurosurg Clin North Am* 11(1):167–185, 2000.
20. Clatterbuck RE, Belzberg AJ, Ducker TB: Intradural cervical disc herniation and Brown-Sequard's syndrome: report of three cases and review of the literature, *J Neurosurg* 92(suppl 2):236–240, 2000.
21. Collignon FP, Cohen-Gadol AA, Krauss WE: Circumferential decompression of the foramen magnum for the treatment of syringomyelia associated with basilar invagination, *Neurosurg Rev* 27(3):168–172, 2004.
22. Covert S, Gandhi D, Goyal M, et al: Magnetic resonance imaging of intramedullary meningioma of the spinal cord: case report and review of the literature, *Can Assoc Radiolog J* 54(3):177–180, 2003.
23. Curry WT, Hoh BL, Amin-Hanjani S, Eskandar EN: Spinal epidural abscess: clinical presentation, management, and outcome, *Surg Neurol* 63(4):364–371, 2005.
24. Davis DP, Wold RM, Patel RJ, et al: The clinical presentation and impact of diagnostic delays on emergency department patients with spinal epidural abscess, *J Emerg Med* 36(3):285–291, 2004.
25. Drummond KJ: Spinal abscess. In Kaye AH, Black ML, editors: *Operative neurosurgery,* New York, 2000, Churchill Livingstone.
26. Dubendorf P: Personal communication, June 5, 2006.
27. Evans BK: HIV infection and diseases of the spinal cord, nerve roots, peripheral nerves and muscle. In Samuels MA, Feske SK, editors: *Office practice of neurology,* Philadelphia, 2003, Churchill Livingstone.
28. Fearnside MR: Decompressive cervical laminectomy. In Kaye AH, Black ML, editors: *Operative neurosurgery,* New York, 2000, Churchill Livingstone.
29. Feigenbaum F, Henderson FC: Cervical graft options. In Batjer HH, Loftus CM, editors: *Textbook of neurological surgery,* Philadelphia, 2003, Lippincott Williams & Wilkins.
30. Forrest GP, Dubin A: The patient undergoing rehabilitation for neurological disorders. In Popp AJ, editor: *A guide to the primary care of neurological disorders,* Park Ridge, IL, 1998, American Association of Neurological Surgeons.
31. Geckle DS, Hlavin ML: Spondylosis and disc disease. In Samuels MA, Feske SK, editors: *Office practice of neurology,* Philadelphia, 2003, Churchill Livingstone.
32. Guiot B, Fessler RG: Endoscopic discectomy. In Kaye AH, Black ML, editors: *Operative neurosurgery,* New York, 2000, Churchill Livingstone.

33. Heros RC, Heros DO, Schumacher JM: Principles of neurosurgery. In Bradley WG, editor: *Neurology in clinical practice,* Philadelphia, 2004, Butterworth Heineman.

34. Hida K, Shirato H, Isu T, et al: Focal fractionated radiotherapy for intramedullary spinal arteriovenous malformations: 10-year experience, *J Neurosurg* 99(S1):34–38, 2003.

35. Hilton EL, Henderson LJ: Neurosurgical considerations in posttraumatic syringomyelia, *AORN J* 77(1):141–144, 146–148, 2003.

36. Iwasaki Y, Hida K, Koyanagi I, Abe H: Reevaluation of syringosubarachnoid shunt for syringomyelia with Chiari malformation, *Neurosurgery* 46(2):407–412, 2000.

37. Jaksche H, Schaan M, Schulz J, Boszczyk B: Posttraumatic syringomyelia—a serious complication in tetra- and paraplegic patients, *Acta Neurochir* 93(S):165–167, 2005.

38. Jonsson B, Stromqvist B: Significance of a persistent positive straight leg raising test after lumbar disc surgery, *J Neurosurg* 91(suppl 1):50–53, 1999.

39. Joshi SM, Hatfield RH, Martin J, Taylor W: Spinal epidural abscess: a diagnostic challenge, *Br J Neurosurg* 17(2):160–163, 2003.

40. Kara B, Tulum Z, Acar U: Functional results and the risk factors of reoperation after lumbar disc surgery, *Eur Spine J* 14(1):43–48, 2005.

41. Kase CS, Estol CJ: Vascular malformations. In Samuels MA, Feske SK, editors: *Office practice of neurology,* Philadelphia, 2003, Churchill Livingstone.

42. Kelley NC: Osteomyelits. In Smith DS, Sullivan LE, Hay SF, editors: *Field guide to internal medicine,* Philadelphia, 2005, Lippincott Williams & Wilkins.

43. Kilmo P Jr, Schmidt MH: Surgical management of spinal metastases, *Oncologist* 9(2):188–196, 2004.

44. Kleeman TJ: Spinal fusion and bone morphogenetic protein, January 8, 2004. Available at www.spineuniverse.com/displayarticle.php/article1708.html (accessed November 20, 2005).

45. Koyanagi I, Iwasaki Y, Hilda K, Houkin K: Clinical features and pathomechanisms of syringomyelia associated with spinal arachnoiditis, *Surg Neurol* 63(4):350–355, 2005.

46. Krings T, Mull M, Gilsbach JM, Thron A: Spinal vascular malformations, *Eur Radiol* 15(2):267–278, 2005.

47. Kuo J, Fishgrund J, Biddinger A, Herkowitz H: Risk factors for spinal epidural hematoma after spinal surgery, *Spine* 27(15):1670–1673, 2002.

48. Kuo JS, Licholai GP, Woodard EJ: Anterior cervical vertebral resection and stabilzation. In Kaye AH, Black ML, editors: *Operative neurosurgery,* New York, 2000, Churchill Livingstone.

49. Lopez JR: The use of evoked potentials in intraoperative neurophysiologic monitoring, *Phys Med Rehabil Clin North Am* 15(1):63–84, 2004.

50. Maher De Leon ME, Schnell S, Rozental JM: Tumors of the spine and spinal cord, *Semin Oncol Nurs* 14(1):43–52, 1998.

51. Manthis JM, Ortiz AO, Zoarski GH: Vertebroplasy versus kyphoplasty: a comparison and contrast, *Am J Radiol* 25(5):840–845, 2004.

52. Maus TP, Thielen KR, Wald JT: Percutaneous methylmethacrylate vertebroplasty (in press).

53. Moorhead S, Johnson M, Maas ML: *Nursing Outcomes Classification (NOC) Iowa Outcomes Project,* St Louis, 2004, Mosby.

54. Van Goethem JW, van den Hauwe L, Ozsarlak O, et al: Spinal tumors, *Eur J Radiol* 50(4):159–176, 2004.

55. New KC, Friedman AH: Intramedually tumors and tumors of the cauda equina. In Rengachary SS, Ellenbogen RG, editors: *Principles of neurosurgery,* St Louis, 2005, Elsevier Mosby.

56. Ohaegbulam C, Eichler M: Spinal cord tumors. In Samuels MA, Feske SK, editors: *Office practice of neurology,* Philadelphia, 2003, Churchill Livingstone.

57. Osenbach RK, Burchiel KJ: Pain management: general principles. In Crockard A, Hayward R, Hoff JT, editors: *Neurosurgery,* London, 2000, Blackwell Science.

58. Osenbach RK, Pradhan A: Brain and spinal abscess. In *Principles of neurosurgery,* St Louis, 2005, Elsevier Mosby.

59. Ottentacher KJ: The reliability of the functional independence measure, *Arch Phys Med Rehabil* 77(12):1226–1232, 1996.

60. Pandit HG, Sonsale PD, Shikare SS, Bhojraj SY: Bone scintigraphy in tuberculous spondylodiscitis, *Eur Spine J* 8(3):205–209, 1999.

61. Parkinson JF, Sekhon LH: Spinal epidural abscess: appearance on magnetic resonance imaging as a guide to surgical management. Report of five cases, *Neurosurg Focus* 17(6):E12, 2004.

62. Pereira CE, Lynch JC: Spinal epidural abscess: an analysis of 24 cases, *Surg Neurol* 63(S1):S26–S29, 2005.

63. Poirrier GP, Oberleitner MG: *Clinical pathways in nursing: a guide to managing care from hospital to home,* Springhouse, PA, 1999, Springhouse Corp.

64. Popovic EA: Decompressive thoracic laminectomy. In Kaye AH, Black ML, editors: *Operative neurosurgery,* New York, 2000, Churchill Livingstone.

65. Possick SE: Tuberculosis. In Smith DS, Sullivan LE, Hay SF, editors: *Field guide to internal medicine,* Philadelphia, 2005, Lippincott Williams & Wilkins.

66. Potter K, Saifuddin A: Pictorial review: MRI of chronic spinal cord injury, *Br J Radiol* 76(905):347–352, 2003.

67. Profeta G, de Falco R, Ianniciello G, et al: Preliminary experience with anterior cervical microdiscectomy with interbody titanium cage fusion (Novus CT-Ti) in patients with cervical disc disease, *Surg Neurol* 53(5):417–426, 2000.

68. Pui MH: Gadolinium-enhanced MR angiography of spinal arteriovenous malformation, *Clin Imaging* 28(1):28–32, 2004.

69. Quenones-Hinojosa A, Woodard EJ: Lumbar microdiscectomy. In Kaye AH, Black ML, editors: *Operative neurosurgery,* New York, 2000, Churchill Livingstone.

70. Reindl R, Steffen T, Cohen L, Aebi M: Elective lumbar spinal decompression in the elderly: is it a high-risk operation? *Can J Surg* 43(1):43–46, 2003.

71. Riina HA, Soni D, Stieg PE: Surgical treatment of spinal arteriovenous malformations. In Batjer HH, Loftus CM, editors: *Textbook of neurological surgery,* Philadelphia, 2003, Lippincott Williams & Wilkins.

72. Rodesch G, Lasjaunias P: Spinal cord arteriovenous shunts: from imaging to management, *Eur J Radiol* 46(3):221–232, 2003.

73. Rodesch G, Hurth M, Alvarez H, et al: Angio-architecture of spinal cord arteriovenous shunts at presentation. Clinical correlations in adults and children. The Bicetre experience on 155 consecutive patients seen between 1981–1999, *Acta Neurochir* 146(3):217–226, 2004.

74. Rolak LA: Brain and spinal abscess. In Samuels MA, Feske SK, editors: *Office practice of neurology,* Philadelphia, 2003, Churchill Livingstone.

75. Rosenbaum RB, Ciaverella DP: Disorders of bones, joints, ligaments, and meninges. In Bradley WG, editor: *Neurology in clinical practice,* Philadelphia, 2004, Butterworth Heinemann.

76. Sala F, Niimi Y, Krzan MJ, et al: Embolization of a spinal arteriovenous malformation: correlation between motor evoked potentials and angiographic findings; technical case report, *Neurosurgery* 45(4):932–937, 2000.

77. Schaller B: Failed back surgery syndrome: the role of symptomatic segmental single-level instability after lumbar microdiscectomy, *Eur Spine J* 13(3):193–198, 2004.

78. Schiff D, Wen P: Cancer and the nervous system. In Bradley WG, editor: *Neurology in clinical practice,* Philadelphia, 2004, Butterworth Heinemann.

79. Siddiq F, Chowfin A, Tight R, et al: Medical vs surgical management of spinal epidural abscess, *Arch Intern Med* 164(22): 2409–2412, 2004.

80. Sklar EM: Neuroimaging. In Bradley WG, editor: *Neurology in clinical practice,* Philadelphia, 2004, Butterworth Heinemann.

81. Sorensen P: Spinal epidural abscesses: conservative treatment for selected subgroups of patients, *Br J Neurosurg* 17(6):513–518, 2003.

82. Spinasanta S: SPECT scan, June 6, 2005. Available at www.spineuniverse.com/displalyarticle.php/article328.html (accessed November 20, 2005).

83. Stone JL, Lichtor T: Triage and management of neurosurgical emergencies. In Batjer HH, Loftus CM, editors: *Textbook of neurological surgery,* Philadelphia, 2003, Lippincott Williams & Wilkins.

84. Tagliati M: The role of somatosensory evoked potentials in the diagnosis of AIDS-associated myelopathy, *Neurology* 54(7): 1477–1482, 2000.

85. Talbot L: Failed back surgery syndrome, *BMJ* 327:985–986, 2003.

86. Tarlov EC: Cervical nerve root compression: surgical treatment by the posterior approach. In Kaye AH, Black ML, editors: *Operative neurosurgery,* New York, 2000, Churchill Livingstone.

87. Tawk RG, Liu JC: Minimally invasive spine surgery. In Batjer HH, Loftus CM, editors: *Textbook of neurological surgery,* Philadelphia, 2003, Lippincott Williams & Wilkins.

88. Teddy PJ, Lustgarden L: Post traumatic syringomyelia. In Kaye AH, Black ML, editors: *Operative neurosurgery,* New York, 2000, Churchill Livingstone.

89. Thielen KR: Vertebroplasty: a new option for compression fractures (in press).

90. Tropiano P, Huang RC, Girardi PF, Marnay T: Lumbar disc replacement: preliminary results with ProDisc II after a minimum follow-up period of 1 year, *J Spinal Disord Tech* 16(4):362–368, 2003.

91. Valiante TA, Fehlings MG: Primary tumors of the spinal cord, root, plexus, and nerve sheath. In Noseworthy JH, editor: *Neurological therapeutics: principles and practice,* New York, 2003, Martin Dunitz.

92. Van Ooij A, Oner FC, Cumhur AJ: Complications of artificial disc replacement: a report of 27 patients with the SB Charite Disc, *J Spinal Disord Tech* 16(4):369–383, 2003.

93. Verma A, Solbrig MV: Bacterial infections. In Bradley WG, editor: *Neurology in clinical practice,* Philadelphia, 2004, Butterworth Heinemann.

94. Vucetic N: Diagnosis and prognosis in lumbar disc herniation, *Clin Orthop* 361:116–122, 1999.

95. Weisz RD, Errico TJ: Spinal infections: diagnosis and treatment, *Bull Hosp Joint Dis* 59(1):40–46, 2000.

96. Wolfla CE: Lumbar disc herniation. In Rengachary SS, Ellenbogen RG, editors: *Principles of neurosurgery,* Philadelphia, 2005, Elsevier Mosby.

97. Wyatt LH: Spine cancer: a summary and review, *Australas Chiropr Osteopat* 12(1):9–17, 2004.

98. Yalamanchili M, Lesser GJ: Malignant spinal cord compression, *Curr Treat Options Oncol* 4:509–516, 2003.

99. Yoshikawa TT: Tuberculosis in aging adults, *J Am Geriatr Soc* 40:178–187, 1992.

CHAPTER 15

ANNE G. MIERS

Peripheral Nerve Disorders

The **peripheral nervous system (PNS)** refers to the motor and sensory nerves and ganglia outside the cranial cavity and vertebral column. The PNS consists of the 12 paired cranial nerves, the 31 paired spinal nerves, and their branches (see Chapter 1). The axons of these nerves, which travel to and from the brainstem and spinal cord, may become diseased, injured, compressed, or severed by a multitude of causes, resulting in degeneration. This chapter focuses on peripheral nerve injury, peripheral nerve tumors, inflammatory demyelinating polyradiculoneuropathies, and chronic neuropathies. It includes a review of the more common etiologies of peripheral nerve dysfunction and a discussion of the assessment and clinical management parameters for care and case management. The chapter concludes with special sections on the common peripheral nerve disorders of carpal tunnel syndrome and thoracic outlet syndrome.

ETIOLOGY

Individual spinal nerves form **plexuses,** or interconnecting networks, of nerves. These plexuses, in turn, innervate specific areas of the body and form the major peripheral nerves. The PNS is thus an intricate web of nerves; damage to this web results in loss of movement and sensation in the area innervated distal to the lesion, making such damage a complicated and complex disorder.

A neuropathy may occur at the level of the spinal nerves, roots, or plexus before peripheral nerve formation, or at the peripheral nerves themselves. Terms related to neuropathy include the following:

- **Peripheral neuropathy** is a general term denoting a primary loss or destruction of the nerve cell bodies with resultant degeneration of their entire peripheral axon.[3] These neuropathies may be single or multiple, symmetric or asymmetric.
- **Mononeuropathies** are localized disorders of single peripheral nerves that are often due to entrapment or to trauma.
- **Polyneuropathies** are generalized and involve the entire PNS. Polyneuropathies are symmetric, multiple lesions commonly caused by degenerative, infectious, toxic, metabolic, or hereditary diseases.
- **Neuralgias** are painful conditions that result from an infection or disease that damages a peripheral nerve.

- **Radiculopathy** is a disease of the spinal nerve roots.

There are more than 100 known conditions associated with disorders of the PNS. Symptoms and signs of PNS damage may come on acutely or manifest themselves over a relatively long course of weeks to months. Because of this time factor, as well as the sheer number of associated disorders, a single, exact cause is often difficult to determine. Moreover, multiple and mixed factors may contribute to any one disorder. Some of the more common etiologies of PNS disorders include drugs, toxins, metabolic disorders, immune states, and genetic causes. Genetic causes are linked to numerous defective chromosomes.

One way to classify the causes of PNS injuries is to divide them into penetrating and nonpenetrating types. **Penetrating** injuries result in partial or complete discontinuity of the nerve. Injection injuries and blast injuries are other examples of penetrating injury, although they do not normally cause complete discontinuity of the nerve.[3] **Nonpenetrating** injuries may be traumatic, such as following blunt trauma, or may be nontraumatic due to a wide range of factors. Median nerve injury at the wrist, known as carpal tunnel syndrome (CTS), is a common nonpenetrating injury caused by chronic pressure and ischemia. Tumors can affect peripheral nerves either by extrinsic compression or by intrinsic compression or infiltration. Box 15-1 lists the most common etiologies of PNS disorders.

PATHOPHYSIOLOGY

One of the unique properties of the PNS is its capacity to regenerate. When the fibers are transected, two uneven nerve fragments result. The distal stump is destroyed by wallerian degeneration, but the proximal stump is preserved and can support regeneration.[23] The rate of axonal regeneration is 1 to 5 mm/day. A useful clinical approximation for recovery of motor functions is an overall growth rate of 1 inch per month.[23] The rate is faster more proximal to the cell body and slower more distally. Figure 15-1 illustrates the process of regeneration.

The most basic pathologic processes in disorders of the PNS are wallerian degeneration, axonopathy, and myelinopathy. These are the cellular responses that occur in nerve damage regardless of the etiology.

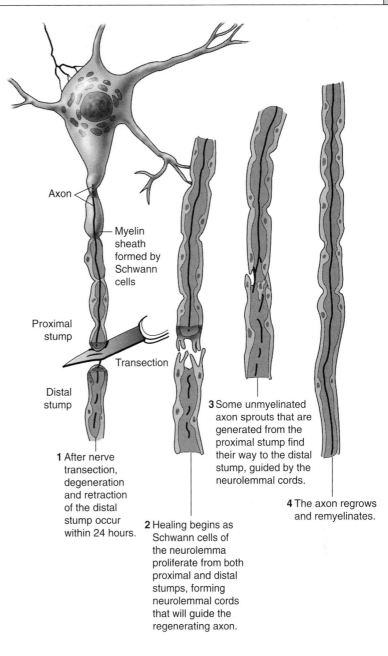

Figure 15-1 Regeneration of a peripheral nerve after injury.
(From Ignatavicius DD, Workman ML: Medical-surgical nursing: critical thinking for collaborative care, St Louis, 2002, WB Saunders.)

Axon

Myelin sheath formed by Schwann cells

Proximal stump

Transection

Distal stump

1 After nerve transection, degeneration and retraction of the distal stump occur within 24 hours.

2 Healing begins as Schwann cells of the neurolemma proliferate from both proximal and distal stumps, forming neurolemmal cords that will guide the regenerating axon.

3 Some unmyelinated axon sprouts that are generated from the proximal stump find their way to the distal stump, guided by the neurolemmal cords.

4 The axon regrows and remyelinates.

Wallerian degeneration, or the breakdown of nerve fibers distal to a lesion, is the most common pathologic process in PNS disorders (Fig. 15-2). The process involves distal degeneration, fragmentation, and phagocytosis of the axon and myelin sheath, which occur after severing of nerve fibers. Motor weakness and sensory loss are immediate in the distribution of the damaged nerve. Because wallerian degeneration does not occur immediately, distal conduction is preserved for several days before disappearing.[3] Motor responses are lost first, and then sensory responses are lost.[3] This degeneration takes place over a 2- to 3-week period after an injury or insult to the nerve. At the end of this time, the empty connective tissue framework of the distal portion of the peripheral nerve is all that remains. The quality of the recovery depends on the degree of preservation of the Schwann cell basal lamina tube and the nerve sheath and surrounding tissue, as well as the distance of the site of injury from the cell body and the age of the individual.[3]

Axonopathy denotes an axonal atrophy and degeneration. Metabolic derangement within the neuron results in distal axonal breakdown. The myelin sheath breaks down at the most distal part of the nerve fiber and progresses toward the nerve cell body. The term for this is **dying-back neuropathy.**[3] The clinical manifestation of this type of damage is a **"stocking-glove"** phenomenon involving sensory loss in the areas of the arms and legs where stockings and gloves are worn. The damage is distal and symmetric, with gradual shading of normal to diminished sensation. In addition to the sensory loss, there is distal muscle weakness and atrophy, and loss of ankle reflexes if the legs are affected. This type of damage occurs with exogenous toxins and

BOX 15-1	**Etiologies of Peripheral Nerve Disorders**

Penetrating: Partial
Gunshot wound
Tumor
Injections
Birth injury
Penetrating: Complete
Fractures
Lacerations
Surgical injury
Birth injury
Tumor
Nonpenetrating
Electrical current
Radiotherapy
Chronic pressure and ischemia
Toxins
Contusions
Friction injuries
Stretch injuries
Occupational palsies
Metabolic imbalances
Tumors

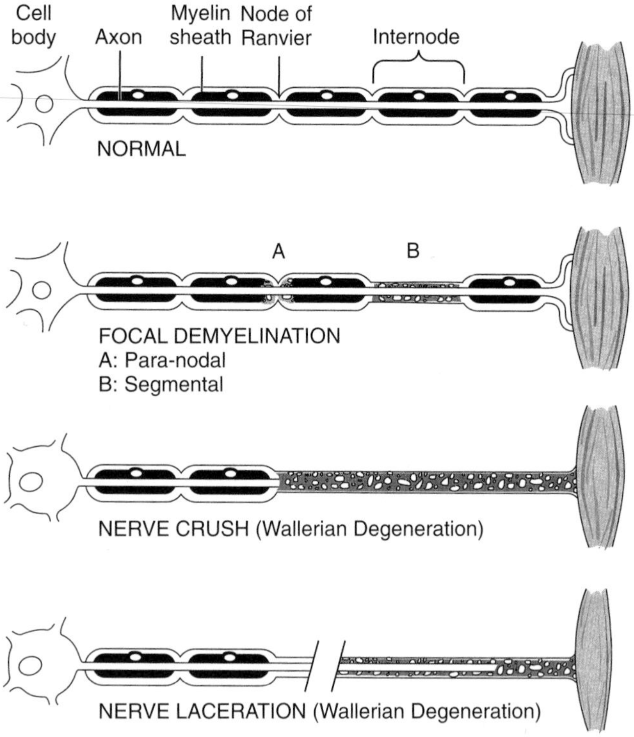

Figure 15-2 Diagram of a single myelinated nerve fiber showing the kinds of damage that may occur with focal demyelinization from either nerve crush or laceration. In either type of injury, there is complete wallerian degeneration from the point of trauma distally. A certain degree of regeneration occurs in the nerve crush lesion, but the quantity depends on the severity and duration of the crush and the extent of damage to the blood supply. Regeneration after a nerve laceration depends on end-to-end repair of axonal tissue, blood supply, and the amount of fibrosis. *(Modified from Stewart JD: Focal peripheral neuropathies, New York, 1987, Elsevier.)*

systemic metabolic disorders, such as diabetes mellitus (DM).[3]

Myelinopathy is segmental demyelination that occurs where the nerve is not directly severed. Slow changes in the myelin sheath or Schwann cells occur with sparing of the axon.[3] A conduction block is usually present, which results in muscle weakness. Relative sparing of temperature and pinprick sensation reflects preserved function of unmyelinated and small-diameter myelinated fibers.[3] Primary and secondary demyelination can occur. Primary damage can be caused by nerve compression or by toxins, whereas secondary changes occur as the result of axonal atrophy or swelling.[3] Repeated episodes of demyelination and remyelination produce proliferation of multiple layers of Schwann cells around the axon, termed an **onion bulb.**[3]

In addition to the cellular response, several delayed pathologic responses can occur as the result of peripheral nerve disorders. These include **regeneration** and the formation of **neuromas.** Neuromas may be of two types: (1) lesions in continuity that may reflect neural injury (with or without recovery); and (2) lesions not in continuity that result in transected stumps. **Pain syndromes** such as causalgia, reflex sympathetic dystrophy, phantom limb pain, and pain connected with regeneration, degeneration, and disuse can all occur as a delayed reaction to peripheral nerve disorders (see Box 15-3 later in this chapter and Chapter 23 for pain syndromes).

PERIPHERAL NERVE INJURY

Peripheral nerve injury may involve partial or total nerve fibers (Fig. 15-3). The injury is classified as follows:

- **Neuropraxia:** a lesion causing a temporary block of nerve conduction without transection of axons.[23] It is generally the result of a mild degree of compression or stretch. Disturbance of function can last from hours to weeks and, rarely, months. There is usually a conduction block in the area of the lesion, with preservation of electrical excitability of the distal nerve segment. The prognosis for complete recovery is good. A common example is "Saturday night palsy," a compression neuropathy of the radial nerve following sleeping on the arm. This type of nerve lesion has a favorable outcome, with recovery often seen within days or weeks.
- **Axonotmesis:** a lesion in which there is a transection of the axon while the nerve sheath remains intact.[23] Because the nerve sheath remains intact, regeneration can occur under optimal conditions; in more severe cases, however, regeneration does not occur spontaneously. Radial nerve palsies associated with humeral fracture are often due to axonotmesis.
- **Neurotmesis:** a nerve lesion with complete transection of the nerve fiber and sheath.[23] These

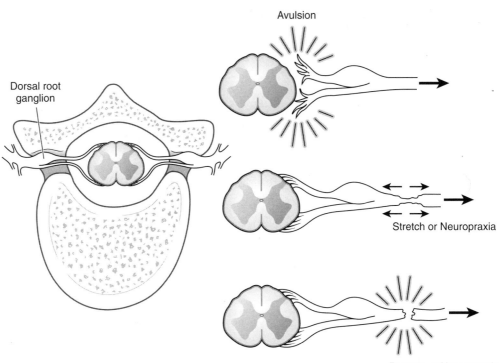

Avulsion

Dorsal root
ganglion

Stretch or Neuropraxia

Rupture or Neurotmesis

Figure 15-3 Peripheral
nerve injury.
*(By permission of Mayo
Foundation for Medical
Education and Research. All
rights reserved.)*

lesions result from injuries with sharp objects, such as knives or broken glass, and with more blunt mechanisms, such as chain saws, propeller blades, automobile metal, and animal bites. Because spontaneous recovery does not occur, surgery is the mainstay of treatment. Nerve grafting is necessary.

There are several classification schemes for identifying nerve injury. Figure 15-4 compares the Seddon and the Sunderland classifications.

Peripheral nerve injuries are often described in terms of their anatomic location. The ulnar, median, and radial nerves and the brachial plexus are the most commonly injured in the upper extremity. The sciatic and fibular (peroneal) nerves are the most often injured in the lower extremity.

Tunnel syndromes and **entrapments** are defined as a focal neuropathy caused by restriction or mechanical distortion of a nerve within a fibrous or fibro-osseous tunnel.[3] Nerves pass through fibrous, osteofibrous, and fibromuscular tunnels from their origin in the spinal cord to their effector organ, risking compression, damage, and impairment of function at any point. Damage may be due to many causes. Table 15-1 shows examples of entrapment neuropathies of the upper and lower limbs.

Upper Extremity

Ulnar Nerve Injuries

The ulnar nerve is one of the terminal branches of the brachial plexus that arise from the medial cord of the brachial plexus. It receives fibers from both cervical (C8) and thoracic (T1) nerve roots and supplies some muscles of the forearm and hand and the skin on the ulnar side of the hand. The ulnar nerve can be palpated as it courses along the groove

between the olecranon process and the medial epicondyle of the humerus, giving rise to the popular term "the funny bone."

Most commonly, the ulnar nerve is compressed or entrapped at the elbow region. This may be due to repetitive microtrauma. The ulnar nerve may also be injured following elbow fractures or dislocations or from improper positioning during surgery.[3]

The weakness in hand and finger muscles leads to weakness in grip. For example, patients with ulnar nerve palsy exhibit difficulty manipulating coins or turning a key in a lock. Ulnar nerve paralysis may lead to clawing of the little and ring fingers. Because of muscle imbalance, the fingers are hyperextended at the metacarpophalangeal joints and the more distal joints are flexed, leading to a clawlike appearance.[22] **Froment's sign** of ulnar palsy is shown in Figure 15-5. The patient grasps a flat object firmly with the thumb and index finger of each hand and pulls vigorously. If flexion of the distal phalanx of the thumb occurs, the test result is positive and indicative of ulnar palsy.[22] Sensory symptoms include loss of sensation over the fifth finger, the ulnar aspect of the fourth finger, and the ulnar border of the palm. With ulnar nerve lesions at the elbow, sensation is also diminished on the dorso-ulnar aspect of the hand.

The ulnar nerve can also suffer entrapment at the wrist in Guyon's canal, which is formed between the pisiform bone and the hook of the hamate bone. The usual cause is chronic or repeated external pressure by tools, bicycle handlebars, the handles of canes, or excessive push-ups.[3] Other causes include degenerative wrist joint ganglia, rheumatoid arthritis, and distal vascular anomalies.[3]

Volkmann's contracture (ischemic contracture) is a serious, persistent flexion contraction of the forearm and

PERIPHERAL NERVE TRAUMA

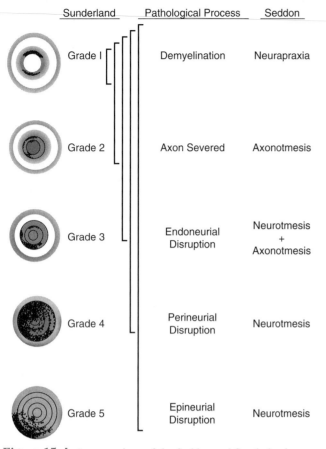

Figure 15-4 A comparison of the Seddon and Sunderland classification systems.
(From Bradley WG: Neurology in clinical practice, Oxford, 2000, Butterworth-Heinemann.)

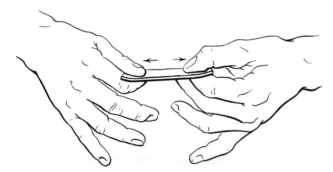

Figure 15-5 Froment's sign of ulnar palsy: positive in the left hand, as indicated by flexion of the terminal phalanx of the thumb.
(From Mayo Clinic Department of Neurology: Mayo Clinic examinations in neurology, ed 7, St Louis, 1998, Mosby.)

hand caused by ischemia. Pressure (e.g., from restrictive dressings or a tight cast) or a crushing injury in the region of the elbow usually precedes the neurovascular compression. The resultant damage can range from permanent fibrosis to muscle degeneration. Clinicians must closely monitor

at-risk patients for the symptoms of pain, pallor, edema, cyanosis, paralysis, and coldness in the hand or arm. Complaints of pain suggesting that a cast or bandage is too tight must not be ignored.

Median Nerve Injuries

The median nerve is one of the terminal branches of the brachial plexus that extend along the radial portions of the forearm and hand. It innervates the palm and radial side of the hand. The nerve may be injured anywhere along its path. For example, the nerve may be injured in the arm by penetration or compression, in the antecubital fossa by an injection injury, or in the forearm by trauma. Complete interruption of the nerve results in an inability to pronate the forearm or flex the fingers. The most common entrapment neuropathy is CTS, which is discussed later in this chapter.

Radial Nerve Injuries

The **radial nerve** is the largest branch of the brachial plexus and arises on each side of the posterior cord. This nerve supplies the skin and extensor muscles of the arm and forearm and may be injured anywhere along its course. Common types and sites of injury include the following:[3]

- Compression in the axilla (often caused by ill-fitting crutches or from the weight of a sleeping partner's head) or in the arm (Saturday night palsy)
- Fractures in the middle third of the humerus

Clinical manifestations of radial nerve injury (also called **radial nerve palsy**) include paralysis of extension of the wrist and fingers (wrist and finger drop) and decreased sensation on the dorsum of the hand.

Brachial Plexus Injuries

The brachial plexus is a network of nerves in the neck that passes under the clavicle and into the axilla, innervating the muscles and skin of the chest, shoulders, and arms. It originates from C5 to C8 and T1 and forms upper, middle, and lower trunks (Fig. 15-6). The results of injury to the brachial plexus are determined by the trunk or nerve cord that is affected.

With trauma, the most common mechanisms for injury relate to stretch, but may also result from compression (e.g., hematoma or tumor), contusion (e.g., gunshot wounds) or direct penetration (e.g., knife wounds). Depending on severity, nerves may be functional or nonfunctional and may be in continuity or discontinuity. Brachial plexus injuries produce a severe neurologic deficit. Frequently, surgery is necessary to improve function. This may consist of primary surgical reconstruction concentrating on the nerve or secondary surgery concentrating on muscle or tendon transfers or bony procedures. With a less profound injury, muscle and tendon transplants are sometimes used.[6]

Two terms generally related to brachial plexus injury are as follows:

- **Rupture:** Individual nerves may be pulled apart (neurotmesis) distal to the dorsal root ganglia (postganglionic injury). Without surgery, recovery will not take place.

TABLE 15-1	Entrapment Neuropathies of the Upper and Lower Limbs		
Nerve	**Site of Compression**	**Predisposing Factors**	**Major Clinical Features**
Upper Limbs			
Median	Wrist (carpal tunnel syndrome)	Tenosynovitis, etc.	Sensory loss, thenar atrophy
	Anterior interosseous	Strenuous exercise, trauma	Abnormal pinch sign, normal sensation
	Elbow (pronator teres syndrome)	Repetitive elbow motions	Tenderness of pronator teres, sensory loss
Ulnar	Elbow (cubital tunnel syndrome)	Elbow leaning, trauma	Clawing and sensory loss of fourth and fifth fingers
	Guyon's canal	Mechanics, cyclists	Hypothenar atrophy, variable sensory loss
Radial	Axilla	Crutches	Wristdrop and finger drop; triceps involved, sensory loss
	Spiral groove	Abnormal sleep postures	Wristdrop, and finger drop sensory loss
	Posterior interosseous	Elbow synovitis	Paresis of finger extensors, radial wrist deviation
	Superficial sensory branch (cheiralgia paresthetica)	Wrist bands, handcuffs	Paresthesias in dorsum of hand
Suprascapular	Suprascapular notch	Blunt trauma	Atrophy of supraspinatus and infraspinatus muscles
Lower trunk of the brachial plexus or C8/T1 roots	Thoracic outlet	Cervical rib, enlarged C7 transverse process	Atrophy of intrinsic hand muscles, paresthesias of hand and forearm
Lower Limbs			
Sciatic	Sciatic notch	Endometriosis, intramuscular injections	Pain down thigh, footdrop, absent ankle jerk
	Hip	Fracture dislocations	
	Piriformis muscle	—	
	Popliteal fossa	Popliteal Baker's cyst	
Fibular	Fibular neck	Leg crossing, squatting	Footdrop, weak evertors, sensory loss in dorsum of foot
Deep fibular	Anterior compartment	Muscle edema	Footdrop
Tibial	Medial malleolus (tarsal tunnel syndrome)	Ankle fracture, tenosynovitis	Sensory loss over sole of foot
Femoral	Inguinal ligament	Lithotomy position	Weak knee extension, absent knee jerk
Lateral femoral cutaneous	Inguinal ligament (meralgia paresthetica)	Tight clothing, weight gain, utility belts	Sensory loss in lateral thigh
Ilioinguinal	Abdominal wall	Trauma, surgical incision	Direct hernia, sensory loss in the iliac crest, crural area
Obturator	Obturator canal	Pelvic fracture, tumor	Sensory loss in medial thigh, weak hip adduction

Adapted From Bradley WG: *Neurology in clinical practice*, Oxford, 2000, Butterworth-Heinemann.

- **Avulsion:** Nerves may be pulled directly from the spinal cord (preganglionic injury), leaving anterior and posterior roots disconnected (see Fig. 15-3).

Upper Plexus Injury. An upper plexus injury typically results from the forced separation of the humeral head and shoulder, resulting from a motorcycle or motor vehicle accident, fall, or birth injury. All of the muscles of the shoulder, except the trapezius, may be involved, as well as the flexor muscles of the elbow. Such injuries often occur in multitrauma situations, and the nerve injury may be misinterpreted as pain from the skeletal injury or assumed to be a rotator cuff pathology.[30] This may lead to delay in treatment or inappropriate treatment.

When an upper plexus injury results from forcible traction in childbirth **(obstetric brachial plexus palsy),** it is commonly called **Erb's palsy.** Babies hold the affected limb adducted at the shoulder and extended at the elbow, with the hand pronated. There is sensory loss in a C5 and C6 distribution[6] (see Fig. 2-12). While awaiting spontaneous recovery, the limb may be immobilized for comfort and to reduce inflammation and swelling; physical therapy is necessary to maintain full passive range of motion.

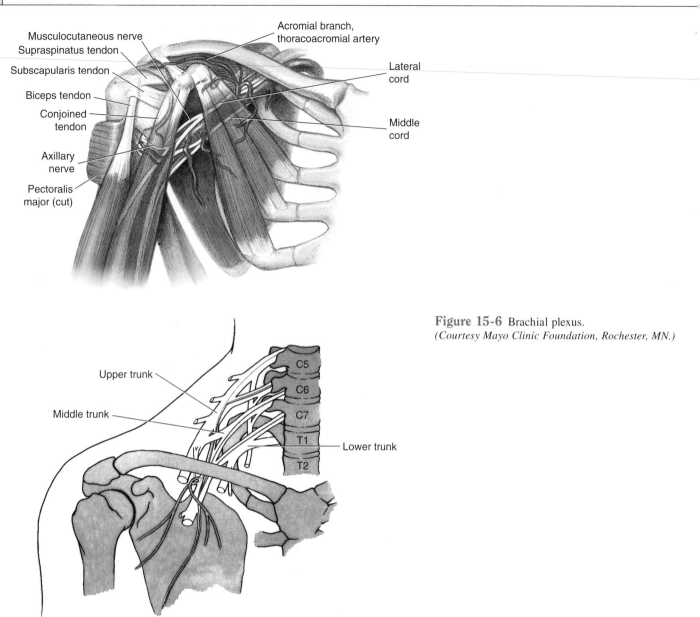

Figure 15-6 Brachial plexus.
(Courtesy Mayo Clinic Foundation, Rochester, MN.)

Lower Plexus Injury. Damage to the lower plexus (C8 and T1) rarely occurs as a type of birth palsy or traction injury separating the upper limb from the trunk. Lower plexus paralysis involves wasting of the small hand muscles and a clawing of the hand. The shoulder and elbow motor function is preserved, but there is weakness in the flexors of the fingers and wrist and sensory loss in the forearm and hand. The weakness and sensory loss occur in a C8 and T1 distribution.[6] A **Horner's syndrome** (ptosis, miosis, anhidrosis, and exophthalmos) is often associated with lower plexus injury due to the proximity of the sympathetic chain near these neural elements.[30] The presence of a Horner's syndrome (see Fig. 16-4) is suggestive of a preganglionic injury.

Complete Brachial Plexus Injury. With a complete brachial plexus injury, depending on the level of the lesion, paralysis may involve all of the muscles of the upper extremity (except the trapezius) and a loss of sensation in the entire hand and forearm. The limb is flaccid and areflexic.[6] In cases where paralysis of the limb is complete, amputation may be indicated.[6]

Lower Extremity

Common Fibular Nerve Injury

The peripheral nerve plexuses that form the **fibular nerve (peroneal nerve)** are formed from the L4 to S2 nerve roots. Because of confusion between the terms *peroneal* and *perineal,* the Federative Committee on Anatomic Terminology has renamed the peroneal nerve the fibular nerve.[3] This nerve can be injured by prolonged traction, leg crossing, application of a tourniquet or cast, and compression during surgery. Clinical manifestations of fibular nerve injury include foot-

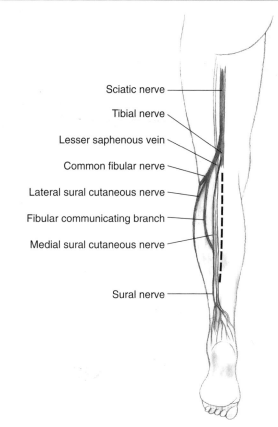

Figure 15-7 Peripheral nerve plexuses. *(Courtesy Mayo Clinic Foundation, Rochester, MN.)*

drop, steppage gait, and sensory loss of the medial aspect of the dorsum of the foot and outer aspect of the leg[3] (Fig. 15-7).

Sciatic Nerve Injury

The **sciatic nerve** is the biggest nerve of the body. It is a long nerve originating in the sacral plexus and extending through the muscles of the thigh, leg, and foot. It has many branches and supplies the hamstrings and all the muscles below the knee. The sciatic nerve may be injured in several places and through several mechanisms. Causes of damage to the sciatic nerve include the following:

- Fractures of the pelvis or femur
- Hematomas in the posterior thigh compartment
- Gunshot or other penetrating wounds
- Injections into the buttocks that are poorly placed
- Compression during childbirth

Clinicians should always use caution and identify the appropriate anatomic landmarks when administering intramuscular (IM) injections. Symptoms and signs of sciatic nerve injury include an inability to flex the knee, paralysis of muscles below the knee, pain across the buttocks and into the thigh, footdrop, and sensory loss of the entire foot.[3]

Assessment

Regardless of the exact cause and location of peripheral nerve injury, a common set of symptoms and signs are definable. Patients may have any or all of the following:[3,22]

- Motor: weakness, loss of dexterity
- Sensory: decreased feeling and loss of two-point discrimination
- Deep tendon reflexes (DTRs): diminished or lost
- Pain: intermittent or constant pain in the involved area at the nerve insertion site (percussion tenderness that is strong immediately after injury is suggestive of rupture; absence of tenderness suggests avulsion)[30]
- Horner's syndrome

If the injury is 2 to 3 weeks old, the patient may also have the following additional symptoms:

- Motor: muscle atrophy and fasciculations
- Skin: color and temperature changes in the affected area

PERIPHERAL NERVE TUMORS

PNS dysfunction can also be caused by tumors. There are several classifications of peripheral nerve tumors; unfortunately, their terminology is not uniform. The classification system that is based mainly on tumor location is described in this chapter. Symptoms may be due to tumors that affect the nerve primarily or secondarily by compression. Tumor removal may be required.

The most common tumors of the peripheral nerves arise from the **nerve sheaths.** The majority of these tumors are slow growing, encapsulated tumors. The benign lesions are either schwannomas (neurilemmomas) or **neurofibromas,** which may be single or multiple. Schwannomas typically arise from a single nerve fascicle and displace the main nerve; in contrast, neurofibromas generally involve several nerve fascicles and usually are more central within the nerve. Therefore schwannomas are easier to resect. When multiple neurofibromas are present, they may be part of a systemic condition known as **neurofibromatosis** or **von Recklinghausen's disease.** Neurofibromatosis is an inheritable condition with skin pigmentary changes (café au lait spots) and nerve sheath tumors. The rare malignant lesions, so-called malignant peripheral nerve sheath tumors, manifest with increasing pain, neurologic deficit, or size of the lesion.[35] They may arise spontaneously or following radiation or transformation from neurofibromas. Schwannomas do not become malignant.

Other types of benign or malignant tumors may affect peripheral nerves intrinsically. An example of a benign lesion would be an intraneural ganglion cyst. This mass is derived from a neighboring joint; cyst fluid may extend within the epineurium of the nerve and displace nerve fascicles, causing compression. Metastatic infiltrations of the peripheral nerves can occur in lymphoma, lymphatic leukemias, and adenocarcinoma.[3] These patients may also have pain, weakness, and sensory loss.

Individual nerves can be compressed or invaded secondarily by growths from adjacent tissue. For example, joint-related cysts (ganglia) may compress a nerve from the outside (in contrast to the intraneural cysts described previously). Other benign lesions (e.g., lipomas) or malignant ones (e.g., sarcomas) also may compress nerves.

INFLAMMATORY DEMYELINATING POLYRADICULONEUROPATHIES

Inflammatory demyelinating polyradiculoneuropathies are acquired and immunologically mediated. They can be classified by their clinical course into two major groups: an **acute inflammatory demyelinating polyradiculoneuropathy (AIDP),** called **Guillain-Barré syndrome,** and **chronic inflammatory demyelinating polyradiculoneuropathy (CIDP)**[3] (see Chapter 9 for Guillain-Barré syndrome).

It is estimated that CIDP represents approximately 20% of all initially undiagnosed neuropathies for which patients are referred to specialized neuromuscular centers.[3] An autoimmune basis is suspected, as with AIDP, but CIDP has a longer clinical course and is rarely associated with preceding infections. There are two patterns of disease associated with CIDP. About 60% of the patients show a continuous or step-wise progressive course over months to years, whereas one third have a relapsing course with partial or complete recovery between recurrences.[3]

To fulfill the diagnostic criteria of CIDP, weakness must be present for at least 2 months. Proximal limb weakness is almost as severe as distal limb weakness.[3] Both upper and lower limbs are affected, although the legs are often more severely involved. Muscle wasting is rarely pronounced. These signs provide helpful clinical clues to distinguish CIDP from axonal neuropathies.[3] Diagnostic criteria are based on clinical features, electrodiagnostic studies, cerebro-spinal fluid (CSF) examination, and results from nerve biopsy.[15] It is important to recognize CIDP in patients with diabetes because, unlike diabetic polyneuropathy, CIDP is treatable.

CHRONIC PERIPHERAL NEUROPATHIES

Metabolic and Toxic Neuropathy

In most neuropathies, the more distal part of the peripheral nerve is affected, secondary to related metabolic changes in the nerve cell and alterations in axonal flow. **Diabetes mellitus (DM)** is the most common cause of metabolic neuropathy. In fact, **diabetic neuropathy** is one of the most common chronic, demyelinating, generalized neuropathies.[10] Metabolic or toxic neuropathies are, for the most part, chronic, progressive diseases.

Disruptions in the peripheral nerve system are common in diabetic patients, particularly those over 40 years of age. There are several different kinds of diabetic neuropathies, including **diabetic amyotrophy** (acute, painful, asymmetric proximal lower limb syndrome), **diabetic pseudotabes** (large-fiber neuropathy), and **diabetic arthropathy** (involves small joints in the feet).[3] Axonal degeneration of unmyelinated nerve fibers occurs early, followed by Schwann cell abnormalities.

Symptoms may vary and can include decreased sensation, diminished or absent ankle DTRs, impaired vibration appreciation, muscle tenderness, or abnormal objective measurements (e.g., nerve conduction studies) without evidence of other causes of neuropathy.[3] With more severe involvement, patients develop variable loss of sensation in the toes, feet, and distal legs; decreased abnormality of muscle stretch reflexes; and autonomic abnormalities and weakness of small foot and ankle dorsiflexor muscles.[10] Classic signs of type 2 diabetes are visual changes with diabetic retinopathy that include symptoms of third cranial nerve palsy without pupillary involvement and paresthesias, a common manifestation of diabetic neuropathies.

Mononeuritis multiplex (multiple mononeuropathies) is also associated with DM and other vascular diseases such as vasculitis. It is believed to have a metabolic and vascular basis.[2] The metabolic changes of diabetes may be responsible for abnormal neuronal and axonal metabolism and subsequent impairment of axonal transport.[3] The vascular changes are being researched, but it is thought that endoneurial hypoxia is produced by decreased blood flow to the nerve and increased vascular resistance.[10] The hypoxia inhibits axonal transport.[3] This neuropathy has an acute onset with asymmetric symptoms. Initially only one peripheral nerve is affected, but gradually other nerves, in a step-by-step fashion, become involved over a period of weeks to months.

Other causes of metabolic and toxic neuropathies include the following:

- Uremia: produces symmetric, sensorimotor polyneuropathy. Dysesthesias, muscle cramps, and restless legs are common symptoms. The neuropathy may stabilize or improve with long-term dialysis.[2]
- Alcoholism: the most common nutrition-related neuropathy; alcoholism causes deficiency in the B-complex vitamins, which are necessary for proper nerve conduction. Axonal degeneration and demyelination of the axons in the legs cause pain, dysesthesias, burning paresthesias, and tenderness and cramps in muscles surrounding the nerves. There is a loss of tendon reflexes, and the legs are always more affected than the arms.[3]
- Drugs: many pharmaceutical agents can cause peripheral neuropathy. Some of the known agents are listed in Table 15-2. Most drug-induced neuropathies will reverse when the offending drug is discontinued.[3]
- Heavy metal intoxication: includes metals such as arsenic, mercury, and lead. Recognition of neurotoxic disorders is difficult when exposure is chronic or symptoms are nonspecific.[1] History taking should include questions regarding exposure to chemicals, and the clinician should be aware of occupations that expose people to metals such as lead (e.g., working in smelting factories and metal foundries; jobs involving demolition, ship building, or manufacturing of batteries or paint).[1] People who take some traditional Chinese medicinal preparations may be exposed to chronic poisoning from arsenic and mercury.[1]
- Anorexia and nutritional deficiency: especially a deficiency in the B-complex vitamins (see "Alcoholism").

In addition, other chronic neuropathies occur in connection with other disorders:

TABLE 15-2	Neuropathies Caused by Drugs	
Drug	**Clinical and Pathologic Features**	**Comments**
Antineoplastic		
Cisplatin	S, DA, N	Binds to DNA; disrupts axonal transport?
Suramin	SM, DA, SD	DA: inhibits binding of growth factors; SD: immunomodulating effects?
Taxoids (paclitaxel, docetaxel)	S, DA	Promote microtubule assembly; disrupt axonal transport
Vincristine	SM, M, DA	Interferes with microtubule assembly; disrupts axonal transport
Antimicrobial		
Chloroquinine	SM, DA	Myopathy
Dapsone	M, DA	Optic atrophy
Isoniazid	SM, DA	Pyridoxine antagonist
Metronidazole	S, DA	
Nitrofurantoin	SM, DA	
Antiviral		
Dideoxynucleosides (dideoxycytidine, dideoxyinosine, stavudine)	S, DA	
Cardiovascular		
Amiodarone	SM, SD	Lysosomal lamellar inclusions, myopathy
Hydralazine	SM, DA	Pyridoxine antagonist
Perhexiline	SM, SD	Lipid inclusions
CNS		
Nitrous oxide	S, DA	Inhibits vitamin B_{12}–dependent methionine synthase; myelopathy synthase; myelopathy
Thalidomide	S, N	
Other		
Colchicine	SM, DA	Myopathy, raised creatine kinase levels
Disulfiram	SM, DA	
Gold	SM, DA	Myokymia
Phenytoin	SM, DA	Asymptomatic in most
Pyridoxine	S, N, DA	Megadoses >300 mg/day
L-Tryptophan	SM, DA	Eosinophilia-myalgia syndrome

From Bradley WG: *Neurology in clinical practice,* Oxford, 2000, Butterworth-Heinemann.
CNS, Central nervous system–active drugs; *DA,* distal axonopathy; *DNA,* deoxyribonucleic acid; *M,* motor; *N,* neuronopathy; *S,* sensory; *SD,* segmental demyelination; *SM,* sensorimotor neuropathy.

- Systemic lupus erythematosus (SLE): A symmetric, subacute, or chronic axonal polyneuropathy with predominant sensory symptoms is most common.[3]
- Scleroderma: Carpal and cubital tunnel syndrome may be present; these neuropathies may be due to an increase in collagen within the nerve.[3]
- Cryoglobulinemia: These immunoglobulins have caused mononeuropathies and distal neuropathies; associated neuropathies may vary in extent of involvement from mild paresthesias to marked motor and sensory changes in the extremities.[3]
- Sjögren's syndrome: Sjögren's syndrome is associated with mild distal sensory neuropathy with symmetric mononeuropathy;[3] the pathogenesis of this neuropathy may be related to blood vessels within the nerve, since vascular and perivascular infiltrates are seen in pathologic studies of patients with this syndrome.
- Human immunodeficiency virus (HIV): Neuropathies associated with HIV may be related to the disease

complex, medications used to combat the disease, or the nutritional imbalances accompanying it.

Inherited Neuropathy

Some patients with neuropathy may have an inherited form of peripheral nerve dysfunction that is of autosomal dominant, recessive or X-linked inheritance.[5] Although vary rare, recognition is important because many require specific therapy. Several generalizations about these inherited forms may be drawn. First, peripheral nerves are involved in each of the disorders. Second, both motor and sensory fibers are commonly affected; however, in certain variants, only motor or sensory neurons are affected. Finally, the genetic patterns of these diseases are being recognized with newer genetic testing.[5]

The two most common forms of **hereditary motor and sensory neuropathy (HMSN)** are as follows:
- Type I: hypertrophic Charcot-Marie-Tooth disease
- Type II: neuronal type of Charcot-Marie-Tooth disease

Both types are inherited as an autosomal dominant trait.[3] Initial symptoms include difficulty in walking, abnormally high lifting of the knees during walking, frequent fatigue, and muscle aches after exercise. Atrophy progresses in the legs, but sensory complaints are uncommon. In a few patients, symptoms may spread to the upper extremities, resulting in loss of fine motor control or tremor. During physical examination these patients exhibit hypoactive reflexes, and about one fourth have thickened peripheral nerves.[3] Other hereditary neuropathies include hereditary neuropathy with liability to pressure palsy (HNPP), amyloidoses, porphyrias, disorders of lipid metabolism, disorders associated with defective deoxyribonucleic acid (DNA) repair, and other idiopathic neuropathies.[3]

Assessment

Peripheral nerve disorders result in motor, sensory, and autonomic losses in the distribution appropriate to the nerve involved.[3] A complete neurologic assessment should be done, including an investigation of patient complaints with attention to the history, motor, and sensory assessment parameters.

History

Document the onset of symptoms, such as acute or chronic sensations of numbness, tingling, and burning, with symptoms noticed first in the distal extremities. Note occupational or daily activities that aggravate the condition.

Motor Parameters

The type and distribution of a motor deficit helps the clinician determine the affected nerve.[3] Assess the motor system by means of inspection and testing of strength, using a head-to-toe approach and comparing sides (right versus left) and extremities (upper versus lower). Measuring extremities with a tape measure helps in the comparisons. Noting minor differences in the circumference of the extremities is an unreliable means of determining atrophy, since asymmetric development of muscle groups is not uncommon.[22] Measurements are helpful, however, in determining progression of atrophy or documenting recovery.

Muscle strength is tested by having the patient move against gravity and resistance.[22] The clinician should observe for muscle contraction and feel the strength exerted. If the patient is unable to move against gravity, the ability to move the extremity with gravity eliminated should be assessed[22] (see Chapter 2 for evaluation of motor strength).

The major motor finding for the patient with a neuropathy is motor weakness, although the degree and distribution depend on the nature and severity of the neuropathy. Muscle cramps, fasciculations, myokymia, and tremor are positive manifestations of motor nerve dysfunction.[3] Motor symptoms in polyneuropathies may produce early distal toe and ankle extensor weakness, resulting in tripping on rugs or uneven ground.

Muscle examination findings vary according to the peripheral nerve disorder and may range from slight weakness to paralysis of the affected extremity.

BOX 15-2	Terms Used to Describe Sensory Changes

- **Dysesthesia:** Unpleasant, abnormal sensation in response to an ordinary, painless stimulus
- **Paresthesia:** Unpleasant sensation, sometimes arising spontaneously without an apparent stimulus; often described as "pins and needles"
- **Allodynia:** Perception of nonpainful stimuli as painful, such as stroking of the skin
- **Anesthesia:** No recognition of external stimuli other than movement of the part or extreme pressure on the part
- **Hypoesthesia:** Diminished recognition of a sharp or dull object on the skin
- **Hypalgesia:** A lessened sensitivity to pain; the opposite of **hyperalgesia**

Adapted from Bosch EP, Smith BE: Disorders of peripheral nerves. In Bradley WG, editor: *Neurology in clinical practice*, Philadelphia, 2004, Butterworth-Heinemann.

Sensory Parameters

First, note the patient's ability to perceive stimuli. Compare sensations in symmetric areas on the two sides of the body. When testing pain, temperature, and touch, compare distal and proximal areas of the extremities.[22] Terms used to describe sensory changes are listed in Box 15-2. At various times during the examination, ask the patient to indicate, with a finger, the exact location of the stimulation. This practice not only sharpens the patient's attention during a relatively monotonous procedure but also may reveal an unsuspected defect in the ability to localize stimuli (**topagnosis**).[22] Clinicians should remember that sensory testing is a challenge because the patient's underlying condition may lead to fatigue, which may produce unreliable and inconsistent results.

Sensory assessment varies according to the exact PNS dysfunction; however, patients commonly describe sensory loss in a specific area. For example, patients with CTS report numbness in their entire hand (that is actually only affecting the radial 3½ digits); patients with diabetic peripheral neuropathies describe loss of sensation in a stocking-and-glove distribution.[3] Because routine sensory conduction studies assess only large, myelinated fibers, such studies may be entirely normal in early compression syndromes or in selective small-fiber neuropathies.[3] Other studies may be necessary, such as quantitative thermal sensory threshold testing or tests for autonomic functions.[3]

Sensory findings are most commonly identified in discrete nerve territories. One of the earliest indications of sensory loss is decreased vibratory sensation, which can be tested with a tuning fork.[22] In patients with diabetes, hardness of the plantar skin has been found to correlate with decreased sensation and severity of neuropathy.

Vibration and Position

Begin with the fingers and toes. If these tests are normal, one can assume that more proximal areas are also normal.[22] Stimuli should be scattered so that most dermatomes and major peripheral nerves are included in the assessment. Vary the pace of testing so that the patient does not merely respond to a repetitive rhythm.[22]

Inspection and Palpation

Examine the nerve by inspection and palpation. Look and feel carefully along the course of the nerve for abnormal masses or for areas that cause unusual tenderness to palpation or percussion.[22] Assess the skin for increased warmth or coolness, redness, pallor, cyanosis, increase or decrease in sweating, atrophy of the skin or hyperkeratosis, and irregular growth of the hair and nails.[22]

Pain

Assess pain using an appropriate pain assessment scale (see Chapter 23). Pain is frequently due to direct insult to the nerve, as with the pain of a brachial plexus injury, but may also be due to muscle imbalance related to the dysfunction. Sensory findings are often mixed with pain. For example, patients with metabolic, toxic, nutritional, or idiopathic peripheral neuropathies typically complain of symmetric sensations of numbness, tingling, burning, tightness, band-like constrictions, and, at times, a feeling of walking on sand or pebbles.[22] **Neuropathic pain** often has a deep, burning, or drawing character that may be associated with jabbing or electrical shooting or lancinating pains.[3]

Peripheral nerve lesions may precipitate the development of pain syndromes; indeed, the more traumatic the injury to the peripheral nerve, the greater the likelihood of a pain syndrome. The more common pain syndromes associated with PNS dysfunction are summarized in Box 15-3.

Autonomic Function

One or multiple organs may be involved. For example, diabetic autonomic neuropathies can manifest themselves in the form of genitourinary, gastrointestinal, or cardiovascular signs and symptoms.[3] Carefully question the patient regarding symptoms related to autonomic function, including the following:[3]

- Bladder or sexual dysfunction: may indicate genitourinary autonomic problems
- Early satiety, anorexia, nausea, or bowel dysfunction: may suggest gastrointestinal autonomic dysfunction
- Postural hypotension, fainting, orthostatic light-headedness, reduced or excessive sweating: associated with cardiovascular dysfunction

Research has shown that patients with diabetic autonomic neuropathy can experience severe intraoperative hypothermia.[20] This is thought to happen because these patients' peripheral neuropathy delays the onset of thermoregulatory vasoconstriction and reduces its efficacy once triggered.[20] These patients need to be monitored closely during and after surgery.

Continual assessments compare current findings with initial baseline analyses. A flow sheet is helpful to document serial assessments of the affected areas.

Neurodiagnostic and Laboratory Studies

When electrodiagnostic studies are carefully performed and adapted to the particular clinical situation, they can play a

---

| BOX 15-3 | **Common Pain Syndromes Associated With Peripheral Nervous System Dysfunction** |

Causalgia
Causalgia is associated with injury to proximal segments of the median, ulnar, and sciatic nerves and the brachial plexus. The patient is protective of the affected extremity, and manipulation of the area results in an explosion of pain. Pain onset is soon after injury and is typically described as burning, piercing, or cutting.

Reflex Sympathetic Dystrophy (RSD)
RSD is associated with injury to the distal portion of an extremity.
Pain does not have the severity of severe, acute causalgia.
Manipulation of the extremity is less likely to cause a burst of pain.

Neuritic Pain (Neurodynia)
Neuritic pain is less severe than either causalgia or RSD.
Pain is usually characterized as deep or throbbing but within the distribution of the nerve.
Unlike causalgia (and sometimes RSD), it rarely spreads to other parts of the affected extremity.

Neuromas
Pain associated with neuromas is extremely difficult to treat because of the damage done to the nerve itself.
Neuromas are associated with amputation, lesions in sensory nerves, or a sensory-motor nerve that cannot be repaired.

Phantom Limb Pain
This type of pain may occur with amputation but also is associated with severe denervation of an extremity (e.g., a brachial plexus injury).
This type of pain is very difficult to treat.

Regeneration Pain
When a nerve regenerates, the patient may experience a shocklike pain in the distribution of the nerve.
Avoiding vibration, percussion, or compression of the affected limb usually limits this pain to a manageable degree.

---

key role in the evaluation by confirming the presence of neuropathy, providing precise localization of focal nerve lesions, and giving information as to the nature of the underlying nerve disease[3] (see Chapter 3). The following neurodiagnostic studies may be ordered:

- Electromyography (EMG) and nerve conduction studies (NCS): Typically performed together, these are the most common neurodiagnostic studies used in the diagnosis, assessment, and reassessment of peripheral nerve disorders. Because wallerian degeneration takes 2 to 3 weeks to occur, EMG is rarely indicated earlier than 3 weeks after the initial onset of clinical symptoms.[30] Severe or progressive neurologic deficit may be a special circumstance in which early use of EMG would be indicated. EMG and NCS are helpful in confirming a diagnosis of peripheral neuropathy and grading it.

- Somatosensory-evoked potentials (SSEPs): Absence with individual nerve stimulation implies root avulsion.[30]
- Motor-evoked potentials (MEPs): Allows the evaluation of the integrity of the ventral motor roots.[30]
- Nerve action potentials (NAPs): Any positive response across a lesion suggests viability or regeneration of axons; flat tracings reflect no capacity to recover.[30]
- Sonography: Helpful to differentiate peripheral nerve tumors from lymph nodes.
- Computed tomography (CT) with myelogram: An imaging modality to test for diagnosing root avulsion.[30]
- Magnetic resonance imaging (MRI): Provides high resolution of mass lesions. Some centers use MRI instead of CT with myelogram in assessing root avulsions.[31]
- Positron emission tomography (PET): PET is being evaluated for distinguishing malignant from benign peripheral nerve sheath tumors.[11]

Treatment

Medical Management

Nonoperative therapy for peripheral nerve lesions is indicated while awaiting spontaneous recovery, if surgery is not feasible, or as a follow-up to surgical intervention. The goals of conservative therapy include the following:[3]

- Improvement of symptoms related to compression
- Avoidance of secondary damage in paralyzed extremities
- Prevention or delay of muscle atrophy with the use of electrotherapy
- Stimulation or regeneration of motor and sensory fibers
- Functional replacement through exercise of the remaining musculature

Conservative measures include observation, immobilization, rest, exercise, ultrasound, heat, massage, steroid injections, and antiinflammatory medications. Trials of medical treatment and combinations of different measures should be monitored to assess the patient's response. Specific medical management parameters include treatment of the following:

- Tunnel syndromes: splinting and rest to relieve compression; used especially at night for approximately 6 months.[3,36] Avoidance of exacerbating positions or activities is important. A trial of antiinflammatory agents and a steroid injection may be applicable.
- Peripheral nerve tumors: small or asymptomatic benign lesions may be followed with repeated clinical examinations and imaging. For malignant lesions, the optimal treatment is still being debated, but usually consists of a combination of surgery, radiotherapy, and chemotherapy.
- Diabetic neuropathies: intensive control of blood glucose levels; management is primarily symptomatic and palliative.[10]

- Chronic inflammatory demyelinating polyradiculoneuropathy (CIDP): prednisone, plasmapheresis, and intravenous (IV) immune globulin have all been shown to be effective treatments. Depending on the severity of the disease, some patients undergoing plasmapheresis may need treatment for months to years.[3] It is important to treat aggressively in order to attain an optimal treatment response as soon as possible, since the longer the disease persists, the more it becomes refractory to treatment.[15]
- Inherited neuropathies: the majority have no specific treatment. Rare ones may need enzyme replacement therapy or bone marrow transplantation.[5]

Surgical Management

Surgical intervention in peripheral nerve lesions is frequently performed for nerve injuries, compression, tumors, and neuropathic pain. Indications for surgery would include lack of recovery of closed nerve injuries that have not recovered to some extent within 3 to 6 months. Open injuries should be explored urgently because severed nerves fare better with early surgery and would not recover otherwise. Patients with symptomatic compression syndromes, tumors, or refractory neuropathic pain may be candidates for surgery. Some patients with neuropathies may be candidates for a nerve biopsy (such as the sural nerve). Surgical techniques for specific peripheral nerve injuries include the following:

- Direct nerve repair: typically only performed after acute management of sharp injury such as from glass or a knife. Two ends of a nerve are directly reapposed.
- Neurolysis: used when a nerve is in continuity and the lesion conducts an NAP across it. Scar is removed from the nerve.
- Nerve grafting: performed when there is a postganglionic rupture or a neuroma in continuity that does not conduct an NAP. The neuroma is then resected. Interpositional grafts are used to span the defect. Sural nerves or other cutaneous nerves are often used for donor nerves.

In the area of brachial plexus injuries, new surgeries are being developed to help patients regain lost function.[30] Priorities for functional return include elbow flexion, shoulder abduction (external rotation) and stability and hand sensibility, then grasp (wrist extension, finger flexion), release (wrist flexion, finger extension), and intrinsic function.[30] Hand function has traditionally been difficult to achieve because of the long distance necessary for reinnervation and slow nature of nerve regeneration to reach fine hand muscles before progressive motor end-plate degeneration occurs.[30] Surgeons continue to search for new techniques to overcome these physiologic barriers. Recovery is slow. It may begin as early as 6 months with some of the new techniques but may take up to 3 years.

Nerve Transfers. Nerve transfers (neurotization) have brought new hope for patients with severe functional loss. The principle of this technique is to use an "expendable" nerve for another function, often permitting nerve repair closer to the

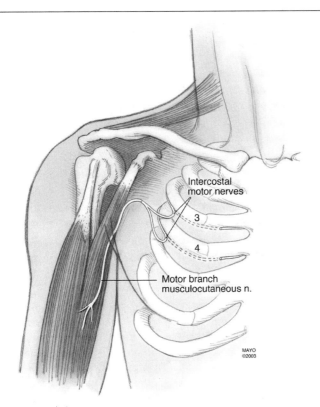

Figure 15-8 Intercostal motor nerve transfer to biceps motor branch.
(By permission of Mayo Foundation for Medical Education and Research. All rights reserved.)

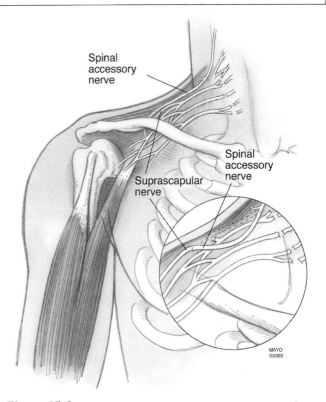

Figure 15-9 Spinal accessory nerve transfer to suprascapular nerve.
(By permission of Mayo Foundation for Medical Education and Research. All rights reserved.)

motor end plate.[30] Nerve transfers can be used in cases of preganglionic injury that would otherwise not be reconstructible with standard nerve surgery. They can also be used in postganglionic lesions in an attempt to provide more rapid and sometimes more reliable recovery of specific vital functions. In addition, they can be used to power free muscle transfer.[30]

Nerve transfers are derived from extraplexal and intraplexal sources. Extraplexal sources include the intercostals and the spinal accessory nerves. These nerves have been found to provide good functional recovery and can be sacrificed with little morbidity. Figure 15-8 shows the transfer of the intercostal nerve to the biceps motor branch, and Fig. 15-9 demonstrates spinal accessory nerve transfer to the suprascapular nerve. The ipsilateral phrenic nerve and the contralateral C7 have also provided newer extraplexal sources of nerves.[30] These types of transfers are being used in several clinical settings.[30]

In cases of upper plexal loss, intraplexal sources of nerves have shown promise. Intraplexal neurotization entails exploiting available branches or fascicles of working donor nerves.[30] A new technique is the transfer of a fascicle of the ulnar nerve to the biceps branch in the arm.[30]

Free Functioning Muscle Transfer. Free functioning muscle transfer technique may be used when irreversible muscle atrophy has occurred, or as part of an early reconstructive procedure combined with other nerve transfers or grafting techniques.[30] Figure 15-10 demonstrates the contralateral gracilis muscle attached to the clavicle and passed subcutaneously to the elbow, where it is secured. Common donor nerves that neurotize the muscle are the spinal accessory and the intercostals (Fig. 15-11). The goal of elbow flexion is a full arc of elbow flexion with an approximate 30-degree extension lag.[30] Very good success rates have been reported.[30]

Reimplantation. Reimplantation of avulsed spinal nerves is being attempted in several centers based on success in animal models. Despite the exciting possibilities of reimplantation, this procedure remains experimental at the current time.[30]

Depending on the amount of recovery, secondary procedures may be helpful in certain situations. They should be considered in all patients but may be most applicable in those patients who do not achieve useful function after primary procedures or in those who were not operated initially.[30] Tendon transfers can be performed to augment or restore function, but can only be performed if donors are available for transfer. Soft tissue procedures may release contractures. Bony procedures such as joint fusion (arthrodesis) may position limbs in more beneficial positions.

Specific surgical interventions for PNS dysfunction include treatment for the following:

- Entrapment syndromes: Neurolysis of the nerve and release of any source of compression is performed.
- Tumors: Resection is done, preserving nerve integrity whenever possible.

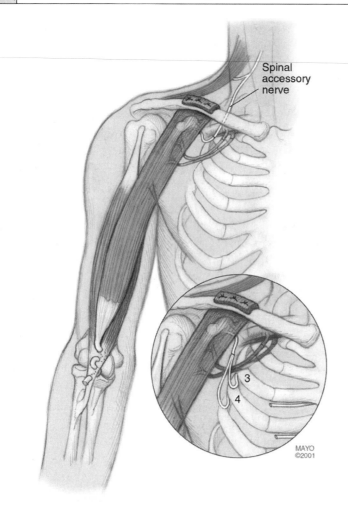

Spinal
accessory
nerve

MAYO
©2001

Figure 15-10 Technique for free functioning muscle transfer for elbow function. Contralateral gracilis muscle attached to clavicle.
(By permission of Mayo Foundation for Medical Education and Research. All rights reserved.)

- Medical neuropathies: Biopsy of a cutaneous nerve (such as the sural nerve) may be performed for diagnostic purposes and potential therapeutic implications.
- Neuropathic pain: Neurolysis, decompressing a neuroma in continuity in a region of scar, may be helpful in relieving pain. Neurectomy, resection of a painful proximal nerve stump (from a previous injury) and burying it deep beneath a muscle, may provide pain relief. Peripheral nerve or spinal cord stimulators, stimuli provided by an implanted device, may provide sensory symptoms that are more pleasing than those experienced usually; over time, the brain can adapt to the new stimulation and the pain may be lessened. Dorsal root entry zone (DREZ), lesions to the spinal cord, may be attempted for refractory deafferentiating pain.[30] Implantable pumps may be implanted for intrathecal delivery of pain medications. Outcomes are not predictable when performing any of these procedures for pain.

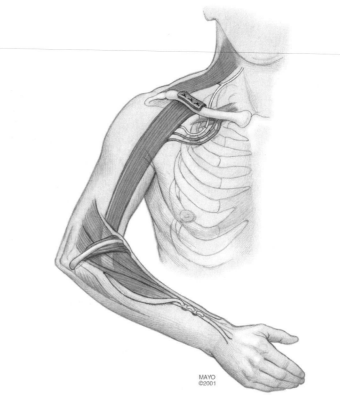

MAYO
©2001

Figure 15-11 Techniques for free functioning muscle transfer for a dual-function elbow flexion and wrist extension.
(By permission of Mayo Foundation for Medical Education and Research. All rights reserved.)

Acute Care

Patients with peripheral nerve disorders may be hospitalized for treatment of acute inflammatory demyelinating polyradiculoneuropathy (AIDP) or CIDP. Care is based on the severity of the disease and the treatment ordered.

Pathways for recovery of the patient with a peripheral nerve disorder, however, most often involve preoperative and postoperative care. These patients are hospitalized for removal of a tumor or a surgical reconstruction, but not usually for a decompression or a routine nerve biopsy, which is done on an outpatient basis.

Preoperative Assessment

The preoperative assessment should include careful documentation of motor, sensory, and autonomic functions. An accurate preoperative baseline neurovascular evaluation of the affected area is essential for postoperative comparison. The essential elements of a neurovascular assessment include the following:[22]

- Amplitude of peripheral pulses
- Skin color and temperature
- Capillary refill
- Sensation
- Movement

Postoperative Care

The goals focus on the preservation of existing function and prevention of further loss of function or complications. The

---

limb may need to be immobilized postoperatively for protection, especially after nerve reconstruction or free muscle grafting. Helping patients attain their optimal level of physical mobility is often a challenge. Collaboration with occupational and physical therapists is invaluable in the clinical management of patients with peripheral nerve dysfunction. These colleagues can assist in recommending orthotic devices and therapy programs for optimal preservation and restoration of function.

Because motor and sensory deficits may put these patients at high risk for injury from falls, the patient's safety also must be protected, especially in the postoperative period. Knowledge of preoperative function assists in the assessment of operative damage due to swelling or blood clots. Carefully orienting the patient to the environment and giving reminders regarding his or her deficits can help prevent further injury.

Postoperative neurovascular compromise is a possible complication that serial neurovascular assessments can help detect. Hematoma and edema are the most common causes and can be minimized with the application of ice bags and elevation of the affected extremity (Box 15-4).

If the patient is hospitalized, standard postoperative management procedures should be used, including coughing, turning, and deep breathing to prevent anesthesia complications and attention to surgical sites for early detection of infection. Often for free muscle flaps, room temperatures are kept at greater than 85° F to promote peripheral vasodilation. Patients must be kept well hydrated, and catheters are often used for urinary drainage. If a skin paddle is present, color assessment is vital. Purple color is abnormal and indicates venous congestion. If intercostal nerves or the phrenic nerve was used as a nerve transfer, there is the potential for pulmonary dysfunction or even pneumothorax. Postoperative instructions are individualized according to the type of disorder and physician preferences.

Pain Management

Pain management is an important part of the long-term management of patients with peripheral nerve dysfunction. Chronic pain of peripheral neuropathies in the lower extremities can actually be relieved by walking if the patient's physical condition permits it.[3] These patients should be advised to wear appropriate shoes and socks, and they may find that changing shoes at midday helps distribute stress and avoid injury.[3] Shoe pads may also help distribute pressure.

All of the principles of good pain management should be employed in the use of analgesics in the treatment of neuropathy pain, especially the use of around-the-clock administration (see Chapter 23). The patient may want to explore complementary treatments to help with pain management, such as imagery and progressive relaxation techniques. If visual imagery is used, it should be practiced several times a day. **Transcutaneous electrical nerve stimulation (TENS),** which controls pain through the application of electrical impulses to the nerve endings, may be especially effective for diabetic neuropathy. Electrodes placed on the skin and attached to a stimulator generate impulses that block transmission of pain signals to the brain. TENS is contraindicated in patients with a demand-type cardiac pacemaker and may cause skin irritation in some patients.

Rehabilitation

Patients with chronic peripheral nerve problems may be admitted to rehabilitation programs for reconditioning, with an emphasis on regaining mobility, building strength, and increasing endurance. Skills that assist in the accomplishment of reconditioning are initially taught and supervised by a therapist. These skills are reinforced by the caregivers and continued when the patient is discharged. Increased independence and mobility may be accomplished through the use of assistive devices for ambulation, such as walkers and canes, as well as wheelchairs for long trips. Rehabilitation is especially helpful for patients with AIDP or CIDP (see Chapter 13).

Home Care

The focus of this stage of care is ensuring safety in the home and protecting skin integrity, noting areas of decreased sensation. Impaired skin integrity is an important concern for any patient with a peripheral neuropathy if sensation in the extremities is altered. The patient should be instructed to lower the setting on his or her water heater and to test the water temperature before entering a bath or shower to prevent burns. Proper foot care should also be stressed.

COMPREHENSIVE PATIENT MANAGEMENT: CHRONIC PERIPHERAL NEUROPATHIES

Health Teaching Considerations

Coping with loss of function and pain is an important focus for health teaching. The clinician should emphasize that rehabilitation may require long-term therapy with adherence to a program where gains may be measured in small improvements and, in some cases, a gradual return of functional abilities. The clinician first teaches the cause of the peripheral nerve disorder, reviews the goals of treatment interventions, and then emphasizes the individual's need to assume as much responsibility as possible for long-term self-management. For patients with inherited neuropathies, the caregiver should provide genetic counseling, prognostic advice, and supportive therapy to improve quality of life and to prevent and treat premature complications.[5]

Risk factors for injury with strategies for prevention are reviewed to assist individuals in learning new and safe ways to perform activities of daily living (ADLs), return to work, and participate in a productive lifestyle as they recover and adapt to their peripheral nerve disorder. Frustration, depression, and chronic pain may require additional counseling and in some cases medications. Verbal and written information should be provided, questions from the individual and family should be addressed, and information on appropriate resources in the community should be provided. Wearing or carrying medical alert identification that outlines the condition is advised, and emergency considerations should be discussed.

Psychosocial Considerations

Peripheral nerve disorders can sometimes lead to disfigurements of the body that cannot be concealed. Neurofibromatosis, for example, can cause multiple lesions that lead to cosmetic disfigurement.[27] Clawhand deformities, Volkmann's contracture, or brachial plexus palsy may cause body image problems. The pain associated with diabetic polyneuropathy has been shown to cause substantial interference in sleep and enjoyment of life and moderate interference in recreational activities, normal work, mobility, general activity, social activities, and mood.[13] An ongoing psychosocial assessment should be done to evaluate the patient's coping level and identify any signs of depression related to pain or the chronic disease state. Interventions might include helping the person identify previously successful coping mechanisms or referral to a rehabilitation psychologist. Occupational counseling is often needed in this population if the neurologic deficit is such that it prevents return to a previous occupation or limits participation in some occupations.

Older Adult Considerations

Considerations for older adult patients include the following:
- Diabetic neuropathy is common among older persons with type 2 diabetes. It is mostly asymptomatic, but there is little improvement with insulin treatment.
- The peak incidence of the development of CIDP is in the fifth and sixth decades.[3]
- Brachial plexus injuries usually are related to high-speed injuries or alcohol use.
- One of the risk factors for falls is increased age. Prevention of injury is a major consideration that requires safety instructions and patient education.

Case Management Considerations

Case management services are usually reserved for patients who require longer follow-up or who have a complicated recovery. After completing a patient assessment and consultation with the health care team, the case manager coordinates services that are needed, with an emphasis on rehabilitation, patient compliance with therapy, and follow-up return visits to health care providers. The case manager might incorporate the following information:

- Total-contact casting of patients with plantar ulcers due to diabetes leads to healing and is a modality that should be considered in treatment.
- CIDP tends to be associated with prolonged neurologic disability and may affect the ability to return to work. Job counseling may be necessary.
- Patients who undergo rehabilitation following hand surgery have a shorter interval before they can return to work.[25]
- Neuropathies caused by toxins related to occupations will require long-term follow-up to ensure that proper care continues.[1]

CARPAL TUNNEL SYNDROME

Carpal tunnel syndrome (CTS), a chronic entrapment peripheral neuropathy, is a common cause of median nerve injury. CTS is widely known as an occupational injury affecting (1) workers such as carpenters and those who use vibrating tools, (2) workers who perform repetitive wrist motions, and (3) workers at risk for trauma to the palm. Industry now recognizes that employees using repetitive wrist motions may develop CTS from compression of the nerve at the wrist[28] (Fig. 15-12). CTS is the most common entrapment syndrome.

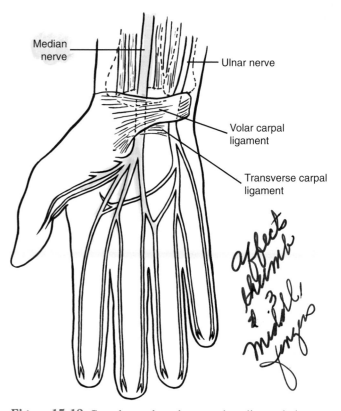

Figure 15-12 Carpal tunnel syndrome and median and ulnar nerve anatomy.
(Courtesy Mayo Clinic Foundation, Rochester, MN.)

Etiology and Incidence

Usually idiopathic in origin, CTS is seen more in middle-aged and older women who have occupations that require extensive use of their hands.[32] The patient may have other predisposing factors that may contribute to the condition (e.g., obesity, arthritis, diabetes mellitus, pregnancy, menses, gout, or other conditions that increase pressure on the median nerve). The prevalence of CTS in the general population was estimated to be 346 cases per 100,000 population per year in 1998.[24]

Pathophysiology

The median nerve, nine flexor tendons, and blood vessels normally pass through the carpal tunnel in the wrist. Any process decreasing the space for the median nerve may compress it and result in CTS. If the structures enlarge (e.g., thickening of the tendon sheaths) or the tunnel boundaries constrict, the median nerve is pinched against the volar transverse carpal ligament. CTS may be unilateral or bilateral. The causes of CTS include tissue swelling from local fractures or dislocations, tissue swelling caused by myxedema, edema related to heart failure or pregnancy, acromegaly, arthritis, gout, fibrosis, direct trauma to the wrist area, and occupational risks of repetitive motion (e.g., a pianist or keyboard operator). On rare occasions CTS can be familial.[3]

Assessment

After completion of a thorough neurologic assessment, it is important to review specific parameters, including history, pain, atrophy, and muscle and sensory testing.

History includes not only one or more of the precipitating factors previously listed, but also usually **nocturnal paresthesias,** or lack of sleep because of aching or tingling or numbness, positional symptoms (such as those related to driving a car), or relief of nocturnal paresthesias by shaking the hands.

The paresthesias are most often confined to the thumb, index, and middle fingers.[3] Because the median nerve is both a motor and a sensory nerve, sensation and muscle control are affected; however, symptoms are typically sensory. Patients may report that dangling their arm over the side of the bed relieves the pain and discomfort. There may also be a history of morning stiffness and other unrelenting symptoms that may have persisted for months or years with a gradual worsening of pain.

Pain may extend up to the elbow or even the shoulder in severe cases. Hypalgesia is a diagnostic symptom.[9]

Thenar atrophy may be observed as the flattening of the muscle at the ball of the thumb.

Muscle testing may reveal difficulty grasping objects or complaints of dropping objects and awkwardness of fine motor function. Weak thumb abduction strength is one of the classic signs associated with CTS.[9] The syndrome is often bilateral and usually of greater intensity in the dominant hand.[6]

Phalen's test requires the patient to sit with elbows resting on a table with the wrists in a flexed position for 30 to 60 minutes. For the **forced wrist flexion test,** the patient approximates and presses the backs of both hands against each other for 60 seconds. If paresthesia and numbness occur in either test, the tests are positive. This test may suggest nerve compression but is not conclusive on its own.[9]

Tinel's sign is positive if the patient reports a tingling sensation along the distribution of the median nerve when the wrist is lightly tapped over the palm or the wrist using a finger or percussion hammer. Tinel's sign may not always be positive in patients with CTS.[9]

Sensory testing uses a pin to prick and map areas of numbness. Two-point discrimination in affected fingers may be greater than in normal digits.

Neurodiagnostic and Laboratory Studies

Positive clinical examinations alone may not be adequate for making the diagnosis of CTS; neurodiagnostic studies may be necessary.[9] Even then, care must be taken to avoid an inappropriate carpal tunnel operation when clinical or electrodiagnostic features are atypical.[38]

- EMG/NCS: Prolonged sensory latency is the earliest finding on NCS. Median nerve conduction velocity may be slowed. Abnormalities in muscles on EMG are usually only seen in more advanced stages. The test may also be within normal limits for some patients with CTS.
- Imaging MRI[18] and ultrasound: These imaging modalities may be used to help diagnose CTS in select cases.[19]

Treatment

Medical Management

Ergonomics, the scientific discipline devoted to the study and analysis of human work, has been applied by industry to jobs that require repetitive motions. This has resulted in job rotation, reassignment, use of robots, and other strategies for prevention of problems such as CTS. However, when CTS does occur, medical management aims at the reduction of symptoms through the following methods:

- Splinting: simple carpal wrist splint to hold the hand in a straight and neutral position
- Elevation: positioning the hand on a pillow at night
- Cold: ice packs
- Rest: avoidance of wrist flexion and weight bearing
- Nonsteroidal antiinflammatory drugs: offer relief for more severe symptoms
- Steroid injections: may increase the response rate with a combination of lidocaine (10 mg) and methylprednisolone (40 mg)[16]
- Alternative therapies: massage therapy has been shown to improve median peak latency and grip strength[12]

Surgical Management

Surgery may become necessary if pain persists despite adequate nonoperative measures or if signs are advanced. The most common surgical procedure is open decompression. With the patient under local anesthesia, a 2-inch incision is made from the palm to the wrist. The entire transverse carpal ligament is released, allowing more room in the tunnel for the median nerve. After completing the procedure, the surgeon closes the incision and applies a bulky dressing. The hand may be placed in a sling or simply elevated for a few days. As the dressings become smaller, finger exercises are encouraged to prevent stiffness.

Since the 1990s, surgeons have also been using an endoscopic procedure.[17] This less invasive technique uses one or two small incisions at the wrist crease or in the middle of the palm (or in both locations) to insert a metal tube. This allows a videoscope to slide into the tube, and the tunnel is cut. The entire surgery takes about 25 minutes. Patients may use the hand in a few days and resume activities in about 2 weeks.

Results from CTS surgery are good or excellent in about 90% of cases. Complications of CTS surgery are rare, although irreversible damage to the nerve has been reported in both open and endoscopic procedures. Endoscopic procedures have a higher risk of transection of the median nerve, especially when done by inexperienced surgeons. Both the older open procedure and the newer endoscopic procedure can result in rare cases (0.03%) of reflex sympathetic dystrophy, hematomas, and wound infections. It is necessary to inform patients before surgery that incomplete relief or recurrence of symptoms can occur with either procedure; however, the advancement in techniques has greatly improved results.[17]

Acute and Postacute Care

Most patients with CTS are treated in outpatient settings or same-day surgery centers. Excellent preoperative preparation and postoperative discharge instructions are needed for positive outcomes for patient recovery.

Relief from pain and return of sensation allow the patient to rest and sleep; therefore measures to promote comfort are priorities of patient management. A study has been done that demonstrates the benefits of wearing splints full time rather than just at night.[36] This information should be included in patient teaching. A review of prescribed medical interventions can be supplemented with patient teaching of the importance of protecting the wrist from unnecessary flexion and weight lifting.

Consultation with a rehabilitation specialist experienced in CTS may provide valuable assistance in evaluating the patient's job requirements and making suggestions to reduce wrist flexion activities. Trials of nonsteroidal medications and close patient follow-up are useful to determine which patients are not getting relief from symptoms and are surgical candidates.

Rehabilitation

As stated earlier, patients who undergo rehabilitation following hand surgery have a shorter interval before returning to work.[25] It has also been shown that a higher percentage of patients with chronic cases of CTS who receive occupational rehabilitation return to work than is the case with patients who receive usual care.

COMPREHENSIVE PATIENT MANAGEMENT: CARPAL TUNNEL SYNDROME

Health Teaching Considerations

Postoperative care instructions include elevation of the hand to avoid venous congestion and edema, neurovascular checks, and the use of a sling to keep the hand elevated. The patient can be taught to make a gentle fist and release immediately after surgery. Printed handouts for wound care, home finger exercises, and activities to prevent stiffness are required. Patients may need assistance with some ADLs, such as buttoning clothes, until the dressing is removed, especially if the dominant hand is involved. Surgery often diminishes pain and paresthesias in the immediate postoperative period: sensation may recover more gradually and advanced atrophy may not recover. By several weeks postoperatively, most patients are able to resume normal activities.

Case Management Considerations

A case manager may be needed for patients who have a complicated recovery and other health care needs in addition to those associated with CTS, especially the older population:

- Studies show that patients who have endoscopic treatment of CTS return to work 42 days earlier than patients treated with the open technique.[33] There may be a slightly higher complication rate for endoscopic procedures if the surgeon is not experienced.[33]
- Pain can recur after surgical release of CTS.[7]
- Job evaluations may require that the patient be retrained for a new job to prevent reinjury of the nerve.

THORACIC OUTLET SYNDROME

Thoracic outlet syndrome (TOS) is a term that consolidates the various disorders associated with compression of the neurovascular structures that traverse the thoracic outlet. TOS is a condition in which the brachial plexus and the subclavian artery and vein are compressed by a cervical or first rib, scalenus anterior muscle, or clavicle[4] (see Fig. 15-6). The general term *thoracic outlet syndrome* includes the following specific syndromes: cervical rib, scalenus anticus, costoclavicular, and hyperabduction syndromes. Pain and paresthesia are the most commonly reported symptoms, with the forearm and hand typically involved. The syndrome may be neurologic or vascular, with the vascular form being the less common but more serious form.

Etiology and Pathophysiology

TOS develops in people who have one or more congenital anomalies that predispose them to develop symptoms. Symptoms sometimes occur spontaneously or may follow trauma of a type that causes chronic muscle spasm in the neck or shoulder region.[4]

Because of the anatomic location and the route that the lower trunk of the brachial plexus and the subclavian artery and vein follow to traverse the thoracic outlet, the artery is subject to compression either statically or dynamically. Congenital anomalies such as a cervical rib, the development of increased muscle bulk, strenuous exercise, trauma, and fractures can be implicated in TOS. Middle-aged women are three times more likely than men to be affected by this mononeuropathy.[4]

Assessment

A complete history and neurologic assessment is completed with focused assessment for the following:

- Skin: color
- Circulation: presence and quality of pulses, especially with hands in different positions
- Raynaud's phenomenon: ischemia of the extremities, especially the fingers, toes, ears, and nose, with severe blanching followed by cyanosis and redness; may also include numbness, tingling, burning, and pain
- Blood pressures: in each arm (a 20 mm Hg difference between arms is significant)[4]
- Edema
- Pain: in the occipital region, neck, shoulder, arm, and hand[6]
- Sensory: paresthesias or numbness in the ulnar distribution
- Motor: determination of strength or weakness of the arm and hand
- Muscle: assessment for muscle atrophy

Patients will often complain of paresthesias in the little and ring fingers, leading to confusion with ulnar nerve compression (cubital tunnel syndrome). Those with thoracic outlet problems will usually identify the locus of their complaint as the medial forearm, little finger, and ring finger.[4]

Many patients will also describe discomfort felt in the posterior hemithorax, anterior chest or breast, and upper arm. This has been confused with angina when experienced on the left side.[34]

Some patients report the feeling that blood is being shut off to the arm. Some will also have acute thrombosis of the subclavian vein, and this must be treated as a medical emergency.[21]

There are several provocative maneuvers that can help in re-creating symptoms and assist in the diagnosis. Figure 15-13 demonstrates the maneuvers described here.

To perform **Adson's maneuver** or the **scalene maneuver,**[34] the clinician has the patient in a sitting position with hands resting in a natural and comfortable position on the thigh. The clinician palpates both radial pulses simultaneously as the patient rapidly and completely fills the lungs by deep inspiration. While holding the breath, the patient hyperextends the neck and then turns the head as far as possible toward one side. Disappearance or reduction of the radial impulse constitutes a positive test. The clinician should also listen for a bruit in the supraclavicular fossa. A palpable thrill may sometimes be felt in the subclavian artery. This test is generally the most useful of this group of tests, but positive results may be obtained in normal subjects.[22]

The patient is asked to move the arm into a position of hyperabduction, or the ball thrower's position, to perform the **hyperabduction maneuver (Wright's maneuver).** The clinician feels the radial pulse while the arm is slowly lifted. In normal subjects the pulse will decrease decidedly or disappear with maximal hyperabduction, and with only moderate degrees of abduction in some.[22] If the radial pulse on the affected side is obliterated with greater ease than is usually the case in normal subjects, the test may have value in diagnosis of the "hyperabduction syndrome."[22]

For the **costoclavicular compressive maneuver,** the patient is asked to thrust the arms downward and backward in an exaggerated military posture. Disappearance or reduction of the radial pulse with the appearance of a subclavian bruit indicates a positive test result. Results are positive in

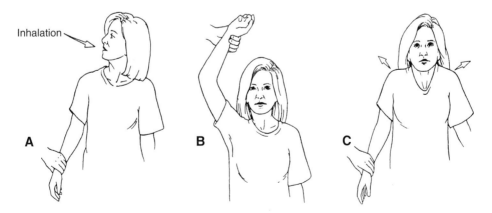

Figure 15-13 Provocative maneuvers used in evaluation of patients with suspected thoracic outlet syndrome. Symptoms must be reproduced for tests to be considered positive. **A,** Adson's maneuver. **B,** Wright's maneuver. **C,** Costoclavicular, or military brace, maneuver.
(Copyright American Academy of Orthopedic Surgeons. From Leffert RD: Thoracic outlet syndrome, J Am Acad Orthop Surg 2[6]:317, 325, 1994. Reprinted with permission.)

the "costoclavicular syndrome," but a positive diagnosis should be based on reproduction of the patient's symptoms in association with a positive reaction to the test.[22]

Some believe that the most reliable test for TOS is the **"elevated arm stress test."**[4] The patient puts both arms in the 90-degree abduction-external rotation position with the shoulders and elbows in the frontal plane of the chest. The patient is instructed to open and close the hands slowly over a 3-minute period. In those with an outlet syndrome, the test reproduces the patient's symptoms.

Percussion over the lower trunk in the neck may produce radiating paresthesias into the hand. This is known as **Tinel's sign.**

Neurodiagnostic and Laboratory Studies

The following neurodiagnostic studies may be ordered:
- Radiologic studies: to examine the neck and chest and to determine the presence or absence of cervical ribs, fractures, arthritis, tumors, or narrowing of the foramina[4]
- Arteriograms and magnetic resonance angiography: to determine vascular abnormalities
- EMG and SSEPs (of the ulnar nerve): to monitor slowing of conduction velocity[34]
- Venography: mandatory in the diagnostic workup for suspected acute thrombosis of the subclavian vein or when venous TOS is suspected[4]
- Open MRI: to allow abduction of the arm, which is not possible in a conventional machine[29]
- Doppler ultrasound and blood flow studies
- Coagulation studies: for patients with embolization or venous occlusion[34]

Treatment

Medical Management
A conservative trial of physical therapy with exercises, weight reduction, and avoidance of activities and postures that aggravate symptoms may provide relief for many patients. The conservative course of treatment should be pursued faithfully for 3 to 4 months unless symptoms are worsened.[8] Failure of this regimen may be an indication for surgical intervention.

Surgical Management
The surgical procedure that is appropriate to eliminate the cause is chosen, and the patient is prepared for surgery. Surgery involves decompression of the neurovascular structures. Typically the scalene muscles are resected. In many cases surgery involves removal of a cervical rib (if present) and at times the first rib. The traditional approach to decompression of the thoracic outlet has been by transaxillary resection of the first rib. Recently, the trend has been toward a more selective and tailored surgical approach via the supraclavicular route.[26] Some surgeons combine these approaches.

Patients usually recover promptly. Complications are relatively rare but may be substantial. They may include injury to the brachial plexus, phrenic nerve, long thoracic nerve, sympathetic chain, and thoracic duct.[26] Other injuries reported are pneumothorax, injury to the subclavian vein or artery, and apical hematoma.[21]

Acute and Postacute Care

In an outpatient or clinic setting, the initial emphasis is on patient education, symptom relief, and instructions on protecting the nerve by avoiding positions and activities that aggravate the condition. The patient can be encouraged to participate in a physical therapy program with exercises, posture control, and reduced weight lifting. Physical therapists will vary the exercises depending on the degree of irritability or the structure in the thoracic outlet. Patients who fail to respond to conservative therapy may be recommended for surgery.

Postsurgical management focuses on vascular assessment, pain control, and monitoring for signs of hemorrhage, pneumothorax, and infection. The affected arm is elevated on pillows and never used for IV routes or blood pressures. Recovery is usually rapid, with the patient experiencing relief from the precipitating symptoms. Range-of-motion (ROM) exercises should be encouraged postoperatively. During the recovery period the patient is told to avoid lifting objects weighing more than 3 to 5 pounds, to avoid strenuous exercises for about 4 weeks, and to return for a follow-up visit in 2 weeks.

Rehabilitation

Rehabilitation may involve outpatient visits to a physical or occupational therapist for assistance with exercises to strengthen muscles and help with using assistive devices for performing ADLs. Therapy is catered to each individual, and adjustments are made to accommodate changes in symptoms and function.[37]

COMPREHENSIVE PATIENT MANAGEMENT: THORACIC OUTLET SYNDROME

Case Management Considerations

Most patients will require only return visits to their health care provider for follow-up. Others, however, may need assistance from the case manager until they have regained function and relief from the pain and discomfort of treatment:
- Laborers with neurogenic TOS are less likely to return to their original occupation. Retraining for a non–labor-intensive occupation may be necessary.[14]
- Approximately 15% of patients derive no benefit from surgery, but those who are carefully selected have good results.

CONCLUSION

Patients with disorders of the peripheral nervous system present many challenges to the neuroscience clinician. Injury to the nerve axons that form an extensive network from the brainstem and spinal cord can result from a multitude of disease processes, causing pain and disability. Pain, paresis, and paralysis, although debilitating, are not life threatening, but patients often endure long periods of discomfort until the diagnosis is confirmed. The diagnostic evaluation to determine the cause is often extensive; however, after the cause is eliminated and treatment is initiated, symptoms can be controlled. Peripheral nerve injuries corrected by therapeutic management or surgery challenge the clinician to keep abreast of ever-changing techniques and to provide care and teaching during short hospital stays or clinic visits.

Acknowledgments

The author acknowledges and thanks Mary Goplen, RN, CNRN, and John Sheski, RN, for their suggestions to revisions of this chapter.

RESOURCES FOR PATIENTS AND CAREGIVERS

Federative Committee on Anatomical Terminology: www.ifaa. lsumc.edu/fcat.htm

REFERENCES

1. Aminoff MJ: Effects of occupational toxins on the nervous system. In Bradley WG, editor: *Neurology in clinical practice,* Philadelphia, 2004, Butterworth-Heinemann.

2. Aminoff MJ: Neurological complications of systemic disease. In Bradley WG, editor: *Neurology in clinical practice,* Philadelphia, 2004, Butterworth-Heinemann.

3. Bosch EP, Smith BE: Disorders of peripheral nerves. In Bradley WG, editor: *Neurology in clinical practice,* Philadelphia, 2004, Butterworth-Heinemann.

4. Brantigan CO, Roos DB: Diagnosing thoracic outlet syndrome, *Hand Clinics* 20(1):27–36, 2004.

5. Burns TM: Inherited neuropathies with known metabolic derangement. In Noseworthy JH, editor: *Neurological therapeutics: principles and practices,* New York, 2003, Martin Dunitz.

6. Chad DA: Disorders of nerve roots and plexuses. In Bradley WG, editor: *Neurology in clinical practice,* Philadelphia, 2004, Butterworth-Heinemann.

7. Concannon MJ, Brownfield MI, Puckett CL: The incidence of recurrence after endoscopic carpal tunnel release, *Plast Reconstr Surg* 105(5):1662–1665, 2000.

8. Crosby CA, Wehbe MA: Conservative treatment for thoracic outlet syndrome, *Hand Clinics* 20(1):43–49, 2004.

9. D'arcy CA, McGee S: Does this patient have carpal tunnel syndrome? *JAMA* 283(3):3110–3117, 2000.

10. Dyck PJ, Rizza RA: Diabetic polyneuropathy. In Noseworthy JH, editor: *Neurological therapeutics; principles and practice,* New York, 2003, Martin Dunitz.

11. Ferner RE, Lucas JD, O'Doherty MJ, et al: Evaluation of (18) fluorodeoxyglucose positron emission tomography ([18]FDG PET) in the detection of malignant peripheral nerve sheath tumours arising from within plexiform neurofibromas in neurofibromatosis 1, *J Neurol Neurosurg Psychiatry* 68(3):353–357, 2000.

12. Field T, Diego M, Cullen C, et al: Carpel tunnel syndrome symptoms are lessened following massage therapy, *J Bodywork Movement Therapies* 8(1):9–14, 2004.

13. Galer BS, Gianas A, Jensen MP: Painful diabetic polyneuropathy: epidemiology, pain description and quality of life, *Diabetes Res Clin Practice* 47(2):123–128, 2000.

14. Goff CD, Parent FN, Sato DT, et al: A comparison of surgery for neurogenic thoracic outlet syndrome between laborers and nonlaborers, *Am J Surg* 176(2):215–218, 1998.

15. Hahn AF: Chronic inflammatory demyelinating polyradiculoneuropathy. In Noseworthy JH, editor: *Neurological therapeutics: principles and practice,* New York, 2003, Martin Dunitz.

16. Helwig AL: Treating carpal tunnel syndrome, *J Fam Pract* 49(1):79–80, 2000.

17. Hoffmeister E: Carpal tunnel syndrome treatment: endoscopic or open carpal tunnel release, *Bone Joint* 11(3):25–26, 29, 2005.

18. Jarvik JG, Kliot M, Maravilla KR: MR nerve imaging of the wrist and hand, *Hand Clinics* 16(1):13–24, 2000.

19. Kele H, Verheggen R, Bittermann H, Reimer S: The potential value of ultrasonography in the evaluation of carpel tunnel syndrome, *Neurology* 61(3):389–391, 2003.

20. Kitamura A, Hoshino T, Kon T, Ogawa R: Patients with diabetic neuropathy are at risk of a greater reduction in core temperature, *Anesthesiology* 92(5):1311–1318, 2000.

21. Leffert RD: Complications of surgery for thoracic outlet syndrome, *Hand Clinics* 20(1):91–98, 2004.

22. Mayo Clinic Neurology Department: *Mayo Clinic examinations in neurology,* ed 7, St Louis, 1998, Mosby.

23. Murry B: Peripheral nerve trauma. In Bradley WG, editor: *Neurology in clinical practice,* Philadelphia, 2004, Butterworth-Heinemann.

24. Nordstrom DL, Destefano F, Vierkant RA, et al: Incidence of diagnosed carpal tunnel syndrome in a general population, *Epidemiology* 9:342–349, 1998.

25. Provinciali L, Giattini A, Splendiani G, Logullo F: Usefulness of hand rehabilitation after carpal tunnel surgery, *Muscle Nerve* 23(2): 211–216, 2000.

26. Sanders RJ, Hammond SL: Supraclavicular first rib resection and total scalenectomy: technique and results, *Hand Clinics* 20(1):61–70, 2004.

27. Schwarz J, Belzberg AJ: Malignant peripheral nerve sheath tumors in the setting of segmental neurofibromatosis: case report, *J Neurosurg* 92(2):342–346, 2000.

28. Shaw Wilgis EF: Treatment options for carpal tunnel syndrome [editorial], *JAMA* 288(10):1281–1282, 2002.

29. Smedby O, Rostad H, Klaastad O, et al: Functional imaging of the thoracic outlet syndrome in an open MR scanner, *Eur Radiol* 10(4):597–600, 2000.

30. Spinner RJ, Shin A, Bishop AT: Update on brachial plexus surgery in adults [hand and wrist], *Curr Opin Orthop* 15(4):203–214, 2004.

31. Taira H, Takasita M, Yoshida S, et al: MR appearance of paraganglioma of the cauda equina: case reports, *Acta Radiol* 41(1):27–30, 2000.

32. Treaster DE, Burr D: Gender differences in prevalence of upper extremity musculoskeletal disorders, *Ergonomics* 47(5):495–526, 2004.

33. Trumble TE, Diao E, Abrams RA, Gilbert-Anderson MM: Single-portal endoscopic carpal tunnel release compared with

open release: a prospective, randomized trial, *J Bone Joint Surg Am* 84-A(7):1107–1115, 2002.

34. Urschel HC, Patel AN: Thoracic outlet syndrome. In Franco KL, Putnam JB, editors: *Advanced therapy in thoracic surgery,* Hamilton, Ontario, 2005, Decker.

35. Valiante TA, Fehlings MG: Primary tumors of the spinal cord, root, plexus, and nerve sheath. In Noseworthy JH, editor: *Neurological therapeutics; principles and practice,* New York, 2003, Martin Dunitz.

36. Walker WC, Metzler M, Cifu DX, Swartz Z: Neutral wrist splinting in carpal tunnel syndrome: a comparison of night-only verse full-time wear, *Arch Phys Med Rehabil* 81(4):424–429, 2000.

37. Wishchuk JR, Dougherty CR: Therapy after thoracic outlet release, *Hand Clinics* 20(1):87–90, 2004.

38. Witt JC, Stevens JC: Neurologic disorders masquerading as carpal tunnel syndrome: 12 cases of failed carpal tunnel release, *Mayo Clin Proc* 75(4):409–413, 2000.

CHAPTER 16

Cranial Nerve Deficits

The 12 pairs of cranial nerves connect to the undersurface of the brain. Most cranial nerves are attached at the brainstem and exit via foramina of the skull. When cranial nerves are compressed, inflamed, or degenerate, their disorders present specific challenges as a result of single or multiple cranial nerve palsies. As a component of the peripheral nervous system, the cranial nerves participate in the regulation of the special senses (smell, vision, hearing, and taste) and of somatosensation and movement of the face and its structures. The cranial nerves take an active part in the control of human responses in interaction with the internal and external environments.[21] Four cranial nerves (CN III, VII, IX, and X) serve specific parasympathetic functions. Protective reflexes involving facial structures are regulated by the interactions of two sets of cranial nerves (CN IX and X, and CN V and VII). The control of speech, swallowing, and balance involves innervation of facial structures by CN V, VII, VIII, IX, X, and XII (see Chapter 1).

In addition to their individual functions, the cranial nerves are important in the identification and localization of intracranial lesions. The **cranial nerve nuclei** are situated in a rostrocaudal pattern in the diencephalon and brainstem (see Chapter 1). Lesions involving these areas are often initially manifested by disorders of function of specific cranial nerves. Expanding lesions may encroach on the pathways of the cranial nerves as they traverse the brain and give rise to single or multiple cranial nerve palsies. Knowledge of the anatomy of these pathways is crucial to the interpretation of assessment data and rapid intervention by the clinician to help prevent catastrophic intracranial events.

This chapter presents information on the pathophysiology of cranial nerve disorders—identifying the disorders and how to manage the care of the affected individual. The chapter begins with a discussion of the protective role of specific cranial nerves in environmental interaction. After this discussion, cranial nerve disorders are discussed singly or, where appropriate, in combination. The reader is encouraged to review those sections of Chapters 1, 2, and 3 of this text that discuss the anatomy, physiology, assessment, and diagnostic testing of the cranial nerves.

This chapter focuses on the protective role of cranial nerves in environmental interaction and the importance of cranial nerve assessment in planning neurologic clinical management in the emergency, acute, and nonacute care settings; the pathophysiology, diagnosis, and treatment of disorders of each of the 12 cranial nerves, with emphasis on trigeminal neuralgia (TN), Bell's palsy and Meniere's

disease; and management of patients experiencing cranial nerve disorders in acute and nonacute care settings, including patient and family health teaching, case management, and resources.

The etiology, pathophysiology, assessment, and treatment of disorders involving the cranial nerves singly or in combination are presented. Management of the patient experiencing each cranial nerve palsy is covered in general; where appropriate, concerns related to specific settings (acute, postacute, nonacute, and rehabilitation) are addressed individually.

PROTECTIVE CRANIAL NERVE REFLEXES

The cranial nerves serve many important functions in human-environmental interaction, but two protective reflexes are especially important. These reflexes are the corneal blink and gag reflexes. Disruption of either the sensory or motor component of these reflexes places the individual at great risk for disability or death.

Because of the caudal location of the nuclei controlling these reflexes, they are among the last protective reflexes to be lost with increased intracranial pressure (IICP) and the first to return as the patient's condition improves. Initial and ongoing assessment of the integrity of these reflexes is crucial in the emergency and critical care assessment of patients at risk for intracranial hypertension or with a diminished level of consciousness (LOC). Subtle changes in reflex response provide the clinician with a guide to the integrity of brainstem function.

CORNEAL BLINK REFLEX

The corneal blink reflex protects visual integrity by causing the individual to blink the eyelids in response to any irritation of the cornea. A clear cornea, free of lesions or opacities, is crucial to maintaining visual acuity.[56]

Pathophysiology

Abnormalities of the corneal blink reflex occur with disorders of the afferent component of the olfactory branch of the **trigeminal nerve** (CN V) or efferent branch of the **facial nerve** (CN VII). To distinguish the nerve involved, the clinician needs to carefully assess the ipsilateral and contralateral responses to sensory stimulation of the patient's cornea. The corneal reflex may be delayed with certain disorders (e.g., posterior fossa and cerebellopontine angle tumors, acoustic neuromas, multiple sclerosis (MS), brainstem strokes, and Parkinson's disease). When absence of the reflex is due to insensitivity of the cornea (CN V involvement), neither eye blinks in response to stimulation on the affected side; both eyes blink when the contralateral cornea is stimulated. If a facial nerve lesion is the cause of an absent reflex, stimulation of the cornea results in loss of blink on the ipsilateral side, whereas the unaffected side blinks regardless of which cornea was stimulated.[5]

Clinical Management

When the patient's ability to protect the cornea is compromised, the clinician must incorporate this protective function of patching and protecting the eye into the patient's care and teaching. All patients with alterations in LOC, brainstem lesions, and disorders of the trigeminal and facial nerves should be assessed routinely for the integrity of the corneal blink reflex. When the blink reflex is impaired or the corneal reflex is absent, the patient has ineffective protection to the eye. Interventions for eye care are presented in Box 16-1.

GAG REFLEX

The gag or pharyngeal reflex is innervated by the sensory and motor components of the **glossopharyngeal nerve** and **vagus nerve.** Absent or diminished gag function places the patient at great risk for pulmonary aspiration and its attendant complications, including aspiration pneumonia, sepsis, and acute respiratory distress syndrome (ARDS). Impaired gag function may be unilateral or bilateral.

Pathophysiology

A variety of disorders, both within and outside the neurologic system, can interfere with the integrity of the gag reflex. For example, the use of local anesthesia of the throat for endoscopic/bronchoscopic procedures is designed to diminish this reflex. Intracranial pathologic conditions, metabolic abnormalities, and general anesthesia may temporarily or permanently abolish the reflex. Lesions involving the glossopharyngeal and vagus nerves (bulbar palsy and syringobulbia) may interfere with the gag reflex, as well as with the actions of swallowing and speaking.

Bulbar palsy is characterized by progressive motor weakness or paralysis from disruption of cranial nerve nuclei located in the lower brainstem. Causes of this disorder include diphtheria, poliomyelitis, and amyotrophic lateral sclerosis (ALS).[1,30] The cranial nerves involved include the trigeminal nerve (CN V), facial nerve (CN VII), glossopharyngeal nerve (CN IX), vagus nerve (CN X), spinal accessory nerve (CN XI), and hypoglossal nerve (CN XII). Manifestations are those of lower motor neuron dysfunction with weakness and flaccid paralysis of the involved muscles. **Syringobulbia** is characterized by the presence of fluid-filled cavities (syrinxes) in the medulla oblongata, usually involving dorsal structures. The condition is generally believed to occur as an upward extension of syringomyelia.[30,54] Manifestations include weakness of the tongue, dysphagia, and dysarthria, as well as a diminished gag reflex. The normal gag reflex may vary and may be reduced in smokers and older adults.

Clinical Management

When the patient's ability to protect the airway is compromised, it is crucial to plan and implement interventions designed to avoid pulmonary aspiration. The clinician must be aware of the variety of causes of diminished gag function and assess susceptible patients for the integrity of the gag reflex. For example, patients recovering from oral endoscopic procedures should remain on NPO status (nothing by mouth) until the gag reflex has fully returned. These patients should not be discharged from the outpatient recovery area until they can manage both liquid and solid intake without the risk of aspiration. When providing postoperative care or especially care to the patient who has had a stroke, the clinician must be cautious in administering liquids and initiating oral feedings. Before offering the patient liquids, the clinician should assess the gag reflex and, if necessary, consult the speech/language pathologist at the hospital regarding types of foods and fluids, patient positioning, and strategies to avoid aspiration if the gag reflex is compromised. Interventions to prevent aspiration are outlined in Box 16-2.

BOX 16-1   Interventions for Eye Care

- Inspect the cornea on a routine schedule (e.g., every 4 hours).
- Gently rinse the cornea with isotonic sterile saline solution every 4 hours and as needed.
- Instill artificial tears every 4 hours and as needed.
- Use a lubricating ointment when sleeping.
- Teach eye assessment and care, use of protective eyewear, and environments to avoid (e.g., dust, flying debris, wind).
- Refer to an ophthalmologist for alterations in the cornea.

BOX 16-2   Interventions to Prevent Aspiration

- Test the bilateral gag reflex.
- Assess the oral cavity and lung sounds every 4 hours and as needed.
- Provide for oral care every 4 hours and as needed.
- If oral feeding is contraindicated, ensure adequate fluid and caloric intake via the enteral/parenteral route.
- Keep suction equipment readily available. Suction the oropharynx as needed; suction nasotracheally if indicated.
- Position the patient to facilitate secretion clearance.
- Consult with a speech therapist for swallowing evaluation and dietary consistency.
- Teach strategies to avoid aspiration, for suctioning technique, and for preferred dietary consistency.

OLFACTORY NERVE DISORDERS

Etiology

The olfactory nerve (CN I) is often skipped in cranial nerve testing. This is unfortunate because CN I is responsible for the following:

- Smell: Primary receptor for the sense of smell
- Taste: Flavor and palatability of food and fluids
- Protective function: Spoiled foods and beverages, toxic fumes, smoke and air pollution
- Pleasurable odors (e.g., baby and mother; evokes memories)
- Potential diagnosis of Alzheimer's disease and other medical conditions

Anosmia, loss of the ability to smell, is associated with extracranial and intracranial pathologic conditions and may be unilateral or bilateral. **Hyposmia** is a diminished ability to smell. **Dysosmia** is defined as a distorted ability to smell. **Hyperosmia** is an exaggerated or abnormal sense of smell (e.g., the patient's report of smelling rotten eggs before a seizure). Upper respiratory tract infections and other local diseases that affect the nasal passageways often result in a reported loss of the sense of smell. Facial trauma involving the nose can either directly or indirectly (e.g., through swelling and ischemia) damage olfactory cells. Intracranial conditions associated with loss of smell include olfactory groove meningiomas, large aneurysms of the anterior cerebral and communicating arteries, space-occupying lesions deep in the frontal lobe, basilar skull fractures of the anterior fossa (cribriform plate of ethmoid bone), meningitis, and concussion. Loss of smell and taste may have a negative effect on nutritional status and personal safety.

Pathophysiology

The anatomy of the olfactory pathways is illustrated in Fig. 16-1. Olfactory cells, located on the nasal and septal walls of the upper nasal cavities, perforate the cribriform plate of the ethmoid bone and enter the olfactory bulb at the base of the frontal lobe. Impulses are conducted along the olfactory tract to the primary olfactory cortex located in the medial temporal lobes.[1]

Lesions that interrupt the reception or conduction of olfactory impulses along this pathway interrupt the sense of smell. Tumors, hematomas, or other space-occupying lesions involving the olfactory cortex may result in an impairment of the sense of smell. Four types of olfactory disturbances have been identified: quantitative alterations, qualitative changes, olfactory hallucinations, and loss of olfactory discrimination.[1] Anosmia, the most common olfactory disorder, can present as a unilateral or bilateral loss of the sense of smell. When anosmia is unilateral, it often goes unrecognized by the individual.

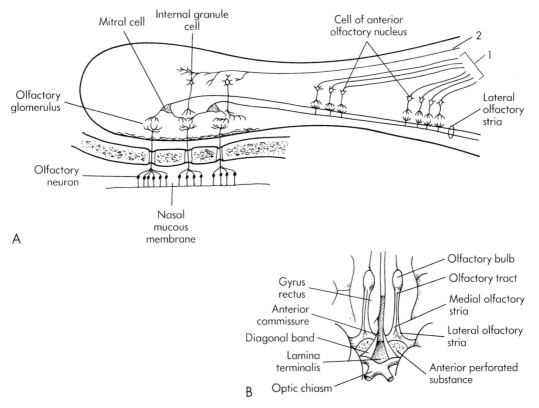

Figure 16-1 Olfactory pathway. **A,** Diagram illustrating the relationships between the olfactory receptors in the nasal mucosa and neurons in the olfactory bulb and tract. Cells of the anterior olfactory nucleus are found in scattered groups, caudal to the olfactory bulb. Fibers from the anterior olfactory nucleus project centrally *(1)*. A fiber from the contralateral anterior olfactory nucleus is labeled *(2)*. **B,** Diagram of the olfactory structures on the inferior surface of the brain.

Assessment

Disorders of the olfactory nerve are manifested by abnormalities or absence of smell. In addition to loss of smell on the affected side, patients with disorders of the olfactory nerve commonly report abnormalities of taste and associated changes in appetite.[1,20] A detailed history includes a description of the dysosmia; time of onset; medical problems with viral or bacterial infections; surgery; head or facial trauma; medications (e.g., chemotherapeutic or thyroid drugs); long-term exposure to toxic conditions; seizure activity; allergies; smoking and drug abuse or intranasal medications; nasal discharge, especially foul-smelling or discolored discharge; and dementia. Each nostril is assessed separately. The ability to taste to discriminate between sweet, sour, bitter, and salty versus flavors like coffee, chocolate, vanilla, strawberry, pizza, licorice, and cola is assessed.[19]

The nasal mucosa is assessed for color, surface texture, swelling, inflammation, exudate, ulceration, epithelial metaplasia, erosion, purulent rhinorrhea, and atrophy. The clinician checks for the presence of polyps or masses, crusting, and dryness. The University of Pennsylvania Smell Identification Test (UPSIT) and other commercial scratch-and-sniff tests can be self-administered, are easy to score, and are reliable. Patients with evidence of infection, lesions, sinus problems, drug abuse, seizures, or serious medical conditions are referred for additional appropriate diagnostic workup. It is thought that up to 90% of individuals with idiopathic Parkinson's disease have a demonstrable olfactory loss, yet fewer than 15% are aware of the problems until tested.[19]

Neurodiagnostic and Laboratory Studies

- Computed tomography (CT) scan: Screens for sinonasal tract inflammatory disorders
- Evoked potential olfactometry: Detects olfactory disorders
- Laboratory studies: Complete blood count (CBC), erythrocyte sedimentation rate (ESR), thiamine level (if alcohol abuse is suspected)
- Neuropsychologic testing: If dementia is evident (Alzheimer's disease)

Treatment

Medical Management

Medical management of dysosmia involves identification and correction of the underlying cause. In the event that an intracranial space-occupying lesion is found, supratentorial craniotomy to resect the lesion may be indicated. Surgical intervention may be needed for problems of blockage or septal deviations.

Clinical Management

Clinical management of the person experiencing anosmia is aimed at preserving appetite and protecting the person from potentially harmful situations that are identified by certain odors.[1,48] Admission to a hospital for anosmia is rare; rather, the clinician is more likely to encounter this patient in a nonacute care setting such as a clinic or primary provider's office.

Specific interventions depend on the individualized needs of the patient. General interventions for altered olfaction are listed in Box 16-3.

| BOX 16-3 | **Interventions for Altered Olfaction** |

- Teach the patient to carefully read labels for contents and expiration dates.
- Teach the patient to have the home heating system and car exhaust system checked routinely for function.
- Suggest the installation of smoke detectors; teach the patient to change batteries twice a year.
- Assess the patient's nutritional status.
- Obtain dietary consultation.
- Prepare and present meals in an appetizing fashion.
- Incorporate food likes into meal planning.
- Weight the patient twice weekly.
- For unplanned weight loss of more than 2 pounds per week, institute calorie counts and reconsult with the dietitian.
- Provide a pleasant environment at mealtime.

COMPREHENSIVE PATIENT MANAGEMENT: OLFACTORY NERVE DISORDERS

Health Teaching Considerations

In planning care for the patient with dysosmia, the clinician must discuss safety factors related to loss of the ability to recognize potentially harmful odors. An evaluation of the patient's occupation and lifestyle is necessary to assist in the identification of situations that increase the patient's risk for injury. Important areas to consider are the type of home heating system; kitchen, laundry, and other appliances; the patient's occupation (e.g., working on motors, exhaust systems, or with chemicals); hobbies and leisure activities; and the use of tobacco products.[48] Patients should be encouraged to stop smoking with referral to a hospital- or community-based program designed for smoking cessation.

Nutritional Considerations

Because patients often report a decreased sensation of taste, nutritional status may be altered in the patient with anosmia. With isolated disorders of the olfactory nerve, the sensation of taste remains intact; the reported loss of taste reflects impairment in the "perception of flavor."[1] The clinician should assess the patient's nutritional status, including usual food patterns and physiologic indexes of nutrition (e.g., weight, serum protein, immune competence), and assess the psycho-emotional effects of anosmia on the patient's appetite. Consultation with a nutritionist should be considered for those patients at risk for nutritional alterations.

OPTIC NERVE DISORDERS

The optic nerves (CN II) originate from the bipolar cells of the retina, carry visual information from the eyes to the brain, and unite to form the optic chiasm where some of the nerve fibers then cross to the opposite side to continue as the optic tracts. Because disorders and conditions of the optic nerves are discussed in other chapters, only a few examples are included in this chapter. **Optic neuritis,** for example, refers to conditions (e.g., MS, inflammation, viruses) and other illnesses that affect the optic nerve and may reduce visual function. Treatment is focused on the underlying disease.

Another example of optic nerve disorders involves herpes zoster (Shingles) that occurs as vesicles on the face with risk of **cranial nerve herpes zoster virus infection (HZVI).** HZVI is usually followed by otologic or ophthalmic sequelae. Otologic complications of varicella-zoster virus (**Ramsay Hunt syndrome**) include the following[58]:

- Facial paralysis
- Tinnitus
- Hearing loss
- Hyperacusis
- Vertigo
- Dysgeusia and decreased tear secretion

There may also be CN V, IX, and X involvement. Infections of the retina with the virus can lead to severe visual impairment. Patients with immunodeficiency/advanced human immunodeficiency virus (HIV) infection carry a higher risk of retinal infection.

After a thorough history and evaluation, gadolinium-enhanced magnetic resonance imaging (MRI) may demonstrate enhancement of the geniculate ganglion and facial nerve. These manifestations are identical to those of Bell's palsy but are more severe and carry a graver prognosis. Therapy includes acyclovir, prednisone, analgesics, and the use of dark glasses because of photophobia.[58]

Etiology

Alterations in vision result from a variety of disorders involving the optic nerve, chiasm, optic tracts, optic radiations, or occipital cortex. Visual abnormalities may affect central or peripheral vision and require immediate investigation to prevent, where possible, permanent visual impairment or blindness. The most common causes of optic nerve dysfunction include disorders of the nerve itself and lesions compressing the nerve, such as frontal lobe tumors and aneurysms of the anterior circulation in the circle of Willis. **Optic gliomas** involve the optic tract and may cause complete unilateral blindness and hemianopia of the opposite eye. Optic atrophy may also occur.

Pathophysiology

Alterations in vision occur with disruption of the visual pathway at any location between the retina and the cortex. The following discussion is limited to specific pathophysiology of the optic nerve anterior to the decussation of the nasal fibers at the optic chiasm.

Optic neuritis is a common cause of acute visual loss. It is typified by sudden onset of visual impairment and pain with eye movements, followed by spontaneous recovery of vision over months. Pathologically, optic neuritis is an acute demyelinating event affecting the optic nerve.

Optic neuritis may result as a consequence of MS, meningitis, encephalitis, nutritional deficiencies (tobacco-alcohol amblyopia), poisonings (e.g., lead, carbon monoxide, methanol, quinine), antitubercular drugs, and ischemia of the nerve from temporal arteritis or atherosclerosis. With neuritis the nerve is inflamed and edematous, resulting in rapid compromise in vision associated with scotomas, visual field losses, and globe pain on movement and palpation. The funduscopic examination reveals the optic disc to be red and edematous with blurred margins. Opacities of the vitreous are often found as the first indication of MS.

Papilledema or swelling of the optic disc generally occurs as a nonlocalizing sign of IICP. Disorders associated with papilledema are intracranial trauma, space-occupying lesions of the brain, pseudotumor cerebri, intracranial infections, intracranial hemorrhages, orbital lesions, systemic hypertension, leukemia, anemia, polycythemia, vitamin A intoxication, and craniofacial synostosis.[49] The mechanism for the development of papilledema is not fully understood; recent investigations suggest a disorder of axoplasmic transport along the axon of the optic nerve.[1] In papilledema the optic disc is swollen with blurred margins and may appear pale to red; venous pulsations are absent.

In rare instances, unilateral papilledema is present on funduscopic examination. When papilledema is associated with atrophy of the optic disc in the opposite eye, **Foster Kennedy syndrome** is present.[1,7,22] This syndrome, with the combination of optic disc pallor and papilledema, is seen in association with tumors of the sphenoid ridge or orbital surface of the frontal lobe, olfactory groove meningiomas, aneurysms of the anterior cerebral or anterior communicating artery, or vascular disease affecting the optic nerve. In this syndrome compression of the ipsilateral optic nerve causes atrophy of the optic disc, whereas IICP from the expanding space-occupying lesion results in contralateral papilledema.[7]

Chronic optic neuritis or papilledema may lead to atrophy of the optic nerve. Optic atrophy can also occur congenitally (Leber's hereditary optic atrophy) and as a consequence of tertiary syphilis; optic nerve injury or tumors; severe systemic blood loss; arteriosclerosis; carotid thrombosis; or poisonings with lead, carbon monoxide, and various industrial chemicals.[49] With optic nerve atrophy the disc turns white or yellow-gray and visual acuity is diminished.

Primary tumors of the optic nerve are most commonly melanocytomas. Other tumor types that arise from the optic nerve include neurocytomas, gliomas, fibromas, and endotheliomas.

Optic nerve trauma occurs with craniofacial trauma. Orbital and eye injuries may be minor or extensive, depending on whether the injury is blunt or penetrating trauma, which may be work related, automobile crash related, or sports related. Trauma may cause blowout orbital fractures, Le Fort fractures, panfacial fractures, and frontobasilar skull fractures.[4]

Assessment

Lesions involving the optic nerve result in impairments in central and peripheral visual acuity. Lesions of the optic nerve lead to **monocular** visual disturbances ranging from diminished visual acuity to blindness. The sudden onset of blindness in an eye is termed **amaurosis.** Patients report a reduction in visual brightness akin to "looking through a shade or veil." **Scotomas,** blind spots in the visual field, are often reported or found on visual examination.

Optic nerve lesions are confirmed by **Marcus Gunn's pupillary sign.**[5] This sign is characterized by an absent response to direct light with a normal consensual light reflex in the affected eye. A positive Marcus Gunn's pupillary response may be seen with injury to the visual tract between the retina and optic chiasm. The clinician tests for this sign by rapidly alternating the light source between the eyes. When the light is directed to the affected eye immediately after it has constricted from consensual reaction, the eye appears to dilate in response to the light. This response is also called the **swinging flashlight sign**[17] or afferent pupillary defect.[1]

Assessment findings for optic neuritis may include the following[25]:

- Afferent pupillary defect
- Marcus Gunn's pupil
- Diminished central visual acuity
- Loss of vision: monocular, but commonly bilateral in children
- Diminished color vision
- Decreased contrast sensitivity
- Visual field abnormalities
- Orbital pain exacerbated by eye movement
- Uhthoff's sign: increase in motor weakness after heat, fever, or exercise

The recommendations for assessment of function and vision after craniofacial trauma may include the following[64]:

- Detailed history, circumstances of the injury, and mechanisms of injury: Questions to ask include "Do you wear glasses?" "Have you ever had eye surgery?" "Do you use eye medications?" "Do you have allergies?" "Are you diabetic?" "Are you hypertensive?" and "Do you have glaucoma?"
- External eye: Careful and complete evaluation of the eyes using sterile gloves, first to inspect the gross position of the eyes and lids to see if the eyes are set equally apart or sunken. The patient should be asked to open and close the eyes against the force of the clinician's fingers. The eyes are gently palpated for pain and tenderness. Sterile cotton is used to assess the corneal reflex and blink response.
- Ophthalmoscopy: Examination of the retina and optic nerve for color, pallor, swelling, hemorrhage, pulsations, and exudate.
- Visual acuity: Can the patient see? An eye chart should be used if the patient's condition permits it. If vision is impaired, counting fingers, hand motions, or light perception may be used. If vision is low, a Sloan chart may be used.
- Color vision: Crude assessment with simple color; sophisticated assessment with color plates or an anomaloscope one-hue test.
- Pupil: Evaluation of shape (irregular suggests trauma), reactivity, and accommodation comparing each eye; right eye with left eye; assessment for diplopia.
- Confrontation: Evaluation of the visual fields. One eye of the patient is covered, and the visual fields are checked, first with the clinician's still finger and then with moving fingers (immobile fingers are more difficult to see).

- Motility: Evaluation of extraocular muscle movements for CN III, IV, and VI.
- Pain: Subjective complaints to touch, light, and movement when opening and closing the eyes.

Neurodiagnostic and Laboratory Studies

- Visual brainstem evoked potential: May be ordered to diagnose the presence of optic neuritis
- CT/MRI: To rule out foreign bodies, hemorrhage, fractures, or orbital damage from trauma, MS, or tumors, or to assist in identification and localization
- Laboratory tests: CBC, syphilis serologies, antinuclear antibody (ANA), ESR
- Light perception: For patients with neurologic signs and symptoms
- Lyme titer: To rule out Lyme disease
- Neuro-ophthalmologic testing: To identify visual defects; includes perimetry and tangent screening

Treatment

Medical Management

The medical management of optic nerve disorders is specific to the etiology of the lesion. After the diagnosis of optic neuritis is confirmed, for example, treatment is usually intravenous (IV) methylprednisolone 250 mg every 6 hours for 3 days, followed by prednisone 1 mg/kg/day for 11 days. More than 75% to 90% of patients recover vision to near baseline or better.[64]

Inflammatory conditions may be treated with a course of steroids, nutritional causes may be treated with vitamin administration and nutritional therapies, and intracranial infections may be treated with appropriate antimicrobial therapy. Because MS is often associated with visual disturbances, see Chapter 20 for a discussion of that disorder.

Surgical Management

Resectable tumors are surgically removed by craniotomy or transsphenoidal hypophysectomy (see Chapter 8). When surgery is required, postoperative care is focused on checking the eyes for vision, swelling, hemorrhage, discharge, increased pain, and signs and symptoms of infection. All orders are clarified with the surgeon (e.g., positioning, application of ice, the need for an eye dressing, the type of dressing [occlusive versus nonocclusive, dry versus wet, special eye patch versus gauze], the frequency of dressing changes, medications to be instilled directly into the eye, and especially indications for calling the surgeon).

Acute Care

Loss of visual acuity is frightening for patients and their families. Management of the patient with optic nerve disorders must focus on the medical or surgical treatment described previously, in collaboration with the health care team. The emotional response of the patient is monitored as therapy is focused to restore and preserve visual acuity.

The setting in which the clinician encounters a person experiencing an optic nerve disorder varies with the nature

BOX 16-4	Interventions for Altered Vision

- Arrange for a safe environment. Maintain objects in expected locations, and remove extra equipment.
- Make adaptive devices available.
- Teach appropriate use and care of adaptive devices.
- Arrange the environment and use natural and artificial light to capitalize on remaining vision.
- Teach the patient to use other senses when appropriate.
- Teach the family the importance of a predictable home environment.
- Teach the patient strategies to scan the entire visual world and capitalize on remaining visual function.
- Refer the patient and family to available community resources and support groups.

of the visual loss (sudden versus gradual) and the medical management of the patient. Interventions for altered vision are listed in Box 16-4. Care should be individualized for the patient's particular visual impairments and the setting in which the patient is encountered (e.g., acute, postacute, nonacute).

COMPREHENSIVE PATIENT MANAGEMENT: OPTIC NERVE DISORDERS

Psychosocial Considerations

Because emotional responses vary with the individual, the clinician needs to consider the wide range of nursing diagnoses applicable to the patient's psychosocial response. Counseling and follow-up are needed to help the patient adjust and adapt to a quality of life with altered vision or visual loss. Large-print books or audio books and other visual-enhancing devices help to decrease the negative psychological feelings with vision loss.

Case Management Considerations

Permanent impairments in central or peripheral visual acuity require significant adjustment by the patient and family. The clinician or case manager must complete an environmental assessment of the home, suggesting strategies to provide a safe, stable environment for the patient. A referral to a vocational counselor may be needed if changes in the patient's occupation are necessary. If visual impairments restrict driving privileges, the case manager may need to make referrals to local associations and organizations that assist with transportation. In addition, referral to occupational therapists and recreational therapists may assist the patient with lifestyle changes. National and local organizations for the visually impaired offer resources and support for patients and families; the case manager should be sure to provide the patient with the name, address, and telephone numbers of these organizations.

OCULOMOTOR SYSTEM DISORDERS

The oculomotor nerve (CN III), trochlear nerve (CN IV), and abducens nerve (CN VI) provide innervation to the six pairs of muscles of eye movement. Because of their combined role in the regulation of ocular movements, these nerves are discussed together as oculomotor system disorders.

Etiology

Disturbances of the oculomotor system can result from a variety of extracranial and intracranial pathologic conditions. Extracranial causes of **ophthalmoplegia** include local and systemic muscle disorders (e.g., myasthenia gravis, thyroid disease). Among the intracranial causes are upper (supranuclear) or lower (nuclear/infranuclear) motor neuron diseases of the oculomotor nerves, head trauma, IICP, and space-occupying lesions (e.g., tumors, aneurysms, abscesses) that compress the ocular pathways.

Pathophysiology

The pathophysiology of oculomotor system palsies includes problems associated with disorders of eye movement, pupillary constriction to light, and innervation of the muscles that elevate the eyelid.

Disorders of Eye Movement

Paresis or paralysis of gaze results from disruption of the neural control of the extraocular muscles. Third-nerve palsies are identified by gaze disturbances of the medial, superior, or inferior rectus or inferior oblique muscles. These gaze disturbances result in an inability to move the affected eye in, up and out, down and out, and up and in, respectively. The oculomotor nerve travels a great distance in the intracranial cavity from its origin in the midbrain to its termination at the eye. Lesions of the nerve itself, as well as compression of the nerve along its course, result in single or multiple gaze disturbances. Common causes of oculomotor nerve compression are tentorial herniation (uncal or central), posterior communicating artery aneurysm, and head trauma.[1,20,30,49] Other common causes of third-nerve palsy are diabetes mellitus (DM) and migraines.[1,20,49]

Palsies of the trochlear nerve interfere with downward and inward movements of the eye. These gaze disturbances, involving the superior oblique muscle, result in diplopia when activities are being performed that require focusing on downward gaze. Visual disturbances are reported when reading or walking down stairs or inclines. The trochlear nerve is often injured as a consequence of head trauma.[1] An occipital impact should alert the health care team to evaluate CN IV for trochlear nerve palsy after an impact to the back of the head. Patients may complain of diplopia and blurred vision.[32]

The abducens nerve innervates the lateral rectus muscle. Damage to the nerve, at its origin, or along its course, results in lateral gaze deviations manifested by complaints of diplopia when looking to the affected side. Common causes of sixth-nerve dysfunction include IICP, meningitis, basilar skull fractures (petrous pyramid), brain tumors, and Wernicke's encephalopathy.[1,20,30,49]

Internuclear ophthalmoplegia (INO) results from injury to the medial longitudinal fasciculus (MLF), resulting in abnormalities of lateral gaze involving the third and sixth cranial nerves. INO is characterized by inability of the affected eye to move medially (adduct) on lateral gaze with nystagmus of the abducting eye. The striking pattern of disconjugate eye movements is referred to as INO because the lesion disconnects the sixth and the third cranial nerve nuclei by causing failure of neural connections in the internuclear pathways—the MLF. The peculiar monocular nystagmus can be either transitory (one or two beats) or sustained.[24] Common causes of INO are small demyelinating plaques of MS, small-vessel infarctions, head trauma, and brainstem vascular insufficiency.[1,5,9,11] INO is one of the characteristic findings used in the diagnosis of MS. Any patient presenting with the motility pattern that characterizes a pure MLF lesion should also have an edrophonium chloride (tension) test done to check for myasthenia gravis (see Chapter 22).

Disorders of Pupillary Constriction

The oculomotor nerve carries the parasympathetic fibers responsible for pupillary constriction and accommodation. As illustrated in Fig. 16-2, the pupillary constrictor fibers originate in the Edinger-Westphal nucleus of the midbrain and join the superior part of the oculomotor nerve as it travels toward the ciliary ganglion. Damage to these fibers results in abnormalities of shape and reactivity of the pupil to light and accommodation. Figure 16-3 illustrates common pupillary abnormalities.

With third-nerve compression, the ipsilateral pupil becomes temporarily ovoid and then dilated and nonreactive to light **(Hutchinson's pupil).** The **Argyll Robertson pupil** demonstrates normal accommodation but absent reaction to light; the pupil is irregular and small. The lesion responsible for these pupillary abnormalities is located in the pretectal neurons above the Edinger-Westphal nucleus.[49] This finding is associated with neurosyphilis, midbrain lesions, DM, and MS.[1,5,9,49] **Adie's pupil** results from degeneration of the ciliary ganglion and its postganglionic parasympathetic innervation to the affected pupil. This pupillary response is identified by an absent to poor response to both light and accommodation.[1,5,9,20,49] Adie's pupil is believed to represent a mild polyneuropathy.[1]

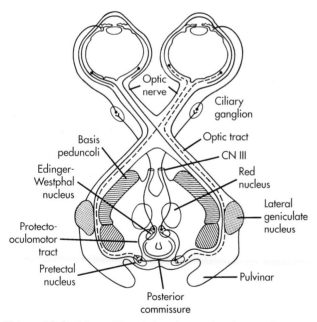

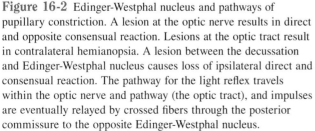

Figure 16-2 Edinger-Westphal nucleus and pathways of pupillary constriction. A lesion at the optic nerve results in direct and opposite consensual reaction. Lesions at the optic tract result in contralateral hemianopsia. A lesion between the decussation and Edinger-Westphal nucleus causes loss of ipsilateral direct and consensual reaction. The pathway for the light reflex travels within the optic nerve and pathway (the optic tract), and impulses are eventually relayed by crossed fibers through the posterior commissure to the opposite Edinger-Westphal nucleus.

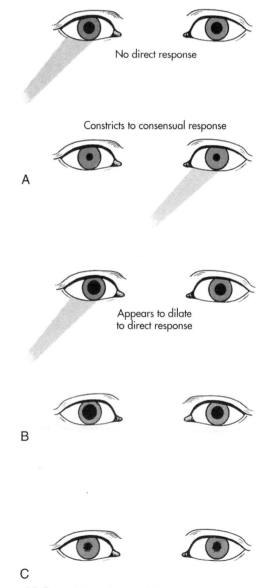

Figure 16-3 Pupillary abnormalities. **A,** Marcus Gunn's syndrome. **B,** Adie's (tonic) pupil. **C,** Argyll Robertson pupil.

Disorders of Eyelid Elevation

Ptosis, or drooping of the upper eyelid, can accompany disorders of the oculomotor nerve (CN III). The fibers that innervate the upper eyelid are located inferiorly in the nerve.[1] In oculomotor ptosis this innervation to the levator palpebrae superioris muscle is damaged, resulting in ptosis. Other causes of ptosis are Horner's syndrome (Fig. 16-4), myasthenia gravis, and muscular dystrophies.[1,5]

Assessment

The most common complaint associated with disorders of the oculomotor system is **diplopia,** or double vision. Diplopia is a troublesome and potentially dangerous problem for patients. The clinician caring for the patient experiencing diplopia must consider the sensory-perceptual alterations that occur and their effect on patient safety, activities of daily living (ADLs), and recreational/leisure activities.

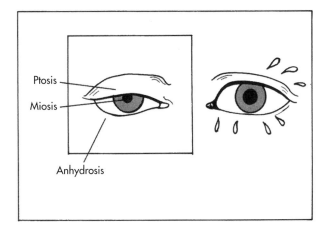

Figure 16-4 Components of Horner's syndrome.

Ptosis, an abnormal condition or one or both upper eyelids in which the eyelid droops because of a congenital or acquired weakness of the levator muscle or paralysis of CN III is assessed by observation to determine if the eyelid droops because of weakness of the levator muscles or paralysis of CN III. A thorough description of the patient's diplopia is obtained to guide examination of CN III, IV, and VI. Further neuro-ophthalmologic assessment is indicated when abnormalities of gaze or pupillary reaction to light are identified. Pupillary abnormalities are discussed earlier, under Disorders of Pupillary Constriction, in the Pathophysiology section.

Disorders of the three cranial nerves responsible for extraocular movement result in gaze deviations identified during testing. Figure 16-5 illustrates the gaze deviations seen with these disorders.

A thorough assessment should be done to identify the effect of the diplopia on the patient's lifestyle. The patient should be asked about changes that have occurred in self-care abilities, recreational and leisure activities, and role performance (e.g., family, job, school). Problems arising in association with the diplopia, such as headache, should be investigated. The cranial nerves are examined, and the findings are documented. Using the information gained through history taking, physical examination, and interpretation of diagnostic tests performed by the neurologist, the clinician can readily identify those problems that require care.

Additional tests that are performed to identify gaze disturbances are the corneal light reflex and the red glass test. In the **corneal light reflex test,** a light source is applied over the bridge of the nose and the patient is asked to fixate on the light as the head is passively moved in all directions. The clinician notes the appearance of the light's reflection on the cornea as the head is moved. In the absence of gaze disturbances, the light's reflection should be symmetric; extraocular muscle weaknesses result in asymmetric reflections of light.[5]

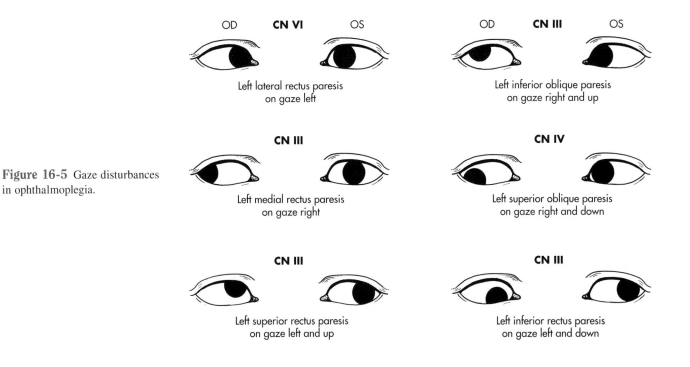

Figure 16-5 Gaze disturbances in ophthalmoplegia.

BOX 16-5	Interventions for Diplopia

- Arrange the environment in a safe, consistent fashion.
- Consider patching the affected eye and rotating every 2 to 4 hours.
- Approach and interact with the patient in a way that minimizes the need to use the involved eye muscle.
- Teach the importance of scanning the entire visual world.
- Provide nonvisual leisure activities to minimize boredom.
- Consult an occupational therapist or therapeutic recreation specialist.
- Teach the family and visitors strategies for approaching the patient.
- Teach the patient strategies to minimize diplopia (e.g., use of head turning and positioning).
- Teach the patient strategies to avoid injuries caused by diplopia (e.g., descending stairs with trochlear nerve palsy).

Treatment

Medical Management

To appropriately treat the patient with a disorder of the oculomotor system, the physician or clinician must identify the cause of the disorder. Compressive and expanding lesions causing oculomotor system palsies require rapid identification and surgical removal. Metabolic imbalances, seen with diabetes or thiamine deficiency, are treated with appropriate replacement therapies. The treatment of MS and myasthenia gravis, neurologic conditions commonly associated with ophthalmoplegia, is thoroughly discussed in Chapters 20 and 22.

Surgical Management

Compressive and expanding lesions causing oculomotor system palsies require rapid identification and surgical removal. Ptosis can be treated surgically by shortening the levator muscle.

Acute Care

The focus is on environmental manipulation, education, and psychosocial support.[48,62] Patching the eye is commonly recommended to minimize the visual disturbances and eye strain associated with diplopia. The clinician should suggest that the patient patch one eye at a time, alternating between eyes every 2 to 4 hours. Additional interventions for diplopia are listed in Box 16-5.

COMPREHENSIVE PATIENT MANAGEMENT: OCULOMOTOR NERVE SYSTEM DISORDERS

Case Management Considerations

The discharge planning and case management needs for the patient with an oculomotor system or pupillary reaction disorder depend primarily on the etiology of the disorder and its resulting medical management. Specific discharge needs related to diplopia focus on continued education to ensure a safe environment and a return to the patient's preferred lifestyle. The patient and family should be cautioned to examine home and work environments for safety. Extra furniture and objects should be removed if their presence increases the patient's risks for falls or collisions. The environment should remain as consistent as possible (e.g., minimize furniture rearrangement).

Patients with trochlear nerve palsies should be instructed to exert extreme care when performing activities that require downward gaze, such as descending stairs, inclines, or uneven terrain.[9,48] Strategies to minimize diplopia, such as covering or patching one eye, should be taught. Referrals for adaptive or corrective eyewear may be indicated.

Recreational and leisure activities should be encouraged, with referral to appropriate counselors as needed. Whether the patient can drive a motor vehicle depends on the severity of the visual disturbance. If driving privileges are curtailed, the patient and family should be assisted in examining the options available in public transportation or referred to local community agencies that help the disabled with transportation needs.

TRIGEMINAL NERVE DISORDERS

The trigeminal nerve (CN V) is one of the largest nerves in the head. It is responsible for sending impulses of touch, pain, pressure, and temperature from the face, jaw and gums, forehead, and periocular region of the eye to the brain. Because the trigeminal nerve is a mixed sensory and motor nerve, disorders involving it can present as sensory abnormalities, motor weakness, or both. The trigeminal nerve has a wide anatomic distribution. As a result of this anatomy, complete disruption of the trigeminal nerve rarely occurs. However, disorders of isolated parts of the nerve, especially the sensory branch, are common.[1] Although a variety of disorders from compression, inflammation, or degeneration involving the trigeminal (fifth) cranial nerve have been identified,[1,30,55] this discussion is limited to the most frequent disorder—**trigeminal neuralgia (TN), or tic douloureux.** TN is a painful condition of the face characterized by recurring episodes of paroxysmal lancinating, intense, stabbing, shock-like pain radiating from the angle of the jaw confined to the somatosensory distribution or branch of the trigeminal nerve (CN V).

Etiology

The exact etiology of TN remains unknown. It has been suggested that the etiology is vascular compression of the central axons of CN V at the level of pontocerebellar region or a hyperactive dysfunctional syndrome. TN may result from the focal demyelination of the trigeminal nerve or ganglia. It has been associated with MS, vascular lesions, and tumors.[1] There are some who believe that with aging, the pulsating artery becomes elongated and comes in contact with the trigeminal nerve root, producing the painful symptoms. Others believe that arachnoiditis may play a role. The annual prevalence of TN is approximately 100 to 200 per 100,000 persons.[59] According to the National Institute of Neurological Disorders and Stroke (NINDS), TN rarely affects anyone younger than 50 and is primarily a disorder of middle-age and older adults (65 to 75 years of age). TN occurs more often in women than in men at a 3 : 2 ratio. Right-sided nerve involvement is found twice as often as left-sided involvement and rarely bilaterally.

The disorder is characterized by sudden, severe, electric shock–like or stabbing pain, typically felt on one side of the jaw or cheek. The brief, paroxysmal episodes of excruciating pain occur most commonly in the distribution of the maxillary or mandibular division of the trigeminal sensory root. The attacks of pain, which generally last several seconds and may be repeated one after the other, may be brought on by stimulation of a **trigger point** somewhere in the distribution of the involved nerve division. The pain can be triggered by talking, brushing teeth, touching the face, shaving, chewing, swallowing, or even a slight breeze to the face. The attacks may come and go throughout the day and last for days, weeks, or months at a time, and then disappear for months or years.

During the painful attack, the face may appear contorted, and it remains in that position until the pain eases—hence the term *tic*.[59] Painful episodes are unilateral and of short duration, generally lasting less than 2 minutes, but can recur. When the recurrences are frequent, the patient may be incapacitated for hours from paroxysmal bouts of the neuralgia. Although the patient is pain free in the period between paroxysms, the anxiety associated with the anticipation of another attack may compromise the patient's ability to cope with this disorder. Narcotic analgesics are not very effective and are rarely prescribed to manage the pain[55]; those patients for whom opioids are prescribed are at risk for narcotic addiction.

Pathophysiology

An identifiable lesion of the fifth nerve contributing to the development of idiopathic TN has not been found. Degeneration of the gasserian ganglion and compression of the fifth nerve by anomalous blood vessels or tumors have been found in some cases of symptomatic TN. In addition, demyelinating lesions of the spinal root of the fifth nerve have been hypothesized to give rise to this disorder. Lesions in the symptomatic form are believed to compress or invade the pathway of the fifth nerve, resulting in microscopic pockets of demyelination. These pockets disrupt normal impulse transmission and give rise to synapses that trigger the pain characteristic of TN.

At the gasserian ganglion, located in a depression of the petrous portion of the temporal bone, the three sensory divisions of the trigeminal nerve merge. The two lower divisions (maxillary and mandibular) are most often implicated in TN. The disorder can progress to involve all three divisions of the fifth nerve. From the gasserian ganglion the sensory root enters the pons. The sensory fibers that carry pain descend in the spinal tract of the trigeminal nerve to terminate in the nucleus of the spinal tract located at the third cervical segment. From here the fibers cross the midline and ascend to the ventral posteromedial nucleus of the thalamus.

Assessment

The diagnosis of TN is based on the description of facial pain given by the patient. In addition to the characteristic pain described previously, the clinician often notes guarding or reluctance of the patient to touch the trigger area and limitation of facial movements. Facial and oral hygiene may be compromised if hygienic activities serve as pain triggers. The patient may be undernourished if oral movements provoke pain episodes.

After a thorough neuroassessment is completed, a routine medical evaluation can be performed to rule out other medical conditions. An MRI scan of the brain is indicated, even if there is no loss of sensation or other abnormality. The value of a dental evaluation is uncertain.[59] Some patients have had one or more, or even all, of their teeth extracted when dental problems were initially suspected.

Other causes of facial pain must be considered in the assessment. Other disorders to be considered include diseases of the teeth, sinuses, and jaw; herpes zoster and other inflammatory disorders; atypical facial pain; cluster headache; craniocerebral trauma; tumors; and systemic immune diseases.[1,30,55] Several cases of pre-TN have been reported.[23] This condition is associated with dull, continuous, aching facial pain located in the upper or lower jaw that later develops into the classic paroxysmal pain of TN. Identification of this condition is important for prompt treatment and prevention of unnecessary dental surgery.

Older adults may present with vague, nonspecific, insidious complaints as opposed to the "classic presentation" described previously. When assessing older adults, clinicians should be aware of "other" causes of facial pain with similar presentations. Preexisting pain could be related to dental disease (acute or chronic), temporal arteritis, glaucoma, and depression. With aging, pain-free remissions shorten in duration. Because of alterations in pharmacokinetics and a higher incidence of polypharmacy, older adults are at increased risk for drug toxicity and drug interactions in the treatment of TN.

Treatment

Medical Management
Treatment of TN often begins with the administration of either carbamazepine (Tegretol) 200 to 1200 mg/day in two divided doses, or phenytoin (Dilantin) 300 to 500 mg/day. These anticonvulsant drugs are believed to inhibit synaptic transmission in the spinal nucleus of the trigeminal nerve.

Carbamazepine is initially administered as a 100-mg dose twice daily. The dose is increased by 100 mg every 12 hours until the pain is relieved, signs of toxicity appear, or a maximum daily dose of 1200 mg has been reached.[55] After pain control is achieved, the dosage of carbamazepine is tapered; maintenance doses are 200 to 400 mg twice a day. While the patient is receiving carbamazepine therapy, the clinician must monitor the patient for side effects, especially

BOX 16-6	**Pharmacotherapy for Trigeminal Neuralgia: Clinical Concerns**

Carbamazepine
- Administer with meals to lessen nausea.
- Monitor WBC and platelet count; discontinue for dropping counts.
- Monitor for CNS side effects, especially drowsiness, vertigo, and ataxia; teach patient to avoid activities requiring alertness if CNS side effects occur.
- Avoid in patients with known allergy to tricyclic antidepressants and those on MAOIs.
- Discontinue administration if skin rash or hepatic damage develops.
- Teach patient drug is not an analgesic and should not be used for other pain.
- Teach patient photosensitivity precautions.
- Suggest ways to minimize dry mouth.
- Store drug in a cool, dark place.
- Obtain careful drug history; has interactions with several drugs.

Phenytoin
- Administer same brand of drug (bioavailability varies among brands).
- Monitor for CNS side effects, especially nystagmus, ataxia, and slurred speech.
- Advise women of risk of hirsutism.
- Obtain careful drug history; has interactions with many drugs.
- Administer with meals to lessen GI upset.
- Monitor for folic acid and vitamin D deficiencies.

WBC, White blood cell; *CNS,* central nervous system; *MAOIs,* monoamine oxidase inhibitors; *GI,* gastrointestinal.

those associated with suppression of the hematologic system. Important management considerations are listed in Box 16-6.[8,12]

In addition to its preventive use, IV or oral phenytoin may be used to interrupt acute attacks of TN.[55] Daily dosages range from 300 to 500 mg, with reports of as much as 700 mg/day required to control pain episodes.[55] At this high dosage range, side effects often preclude continued administration. As with carbamazepine, interventions in the administration of phenytoin center on identification of early signs of drug intolerance (see Box 16-6).

If carbamazepine and phenytoin are ineffective in the control of TN, gabapentin (Neurontin), valproic acid (Depakene), clonazepam (Topamax), baclofen (Lioresal), oxcarbazepine (Trileptal),[67] or pimozide (Orap)[37] may be tried. Pilot studies treating TN with botulinum-A neurotoxin (BoNT/A) have resulted in pain reduction with no major side effects, indicating a need for further placebo-controlled clinical trails.

Approximately two thirds of the patients with TN respond initially to pharmacotherapy. Many of these patients eventually are weaned from the drugs; the maintenance dose of the drug is restarted only if attacks recur. The remaining patients need surgical intervention to control their pain.

Surgical Management

Patients who do not respond to drug therapy are candidates for surgical treatment of TN.[44] Distal nerve blocks or ablative procedures generally are not recommended because of a high incidence of early recurrence.[59] A wide variety of surgical approaches have been used to treat TN (e.g., removal of the trigeminal ganglion on the posterior portion of the nerve, microvascular decompression, radiofrequency retrogasserian rhizotomy, percutaneous glycerol rhizotomy [chemoneurolysis], and percutaneous balloon microcompression).

Gamma Knife Radiosurgery. **Gamma knife radiosurgery** is an option for patients with either unilateral or bilateral TN who are considered appropriate candidates by the health care team after a thorough evaluation. A radiosurgery dose of 70 to 80 Gy is delivered to the trigeminal root entry zone approximately 2 to 4 mm anterior to the junction of the pons and trigeminal nerve with a single 4-mm collimator helmet (see Chapter 8). Patients have complete or partial relief with no morbidity. Radiosurgery, therefore, seems to be an effective approach for medically or surgically refractory TN.[34]

Radiofrequency Retrogasserian Rhizotomy. Radiofrequency rhizotomy (RFR) is designed to produce a sensory defect in the affected divisions of the trigeminal nerve. It is generally performed in the radiology department. The patient is placed in the supine position.[27,47] Intraoperative three-dimensional (3-D) CT scanning can be used to guide the trajectory of the needle puncture of the foramen ovale with the goal of providing the success rate of puncture and to enhance safety. A needle is guided into the trigeminal root using local anesthesia with IV sedation (Fig. 16-6).[15] After proper placement has been confirmed through reproduction of the patient's pain with thermal stimulation, the patient is anesthetized using ultrashort-acting IV agents, e.g., methohexital sodium (Brevital). Thermocoagulation of as many as 2 to 5 lesions can be made using a radiofrequency current at a temperature of 60° to 75° C for durations of approximately 60 to 90 seconds depending on the patient's pain distribution and age.[51] During application of the current, erythema in the distribution of the affected division appears. This observation is associated with a durable lesion in the division with resultant sensory deprivation.[47] After the current is delivered; the patient is awakened and tested for adequate sensory loss. Repeat applications of the current may be needed to ensure satisfactory destruction of involved fibers. With repeat applications the patient is again briefly anesthetized while the radiofrequency current is reapplied. The thermocoagulation destroys C fibers and A-delta fibers that conduct pain stimuli while preserving larger myelinated touch fibers.

With RFR the hospital stay is short (ambulatory or overnight). The benefits include less risk than is generally associated with general anesthesia, preservation of motor function, preservation of touch sensation, and prolonged relief of pain.

As with the other two percutaneous surgical treatments (glycerol rhizolysis and percutaneous microcompression), sensory disturbances are reported after RFR. These disturbances include anesthesia, hypesthesia (decrease in normal feeling or numbness), paresthesia (new or additional feelings such as "pins and needles"), and dysesthesia (disturbing sensory changes).[38] Sweet[63] has reported a combined dyses-

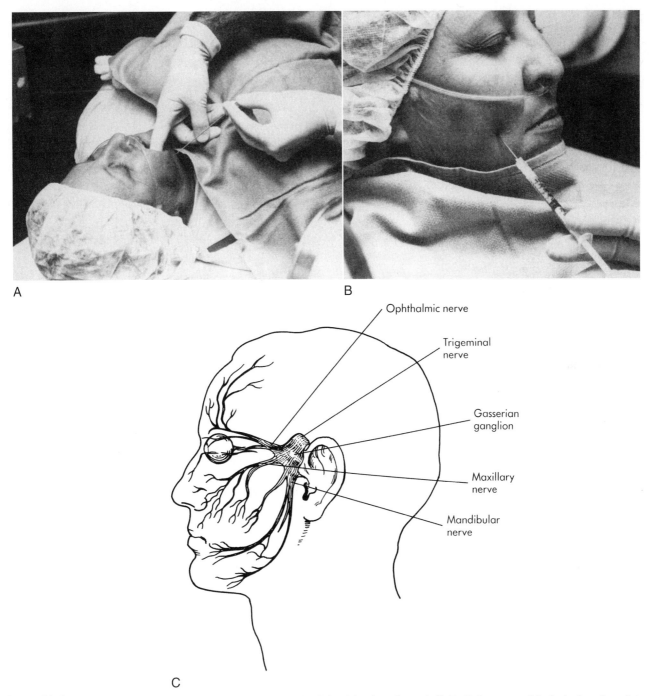

Figure 16-6 **A,** Patient with TN having a needle placed. **B,** Physician injecting glycerol. **C,** Radiofrequency rhizolysis: location of the gasserian ganglion. The electrode is inserted through the cheek and foramen ovale to the gasserian ganglion, so that a lesion is created electrically for control of pain.

thesia rate of 18% after RFR; 13% of these patients did not require pharmacologic agents to control the dysesthesia, and the remaining 5% of patients received drug therapy. In addition to sensory disturbances, patients experience brief periods (3 to 9 months) of weakness of the masseter and pterygoid muscles after this procedure.

Potential Complications

Complications of RFR may include hematoma formation at the needle insertion site in the cheek, loss of or a decreased corneal blink reflex (2% to 6% of patients), neuropathic keratitis, meningitis, temporal lobe abscess, ocular nerve palsies (especially of the sixth nerve), carotid artery injuries, analgesia/anesthesia dolorosa, and rarely, death.[23,34,43,47] A proportion of patients experience a recurrence of painful neuralgia after initial successful RFR. The recurrence rate increases over time; at 5 years 21% to 28% of patients require reoperation.[63]

Percutaneous Glycerol Rhizotomy.

Percutaneous glycerol retrogasserian (GR) injection is designed to provide symptomatic relief from the pain associated with TN. GR uses the same operative approach as RFR as a minimally invasive technique often used for patients not considered good surgical candidates. The needle position is confirmed, and small doses of glycerol are injected into the cistern. The total glycerol dose ranges from 0.3 to 0.5 ml.[46,57] Glycerol is believed to destroy the demyelinated sections of the rootlets involved in triggering the pain of TN.[2]

The advantages of GR are similar to those of RFR in that the hospital stay is short (usually same-day procedure or overnight admission) and local anesthesia with sedation is used. The success rate reported with GR ranges from 80% to 90% in centers that perform the procedure frequently.[38,57] In addition, there is less likelihood of loss of corneal sensation, less pain associated with this procedure, and less facial numbness as a consequence of the procedure.[46,57]

The median pain-free, medication-free interval after GR is reported to be between 16 months and 2 years,[46,57] with neuralgia recurrence rates of approximately 29%.[57] Resumption of pharmacologic therapy, repeat GR, or performance of another surgical procedure is indicated when return of symptoms becomes problematic for the patient.

Potential Complications

Complications after GR may include facial numbness; morbidity; bleeding, bruising, or swelling at the needle insertion site; a delay of as long as 2 weeks in the relief of pain; hypesthesia, paresthesia, or dysesthesia; a decreased corneal blink reflex and diplopia; herpes simplex; and meningitis.[2,46,57]

Percutaneous Balloon Microcompression. Percutaneous balloon microcompression, a technically simple, nonpainful procedure for the treatment of TN, was introduced in 1978. The patient is placed in the supine position on the operating room (OR) table with the head in neutral position. With the patient under brief general anesthesia, Meckel's cavity is entered through the cheek and foramen ovale using a small balloon catheter. After the catheter is in position, the balloon is inflated with contrast material. Balloon inflation with 0.6 to 1.1 ml of the contrast material is maintained for 1 minute, after which time the contrast material is aspirated, the catheter is withdrawn, and pressure is applied to the cheek puncture site.[25,26] The entire procedure takes 15 minutes. To limit the hypertensive response associated with balloon inflation, inflation times are limited to 1 minute and the patient may be pretreated with sodium nitroprusside.[39] Atropine can be used to treat symptomatic bradycardia.[38]

The advantages of balloon microcompression are similar to those of RFR and GR. The hospital stay is short (same-day procedure or overnight admission), and brief general anesthesia without the need for endotracheal intubation is used. This procedure can be used to treat neuralgia arising from the ophthalmic division with less concern for loss of corneal sensation.[39] A successful procedure is associated with hemifacial numbness (hypesthesia) on the operative side. In addition, transient ipsilateral masseter muscle weakness (lasting as long as 3 months) is present.

Neuralgia recurs in 10% to 20% of patients at 1 to 4 years after balloon microcompression,[38,39] in 20% of patients at 5 years, and in 28% of patients at 10 years.[38] The duration of the hypesthesia is closely correlated with the length of the pain-free interval. Patients who were previously unresponsive to carbamazepine therapy are often successfully treated with this drug when neuralgia recurs after balloon microcompression.[38]

Potential Complications

Complications associated with balloon microcompression may include cardiovascular instability during balloon inflation (stepwise increases in blood pressure or bradycardia), bleeding through the cannula, herpes simplex, transient decreases in corneal sensitivity, ocular nerve palsies with diplopia, dysesthesias, paresthesias, cheek hematoma, and meningitis.[39]

Microvascular Decompression. When anomalous vessels are believed to be the cause of TN, microvascular decompression (MVD) of the nerve with repositioning of the vessels is a highly accepted and effective procedure.[6] The goal of MVD is to provide a permanent cure by decompressing the trigeminal root from its offending vessel(s)—in most cases one or several elongated arteries. This procedure requires that the patient undergo a posterior fossa craniotomy under general endotracheal anesthesia. The patient is usually placed in the lateral decubitus position, although a modified sitting position may be used.[50] The neurosurgeon uses the operating microscope to identify and reposition the vessels while leaving the nerve undisturbed. The superior cerebellar artery (SCA) is the most commonly conflicting vessel.[61] Endoscopy may be used as an adjunctive imaging modality to microscopy to confirm nerve-vessel conflicts and to assess the adequacy of decompression.[33]

The advantages of this procedure include preservation of the trigeminal nerve with relief of pain and no dysesthesias. Disadvantages are associated with general anesthesia and a major surgical procedure. Mortality and major morbidity (e.g., stroke) rates of 1% respectively are associated with MVD.[38] Pain recurrence rates of between 4% and 47% at as long as 8 years after surgery have been reported.[38] If anomalous vessels are not found, the surgeon may destroy part of the nerve to minimize pain, leaving the patient with sensory abnormalities and recurrent pain.[2,36] The use and advantages of the endoscope to visualize the structures within the cerebellopontine (CP) angle have been trialed. This newer procedure will determine if the technique of endoscopic vascular decompression (EVD) can supplement the microscope to improve localization and success rates and decrease complications.

Acute and Postacute Care

The management of the patient diagnosed with TN depends on the setting in which the patient is encountered and the type of treatment the patient is receiving. Generally, patients receiving drug therapy are encountered in the nonacute setting unless complications associated with the drug necessitate hospital admission. Conversely, the patient undergoing surgical treatment is encountered in the acute or postacute setting.

When surgical treatment of TN is selected, the patient is admitted to the hospital for short-stay or extended-stay surgery. The clinical management associated with these procedures is presented here.

Short-Stay Surgical Procedures. The percutaneous procedures (RFR, GR, and balloon microcompression) are most commonly performed as a same-day procedure or with an overnight admission. The preoperative preparation of patients is generally accomplished in the neurosurgeon's office or through a hospital-sponsored preoperative preparation program for ambulatory surgery. This preparation should include a description of the procedure and its benefits and risks consistent with standards for informed consent. It is especially important to describe the sensory and motor deficits that follow each procedure. The patient should anticipate ipsilateral hypesthesia or paresthesia after the procedure. The patient should understand that this sensory alteration indicates successful nerve destruction. In addition, temporary masseter weakness may affect chewing, swallowing, and speaking.

Preoperative Care

Because these procedures are performed using local anesthesia with IV sedation and brief periods of unconsciousness, the activities should be explained to the patient. These explanations should be reinforced during the actual procedure. Because patient positioning and cooperation are essential in needle localization, the patient should also be taught what to expect during surgery.

Before the procedure the clinician obtains a history of the patient's neuralgia, including precipitating factors and typical pain triggers and patterns. A neurologic examination is done with special attention to the condition of the cornea and mouth; care is exercised to avoid trigger areas during the examination. Attention should be directed to the patient's preoperative nutritional, emotional, and physical state, since each of these areas may be compromised by self-imposed limitations to avoid neuralgic episodes.[15] Problems identified on preoperative assessment must be addressed during postoperative care and discharge teaching.

Postoperative Care

After the procedure the patient must be maintained in the position ordered by the neurosurgeon for the specified period of time. For example, GR requires that an upright, seated position with the head flexed and turned slightly to the ipsilateral side be maintained for approximately 1 to 2 hours postoperatively,[2,57] sometimes followed by 5 to 6 hours of strict bed rest with 60-degree elevation of the head of the bed.[46] To minimize swelling at the percutaneous needle insertion site, ice packs are applied. Routine postoperative vital and neurologic signs are obtained according to the institution's policy. Special attention must be directed to ascertaining the presence of the corneal blink reflex and condition of the cornea and determining areas of diminished facial sensation. Oral intake is resumed when sensation has returned to the buccal cavity; a soft diet is ordered, and excessively hot or cold foods and beverages are avoided. Chewing on the nonoperative side is recommended.[2]

Discharge and Health Teaching

The patient meets the criteria for discharge when buccal/facial sensation has returned, vital signs are stable, oral intake has resumed, and the patient has voided. Teaching before discharge centers on the expected effects of the procedure and potential complications.

The expected and obtained sensory changes need to be reinforced for the patient and family. Anesthesia, hypesthesia, paresthesia, or dysesthesia follow all percutaneous surgical procedures. Patients' abilities to cope with these sensory alterations will be affected by their preoperative understanding of anticipated surgical results, prior experience in surgical treatment for their neuralgia, and careful reexplanation and reinforcement of the expected effects of their surgery. The use of empathetic therapeutic communication strategies is imperative in facilitating the patient's adjustment to sensory and motor losses after surgery.

Because sensation to the affected area is compromised, the patient must be taught to protect this area from injury and inspect it frequently for signs of injury (e.g., protective goggles or eyewear and irrigating the eye). If the patient would be unable to experience oral pain, visits to the dentist or dental hygienist regularly (every 6 months) are recommended for early detection of a toothache or dental caries. Care specific to loss of the protective corneal blink reflex is presented earlier in this chapter. The patient is expected to use adaptive strategies to prevent injury and infection. To accomplish this outcome, the patient should be taught to avoid beverages and foods that are excessively hot or cold; use care while chewing to prevent biting the involved side of the mouth and chew on the unaffected side; frequently inspect the oral cavity, especially after eating; frequently perform oral hygiene (on awakening, after meals, and at bedtime), including careful flossing between the teeth to remove accumulated food particles; protect the involved area from environmental extremes of cold, heat, and wind; avoid scratching and rubbing the skin over the involved area; and for men, use care when shaving.[2,48]

Patients should be provided with the name and telephone number of the neurosurgeon in case problems occur after discharge. The clinician should review when to call the neurosurgeon immediately (e.g., for high fever or severe headaches) and when problems can wait for the next office visit (e.g., development of herpes simplex lesions).[2,36] The patient is given an appointment for follow-up care 1 to 2 weeks after surgery. Same-day and short-stay surgical procedures limit the available time a clinician has to interact with the patient. Clinicians practicing in these settings should consider developing an outreach or follow-up telephone program to identify problems or concerns experienced by patients after discharge. These programs could be coordinated with clinicians practicing in the neurosurgeon's office or clinic. Programs such as these provide the patient with access to continued professional clinical management during the adjustment period after surgery. They also give the clinician the opportunity to evaluate teaching effectiveness in preparing the patient for postoperative lifestyle changes. In addition, written discharge instructions are a valuable resource for the patient and family.

Acute Care Extended-Stay Surgical Procedures. When the patient has been scheduled for microvascular decompression, principles of clinical management after posterior fossa (infratentorial) surgery are followed (see Chapter 8). While providing postoperative care to the patient, the clinician must pay particular attention to the integrity of the trigeminal nerve and monitor the patient for the recurrence of pain. Known trigger points and their stimuli should be avoided in positioning, hygienic care, and environmental control. Postoperatively, the patient is transferred to the intensive care unit (ICU) and extubated as soon as he or she is awake. Monitoring is continued overnight, and the patient is transferred to nonacute care the next day.

Postprocedure Assessment

After treatment for TN, the assessment may include the following:

- Neurologic pain: Comparison with pretreatment pain to evaluate the degree of relief of facial pain
- CN V: Comparison with the pretreatment motor and sensory status
- Ability to chew, swallow, and resume a routine diet
- Cornea: Changes or damage related to the procedure
- Speech: Changes in normal speech or language
- Cerebrospinal fluid (CSF) leak
- Infection
- Hearing: Changes or decrease in acuity

Potential Complications

Complications may include visual or ocular complaints. Potential complications to monitor include CSF leak, infection (meningitis), normal pressure hydrocephalus (NPH), corneal anesthesia, neurotrophic keratitis, optic neuropathy, ocular motor cranial neuropathies, decrease in hearing caused by blood in the middle ear, otitis, delayed wound healing, recurrence of pain, or failure to obtain pain relief.[61]

Nonacute Care for Extended Stay. Management of patient care requires careful monitoring and assessment for the following[61]:

- Neuralgic pain. Assessment includes triggering stimuli and trigger points.
- Diet. A normal diet is resumed.
- Activity. Progressive ambulation is begun as tolerated.
- Analgesics for headache. If the headaches are severe, a CT scan is done before analgesics are given.
- Anticonvulsants. These are prescribed for 10 days, until the air in the subarachnoid spaces has been resorbed.
- Mild hyperthermia. This is presumed to be due to CSF depletion, air accumulation, and reactions to the implanted prosthesis.
- Suture removal/dressing. Sutures are removed after several days, followed by application of a new compressive dry dressing.
- Discharge. Patients with an uncomplicated course are discharged when stable.
- Medications. Patients who keep having some paroxysmal pain in their face will stay with their previous treatment, but at lower doses.
- Postoperative return physician visit. Patients return for a follow-up visit 2 months after discharge unless they have recurrence of pain.

Effectiveness of treatment, and strategies used in coping are related to the patient's knowledge of his or her prescribed medications. A thorough patient assessment should be performed to assist in the identification of complications of the neuralgia (e.g., undernourishment, poor oral hygiene, corneal irregularities) and side effects of drug therapy.

Interventions used in the nonacute setting typically center on medication monitoring and teaching, control of pain, and psycho-emotional support. Concerns associated with medication monitoring and teaching are outlined in Box 16-6.

Pain Management

Strategies to assist the patient with pain control must consider the need for the patient to maintain an adequate nutritional intake and ideal body weight and to maintain oral and facial hygiene. Analgesic medications are not useful in the management of TN. It is important for the patient to report the effectiveness of the prescribed medications so that the dosage may be adjusted appropriately (see Chapter 23).

Oral Hygiene

Brushing should be performed routinely with a soft toothbrush. Dental professionals can offer suggestions for oral hygiene to minimize the risk of triggering a painful episode and to maximize oral health.

COMPREHENSIVE PATIENT MANAGEMENT: TRIGEMINAL NERVE DISORDERS

Health Teaching Considerations

TN may be a chronic disorder for some patients. Evidence demonstrates that with aging, remissions become shorter. Patients and families must understand the natural history of this disorder, common patient responses, and available treatment options. In addition, medication teaching, self-care, and nutrition teaching are needed (see Nonacute Care for Extended Stay).

Nutritional Considerations

Although eating and hygiene may be avoided during a painful episode, the patient must engage in these activities during remissions. A nutritional consultation with a registered dietitian is helpful in determining minimum daily caloric intake. Strategies to avoid triggering pain include chewing small portions, chewing on the unaffected side, and avoiding foods and beverages at temperature extremes.

Psychosocial Considerations

Psychosocial responses in TN depend on the premorbid personality, coping strategies, and support system of the patient. Studies have found depression to be common in persons suffering from chronic facial pain.[41] The appearance of depression is related to ineffective pain relief. Individualized support, along with referral to national and local support organizations, may be helpful to patients with TN or chronic pain.

Case Management Considerations

Before leaving the setting in which clinical management is provided, the patient should receive information on available community support groups for people with TN or chronic pain. When appropriate, the clinician or case manager should provide referrals to mental health counselors, dietitians, and community health care providers.

FACIAL NERVE DISORDERS

Although the seventh cranial nerve carries mixed fibers, disorders associated with the nerve are primarily motor-related problems. The most frequent type of peripheral facial paresis is **Bell's palsy.** This idiopathic neuropathy disorder of CN VII is discussed in detail in this section. For a review of other causes of facial palsy, see Adams and Victor,[1] Haymaker and Kuhlenbeck,[30] or Rowland.[55]

Etiology

Bell's palsy, or idiopathic facial paralysis, is a disorder of unknown etiology in up to 75% of cases. The annual incidence is about 15 to 40 per 100,000, with an increasing incidence seen with increasing age. High-risk patients include pregnant women and patients with DM or MS.[10] It has been associated with a preceding viral infection[1]; inflammation associated with exposure of the face to cold, wind, or drafts[55]; and a hereditary factor.[30]

This common disorder of the facial nerve affects individuals of all ages and both sexes. It is reported to occur more often in young adults, older adults, and people with diabetes, hypertension, and lipid abnormalities.[66] Some reports have not found an increase during pregnancy.[1,30] An association between second-stage Lyme disease and manifestations of Bell's palsy has been reported.[45,52] Reactivation of latent herpes virus accounts for many cases but is difficult to document. A small number of patients report a positive family history of Bell's palsy.

Bell's palsy is characterized by CN VII dysfunction involving all distal branches. It is characterized by the sudden occurrence of unilateral facial paralysis that peaks within 2 to 5 days and resolves gradually over 1 to 2 months. Some individuals report pain behind the ear on the affected side 1 to 2 days before the onset of paralysis. Sensory fibers generally are involved, with taste impaired for as long as 2 weeks. Involvement of the muscles that supply the ear is characterized by **hyperacusis,** or distortions of sound.

The recovery process is completed within 2 months in approximately 80% to 85% of affected individuals. Evidence of denervation on electromyography (EMG) (reaction of degeneration [RD]) is associated with a longer recovery process and the potential for incomplete nerve regeneration.

Pathophysiology

The facial nerve originates in the pons (see Chapter 1). Its branchial motor fibers exit the brainstem at the level of the cerebellopontine angle to enter the internal auditory meatus on the opposite side. These fibers travel through the geniculate ganglion, where they enter the facial canal, eventually leaving the skull through the stylomastoid foramen. Distal to this foramen is the large nerve fibers that branch into small fibers supplying the muscles of facial movement. Lesions in

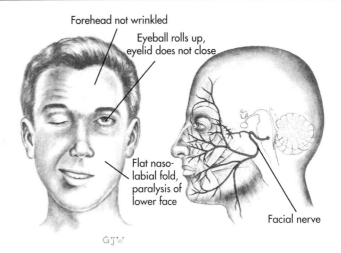

Figure 16-7 Bell's palsy: facial characteristics. *(From Chipps E, Clanin N, Campbell V:* Mosby's clinical series: neurologic disorders, *St Louis, 1992, Mosby.)*

the vicinity of the stylomastoid foramen have been identified during surgical exploration.[30]

Complete paralysis of the nerve results in loss of motor, sensory, and parasympathetic function ipsilateral to the lesion. Motor paralysis is characterized by complete loss of voluntary and automatic expression over the affected hemiface. The involved side of the face is immobile during attempts at expression. There is flattening of the nasolabial fold, sagging at the corner of the mouth, and displacement of the lips toward the unaffected side. The forehead flattens, and the eyebrows lose their symmetry. The palpebral fissure widens (Fig. 16-7). On attempts at eye closure, **Bell's phenomenon** is seen. This phenomenon is characterized by rotation of the affected eyeball in an upward position with inability to close the lid. Loss of blinking results in the collection of tears in the lower lid (epiphora). The ipsilateral corneal blink reflex is absent.

The loss of facial nerve function presents many challenges for the patient. Loss of expression interferes with communication, complicating the dysarthria that accompanies attempts to speak. Tearing and drooling occur on the affected side, because the patient is unable to control the flow of tears and saliva. Eating and drinking are compromised by the paralysis of facial muscles that assist with oral intake; loss of taste over the anterior part of the tongue may further interfere with the patient's eating patterns.

Assessment

The diagnosis of Bell's palsy is based on findings from the examination of the patient. Occasionally EMG is performed to confirm the diagnosis or determine the course of the recovery process. Bell's palsy is characterized by abrupt onset with complete or unilateral facial weakness or facial asymmetry at rest and with movement. The assessment includes observing for a tightening of the facial muscles, deepening nasolabial fold, reduced palpebral fissures, blepharospasm, asymmetric smile, numbness or pain around the ear, reduction in taste, hypersensitivity to sounds, and inability to perform requested facial movements on the involved side. If the sensory routes are involved, taste over the anterior two thirds of the ipsilateral side of the tongue is absent. The clinical manifestations seen with this disorder are described in the Etiology and Pathophysiology sections.

A thorough assessment is done to document a baseline and to facilitate the identification of the patient's response to the episode of Bell's palsy. Particular attention should be given to the patient's nutritional status, oral hygiene, integrity of the corneal blink reflex, quality of speech, and psycho-emotional response. A baseline evaluation of facial muscle motor function should be obtained, with periodic reevaluation conducted during the course of the palsy.

Neurodiagnostic and Laboratory Studies

Diagnosis of Bell's palsy is largely one of exclusion. In addition to a thorough history and evaluation to distinguish Bell's palsy from other facial paralysis, the following diagnostic studies may be ordered:

- EMG: May be performed 10 days to 2 weeks after onset to determine the presence of nerve degeneration. When RD is present, both the nerve and the muscle fail to respond to faradic current. The nerve response to galvanic current is initially absent, and the muscle demonstrates irritability. These findings, consistent with RD, are prognostic indicators for a poor outlook for full recovery.[30]
- Routine laboratory studies: As needed.

Treatment

Surgical Management

The therapeutic value of surgical decompression of the facial nerve is controversial. Rowland[55] has noted that some otologists perform the operation at 6 weeks after onset if paralysis is slow to resolve.

Acute Care

Treatment with corticosteroids and antivirals is weighed against the knowledge that in some cases, Bell's palsy may resolve spontaneously without treatment over a period of 6 months. Studies are underway to compare the effectiveness of botulinum toxin injections with traditional therapies or trials with combination therapy. In older adults or individuals with severe paresis or paralysis, treatment begins in the first days of the disease. Overall management of the patient with Bell's palsy is directed toward the prevention of complications and provision of psycho-emotional support. Several outcomes are expected in care provided to prevent complications. Measures to avoid corneal damage are necessary until voluntary and spontaneous eye closing returns. Clinical management to prevent corneal damage is found in Box 16-1.

Weight loss and undernourishment must be prevented. The clinician needs to be sensitive to the patient's embarrassment when the patient experiences drooling and difficulty chewing and swallowing. Strategies to prevent nutritional complications include recommending a soft diet; suggesting small, frequent meals; and chewing on the uninvolved side. Some patients may prefer privacy during eating. Because eating is an important time for socialization, the clinician may suggest dining with others in whose presence the patient is comfortable and relaxed.

Unless facial paralysis is a complication of an acute disorder, the clinician generally encounters patients experiencing an episode of Bell's palsy in the nonacute care setting. As with all idiopathic disorders, the treatment of Bell's palsy is directed toward symptom relief and prevention of complications. Without treatment, improvement is noted within 3 weeks in 85% of patients.[10] Therapies currently used include administration of steroids and vasodilators, physical therapy, electrotherapy, and surgical decompression of the nerve. No one form of therapy has proved superior in improving outcome.

If herpes simplex is accepted as the cause, treatment consists of a 10-day course of valacyclovir (Valtrex) 400 mg orally five times per day and steroids (prednisone 60 mg/day orally for 5 days and tapered). This therapy has been shown to hasten the recovery and to lessen the ultimate degree of dysfunction.[10] Vasodilator agents are occasionally used to improve circulation to the facial nerve.

Massage, exercise, and support of the facial musculature are used to control symptoms and prevent sagging or contracture of affected facial muscles. Warm, moist heat application improves circulation and soothes painful facial muscles. Mild analgesics may also be prescribed. Electrical stimulation of the muscle is thought to maintain tone and prevent atrophy. When the acute stage of the disorder is over, physical therapy may be used to strengthen the affected muscles. The patient is instructed to practice facial movements several times a day in front of the mirror. Movements to be practiced include blowing, smiling, pursing the lips, wrinkling the brow, and forcibly closing the eyelids.

Potential Complications. Complications of Bell's palsy are associated with incomplete recovery of nerve function, faulty reinnervation of effectors, and recurrence of the disorder. Incomplete recovery occurs in 10% to 25% of cases of Bell's palsy[22] and is associated with contractures of the facial muscles, clonic facial spasms, and tics. Crocodile tears phenomenon (tearing associated with eating) and abnormal associated movements are believed to result from faulty reinnervation of effector glands and muscles during nerve regeneration. The recurrence rate for Bell's palsy is approximately 7%.[30]

Ramsay Hunt Syndrome. **Ramsay Hunt syndrome** is another disorder of CN VII with a facial palsy. This lesser-known neurologic condition results from invasion of CN VII and the geniculate ganglion by varicella-zoster virus. The syndrome is relatively common in older children and vaccination can prevent or reduce the occurrence.[29] Patients may complain of the following:

- Severe ear pain
- Facial nerve (CN VII) palsy or paralysis or weakness of the ipsilateral side of the face
- Decreased tearing on the affected side
- Hyperacusis
- Decreased taste on the anterior two thirds of the tongue

- Vesicles over the tympanic membrane and along the posterior aspect of the external auditory meatus (sensory distribution of CN VII)
- Vertigo
- Hearing loss
- Mild, generalized encephalitis

There are reports of older patients presenting with small, circumscribed eruptions and pain in the ear and with erosions on the tongue with loss of taste.[3] Vertigo may last for days or weeks but usually resolves. The facial paralysis may be permanent. The hearing loss may be partial or total. Treatment with corticosteroids has been the primary therapy.

COMPREHENSIVE PATIENT MANAGEMENT: FACIAL NERVE DISORDERS

Health Teaching Considerations

All patients with facial nerve disorders should be taught about prescribed medications and therapies. Depending on the duration of steroid therapy, the patient needs to be taught the side effects and critical administration concerns related to prolonged use of corticosteroids. The clinician must explain measures designed to promote comfort and minimize muscle atrophy, including heat application, facial splints, and facial exercises. Return demonstrations or explanations assure the clinician that the patient understands the prescribed techniques.

In Bell's palsy most cases are self-limiting. Complete recovery can generally be expected within 2 to 3 months after the onset of paralysis. Educating the patient and family about the natural course of the disorder is important in promoting effective coping and for timely identification of potential complications. The patient should receive appropriate teaching on medications, facial exercise, and symptom control (see earlier discussion). Return explanations and demonstrations by the patient ensure that teaching has been effective. This is especially important in the prevention of facial muscle atrophy and contractures through appropriately performed facial exercises.

Psychosocial Considerations

Psychosocial support is imperative in promoting adaptive coping by the patient with a facial nerve disorder. The combined loss of articulate speech and facial expression serves to impair communication. Lohne and colleagues described reactions by others to facial disfigurement associated with facial paralysis as heightened attention, horror, anxiety, rejection, and excessive sympathy.[40] In their study, patients experienced social anxiety, disturbed self-concept, and depression as a result. Follow-up appointments or referrals to counselors should be offered to all patients when psychologic difficulties are suspected.

Case Management Considerations

It is unusual for a patient to be hospitalized for the nonsurgical treatment of a facial disorder, including Bell's palsy. If decompressive surgery has been performed, the discharge considerations are consistent with those described for the patient after cranial surgery (see Chapter 8). Case management may not be necessary except for complex or complicated cases.

ACOUSTIC NERVE DISORDERS

Disorders of the eighth cranial nerve can involve both the cochlear and vestibular branches, or either branch in isolation. Cochlear involvement presents with **tinnitus** and hearing impairments of sensorineural origin. Lesions involving the organ of Corti, cochlear nerve, secondary connections within the brainstem or thalamus, or primary and secondary auditory cortex are responsible for these impairments (see Chapter 7). The hearing loss is characterized by decreased bone conduction of sound and partial loss of perception of high-pitched tones. Other findings are loudness recruitment, hyperacusis, paracusis, impaired speech discrimination, and tinnitus. Examples of conditions associated with sensorineural hearing losses are cerebellopontine angle tumors, MS, labyrinthitis and other infections of the middle and inner ear, basilar skull fracture of the middle fossa, congenital defects, chronic exposure to intense noise, ototoxic agents (e.g., mycin antibiotics and acetylsalicylic acid), and aging.[30,55]

When the vestibular branch of the eighth nerve is involved, equilibrium is impaired and the patient will report varying degrees of **vertigo. Nystagmus** is present, and ocular movements are impaired.

The discussion here focuses on classic Meniere's disease, a vestibular disorder that can cause proprioceptive dysfunction. Classic Meniere's disease is one of the most common disorders of the eighth cranial nerve. This chronic disorder is estimated to affect 1 to 2 persons per 10,000 population. An individual with classic Meniere's disease can experience loss of proprioception during an acute attack so that they are unable to stand or walk.

Etiology

[handwritten: CN 8th nerve involvement only]

The cause of classic Meniere's disease remains unknown. Men are affected more often than women (2:1 to 3:1 ratio); onset is generally between the fourth and sixth decades.[30,65]

Classic Meniere's disease is characterized by paroxysmal attacks of vertigo associated with tinnitus and sensorineural hearing loss. The duration of an attack can vary from minutes to several hours; attacks occur days to months apart. During an attack the patient usually experiences nausea, vomiting, diaphoresis, and feelings of fullness and pressure in the involved ear. Horizontal and rotational nystagmus toward the involved ear is present. Between attacks the patient is free of vertigo; however, tinnitus, hearing loss, and nystagmus persist.

Pathophysiology

Classic Meniere's disease presents as the following four paroxysmal symptoms:[28]

- Tinnitus: Appears as two types—between attacks as a ringing noise and during the attack as a multifrequency noise like a roar, hiss, or buzz.
- Monaural fullness: Described as a sensation of the ear being full of water, beginning a day or two before the attack.
- Fluctuating hearing: Normal at the onset of the condition, with a reduction in hearing with each attack (this reduction resolves a day or two later). After a multiple attack, hearing declines and may develop into permanent sensorineural pattern deafness.
- Vertigo: Episodic.

Endolymphatic dilation (hydrops), or the clinical picture just described, is sometimes called the "hydrops" symptom complex, inferring that the mechanism is related to dilation and rupture of the endolymphatic compartment of the inner ear, although it is not known if hydrops is the cause of the patient's symptoms.[65] Hydrops, the accumulation of fluid in the endolymphatic space, is usually unilateral. Fluid accumulation results from either overproduction or impaired reabsorption of endolymph.

Several theories have been postulated to explain the development of endolymphatic hydrops. The most recent theory postulates an autoimmune etiology evidenced by the presence of higher levels of circulating immune complexes in patients with Meniere's disease.[17] Mechanical blockage of the cochlea and endolymphatic ducts, vasospasm of inner ear vessels associated with autonomic imbalances, abnormal salt metabolism, allergy, vitamin deficiencies, and emotional disorders are common theories. It is believed that vertiginous attacks result from rupture of the labyrinth, allowing endolymph to leak into the perilymph and disrupt vestibular sensorineural function.[1,30]

Assessment

Diagnosis of Meniere's disease is based on the history and audiometric testing. Typically the patient reports disabling attacks of vertigo described as a feeling of whirling or spinning. The attacks may occur suddenly or gradually and are often preceded by a sensation of fullness or pressure; low-pitched, roaring tinnitus; and impaired hearing in the involved ear. Associated findings during an attack are described previously. Between attacks the patient is free of vertigo, although tinnitus may persist, and with repeated attacks hearing loss becomes permanent.

Neurologic examination during an attack is positive for nystagmus as described previously. Caloric testing reveals abnormalities of the oculovestibular system; responses to cold and warm water irrigation of the affected ear are diminished or lost. With the exception of eighth-nerve deficits, the remainder of the neurologic examination is normal.

The assessment of the patient with Meniere's disease focuses on the patient's response to this chronic, occasionally disabling disorder. The clinician should obtain a description of the attacks and the strategies the patient uses for coping during attacks. The presence and extent of hearing loss and tinnitus should be determined.

Neurodiagnostic and Laboratory Studies

- Audiometry
- Electrocochleography
- Electronystagmography (ENG)
- CT/MRI
- Auditory brainstem evoked potentials: May be ordered to rule out other causes of dizziness and vertigo
- Blood tests: Fluorescent treponemal antibody (FTA), ANA, CBC, fasting blood sugar—to identify treatable causes[28]

Treatment

Medical Management

Treatment of Meniere's disease depends on the severity of the attacks. Initially, diet modifications, lifestyle changes, and pharmacologic therapy are ordered. A low-salt diet is prescribed, with a goal of minimizing the production of endolymph. For more severe cases a strict salt-free, neutral-ash diet (Furstenberg diet) is recommended. The restrictions associated with this diet are described by DeWeese and Saunders.[18]

Because of the vasoconstricting effect of nicotine, patients with Meniere's disease are instructed to stop smoking. Caffeine and alcohol limits are suggested, and the patient is cautioned to avoid the use of over-the-counter (OTC) decongestants. Positions and environments known to trigger an attack should be avoided.

Primary drugs used for symptom control include antihistamines (dimenhydrinate, buclizine hydrochloride, and meclizine hydrochloride) and anticholinergics (propantheline and glycopyrrolate).[12] Oral administration of prednisone, inner ear perfusion by intratympanic injection of dexamethasone, transtympanic injection of gentamicin, and other therapies are under study. Pharmacologic agents are prescribed to control symptoms and to terminate acute attacks. Ammonium chloride, administered in 2-g doses three times a day, is used to control vertigo. Diuretics may also be ordered in an effort to correct inner ear fluid imbalances. The efficacy of these prophylactic therapies (both diet and drugs) in treating Meniere's disease has not been established.[1] Anxiolytics may be used when alternative strategies to control anxiety are ineffective. Gentamicin treatment is growing in popularity. Vestibular suppressants are listed in Table 16-1.

Vasodilators are also used to control the symptoms of Meniere's disease. Nicotinic acid is the drug of choice. Other vasodilators prescribed include tolazoline hydrochloride (Priscoline) and nicotinyl alcohol (Roniacol).

Treatment during an acute attack is aimed at terminating the attack and controlling associated symptoms. Bed rest in a comfortable position is often all that is needed. Subcutaneous atropine 0.2 mg, IV epinephrine 0.3 ml given slowly, IV diazepam, and dilute histamine diphosphate (2.75 mg diluted in 250 to 500 ml of 5% dextrose in water) have been used to terminate attacks.[13,53,65] Antiemetics are used to treat nausea and vomiting (Table 16-2).

TABLE 16-1   Vestibular Suppressants*

Drug	Dose	Adverse Reactions	Pharmacologic Class and Precautions
Meclizine (Antivert, Bonine)	12.5–50 mg q4–6h	Sedating; precautions in prostatic enlargement, glaucoma	Antihistamine Anticholinergic
Lorazepam (Ativan)	0.5 mg twice daily	Mildly sedating Drug dependency	Benzodiazepine
Clonazepam (Klonopin)	0.5 mg twice daily	Mildly sedating Drug dependency	Benzodiazepine
Scopolamine (Transderm-Scop)	0.5 mg patch every 3 days	Topical allergy with chronic use; precautions in glaucoma, tachyarrhythmias, prostatic enlargement	Anticholinergic
Dimenhydrinate (Dramamine)	50 mg q4–6h	Same as meclizine	Antihistamine Anticholinergic
Diazepam (Valium)	2–10 mg (1 dose) given acutely orally, intramuscularly, or intravenously	Sedating Respiratory depressant Drug dependency Precautions in glaucoma	Benzodiazepine

From Goetz CG, Pappert EJ: *Textbook of clinical neurology,* Philadelphia, 1999, WB Saunders.
*Doses listed are used in adults. Drugs are arranged in order of preference.

TABLE 16-2   Antiemetics*

Drug	Usual Dose	Adverse Reactions	Pharmacologic Class
Droperidol (Inapsine)	2.5 or 5 mg sublingually or IM q12h	Sedating Hypotension Extrapyramidal	Dopamine antagonist
Meclizine (Antivert, Bonine)	12.5–50 mg PO q4–6h	Sedating Precautions in glaucoma, prostate enlargement	Antihistamine and anticholinergic
Metoclopramide (Reglan)	10 mg PO three times daily or 10 mg IM	Restlessness or drowsiness Extrapyramidal	Dopamine antagonist
Ondansetron (Zofran)	4–8 mg PO single dose	Hypotension	5-HT$_3$ antagonist
Prochlorperazine (Compazine)	5 mg or 10 mg IM or PO q6–12h or 25 mg rectally q12h	Sedating Extrapyramidal	Phenothiazine
Promethazine (Phenergan)	12.5–25 mg PO q6–8h or 12.5–25 mg rectally q12h 12.5 mg IM q6–8h	Sedating Extrapyramidal	Phenothiazine
Trimethobenzamide (Tigan)	250 mg PO three times daily or 200 mg IM three times daily	Sedating Extrapyramidal	Similar to phenothiazine
Thiethylperazine (Torecan)	10 mg PO, up to three times daily or 2 ml IM, up to three times daily	Sedating	Phenothiazine

From Goetz CG, Pappert EJ: *Textbook of clinical neurology,* Philadelphia, 1999, WB Saunders.
*Doses listed are used in adults.

Surgical Management

Approximately 10% to 20% of patients fail to respond to medical therapy and are candidates for surgery. Before selecting surgical treatment, patients need to know that the disease often spontaneously disappears after a few years.[60]

The preferred surgical procedure for the treatment of Meniere's disease is controversial because of the great vari-ability of outcomes. Procedures performed include general destructive surgeries (labyrinthectomy), selective destructive surgeries (vestibular neurectomies), and operations for endolymphatic sac decompression.

Destructive procedures result in the loss of partial or complete function of the acoustic nerve. Procedures that completely destroy the labyrinth are reserved for patients with unilateral disease, intractable vertigo, and rapidly progressive hearing loss. The labyrinth is approached through the external auditory canal, the semicircular canals are removed or destroyed, and the inner ear is packed with a streptomycin-soaked pack. After general destructive procedures the patient experiences vertigo, which resolves within 1 month; disorders of balance may remain as permanent sequelae.

Selective destructive procedures are considered to be the most effective procedures for controlling vertigo and preserving hearing.[31,45] These procedures include midfossa vestibular neurectomy, posterior fossa retrolabyrinthine neurectomy, and transmeatal cochleovestibular neurectomy. Various surgical approaches are used with these procedures to isolate the eighth cranial nerve and its divisions for destruction. Endolymphatic sac surgery has not been shown to offer significant improvement for the patient. A mastoidectomy is performed, in which the endolymph is directed into the subarachnoid space. Some improvement in vertigo is initially experienced in 80% of patients; however, within 5 years half of these patients experience a recurrence of vertigo.

Acute and Nonacute Care

Unless surgical treatment has been selected, the clinician generally encounters the patient with Meniere's disease in the nonacute care setting. For a discussion of care of the patient after craniotomy, see Chapter 8.

Therapies that the physician has prescribed should be reviewed to determine the patient's level of knowledge regarding diet, drugs, and recommended lifestyle changes. The use of OTC preparations for treating colds and allergy symptoms should be determined. Because stress and fatigue are known to exacerbate episodes of Meniere's disease, the patient should be questioned about current sources of stress and rest/activity patterns. Information should be obtained about the patient's habits in relation to smoking, alcohol, and caffeine intake.

The eighth-nerve function should continue to be assessed. To identify the extent of hearing loss, the clinical evaluation should be compared with a review of the results of audiometric and other diagnostic tests.

COMPREHENSIVE PATIENT MANAGEMENT: ACOUSTIC NERVE DISORDERS

Health Teaching Considerations

Safety, hearing loss, education, medications, and psychosocial considerations are the cornerstones of management of the patient with Meniere's disease.

Safety

A safe environment protects the patient from injuries that may result during an attack of vertigo and from hearing losses associated with disease progression. Generally, quiet, dark environments are soothing during a vertiginous attack.

The patient almost invariably lies down to achieve a comfortable position. When an attack occurs, the patient should stop all activities and lie down in a position that minimizes the vertigo. Sudden movements should be avoided. If the patient is hospitalized, all side rails should be up and the call light should be easily reachable. Activities necessary to care for the patient should be grouped, carried out quietly, and planned to require minimal position changes by the patient. If the patient is driving when an attack begins, he or she should slowly pull the motor vehicle over to the side of the road. The patient should be instructed to assume a comfortable position and remain still until the symptoms subside. A medical alert bracelet or other device is beneficial for alerting others to the disorder.

Hearing Loss

For significant hearing impairments, the patient should be referred for hearing aid evaluation. Strategies to improve hearing should be explored, including the use of white-noise machines to minimize tinnitus. The clinician should be sure to note the hearing loss in the patient's care plan, along with mutually agreed-on strategies to enhance hearing.

Education

Health teaching is multidimensional. Required lifestyle changes need to be reviewed. Referral to a smoking cessation program may be helpful for the patient who is experiencing difficulty in stopping smoking. Alcohol, caffeine, and OTC decongestants should be avoided. Stress-reduction strategies should be explored for patients with high stress levels. The patient should be cautioned against participating in activities known to trigger vertigo, such as amusement rides and climbing activities. Until the symptoms are controlled, driving is prohibited. The patient must rely on family or friends for transportation. If necessary, the clinician should explore community transportation options for the patient.

Medications

Medication teaching should include the name, dose, schedule, actions, and side effects of all prescribed drugs. It is important that the patient take "as-needed" medications as soon as any symptoms signal an attack. Specific concerns associated with anticholinergic and antihistamine agents are described in Table 16-1. Because medications may mask the signs of the disease during diagnostic testing, the patient needs to be taught to discontinue all medications during testing.

Nutritional Considerations

The patient and the primary meal preparer in the family must understand dietary restrictions. A consultation with a registered dietitian is recommended for teaching and meal suggestions for the patient with either a low-salt diet or the Furstenberg diet. Because niacin improves blood flow to the vestibular apparatus, foods high in niacin should be incorporated into meal planning. Examples of dietary sources of niacin are whole-grain and enriched breads and cereals, poultry, fish, and meat.

Psychosocial Considerations

The psycho-emotional sequelae of Meniere's disease include depression,[14] attack-associated feelings of depersonalization,[26] social isolation,[13] and high levels of anxiety and stress from the unpredictability of attacks. Reassurance and psychologic support for the patient are critical clinical interventions. Family members, employers, co-workers, friends, and others who are in regular contact with the patient need to be informed about the disorder so that they avoid suspecting problems such as malingering or substance abuse. Uncontrolled anxiety may respond to a short course of anxiolytic drug therapy in conjunction with stress-reduction strategies. When necessary, the patient should be referred to a mental health provider for counseling. The clinician should discuss the natural course of Meniere's disease with the patient; often an understanding of the self-limiting nature of the disease assists with coping.

Case Management Considerations

The patient with Meniere's disease needs to be aware of available national and community supports. Meniere's Network gives patients referrals to self-help groups and related services. The patient needs to be aware of the cause, treatment, and expected outcome of therapy for long-term follow-up. Diplopia can be a troublesome and potentially dangerous problem. After discharge, the individual must consider the sensory-perceptual alterations that can occur and their effect on safety, ADLs, and recreational/leisure activities.

GLOSSOPHARYNGEAL NERVE DISORDERS

The ninth and tenth cranial nerves are often considered together because of their close spatial relationship and common participation in the protective gag reflex. Isolated disorders of these nerves are uncommon but do occur. A discussion of the causes of a diminished or absent gag reflex and clinical management of the patient is found earlier in this chapter.

Glossopharyngeal neuralgia (GPN) is an uncommon disorder or syndrome, similar to TN that occurs 5% as often, with the onset typically in the fourth to fifth decade. GPN is described as a paroxysmal pain condition of the throat, tonsillar region, and ear. The duration of the pain attack is shorter than in TN, but the attacks are more severe. Symptoms consist of brief, recurrent, stabbing pains lasting only a few seconds to a couple of minutes. The incidence is only 0.7 per 100,000 population.[31] Men are affected more often than women. The pain, similar in character to that of TN, is located in the sensory distribution of the glossopharyngeal and, occasionally, vagus nerve, located at the base of the tongue, tonsils, ear, or angle of the jaw and triggered by talking, chewing, laughing, swallowing, and coughing.[31] When the vagus nerve is involved, the term **vagoglossopharyngeal neuralgia** is often used.

From the trigger sites the pain radiates along the distribution of the nerve to the angle of the jaw and the ipsilateral ear. Cardiac slowing, evidenced by bradyarrhythmias or the sudden onset of cardiac asystole, may occur with vagus nerve involvement.

The etiology of this disorder is unknown. Other causes of pain in the distribution of these nerves are peritonsillar abscess, tumors involving the oropharynx, posterior fossa tumors, and vertebral artery aneurysms.

There are reports of unusual GPN caused by compression of a herniated cerebellar tonsil secondary to Arnold-Chiari type I malformation. Lower cranial nerve deficits that result from direct brainstem compression, stretching, or syringobulbia are comparatively common in patients with Arnold-Chiari type I malformation. This allows CN IX to become compressed or sandwiched between a cerebellar tonsil and a vertebral artery. Patient complaints may include pain in the lower jaw, base of the tongue, or pharynx that radiates to the ear. The neurologic examination may be normal. MRI scanning helps to identify the cerebellar tonsillar herniation in combination with Arnold-Chiari type I malformation. Surgical treatment to resect the cerebellar tonsil has provided relief of pain and symptoms.[35]

Assessment

Diagnosis is based on the description of the pain provided by the patient and the absence of demonstrable neurologic defects involving CN IX and X on physical examination and radiologic testing.

Treatment

Medical Management

Treatment is similar to that used for TN. Carbamazepine, baclofen, phenytoin, or a combination is tried initially and continued if symptoms are controlled (see Box 16-6 for major concerns in the administration of these drugs).

Surgical Management

When the symptoms are not controlled with pharmacotherapy, surgical resection of the glossopharyngeal nerve is performed through a posterior fossa craniotomy (see Chapter 8). After surgery the affected side is permanently anesthetized, with loss of the ipsilateral gag reflex and taste over the posterior third of the tongue.

Acute and Nonacute Care

The overall management of the patient with GPN parallels care of the patient with TN. Typically, this patient is encountered in the nonacute setting. If surgical resection of the nerve is performed, the postoperative care is that of the patient after posterior fossa craniotomy (see Chapter 8).

Care for the patient with GPN is similar to that provided to the patient with TN. In addition, measures to protect the airway must be implemented if the integrity of the gag reflex is in question. A swallowing evaluation by a speech/language pathologist should be obtained if swallowing is impaired.

VAGAL NERVE DISORDERS

The symptoms of vagal nerve (CN X) disorders depend on the location of the offending lesion. Lesions may compress or arise at any location along the course of the nerve from its nuclei in the brainstem through its thoracic course and terminal fibers. Damage may result from infections, tumors, syringobulbia, vascular disease, or ALS. Some authors have stated that complete bilateral paralysis of the tenth nerve is incompatible with life; however, cases have been reported of complete destruction of the nerve distal to the medullary nuclei (especially the dorsal motor nucleus) in surviving individuals.[1]

Lesions that completely interrupt the intracranial course of the nerve result in ipsilateral paralysis of pharyngeal and laryngeal structures, evidenced by hoarseness, dysphagia, and lack of movement on phonation. The ipsilateral gag reflex is absent. Autonomic function is not compromised. Extracranial lesions generally result from thoracic disease or tumors of the nerve itself. These lesions, located distal to the pharyngeal fibers of the nerve, present with hoarseness unaccompanied by dysphagia. Signs of involvement of the ninth, eleventh, and twelfth cranial nerves, along with symptoms of Horner's syndrome (ptosis, miosis, and anhidrosis), may be present.

Dabir, Piccone, and Kittle have described the occurrence of mediastinal vagal neurilemoma with asymptomatic presentation.[16] The tumors are generally found on chest x-ray examination, although symptoms of mediastinal compression and recurrent laryngeal nerve involvement may be present. Usually benign, the tumors are surgically excised.

Treatment

The management of the patient with a vagal nerve disorder requires familiarity with principles of care after thoracic surgery. In addition, the integrity of the thoracic course of the vagal nerve requires frequent assessment. The clinician should monitor for inspiratory stridor, dyspnea, hoarseness, and dysphonia. Equipment for emergency intubation and tracheotomy must be readily available. Patients who experience swallowing or speech disturbances postoperatively should be evaluated by a speech/language pathologist.

SPINAL ACCESSORY NERVE DISORDERS

Lesions of the spinal accessory nerve (CN XI) present as motor weakness involving the sternocleidomastoid and upper trapezius muscles. The most common cause of spinal accessory nerve palsy is damage to the nerve from trauma or surgery involving the neck. Less common causes of palsies include syringomyelia, poliomyelitis, ALS, and tumors; idiopathic spinal accessory nerve palsy has also been described.

Pathophysiology

Neck surgery and trauma may damage the nerve by a variety of mechanisms. These mechanisms include compression of the nerve by an expanding lesion, stretch injury, ischemia, and direct injury during attempts at cannulation of the jugular vein. When the eleventh nerve is damaged, motor innervation to the trapezius and sternocleidomastoid muscles is compromised. Complete lesions result in an inability to shrug, with drooping of the affected shoulder (trapezius muscle) and weakness on turning of the head to the opposite side (sternocleidomastoid muscle).

Assessment

The spinal accessory nerve is evaluated by determining the strength of the innervated muscles. When weakness is demonstrated, nerve conduction studies and EMG may be used to further define the lesion.

Treatment

Acute and Nonacute Care

Most patients with CN XI palsy are encountered in the nonacute care setting. Treatment of spinal accessory nerve palsy involves physiotherapy, electrical stimulation, and where appropriate, treatment of the underlying cause. Physiotherapy is designed to strengthen the surrounding shoulder abductors to compensate for the weak trapezius muscle and maintain range of motion (ROM) of the neck and shoulder muscles.[42] Atrophy of the affected muscles is avoided by electrical stimulation therapy during the nerve regeneration period.

Because weakness of the neck and shoulder muscles may interfere with the patient's ability to perform ADLs, the clinician must assess self-care performance. The patient should be asked to describe any problems experienced as a result of shoulder weakness. The clinician should observe the patient during activities that require the affected arm to be lifted (e.g., eating if the dominant side is involved, combing hair, brushing teeth). Resistance testing of the muscles supplied by the nerve can identify slight paresis that may interfere with activities requiring prolonged muscle contraction (e.g., carrying objects).

Management of this patient is designed to promote recovery of muscle tone and strength and to help the patient adapt to identify self-care deficits. In consultation with the physical therapist, the patient should perform exercises to preserve and recover function in the affected muscles on a scheduled basis. The patient should be encouraged to repeat these exercises independently several times throughout the day.

The clinician should explore strategies to minimize self-care deficits, especially when the injury is to muscles on the dominant side. An occupational therapy consultation may be needed when performance of ADLs is compromised.

COMPREHENSIVE PATIENT MANAGEMENT: SPINAL ACCESSORY NERVE DISORDERS

Health Teaching Considerations

Health teaching is a critical part of the recovery process. The clinician should demonstrate home neck physiotherapy exercises and strategies for self-care to the patient. Successful return demonstration assures the clinician that the patient understands the treatment regimen that has been prescribed. If the palsy causes temporary or permanent disability, referral to a vocational counselor may be needed for job retraining. Follow-up for compliance, adaptation, and coping with the disorder may be necessary.

HYPOGLOSSAL NERVE DISORDERS

Isolated lesions of the hypoglossal nerve (CN XII) are uncommon. With unilateral interruption, motor innervation to one side of the tongue is lost, with paralysis of unilateral tongue movements. Denervation results in wrinkling, atrophy, fasciculations, and fibrillations on the affected side. Bilateral lesions result in complete paralysis of the tongue and severely impair food handling, swallowing, and word formation. Respiratory distress may result from posterior displacement of the tongue with obstruction of the upper airway.

The causes of twelfth-nerve palsies are similar to causes of disorders of the other bulbar cranial nerves. Vascular insufficiency, tumors, syringobulbia, ALS, pseudobulbar palsy, and poliomyelitis have been identified as occasional causes of twelfth-nerve involvement either at its intracranial nucleus or along its course.

Pathophysiology

When the hypoglossal nerve is damaged, the patient is unable to protrude, retract, or elevate the tongue. In addition, paralysis of the hypoglossus muscle inhibits adduction of the tongue, preventing the upper surface from becoming convex. Supranuclear (cortical) lesions result in contralateral weakness, and lesions of the nerve itself cause ipsilateral weakness.

Assessment

Unilateral lesions of the twelfth nerve result in deviation of the tongue toward the affected side on protrusion. When resting in the buccal cavity, the tongue curves toward the unaffected side, and tongue movements within the mouth are impaired.

Treatment

Acute and Nonacute Care

The management of hypoglossal nerve disorders is primarily dictated by the cause and manifestations of the lesion. Impairments of food handling, swallowing, speaking, and airway patency require active intervention to prevent complications and optimize the patient's lifestyle. Although these interventions are ordered by the physician, the speech and language pathologist is the primary provider of this care.

In consultation with the physiatrist and speech/language pathologist, the clinician can assist patients with hypoglossal nerve disorders in performing ADLs, such as eating, swallowing, and talking, and provide psycho-emotional support. The assessment of the patient with twelfth-nerve palsy includes determinations of the patient's nutritional state, ability to protect the upper airway, ability to communicate, integrity of the tongue, and psychologic state or mood. Identification of problems in these areas assists the clinician in formulating nursing diagnoses and individualizing the patient's care.

The focus of care for the patient with a CN XII disorder centers on the prevention of airway maintenance complications, inadequate nutrition, aspiration, speech problems, psychosocial problems, and lack of knowledge concerning interventions.

Airway. Airway protection must be provided to those patients with bilateral twelfth-nerve lesions. Proper positioning to keep the tongue forward in the buccal cavity reduces the risk of upper airway obstruction. The decision to use an upper airway adjunct should be based on safety factors. A nasal trumpet airway is usually well tolerated by patients and generally does not stimulate the gag reflex. Use of this adjunct during sleep may be necessary. The patient should be taught how to insert, remove, and care for the airway if used at home.

Aspiration. Swallowing difficulties may lead to aspiration or malnutrition. A speech/language pathologist should be consulted for a swallowing evaluation. The speech therapist offers suggestions for food consistency, positioning during eating, and swallowing exercises. In addition, the clinician needs to monitor the patient's nutritional and pulmonary status. Because most of these patients are encountered in a nonacute care setting such as a clinic or physician's office, clinical management at each encounter includes auscultating the lungs, weighing the patient, and reviewing laboratory data indicative of the patient's nutritional status. Consulting a registered dietitian for food selection and meal preparation strategies may be beneficial.

Speech. Difficulties with speech articulation are frustrating for the patient. Again, the speech/language pathologist will suggest exercises and strategies to improve motor speech. The patient should be encouraged to speak slowly. The clinician should look at the patient during speech so that the patient's lip movements can assist with word understanding. Alternative communication methods should be offered when understanding the patient is difficult or speaking excessively tires the patient. The hospitalized patient should have the call light within easy reach; activation of the call light requires staff to go to the patient's room to identify the patient's need.

Rehabilitation

Rehabilitation is directly related to the cranial nerve deficit. Medical care may result in satisfactory recovery, and in some cases surgical intervention is necessary. Complex cases may require a period of rehabilitation to restore function. A physiatrist, as head of the rehabilitation team, can evaluate the patient and prescribe a plan of care to be followed at home.

COMPREHENSIVE PATIENT MANAGEMENT: HYPOGLOSSAL NERVE DISORDERS

Health Teaching Considerations

The patient and family must be knowledgeable about CN XII palsy and its associated impairments. Teaching is tailored to the presence and extent of impairments of the individual patient. Measures to protect the airway and strategies for food preparation, swallowing, and speaking are taught as needed. The patient and family should be knowledgeable regarding procedures to clear an obstructed upper airway; this can be accomplished by referral to local agencies and hospitals that provide cardiopulmonary resuscitation (CPR) training.

Psychosocial Considerations

The psychosocial sequelae of hypoglossal nerve disorders depend on the personality of the patient and the extent to which the disorder has impaired talking and eating. Dysarthria may hinder the patient's articulation of feelings. The clinician must allow time for patients to share their feelings. A private, nonhurried environment should be provided. Patience is necessary during the patient's speech attempts. Nonverbal forms of communication, including touch, should be used when necessary.

Case Management Considerations

The role of case manager is limited to those cases where the patient may be older, has extensive medical and postoperative needs, and requires follow-up care after discharge from the physician or hospital.

CONCLUSION

Patients with cranial nerve palsies are encountered in the nonacute care setting, as well as in acute care settings. Because contact with these patients may be limited, clinicians must develop written teaching materials that patients can use to learn about their cranial nerve disorder and its treatment. In the event that patients with cranial nerve palsies are hospitalized for treatment of the cranial nerve palsy or an unrelated disorder, the clinician needs to evaluate the patient's understanding of the disorder and its treatment. The clinician must identify strategies the patient currently uses to control the disorder so that they can be continued in the acute care setting.

As medical science continues to investigate the cause of cranial nerve palsies, new theories of etiology and new treatment methods will become available. Clinicians' knowledge must remain current so that they can deliver optimal patient care.

Most of the cranial nerve disorders have been discussed individually in this chapter. It is common for cranial nerve palsies to occur in combination because of the anatomic proximity of the nerve nuclei and tracts. Mixed disorders should be suspected when clinical manifestations of more than one nerve disorder are present. The management of the patient with mixed or multiple cranial nerve palsies will be a combination of the strategies suggested for individual disorders.

RESOURCES FOR PATIENTS AND CAREGIVERS

American Chronic Pain Association: www.theacpa.org
National Chronic Pain Outreach Association: www.chronicpain.org
National Foundation for the Treatment of Pain: http://paincare.org
Trigeminal Neuralgia Association: www.tna-support.org

REFERENCES

1. Adams RD, Victor M: *Principles of neurology,* ed 8, New York, 2005, McGraw-Hill.
2. Adler RJ: Trigeminal glycerol chemoneurolysis: nursing implications, *J Neurosci Nurs* 21(6):337–341, 1989.
3. Aframian D, Ben-Oliel R, Sharav Y: Ramsay Hunt syndrome—differential diagnosis, pathogens, and therapy, *Harefuah* 136(4):278–280, 1999.
4. Amrith S, Saw SM, Lim TC, Lee TK: Ophthalmic involvement in cranio-facial trauma, *J Craniomaxillofac Surg* 28(3):140–147, 2000.
5. Barrows HS: *Guide to neurological assessment,* Philadelphia, 1980, JB Lippincott.
6. Bederson JB, Wilson CB: Evaluation of microvascular decompression and partial sensory rhizotomy in 252 cases of trigeminal neuralgia, *J Neurosurg* 71(3):359–367, 1989.
7. Bender MB, Rudolph SM, Stacy CB: The neurology of the visual and oculomotor systems. In Baker AB, Baker LH, editors: *Clinical neurology,* vol 1, Philadelphia, 1982, Harper & Row.
8. Blake GJ: Carbamazepine for trigeminal neuralgia and pain, *Nursing 91* 21(3):102, 1991.
9. Bishop BS: Pathologic pupillary signs: self-learning module, part 2, *Crit Care Nurs* 11(7):58–67, 1991.
10. Brackmann DE, Fetterman BL: Cranial nerve VII. In Goetz CG, Pappert EJ, editors: *Textbook of clinical neurology,* Philadelphia, 1999, WB Saunders.
11. Burde RM: Eye movements. In Eliasson SG, Prensky AL, Hardin WB, editors: *Neurological pathophysiology,* ed 2, New York, 1978, Oxford University Press.
12. Clark JB, Queener SF, Karb VB: *Pharmacological basis of nursing practice,* ed 3, St Louis, 1990, Mosby.
13. Cleveland PJ, Morris J: Meniere's disease: the inner ear out of balance, *RN* 53(8):28–32, 1990.
14. Coker NJ, Coker RR, Jenkins HA, Vincent KR: Psychological profile of patients with Meniere's disease, *Arch Otolaryngol Head Neck Surg* 115:1355–1357, 1989.
15. Conway-Rutowski BL: *Carini and Owen's neurological and neurosurgical nursing,* ed 8, St Louis, 1982, Mosby.
16. Dabir RR, Piccone W, Kittle CF: Intrathoracic tumors of the vagus nerve, *Ann Thorac Surg* 50:494–497, 1990.
17. Derebery MJ, Rao VS, Siglock TJ, Linthicum FH, Nelson RA: Meniere's disease: an immune complex-mediated illness? *Laryngoscope* 101(3):225–229, 1991.
18. DeWeese DD, Saunders WH: *Textbook of otolaryngology,* ed 6, St Louis, 1982, Mosby.
19. Doty RL: Cranial nerve I: olfactory nerve. In Goetz CG, Pappert EJ, editors: *Textbook of clinical neurology,* Philadelphia, 1999, WB Saunders.
20. Dyck PJ: Diseases of the peripheral nervous system. In Beeson PB, McDermott W, editors: *Textbook of medicine,* ed 4, Philadelphia, 1975, WB Saunders.

21. Ellenberger C: The visual system. In Eliasson SG, Prensky AL, Hardin WB, editors: *Neurological pathophysiology,* ed 2, New York, 1978, Oxford University Press.

22. Fetell MR, Stein BM: Tumors of the meninges. In Rowland LP, editor: *Merritt's textbook of neurology,* ed 8, Philadelphia, 1989, Lea & Febiger.

23. Fromm GH, Graff-Radford SB, Terrence CF, Sweet WH: Pre-trigeminal neuralgia, *Neurology* 40:1493–1495, 1990.

24. Goodwin J: Cranial II, IV, and VI: the oculomotor system. In Goetz CG, Pappert EJ, editors: *Textbook of clinical neurology,* Philadelphia, 1999, WB Saunders.

25. Granadier RJ: Ophthalmology update for primary practitioners. I. Update on optic neuritis. *Dis Mon* 46(8):508–532, 2000.

26. Grigsby JP, Johnston CL: Depersonalization, vertigo, and Meniere's disease, *Psychol Rep* 64:527–534, 1989.

27. Guin PR: Radiofrequency lesions—a treatment for trigeminal neuralgia, *J Neurosurg Nurs* 14:192–194, 1982.

28. Hain TC, Micco A: Cranial nerve VIII: vestibulocochlear system. In Goetz CG, Pappert EJ, editors: *Textbook of clinical neurology,* Philadelphia, 1999, WB Saunders.

29. Hato N, Kisaki H, Honda N, Gyo K, Murakami S, Yanagihara N: Ramsay Hunt syndrome in children, *Ann Neurol* 48(2):254–256, 2000.

30. Haymaker W, Kuhlenbeck H: Disorders of the brainstem and its cranial nerves. In Baker AB, Baker LH, editors: *Clinical neurology,* vol 3, Philadelphia, 1976, Harper & Row.

31. Hermananowicz N, Truong DD: Cranial nerves IX (glossopharyngeal) and X (vagus). In Goetz CG, Pappert EJ, editors: *Textbook of clinical neurology,* Philadelphia, 1999, WB Saunders.

32. Hoya K, Kirino T: Traumatic trochlear nerve palsy following minor occipital impact—four case reports, *Neurol Med Chir* 40(7):358–360, 2000.

33. Jarrahy R, Berci G, Shahinian HR: Endoscope-assisted microvascular decompression of the trigeminal nerve, *Otolaryngol Head Neck Surg* 123(3):218–223, 2000.

34. Kannan V, Deopujari CE, Misra BK, Shetty PG, Shroff MM, Pendse AM: Gamma-knife radiosurgery for trigeminal neuralgia, *Australas Radiol* 43(3):339–341, 1999.

35. Kanpolat Y, Unlu A, Savas A, Tan F: Chiari type I malformation presenting as glossopharyngeal neuralgia: case report, *Neurosurgery* 48(1):226–228, 2001.

36. Kirkland J, Williams A: Trigeminal neuralgia: approaches to nursing care, *J Neurosurg Nurs* 15(3):149–153, 1983.

37. Lechin F, van der Dijs B, Lechin ME, Amat J, Lechin AE, Cabrera A, Gomez F, Acosta E, Arocha L, Villa S: Pimozide therapy for trigeminal neuralgia, *Arch Neurol* 46(9):960–963, 1989.

38. Lichtor T, Mullan JF: A 10-year follow-up review of percutaneous microcompression of the trigeminal ganglion, *J Neurosurg* 72:49–54, 1990.

39. Lobato RD, Rivas JJ, Sarabia R, Lamas E: Percutaneous microcompression of the gasserian ganglion for trigeminal neuralgia, *J Neurosurg* 72:546–553, 1990.

40. Lohne V, Bjornsborg E, Westerby R, Heiberg E: Effects of facial paralysis after acoustic neuroma surgery in Norway, *J Neurosci Nurs* 19(3):123–131, 1987.

41. Marbach JJ, Lund P: Depression, anhedonia and anxiety in temporomandibular joint and other facial pain syndromes, *Pain* 11:73, 1981.

42. Marini SG, Rook JL, Green RF, Nagler W: Spinal accessory nerve palsy: an unusual complication of coronary artery bypass, *Arch Phys Med Rehabil* 72(3):247–249, 1991.

43. Marshall SB, editor: *Neuroscience critical care: pathophysiology and patient management,* Philadelphia, 1990, WB Saunders.

44. McKinnis AT: Vestibular neurectomy, *AORN J* 50(4):787–797, 1989.

45. Mounts P: Lyme disease may underlie Bell's palsy, *Nurse Pract* 15(6):7, 1990 (letter to the editor).

46. North RB, Kidd DH, Piantadosi S, Carson BS: Percutaneous retrogasserian glycerol rhizotomy: predictors of success and failure in treatment of trigeminal neuralgia, *J Neurosurg* 72(6):851–856, 1990.

47. Onofrio BM: Radiofrequency percutaneous gasserian ganglion lesions: results in 140 patients with trigeminal pain, *J Neurosurg* 42:132–139, 1975.

48. Pallett PJ, O'Brien MT: *Textbook of neurological nursing,* Boston, 1985, Little, Brown.

49. Pau H: *Differential diagnosis of eye diseases,* ed 2, Stuttgart, Germany, 1988, Thieme Medical Publishers (Blodi FC, translator; original work published 1974).

50. Pollack IF, Jannetta PJ, Bissonette PAC: Bilateral trigeminal neuralgia: a 14 year experience with microvascular decompression, *J Neurosurg* 68:559–565, 1988.

51. Poole M: Percutaneous electrocoagulation for tic douloureux, *AORN J* 24(5):87, 1976.

52. Rakowski J: Lyme disease may underlie Bell's palsy, *Nurse Pract* 15(6):7, 1990 (letter to the editor).

53. Riley MK: *Nursing care of the client with ear, nose and throat disorders,* New York, 1987, Springer.

54. Robinson L, Bisnaire D: Syringomyelia and syringobulbia: pathophysiology, surgical treatment, and nursing implications, *J Neurosci Nurs* 22(2):69–75, 1990.

55. Rowland LP: Injury to cranial and peripheral nerves. In Rowland LP, editor: *Merritt's textbook of neurology,* ed 8, Philadelphia, 1989, Lea & Febiger.

56. Rudy EB: *Advanced neurological and neurosurgical nursing,* St Louis, 1984, Mosby.

57. Sahni KS, Pieper DR, Anderson R, Baldwin NG: Relation of hypesthesia to the outcome of glycerol rhizolysis for trigeminal neuralgia, *J Neurosurg* 72(1):55–58, 1990.

58. Sharief M, Swash M: Viral infections of the nervous system. In Swash M, editor: *Outcomes in neurological and neurosurgical disorders,* Cambridge, 1998, Cambridge University Press.

59. Silberstein SD, Young WB: Headache and facial pain. In Goetz CG, Pappert EJ, editors: *Textbook of clinical neurology,* Philadelphia, 1999, WB Saunders.

60. Silverstein H, Smouha E, Jones R: Natural history vs. surgery for Meniere's disease, *Otolaryngol Head Neck Surg* 100(1):6–16, 1989.

61. Sindou M: Microvascular decompression for trigeminal neuralgia. In Kaye AH, Black PM, editors: *Operative neurosurgery,* London, 2000, Churchill Livingstone.

62. Sparks SM, Taylor CM: *Nursing diagnosis reference manual,* Springhouse, Pa, 1991, Springhouse.

63. Sweet WH: The treatment of trigeminal neuralgia (tic douloureux), *N Engl J Med* 315:174–177, 1986.

64. Varma R, editor: *Essentials of eye care,* Philadelphia, 1997, Lippincott-Raven.

65. Weitzman ED, Fry JM: Meniere syndrome. In Rowland LP, editor: *Merritt's textbook of neurology,* ed 8, Philadelphia, 1989, Lea & Febiger.

66. Wollenberg SP: Primary care diagnosis and management of Bell's palsy, *Nurse Pract* 14(12):14–18, 1989.

67. Zakrzewska JM, Patsalos PN: Oxcarbazepine: a new drug in the management of intractable trigeminal neuralgia, *J Neurol Neurosurg Psychiatry* 52(4):472–476, 1989.

CHAPTER 17

Stroke Management

Acute ischemic stroke (AIS) is a **brain attack**—a sudden neurologic event that is a medical emergency. AIS can be described according to the different categories and mechanisms of injury to the brain, the type of lesion that it causes, and the location. The distinction can be made between large vessel disease from atherosclerosis that may result in a thrombosis or an embolic occlusion secondary to cardiac disease. Small vessel disease may result in a lacuna. AIS is almost always precipitated by a preexisting condition including, but not limited to, vascular disease, atherosclerosis, heart disease, AF, hypercoagulable states, hypertension, obesity, diabetes mellitus (DM), or sickle cell disease. Stroke prevention must focus early in life on the precipitating conditions that cause strokes. Until we are successful in preventing the causes of stroke, health care providers will continue to be challenged to treat and improve the outcomes for thousands of stroke survivors. The problem is likely to get worse because half of Americans age 55 to 65 have hypertension and 2 in 5 are obese. Such pervasive risk factors will likely herald an increased incidence of stroke in the 76 million baby boomers (born between 1946 and 1964) who are now reaching age 60.[34] By all accounts, this group is considered to be at greater risk of stroke than their predecessors.

Strokes are preventable and treatable. Strokes should be treated with the same urgency as a myocardial infarction (MI). Unfortunately, the public fails to recognize the onset of common signs and symptoms of stroke in time to access available treatment. Only a small minority of stroke victims receive available treatment each year,[39] with 3% of stroke patients able to take advantage of acute stroke treatment with tissue plasminogen activator (tPA)—the "clot busting" drug, or the newest treatment with a mechanical device for endovascular embolectomy. This is due to a number of factors, the most important being that patients seldom arrive to the emergency room within the timeframe necessary to administer the interventions safely. Education for the public needs to include steps for stroke prevention, signs and symptoms, the need to call 911 at the onset of symptoms, and the time-limited treatment window for acute intervention. Time is brain (tissue), and every minute counts.

An estimated 50% of stroke deaths happen before the patient arrives at the hospital. Health care professionals, including nurse clinicians, face an enormous challenge in bringing public awareness to a point where the focus on stroke treatment can be prevention and early intervention.

Therefore, it is important to understand all aspects of caring for stroke patients from emergent care to restorative care.

The intent of this chapter is to review the anatomy and physiology of AIS; define terms; describe syndromes; review assessment, treatment, and management; and describe the role of clinicians in acute, nonacute, rehabilitative, long-term, home care, and case management settings. A final section describes the role of prevention and a stroke risk screening tool.[6] The conclusion discusses the impact that stroke will have on the future of the health care delivery system.

RISK FACTORS

Primary care providers should identify predisposing risk factors for stroke and act to increase awareness and knowledge for stroke prevention. **Nonmodifiable risks,** such as family history, age, gender, and race cannot be altered. The health care provider must focus on those **modifiable risk factors** for stroke prevention that are amenable to change or treatment. These include hypertension, diabetes, abnormal lipids (hypercholesterolemia and hyperlipidemia), cigarette smoking, heavy alcohol consumption, obesity, and physical inactivity. Other risk factors may include AF, substance abuse (particularly stimulants such as methamphetamine and cocaine), and poor diet.

Hypertension is the principal risk factor for both AIS and hemorrhagic stroke. Hypertension deserves special attention throughout an individual's lifetime. The American Heart Association (AHA) defines normal blood pressure as less than 120/80 mm Hg and high blood pressure as[28]:

- Systolic pressure of 140 mm Hg or higher; diastolic pressure of 90 mm Hg or higher
- Taking antihypertensive medicine
- Being told at least twice by a physician or other health care professional that you have high blood pressure

A new definition of hypertension from a cardiology perspective is defined as:

A progressive cardiovascular syndrome arising from complex and interrelated etiologies. Early markers of the syndrome are often present before blood pressure elevation is observed; therefore hypertension cannot be classified solely by discrete blood pressure thresholds. Progression is strongly associated with functional and structural cardiac and vascular abnormalities that damage the heart, kidneys, brain, vasculature, and other organs, and leads to premature morbidity and death.[32]

Diabetes has been associated with multiple lacunar infarcts and is frequently encountered in AIS. It is important for individuals with diabetes to maintain tight hyperglycemic control, as well as control their blood pressure. Currently the American Diabetes Association (ADA) recommends that all patients with diabetes and hypertension be treated with a regimen consisting of either angiotensin-converting enzyme (ACE) inhibitors or an angiotensin receptor blocker (ARB). Rigorous control of lipids is also recommended.

Abnormal lipids can be treated with statins that are now considered effective in risk reduction for hypercholesterolemia. Statins may have additional benefits beyond lowering of cholesterol in the prevention of stroke. Readers are directed to review the National Cholesterol Education Program (NCEP) Expert Panel on Detection, Evaluation, and Treatment of High Blood Cholesterol in Adults, National Institutes of Health (NIH) Publication No. 01-3670.

Cigarette smoking is a major risk factor for stroke and may double the risk because of the effect of stenosis on blood vessels and other factors affecting the cerebral vascular system. Secondhand smoke or passive smoke from other smokers is also an important risk factor to consider for those who live or work with someone who smokes. Clinicians should counsel smokers to quit smoking and investigate local smoking cessation programs or recommend or prescribe a medication regimen that is most acceptable to the patient.

Heavy or chronic alcohol consumption is now recognized as a risk factor for stroke. Excessive drinking has been linked to hypertension and other conditions in addition to atrophy of the brain over a period of time. The accepted level of consumption for men is no more than two drinks per day and one drink for nonpregnant women.

Obesity has become increasingly problematic as a major health risk in the United States as well as a risk factor for stroke. Obesity as a risk factor for stroke is complex and in some individuals is in combination with hypertension, diabetes, and elevated cholesterol. Clinicians should initiate weight reduction in individuals who are obese and have a waist circumference larger than 35 inches for women or larger than 40 inches for men through diet, lifestyle changes, daily exercise, and counseling.

The sedentary lifestyle of Americans has been linked to many health problems, including stroke. Regular exercise improves overall health and can reduce the risk of stroke. An established exercise routine of physical activity for at least 30 minutes each day or at least three times per week can be considered to reduce the risk of stroke and improve recovery for patients who have suffered a stroke.

Researchers investigating "migraine with aura and stroke" pointed out that in their study, stroke patients tended to be obese, hypertensive, and smokers. Weight loss, exercise, and a discussion of the risks associated with oral contraceptive use is warranted with appropriate patients.[32] Research suggests that retinopathy, as determined by retinal photography, is an independent predictor of stroke or stroke-related death

in older adults without diabetes. The blood vessels in the eye share similar anatomic characteristics and other characteristics with the blood vessels in the brain. It is exciting to think that such a fairly simple procedure could predict stroke. However, according to the researchers this assessment protocol needs a more simplified grading system to have clinical utility.[63]

Sleep-related breathing disorders and snoring may be other risk factors for stroke. People with sleep apnea are at a higher risk for stroke than those without this condition and should be treated to help reduce their risk. Smoking and secondhand smoke are increasingly recognized as risk factors for stroke because the products of tobacco combustion are absorbed into the systemic circulation, with all blood vessels and organs exposed to tobacco toxins. Hence the warning: "The more you smoke the more you stroke." Nicotine is a vasoconstrictor that can induce hypertension, increase inflammation, and alter many other mechanisms in the body.

Women's risk factors for stroke increase during pregnancy, childbirth, postpartum, and menopause and are associated with hormonal fluctuations. Women using birth control patches should be aware of potential risks and problems of blood clots and stroke that may be brought on by hormones released from such patches.

In general, blacks and Hispanics have a greater risk for stroke than whites. Hospital admissions for stroke are increasing for blacks, who tend to have an increased length of stay, experience stroke at an earlier age, and have worse outcomes and higher mortality rates compared with whites. For individuals at risk, a stroke may occur at a particular time of stress when triggers create an excessive response by the sympathetic nervous system. Mental stress may trigger the premature onset of stroke by causing transient changes in blood clotting and in the function of cells lining blood vessels.[4]

INCIDENCE

According to the AHA, each year there are an estimated 700,000 new or recurrent strokes.[28] Approximately 500,000 are first attacks and 200,000 are recurrent attacks. Stroke is the third leading cause of death in the United States, ranking behind "diseases of the heart" and all forms of cancer. Stroke is one of the leading causes of severe, long-term disability.[28] Strokes kill nearly 275,000 people annually. Of all strokes, 88% are ischemic, 9% are intracerebral, and 3% are subarachnoid hemorrhage (SAH). Each year about 40,000 more women than men have a stroke.[18] Because women live longer than men, more women than men die of stroke each year. Twice as many women die of stroke as breast cancer.[28]

On average, every 45 seconds, someone in the United States has a stroke. Every 3 minutes, someone dies of a stroke.[28] The incidence, morbidity, mortality, and costs of stroke are staggering. It is estimated that stroke-related costs totaled $57 billion in 2005.[26] Of the 700,000 new strokes each year, 15% to 30% of individuals who survive will be permanently disabled.[15] The following **public health burden** of stroke must be recognized[40]:

- Mortality: 700,000 new or recurrent strokes each year.
- Known risk factors: Many are often ignored.
- Knowledge: Individuals with the highest risk of stroke and incidence of stroke are the least knowledgeable about warning signs and risk factors. These populations include individuals older than 75 years of age, blacks, and men.
- Disparities in access to care: Access varies by geographic location, race or ethnicity, gender, and age. In addition, an estimated 42.4 million individuals are uninsured with millions more underinsured.
- Economic burden and lifetime costs: The mean lifetime cost of ischemic stroke in the United States is estimated at $140,048. In 2004, the total estimated direct cost of stroke was $53.6 billion.
- Future trends: The U.S. population is expected to increase by 27% from 280 million to 356 million. The higher-risk populations of blacks and individuals 65 years and older are projected to increase by 40% and 27% respectively. More than 44.7 deaths per 100,000 population from ischemic stroke are projected in 2032.

FDA-APPROVED TREATMENTS

In 1996, the U.S. Food and Drug Administration (FDA) approved thrombolytic therapy using Activase (a tissue plasminogen activator [tPA]) as effective for the treatment of AIS. tPA is considered a "clot buster."[57,58] A decade later, only 3% to 4% of stroke victims in the United States are treated with tPA.[66]

In 2004, the Merci Retriever was cleared by the FDA for mechanical thrombolectomy for the direct removal of blood clots from patients experiencing AIS.[77] The MERCI (Mechanical Embolus Removal in Cerebral Ischemia) Trial evaluated this new device that is used in conjunction with the Merci Microcatheter and the Merci Balloon Guide Catheter techniques.[38] This sets the stage for many more stroke victims to receive acute interventional therapy. To be eligible, patients must present to hospitals equipped and staffed to render this therapy. Organizing regional networks linking primary care hospitals and physicians to comprehensive stroke centers staffed and capable of providing the entire spectrum of acute stroke intervention will be essential in substantially increasing the number of stroke victims who actually receive interventional therapy.[66]

Current Stroke Management

When administered through an intravenous (IV) line within 3 hours of the onset of witnessed stroke symptoms, tPA (IV tPA) can dissolve the clot obstructing blood flow to the brain. Large-scale trials have demonstrated the benefits of intraarterial thrombolytic therapy (tPA) delivered within 6 hours of symptom onset. The window for intraarterial tPA may be longer than for IV tPA, as long as 6 hours or more. Intraarterial tPA may not be readily available in all communities and is often limited to large academic centers.

Interventionists, with an experienced stroke team, may use a technique to deliver tPA via an artery to directly lyse the clot. Intraarterial tPA may prove to be safer in individuals at greater risk for bleeding. In some cases, the interventionist may use a combination of IV tPA and intraarterial tPA, or tPA in combination with the mechanical clot retriever to obtain the best outcome. More lives could be saved and disability could be dramatically reduced if individuals with a suspected stroke arrived within the therapeutic window to be evaluated for these treatment options.

Just as hypertension is no longer considered to have a single profile or prognosis, health care professionals recognize the stroke syndrome as a neurologic disorder that has different causes, different symptoms, and different prognoses. Thus the planning and management for an individual with a stroke is complex.

Specialized Stroke Centers

According to the American Stroke Association (ASA) and the Brain Attack Coalition (BAC), specialized stroke centers improve outcomes. The stroke center concept is designed to expedite treatment so that more patients can take advantage of tPA and other new treatments. A stroke center consists of a comprehensive stroke service that offers infrastructure to bring patients as quickly as possible to the stroke center for immediate diagnosis and treatment as well as early rehabilitation. It refers patients for appropriate treatments, rehabilitation, and secondary prevention. A stroke center offers not only acute stroke unit services, but also 24-hour availability of laboratory, neuroradiology, and ultrasonographic diagnostic services, as well as neurosurgical and cardiologic services.[54] A stroke center is similar in design to cardiac and trauma centers. Helicopters may be needed to transport patients to a stroke center for specialized treatment in the same way trauma patients are transported for life-saving interventions. Not every hospital has the luxury of a stroke center, but every hospital that offers emergency treatment for stroke needs a stroke plan.

DEFINITIONS AND CLASSIFICATION

Stroke refers to the acute neurologic impairment that follows an interruption in blood supply to a specific region of the brain.[15] A **stroke** is an abrupt development of a focal neurologic deficit as a consequence of a local disturbance in the cerebral circulation. A stroke is an irreversible brain injury resulting from cerebral ischemia.[70] A clot (infarct) that obstructs or occludes an artery in the brain deprives that area of blood and causes AIS (Fig. 17-1). The most recent definition of a stroke requires either symptoms lasting longer than 24 hours or imaging of an acute clinically relevant brain lesion in patients with rapidly vanishing symptoms. Ischemic stroke rarely leads to death within the first hour, compared with hemorrhagic strokes that can be fatal.

Transient Ischemic Attack

It is being increasingly recognized that trying to distinguish between an ischemic stroke and a **transient ischemic attack**

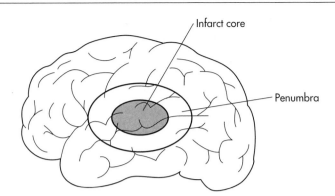

Figure 17-1 Brain attack. In the area of infarction, or ischemic core *(gray center area)*, blood flow may be reduced to a low of 0 to 20 ml/100 g of brain/min. This core is surrounded by the ischemic penumbra, where blood flow is reduced to approximately 20 to 45 ml/100 g of brain/min. Cells in the ischemic penumbra may only be stunned and may be salvageable with early treatment.
(Courtesy Alberto Iaia, MD.)

(TIA) is less important than addressing the pathophysiology of the events and employing prevention strategies. The AHA and ASA published new *Guidelines for Prevention of Stroke in Patients with Ischemic Stroke or Transient Ischemic Attack.*[67] According to the ASA, the new definition of TIA is a "brief episode of neurological dysfunction caused by a focal disturbance of brain or retinal ischemia, with clinical symptoms lasting less than 1 hour, and without evidence of infarction."[67] Several categories and descriptions of stroke have been used to describe the sudden interruption of blood to the brain resulting in focal neurologic deficits. Ischemic stroke is classified into various categories according to the presumed mechanism of the focal brain injury and the type of localization of the vascular lesion. The new classic categories are[67]:

- Large artery disease, which may be extracranial or intracranial
- Embolism from a cardiac source
- Small-vessel disease
- Other determined causes (e.g., dissection, hypercoagulable states, or sickle cell disease)
- Infarcts of undetermined origin

The majority (80%) of TIAs last only 5 to 10 minutes.[44,54] TIA is a serious medical event that serves as a "red flag" and warning sign that a major stroke may occur in the near future and is the most important predictor of an impending brain infarction.[15] TIAs continue to be one of the most controversial and underreported developmental stroke syndromes in terms of their incidence, treatment, and diagnosis.[37] Seizures, migraine, syncope, isolated dizziness, and transient memory disturbance are common disturbances that may be confused with TIA. These spells have no proven atheromatous basis, and the treatments and outcomes differ significantly from those of TIA. The concept of TIA is based on an atherothrombotic and carotid stenosis etiology.[54] The distinction

between TIA and AIS has become less important, and preventive approaches are applicable to both. TIAs are often a precursor to a major stroke and typically occur just hours or days before a stroke, leaving a small window for preventive efforts. One study found that 17% of TIAs occurred on the day of stroke, 9% on the previous day, and 43% sometime during the preceding week. However, in this study, researchers were unable to identify any characteristics or risk factors that predicted which patients would have a short interval between TIA and stroke.[64]

A TIA itself may be as mild as a brief loss of vision in one eye that is hardly noticed by the patient or as serious as a full-blown stroke syndrome. TIAs reach a maximum intensity almost immediately; by the time a health care provider evaluates the individual, the neurologic exam is negative and nonfocal. A person who has had one or more TIAs is over nine times more likely to have a stroke.[24] People are very likely to ignore a TIA, believing that "if you ignore it, it didn't happen."

Diagnostic Studies

The advent of magnetic resonance imaging (MRI) and better computed tomography (CT) images has allowed the visualization of "silent" strokes or TIAs whose symptoms have cleared but have left an unmistakable image of ischemia in the brain. Identifying the etiology using the ABCs (arterial, blood, and cardiac) helps to rule out other causes, such as seizure, arrhythmia, hypoglycemia, intracerebral hemorrhage (ICH), tumor, migraine, and demyelinating diseases. New diagnostic techniques have shown that 60% of patients with a TIA may have some definite evidence of brain infarction.[15]

Other studies may include transthoracic echocardiography (TTE), transesophageal echocardiography (TEE), carotid duplexes, transcranial Doppler (TCD) studies, noninvasive imaging studies of the brain and vasculature, and angiograms. Laboratory studies to consider include a complete blood count (CBC); prothrombin time/partial thromboplastin time (PT/PTT); serum glucose; lipid profiles; and, in some cases, protein C, protein S, homocysteine (Hcy), activated protein C (APC) resistance, factor V Leiden mutation, prothrombin gene mutation 20210, anticardiolipin antibody, and lupus anticoagulant. Vitamin B_{12} and folate levels should be obtained if the Hcy level is abnormal. The cardiac evaluation may include an electrocardiogram (ECG), a transthoracic two-dimensional (2-D) echo, and TEE to search for causes of arrhythmia or emboli. Noninvasive carotid duplex Doppler ultrasonography quantifies the percentage of stenosis and plaque formation to determine which patients are candidates for angiography or magnetic resonance angiography (MRA) and carotid endarterectomy (CEA) or stent.

Treatment Options

Treatment of TIAs is directed at the underlying causes. Interventions include lowering high blood pressure, cholesterol levels, and weight. Medications (e.g., oral anticoagulants [warfarin] and antiplatelet agents [aspirin, ticlopidine, and clopidogrel]) and surgery (CEA or stenting) are considered secondary therapy.[76] These interventions may significantly reduce the risk of stroke depending on test results. Surgery may offer benefits beyond that of aspirin therapy in some cases.

Other Types of Stroke

Hypoperfusion is a more global pattern of brain infarction that results from low blood or intermittent periods of no flow. Hypoperfusion often occurs in patients who recover cardiac function after sudden cardiac arrest. Other common causes include acute MI with significant loss of pump function and hemodynamically unstable arrhythmias.[15]

A **small vessel disease** (e.g., **lacunar stroke**) is defined as occlusion of very small arteries in the brain, which may result in stroke symptoms but may not show up on a CT or MRI scan. Lacunar infarcts may account for up to 13% to 20% of strokes and often occur in individuals with DM and hypertension. Lacune refers to a small, deep infarct attributable to a primary arterial disease that involves a penetrating branch of a large cerebral artery. Most autopsy-documented lacunar infarcts are small, ranging from 0.2 to 15 mm^3 in size. Lacunes predominate in the basal ganglia, especially the putamen, the thalamus, and the white matter of the internal capsule and pons and may be largely asymptomatic.[48]

A **pure motor stroke** or **pure motor hemiparesis** is one of the most common lacunar syndromes. The classic "homunculus" view helps to correlate the location and clinical presentation of a pure motor lacunar syndrome that may be seen in patients in whom the stroke affects only the face, arm, or leg. Lacunar strokes usually have mild severity with symptoms resolving without need for thrombolytic therapy. Improvement is expected in many of the individuals experiencing a pure motor stroke.

Pure sensory stroke is assumed to be caused by infarction of the sensory pathways (e.g., those in the brainstem or thalamus). The pure motor stroke disturbances in sensation may extend over one entire side of the body. Individuals usually return to normal function after lacunar stroke syndrome. Other lacunar syndromes may include ataxic hemiparetic stroke and clumsy hand syndrome. After the correct diagnosis is made to distinguish lacunar stroke from other more life-threatening AIS, both the stroke symptoms and the underlying disease state (usually hypertension and/or DM) are treated. Lacunar infarcts may have little effect on cognition, memory, speech, or level of consciousness (LOC).[48] Thrombotic stroke and embolic stroke are discussed in Pathophysiology.

PATHOPHYSIOLOGY

The brain is exquisitely sensitive to brief interruptions in the supply of oxygenated blood. Irreversible brain cell death and cellular necrosis begin to occur within 3 to 5 minutes of interruption. **Encephalomalacia** or "brain softening" is a condition first described by Morgagni in the late seventeenth century.[52] Ischemic cerebral infarcts may appear pale without blood or, in congested areas, filled with blood extravasated from many small vessels. These congested areas are possibly a result of bleeding from newly established collateral circulation that surrounds the necrosed tissue.[5] Hemorrhagic infarcts reabsorb but leave behind vacuoles that are either filled with serous fluid or empty where the bleeding mass has caused physical disruption of the ischemic area. On imaging, the central core called the **necrotic core** is visualized and cannot be restored. The blood flow in the region of the cerebral tissue surrounding the necrotic core is compromised and is referred to as the **ischemic penumbra.** The neurons of the brain tissue in the ischemic penumbra are hypoperfused, but not irreversibly injured. They are "stunned" or ailing neurons that can be saved if treatment is initiated within 3 hours, such as with IV tPA (see Fig. 17-1).

The brain's response to acute ischemia is influenced by the extent and size of the injury, the degree of reduction in blood flow, and the duration of the loss of blood flow. Cerebral blood flow (CBF) is approximately 50 to 55 ml/100 g of brain/min. If CBF drops to 18 ml/100 g of brain/min, synaptic transmission fails; at 8 ml/100 g of brain/min, irreversible cell death is likely. Researchers continue intense studies on the range between damaged function and cell death. It is in this range where intervention might save the "sick" brain and allow it to recover. The involved areas are often found around the infarcted area or penumbra as well as and possibly the opposite hemisphere (**diaschisis**) and in edematous areas of the brain. Collateral circulation is limited to the anterior circulation.

In AIS, a core of profoundly ischemic tissue is surrounded by a much larger penumbra of less ischemic tissue that is recruited progressively with time into the infarct—the so-called "ischemic cascade." In short, the starving, swollen brain cells cease the electrical activity that characterized their function and they die. This extends the area of infarction. Once again: *Time is brain.* Thus, it is essential to remove the clot that is obstructing the CBF, recannulate the vessel, and reperfuse the brain as quickly as possible.

Thrombolic Stroke

Thrombolic events are responsible for about 75% of strokes. **Large artery disease** from **atherosclerotic stroke** occurs when an acute clot occludes an artery. These occlusions most commonly occur at the carotid bifurcation of the internal and external carotid arteries and in vertebral arteries at their junction with the basilar arteries. Thrombotic strokes are caused by large vessel disease that alters the endothelial lining of the artery. Endothelial damage within the vessel lining produces clusters of fatty acid deposits called **plaques,** which change blood flow dynamics. The buildup of plaque causes the formation of microemboli composed of platelets and fibrin. Furthermore, the fatty acid damages the arterial wall itself, causing craters and ulceration of the vessel wall. Platelets accumulate at the site and with further buildup of platelet aggregation form a thrombus. Blood pressure may escalate into a turbulent flow that further damages the vessel wall, often with the creation of an ulcer that can bleed and release small emboli or other particles. This release of debris into the vessel lumen travels to the brain circulation and closes off normal flow. It is rare for plaques to form in cerebral vessels distal to their first branching (Fig. 17-2).

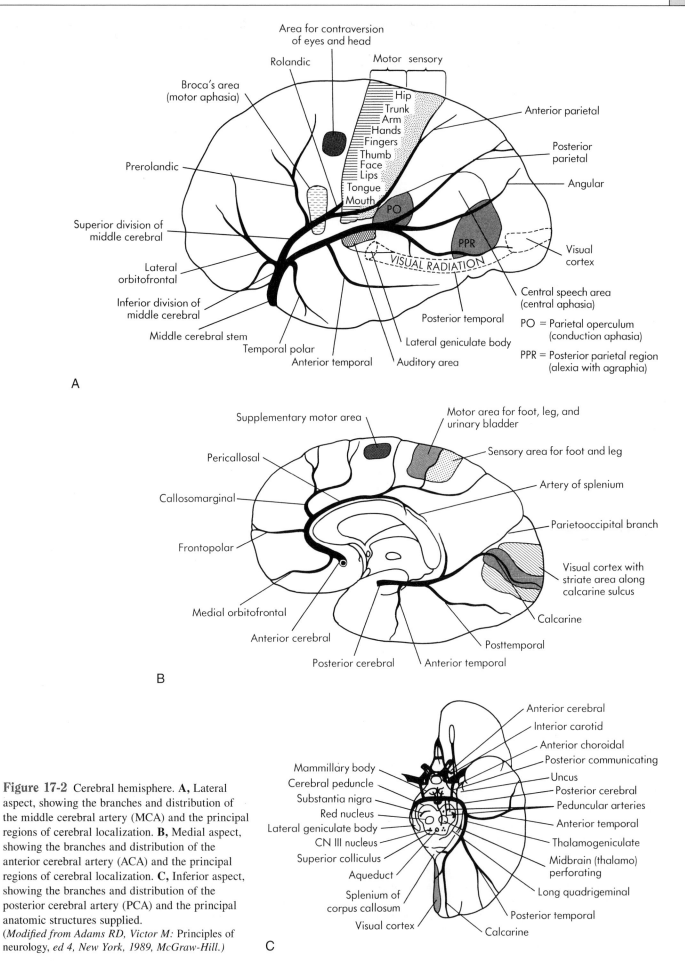

Figure 17-2 Cerebral hemisphere. **A,** Lateral aspect, showing the branches and distribution of the middle cerebral artery (MCA) and the principal regions of cerebral localization. **B,** Medial aspect, showing the branches and distribution of the anterior cerebral artery (ACA) and the principal regions of cerebral localization. **C,** Inferior aspect, showing the branches and distribution of the posterior cerebral artery (PCA) and the principal anatomic structures supplied.
(*Modified from Adams RD, Victor M: Principles of neurology, ed 4, New York, 1989, McGraw-Hill.*)

TABLE 17-1	Clinical Manifestations of the Various Causes of Stroke
Cause	Clinical Manifestations
Thrombosis	Tends to develop during sleep or within 1 hour of arising
	Ischemia is produced gradually; therefore the clinical manifestations develop more slowly than those caused by hemorrhage or emboli
	Relative preservation of consciousness
	Hypertension
Embolism	No discernible time pattern, unrelated to activity
	Clinical manifestations occur rapidly, within 10–30 sec, and often without warning
	May have rapid improvement
	Relative preservation of consciousness
	Normotension
Hemorrhage	Typically occurs during active, waking hours
	Severe headache and nuchal rigidity occur (if patient is able to report manifestations)
	Rapid onset of complete hemiplegia, occurs over minutes to 1 hour
	Usually results in extensive, permanent loss of function with slower, less complete recovery
	Rapid progression to coma

From Black JM, Hawks JH: *Medical-surgical nursing: clinical management for positive outcomes,* ed 7, St Louis, 2005, WB Saunders.

White clot thrombi are made up of platelets recruited when the atheromatous plaque ruptures and contains little fibrin. White clot thrombi, therefore, may not be as responsive to thrombolytic therapy as antiplatelet therapy. **Red clot thrombi,** on the other hand, contain fibrin and are usually associated with venous clots that can completely occlude the vessel. Red thrombi would therefore be more responsive to thrombolytic pharmacologic agents.

The vascular distribution or territory of AIS includes infarction of the middle cerebral artery (MCA) approximately 60% of the time, anterior cerebral artery (ACA) about 10% of the time, and posterior cerebral artery (PCA) circulation about 10% to 15% of the time. It was once taught that the sudden onset of a clinical deficit was typical of embolism and that a nonsudden onset would be more typical of thrombosis. Numerous case examples have now amply demonstrated that a sudden onset may occur with either condition[68] (Table 17-1).

Embolic Stroke

Embolic strokes are caused by emboli that may arise from the heart or extracranial arteries. A portion of the clot breaks free from its origin and lodges in a cerebral vessel. Atrial fibrillation (AF) and valvular abnormalities are associated with cardiogenic emboli. Valvular thrombi from mitral stenosis, endocarditis, and prosthetic valves also contribute to embolic strokes. **Cardiac emboli** account for approximately 14% of strokes and occur most often with cardiac disease. Mural thrombi after MI, prosthetic valvular disease, cardiomyopathy, infectious endocarditis, and rheumatic heart disease are among the predisposing factors in the development of cardiac emboli. Arrhythmias, notably AF, are also known to predispose individuals to cardiac emboli and increase the risk of stroke up to five times that of the well population. In older adults, more than 30% of strokes are thought to be related to the presence of AF.[36] The inefficient cardiac output caused by the fibrillation of the heart allows blood to pool in the ventricles, where it then forms intravascular material or clots that stick to the ventricular wall. When a rare efficient heartbeat suddenly empties the ventricular chamber, the clots flow through the aorta and are sent outward. A clot then lodges in the cerebrovasculature, which is too small to allow the clot to pass (e.g., bifurcation or natural curves of vessels), and occludes a distal site. Ischemia and stroke symptoms usually follow. A column of blood develops around the emboli and gradually increases into a fibrin-platelet complex.

Patients with cardioembolic strokes have the poorest survival rate, experience more severe neurologic deficits at the time of stroke, and have poorer functional outcomes compared with other types. These patients are nearly four times more likely to die within 30 days after a stroke.[61]

Neurovascular Stroke Syndromes Caused by Occlusion or Stenosis

Stroke syndromes have classically been described according to the distribution of the vessels that supply particular areas of the brain. The ability to closely map the brain regions and characterize their functional relationships has contributed to understanding both the similarities and differences in clinical presentation among stroke survivors who have had apparently similar vascular events. Table 17-2 outlines the major syndromes according to location of the vessel, area of the brain most commonly infarcted by occlusion of the vessel, and common signs and symptoms noted by category of modality (e.g., motor, sensory); it should also help in understanding the various combinations of symptoms that do not commonly appear together but can be explained by the distribution of the vessel involved (see Fig. 17-2).

Understanding the common stroke syndromes can help target the approach to assessment and can prioritize interventions in the acute setting. As the patient recovers, the ability to understand the anatomic location optimizes the best management and recovery.

TABLE 17-2	Stroke Syndromes Secondary to Occlusion or Stenosis	
Location/Vessel	**Area of Brain Infarcted**	**Signs and Symptoms**
Anterior and Central Circulation	NOTE: The internal carotid artery enters the circle of Willis and supplies the lateral anterior and central portions of the cerebral hemispheres through the MCA and the paramedial frontal lobe superior to the corpus callosum through the ACA; penetrating branches serve the deeper layers of the hemispheres	
Internal carotid artery	If collateral circulation is intact, there is commonly no infarction; if infarcted, it is in the same area as the MCA	Arterial pressure may be low in the retina Bruits over the internal carotid artery Possible retinal emboli History of TIA Positive noninvasive studies
MCA (most common area); either stem or branches of MCA	Cortical motor area (face, arm, leg) and/or posterior limb, internal capsule, corona radiata Cortical sensory area (face, arm, leg) and/or posterior limb of internal capsule Broca's area and deep fibers in the dominant hemisphere Broca's area and deep fibers in the nondominant hemisphere Optic radiations deep in the temporal lobe Location not known Posterior limb or internal capsule and adjacent corona radiata Penetrating branches of MCA (lenticulostriate branches) into the basal nuclei	*Motor:* contralateral hemiparesis or hemiplegia, greater in face and arm than leg *Sensation:* contralateral loss in same distribution as motor loss *Speech:* expressive (motor) disorder with anomia (left hemisphere most commonly affected) with nonfluent aphasia and some comprehension defects *Speech:* dysarthria *Vision:* contralateral homonymous hemianopsia or quadranopsia *Motor:* mirror movements *Respirations:* Cheyne-Stokes respirations, contralateral hyperhidrosis, occasional mydriasis *Motor:* pure motor hemiplegia *Motor:* varying degrees of contralateral weakness of face, arm, or leg *Sensory:* little or no loss; if present, contralateral following the motor distribution *Speech:* transcortical sensory aphasia (communicating pathways are interrupted) *Perception:* transient visual and sensory neglect on the left if a right lesion
ACA (least common area)	Proximal segment: corona radiata (rarely) Main stem (complete occlusion is uncommon; thus areas affected differ, and collateral circulation may alleviate signs or symptoms); medial aspect of frontal lobes, caudate nucleus, and corpus callosum are supplied by the ACA	*Motor:* when present, a mild contralateral hemiparesis (greater in leg); with bilateral occlusion of ACA, cerebral paraplegia in both legs can occur *Motor:* contralateral paralysis or paresis (greater in foot and thigh); mild upper extremity weakness *Sensory:* mild contralateral lower extremity deficiency with loss of vibratory and/or position sense, loss of two-point discrimination *Speech:* may have transcortical motor and sensory aphasia if left hemisphere
Posterior Circulation	NOTE: The posterior circulation includes the PCA, the vertebral arteries, and the basilar artery; the anatomic territory covered includes the posterior aspects of the hemispheres, the central areas of the thalamus and midbrain, and the brainstem; occlusion of the vessels is most commonly by emboli; effects of infarct in these vessels and their penetrating vessels can be specific or devastatingly global; many complex syndromes have been identified (see the original sources from which this table is compiled or basic neurology texts [e.g., Kandel] for detailed descriptions)	
Vertebral arteries	Medulla and spinal cord tracts, anterior spinal artery and penetrating branches (medial medullary syndrome)	*Motor:* contralateral hemiparesis (face spared) and/or impaired contralateral proprioception; flaccid weakness or paralysis of the tongue and/or dysarthria

Continued

TABLE 17-2   Stroke Syndromes Secondary to Occlusion or Stenosis—cont'd

Location/Vessel	Area of Brain Infarcted	Signs and Symptoms
Basilar artery three sets of branching	Midline structures of pons (paramedian branches); three general infarction syndromes are common: (1) medial inferior pontine syndrome, (2) medial midpontine syndrome, and (3) medial superior pontine syndrome	*Motor:* contralateral hemiparesis or hemiplegia, ipsilateral lower motor neuron facial palsy, "locked-in syndrome" *Sensory:* contralateral loss of vibratory sense, sense of position with dysmetria, loss of two-point discrimination, impaired rapid alternating movements *Visual:* inferior pontine: diplopia; impaired abduction of ipsilateral eye: internuclear ophthalmoplegia; medial superior: diplopia, internuclear ophthalmoplegia, skewed deviation
	Corticospinal and corticobulbar tracts in pons, sensory tracts of medial and lateral lemnisci, vestibular nuclei, inferior and middle cerebellar peduncles, cranial nerve nuclei and/or fibers, cerebellar connections in tectum, descending sympathetic pathways, central brainstem, pontine tegmentum (vertebral basilar syndrome)	*Motor:* upper motor neuron type of weakness: paralysis in combinations involving face, tongue, throat, and extremities; dysphagia, facial weakness, dysmetria, ataxia (either trunk or extremities), weak mastication muscles *Sensation:* combinations of impaired sensation (vibratory, two-point, position sense, pain, temperature), facial hypesthesia, anesthesia of CN V
PCA	Central territory (thalamic area, dentothalamic tract, cerebral peduncle, red nucleus, subthalamic nucleus, and CN III)	*Motor:* contralateral hemiplegia with possible dysmetria, dyskinesia, hemiballism or choreoathetosis, dystaxia, cerebellar ataxia, and tremor; contralateral upper motor neuron palsy; several syndromes are associated: (1) Weber's: CN III palsy and contralateral hemiplegia; (2) thalamoperforate syndrome: superior, crossed cerebellar ataxia or inferior crossed cerebellar ataxia with CN III palsy (Claude's syndrome), (3) decerebrate attacks *Sensory:* contralateral sensory loss of all modalities without agraphia *Function:* prosopagnosia (inability to recognize familiar faces), topographic disorientation, memory deficits, alexia, inability to read, color anomia *Level of consciousness:* in bilateral PCA syndromes, coma with absent doll's eyes or loss of alertness may occur; if tegmentum of midbrain near hypothalamus and third ventricle is damaged, akinetic mutism may occur
Small Vessel Disease	NOTE: Small penetrating vessels in brain parenchyma that supply areas near the basal ganglia are most vulnerable to infarction, although any small vessels can occlude deep in the brain and cause injury, producing neurologic signs or symptoms; such infarcts are commonly called *lacunes* ("small pit or hollow"), a term that is changing in meaning; they can be caused by emboli but are most commonly associated with microatheromas; although they can be found in otherwise healthy people, those with concurrent atherosclerosis, hypertension, and/or diabetes have a higher incidence of this type of infarct	
	Internal capsule, most commonly	*Motor:* contralateral hemiparesis on a single side, with equal deficit in face, arm, and leg; often unaccompanied by detectable signs of sensory, visual, and speech loss, depending on location; old term is *pure motor stroke,* although evidence suggests that other neurologic signs are present but overlooked because of low intensity
	Thalamus, most commonly	*Sensory:* complete or partial loss in face, arm, trunk, and leg that appears exactly in midline; may be accompanied by pain, hypesthesias, and uncomfortable sensations

Data from Adams RD, Victor M: *Principles of neurology,* ed 4, New York, 1989, McGraw-Hill; Bronstein KS, Popovich JM, Stewart-Amidei C: *Promoting stroke recovery: a research-based approach for nurses,* St Louis, 1991, Mosby; Kandel ER, Schwartz JH, Jessell TM: *Principles of neural science,* ed 3, New York, 1991, Elsevier; and Millikan CH, McDowell F, Easton JD: *Stroke,* Philadelphia, 1987, Lea & Febiger.
MCA, Middle cerebral artery; *ACA,* anterior cerebral artery; *TIA,* transient ischemic attack; *PCA,* posterior cerebral artery.

Initial Recognition of Stroke Event

The initial recognition of a stroke often begins with a bystander, family member, or casual observer who reports that an individual is no longer acting normal. Time is critical. The 3-hour treatment window starts with the initial recognition and onset of symptoms. The patient should be transported to the nearest facility that is best equipped for a higher level of stroke treatment for accurate and rapid diagnosis. Immediate interventions may minimize the extent of the brain damage and maximize or improve functional outcomes.

According to the National Institute of Neurological Disorders and Stroke (NINDS), the faster a stroke patient gets to the hospital, the better the chances for recovery. NINDS found that patients who received tPA within 90 minutes of the onset of stroke symptoms improved more at 24 hours than did those who received treatment later than 90 minutes but within the recommended 3-hour treatment window. Patients treated within 90 minutes demonstrated improved outcomes after 3 months. Investigators from NINDS urge continued efforts to treat stroke patients as quickly as possible within the 3-hour window. The clot becomes larger and more organized with the passage of time; this larger clot burden is considerably more difficult to lyse. In addition, areas with prolonged ischemia have greater endothelial damage after reperfusion, which may increase the extent of infarcted tissue and escalate the potential for delayed hemorrhage.[13]

PREHOSPITAL CARE

An emergency is an unforeseen serious medical condition requiring immediate attention if left untreated. *A stroke is a medical emergency.* The patient, bystander, or family member should immediately call 911 and not delay treatment.[8] The AHA promotes the concept of stroke as a medical emergency with measures referred to as the seven-step chain of **D**etection, **D**ispatch, **D**elivery, Emergency Department **D**oor, **D**ata, **D**ecision, and **D**rug treatment within the 3-hour time limit.

Quality emergency medical services (EMS) management of stroke patients treats AIS with the same emphasis as an acute heart attack or acute trauma, recognizing that "time lost is brain lost." This care is a result of extensive training of EMS personnel throughout the United States. The EMS system serves as the initiator of appropriate treatment for stroke management. When a 911 call is received, the dispatcher provides prearrival information to the caller and determines the closest unit to respond for the transport destination. The call can be dispatched to first responders, emergency medical technicians (EMTs), EMT-paramedics, or prehospital registered nurses (RNs) with backup from medical command physicians. The EMS system may include Quick Response Services (QRSs), Basic Life Support (BLS) services, Advanced Life Support (ALS) services, or Air Ambulance services for immediate response. The EMS "run time" for a "brain attack" is modeled after the acute MI model.

Early recognition of stroke symptoms with rapid assessment of the individual is needed to accurately identify patients with signs and symptoms of AIS (Table 17-3). The 1-minute Cincinnati Prehospital Stroke Scale (CPSS) (Table 17-4) is an example of a three-item stroke neurologic exam used in the prehospital setting to assess the presence of facial droop (palsy), arm drift (weakness), and abnormal speech in identifying patients with a suspected stroke. The Los Angeles Prehospital Stroke Screen (LAPSS) is another tool used in the field.[41] Early hospital notification with two-way communication between the EMS in the field and physicians in the emergency department (ED) provides triage and dispatch instructions, helps to expedite rapid transportation to the receiving primary stroke treatment center, establishes the time of first stroke symptoms, gives an estimated time of arrival (ETA), and alerts the ED to activate the stroke response team. Documentation from the scene is important information for inclusion or contraindications of tPA therapy. Examples may include an EMS report of a patient who went to bed functioning normally and the stroke began during sleep, or an individual who lived alone and was found unresponsive. In cases like this, the responders are unable to determine the exact time of stroke onset and the individual would not meet the established criteria for tPA.

EMERGENCY CARE

Initial Emergent Assessment and Management

The ED is the point of first contact for the majority of patients admitted for stroke. The ED also serves as the base command center for the EMS. ED personnel should be experienced and competent with AIS to quickly assess and make treatment and management decisions appropriate for each patient. The immediate care starts with the triage nurse as the first contact for general ED assessment. The triage nurse should record the time of witnessed stroke onset and whether the patient arrives by ambulance, helicopter, or family transportation.

Initial care includes rapid assessment and neurologic evaluation to determine what treatments should be implemented, with a goal of completing the following interventions within the first 10 minutes:

- Record the patient's chief complaint
- History should include present illness, addressing stroke symptoms, any cardiac disease, seizures or epilepsy, migraine headaches, use of anticoagulants, or trauma
- Telemetry: continuous cardiac monitoring
- ABCs (airway open, breathing and respiratory rate, and circulation with pulse check)
- Vital signs to be repeated every 15 minutes
- 12-lead ECG
- Glucose testing by finger stick (treat if indicated)
- Oxygen via nasal cannula
- IV access with insertion of 2 large-bore lines (one with heplock)
- Blood specimens drawn for routine stroke laboratory tests and analysis while tPA or other options are being considered
- Estimated weight

TABLE 17-3　Clinical Manifestations of Stroke Associated With Area of Brain Affected

	Middle Cerebral Artery	Anterior Cerebral Artery	Posterior Cerebral Artery	Internal Carotid Artery	Vertebrobasilar System	Anteroinferior Cerebellar (Lateral Pontine) Artery	Posteroinferior Cerebellar Artery
Motor changes	Contralateral hemiparesis or hemiplegia, face and arm deficits greater than leg	Contralateral hemiparesis, foot and leg deficits greater than arm, footdrop, gait disturbances	Mild contralateral hemiparesis (with thalamic or subthalamic involvement) Intention tremor	Contralateral hemiparesis with facial asymmetry	Alternating motor weaknesses Ataxic gait, dysmetria (uncoordinated actions)	Ipsilateral ataxia Facial paralysis	Ataxia Paralysis of larynx and soft palate
Sensory changes	Contralateral hemisensory alterations Neglect of involved extremities	Contralateral hemisensory alterations	Diffuse sensory loss (thalamic)	Contralateral sensory alterations	Contralateral hemisensory impairments	Ipsilateral loss of sensation in face, sensation changes on trunk and limbs	Ipsilateral loss of sensation in face, contralateral on body
Visual or ocular changes	Homonymous hemianopia Inability to turn eyes toward affected side	Deviation of eyes toward affected side	Pupillary dysfunction (brainstem) Loss of conjugate gaze, nystagmus Loss of depth perception Cortical blindness Homonymous hemianopia	Homonymous hemianopia Ipsilateral periods of blindness (amaurosis fugax)	Double vision Homonymous hemianopia Nystagmus, conjugate gaze paralysis	Nystagmus	Nystagmus
Speech changes	Dyslexia, dysgraphia, aphasia	Expressive aphasia	Perseveration Dyslexia	Aphasia if dominant hemisphere is involved	Dysarthria		Dysarthria
Mental changes	Memory deficits	Confusion, amnesia Flat affect, apathy Shortened attention span Loss of mental acuity	Memory deficits		Memory loss Disorientation		
Other changes	Vomiting may occur	Apraxia (inability to carry out purposeful movements in nonaffected areas) Incontinence	Visual hallucinations	Mild Horner's syndrome Carotid bruits	Drop attacks Tinnitus, hearing loss Vertigo Dysphagia	Horner's syndrome Tinnitus, hearing loss	Horner's syndrome Hiccups and coughing Vertigo Nausea, vomiting

Modified from Black JM, Hawks JH: *Medical-surgical nursing: clinical management for positive outcomes*, ed 7, St Louis, 2005, Elsevier Saunders.

TABLE 17-4	The Cincinnati Prehospital Stroke Scale*
Facial Droop:	Have patient smile or show teeth
Normal	Both sides move equally
Abnormal	One side does not move as well
Arm Drift:	Patient closes eyes and holds both arms out
Normal	Both sides move equally
Abnormal	One side does not move as well
Speech:	Have patient say "you can't teach an old dog new tricks."
Normal	Patient uses correct words without slurring
Abnormal	Slurs words, uses inappropriate words, or is unable to speak

From Mohr JP, Choi DW, Grotta JC, Wolf P, editors: *Stroke: pathophysiology, diagnosis, and management,* ed 4, Philadelphia, 2004, Churchill Livingstone.

*Any one or more abnormal findings is suggestive of acute stroke.

If the stroke team has not been previously alerted when the ED was notified by the EMS, the stroke team should be activated. The ED physician is informed of the initial findings with a goal of completing the physician assessment within 10 minutes. This includes a review of the patient's history and oxygenation status, time of stroke onset, and review of the laboratory studies per the written ED protocols. When AIS is suspected, the ED physician communicates with the stroke team the need for a stat CT scan of the head.[15]

Reassessment of the stroke patient is performed at frequent intervals with careful documentation. The **time of onset** of the first stroke symptoms dictates if the patient meets the 3-hour timeframe for tPA eligibility. If patients or family members are unable to accurately state the exact time of the stroke symptom onset, bystanders or family can be asked what time the patient was last observed functioning normally. The neurologic evaluation includes mental status assessment, Glasgow Coma Scale, pupil check, cranial nerve II to XII assessment, motor/sensory status, deep tendon reflexes (DTRs), and respiratory evaluations completed and documented as part of the ED baseline assessment (see Chapter 2).

The clinical judgment of a well-seasoned emergency physician, neurologist, or other stroke expert is the first step in accurately diagnosing and successfully treating a stroke syndrome.[25] Smaller institutions that do not have 24-hour stroke teams and are unable to provide state-of-the-art stroke treatment may use telemedicine to offer on-site stroke care.

The differential diagnosis for AIS includes ruling out an ICH (see Chapter 18). ICH may present in an identical manner to AIS, especially in the very early stages, and should be ruled out before any treatment. Even vague symptoms (e.g., isolated vertigo) may sometimes be a warning of a stroke.[44] The clinical presentation of the stroke patient is usually a sudden onset of focal cerebral dysfunction that may include the following:

- Loss of consciousness, syncope (transient loss of consciousness), confusion, disorientation, memory loss, delirium that may progress to stupor or coma
- Headache: Intense and described as "the worst headache of my life" (may indicate a hemorrhagic stroke)

- Pain: Neck pain with nuchal rigidity; facial pain
- Speech and language: Aphasia, slurred speech, difficulty understanding and following commands
- Motor problems: Ataxia; weakness of the face, arm, or leg; limb paralysis
- Sensory problems: Paresthesia, unilateral sensory loss, hearing loss
- Cranial nerve palsies: Facial, asymmetric
- Hypertension: Cardiac arrhythmias and elevated blood pressure
- Visual changes, diplopia, hemianopsia, photophobia
- Cerebellar problems: Vertigo, dizziness
- Nausea/vomiting and the potential for aspiration
- Seizures following AIS or hemorrhagic stroke

Hospitals should have preestablished policies to streamline assessment and prevent errors. Protocols ensure that patients with a suspected stroke are appropriately triaged in the ED and evaluated emergently per a "code stroke" because "time is brain." Policies can define the role for each member of the health care team and can provide guidelines for a rapid neurologic evaluation. Protocols may require the details of a patient's history significant for the presence of a stroke, blood pressure perturbations, and any other clues helpful to the differential diagnosis of stroke. Emergencies other than hemorrhagic stroke are to be ruled out (e.g., central nervous system [CNS] trauma, CNS infections [meningitis, encephalitis, or abscess], cerebral tumors, seizures or epilepsy, metabolic disorders [hyperglycemia or hypoglycemia, hyponatremia], cardiac emergency, migraine headache, Todd's paralysis, drug or alcohol overdose).

One report found that many patients with mild strokes worsen without tPA treatment, prompting them to state that based on their data, a reevaluation of the stroke severity criteria for IV tPA administration may be warranted. The team advised further studies before changes are made but warned that they patients who look "too good to treat" may in fact worsen or even die.[47] In such cases, it is important to note that the time of onset is measured from the initial symptoms and not the point of symptom worsening. After the patient with suspected AIS arrives in the ED, the NINDS Consensus Conference recommends that evaluation "targets" or written guidelines be in place for diagnosis and treatment.

Continued Assessment

A completed medical and surgical history and assessment for stroke risk factors is collected. This should include collection of data regarding cardiovascular conditions, hypertension, smoking, oral contraceptive use, obesity, diet, medications, uncontrolled diabetes, and substance abuse. The physical and neurologic examination helps to identify stroke symptoms and determine the vascular distribution responsible for the deficit.

The assessment and diagnostic studies are also needed to determine (1) the location, type, and severity of the lesion within the vessel; (2) the state of the blood and serum that flow through the vessels; and (3) the state of the brain in the region of the symptoms (i.e., normal but threatened, reversibly injured, or dead). Approximately 5% of patients with AIS present with a seizure and up to 30% have a headache.

The symptoms of AIS vary based on the location of the stroke and the collateral blood supply.[44]

Fortunately, diagnostic tools are now available to help the clinician with an accurate diagnosis. Combined with a careful history and physical examination, diagnostic tools can guide the direction of intervention and management at all stages of recovery. Specific modalities are discussed later in this chapter under medical management for the specific stages of recovery.

The comprehensive assessment includes the following:
- ABCs of critical care, gag reflex, and ability to control the tongue and secretions
- Report from EMS, police, family, and bystanders who accompany patient
- Past medical and stroke history
- Exact time of symptom onset
- Brief physical and baseline neurologic examination, including LOC using the Glasgow Coma Scale and repeated every hour (see Chapter 2) and radiographic findings to determine the type of stroke (AIS versus hemorrhagic) (see Chapter 3)

- Baseline National Institutes of Health Stroke Scale (NIHSS) for level of stroke severity; repeat every 15 minutes (Table 17-5) (NIHSS score indicates stroke severity: 0-1 is normal; 1-4, minor stroke; 5-15, moderate stroke; 15-20, moderately severe stroke; greater than 20, severe stroke[44])
- Hunt and Hess Scale if hemorrhagic stroke is suspected (see Chapter 18)

The **NIHSS** is a standardized neurologic examination for patients with AIS. The completed examination measures neurologic function and helps to determine the level of stroke severity. In the absence of exclusion factors, patients with AIS should be considered a candidate to receive tPA if they have an NIHSS score of greater than 4 and less than 22 and a sustained neurologic deficit that is not improving[31] (see Table 17-5). The patient's NIHSS score is discussed with the patient and family along with treatment options (including the risks and benefits of tPA if the patient is a suitable candidate).

Symptoms such as **Todd's paralysis** or postictal paralysis from a seizure can mimic a stroke. After a seizure, it is not

TABLE 17-5	National Institutes of Health Stroke Scale Assessment Items		
Item Assessed		**Score**	
1a. Level of consciousness	0 = Alert	2 = Not alert	
	1 = Not alert, unarousable	3 = Unresponsive	
1b. Level of consciousness questions	0 = Answers both questions correctly	2 = Answers neither correctly	
	1 = Answers one question correctly		
1c. Level of consciousness commands	0 = Performs both tasks correctly	2 = Performs neither task	
	1 = Performs one task correctly		
2. Gaze	0 = Normal	2 = Total gaze paresis	
	1 = Partial gaze palsy		
3. Visual fields	0 = No visual loss	2 = Complete hemianopia	
	1 = Partial hemianopia	3 = Bilateral hemianopia	
4. Facial palsy	0 = Normal	2 = Partial paralysis	
	1 = Minor paralysis	3 = Complete paralysis	
5. Motor arm	0 = No drift	3 = No effort against gravity	
	1 = Drift before 10 sec	4 = No movement	
	2 = Falls before 10 sec	9 = Amputation, joint fusion	
6. Motor leg	0 = No drift	3 = No effort against gravity	
	1 = Drift before 5 sec	4 = No movement	
	2 = Falls before 5 sec	9 = Amputation, joint fusion	
7. Limb ataxia	0 = Absent	2 = Two limbs	
	1 = One limb	9 = Amputation, joint fusion	
8. Sensory	0 = Normal	2 = Severe to total loss	
	1 = Mild to moderate loss		
9. Language	0 = Normal	2 = Severe aphasia	
	1 = Mild aphasia	3 = Mute or global aphasia	
10. Dysarthria	0 = Normal	2 = Severe, unintelligible	
	1 = Mild to moderate slurring	3 = Intubated or other physical barrier	
11. Extinction and inattention	0 = Normal	2 = Severe	
	1 = Mild		
12. Distal motor function*	0 = Normal	2 = No voluntary extension after 5 sec	
	1 = Some extension after 5 sec		

Data from Lyden P et al: Improved reliability of the NIH Stroke Scale using video training, NINDS tPA Stroke Study Group, *Stroke* 25:2220-2226, 1994; National Institute of Neurological Disorders and Stroke t-PA Stroke Study Group: Tissue plasminogen activator for acute ischemic stroke, *N Engl J Med* 333:1581-1587, 1995.
*Additional item, not part of NIHSS, used in the NINDS t-PA Stroke Trial.

uncommon to have focal dysfunction of the area of the brain that was involved. Typically, seizures present with "positive" symptoms (e.g., tonic or clonic activity), eye deviation, or other symptoms such as weakness or drop attacks. The patient having only a seizure will progressively improve over time. If the onset of the seizure was not witnessed, ruling out a seizure as the precipitating factor can be difficult and it is often best to assume that the patient has had a stroke and treat appropriately.[51]

Acute Emergent Management

As part of admission to and treatment in the ED, the patient may receive emergent management that can include thrombolytic therapy, anticoagulation, angioplasty, or stent placement. It is common to involve a multidisciplinary team that includes neurologists, radiologists, emergency physicians, and other specialists who understand the need to move quickly, much like a trauma team or cardiac team that treats MI. Proper management to prevent complications with frequent physiologic monitoring, vital signs, neuroassessment, and detection of signs and symptoms that indicate cerebral bleeding should be ensured.[31]

The initial evaluation, emergency supportive care, and urgent CT scan are important to differentiate among AIS, hemorrhagic stroke, and other diagnoses. The appropriate protocols and guidelines are implemented when the patient returns from radiology and the results of the noncontrast CT scan are known. **Diffusion-perfusion MRI scanning** is being performed in some stroke centers as a diagnostic tool to better select patients who may benefit from intervention despite time of onset by allowing assessment of the degree of cell death in the penumbra (see Fig. 17-1). If the CT scan demonstrates a bleed, a neurosurgery consultation is called. Based on whether or not there is a bleed versus evidence of an infarction, the thrombolytic or nonthrombolytic protocol is initiated. AIS or hemorrhagic stroke standing orders are initiated, the patient is ordered to have nothing by mouth (NPO), and oxygen at 2 L/min is administered based on an oxygen saturation of less than 90%. If the patient is a candidate for thrombolytic therapy, the algorithm for tPA is initiated.

Neurosurgical Consult for Subarachnoid Hemorrhage

If a SAH is suspected, a neurosurgeon should be consulted to evaluate the patient and determine if the patient has a hemorrhagic stroke. If the initial CT scan indicates an SAH, the patient may require a lumbar puncture (LP) to test the cerebrospinal fluid (CSF) for red blood cells (RBCs) (see Chapter 18).

NEURODIAGNOSTIC AND LABORATORY STUDIES

The following neurodiagnostic and laboratory studies are part of the ongoing stroke assessment:

- 12-lead ECG: Must be completed and reported immediately
- CT: Urgent noncontrast CT scan of the head in the thrombolytic candidate to rule out hemorrhage
- Diffusion-weighted MRI image: Show the necrotic core area affected and the penumbra (see Fig. 17-1)
- Lateral C-spine: For patients who are comatose or present with a history of trauma
- Blood tests: Stroke panel should include a CBC with coagulation screen: platelet count, PT/international normalized ratio (INR), and activated partial thromboplastin time (APTT); glucose, creatinine, and chemistry screen with a turn around time (TAT) that provides results in 15 minutes; type and screening for patients that may have a hemorrhagic stroke or receive tPA
- Urinalysis: A total urinalysis with multiple routine tests
- Pregnancy tests: For appropriate female patients to detect human chorionic gonadotropin (hCG) that appears in the urine of pregnant women as early as 10 days after conception
- Chest x-ray: For patients with suspected cardiac diseases, pulmonary edema, or aspiration
- Glucose finger stick: For quick evaluation and treatment
- Routine laboratory studies: Electrolytes
- Serum blood glucose: To rule out metabolic problems
- Oxygenation/ventilation: For patients receiving oxygen, obtain baseline oxygen saturation percentage and continuous pulse oximetry for monitoring oxygen saturation levels
- LP: May obtain after CT has ruled out increased intracranial pressure (IICP) (CT may not rule out high ICP for patients with a high suspicion of SAH; if an LP is performed, the patient will no longer be a candidate for thrombolytic therapy; there is no need to perform an LP if the CT shows SAH[46])
- Angiography: Emergently if patient is diagnosed with SAH and requires emergent surgery
- Toxicology Screen: Drug and substance screening for patients suspected of drug or alcohol abuse

Additional studies may include single photon emission computed tomography (SPECT), xenon CT, heart studies (transthoracic or transesophageal echocardiography), carotid artery ultrasound (duplex testing), TCD, and ECG. The PLAC test, cleared by the FDA, provides a quantitative determination of lipoprotein-associated phospholipase A2 (Lp-PLA2) in plasma. Increased Hcy blood levels are associated with increased stroke risk. Hcy appears to promote the progression of atherosclerosis by causing endothelial damage. Smoking and hypertension are associated with increased Hcy levels.

CT scan without contrast remains the mainstay in AIS and is completed and read by radiologists/neurologists or a qualified ED physician. A CT scan is sensitive for detection of 90% of SAH within the first 24 hours of bleeding.[78] For parenchymal imaging; an MRI scan that uses diffusion techniques sensitive to ischemia and that uses susceptibility techniques sensitive to hemorrhage is the preferred imaging modality in some of the larger hospitals that have this capability. Susceptibility-weighted MRI scans are increasingly supplanting CT scans (see Chapter 3). Diffusion-weighted imaging (DWI) that discloses areas of diminished CBF, intracranial hemorrhage, early ischemic changes, and the ischemic penumbra is available in some centers that treat AIS and may ultimately help guide the selection of patients for acute treatment with thrombolysis or neuroprotectives.

After diagnosis of AIS, additional testing may include positron emission tomography (PET), which is usually available only in large medical centers as an experimental model and is used infrequently to determine the size of the metabolic loss. Other studies may include digital subtraction angiography (DSA) and noninvasive blood flow studies including carotid artery ultrasound, carotid Doppler sonography, thermography, and ophthalmodynamometry to study the vascular tree leading to the brain. Cardiac causes of disease may be investigated with testing (e.g., ECG, cardiac enzyme elevation, or echocardiography) to rule out arrhythmias, valvular or structural abnormalities of the heart, and MI. Hematologic studies may be conducted for problems with viscosity to include coagulation studies or cellular configuration (e.g., sickle cell disease). Electroencephalograms (EEGs) are rarely of any diagnostic use unless the patient experiences seizure activity.

TREATMENT

Medical Management

Many hospitals today offer patients diagnosed with AIS state-of-the art EDs with highly qualified stroke teams or stroke units that have been certified by the Joint Commission on Accreditation of Healthcare Organizations (JCAHO). JCAHO certification is designed to provide comprehensive stroke management to include short- and long-term rehabilitation interventions for recovery.

Sedatives and opioids should be avoided because they decrease alertness and confound the neurologic assessment.[53] It has been estimated that approximately 80% of patients with AIS are hypertensive. Treatment protocols for these patients are used to limit the size of the infarct, prevent and treat complications, and prevent extension or recurrences.

Pharmacologic Thrombolytics for Acute Ischemic Stroke

In 1996 the FDA approved the recombinant tPA alteplase (Activase), which acts as a thrombolytic by binding to the fibrin in a thrombus and converting entrapped plasminogen to plasmin. This process initiates fibrinolysis and decreases clotting time. The IV drug's half-life is 5 to 35 minutes.[56] Thrombolytic therapy (e.g., tPA) has the potential to dissolve the clot, recanalize the occluded artery, and restore the blood flow to the ischemic penumbra. TPA is the only FDA-approved drug that can be administered to reverse the effects of a stroke if given within the first 3 hours. Beyond 3 hours, if the occluded artery is opened, revascularization of the core necrotic tissue can increase the risk of cerebral edema and hemorrhage.[2] It is important to carefully screen suspected stroke patients and use well-defined written protocols that are consistently maintained by all treating providers who treat AIS with tPA (Box 17-1).

Thrombolysis should not be implemented unless the stroke diagnosis is established by a physician with expertise in stroke and a brain CT is assessed by a physician with expertise in reading this imaging study. Before thrombolysis is given, exclusion and inclusion criteria should be used to determine if the patient is a candidate (Box 17-2). Treatment with tPA if the blood pressure is above 185/110 can be initiated if the blood pressure is managed first using standard regimens, which may include Cardene, nitroglycerin paste (Nitro-Bid), labetalol (Trandate), or enalapril (Vasotec).[56]

TPA should be ordered from the pharmacy and delivered within 10 minutes for immediate administration. Blood pressure parameters are closely monitored and guidelines for treatment strictly followed. Although the incidence of hemorrhage is low, consideration of bleeding must always be part of the close monitoring. Patients who have been taking anticoagulants may not be eligible for thrombolytic therapy because of the high risk for cerebral hemorrhage. The lytic action of tPA occurs as the plasma protein (plasminogen) is converted to plasmin (fibrinolysin), whose enzymatic action digests fibrin threads and fibrinogen thereby lysing the clot. Activase has the advantage of a short half-life, does not reduce overall fibrinogen concentration to the same degree as other thrombolytics, and has nonantigenicity.[56]

Although tPA is clot specific, hemorrhage remains a possible side effect. The greatest usefulness of the drug in stroke therapy is in early intervention.[13] Its value is doubtful after 3 hours, and it carries an increased risk of hemorrhagic transformation of the ischemic area or of induced hemorrhage in the vessels beyond the occlusion. This puts the patient at increased risk for further neurologic damage.

The patient's weight is recorded and two IV lines must be in place before administrating tPA. The manufacturer's current recommended IV dose is 0.9 mg/kg of body weight, with 10% administered as a bolus over 1 to 2 minutes and the remaining 90% infused over 60 minutes not to exceed 90 mg following the inclusion and exclusion criteria (Fig. 17-3; see also Box 17-2). For continued recovery, the patient is admitted to a stroke unit or intensive care unit (ICU) for close monitoring of vital signs, neurologic and cardiovascular status to detect any signs of deterioration suggesting hemorrhage, reocclusion, or complications.

A study was done with patients diagnosed with AIS caused by occlusion of the MCA. They were treated with IV tPA within 3 hours after the onset of symptoms and also received continuous **2-MHz TCD ultrasonography.** The objective was to determine if ultrasonography could enhance the thrombolytic activity of tPA. Patients treated with this combination had a nonsignificant trend toward an increased rate of recovery compared with patients treated with a placebo.[1]

After transfer from the ED, post-tPA orders commonly include avoiding the administration of aspirin, heparin, or warfarin for the next 24 hours. The patient should be closely monitored for early signs of neurologic deterioration, which may include tachycardia, increased respiratory rate, decreased

BOX 17-1   TPA Stroke Study Group: Protocol Guidelines*† for the Administration of rt-PA to Patients With Acute Ischemic Stroke

These Protocol Guidelines represent only one possible approach to the treatment of eligible patients with acute ischemic stroke. Health care practitioners and institutions will need to exercise their own professional judgment in creating or adopting treatment protocols or guidelines, as well as in the treatment of each individual patient.

1. Eligibility for IV treatment with rt-PA
- Age 18 years or older.
- Clinical diagnosis of ischemic stroke causing a measurable neurologic deficit.
- Time of symptom onset well established to be less than 180 minutes before treatment would begin.

2. Patient selection: contraindications[c] and warnings[w]
- Evidence of intracranial hemorrhage on pretreatment computed tomography (CT).[c]
- Only minor or rapidly improving stroke symptoms.[w]
- Clinical presentation suggestive of subarachnoid hemorrhage, even with normal CT findings.[c]
- Active internal bleeding.[c]
- Known bleeding diathesis, including but not limited to:
  Platelet count less than 100,000/mm³.[c]
  Receipt of heparin within 48 hours and an elevated activated partial thromboplastin time (aPTT) (greater than upper limit of normal for laboratory).[c]
  Current use of oral anticoagulants (e.g., warfarin sodium) or recent use with an elevated prothrombin time (PT) greater than 15 seconds.[c‡]
- Major surgery or serious trauma excluding head trauma in the previous 14 days.[w]
- Intracranial surgery, serious head trauma, or previous stroke within 3 months.[c]
- History of gastrointestinal or urinary tract hemorrhage within 21 days.[w]
- Recent arterial puncture at a noncompressible site.[w]
- Recent lumbar puncture.[w]
- On repeated measurements, systolic blood pressure greater than 185 mm Hg or diastolic blood pressure greater than 110 mm Hg at the time treatment is to begin, and aggressive treatment required to reduce blood pressure to within these limits.[c]
- History of intracranial hemorrhage.[c]
- Abnormal blood glucose level (less than 50 or greater than 400 mg/dl).[w]
- Post-myocardial infarction pericarditis.[w]
- Seizure observed at the same time the onset of stroke symptoms was observed.[w]
- Known arteriovenous malformation or aneurysm.[c]

3. Treatment
- rt-PA 0.9 mg/kg (maximum of 90 mg) infused over 60 minutes with 10% of the total dose administered as an initial IV bolus over 1 minute.

4. Sequence of events
- Determine whether time is available to start treatment with rt-PA before 3 hours.
- Draw blood for tests while preparations are made to perform noncontrast CT scan.
- Start recording blood pressure.
- Perform neurologic examination.

- Perform CT scan without contrast.
- Determine whether CT scan shows evidence of hemorrhage.
  If patient has severe head or neck pain or is somnolent or stuporous, be sure there is no evidence of subarachnoid hemorrhage.
  If there is a significant abnormal lucency suggestive of infarction, reconsider the patient's history, because the stroke may have occurred earlier.
- Review required test results.
  Hematocrit
  Platelets
  Blood glucose
  PT or aPTT (in patients with recent use of oral anticoagulants or heparin)
- Review patient selection criteria.
- Infuse tPA.
  Give 0.9 mg/kg, 10% as a bolus, intravenously.
  Do *not* use the cardiac dose.
  Do *not* exceed the 90-mg maximum dose.
  Do *not* give aspirin, heparin, or warfarin for 24 hours.
- Monitor the patient carefully, especially the blood pressure.
- Monitor neurologic status.

5. Adjunctive therapy
- Do not administer concomitant heparin, warfarin, or aspirin during the first 24 hours after symptom onset. If heparin or any other anticoagulant is indicated after 24 hours, consider performing a noncontrast CT scan or other sensitive diagnostic imaging method to rule out any intracranial hemorrhage before starting an anticoagulant.

6. Blood pressure control
- Pretreatment
  Monitor blood pressure every 15 minutes. It should be less than 185/110 mm Hg.
  If blood pressure is greater than 185/110, treat with nitroglycerin paste and/or one or two 10- to 20-mg doses of labetalol given in an IV push within 1 hour. If these measures do not reduce blood pressure to less than 185/110 mm Hg and keep it down, do not treat with rt-PA.
- During and after treatment
  Monitor blood pressure for the first 24 hours after starting treatment:
    Every 15 minutes for 2 hours after starting the infusion, then
    Every 30 minutes for 6 hours, then
    Every hour for 18 hours
  If diastolic blood pressure is greater than 140 mm Hg, start an intravenous infusion of sodium nitroprusside (0.5 to 10 mcg/kg/min).
  If systolic blood pressure is greater than 230 mm Hg and/or diastolic BP is 121 to 140 mm Hg, give labetalol 20 mg intravenously over 1 to 2 minutes. The dose may be repeated and/or doubled every 10 minutes, up to 150 mg. Alternatively, after the first bolus of labetalol, an intravenous infusion of 2 to 8 mg

Continued

BOX 17-1	TPA Stroke Study Group: Protocol Guidelines*† for the Administration of rt-PA to Patients With Acute Ischemic Stroke—cont'd

labetalol per minute may be initiated and continued until the desired blood pressure is reached. If satisfactory response is not obtained, use sodium nitroprusside.

If systolic blood pressure is 180 to 230 mm Hg and/or diastolic blood pressure is 105 to 120 mm Hg on two readings 5 to 10 minutes apart, give labetalol 10 mg intravenously over 1 to 2 minutes. The dose may be repeated or doubled every 10 to 20 minutes, up to 150 mg. Alternatively, after the first bolus of labetalol, an intravenous infusion of 2 to 8 mg labetalol per minute may be initiated and continued until the desired blood pressure is reached.

- Monitor blood pressure every 15 minutes during the antihypertensive therapy. Observe the hypotension.
- If, in the clinical judgment of the treating physician, an intracranial hemorrhage is suspected, the administration of rt-PA should be discontinued, and an emergency CT scan or other diagnostic imaging method sensitive for the presence of intracranial hemorrhage should be obtained.

7. **Management of intracranial hemorrhage**
- Suspect the occurrence of intracranial hemorrhage after the start of rt-PA infusion if there is any acute neurologic

deterioration, new headache, acute hypertension, or nausea and vomiting.
- If hemorrhage is suspected, do the following:
Discontinue rt-PA infusion unless other causes of neurologic deterioration are apparent.
  Perform immediate CT scan or other diagnostic imaging method sensitive for the presence of hemorrhage.
Draw blood for PT, aPTT, platelet count, and fibrinogen, and type and crossmatch (may wait to do actual type and crossmatch).
Prepare for administration of 6 to 8 units of cryoprecipitate containing factor VIII.
Prepare for administration of 6 to 8 units of platelets.
- If intracranial hemorrhage is present, do the following:
Obtain fibrinogen results.
Consider administering cryoprecipitate or platelets if needed.
Consider alerting and consulting a hematologist or neurosurgeon.
Consider decision regarding further medical and/or surgical therapy.
Consider second CT scan to assess progression of intracranial hemorrhage.
- Plan for access to emergent neurosurgical consultation.

Courtesy Genentech, Inc, South San Francisco, CA.
*This protocol is based on research supported by the National Institute of Neurological Disorders and Stroke (NINDS) (N01-NS-02382, N01-NS-02374, N01-NS-02377, N01-NS-02381, N01-NS-02379, N01-NS-02373, N01-NS-02378, N01-NS-02376, N01-NS-02380).
†Reference should also be made to the manufacturer's prescribing information for alteplase (Genentech, Inc, South San Francisco, Calif).
‡In patients without recent use of oral anticoagulants or heparin, treatment with rt-PA can be initiated before the availability of coagulation study results but should be discontinued if either the prothrombin time is greater than 15 seconds or the partial thromboplastin time is elevated by local laboratory standards.

BOX 17-2	Exclusion Criteria for Intravenous rt-PA Therapy for Acute Ischemic Stroke

- Current use of oral anticoagulants or prothrombin time greater than 15 seconds
- Use of heparin in previous 48 hours and a prolonged partial thromboplastin time
- Platelet count less than 100,000/mm³
- Another stroke or serious head injury in previous 3 months
- Major surgery within preceding 14 days
- Pretreatment systolic blood pressure greater than 185 mm Hg or diastolic blood pressure greater than 110 mm Hg
- Rapidly improving neurologic signs
- Isolated, mild neurologic deficits, such as ataxia alone, sensory loss alone, dysarthria alone, or minimal weakness
- Prior intracranial hemorrhage
- Blood glucose level less than 50 mg/dl or greater than 400 mg/dl
- Seizure at onset of stroke
- Gastrointestinal or urinary bleeding within preceding 21 days
- Recent myocardial infarction

From Urden LD, Stacy KM, Lough ME: *Thelan's critical care nursing: diagnosis and management,* ed 4, St Louis, 2002, Mosby.

blood pressure, pupillary changes, hypertension, onset of headache, nausea and vomiting, and bradycardia. If a cerebral hemorrhage is suspected, the attending physician should be notified and the tPA discontinued. Appropriate laboratory work should be drawn for stat analysis and the patient prepared for an emergent CT scan.

Intraarterial thrombolytics (IATs) are another alternative treatment for dissolving the clot that is obstructing CBF in carefully selected patients with AIS caused by large cerebral vessel occlusion, e.g., the MCA or basilar artery. An NIHSS score over 10 is used in some centers for patient-selection criteria. The window of therapy may be extended up to 6 hours, or beyond in some cases, for experimental intraarterial administration of thrombolytics. Drugs used include the recombinant tPA reteplase (Retavase), which is water soluble with a serum half-life of 13 to 16 minutes and is not weight adjusted, or the recombinant tPA alteplase (Activase), which is weight adjusted.[62] Treatment with IAT can be initiated as long as $6\frac{1}{2}$ hours after symptom onset; the earlier the recanalization, the better the outcome.

Benefits of IAT include the direct infusion of higher local concentrations of the thrombolytic to the lesion site with lower systemic drug concentration. Disadvantages include the risks associated with the procedure and the risk of hemorrhagic transformation.[42] In centers where this expertise is available, patients who are confirmed eligible undergo this

Suspected Acute Stroke Emergi-path

This Emergi-path is to be used as a documentation and patient care guide

OUTCOME GOALS:	1. Rapid identification of patients potentially qualifying for acute stroke therapy upon ED arrival
	2. Head CT done as a top priority
	3. Rapid notification of Stroke Team for patients qualifying for acute onset stroke therapy
	4. Stroke treatment offered to patient within a timely manner
RESPONSIBLE PERSON	**PERTINENT INFORMATION TO DOCUMENT**
NURSING PERSONNEL	Chief Complaint: Sudden onset numbness, weakness, difficulty speaking, severe headache, visual changes, or uncoordination
ASSESSMENT	Pertinent History:
	Age, Onset time (last time patient was known to be normal), Symptoms
	Hx: CAD, Coagulopathy, Cardiac arrhythmias
	Primary Care Provider (PCP)
	Medications/Allergies
INTERVENTIONS	Place immediately in a treatment room; notify staff MD/primary RN of potential acute onset stroke patient
	Attach cardiac monitor
	Oxygen 2-4 L NP
	Initiate Social Services for family (PRN)
	Alert CT/radiology department
	Initiate IV & send labs (see below). A 2nd IV should be established after CT if requested by the Stroke Team
	Obtain a 12 lead EKG (can be done after CT)
	Monitor BP q 15 minutes
	Neuro checks q 15 minutes including patient's ability to move each limb against gravity
PHYSICIAN	Time seen by physician.
Chief complaint	Review: History, Age, Time of symptom onset, VS, Medications, Allergies
History & Physical	Directed H&P (include ability to hold limbs against gravity [drift], visual fields, EOMs, presence of neglect)
INTERVENTIONS	Rapidly contact the Stroke Team if deficits are present and stroke onset is <24 hrs. (Pager 12600). Also contact the Stroke Team for pediatric patients, and for patient/family requests for stroke eval or treatment when the ED physician does not feel it is indicated.
	Stat head CT without contrast (Top priority). Stroke Team will review CT films
	Labs to include: CBC-diff; PT/PTT, INR; electrolyte, liver, & renal panels; glucose; UA; urine HCG (for female patients of childbearing age)
	Chest X-ray (can be done after CT; should not delay t-PA treatment)
	Code intervention determined & advance directives reviewed
If CT of head shows:	**1. CT shows no stroke or early acute ischemic stroke**
	Stroke treatment medical therapies are offered
	<3 hour t-PA or investigational tx - Stroke Team will evaluate
	STROKE TEAM MEMBERS WILL PREPARE AND ADMINISTER DRUGS FOR ACUTE STROKE TREATMENT
	Oregon Stroke Center guidelines for IV t-PA in acute ischemic stroke patients (see back of sheet).
	2. CT shows intracranial or subarachnoid hemorrhage
	Request neurosurgical evaluation for possible surgery
	Reverse any anticoagulants

Authors: Developed in collaboration with OHSU ED staff and Oregon Stroke Center staff

Figure 17-3 Suspected Acute Stroke Emergi-path is to be used as a documentation and patient care guide.
(Courtesy Oregon Health Sciences University Hospital, Portland, OR.)

procedure in either the cardiac catheterization lab or in the interventional radiology department. An interventional physician performs the standard femoral approach to perform diagnostic cerebral angiography to identify the occluded vessels. The next step is to continue with a bolus infusion into the clot. The tip of the catheter is inserted into the thrombus via a microcatheter. Heparin may be administered with an IV bolus of 2000 units followed by 500 units per hour during the procedure. A follow-up angiogram is used to determine the success of the procedure. With the sheath left in place, patients recover in the ICU with vigilant monitoring of vital signs and neurologic checks (using the NIHSS) for early detection of bleeding. Of particular concern is blood pressure management for adequate perfusion and dangerous levels of blood pressure fluctuations. After the sheath is removed the following day, the heparin is discontinued and the patient is closely observed as the coagulation is reversed back to normal.[79]

Mechanical Thrombolectomy

Mechanical thrombolectomy is the newest FDA-approved treatment for AIS using the Merci Retriever.[45] This tiny corkscrew-like device was approved by the FDA in August 2004 to remove clots from an artery in the brain of patients experiencing ischemic stroke.[71] Inclusion criteria may include patients with a diagnosis of ischemic stroke older than 18 years of age with an NIHSS score greater than 8 who are ineligible for IV tPA or who fail IV tPA and arrive in the ED within 8 hours of symptoms. Many hospital centers with highly skilled stroke teams are able to perform the three-step process: (1) engage, (2) capture, and (3) remove the clot (Fig. 17-4).

First a diagnostic angiography is performed to identify the proximal arterial occlusion for recanalization. Using sterile technique, the physician inserts the Merci Balloon Guide Catheter through a small incision in the femoral artery in the groin into the anterior or posterior circulation. Under x-ray guidance, the catheter is maneuvered up through the carotid artery. A guidewire and the Merci Microcatheter are deployed just beyond the clot. The physician carefully ensnares the clot. When the clot is captured, the balloon guide catheter is inflated to temporarily stop the flow while the clot is gently withdrawn and pulled into the guide catheter for removal from the body via the groin site. The balloon is deflated and arterial blood flow is restored to perfuse the brain and prevent neuronal death. A maximum of six retrieval attempts in the same vessel is recommended to prevent damage to the vessel. A final angiogram is performed, the sheath is removed and the site closed with standard protocols, and a small dressing is applied. Combination therapy with IATs and mechanical clot disruption, based on the physician's best judgment, may be necessary in emergency or special circumstances when pharmacologic thrombolysis alone is ineffective or the patient is a poor candidate for IV thrombolytics.

Follow-up management includes monitoring neurologic status for deterioration, blood pressure changes, signs and symptoms of intracerebral bleeding, bleeding or hematoma at the femoral catheter insertion site, and other patient-specific parameters. Posttreatment angiographic images can be used to evaluate successful recanalization before patient discharge.[62]

Surgical Management

Surgical options of use in preventing further stroke and/or improving CBF may include CEA, carotid or intracranial stent placement, carotid or intracranial vessel angioplasty, and extracranial-to-intracranial bypass. The repair of aneurysms and atrioventricular malformations and the removal of intracranial hematomas may also require intracranial surgical procedures (see Chapters 8 and 18).

Carotid Endarterectomy

Narrowing of the internal carotid at the carotid bifurcation in the neck from atherosclerosis is a common cause of TIA and stroke. CEA is the most commonly performed surgery involving the arteries, with an estimated 130,000 procedures performed every year in the United States. CEA is performed most often on men 75 to 84 years of age. Age is a factor as is comorbidity. A clinical practice guideline published in the November 2005 issue of *Neurology* found that there is scientific evidence to support the use of CEA to reduce future stroke risk. Authors reviewed literature from 1990 to 2004 and found that CEA is effective for patients with severe stenosis and recent symptoms of stroke or TIA; it may also be considered for patients with moderate stenosis and recent symptoms of stroke.[11] The North American Symptomatic Carotid Endarterectomy Trial (NASCET) released in 1994 showed a 17% reduction in the occurrence of ipsilateral strokes between surgical and nonsurgical groups of patients with more than 70% stenosis who were symptomatic from their lesions.[21,22] The European Carotid Surgery Trial (ECSR) reported a nonsurgical stroke occurrence risk of 16.8% versus a 10.3% risk for those who had undergone CEA.[21,22] The evidence amassed from these two large trials suggests that patients with lesions producing a focal hemispheric or retinal ischemia symptomatology will benefit from CEA when the surgeon can achieve a perioperative morbidity and mortality rate of 3% or less. Within these limits, NASCET reported a 65% relative risk reduction and a 17% absolute risk reduction. There is, therefore, robust evidence to recommend CEA if there is more than a 70% stenosis that produces focal symptoms. Patients with 50% to 69% stenosis should be considered for CEA if they have hemispheric events rather than simply TIA.

The aspirin and CEA trial determined that medical care is superior to CEA for asymptomatic patients.[3] Some studies have estimated that as many as 10% of patients may have narrowing after CEA—some within the first year. Subsequently, the risk may be about 1% per year for restenosis.

CEA has been used immediately after stroke to prevent progressing stroke, in symptomatic patients with recurrent TIAs, and in asymptomatic patients with known carotid stenosis. The indications for considering CEA in symptomatic patients with carotid occlusion are complex plaque or significant carotid stenosis detected by acceptable imaging techniques. CEA is depicted in Fig. 17-5. Assessment for carotid stenosis includes auscultating for a bruit. A **bruit** is a blowing

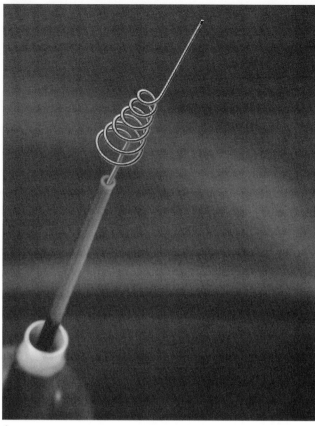

A

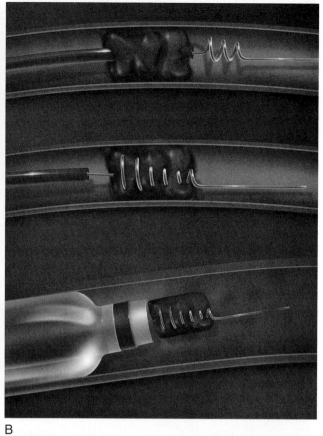

B

Figure 17-4 The Merci Retriever: Find it, engage it, retrieve it. **A,** Merci corkscrew. **B,** Merci clot retriever. **C,** Merci application. *(Courtesy Concentric Medical, Mountain View, CA.)*

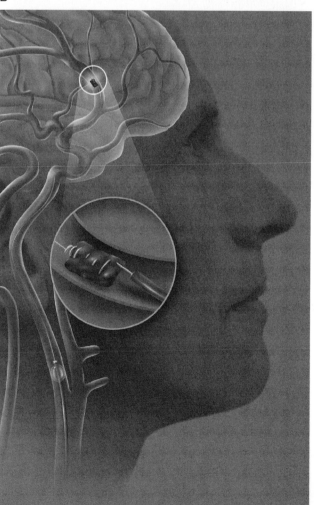

C

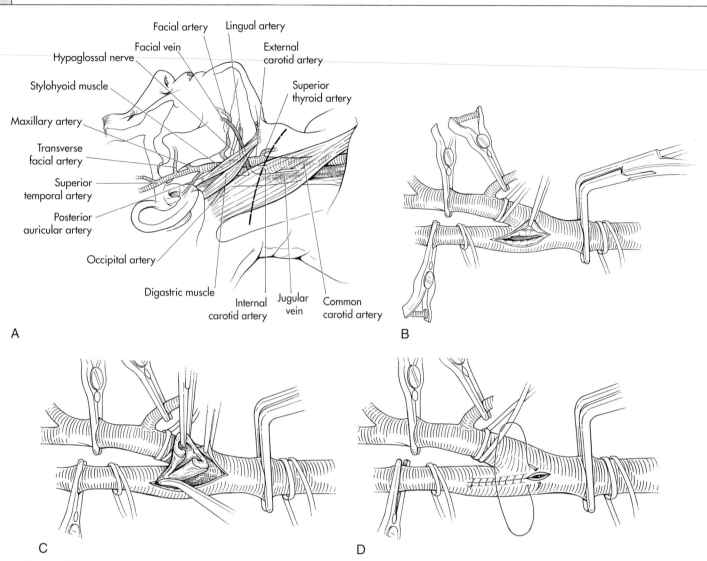

Figure 17-5 CEA. **A,** Relationship of incision to carotid bifurcation in the neck. **B,** Dissection. **C,** Removal of atheroma. **D,** Surgical closure. *(From Kaye AH, Black P:* Operative neurosurgery, *New York, 2000, Churchill Livingstone.)*

or swishing sound that may be detected when auscultating the carotid artery. Bruits are the result of blood flowing through a narrow or occluded artery when carotid stenosis is present.

The goal of CEA is to reestablish adequate CBF and prevent cerebral ischemic events secondary to emboli from atheromatous plaques.[21] Before surgery, the patient may undergo a Doppler/duplex ultrasound test to demonstrate the severity of the carotid stenosis, a four-vessel arteriogram, MRA to image the carotid arteries, a brain MRI or CT scan, and routine laboratory studies (see Chapter 3).

Before the surgery, patients may receive antiplatelet agents (e.g., aspirin, Plavix).[74] A local or general anesthetic is used, with a general anesthetic favored by most surgeons. The patient is usually placed in the supine position with the neck slightly hyperextended and a shoulder roll placed on the side of the surgical procedure. Intraoperative EEG monitoring, TCD, somatosensory evoked potentials (SSEPs), and other monitoring devices may be used to detect ischemia. The neck incision is typically made along the border of the sterno-cleidomastoid muscle area and is carried down to the platysma and fascia. The hypoglossal nerve is identified for protection during surgery. As the common carotid is exposed, 0.5 ml of 2% lidocaine is used to anesthetize it and prevent bradycardia and hypotension during manipulation of the carotid bifurcation. When the atheromatous plaque is fully visualized, it is dissected away from the wall of the artery proximally and distally, from the beginning and along the length of the plaque. Careful dissection is needed to prevent an "intimal flap," which can occlude the vessel postoperatively (see Fig. 17-5). Closure is complete after the vessel has been flushed of any debris and the arteriotomy is closed; in some cases a drain may be inserted and left in overnight.[21]

Postoperative risks include hemodynamic instability, hypotension and/or hypertension, bradycardia, neurologic changes, bleeding, neck hematoma, postoperative stroke, and cardiac adverse events, particularly for patients with a history of cardiac disease.[22] For these reasons, the patient must be closely monitored, usually in an intensive care setting, immediately postoperatively. Pathways for shorter hospital stays of only one or more days are becoming routine unless the patient has comorbidities that require additional services.[35]

Carotid Stenting

Carotid stenting is now available as a less invasive alternative to CEA for carotid stenosis. Early results recommend caution and an awareness of the potential risks and benefits. In March 2005, however, Medicare recognized the value of carotid stenting in symptomatic patients with greater than 70% carotid stenosis, citing research done by Brooks and colleagues, which indicated that, in this patient population, stenting is as effective as CEA in the hands of a surgeon with a morbidity and mortality rate of less than 3% with CEA.[9] Typically, the femoral artery is cannulated with the Seldinger technique and a standard guidewire is passed. Angiography is performed to determine the length and severity of the lesion, and an appropriate size stent is deployed.[16] The procedure involves guiding a catheter into the carotid or vertebrobasilar artery to insert a tubular mesh stent that expands to widen the blocked artery. The goal is to open the occlusion and restore blood flow to the area. TPA may be used to lyse the clot as well. This alternative may be preferred for patients who have cardiac and other disease and are considered poor candidates for surgical intervention. Deficits that should be monitored for during the first 24 hours after the procedure include hypotension, confusion, dysphasia, dysarthria, weakness, hemiparesis, sensory loss, and ipsilateral or contralateral carotid artery stenosis.

Percutaneous Transluminal Angioplasty

Percutaneous transluminal angioplasty (PTA) is being assessed as an alternative to carotid surgery for patients with carotid stenosis. More reports will provide outcomes from this balloon inflation procedure to compare problems with microembolism and plaque disruption. If proven successful, the advantages for the patient would be avoidance of the neck incision and general anesthesia, shorter hospitalization, and faster recovery with less potential for complications.[14] This procedure may also be combined with stent placement.

Cerebral Revascularization: External Carotid to Internal Carotid Bypass

The superficial middle temporal artery (MTA) to MCA bypass graft is a type of graft used to restore circulation to the brain after occlusion. This procedure is not performed as frequently today. The goal of surgery is to supplement brain blood flow, replace brain blood flow, and/or eliminate the CNS as a target for embolization. Bypass surgery using the occipital to posteroinferior cerebellar artery (PICA) or carotid-saphenous vein to PICA has relieved vertebrobasilar ischemia caused by bilateral distal vertebral artery occlusion. The primary complication of this surgery is the development of cerebellar hemorrhage that causes compression and may lead to coma and death. Clinicians must be alert to impending signs of cerebellar compression and intervene immediately.

Preoperative studies include a CT and/or MRI scan, xenon CT scan, SPECT, MRA, CT angiography, angiography, Amytal testing, balloon-occlusion testing, TCD, duplex scan-

ning of the extracranial carotid artery, oculoplethysmography (OPG), PET, and EEG. After the risks and benefits of surgery have been fully explained and understood, the surgery is planned with anesthesia. The patient is positioned with the head rotated approximately 90 degrees laterally. The head is prepared and marked for the craniotomy (see Chapter 8). The incision is made over the superficial temporal artery (STA) and the delicate task of isolating the vessels to join a branch of the STA to a branch of the MCA is begun.

After the procedure, the clips used to occlude blood flow during the procedure are released, the vessels are inspected for oozing or leaking, and the wound is closed.[55] Patients recover in an ICU for routine craniotomy recovery. Special considerations include monitoring for bleeding, checking the patency of the revascularized vessels with a portable Doppler, maintaining blood pressure within specific parameters, and monitoring for changes in neurologic status for evidence of ischemia. Careful attention to the dressing will prevent compromise of the anastomosis site. Potential complications include infarction, bleeding, hydrocephalus, infection, and vasospasm. An early patency rate of 96% to 99% can be achieved with long-term rates approaching 95%.[55] Patients may be prescribed anticoagulation therapy after surgery. Follow-up management is recommended for preventive care.

Other Treatment Options

Laser treatment has been performed on a small group of patients with results indicating that the laser may eventually be an important treatment to dissolve stroke-causing blood clots in the carotid arteries. For this treatment, a pulsed dye laser system with laser energy is delivered to the clot via a quartz optical fiber that sits inside a large plastic catheter. The catheter is positioned at the clot, and the laser beam clears away the gelatinous clot in a short time without damaging the artery walls. Mechanical techniques such as laser therapy are under investigation along with vacuum-based systems and ultrasound devices that are designed to work faster than chemically based methods.[30]

The development of an **endovascular photoacoustic recanalization laser** is being tested experimentally as a less risky alternative for AIS. The laser produces a mechanical thrombolysis rather than pharmacologic lysis. The tip of the laser is placed directly into the clot and emits light energy that emulsifies the clot. Even though there is the risk of embolization, pioneer efforts with laser therapy may help it become another alternative for stroke treatment.

Some stroke patients who receive therapy may appear to have changes in their neurologic status after treatment. Close observation and monitoring are needed to alert the health care team to any change in the patient's neurologic status. Some of these changes may be attributed to the causes listed in Box 17-3.[47]

STROKE UNITS

The purpose of a stroke center is to provide optimal, rapid, and efficient care to stroke patients. Having stroke unit and

BOX 17-3	Possible Causes for Changes in Neurologic Status After Treatment for Stroke

- Thrombus propagation
- Occlusion of a stenotic artery because of thrombus
- Recurrent embolism
- Hemorrhagic transformation
- Failure of collateral blood supply
- Hypoperfusion caused by systemic hypotension
- Hypovolemia or decreased cardiac output
- Hypoxia
- Cerebral edema
- Herniation
- Seizures
- Medication effects
- Medical conditions (e.g., pneumonia, PE, MI, CHF, electrolyte imbalance, urosepsis)

PE, Pulmonary embolism; *MI,* myocardial infarction; *CHF,* congestive heart failure.

neurologic expertise can reduce complications and improve outcomes. A **Primary Stroke Center (PSC)** is a facility that is able to initially stabilize and treat most stroke patients. **Primary Stroke Center Certification** was developed by the JCAHO in collaboration with the ASA as a voluntary accreditation process with 12 key components. These components include:

- Stroke team management
- EMS
- Written protocols for care
- ED management involvement
- Formation of a stroke unit
- Neurological and neurosurgical services
- Naming a stroke center director
- Neuroimaging
- Laboratory services
- Monitoring outcomes
- Outcome and quality improvement (QI)
- Continuing medical education (CME)

There are 10 items that JCAHO monitors as part of the Standardized Stroke Measure Set (see JCAHO's website, listed in the Resources section). In 2005, there were 150 JCAHO designated PSCs in the United States. In 2006, the AHA and ASA published *Guidelines for Prevention of Stroke in Patients with Ischemic Stroke or Transient Ischemic Attack.*[67] These guidelines are available at http://stroke.ahajournals.org/cgi/reprintframed/37/2/577? (Table 17-6).

Types of therapies that a PSC could administer include IV tPA and blood pressure therapies. Heparin has been shown of no value in stroke treatment and might be used for deep vein thrombosis (DVT) prophylaxis only in the absence of other options or high-risk and emergent treatment of IICP. Other important components include a **stroke team,** a center director, rapid CT availability, rapid laboratory tests, educational programs, written protocols, involvement of the EMS, and QI programs. The stroke center concept is rapidly gaining momentum around the country to provide efficient and modern care to patients everywhere in the United States. Neuroscience clinicians are the backbone and driving force

to form this network of hospitals to treat AIS, test new therapies, and promote stroke prevention.

Acute Care

The patient diagnosed with AIS is triaged, diagnosed, and treated emergently in the ED. Appropriate treatment interventions are completed and the patient is closely monitored for vital signs, cardiac status, and oxygenation. A swallowing evaluation can be initiated in the ED while the patient is NPO. IV access with normal saline (NS) at 60 ml/hr is routine. Urinary indwelling catheters are optional at this time. The ED orders and protocols are completed and the patient transferred to the stroke unit or ICU to follow written protocols or pathways. It is critical that no anticoagulants or antiplatelet agents (heparin, warfarin, or aspirin) are given for 24 hours after tPA to prevent bleeding. During the first 24 to 48 hours of hospitalization, indications for admission to an ICU consist of the following[15]:

Inability to protect the airways

- Need for intensive cardiovascular monitoring to maintain mean arterial pressure (MAP) 90 to 100 mm Hg or normal systolic level for patient; titrate fluids and vasoactive agents as needed; arterial pH 7.3 to 7.5
- Need for intensive respiratory monitoring with arterial PCO_2 30 to 35 mm Hg
- Neurologic monitoring for ongoing neurologic deterioration related to cerebral edema or reperfusion
- Ischemic stroke at high risk for neurologic deterioration
- Treatment with IV or intraarterial thrombolytic agents with aggressive blood pressure management and observation for signs and symptoms of hemorrhage
- Sedation: morphine or diazepam (Valium) as needed
- Anticonvulsants as needed (see Chapter 24)
- Maintain blood chemistries within normal limits (WNL)
- Maintain normothermia
- Nutritional support within 24 hours after clearance by dysphagia screening
- Immobilization: neuromuscular paralysis as needed
- Management of ICP if needed (see Chapter 10)
- Standard of care: Patients receiving IV or intraarterial tPA are monitored during and after the procedure in an ICU

Assessment

The findings on neurologic assessment will reveal clinical findings and neurologic changes in relation to the area of the brain that is injured. The patient may exhibit focal or global signs and symptoms. The Glasgow Coma Scale score or LOC in patients with stroke may range from alert and oriented to a comatose state (see FOUR score in Chapter 2). After establishing an admission baseline, the focused assessment may include the following:

- Neurologic assessment: Performed hourly for the first 4 hours, every 2 hours for the next 8 hours, and every 4 hours thereafter (A change in status could necessitate assessment every 15 minutes)
- TPA protocol: All tPA recipients have specific assessment guidelines for early detection of an

TABLE 17-6	Guidelines for Prevention of Stroke in Patients With Acute Ischemic Stroke or Transient Ischemic Attack
Risk Factor	**Treatment Recommendations**
Hypertension: high blood pressure is 140/90, and normal blood pressure is less than 120/80; goals should be tailored to each patient.	Lifestyle modifications such as increased physical activity, weight management, and eating a heart-healthy diet can help reduce blood pressure. Reducing the systolic pressure by 10 mm Hg and the diastolic pressure by 5 mm Hg has proven beneficial. Although the best drug combination isn't known, evidence supports using diuretics alone or by combination of diuretics and an angiotension-converting enzyme (ACE) inhibitor. Just like the goals, choice of drugs should be individualized to patients depending on the particular characteristics.
Diabetes: Patients with diabetes must tightly control blood pressure and lipids (cholesterol and triglycerides). Glucose should be controlled to near-normal levels.	The goal of HbA1c, a test that measures blood sugar control over time, is less than 7%. More rigorous control of blood pressure should be considered in all patients with diabetes. Although all major classes of antihypertensives are suitable for blood pressure control, most patients will require more than one agent. ACE inhibitors and angiotensin receptor blockers (ARBs) are more effective in reducing the progression of renal disease and are recommended as first-choice medications. Lipids (e.g., cholesterol) should be rigorously controlled. Glucose control is recommended to near-normoglycemic levels among diabetics with AIS or TIA to reduce microvascular complications.
Cholesterol: Patients with high cholesterol and coronary artery disease or atherosclerosis should follow lifestyle modifications, dietary guidelines, and medication recommendations according to National Cholesterol Education Program (NCEP) III(ATP III) guidelines.	Statin drugs are recommended; the goal is an LDL-C of less than 100 mg/dl for those with coronary heart disease (CHD) or atherosclerotic disease and an LDL-C of less than 70 mg/dl for individuals at very high with multiple risk factors. Patients whose stroke or TIA was likely caused by atherosclerosis may still be treated with statins for those without elevated cholesterol levels. Patients with a low HDL-C (under age 40 for men or age 50 for women) may be considered for treatment with niacin or gemfibrozil, an antihyperlipidemic.
Smoking	Advise patients to stop smoking. Avoid secondhand smoke. Counseling, nicotine products, and oral smoking cessation programs can be effective in helping smokers to quit.
Alcohol	Heavy drinkers should eliminate or reduce their alcohol consumption. No more than two drinks per day for men; one drink per day for nonpregnant women.
Obesity	A weight-reduction and management program to reach a body mass index (BMI) goal of from 18.5 to 24.9 kg/m^2 or a waist circumference of less than 35 inches for women and less than 40 inches for men.
Physical inactivity	Recommend at least 30 minutes of physical activity daily. Patients with one or more disabilities may benefit from a supervised therapeutic exercise regimen.

Modified from Sacco RL, Adams R, Albers G, et al: Guidelines for prevention of stroke in patients with ischemic stroke or transient ischemic attack, *Stroke* 37(2):577-617, 2006; http://stroke.ahajounrals.org/cgi/reprintframed/37/2/577? (accessed August 2006); and *Stroke Connection,* July/August, 26-27, 2006.

intracranial bleed, which may include decrease in Glasgow Coma Scale score, vomiting, headache, hematuria, gastrointestinal (GI) bleed, abdominal pain, ecchymosis, hematoma, or bleeding from IV sites
- NIHSS: Administered per protocol every 12 hours to assess stroke deficit and any neurologic changes (see Table 17-5).
- Continuous ECG monitoring: Performed after completion of a 12-lead ECG
- Pulse oximetry
- Vital signs: Noninvasive and invasive with arterial line if needed for close control of blood pressure and arterial blood gas (ABG) studies
- Pulmonary artery catheter, if needed, to monitor cardiac output
- EEG monitoring: If needed to detect and treat seizures
- TCD: To monitor for vasospasm

- Cardiac monitoring because catecholamine release may trigger arrhythmias
- Meningeal signs may appear when there is blood in the subarachnoid space
- Symptoms of hydrocephalus may result from hemorrhage with decreased LOC and cranial nerve deficits
- Dysphagia screening: Perform on all AIS patients before giving food or drink

According to the Agency for Healthcare Research and Quality (AHRQ), 27% to 50% of stroke patients develop dysphagia, to include aspiration pneumonia (43% to 54%) and malnutrition (37%) that increased length of hospital stay. Clinicians and physicians may be taught formal screening procedures for assessing dysphagia. Otherwise, the speech therapist should be consulted to evaluate the patient, because 70% of all dysphagia is "silent." In some hospitals dysphagia screening is initiated while the patient is in the ED.

Interventions

Interventions in acute care include:
- Bowel and bladder: Indwelling urinary catheter should be avoided to prevent urinary tract infection (UTI)
- DVT/pulmonary embolism (PE): Use of intermittent compression device (ICD) unless anticoagulated
- Fall precautions: Assessment and following of hospital policy (A fall by a patient who is anticoagulated could be fatal)
- Head of bed: Elevation to 30 degrees to avoid aspiration

Fluid management may be continued with IV isotonic solutions. Glucose solutions are not recommended. Hyperglycemia in AIS patients increases cerebral infarct size and worsens neurologic outcome with and without preexisting DM. Hyperglycemia results from metabolic alterations in glucose metabolism and is common in stroke patients. Strict control of hyperglycemia with intensive insulin therapy has been shown to dramatically decrease hospital morbidity and mortality, inpatient stays, hospital costs, and most importantly neurologic injury.[60] The routine use of aspirin or clopidogrel (Plavix) within 48 hours of stroke may be ordered to reduce the risk of recurrent strokes or early death.[53] The patient should be kept normothermic.

Potential Complications After Stroke Treatment

The most important and significant potential complication after treatment for stroke is hemorrhage. Hemorrhage may occur secondary to thrombolytic therapy or reperfusion injury. It occurs most commonly in the brain distal to the occlusion. Close monitoring is needed to quickly identify and rapidly respond to complications that may include cerebral edema, IICP, respiratory distress, hydrocephalus, seizures from injury to the brain (which complicate the stroke), MI that may be caused by decreased myocardial perfusion, DVT, PE, skin breakdown with pressure ulcers, dehydration, hyponatremia, incontinence, congestive heart failure (CHF), metabolic abnormalities, and infections (e.g., pneumonia from aspiration, UTI). It is now known that pathologic changes in the CNS begin when perfusion pressure drops.

Subcutaneous unfractionated heparin, low-molecular-weight heparins, and heparinoids may be considered for DVT prophylaxis in at-risk patients with AIS, recognizing that nonpharmacologic treatments for DVT prevention exist. The risk of these agents must be weighed against the risk of systemic and ICH.[3]

Complications may include cranial nerve deficits, occasional MI, and, rarely, subsequent stroke. Immediate investigation is mandated for any neurologic or cardiac deterioration. Feeding tube complications may be significant for patients with a decreased LOC and at risk for aspiration. The potential risk for UTI, pneumonia, pressure ulcers, seizures, and GI bleed should alert clinicians to monitor closely for the earliest signs and symptoms. Hydrocephalus may complicate recovery in a small number of individuals.

Pain Management. Pain is common after a stroke and requires a thorough assessment to determine the source, severity, and potential to interfere with recovery as a major disability. Routine pain management based on individual needs for AIS is usually adequate. A stroke in the region of the thalamus or brainstem can cause more pronounced pain. During recovery and rehabilitation, pain assessment should be evaluated and treated to locate the source and type of pain (e.g., nociceptive, neuropathic) (see Chapter 23). Pain can be secondary to musculoskeletal changes, contractures, extreme fatigue, spasticity, or injury sustained at the time of stroke. Musculoskeletal pain is common and may involve the shoulders and hands. Limb pain can be managed with analgesics, antiinflammatory medications, and physical modalities, including range of motion (ROM) exercises and orthotic devices for support.[16]

Central post-stroke pain (CPSP) caused by a thalamic lesion is estimated to occur in 8% to 16% of patients. CPSP is an example of **neuropathic** pain. Symptoms include paroxysmal burning, hyperpathia (heightened painful response to noxious stimuli), and allodynia (interpretation of normally nonpainful stimuli as painful). The clinical features of CPSP may be vague and difficult for the individual to describe, poorly localized, and worse when touched.[10] Modalities include desensitization techniques, transcutaneous electrical nerve stimulation (TENS) unit, acupuncture, biofeedback, and relaxation techniques. Pharmacologic interventions include acetaminophen, nonsteroidal antiinflammatory drugs (NSAIDs), and anticonvulsants such as gabapentin or lamotrigine. Other pain medications may include opioids, tramadol (Tramal), antispasm medications, and topical lidocaine or capsaicin. Antidepressants are commonly prescribed for CPSP and may facilitate endogenous inhibition of pain. First-line agents include gabapentin, topical lidocaine, antidepressants, tramadol, and opioids.[10]

Hemiplegic shoulder pain (HSP) occurs in 16% to 84% of stroke survivors. HSP results in an increased length of stay and a reduced quality of life. HSP can be caused by subluxation, rotator cuff disorders, adhesive capsulitis, impingement syndrome, tendonitis, or complex regional pain syndrome. Clinicians can pay attention to positioning and therapists can offer taping, therapeutic exercises with ROM, or functional electrical stimulation (FES). Botox injections and oral spasticity medications (e.g., baclofen) are additional interventions. In extreme cases, surgical interventions for rotator cuff repair, muscle release, and other procedures may offer relief.

Health Teaching. Patient and family education focuses on the original medical conditions and risk factors that may have contributed to the patient's stroke. These include issues such as uncontrolled hypertension and diabetes, risky behaviors, unhealthy lifestyle, poor diet, smoking, and excessive alcohol consumption. Reinforcement to seek immediate medical care for the signs and symptoms of a stroke is crucial because of the known increased morbidity and mortality from a second stroke. Verbal and written information that shows how to modify and eliminate risk factors to prevent subsequent strokes should be provided as soon as appropriate. Teaching may include a review of new medications and rehabilitation. Teaching also includes preventive treatment with medications that may be prescribed for life and that require close follow-up with the patient's health care provider to monitor total compliance and possible side effects.

Nutritional Considerations

Patients often experience **dysphagia** (difficulty swallowing) after a stroke. These symptoms often go unrecognized. Failure to detect dysphagia can lead to dehydration, malnutrition, aspiration pneumonia, or even death. The incidence of pneumonia is decreased in hospitals with formal dysphagia screening programs for all patients with AIS. A swallowing evaluation should be performed before oral intake.[29] Algorithms can facilitate early swallowing assessment. Dysphagia management delays may lead to aspiration pneumonia, a life-threatening complication.[80] Assessment may include the following:

- Dysphagia: Monitor for dysphagia and respond quickly if the patient appears to suffer from coughing or has a wet-sounding and gurgling voice during or after eating or drinking
- Weight: Weigh frequently to determine weight loss because of slow eating or repetitive bouts of pneumonia
- Aspiration: Use aspiration precautions with the patient seated upright when eating or out of bed
    Patients should also be considered for the following:
- Decreased or absent gag reflex: This increases the risk of aspiration and subsequent pneumonia

- Congestion after oral intake: Does the patient have identifiable voice changes with breathy, strangled, or hoarse voice?
- Swallow: Does the patient have a swallow as evidenced by the rise and fall of the larynx?
- Cough: Can the patient cough on demand versus coughing on his or her own secretions?
- Duration: Is the patient slow in eating, taking multiple swallows of a single mouthful of food?
- Fatigue factor: Is the patient too tired to eat and exhibits shortness of breath while eating?

In general, dysphagia is more severe when there is brainstem injury or a prolonged coma. The existence and extent of swallowing impairment depends on the site and extent of the stroke. In most cases, bilateral cerebral dysfunction is required for marked and prolonged impairment in the ability to eat.

Enteral Tube Feedings. Enteral feedings are usually required if oral nutrition is inadequate because of alterations in the LOC, documented aspiration, or dysphagia. Several factors affect the decision to begin enteral feedings. These include the presence of a treatable underlying disease, an inability to eat sufficient quantities of food, and a functioning GI tract. In contrast to many other hospitalized patients at risk for malnutrition, the neurologic patient generally has a normal GI tract and therefore is often an ideal candidate for enteral nutrition. After the decision has been made to feed a patient enterally, the site and route of nutrient delivery must be decided. The risk of aspiration and the anticipated amount of time the patient will require tube feedings are pivotal considerations.

Routes of Administration. Tube feeding can be delivered into the stomach or directly into the small intestine (duodenum or jejunum) (Table 17-7). The pyloric sphincter is the barrier between the stomach and duodenum and prevents the reflux of foodstuffs into the stomach. The primary reason for postpyloric tube feeding in the neurologic patient is the high risk for aspiration. The risk for aspiration is high when there is an absent gag or cough reflex or delayed gastric emptying. **Gastric feedings** can be administered by either nasogastric or gastrostomy tube. The anticipated amount of time the patient will require tube feedings is the primary factor. **Nasogastric feedings** are for short-term feedings in which

TABLE 17-7	Techniques of Feeding Administration	
Technique	**Rate of Administration**	**Comments**
Bolus (syringe method)	Rapid infusion (less than 10 min/feeding) 4–6 feedings/day, usually given 3–4 hours apart 250–500 ml/feeding	Associated with frequent GI complications Not recommended for patients at high risk for aspiration
Intermittent	Slow gravity drip (using a feeding bag) 4–6 feedings/day given over 30 minutes to 1 hour Less than 400 ml/feeding	Fewer GI complications than with bolus method but prone to accidental bolus
Continuous	Pump-assisted or slow gravity drip Formula infused over 16–24 hours/day In general, less than 150 ml/hour	Associated with fewer GI complications Required for small-bowel feedings

GI, Gastrointestinal.

the patient has a relatively low risk for aspiration. The best tubes are small-bore enteral feeding tubes, which are less irritating and may reduce the risk for aspiration because they produce less compromise of the lower esophageal sphincter.

Patients who require enteral feedings on a long-term basis (more than 2 to 3 months) should have a **gastrostomy tube** placed. Patient comfort and reduced risk of tubes being dislodged or pulled are two major advantages of a gastrostomy tube. Gastrostomy tubes can be placed either surgically or via endoscopy. The **percutaneous endoscopic gastrostomy (PEG)** has several advantages. It does not require the use of a general anesthetic, it is less costly, and feedings can be initiated within 24 hours after tube placement. In addition, the equipment can be placed at the bedside, which can be a major advantage in the ICU.

If postpyloric tube feeding is required, nasoduodenal or nasojejunal tubes can be placed provided the duration of feeding is anticipated to be less than 2 to 3 months. These tubes can be placed under endoscopy or fluoroscopy to ensure proper placement. Many available tubes have weighted tips that are designed to help the tube pass into the small intestine. These are often given with gastric motility stimulants and with the patient lying on the right side to aid tube passage. These tubes often remain in the stomach after attempts at placement. A major disadvantage of nasointestinal tubes is that they can easily become dislodged and thus become nasogastric tubes. If a patient requires long-term enteral nutrition and is at high risk for aspiration, a gastrostomy tube should be placed and a jejunostomy tube should be passed through the gastrostomy tube (gastrojejunostomy). This provides a separate gastric port to check for regurgitation, provide gastric suction, or administer medications. Jejunostomy tubes also can be placed surgically. Needle catheter jejunostomy tubes are used less often because they have an extremely narrow lumen and are therefore prone to clogging.

Techniques of Feeding Administration. Patients who are fed directly into the stomach have several options of administration: bolus, intermittent, or continuous infusion. Patients requiring small bowel feedings are limited to continuous infusion.

Postacute and Nonacute Care

Assessment

Not all stroke survivors require intensive care intervention. For those who do, early mobilization; passive exercise to maintain joint mobility; cognitive retraining and socialization; improved nutrition; prevention of pressure sores and contractures; and maintenance of normal eating, elimination, and grooming habits should begin immediately. Discharge planning should begin at once. Family assessment should start with the first encounter. Interventions and management may vary but should be tailored for each patient in accordance with the following information.

Routine postoperative step-down and nonacute care is provided overnight and may include the following[32]:
- Neuroassessment and vital signs: Monitor every hour for 12 to 18 hours and notify the surgeon of any neurologic deterioration

- Blood pressure: Monitor and report abnormalities based on ordered parameters; administer and titrate antihypertensive drugs as ordered
- Pulse: Monitor for bradycardia and administer drugs (e.g., atropine) per protocol
- Postoperative bleeding: Monitor and report immediately
- Incision: Monitor for hemorrhage or bleeding and apply pressure until the surgeon arrives
- Airway and breathing: Observe closely and monitor for neck swelling, airway obstruction, or stridor
- Intake and output (I&O): Monitor fluid deficit and overload
- Pain management: Follow physician preference based on individual patient needs
- Activity: Perform a fall assessment and then allow the patient out of bed as tolerated with safety precautions; elevate the head of the bed at least 30 degrees unless ordered otherwise
- Anticoagulant: Use depends on physician's preference
- Diet: Provide as tolerated; patient may require a special diet (e.g., low fat)

After the stroke survivor becomes medically stable, the nursing care emphasis changes. Constant vigilance for changes in neurologic and vital function status continues throughout the acute and rehabilitation phases of recovery because stroke patients have a high risk for rebleeding, new embolic events, and other life-threatening events (e.g., MI, pneumonia, DVT, PE, cardiac or respiratory arrest). The emphasis is now on increasing mobility, endurance, and learning to prepare the patient for active rehabilitation and/or a return to the community.

Health Teaching

General health teaching needs initiated in the acute phase are reinforced. Teaching may differ for the patient and family based on the type of stroke. The following are general patient teaching needs during postacute and nonacute care:
- Explain the physical and mental changes thereby reducing anxiety, promoting coping, engendering motivation to get well, and forestalling depression.
- Help the patient understand the procedures or regimens being used, as well as their rationale or need.
- Begin rehabilitation education and promote patient involvement in recovery so the patient learns team approaches to care.
- Develop strategies to mobilize positive coping mechanisms or adapt previously successful coping mechanisms.
- Help the patient understand the stroke experience and its potential effects on the future. Address the patient's fears and lack of correct information and identify resources.

Families have similar needs. In some cases, they have higher levels of cognitive functioning than the patient in the very acute phase. Therefore the content and depth of the teaching may differ. In addition, the family needs to (1) be made part of the rehabilitation team and learn their role, (2) have help in learning about changes that the stroke will cause in their social and personal roles, (3) identify the available personal and community resources, and (4) have help in handling the fears and stresses produced by their changed status.

Nutritional Considerations

Nutrition is a primary concern at this stage of recovery. Stroke survivors have many sources of altered nutritional patterns. Nearly one third of stroke survivors experience swallowing problems, difficulty chewing, difficulty with pocketing of food, aspiration, GI bleeding, or malnutrition.

The clinician should assess the patient's nutritional status, personal preferences, and needs. From this assessment, the clinician should develop a plan with the nutritionist to provide an optimal caloric supply. Hypermetabolic states may require total parenteral nutritional (TPN) supplements or oral supplementary feedings. Feeding complications may necessitate supplemental caloric intake. This need may continue for several months.

Small meals of preferred foods should be offered in a pleasant, unhurried atmosphere. Dignity and privacy are needed while the patient is relearning eating tasks. In addition, allowing the patient to help in the process of opening containers and cutting foods aids in fostering independence. Families often can provide the socialization needed to increase appetite and simultaneously aid in the prolonged feedings. Rather than adhering to a strict temporal schedule for the sake of convenience, meal scheduling should be flexible so that food is presented when the stroke survivor is hungry. Getting the patient up and out of bed to eat improves appetite, but presenting food after long, tiring periods of exercise or sitting may reduce it.

The clinician should check the temperature of food to prevent the patient from burning his or her mouth or tongue when feeding and to increase pleasure by ensuring that foods are served at the appropriate temperature. The clinician should check whether the food is appropriate for the diet ordered and whether the intake recording is accurate.

The patient's head is positioned forward and to the unaffected side, and food is placed toward the back of the mouth to aid in moving the food bolus to the pharynx. Offering small bits of food or foods with thicker consistency rather than clear, thin liquids may reduce choking. In patients with facial weakness, the clinician should check the mouth for "pouched" food in the cheek, assess for pieces of unswallowed food that may later be aspirated, and assess for lesions or dentition that interferes with chewing.

Disability in the dominant hand requires new spatial and motor learning. Neglect caused by the infarct may further inhibit learning the new skills. The clinician should assess the patient's coordination, tremor, muscular strength, smoothness of movement, and ability to find and use utensils. If a patient needs to learn new eating skills, he or she may be unable to eat without repeated cueing and supervision. Supervision during feeding is necessary until patients have an established eating habit. Encouragement during meals helps socialization and makes supervision more acceptable. An occupational therapist can be particularly helpful in choosing useful assistive devices when needed.

Prevention of choking and aspiration are the primary goals of acute care. As the stroke survivor begins to recover, measures to increase appetite and intake are important adjuncts. Changes in appetite are in part centrally mediated and may be directly affected by the infarcted area. More commonly, a loss of appetite is secondary to difficulty in swallowing, a loss of smell or taste, increased choking, the loss of the gag reflex, a change in the food presented, an acute illness response, and frustration with trying to relearn how to feed oneself. Poor dentition may affect appetite. Therefore the clinician should provide oral hygiene to prevent mucosal and tongue lesions. Cognitive or behavioral deficits can cause poor intake through problems with attentional deficits, confusion, distractibility, and inability to concentrate. Depression also may cause a loss of appetite.

A recent study to evaluate the nutritional value and health benefits of fruit and vegetable consumption on risk of stroke studies in North American, Europe, and Japan supports the recommendation to eat fruit and vegetables to lower the risk of stroke. In contrast, there was no significant reduction in stroke rates with only vegetable consumption.[17]

Before adding any herbal supplements to their regimen, patients recovering from stroke should discuss the use of herbal supplements with their health care providers and/or nutritionist. Herbal supplements are being used by an increasing number of patients who typically do not share this information with their treating providers. The addition of garlic or feverfew, for example, has been found to inhibit platelet aggregation, whereas ginkgo biloba enhances the effect of warfarin/aspirin.[20] An estimated 10.8 million Americans take ginkgo biloba daily.[7]

General Care

Bowel and Bladder Management. Incontinence is one of the strongest predictors of institutionalization after stroke. Stroke survivors can learn bladder and/or bowel retention and control through careful toileting routines, appropriate stool softeners and suppositories, hydration, diet, and exercise. Bladder incontinence is usually caused by an uninhibited neurogenic bladder that results from damage to the cerebral cortex. Urinary frequency, urgency, and reflex voiding characterize the lack of inhibitory control caused by stroke. Wetness, prolonged sitting and lying, and an inability to care for the skin in the perineal area predispose these patients to decubitus ulcers, which can seriously curtail the rehabilitation process. The use of an indwelling urinary catheter, which can increase the risk of infection, should be avoided.

Safety. Immobile neurologic patients are in danger of injury from falls, perceptual accidents (e.g., bumping into furniture or door frames), accidents of all sorts, and errors of judgment and cognition (e.g., wandering, impulsivity). The clinician should complete a fall assessment and adhere to hospital policies for fall prevention. Seizure activity puts the patient at risk for injury.

Spatial disorders resulting from stroke present as safety factors and may interfere with the patient's ability to determine where he or she is in space. Spatial disorders are caused by altered perception, transmission, or integration of external input. Tactile alterations may produce an inability to feel pain, heat, touch, or joint position or may cause a decreased awareness of these sensations. **Anosognosia,** a condition caused by parietal lesions of the nondominant side, may lead the stroke survivor to deny the stroke, especially on the contralateral side. Most often this is labeled as **"neglect"** and is seen when the patient ignores the left side of the body, disclaims the arm and leg as part of the body, or does not recognize objects to the left even though vision is unimpaired.

Apraxias occur when voluntary motor activities are not completed on command in the presence of normal coordination, sensation, comprehension, and attention. This is a loss of the perception of the use of an object, or an inability to perform purposeful acts, even though it is understood (e.g., grooming the hair with a comb and instead using a toothbrush). Patients can sometimes carry out the activity when given an object (e.g., a comb) that they recognize.

Clinical Management for Secondary Prevention of Stroke

Medications to prevent recurrent ischemia involve antihypertensives, anticoagulation, and blood thinners (antiplatelet and antithrombotic agents).

Antihypertensives. Hypertension is the leading contributor to the causes of stroke. The management of blood pressure is controversial. The management of hypertension should depend on the cause of AIS. Elevated blood pressure may be a compensatory mechanism to perfuse the brain and to open and maintain collateral circulation. This type of blood pressure elevation is transient and usually declines without treatment. Unless the patient is dramatically hypertensive, conservative treatment is recommended. The head of bed can be elevated and short-term, titratable agents used (e.g., sodium nitroprusside, labetalol, nicardipine, esmolol). They are usually started with very low doses and titrated according to desired parameters to achieve a slow and modest reduction in blood pressure to avoid decreased cerebral perfusion.

Diuretics should be avoided except in the setting of acute and compromising heart failure.[59] The use of sublingual nifedipine should be avoided because of its unpredictable hypotensive effect. Treatment is imperative for hypertensive emergencies with systolic pressure greater than 230 mm Hg or diastolic pressure greater than 140 mm Hg.

It has been suggested that the right hemisphere may be the site for sympathetic cardiac autonomic control. Changes noted in the blood pressure of patients with AIS in the right hemisphere have been observed to have greater increases in sympathetic discharge. The left hemisphere may possibly influence some of the parasympathetic responses.

Anticoagulation. Because anticoagulants and antiplatelet agents are effective in long-term care and because most strokes are secondary to clot formation, there has been a strong interest in the use of anticoagulant, antiplatelet, and other medications for preventive management in stroke (Fig. 17-6). Anticoagulant drugs act at the tissue level where injury to the vessel wall produces a clotting cascade, including platelet activation and activation of thrombin by proteins C and S. These drugs interfere with clot formation. By understanding the clotting cascade, the clinician will better understand where and how each of the drugs to be described works and the type of management that must be given in administering and monitoring them.

Although the current data show that rapidly acting antithrombotic agents have a limited role in the immediate treatment of patients with AIS, research continues. There is some evidence that fixed, subcutaneous unfractionated heparin reduces early recurrent ischemic strokes; however, this benefit is negated by a concomitant increase in the occurrence of hemorrhage. Therefore, the use of subcutaneous unfractionated heparin is not recommended for decreasing the risk of death or stroke-related morbidity or for preventing early stroke recurrence. IV unfractionated heparin or high-dose low-molecular-weight heparin/heparinoids are not recommended for any specific subgroup of patients with AIS that is based on any presumed stroke mechanism or location.[3]

Aspirin is one of the most frequently studied antiplatelet options. Aspirin decreases the synthesis of thromboxane A_2 (a powerful vasoconstrictor and platelet aggregator) in the platelet arachidonate pathway. The platelets are irreversibly affected and the amount of time before the antiaggregate effect ceases depends on platelet turnover (approximately 10 days). The use of aspirin early in treatment is beneficial for a wide range of patients. Its prompt use should be routinely considered for all patients with suspected AIS, mainly to reduce the risk of early recurrence.[12] Recent guidelines recommend that patients with AIS presenting within 48 hours of symptom onset should be given aspirin (160 to 325 mg/day) to reduce stroke mortality and decrease morbidity, provided there are no contraindications (e.g., allergy or GI bleeding is absent and the patient has not been or will not be treated with tPA).[3]

Aspirin has been shown to reduce the risk of stroke or death by about 30%. It may be started during acute care and in combination with or instead of antithrombotic drugs (heparin and warfarin sodium). The major aspirin clinical trials (Ticlopidine Aspirin Stroke Study [TASS], Canadian American Ticlopidine Study [CATS]) agree that the use of aspirin reduces subsequent TIAs by approximately 20% to 22%.[23,27] Daily doses of 325 mg/day may be prescribed. A low dose of aspirin (75 mg/day) is tolerated better and is as effective in some cases. A dose of 25 mg/per day may be effective in selected situations. The Warfarin-Aspirin Symptomatic Intracranial Disease (WASID) Study stopped the trial early because patients receiving warfarin had a higher rate of adverse events and the warfarin therapy proved to be no more effective than high-dose aspirin. Other clinicians have added that warfarin was not even effective as backup in preventing a second stroke after aspirin therapy failed to prevent a first stroke. Based on the WASID trial, experts recommend using aspirin in place of warfarin for intracranial stenosis.[69]

Patients must be taught about the adverse effects so they know when to notify their health care provider. In one study, stroke survivors who stopped taking their daily prescribed aspirin tripled their risk of having another stroke within the month, suggesting that patients and health care providers should be informed about this potential risk, with more research needed.[33] The risks of aspirin therapy include GI bleeding and intracranial bleeding.

Clopidogrel (Plavix) is an antiplatelet agent or platelet aggregation inhibitor. Recommendations of up to a once-

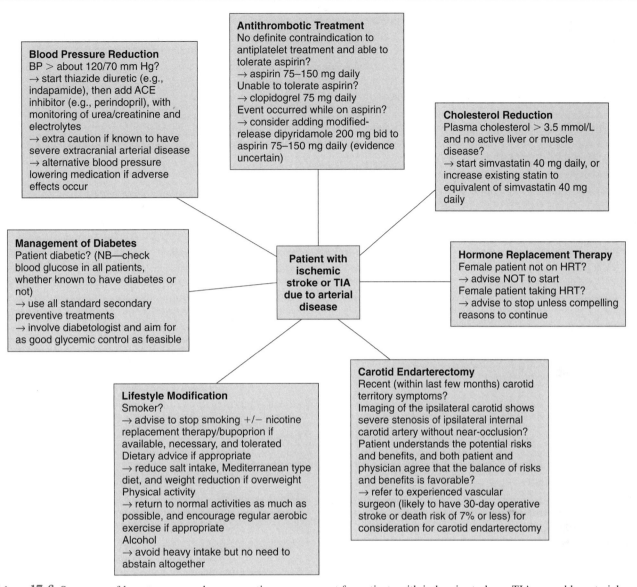

Figure 17-6 Summary of long-term secondary prevention management for patients with ischemic stroke or TIA caused by arterial disease.
(From Mohr JP, Choi DW, Grotta JC, Wolf P, editors: Stroke: pathophysiology, diagnosis, and management, ed 4, Philadelphia, 2004, Churchill Livingstone, p 1146.)

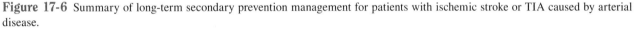

daily dosing of one 75-mg/day tablet (with or without food) may be prescribed to reduce the risk of stroke in high-risk patients.[56] Blood work to measure liver function and blood studies are necessary for patients with past liver disease and for long-term therapy (e.g., aspartate aminotransferase [AST], alanine aminotransferase [ALT], bilirubin, creatinine, CBC, hematocrit [HCT], hemoglobin [Hb], and PT).[56] Rash and diarrhea are the major adverse effects of clopidogrel.

Aggrenox, an antiplatelet drug (25 mg aspirin/200 mg extended-release dipyridamole) has been approved by the FDA to help reduce the risk of stroke in some patients after ischemic stroke or TIA caused by thrombosis. The antithrombotic action is the result of additive antiplatelet effects.[55] Earlier studies were convincing that Aggrenox was better than aspirin alone in preventing the risk of a recurring stroke.

Side effects include headache, abdominal pain, dizziness, and nausea.

Other Pharmacologic Interventions

Anticonvulsants

The use of **anticonvulsants** for seizure control must be carefully evaluated. The rate of epileptic seizures in the acute setting is estimated to be between 4% and 15%. These early seizures within the first 3 days may be attributed to expressions of acute cytotoxic or metabolic events from the ischemia. Seizures may range from a single seizure to uncontrolled status epilepticus. Antiepileptic therapy (e.g., phenytoin, lorazepam) is advised (see Chapter 24).

Neuroprotectants

The administration of neuroprotective drugs early after symptom onset to block the release of excitatory amino acids has been studied. During cerebral ischemia, there is excessive activity of excitatory amino acids, especially glutamate. The activation of glutamate receptors leads to a marked increase in intracellular calcium, which in turn leads to the activation of intracellular enzymes and neuronal death—the excitotoxic cascade. Glutamate receptors are attractive targets for neuroprotective drugs because glutamate plays a central role in the excitotoxic cascade. Several approaches to protection have failed in clinical trials. Recovery could be improved if patients could receive neuroprotective drugs immediately after the onset of stroke. There is great hope that future research efforts will provide treatment.[47]

ALERT: **Ginkgo biloba,** an herb, is the world's oldest living species and has a history of more than 200 million years. Ginkgo has been purported to increase blood flow by vasodilating arteries, capillaries, and veins; to act as a platelet activating factor antagonist; and to prevent membrane damage caused by free radicals. The bulb of the *Allium sativum,* or **garlic,** has been found to prolong bleeding and clotting time, increase fibrinolytic activities, and inhibit collagen-induced platelet aggregation. Warfarin (Coumadin) therapy can be exacerbated by these two herbs. Therefore, patients should be advised to stop taking them before procedures and while undergoing anticoagulation therapy.

Rehabilitation

Stroke rehabilitation is one of the most common rehabilitation diagnoses. Multiple treatment options to return the individual back to a functioning level may involve physical therapy, occupational therapy, speech therapy, cognitive and respiratory therapy, psychiatry and psychology services, nutrition, education, and aquatic and recreational therapies.[19] Age-related decline in muscle mass and decreased upper and lower body strength and endurance can create difficulties for older adults after stroke. The rehabilitation plan of care includes specific rehabilitation techniques, drug treatment, and stroke awareness for secondary stroke prevention. Having a stroke is one of the most significant risk factors for having another stroke.

Hemiplegia can be the most disabling primary neurologic disorder caused by stroke, followed by spasticity and aphasias. Neurologic fatigue syndrome or poststroke fatigue may limit intensity and frequency of participation. Patients recovering from stroke may continue to have preexisting medical conditions that originally contributed to their stroke (e.g., cardiac disease) that may inhibit participation or cause more complications than the stroke. Other painful conditions, such as osteoarthritis, can interfere with stroke rehabilitation and recovery. Physical therapy, occupational therapy, speech therapy, and neuropsychological testing can be performed after the acute phase to relearn lost motor activities; relearn activities of daily living (ADLs); relearn language and communication skills; and evaluate and treat memory, executive function, intelligence, and emotional and other behaviors. The combination of rehabilitation, **spontaneous recovery,** and the **plasticity** of the brain to take over lost functions promotes recovery for stroke survivors to regain some or all lost functions.

Steps to Recovery

Poststroke depression is well recognized with symptoms of sadness, anhedonia (inability to experience pleasure), feelings of worthlessness, agitation, or even suicide. Results of testing are used to plan for recovery and integration back to home and community.

Stroke rehabilitation begins during the acute hospitalization at the time of diagnosis and after stabilization of life-threatening problems. A physical conditioning program is implemented to regain prestroke functioning, prevent complications of immobility, and restore the individual to the highest level of function (see Chapter 13). The AHA and the ASA endorse stroke rehabilitation guidelines developed by the Veterans Administration (VA) Department of Defense (DOD).[73] The guidelines promote the concept that patients do better with a well-organized approach to postacute stroke care in a multidisciplinary rehabilitation setting or stroke unit. This rehabilitation process should begin with early evaluation with the NIHSS; aggressive rehabilitation as soon as possible after diagnosis; swallowing evaluation for dysphagia, which can cause pneumonia and death; active prevention of secondary stroke; and aggressive prophylaxis against venous thrombi.

Evaluation by members of the rehabilitation team promotes early spontaneous recovery from stroke and includes a rehabilitation plan of care. A stroke multidisciplinary team includes nurses, physicians, physical therapists, occupational therapists, kinesiotherapists, speech/language therapists, psychologists, recreational therapists, patients, and family members or caregivers. Problems to be addressed include cognition, weakness/paresis/paralysis, balance and coordination, language (aphasia), dysarthria, and neglect. Early rehabilitation for 3 or more weeks in an organized stroke unit not only shortens the patient's time in the hospital but also increases the rate of discharge to the patient's own home. The incidence of pneumonia as a complication also decreases. Early rehabilitation seems to be highly advantageous. Therefore, it is recommended that the rehabilitation staff be involved—even in the acute phase of stroke in the stroke unit.[75]

The following are the goals of stroke rehabilitation[26]:
- Prevent complications
- Minimize impairments
- Improve and maximize function
- Achieve maximal self-sufficiency
- Improve quality of life
- Control risk factors
- Modify social and vocational environment

Athletes and musicians recover from stroke faster than others because they may have hypertrophy of the motor portion of the brain. They know how to train and are extremely motivated to get back to normal by practicing with vigor and commitment.[43] All patients should be encouraged to become active participants and take charge of their recovery.

Because stroke survivors are often deconditioned and predisposed to a sedentary lifestyle that limits performance of ADLs, increases the risk of falls, and may contribute to a heightened risk for recurrent stroke, participation in exercise training and physical activity is needed.

Spasticity

Spasticity may affect up to 65% of stroke survivors. It is a velocity-dependent disorder of muscle tone; that is, the faster an extremity is moved, the greater the tone or resistance exhibited by the muscles. It is speculated that spasticity is a result of injury to the reticulospinal or corticospinal tracts or results from an imbalance between inhibitory and excitatory mechanisms.[72] Spasticity may begin days to weeks after the stroke. It may appear only in a few muscle groups or may be generalized and involve multiple muscle groups. Hypotonic or flaccid muscles start to regain muscle tone, gradually emerging as spasticity. Spasticity that is present in the lower extremities can interfere with ambulation[72] (see Chapter 13). Treatment for spasticity begins with noninvasive interventions (e.g., stretching, ROM) and progresses to more invasive modalities to include surgery.

Home Care

Stroke patients are especially vulnerable after they leave the acute care hospital or rehabilitation setting. A support group of peer survivors and families provides social support and opportunities to express thoughts and feelings to others who understand the needs that many stroke survivors experience after hospitalization. Meetings with special guest speakers and health care professionals who can offer education and coping strategies are helpful.

Stroke survivors can experience a variety of problems at home. The disabilities caused by stroke (e.g., paralysis and paresis, aphasia, dysphagia, ataxia, perceptual and behavioral deficiencies) can severely limit activity when added to premorbid deconditioning and chronic diseases such as diabetes, hypertension, arthritis, and cardiac disease. A speech pathologist can evaluate the patient's speech/language and ability to understand by testing verbal expression, writing ability, reading, and understanding of verbal expression. A physical therapist or occupational therapist can arrange a home visit to evaluate the physical changes related to movement and function in the home setting.

Home care of the disabled older adult is fragmented and is often unavailable. Caregivers often note that the decline is especially evident during the long-term care of patients who are no longer receiving outpatient therapies. After daily therapies are discontinued because the stroke survivor is no longer improving in function, caregivers (informal and formal) and stroke survivors cease these exercises; as a result, mobility is decreased. Rather than maintaining the level of function they have achieved, they begin to lose their abilities and enter a "sine wave" pattern of deconditioning, acute illness (usually pneumonia, decubitus ulcers), hospitalization, reinitiation of therapies, cessation of therapy because of plateau patterns, and acute illness.

This cycle is costly in both human and financial terms. Social isolation causes decreased stimulation and deteriorating mental health. Caregiver role strain (secondary to role changes, dependency needs of the stroke survivor, social isolation, and physical and mental fatigue) is a prominent feature of long-term care, especially in the home. The stroke survivor may not be able to ambulate 6 months or more after discharge from the acute facility. Devices to increase mobility often remain unused. The patient experiences deconditioning, contractures, and other evidence of deteriorating function. Coordinating services and nutrition in the home after hospital discharge can increase and maintain a patient's functional level, result in greater patient and family satisfaction, and require less use of acute care hospitals and nursing homes.

Malnutrition and dehydration are common in older adults with stroke. In addition to nutritional barriers, mobility problems further complicate the picture. An inability to toilet independently leads older adults to drink less fluid. Shopping and food preparation are impeded and safety in cooking areas decreases. The patient quickly becomes dehydrated and malnourished when he or she has no food to prepare, is unable to cook, and has difficulty chewing and swallowing (Box 17-4). Readmission to the hospital can become cyclical.

COMPREHENSIVE PATIENT MANAGEMENT

Older Adult Considerations

Stroke is clearly associated with age. Age is considered by some as a reason not to treat with IV tPA. TPA may not increase the risk of intracranial bleeding in those age 80 years and older. Although outcome may be worse compared with younger patients, it may be justifiable to use tPA in carefully selected old and very old patients using established protocols.

The 2000, the U.S. Census reported a 35% growth in the number of individuals 100 years of age and older, a 45% increase in the 90 to 94 age-group, and a 26% growth in the 80 to 84 age-group.[28,34] These figures on longevity play a big role in the number and needs of older adult stroke survivors. Their needs are similar to those of all other neurologically impaired older adults. They may have multiple concurrent medical diseases or disabilities (e.g., arthritis, Parkinson's disease, dementia) and medication regimens that are interactive and difficult to monitor. Their hospitalization can possibly be lengthened. The limitations in ADLs and instrumental ADLs (IADLs—basic activities necessary to live in the community) imposed by the stroke may be intensified by preexisting conditions such as musculoskeletal problems, dementia, or mental health problems. The stroke may be the final straw that changes their lifestyle to complete dependency.

Even with less severe consequences, stroke survivors attempting to adjust face the facts that both partners are often older, the physical demands of stroke patients can be very great for the aging caregiver, and failing mental capacities produce safety concerns. Financial problems also may be a deterrent to ongoing recovery. Limited income, a fragmentation of financial resources among state and federal agencies, and an inability to travel to offices or resources where financial problems can be addressed are among the more subtle barriers.

An estimated 30% of stroke survivors may have a second stroke within a year and 50% may suffer fatal strokes within 5 years.[28] Older adults have a higher incidence of concurrent heart disease, more rigid and fragile blood vessels, less

| BOX 17-4 | Home Care Nutritional Assessment |

Ideally, nutritional assessment and counseling is performed by a nutrition expert. Clinicians should be aware of and participate in this assessment. The patient's four stages of swallowing are evaluated by a nutritionist or speech pathologist:

1. Anticipatory: Voluntary decision on what to eat and when
2. Oral: Voluntary manipulation to break down food into smaller size
3. Pharyngeal: Involuntary reflexive protective action to propel the food bolus through the pharynx (the throat)
4. Esophageal: Involuntary guarding against the reflux of food and transporting the food bolus through the esophagus into the stomach

At a minimum, the initial nutritional assessment should include a swallowing evaluation to determine any impairment of the stages of deglutition (the act of swallowing), as well as the following:

- Review of usual weight range, with recent gain or loss
- Calculation of the desired weight and the necessary caloric intake and output to maintain it

- Review of a daily diet with emphasis on food preferences and methods of preparation
- Determination of level of education about nutrition, level of interest in participating in nutritional management, and understanding of present nutritional problems and their effect on health
- Neurologic and cranial nerve assessment of ability to chew, swallow, gag, taste, and smell food, as well as assessment of incoordination, mental status, neglect or inattention deficits, and perceptual and sensory deficits
- Physical assessment of skin, mucous membranes, physical proportions, lesions or rashes, bruises, sensory and perceptual deficits, cranial nerve deficits, muscle wasting or atrophy, and laboratory tests (e.g., HCT/Hb, electrolytes, lipids)
- History of concurrent diseases that may affect metabolism or nutrition (e.g., diabetes, ulcer disease, ulcerative colitis)
- Evaluation of oral hygiene, dentition, mouth, gums, and history or presence of GI problems
- Identification of options for help in shopping and preparing meals after discharge

HCT, Hematocrit; *Hb*, hemoglobin; *GI*, gastrointestinal.

vigorous circulation, and an increased incidence of systolic hypertension—all of which increase their risk of further stroke or death. This threat intensifies the normal losses of aging. Thus, the psychologic responses of depression, apathy, and anxiety are common.

Patients 80 years or older with AIS should be carefully evaluated. They should be considered for treatment with a tPA and not be excluded simply because of their age. In older adults, there is an increased risk of bleeding with thrombolytic therapy. Patients must be carefully selected and monitored.[56]

Defining normal blood pressure in older adults can be challenging. Generally systolic blood pressure below 120 mm Hg is considered normal as is diastolic blood pressure below 80 mm Hg. Prehypertension is a systolic pressure of 120 to 139 mm Hg and diastolic pressure of 80 to 89 mm Hg; hypertension is a systolic pressure of 140 mm Hg or higher and diastolic pressure of 90 mm Hg or higher. When both systolic and diastolic pressures are elevated, there is generally increased peripheral resistance. A 10 mm Hg difference between the right and left arm is abnormal. Orthostatic hypotension occurs when there is a drop between supine and standing blood pressure of 20 mm Hg systolic and 10 mm Hg diastolic.[50] Measuring blood pressure at frequent intervals and keeping a log is recommended for older adults taking prescription antihypertensive medications after stroke for prevention of recurrent strokes.

Case Management Considerations

Case management is most successful when initiated as early as possible and used throughout the entire course of the brain attack or stroke. The case manager may be the only health care professional consistently working with the patient and family throughout the illness. Prompt discharge, combined with home rehabilitation, appears to translate into motor and functional gains and a greater degree of function and satisfaction, which translates into better physical health.[49] It is imperative that the case manager become familiar with all available stroke services. The case manager should always select rehabilitation services that are accredited by the Commission on Accreditation of Rehabilitation Facilities (CARF) for quality programs. After the routine assessment, development of a plan of care and approval by the payer, traditional stroke case management focuses on providing assistance to poststroke clients for the prevention of complications, health teaching, and rehabilitation.

The goals of case management are to improve the patient's health and outcomes, coordinate a cost-effective plan of recovery and rehabilitation, and provide continuity of care to eliminate duplication of services. Teaching includes information about preventive drug therapy, blood pressure control, the need to change negative lifestyles, weight reduction, healthy diet/nutrition, smoking cessation, diabetes control, increased physical exercise, and regular checkups with health care providers to prevent another stroke.

Complications and Outcomes

Functional scales help the case manager assess the patient's complications and functional outcome after a stroke. **Functional disability (FD)** refers to limitations in performing independent living tasks. FD distinguishes the daily activities necessary to function personally and in the community in other major social roles. **Instrumental activities of daily**

BOX 17-5 Modified Rankin Scale

0   No symptoms at all
1   No significant disability despite symptoms; able to carry out all usual duties and activities
2   Slight disability; unable to carry out all previous activities but able to look after own affairs without assistance
3   Moderate disability; requires some help but able to walk without assistance
4   Moderately severe disability; unable to walk without assistance but able to attend to own bodily needs without assistance
5   Severe disability; bedridden, incontinent, and requires constant nursing care and attention

living (IADLs) include basic activities necessary to live in the community (e.g., shopping, managing finances, housekeeping, meal preparation). The **Modified Rankin Scale** is a global assessment of patient function, with 0 representing no disability and 5 indicating severe disability[44] (Box 17-5).

The following potential complications may accompany stroke and should be monitored[26]:

- Skin breakdown: This condition may result from abnormalities in sensation, tone, mobility, bowel, or bladder or nutrition. It is relieved by repositioning every 2 hours, use of a pressure-reducing bed and chair, improved nutrition and hydration, and barrier creams.
- Edema: This condition is controlled with compression stockings, edema gloves (Isotoner), positioning with elevation, nutrition (albumin), retrograde massage, and diuretics.
- Contractions: This condition is treated with ROM exercises performed by the therapist or family.
- DVT: The peak incidence is in the first week. Doppler, ultrasound, and impedance plethysmography or venography testing may be needed to rule out this condition. DVT is treated with subcutaneous heparin and pneumatic compression boots.
- Dysphagia and aspiration: This is a major risk factor and is a cause of morbidity and mortality. Strategies to manage the risk of aspiration and pneumonia should be developed with a speech therapist and nutritionist.
- Seizures: A neurologist should be requested to predict the risk for seizures and to prescribe anticonvulsants if needed. Their incidence is greater in hemorrhagic stroke.
- Infections: UTIs are common. Urosepsis is often associated with an indwelling urinary catheter.
- Bladder incontinence: During the first month, 50% to 70% of the episodes of urinary incontinence occur; 15% of individuals will continue to experience urinary incontinence after 6 months. Interventions include regulation of fluids, timed voidings, and checks of postvoid residuals using a portable bladder scan. Catheterizations may be started on an every-4-hour schedule. Medications may include oxybutynin (Ditropan) and bethanechol (Urecholine).

- Bowel incontinence: This condition occurs in 31% of stroke patients but usually resolves in 2 weeks. Severe constipation is prevented by the use of stool softeners, suppositories, or fiber. Severe diarrhea is prevented by diluting feedings, if they are too concentrated.
- Depression: This condition occurs in 40% of patients and is often underdiagnosed. Consult with a psychiatrist. Observe the patient for symptoms such as refusal to eat, poor sleep, and frequent crying spells. Consider counseling for the family.
- Falls: One third of stroke patients fall at least once during their rehabilitation and 2% to 4% may suffer a serious injury. Patients at higher risk for falls are those with the following characteristics: right hemisphere stroke, neglect, visuospatial deficits, impulsivity, bilateral strokes, male gender, poor performance of ADLs, urinary incontinence, and the use of sedatives and diuretics. Implement a fall-prevention program that includes adequate monitoring and supervision; fall-prevention education for caregivers and family; patient training to maximize strength, balance, and cognition; minimal use of sedatives and diuretics; and devices such as special beds and alarms for the bed and chair. Restraints are used as a last resort and include bars, a Posey vest belt, wrist restraints, or mitts.
- Spasticity: Use of antispasticity medications (e.g., baclofen, dantrolene [Dantrium], tizanidine [Zanaflex], diazepam [Valium], clonidine and injections of botulinum toxins [Botox] or phenol)[56] as ordered. ROM exercises, serial casting, splinting, heat and cold as appropriate, and electrical stimulation can also be helpful (see Chapter 13).
- Aphasia: Use communication devices, oral motor strengthening, and speech therapy (see Chapter 13).

Monitoring Home Care Management

Home care for patients with stroke usually requires providing special equipment, administering medications, drawing blood for laboratory studies, monitoring blood pressure, and developing nutrition and psychosocial parameters. Medication compliance is important because drugs such as anticoagulants, antihypertensives, statins or cholesterol-lowering drugs may be prescribed for life. Rehabilitation may be limited to only 6 weeks, which leaves the patient without a home plan and special equipment for functional restoration and exercises. The case manager must often act as a patient advocate and appeal to third-party payer limitations by describing the patient's progress and future potential to overcome deficits if more therapy is provided. The case manager should focus on any problems of swallowing, aspiration, and potential for pneumonia, which could lead to rehospitalization and further debilitation. Skin care and safety from falling should be stressed to those with hemiparesis or hemiparalysis. Good nutrition and adequate hydration aid in recovery and in regaining energy for rehabilitation. Individuals who have suffered a stroke are at an even higher risk for future strokes. With cooperation from the patient and family, the case manager's plan of care must include every possible prevention strategy to help the patient avoid a future stroke.

Reports of a fall require an assessment and appropriate referral for prompt diagnosis of injuries and treatment. Information should be recorded regarding the individual's medications, activity at the time of the fall, and concurrent events (e.g., symptoms of light-headedness, dizziness, palpitations, apnea, chest pain, disorientation, vertigo, syncope, loss of consciousness, incontinence). The assessment findings should include vital signs, AF, mental status, sundowning, memory deficits, aphasia, onset of new pain, vision and visual fields, auditory deficits, evidence of bruises, edema, arthritis, impaired gait and balance, ambulation skills, and safe stair climbing ability.

Caregiver Support. The case manager may be in the best position to observe caregiver fatigue and related problems. Planned respite care from the church, family, friends, or community agencies is the safety net. Family members may experience feelings of guilt or neglect of responsibility if they take a day off or a vacation. Planned periods of time away from the stroke survivor give them "permission" to be away and provide them with the opportunity to look forward to returning to the home and the stroke survivor.

Disease Management. Today's case managers should consider disease management that focuses on reducing the incidence of stroke for their clients. The ability to identify individuals at risk and their risk factors is the first important step in the process of stroke reduction. Case managers who have electronic database systems can use them to identify clients who are either older than 55 years of age or younger than 55 years of age with one or more risk factors (e.g., hypertension, DM). Preventive strategies can be implemented with the information gleaned from this process.

The case manager should develop an educational and screening program that is part of the office, clinic, or home visits. After completion of the screening, the names of all clients found to be at moderate or high risk who have not experienced a stroke are collected and enrolled in a stroke prevention program that features a reduction of their risk factors. A log is provided for each individual and is reviewed by the case manager. This log records weight, blood pressure, pulse, and activities. Those with high risk factors (e.g., hypertension, smoking, DM, obesity, carotid stenosis, heart disease, AF, excessive drinking, other health problems) are given written material and offered classes or special sessions for individualized plans to reduce their risk of stroke. Individuals with significant risk factors are referred for consultation with a specialist (e.g., a cardiologist for heart disease; a neurologist for anyone who reports TIAs, a past history of carotid artery disease, or stroke). Faced with the prospect of having a stroke versus adhering to their new health plan, individuals are offered a choice they cannot refuse.[5]

Quality of Life Considerations

Behavioral, Psychologic, and Cognitive Problems

Ischemic brain damage can clearly result in neurobehavioral and psychologic changes that range from small adjustment reactions to devastating combinations of mood, affect, and psychotic disorders. The literature often describes these changes as "syndromes" to provide a way of dealing with them clinically. The most common forms of behavior and mood changes seen in the stroke population are discussed in the following sections.

Confusional States and Delirium

The global response of the brain to injury includes confusional states and delirium, which reflect disordered attention. These patients usually experience acutely altered sensorium, with poor recent memory; poor concentration; an inability to pay attention; and possibly delusions, hallucinations, or frank delirium. Occlusions that are localized or isolated in the posterior division of the MCA may produce transient confusion with only subtle focal neurologic findings. Older adults are particularly at risk for confusional states because of translocation deficits that result from a sudden movement from home to hospital. The right hemisphere may have a central role in attentional processing; therefore, prolonged confusional states may be observed after large frontal, parietal, or frontoparietal infarcts of the right hemisphere. Other focal areas that may be responsible are the calcarine gyrus, medial structures of the temporal lobe, and the hippocampus in particular.

The confusional episodes from stroke and/or hospitalization usually resolve without treatment. However, caregivers must be alert to the fact that medications can cause confusional states and, more seriously, that combinations of brain ischemia, translocation syndromes in older adults, and medication changes can cause devastating and frightening confusional states. Paranoid responses, combative behavior with fearful components, withdrawal, excessive compliance, or psychotic symptoms may be seen. A common response of professionals is to physically or chemically restrain confused or delirious patients without adequate assessment and management of the factors that may be producing the behavior. Restraint often aggravates the behavior and is unsafe and unsuccessful. Caregivers should be taught to seek the underlying cause of the problem and remove the stimulus if possible.

Depression and Anxiety

Major depression is common after stroke, and stroke patients may experience more depression than other individuals with comparable disabilities. Depression can impede the recovery process. A 30% incidence of clinically significant depression in stroke patients has been reported. The prevalence of major depression in these patients varies from 30% to 40%.[65] Increased depression and combinations of depression and anxiety are often reported in relation to the location of the brain lesion. Relatively little is known about depression in patients with stroke who have the confounding problems of cognitive impairment and aphasias that render these patients unable to express their feelings appropriately. Patients recovering from stroke should be evaluated for disabilities, cognitive impairment, and speech deficits that may contribute to severe depression, poor rehabilitation outcome, or even suicide.

Providers of stroke care have long thought that right-sided lesions produce euphoria, whereas left-sided lesions produce catastrophic, depressive responses. It has been theorized that the right hemisphere is more active during sad mood states, that it is activated by negative emotional stimuli, and that it processes negative and adversive input. Depression and anxiety states clearly do occur in stroke patients with deficits in either hemisphere, are difficult to detect and treat, and may have a biologic and/or psychosocial mechanism or multifactorial origin.

Depression and anxiety may have different patterns of appearance during stroke recovery, with some patients responding to antidepressants and others responding to psychoactive medications. Early depression with a physiologic basis may be responsive to treatment. Patients may experience more functional gain throughout the total recovery period if the depression is avoided. Early detection and treatment are important.

Stroke survivors with severe depression and depressed family members should be periodically screened for suicidal thought content, as well as method and intent, for suicide prevention. Undetected depression can lead to serious, preventable problems in rehabilitation and functional recovery. Older adults who are incontinent often experience shame, disgust, embarrassment, and a reduced social life, which may lead to depression. The degree of depression is usually linked to the severity of the incontinence. Referral to appropriate mental health providers is appropriate for prevention of severe depression and for treatment.

Dementia

Cerebrovascular disease, particularly stroke, is a major cause of dementia.[65] One of the major causes of dementia may no longer be Alzheimer's, but rather small "silent" strokes that cause senility as the individual ages. Aggressive early treatment of TIAs and high blood pressure—during middle age rather than when patient shows signs of dementia—is the goal of preventive care. Dementia can occur before, with, or after an ischemic insult. In focal infarcts of the posterior cerebellar arteries, persistent memory loss may occur and resemble amnestic syndrome or dementia. Frontal infarcts and focal infarction of the angular gyrus region may also result in dementia-like symptoms. Stroke survivors with focal insults are unable to learn new tasks and experience variable short-term memory loss and "patchy" cognitive losses. Their symptoms are notable in that they do not progress. CT and MRI findings usually show focal lesions, and the clinician is alerted to the ischemic cause by the abrupt onset and lack of premorbid dementia symptoms.

The dementia associated with brain softening secondary to repeated ischemic events is commonly labeled **multi-infarct dementia (MID).** A constellation of signs and symptoms may be present, with a prominence of hypertension, a stepwise progression of the dementia (with periods of nonprogression), and often a series of minor neurologic events revealed on history. CT and MRI scans show multiple small infarcts (usually in the deep gray matter) but no classic cortical atrophy and ventricular achalasia.

Binswanger's disease, a rare and rapidly declining dementia (1- to 2-year course) is caused by chronic ischemia or small-vessel atherosclerosis with concurrent hypertension.

Patients with this dementia are typically 60 to 80 years of age and show diffuse bilateral corticospinal dysfunction, abnormal reflexes, and often seizures. Diagnosis is made on autopsy, but the patient usually has concurrent widespread atherosclerotic vessel disease, which helps in making the clinical diagnosis.

Although the overall behavioral and cognitive responses (e.g., forgetfulness, wandering, poor personal hygiene) appear similar to Alzheimer's disease, the progression of MID is often slower and both personality and selected cognitive functions may be intact. Depression may be more common in patients with MID than in patients with Alzheimer's disease. Depression should be treated to improve recovery.

Hemispheric Asymmetry and Behavior

The brain is divided into two hemispheres. In stroke, behavior is related to the affected hemisphere (Box 17-6).

It is important to recognize the location of the stroke lesion(s) and the behaviors controlled by that part of the brain. If the patient has receptive language deficits, the clinician should instruct the patient to follow simple commands (e.g., "blink your eyes"). Questions should be asked that allow the patient to nod or answer "yes" or "no." The patient should be challenged to match words, letters, and pictures of objects and be encouraged to read aloud.

For expressive language deficits, the patient is asked to repeat vowels and simple words and to name objects. Several choices that can be expressed verbally are provided (e.g., "Do you want to brush your teeth now?"). The patient is given a pen and paper to write letters, words, and sentences and to copy simple designs. The clinician should show patience and give generous praise.

Personality Changes

Common behaviors that reflect changed premorbid personality types include increased irritability; aggressiveness; disinhibition of language and thought content; outbursts of temper; sudden withdrawal; overwhelming sadness and negativity; abusive or combative actions; increased drug or alcohol use with resultant disorganized behavior; and behaviors such as stealing, disrobing in public, or uncontrolled laughing, crying, or swearing (usually associated with the area of brain damage). Although these behaviors are fatiguing, they are not necessarily dangerous. They are, however, upsetting to the stroke survivor who may sense a lack of control over the behavior, thus making social situations incredibly difficult, creating family conflicts, and producing negative responses in formal and informal caregivers. The family needs time to grieve the loss of the person they knew and to accept the person who returns to the family after the stroke.

STROKE PREVENTION

Stroke may be prevented. Strategies to reduce the risks of stroke work. Every patient encounter can be an opportunity to teach stroke prevention and review with patients their "stroke risk profile" and how they can reduce each condition

BOX 17-6	Brain Hemisphere Deficits From Stroke

Left Hemisphere Deficits
- Paralysis/paresis of right side of body
- Catastrophic reaction
- Aphasia (sensory or receptive): Difficulty understanding speech or written material
- Aphasia (expressive or motor): Difficulty speaking or writing
- Major depression (left anterior frontal lobe or basal ganglia)
- Minor depression (left or right parietooccipital lobe)
- Dysarthria
- Apraxia
- Problems performing common tasks
- Perseverations
- Emotional lability
- Slow and cautious behavior; tendency for disorganization
- Impaired short-term memory
- Poor attention span
- Slow response time
- Anxiety and hesitancy

Right Hemisphere Deficits
- Paralysis/paresis of left side of body
- Indifference, anxiety, hostility, and egocentrism
- Possible display of unsafe behavior related to unawareness of deficits
- Possible disorientation
- Spatial/perceptual problems
- Quick impulsive behavior; overestimation of abilities
- Impaired short-term memory
- Impaired attention span
- Impaired scanning and tracking
- Impaired intonation and stress
- Masked facies or lack of facial expression
- Impaired conversational skills
- Poor eye contact
- Decreased awareness of illness
- Impaired high-level thought processes

Data from Cummins RO: *Acute stroke,* Dallas, Tex, 2003, American Heart Association, American Stroke Association—A Division of American Heart Association; Love BB, Biller J: Neurovascular system. In Goetz CG, Pappert EJ, editors: *The textbook of clinical neurology,* Philadelphia, 1999, WB Saunders; and Sacco RL, Toni S, Mohr JP: Classification of ischemic stroke. In Mohr JP, Choi DW, Grotta JC, Wolf P, editors: *Stroke: pathophysiology, diagnosis, and management,* ed 4, Philadelphia, 2004, Churchill Livingstone.

that increases their risks. The aging of the American population, coupled with the baby boom generation of 78 million Americans who are approaching the age for risk of stroke, will escalate the incidence of stroke. The resources of the health care system will be stretched to the limits. Steps must be taken now to implement preventive care to save lives and prevent strokes.

Stroke Awareness

The public has little knowledge about strokes. Many Americans are unable to describe the risk factors or recognize the early warning signs of stroke (Fig. 17-7). Some stroke experts believe that up to 80% of strokes can be prevented by modifying the risk factors associated with stroke. One of the most important benefits of educating the public is the fact that another person, friend, or family member is usually the one most likely to recognize the signs of a stroke and call 911. Bystanders can be taught to recognize a stroke by asking three simple questions:
- Ask the individual to smile.
- Ask him or her to raise both arms.
- Ask the individual to speak a simple sentence (e.g., "It is sunny out today.")

The bystander should call 911 immediately if the individual has trouble with any of these tasks.

Get With The Guidelines (GWTG) is the ASA's process for QI, to improve stroke treatment and to prevent future strokes and cardiovascular events. GWTG focuses on protocols to ensure that patients are treated and discharged on appropriate medications and with risk modification counseling (see Resources to access GWTG).

Clinicians' Role in Stroke Prevention

The public needs education on the risk factors of stroke and steps that they can take to reduce their risks. Using the Stroke Risk Screening (SRS) tool (see Fig. 17-7), clinicians can screen and identify individuals who have hypertension, heart disease, diabetes, smoke, and have other risk factors. Clinicians as health educators and advocates are key to teaching dietary and lifestyle changes for risk factor modification. Education on the early warning signs of stroke and on the emergent need to call 911 will ensure patients the best chance for optimal outcome if they suddenly experience any of the following:
- Numbness or weakness of the face, arm, or leg on one side of the body
- Confusion; difficulty speaking or understanding speech
- Severe headache
- Trouble seeing or loss of vision in one or both eyes
- Trouble walking, loss of balance or coordination, or dizziness

CONCLUSION

Many new drugs and technological interventions will be researched and developed to treat AIS. Stroke teams will staff primary and comprehensive stroke units with trends towards regional networks to offer every stroke patient the best treatment and the latest rehabilitation therapies. *Best practices* have been described as a service, function, or process that has been fine-tuned, improved, and implemented to produce superior outcomes that meet or set new standards.

STROKE RISK SCREENING

Site and address of screening: _____   Date: ____/____/____

PART I - STROKE RISK SCREENING TOOL

	YES	NO

1. Have you ever been told that you have high blood pressure? .... ____ ____ **SKIP TO Q.3**
2. If you take medication for high blood pressure, do you frequently miss doses?.................................. ____ ____
3. Do you have a history of irregular heart beat also called atrial fibrillation? .... ____ ____
4. Have you ever been told that you have a narrowing of the arteries (carotid) in the neck? .... ____ ____
5. Have you had a heart attack, heart by-pass surgery, angioplasty or another heart disease?.................. ____ ____
6. Have you had a previous stroke or mini-stroke (TIA)? .... ____ ____
7. Do you have diabetes? .... ____ ____
8. Do you smoke cigarettes regularly, or have you smoked cigarettes in the past 5 years?..................... ____ ____
9. Has a family member had a stroke, heart attack or hemorrhage (rupture) of a blood vessel in the brain? .... ____ ____
10. Do you drink more than 2 ounces of alcohol daily (e.g., 2 drinks of liquor, 2 glasses of wine or 2 beers)?............ ____ ____
11. Have you ever been told that you have abnormal lipids or cholesterol levels? .... ____ ____
12. Do you exercise less than 30 minutes daily or have any type of physical activity less than 3 times a week?.......... ____ ____
13. Do you, or immediate members of your family, have Sickle Cell disease? .... ____ ____
14. Do you use any of the following drugs: Cocaine, Crack, Heroin, Speed, Amphetamines, diet pills or Ecstasy?..... ____ ____
15. Are you more than 20 pounds over your target weight? .... ____ ____
16. If you are a woman, do you smoke cigarettes **and** take birth control pills?.................................... ____ ____

Add the number of "yes" responses in questions 1-16 to find your Health History Risk Score = [____]

	YES	NO

17. Measure blood pressure (BP) in arm in sitting position: _____(systolic)/_____(diastolic)

   Is highest systolic BP >**130 OR** is highest diastolic BP >**85**? .... ____ ____
18. Check radial pulse x 60 seconds: _____ beats per minute. Is radial pulse **irregular**?................... ____ ____

Add the number of "yes" responses in questions 17-18 to find your Clinical Risk Score = [____]

Add your Health History Risk Score to Clinical Risk Score to equal the Brain Attack/Stroke Risk Score = [____]

If Your Age is:	and your **Brain Attack/Stroke Risk Score** is:	Risk for Brain Attack/Stroke is:
<55 years	0	LOW
>55 years	0	LOW
>55 years	2	MODERATE
>55 years	≥3	HIGH
>65 years	1	MODERATE
>65 years	≥2	HIGH
Any age	>2	MODERATE
Any age	≥3	HIGH

Follow-up:
If Risk for Brain Attack/Stroke is **LOW**, this assessment should be shared with your healthcare provider/doctor during the next visit.
If Risk for Brain Attack/Stroke is **MODERATE**, notify healthcare provider/doctor within one week of the results of this screening and request an appointment for evaluation and care to prevent stroke.
If Risk for Brain Attack/Stroke is **HIGH**, call healthcare provider/doctor **today** with the results of this screening and request an appointment for evaluation and care to prevent stroke.

ALL PERSONS SCREENED FOR RISK FACTORS SHOULD BE EDUCATED ABOUT WARNING SIGNS OF BRAIN ATTACK/STROKE.
IF ANY OF THESE WARNING SIGNS OCCUR, CALL "911" IMMEDIATELY AND SEEK TREATMENT AS SOON AS POSSIBLE.

Figure 17-7 Stroke Risk Screening tool. This tool may be duplicated for use in clinical practice.
(Courtesy Neuroscience Nursing Consultants, Ellen Barker, MSN, APN, CNRN.)   *Continued*

> **SIGNS OF BRAIN ATTACK/STROKE:**
> - **Sudden weakness or numbness.**
> - **Sudden change in vision.**
> - **Sudden difficulty speaking.**
> - **Sudden unusual headache.**
> - **Sudden dizziness.**

PART II - DEMOGRAPHICS

Name: (last) _____ (first) _____ (middle initial) _____

Gender: ☐ Male ☐ Female

Highest Level of Education: ☐ Elementary   ☐ College

☐ High School   ☐ Post Graduate Training

Address: _____

City: _____ State: _____ Zip: _____ County: _____

Telephone (home): _____/_____ (work): _____/_____

Best Time To Call: _____ AM/PM

Date of Birth: _____/_____/_____   Age Today: _____

Do you have a healthcare provider/doctor? .... ☐ Yes ☐ No

Have you seen your healthcare provider/doctor within the past year? .... ☐ Yes ☐ No

Do you have healthcare insurance? .... ☐ Yes ☐ No

Ethnicity/Race: ☐ African-American/Black ☐ Caucasian/White ☐ Hispanic/White ☐ Hispanic/Non-White

☐ Asian/Pacific Islander ☐ Native Indian/Alaskan   ☐ Other

To help educate people about the risk of Brain Attack/Stroke, it is important for DSI to understand what participants think and learn about the information they receive. Can we contact you by phone in the next 3 to 6 months for this purpose?

☐ Yes ☐ No

Did you view our stroke video today?

☐ Yes ☐ No

I have received a screening for the risk of Stroke and agree to follow up with the recommendations. I understand this is only a screening. I agree that this data can be entered into a database for research without identifying me by name. Screeners agree to abide by all federal and state laws and regulations, including but not limited to, The Health Insurance Portability and Accountability Act of 1996 (HIPPA), as amended, to protect confidentially any and all private health information obtained in the course of this stroke risk screening.

(Signature of Participant) _____   (Signature of Healthcare Provider) _____

Note: This Stroke Risk Screening Tool has been modified 01/27/04 by Ellen Barker, MSN, APN, CNRN, Neuroscience Nursing Consultants, Greenville, DE. For complete information visit the website: www.neuronurse.com. There is no copyright. Permission is not needed for copying.

Figure 17-7, cont'd

As health care professionals continue to care for today's stroke survivors, they must work diligently to prevent tomorrow's strokes using the effective strategies and best practices described throughout this chapter. All stroke teams, emergency protocols, and stroke units for emergent treatment will have limited success unless the public can be educated about stroke and unless stroke victims can be transported to the hospital in time. Everyone needs to learn and remember that *time is brain.*

Stroke statistics will improve as new prevention and treatment modalities are discovered. Health teaching for stroke prevention, prompt recognition of the warning signs of stroke by the public, and improved hospital stroke management will hopefully reverse the outcomes of many patients discharged today with poor nutritional status, poor functional status, persistent vegetative state, poststroke dementia, and medical complications with an unacceptable high morbidity and mortality.

RESOURCES FOR STROKE

Academy of Aphasia: 617-495-4342
Advanced Recovery Rehabilitation Center: www.AdvancedRecovery.org
AHA Stroke Connection (formerly the Courage Stroke Network): 800-553-6321
American Academy of Neurology: www.aan.com
American Heart Association: www.americanheart.org
American Stroke Association: www.strokeassociation.org
Brain Attack Coalition: www.stroke-site.org
Family Caregiver Alliance: www.caregiver.org
Get With the Guidelines (GWTG)-Stroke: guidelineinfo@heart.org; 888-526-6700
Guidelines for Prevention of Stroke in Patients with Ischemic Stroke or Transient Ischemic Attack, *Stroke* 37(2):577–617, 2006.
Helpful Products for Stroke Survivors and Caregivers: 800-787-6537
Internet Stroke Center: http://strokecenter.org
Joint Commission on Accreditation of Healthcare Organizations (JCAHO): http://jcaho.org
List of Professional Society Guidelines for Stroke Treatment: www.stroke-site.org/guidelines/guidelines.html
National Aphasia Association: www.aphasia.org
National Easter Seal Society: 800-787-6537
National Institute of Neurological Disorders and Stroke: www.ninds.nih.gov
National Stroke Association: www.stroke.org
National Institutes of Health Stroke Scale training and testing online (free): www.strokeassociation.org/presenter.jhtml.identifier=3023009
PLAC Test: www.plactest.com
Recovering After a Stroke, AHCPR Pub No 95-0664; 800-358-9295
The Road Ahead: A Stroke Recovery Guide, ed 4, National Stroke Association; 800-STROKES; www.stroke.org; info@stroke.org
Speech and Language Recovery After Stroke: www.StrokeSoftware.com
Stroke Clubs International: 409-762-1022

REFERENCES

1. Alexandrov AV, Molina CA, Grotta JC, et al: Ultrasound-enhanced systemic thrombolysis for acute ischemic stroke, *N Engl J Med* 35(21):2170–2178, 2004.
2. Al-Khoury L, Lyden PD: Intravenous thrombolysis: In Mohr JP, Choi DW, Grotta JC, Wolf P, editors: *Stroke: pathophysiology, diagnosis, and management,* ed 4, Philadelphia, 2004, Churchill Livingstone.
3. *Anticoagulants and antiplatelet agents in acute ischemic stroke,* Report of the Joint Stroke Guideline Development Committee of the American Academy of Neurology and the American Stroke Association (a division of the American Heart Association), July 2002, National Guideline Clearinghouse, http://www.guideline.gov; accessed March 2006.
4. Barclary L: Negative emotions may trigger ischemic stroke, *Neurology* 63(12):2006–2010, 2004.
5. Barker E: Case management: disease management for stroke victims, *Inside Case Manag* 6(10):1–12, 2000.
6. Barker E: *Modified stroke risk screening tool,* Greenville, Del, 2001, Neuroscience Nursing Consultants.
7. Brinker F: *Herb contraindications and drug interaction,* Sandy, Ore, 1998, Eclectic Medical Publications.
8. Broderick JP, Pancioli AM: Prehospital care of the patient with acute stroke. In Mohr JP, Choi DW, Grotta JC, Wolf P, editors: *Stroke: pathophysiology, diagnosis, and management,* ed 4, Philadelphia, 2004, Churchill Livingstone.
9. Brooks WH, McClure RR, Jones MR, Coleman TC, Breathitt L, White CJ: Carotid angioplasty and stenting versus carotid endarterectomy: randomized trial in a community hospital, *J Am Coll Cardiol* 38(6):1589–1595, 2001.
10. Brown B: *Pain management of the stroke patient,* 4th Annual Cerebrovascular Update 2005, Prevention Strategies and Management of Acute Stroke, Philadelphia, March 18–19, 2005, sponsored by Thomas Jefferson University.
11. Chaturvedi S, Bruno A, Feasby R, Holloway R, Benavente O, Cohen SN, Cote R, Hess D, Saver J, Spence JD, Stern B, Wilterdink J: Carotid endarterectomy—an evidence-based review, Report of the Therapeutics and Technology Assessment Subcommittee of the American Academy of Neurology, *Neurology* 65:794–801, 2005, http://www.aan.com/professionals/practice/guideline/index/cfm; accessed March 2006.
12. Chen ZM, Sandercock P, Pan HC, Counsell C, Collins R, Liu LS, Xie JX, Warlow C, Peto R: Indications for early aspirin use in acute ischemic stroke: a combined analysis of 40,000 randomized patients from the Chinese acute stroke trial and the international stroke trial on behalf of the CAST and IST collaborative groups, *Stroke* 31(6):1240–1249, 2000.
13. Clark WM, Lutsep HL: Medical treatment strategies: intravenous thrombolysis, neuronal protection, and anti-reperfusion injury agents, *Neuroimaging Clin N Am* 9(3):465–473, 1999.
14. Crawley F, Stygall J, Lunn S, Harrison M, Brown MM, Newman S: Comparison of microembolism detected by transcranial Doppler and neuropsychological sequelae of carotid surgery and percutaneous transluminal angioplasty, *Stroke* 31(6):1329–1334, 2000.
15. Cummins RO: *Acute stroke,* Dallas, Tex, 2003, American Heart Association, American Stroke Association—A Division of American Heart Association.
16. Current status of carotid stenting, *Stroke Clinical Updates* 9(5):1–4, 1999.
17. Dauchet L, Amouyel P, Dallongeville J: Fruit and vegetable consumption and risk of stroke: a meta-analysis of cohort studies, *Neurology* 65(10):1193–1197, 2005.

18. *DiaDexus and the Methodist DeBakey Heart Center announce publication of data in JAMA's* Archives of Internal Medicine *demonstrating 11-fold increase in stroke risk associated with elevated Lp-PLA$_2$ and CRP,* http://diadexus.com/press_room/11_28_05.shtml; accessed November 2005.

19. Dobkin BH: Rehabilitation and recovery of the patient with stroke. In Mohr JP, Choi DW, Grotta JC, Wolf P, editors: *Stroke: pathophysiology, diagnosis, and management,* ed 4, Philadelphia, 2004, Churchill Livingstone.

20. Evans V: Herbs and the brain: friend or foe? The effects of gingko and garlic on warfarin use, *J Neurosci Nurs* 32(4):229–232, 2000.

21. Fessler RD, Diaz FG: Carotid endarterectomy. In Kaye AH, Black PM, editors: *Operative neurosurgery,* London, 2000, Churchill Livingstone.

22. Findlay JM, Marchak BE: Carotid endarterectomy. In Mohr JP, Choi DW, Grotta JC, Wolf P, editors: *Stroke: pathophysiology, diagnosis, and management,* ed 4, Philadelphia, 2004, Churchill Livingstone.

23. Gent M, Blakely JA, Easton JD, Ellis DJ, Hachinski VG, Harbison JW, Panak E, Roberts RS, Sicurella J, Turpie AG: The Canadian American Ticlopidine Study (CATS) in thromboembolic stroke, *Lancet* 1(8649):1215–1220, 1989.

24. Glossary: acute stroke treatment terms, *Stroke Connection Magazine,* May/June 1999, pp 8–9.

25. Gorman MJ, Levine SR: Acute stroke care early in the 21st century, *J Stroke Cerebrovasc Dis* 8(3):108–110, 1999.

26. Hall TR: *Stroke rehabilitation and outcomes,* Paper presented at the Maryland General Bryn Mawr Rehab Regional Network, Baltimore, Md, November 14, 2001.

27. Hass WK, Easton JD, Adams HP Jr, Pryse-Phillips W, Molony BA, Anderson S, Kamm B: A randomized trial comparing ticlopidine hydrochloride with aspirin for the prevention of stroke in high-risk patients, Ticlopidine Aspirin Stroke Study Group, *N Engl J Med* 321:501–507, 1989.

28. *Heart Disease & Stroke Statistics—2005,* Dallas, Tex, 2005, American Stroke Association/American Heart Association.

29. Hinchey D: Dysphagia screening after stroke prevents pneumonia, *Stroke* 36:1972–1976, 2005.

30. Hogan H: Laser blasts stroke clots, *Biophotonics Int* 7(2):26, 2000.

31. Hospital focus, *RN* 63(7):24, 2000.

32. *Hypertension highlights,* Medscape, posted October 20, 2005.

33. Ignore daily aspirin, triple your stroke risk, "Stroke Notes," *Stroke Connection,* May/June, 2005.

34. Incidence of U.S. stroke up, *Case Manager* 11(2):6, 2000.

35. Kallenbach AM, Rosenblum J: Carotid endarterectomy: creating the pathway to 1-day stay, *Crit Care Nurse* 20(4):23–36, 2000.

36. Kannel WB, Wolf PA, McGee DL, Dawber TR, McNamara P, Castelli WP: Systolic blood pressure, arterial rigidity and risk of stroke: the Framingham study, *JAMA* 245(12):1225–1229, 1981.

37. Karp HR, Heyman A, Heyden S, Bartel AG, Tyroler HA, Hames CG: Transient cerebral ischemia: prevalence and prognosis in a biracial rural community, *JAMA* 225(2):125–128, 1973.

38. Katz JM, Gobin YP, Segal AZ, Riina HA: Mechanical embolectomy, *Neurosurgery Clin N Am* 16(3):463–474, 2005.

39. Kenton DF: Advocacy and research, making a difference, *Stroke Connection Magazine* Jan/Feb:2, 1999.

40. Kenton EJ: *Public health burden of stroke,* Improving stroke care at your hospital, Presentation April 14, 2004, American Stroke Association, A Division of American Heart Association.

41. Kidwell CS, Schugert GB, Eckstein M, Starkman S: Design and retrospective analysis of the Los Angeles prehospital stroke screen, *Prehosp Emerg Care* 2(2):267–273, 1998.

42. Kohnert SF: Major mechanistic differences explain the higher clot lysis potency of reteplase over alteplase: lack of fibrin binding is an advantage for bolus application of fibrin-specific thrombolytics, *Fibrinolysis & Proteolysis* 11(3):129–135, 1997.

43. Levine P: Path of recovery, *Adv Phys Ther* 16(4):37–38, 138, 2005.

44. Lewandowski CA, Libman R: Acute presentation of stroke, *J Stroke Cerebrovasc Dis* 8(3):117–126, 1999.

45. Liebeskind DS: Acute therapy and clinical research in the post-MERCI approval era, National Stroke Association, *Stroke Clinical Updates* XV(3):1–3, 2005.

46. Love BB, Biller J: Neurovascular system: In Goetz CG, Pappert EJ, editors: *The textbook of clinical neurology,* Philadelphia, 1999, WB Saunders.

47. *Many patients with mild strokes worsen without TPA treatment,* Reuters Health Information, http://www.medscape.com; accessed December 18, 2005.

48. Marti-Vilalta JL, Mohr JP: Lacunes. In Mohr JP, Choi DW, Grotta JC, Wolf P, editors: *Stroke: pathophysiology, diagnosis, and management,* ed 4, Philadelphia, 2004, Churchill Livingstone.

49. Mayo NE, Wood-Dauphinee S, Cote S, Gayton D, Carlton J, Buttery J, Tamblyn R: There's no place like home: an evaluation of early supported discharge for stroke, *Stroke* 31(5):1016–1023, 2000.

50. *Measuring vital signs in elderly people,* http://www.medscape.com/viewprogram/4638; accessed November 5, 2005.

51. Messe SR, Levine SR: *Acute ischemic stroke treatment: use of intravenous tissue plasminogen activator,* http://www.medscape.com; accessed December 5, 2005.

52. Millikan CH, McDowell F, Easton JD: *Stroke,* Philadelphia, 1987, Lea & Febiger.

53. Mitsias P: Ischemic stroke management in the critical care unit: the first 24 hours, *J Stroke Cerebrovasc Dis* 8(3):151–159, 1999.

54. Mohr JP, Gautier JC: Internal carotid artery disease. In Mohr, JP, Choi DW, Grotta JC, Wolf P, editors: *Stroke: pathophysiology, diagnosis, and management,* ed 4, Philadelphia, 2004, Churchill Livingstone.

55. Morgan MK, Morgan DK: Cerebral revascularization. In Kaye AH, Black PM, editors: *Operative neurosurgery,* London, 2000, Churchill Livingstone.

56. *Mosby's 2005 drug consult for nurses,* St Louis, 2005, Mosby.

57. National Institute of Neurological Disorders and Stroke, http://www.ninds.nih.gov/health_and_medical/disorders/stroke.htm; accessed March 2006.

58. National Institute of Neurological Disorders and Stroke rt-PA Stroke Study Group: Tissue plasminogen activator and acute ischemic stroke, *N Engl J Med* 333:1581–1587, 1995.

59. Pancioli AM, Broderick JP: Prehospital and emergency department care of the patient with acute stroke: In Mohr JP, Choi DW, Grotta JC, Wolf P, editors: *Stroke: pathophysiology, diagnosis, and management,* ed 4, Philadelphia, 2004, Churchill Livingstone.

60. Paolino AS, Garner KM: Effects of hyperglycemia on neurological outcome in stroke patients, *J Neurosci Nurs* 37(3):130–135, 2005.

61. Petty GW, Brown RD, Whisnant JP: Ischemic stroke subtypes: a population-based study of functional outcome, survival, and recurrence, *Stroke* 31(12):1062–1068, 2000.

62. Qureshi AI, Siddiqui AM, Suri MFK, et al: Aggressive mechanical clot disruption and low dose intraarterial third generation thrombolytic agent for ischemic stroke: a prospective study, *Neurosurgery* 51(5):1319–1329, 2002.

63. *Retinopathy independently linked to stroke in nondiabetes,* Reuters Health Information, http://www.medscape.com/viewarticle/514307; accessed November 5, 2005.

64. Rothwell PM, Warlow CP: Timing of TIAs preceding stroke: time window for prevention is very short, *Neurology* 64(5):817–820, 2005.

65. Rundek T, Sacco RL: Outcome following stroke. In Mohr JP, Choi DW, Grotta JC, Wolf P, editors: *Stroke: pathophysiology, diagnosis, and management,* ed 4, Philadelphia, 2004, Churchill Livingstone.

66. Rymer MM, Thrutchley DE: Organizing regional networks to increase stroke intervention, *Neurol Res* 27(supplement 1):S9–16, 2005.

67. Sacco RL, Adams R, Albers G, et al: Guidelines for prevention of stroke in patients with ischemic stroke or transient ischemic attack, *Stroke* 37(2):577–617, 2006.

68. Sacco RL, Toni S, Mohr JP: Classification of ischemic stroke. In Mohr JP, Choi DW, Grotta JC, Wolf P, editors: *Stroke: pathophysiology, diagnosis, and management,* ed 4, Philadelphia, 2004, Churchill Livingstone.

69. Schuster L: Warfarin no more effective than aspirin for intracranial arterial stenosis, *Neurol Today* May, 2005.

70. Sharp FR: Neurochemistry and molecular biology. In Mohr JP, Choi DW, Grotta JC, Wolf P, editors: *Stroke: pathophysiology, diagnosis, and management,* ed 4, Philadelphia, 2004, Churchill Livingstone.

71. Smith WS, Sung G, Starkman S, et al: Safety and efficacy of mechanical embolectomy in the acute ischemic stroke: results of the MERCI trial, *Stroke* 36(7):1432–1438, 2005.

72. *Stroke and rehabilitation: understanding the impact of spasticity,* Littleton, Colo, 2000, Medical Education Resources.

73. *Stroke rehabilitation guidelines,* http://stroke.ahajournals.org.cgi/content/full/36/9; accessed March 2006.

74. Taylor DW, Barnett HJ, Haynes RB, Ferguson GG, Sackett DL, Thorpe KE, Simard D, Silver Fl, Hachinski V, Clagett GP, Barnes R, Spence JD: Low-dose and high-dose acetylsalicylic acid for patients undergoing carotid endarterectomy: a randomized controlled trial: ASA and carotid endarterectomy (ACE) trial collaborators, *Lancet* 353(9171):2179–2184, 1999.

75. Toyota A: Early rehabilitation for stroke patients, *J Stroke Cerebrovasc Dis* 9(suppl 2):109–110, 2000.

76. Transient ischemic attacks—limit one per person! *Stroke Clinical Updates* 10(2):1–6, 2000.

77. Versnick EJ, Do HM, Albers GW, Tong DC, Marks MP: Mechanical thrombectomy for acute stroke, *AJNR* 26(4):875–879, 2005.

78. von Kummer R, Patel S: Neuroimaging in acute stroke, *J Stroke Cerebrovasc Dis* 8(3):127–138, 1999.

79. Wechsler L: Long-term follow-up with patients treated with intra-arterial urokinase for acute stroke, *J Stroke Cerebrovasc Dis* 9(5):213–217, 2000.

80. Werner H: The benefits of the dysphagia clinical nurse specialist role, *J Neurosci Nurs* 37(4):212–215, 2005.

Management of Aneurysms, Subarachnoid Hemorrhage, and Arteriovenous Malformation

ANEURYSMS

Intracranial aneurysms are a fairly common condition, remaining asymptomatic until the time of rupture.[75] Subarachnoid hemorrhage (SAH) associated with aneurysmal rupture accounts for 5% to 10% of all strokes (arteriovenous malformation [AVM] accounts for up to 17%) and is a potentially lethal and devastating event with a morbidity rate as high as 50% and a mortality rate of 25%.[30,73] Many patients who survive the initial hemorrhage develop permanent disabilities. This chapter includes content for effective acute management of patients following aneurysmal, vascular, and AVM care and follow-up treatment. Because cerebral bleed related to these conditions can be life threatening, a multidisciplinary team with the knowledge and skills to quickly diagnose and effectively treat these disorders is essential.

Incidence and Prevalence

The National Hospital Discharge Survey of 1990 reported 25,000 patients with SAH in the United States in 1 year,[18] with an additional 12% of persons with SAH not receiving prompt medical attention because of misdiagnosis.[30] The prevalence of aneurysmal SAH in the United States probably exceeds 30,000 persons per year. Population-based studies have shown that the incidence rates for SAH vary from 6 to 16 per 100,000, with the highest rates consistently reported in Finland and Japan.[5,15]

Despite the improvements in diagnosis, management, and preventive measures, the incidence of SAH, or **hemorrhagic stroke,** has not declined over time, unlike other types of stroke. The incidence of SAH increases with age (mean age of approximately 50 years) and is higher in women than in men.[29] The available data also suggest that African Americans are at higher risk than Caucasians.[4]

Risk Factors

An **aneurysm** is defined as an abnormal localized dilation of any blood vessel.[72] Because of the histopathologic and hemodynamic characteristics of cerebral blood vessels, cerebral aneurysms most commonly occur in arteries that supply blood to the brain. The incidence of intracranial aneurysms is about 8% in persons with two or more relatives who have had an SAH or an aneurysm.[61,64] Compared to other family members, the siblings of affected persons have a higher risk of developing aneurysmal SAH.[6] Smoking is a consistent and strong risk factor for SAH. Longstreth and colleagues[40] observed that the risk of SAH among smokers was greatest within 3 hours after smoking a cigarette. The use of alcohol or binge drinking may also be a risk factor for SAH. Binge drinking, stimulants, and drug abuse may also be short-term risk factors. Diabetes does not appear to be a risk factor for SAH.[1]

Pathophysiology

The majority of aneurysms (85%) occur in the anterior circulation with the remaining 15% in the posterior circulation. Intracranial aneurysms are classified as saccular, fusiform, or dissecting. Approximately 90% are saccular (berry aneurysms), which are responsible for most of the morbidity and mortality caused by subarachnoid hemorrhage.[78] Saccular aneurysms develop from defects in the muscular layer (tunica muscularis) of arteries. Changes in internal elastic membrane, lamina elastica interna, weaken the vessel walls, making them less resistant to changes in intraluminal pressure.[65] These changes frequently develop at sites of bifurcation of blood vessels, where blood flow is most turbulent with greatest shear forces against the arterial wall[28] (Fig. 18-1).

Aneurysm Classification

Saccular aneurysms, or **berry aneurysms,** are the most common type. They usually have a well-defined neck and frequently form in first- and second-order arteries originating from the cerebral arterial circle (circle of Willis) at the base of the brain. **Multiple aneurysms** develop in 30% of affected patients.[52] **Giant aneurysms** may be greater than 25 mm in size and may involve more than one cerebral

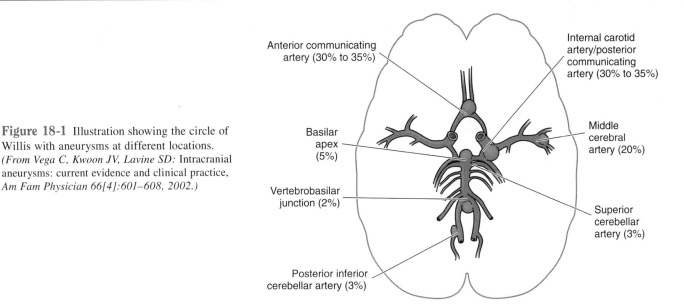

Figure 18-1 Illustration showing the circle of Willis with aneurysms at different locations. *(From Vega C, Kwoon JV, Lavine SD:* Intracranial aneurysms: current evidence and clinical practice, *Am Fam Physician 66[4]:601–608, 2002.)*

artery. **Fusiform aneurysms** develop from ectatic, tortuous cerebral arteries, most often in the vertebrobasilar system, and may grow to 2.5 cm or larger in diameter. They cause symptoms of cranial nerve or brainstem compression, not commonly associated with SAH. **Dissecting aneurysms** may appear as an elongated dilation and are the result of cystic medial necrosis or traumatic arterial tear when blood is forced between layers of the arterial wall, allowing blood to enter into a false track.

Clinical Manifestations

Presenting Symptoms
Subarachnoid hemorrhage is a medical emergency. It is imperative that physicians, nurses, and emergency medical personnel recognize the clinical manifestations of SAH and institute immediate diagnostic and therapeutic measures. Contemporary treatment for SAH is highly specialized and warrants rapid referral to centers with appropriate facilities.

The typical clinical presentation of aneurysmal SAH is one of the most distinctive and dramatic in medicine. The history of abrupt onset of a severe headache, often described by patients as the "worst headache" ever experienced, is characteristic of this disorder.[38] The onset of such headaches may or may not be associated with a stiff neck, brief loss of consciousness, nausea and/or vomiting, and focal neurologic deficits (including cranial nerve palsies). Despite the characteristic history, misdiagnosis of SAH is common.[44]

Patients sometimes have a history of recent, unusually severe, sudden headache in the prior days or weeks. This is called the "warning headache" and is unlikely to be recognized as SAH. Diagnosis of the "warning leak" before a catastrophic rupture may be lifesaving and requires a high index of suspicion.[39]

Symptoms
- Sudden severe headache, with or without alteration of consciousness, may or may not occur during exertion

- Often associated with vomiting
- May be associated with photophobia, drowsiness, restlessness, and agitation
- Sometimes patients have low back pain and bilateral radicular leg pain due to migration of blood in cerebrospinal fluid (CSF) down the thecal sac and the irritation of lumbar roots

Signs
- Neck stiffness in many patients
- Positive Kernig's sign (passive extension of the knee results in pain due to irritation of the lumbar nerve roots) in some patients
- Impaired level of consciousness in some patients
- Subhyaloid hemorrhages on optic funduscopy are seen in some patients with aneurysmal SAH
- The most common focal neurologic sign in acute SAH due to an aneurysm is cranial nerve (CN) III palsy with ptosis, pupillary dilation, and impaired extraocular movements (due to a posterior communicating artery aneurysm compressing the third nerve)

The most commonly used clinical grading systems for SAH are the Hunt-Hess classification (Table 18-1) and the World Federation of Neurosurgeons (WFNS) SAH scale (Table 18-2).

Neurodiagnostic and Laboratory Studies

Computed Tomography
Nonenhanced cranial computed tomography (CT) is the initial diagnostic study in patients with suspected SAH. Enlargement of the temporal horns may occur after SAH in the absence of increases in other parts of the ventricular system. Prominent temporal horns, visible on CT in a patient with a history suggestive of SAH, warrant lumbar puncture or angiography (or both). The amount and location of subarachnoid blood on CT gives important prognostic information about vasospasm and outcomes after SAH,

TABLE 18-1	Hunt-Hass Classification of Neurologic Status After Subarachnoid Hemorrhage[27]
Category	**Criteria***
Grade I	Asymptomatic or minimal headache and slight nuchal rigidity
Grade II	Moderate to severe headache, nuchal rigidity, no deficits other than cranial nerve palsy
Grade III	Drowsiness, confusion, or mild focal deficits
Grade IV	Stupor, moderate to severe hemiparesis, possibly early decerebrate rigidity and vegetative disturbances
Grade V	Deep coma, decerebrate rigidity, moribund appearance

*Serious systemic diseases such as hypertension, diabetes, severe arteriosclerosis, chronic pulmonary disease, and severe vasospasm seen on arteriography result in placement of the patient in the next less favorable category.

TABLE 18-2	World Federation of Neurosurgeons (WFNS) SAH Scale[20]	
WFNS Grade	**GCS Score**	**Motor Deficit**
I	15	Absent
II	14–13	Absent
III	14–13	Present
IV	12–7	Present or absent
V	6–3	Present or absent

GCS, Glasgow Coma Scale; *SAH*, subarachnoid hemorrhage.

TABLE 18-3	Fisher's CT Grades of Subarachnoid Hemorrhage[21]

Grade 1 = normal scan
Grade 2 = less than 1 mm thickness of blood
Grade 3 = more than 1 mm thickness of blood
Grade 4 = any, with ventricular or ICH blood

CT, Computed tomography; *ICH*, intracranial hemorrhage.

which are uniformly graded using Fisher's grading scale (Table 18-3).

Lumbar Puncture

Lumbar puncture (LP) is used to diagnose SAH when the CT scan is normal and there is strong clinical suspicion. If clinical features and CT findings are suggestive of SAH, there is no need for an LP.

ALERT: The contraindications to an LP include coagulation or bleeding disorders, raised intracranial pressure (ICP), intracranial hemorrhage (ICH), and local infection at the puncture site.

Risks of an LP include neurologic deterioration from aneurysm rebleeding or from cerebral herniation. CT scan of the head should always be performed before LP.

Catheter-Based Angiography

Catheter-based cerebral angiography remains the diagnostic test of choice for patients with spontaneous SAH and should be performed in patients who are candidates for further treatment. Catheter angiography is a minimally invasive procedure during which a small tube is threaded through the body to the area being studied. The tube is used to inject a special dye that highlights the blood vessels and makes them visible on the scanned images. Recently, the usefulness of computed tomographic angiography with intravenously administered contrast material for preoperative evaluation has been advocated.[32]

Computed Tomographic Angiography

Computed tomographic angiography (CTA) with intravenously administered contrast material for preoperative evaluation is being increasingly used in the management of intracranial aneurysms.[32] CTA may allow better delineation of the aneurysm neck, shape, and orientation (its relationship to the parent artery and important adjacent bone structures).[17] CTA uses a simple injection in the arm to place the contrast. CTA uses a CT scanner to create the images of blood vessels. This method is less time consuming and causes less discomfort but may need large amounts of contrast material to obtain high-quality images.

Magnetic Resonance Angiography

Magnetic resonance angiography is another noninvasive imaging modality that is based on the detection of blood flow within the cerebral vessels. Its primary advantage is that it can provide very thin, submillimeter source images that can be reconstructed three-dimensionally. The main disadvantages of this technique include prolonged acquisition time and flow and patient motion artifacts.

Assessment

An initial brief neurologic assessment, including level of consciousness, cranial nerves, and motor function, is prudent. This determines the necessity of emergent surgical intervention such as the placement of an external intraventricular drain and evacuation of intracerebral hematoma.

A complete history, including as much documentation as possible of the history leading up to the event of the ruptured aneurysm and SAH, helps in the differential diagnosis and treatment. Document smoking history. This is followed by a complete neurologic assessment. Initial emergency care includes assessment of adequacy of the airway, breathing, and circulatory function.

The nurse clinician collects pertinent information and performs an assessment to document the following:
- Headache: described as "the worst headache of my life"
- Pain assessment: neck pain; pain above and behind the eye
- Pupillary check: unequal; dilated; loss of pupillary reaction; disconjugate gaze; gaze preference; diplopia
- Motor status: hemiplegia; hemiparesis
- Sensory status: paresthesia of an arm or leg
- Alterations in consciousness: loss of consciousness

- Cranial nerves: deficits in CNs I to XII, especially CN XII, and swallowing problems; CN III nerve palsy; extraocular movement (EOM) dysfunction of CNs IV and VI
- Speech: aphasias
- Nausea and vomiting
- Meningeal signs: nuchal rigidity and upper back pain; **Kernig's sign; Brudzinski's sign**
- Vital signs: hypertensive
- Anticoagulated: check medication history
- Seizures: witnessed or reported
- Female patient: date of last menstrual period (LMP)

The cerebral bleed can be considered minor, moderate, or severe. Symptoms of an SAH may vary. Some patients' only symptom may be a headache. Others may describe visual defects or a history of recent migraine-like headaches. Approximately 20% of patients with an SAH from a ruptured aneurysm die before they reach the hospital. The bleeds are described as follows:

- **Minor.** Leaking of blood from the aneurysm may cause only a periodic generalized headache, neck discomfort, transient weakness, unilateral paresthesia, visual changes, ptosis, photophobia, transient speech disturbances, or lethargy.
- **Moderate.** Leaking may cause cerebral ischemia with a transient ischemic attack (TIA) and a possible hemiparesis. Vasospasm may be present.
- **Severe hemorrhage.** Sudden hemorrhage may occur with severe headache, pain in the neck, black eye or face, nausea and vomiting, changes in the level of consciousness (LOC), seizures, electrocardiogram (ECG) changes, autonomic dysfunction, nuchal rigidity, positive Brudzinski's and Kernig's signs, and localizing signs (e.g., hemiparesis, paralysis, abnormal posturing, or ophthalmoplegia) (see Chapter 2). Severe hemorrhage is often fatal and may cause the patient to succumb to a comatose state.

Treatment

General Management

The primary goal of aneurysm treatment is to reduce the risk of rebleeding. Other treatments that might decrease the risk of rebleeding are also considered. The administration of **recombinant activated factor VIIa** may promote coagulation and hemostasis at the site of the hemorrhage. Patients who have been receiving warfarin need to have their anticoagulation quickly reversed to prevent hematoma growth. Factor VIIa given intravenously (IV) in a single dose may promote coagulation without activating the systemic coagulation cascade and may help improve patient outcomes. Guidelines for the use of factor VIIa in warfarin-anticoagulated patients with a traumatic or nontraumatic spontaneous intracranial hemorrhage can be found in Chapter 11, Box 11-11.

The decision to treat a patient is based on multiple factors, including neurologic grade, age, location and size of aneurysm, and coexisting medical conditions. After appropriate resuscitation, the patient can be shifted to an area compatible

with his or her clinical condition while awaiting possible transfer or definitive treatment. Patients in stable condition with WFNS grade 13 SAH may be cared for in a general medical nursing unit as long as the clinician performs hourly neurologic assessment.

ALERT: Any deterioration, such as the development or worsening of neurologic deficits and depression of level of sensorium, may be due to rebleeding or complications of SAH and necessitates an urgent CT scan.[46]

Patients who require tracheal intubation or cardiovascular support are managed in the neuroscience critical care unit (NCCU).

Acute Care

SAH carries a high risk of death. Admission to an NCCU for acute critical care is important for serial neurologic assessments and hemodynamic monitoring to prevent potential complications (e.g., vasospasm or rebleeding). Patients are initially maintained on bed rest with the head of the bed elevated in a quiet environment. Routine monitoring of neurologic status every 2 hours and monitoring of vital signs with continuous cardiac monitoring are maintained until the patient is stable and free of complications.

Keeping the patient well hydrated decreases the impact of the spasmodic vessels. In anticipation of postoperative arterial vasospasm and ischemia, volume expanders can be used to counter the effects of vessel narrowing. **Hypertensive, hypervolemic-hemodilution therapy,** or **triple-H therapy (HHH therapy),** is frequently used. Agents used include plasma protein fraction, saline, 3% saline, albumin, and hetastarch. Ideally, hematocrit is maintained in the range of 30% to 40%. Blood volume is measured using central venous pressure (CVP) (10 ± 2 cm H_2O) and pulmonary capillary wedge pressure (PCWP) (15 ± 3 cm H_2O) using a triple-lumen catheter. IV normal saline or colloids are infused at 100 to 400 ml/hr.[27]

Plasmanate 250 ml is administered over 15 to 30 minutes. Some clinicians prefer 3% saline. Pressor agents (e.g., dopamine, phenylephrine) are used to elevate systolic blood pressure and to maintain mean arterial pressure (MAP) in the range of 100 to 110 mm Hg. Improvement is usually observed as cerebral perfusion improves hour by hour under the skilled eyes of the neuroscience clinician, who balances blood pressure and MAP with the volume expanders and observes for complications (e.g., fluid overload, electrolyte imbalances, cerebral edema, congestive heart failure [CHF], and rebleeding). Cardiac output should be kept in the range of 6.5 to 8 L/min.

In addition to the routine postprocedure care discussed in previous sections, there are special considerations for postoperative aneurysmal surgery, requiring monitoring for neurologic changes (e.g., LOC) that might indicate increases in ICP related to bleeding caused by problems with the aneurysm clip, intraoperative mechanical problems that involve occlusion of adjacent vessels, or vasospasm and evolving edema.

Typical admitting orders are shown in Table 18-4.[42]

TABLE 18-4	Typical Admitting Orders for Patients With a Subarachnoid Hemorrhage

Complete blood examination
Electrolytes, BUN, creatinine
Blood gas analysis: ABGs
Urinalysis
ECG
Imaging: computed tomography (CT)
Chest x-ray: PA view
Angiography: four-vessel cerebral angiography
Daily CSF analysis if ventricular drain in place
Close monitoring: cardiac and hemodynamic
Check neurologic status: GCS score, FOUR score, pupillary reflex; report changes in neurologic status or deficits
Fluid intake and output (I&O)
Temperature
Pulse and BP monitoring—invasive monitoring with arterial line (A-line) in poor-grade patients
Central venous pressure (CVP) monitoring in selected patients for fluid management
ICP monitoring in selected patients
Activity level: complete bed rest until the aneurysm is obliterated
Elevate head of bed 30 degrees
Restricted visitors
Graduated compression stocking and intermittent pneumatic compression (IPC)
Foley catheter for poor-grade patients
Nasogastric (NG) tube for intubated patients
Medications: _____
Stool softeners
Laxative of choice or bisacodyl, 5 mg/day orally, 5–10 mg/day rectally
Extract of senna concentration, 1–4 tablets orally one to four times a day
Analgesics—acetaminophen
Intravenous fluids: at least 125 ml/kg/hr
Antiemetics
H_2 blockers (e.g., sucralfate)
Sedatives: lorazepam 2 mg every 8 hours
Anticonvulsants: phenytoin, 15–20 mg/kg body weight as loading dose (<50 mg/min) followed by 5 mg/kg body weight in three
    divided doses
Calcium channel blockers: nimodipine 60 mg every 4 hours for 21 days (from day of ictus)
Antihypertensives: _____
Antiedema measures
Steroids: dexamethasone 4 mg IV every 6 hours

ABGs, Arterial blood gases; *BP,* blood pressure; *BUN,* blood urea nitrogen; *CSF,* cerebrospinal fluid; *ECG,* electrocardiogram; *GCS,* Glasgow Coma Scale; *ICP,* intracranial pressure; *PA,* posteroanterior.

Medical Management

The method of rebleed prevention is surgical or endovascular treatment of the aneurysm. In the interim period, before definitive treatment, the chances of rebleeding may be reduced by avoiding sudden fluctuations in blood pressure.[24,47] The pain of SAH is severe, causing distress, resulting in adrenergic stimulation and systemic hypertension thereby increasing the risk of rebleeding. Hence, pain management is vital in the initial management of SAH. Although codeine and acetaminophen are the most commonly used medications for pain relief, morphine sulfate can also be administered conventionally or by patient-controlled analgesia (PCA).

ALERT: Nonsteroidal antiinflammatory drugs should be avoided because of their antiplatelet properties, which impair clot formation around the ruptured aneurysm thereby increasing the risk of rebleeding.[53]

Regular antiemetic drug treatment should be considered. Patients are likely to develop constipation as a result of being immobile, on restricted diets, and on opioid drugs. Patients should not be allowed to strain during bowel movements and should be given stool softeners or laxatives.

Patients should be monitored in a 30° head-up position while awaiting definitive treatment. Conscious patients should be maintained in a quiet environment.

Maintenance of Adequate Circulating Blood Volume and Systemic Blood Pressure. **Cerebral ischemia** occurs due to inadequate cerebral perfusion pressure (CPP) and contributes to risk of mortality and morbidity related to SAH. In the early stages following SAH, ischemia is due to hypovolemia and disruption in autoregulatory mechanisms. Later, hypoperfusion is exacerbated by cerebral vasospasm. **Cerebral vasospasm** develops between 4 and 14 days after the initial hemorrhage and can be detected by daily transcranial Doppler (TCD) measurements that show increased intraarterial velocity in the affected artery. Vasospasm usually peaks between 7 and 10 days and causes a narrowing of the vessels from spasmogenic reaction or other causes with resultant decreased CPP, ischemia, and clinical deterioration, including infarction. Clinically, patients may exhibit speech or motor deficits with unilateral paresis or paralysis and decreased LOC with a "waxing and waning" pattern. Angiographic diagnosis confirms the vasospasm and the exact location of the artery involved. Triple-H therapy and nimodipine (Nimotop), a calcium channel blocker 60 mg orally every 4 hours for 21 days, are the two most common treatments. Papaverine may be administered intraoperatively by the neurosurgeon to prevent postoperative vasospasm or interventionally if symptoms of vasospasm develop later, requiring the clinician to closely monitor for increased ICP.

Management strategies to maintain adequate CPP consist of maintenance of an adequate circulating blood volume, vasopressors to maintain systemic blood pressure, and the administration of nimodipine to prevent vasospasm.[74]

A majority of patients with SAH are hypovolemic and often hyponatremic, components of **cerebral salt-wasting syndrome.** An understanding of this situation has resulted in the avoidance of fluid restriction in SAH patients. These patients should be maintained on sodium-containing solutions to maintain circulating volume at normal or supranormal levels. Dehydration should be avoided. The common clinical practice is to administer at least 3 L of fluid per day to prevent negative fluid balance. Fluid administration is monitored by frequent fluid balance assessment and central venous pressure (CVP) or pulmonary artery pressure (PAP) monitoring (via an indwelling intravenous catheter, a transesophageal Doppler, or both) in those patients monitored in an intensive care unit (ICU). Vasopressors such as norepinephrine or vasopressin may be required to maintain adequate systolic blood pressure. In the presence of an untreated, ruptured aneurysm, the target systolic pressure should be 110 to 120 mm Hg in the previously normotensive patient and 20% below baseline for patients with hypertension.[76]

Prevention and Treatment of Cerebral Vasospasm. Cerebral

vasospasm is a major cause of death and disability. It develops between 4 and 14 days after the initial hemorrhage and can be detected by daily TCD measurements that show increased intraarterial velocity in the affected artery. Vasospasm is estimated to be three times more common among smokers and usually peaks between 7 and 10 days; it causes a narrowing of the vessels that may be multifactorial with a release of large amounts of calcium, an inflammatory response or spasmogens (serotonin, histamine, or heme), or other causes with resultant decreased CPP, ischemia, and clinical deterioration, including infarction. Clinically, patients may exhibit speech or motor deficits with unilateral paresis or paralysis and decreased LOC with a "waxing and waning" pattern. Angiographic diagnosis confirms the vasospasm and the exact location of the artery involved. Triple-H therapy and nimodipine (Nimotop), a calcium channel blocker, are two of the most common interventions. Nimodipine has an established role in decreasing vasospasm in all grades of SAH.[58,60] A dose of 60 mg should be given every 4 hours orally or via a nasogastric tube. If hypotension

occurs, the dosage regimen may be reduced to 30 mg every 2 hours. Parenteral forms are available for patients who cannot tolerate the drug orally. It should be started at a rate of 1 mg/hr and increased to a maximum of 2 mg/hr if hypotension does not occur.

Papaverine may be administered intraoperatively by the neurosurgeon. Papaverine acts as a smooth muscle relaxant to prevent postoperative vasospasm or interventionally if symptoms of vasospasm develop later, requiring the clinician to closely monitor for increased ICP, decreased cerebral blood flow, and respiratory arrest.

Triple-H therapy (hypervolemia, hypertension, and hemodilution) is aimed at maintaining adequate blood flow through potentially vasospastic cerebral vessels infusing fluids at rates between 100 and 400 ml/hr. This has been shown to improve cerebral perfusion, decrease delayed cerebral ischemia, and improve outcome.[19] Blood pressure is often maintained at approximately 60 mm Hg above baseline but not in excess of approximately 160 mm Hg in an unclipped aneurysm and not to exceed 240 mm Hg in a clipped aneurysm. Because of the increased risk of rupture and the need for invasive monitoring in a critical care area, triple-H therapy is usually initiated after clipping or endovascular treatment of the ruptured aneurysm. Maintaining MAP in the range of 100 to 110 mm Hg can be achieved by increasing the intravenous volume and using pressors. The hematocrit is maintained at greater than 33% so as not to diminish the oxygen-carrying capacity of the cerebral blood flow. Observe for side effects, including pulmonary edema from fluid overload, CHF with close monitoring of heart and breath sounds every 2 hours, rupture of another unclipped aneurysm, myocardial infarction (MI), hypertensive cerebral hemorrhage, and dilutional hyponatremia (sodium <135 mEq/L). Some centers routinely perform a transthoracic ECG before triple-H therapy.

Transfer of Patients With SAH. Transferring a patient to a

specialized center without initial resuscitation is detrimental. Transfer to a neurosurgical center should be carried out rapidly and safely. The patient should be accompanied by experienced medical and nursing staff, drugs, and equipment to treat potential problems during the transfer. Careful assessment by senior emergency department and anesthesia personnel is required to decide whether the patient requires tracheal intubation and ventilation for safe transfer to distant centers. If there is any doubt about the patient's airway or the adequacy of ventilation, an endotracheal tube should be inserted and mechanical ventilation instituted.[76] Patients who decompensate and have severe coexisting medical conditions are often unsuitable for transfer. If the patient has an endotracheal tube, he or she should be given supportive ICU care. Relatives should be informed of the patient's poor prognosis and decide on a course of action in the event of further decline.

Definitive Treatment of Intracranial Aneurysms

Patients with suspected or confirmed asymptomatic or symptomatic intracranial aneurysms should be referred to a neurosurgeon. Treatment options are open craniotomy, endovascular treatment, or carotid artery stenting. Treatment aims at obliteration of the aneurysm that caused the SAH or its exclusion from the circulation, to prevent rebleeding.

Timing of Aneurysm Surgery

Most experts advocate early surgical intervention, preferably within the first 48 hours after hemorrhage.

Surgical Considerations

Once an aneurysm is identified, a surgical decision is made regarding the technique and timing of obliteration. In the past, surgery was often delayed until the second or third week after the initial hemorrhage to avoid the complications of operating on a swollen brain. A postoperative angiogram can confirm good clip placement with total obliteration of the aneurysm and patent cerebral vessels. An intraoperative angiogram can be performed, which allows the neurosurgeon to reposition the aneurysm clip if needed.

The patient's preoperative status, intraoperative events, and behavior of brain during surgery leads the operating team to the postoperative regimen. The majority of postoperative patients are reversed from general anesthesia, extubated, and transported to the ICU or postanesthesia care unit (PACU).

Despite successful obliteration of the aneurysm, patients remain at significant risk for vasospasm, hydrocephalus, and medical complications and should be treated in an intensive care setting for at least 7 to 10 days.

Clipping of an Aneurysm (Surgical Procedure)

The surgical procedure is done under general endotracheal anesthesia. Continuous monitoring of ECG, arterial pressure, CVP, electrolytes, and urine output, as well as arterial blood gas (ABG), is maintained throughout the operative procedure.

Endotracheal intubation should be done gently with minimal pain and discomfort to the patient. The patient is positioned depending on the location of the lesion and surgical approach. The head is usually fixed with a radiolucent head holder for intraoperative angiogram. While preparing for surgery, a mayo stand should be prepared with various types of aneurysm clips and applicators. Most anterior circulation aneurysms are approached with a classical **pterional craniotomy,** for which the patient is positioned supine with head turned to the opposite side by 15 degrees. Arms and legs are protected while the body is covered with a warm blanket. Intermittent pneumatic compression stockings are applied to extremities to prevent thromboembolic events. Pressure points are protected with padding. Undue stretching of the neck should be avoided, especially in older patients. Sometimes the carotid artery is exposed in the neck for proximal control. Pterional craniotomy can be done with limited clipping of the hair with skin incisions just behind the anterior hairline extending from the midline laterally in front of the tragus. The skin is cleansed and prepped using povidone iodine. The skin incision area is infiltrated with 0.5% lidocaine with adrenaline for hemostasis and to reduce pain during incision. While the skin incision is made, the patient will receive mannitol, an osmotic diuretic (1.5 g/kg of body weight) and furosemide (Lasix), a loop diuretic

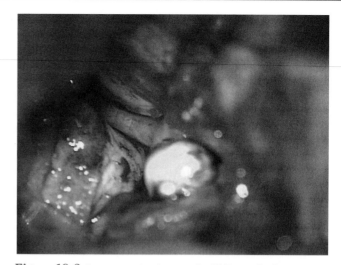

Figure 18-2 Intraoperative image of middle cerebral artery (MCA) aneurysm.
(Courtesy of Dr. Anil Nanda.)

(40 mg). The patient usually receives a dose of broad-spectrum antibiotic as prophylaxis. The skin flap is reflected and the temporalis muscle is separated. A **frontotemporal craniotomy** is done flush with the anterior cranial fossa. The sphenoid ridge is flattened. Under the operating microscope, the dura is opened, exposing the temporal and frontal lobe separated by the sylvian fissure. The sylvian fissure is split wide open, exposing the internal carotid artery, bifurcating into anterior and middle cerebral arteries. Further dissection is carried out depending on the location of aneurysm. In the case of a ruptured aneurysm with SAH, there would be blood clots in the cistern, which should be removed with continuous irrigation of the cistern. Dissection is continued until the aneurysm is identified, exposing the upper and lower border of the aneurysm (Fig. 18-2). The proximal segment of the parent artery should always be exposed before attempting to clip the aneurysm. Before clip application, the surgeon should make sure that all the branches from the artery are preserved. The clip is applied across the neck of the aneurysm, often parallel to the parent artery. If dissection of the aneurysmal sac is difficult, with previous bleeding and adhesions, it is advisable to temporarily occlude the parent artery for safer dissection. After clipping of the aneurysm, the surgeon should carefully assess the adequacy of clipping and look for residual neck, patency of parent artery and branches, and the presence of vasospasm. Successful clipping can be confirmed with an intraoperative angiogram. If the clip needs to be readjusted, it can be done depending on the angiogram findings. The cisterns are copiously irrigated with saline to wash away clots. Meticulous hemostasis is achieved. The patient's blood pressure is maintained at a normotensive level. The dura is closed and dural tacking sutures are used. The bone flap is replaced. The galea and skin are separately closed.

Nonsurgical Treatments

During the past decade, endovascular methods have been refined to treat intracranial aneurysms. The direct oblitera-

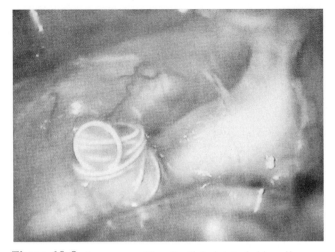

Figure 18-3 Aneurysm with a Guglielmi detachable coil (GDC).

tion of an aneurysm lumen using balloons, microcoils, or carotid artery stenting is now possible. The most popular technique, initially described by Guglielmi and colleagues, uses a soft platinum microcoil called the Guglielmi detachable coil (GDC), which can be detached from the guide wire by electrolysis[37] (Fig. 18-3). The GDC system received U.S. Food and Drug Administration (FDA) approval in 1995 for treatment of surgically high-risk aneurysms. The technique is considered minimally invasive as compared with an open craniotomy and offers patients an alternative to surgery and a reduced hospital length of stay (LOS). It also gives the patient with a poor medical condition or neurologic grade another avenue of treatment.

This successful microcoil is available in a variety of shapes, sizes, and lengths that are magnetic resonance imaging (MRI) compatible and FDA approved. In current practice, endovascular techniques are best suited for posterior fossa aneurysms because of the higher surgical risks associated with these aneurysms. Potential complications of endovascular treatment include rupture of aneurysm, cerebral hemorrhage, anticoagulation complications and vasospasm to distal vessels, ischemia, infarction, or stroke.[57]

The International Subarachnoid Aneurysm Trial (ISAT) published results in 2005 showing the relative efficacy of surgical clipping versus coiling in 2143 patients with ruptured intracranial aneurysms suitable for both treatments. In this study, endovascular coiling is more likely to result in independent survival at 1 year than neurosurgical clipping. Despite a low incidence of late rebleeding, it is more common after endovascular coiling than after neurosurgical clipping.[51]

Treatment options for an intracranial aneurysm are no longer limited to craniotomy with aneurysm clip occlusion. Technical advances in the field of endovascular neurosurgery continue to rapidly evolve, providing the opportunity to integrate microsurgery and endovascular treatment to assess each aneurysm for the best treatment option and outcome.[3] This emphasizes the need for a center-based multimodality approach in the management of cerebral aneurysms.

Preparation of the patient for endovascular treatment includes the following:
- Bilateral groin preparation
- Introduction of indwelling urinary catheter
- Maintenance of IV line
- Insertion of an arterial line (A-line)
- Fully heparinized patient
- ECG and electroencephalogram (EEG) monitoring
- Keeping the patient awake to assess neurologic status

Postoperative management includes the following:
- Head elevation 30 degrees
- Peripheral vascular check
- Monitoring of the sheath, which may be left in place for a short period, in case the patient returns emergently
- Close monitoring of prothrombin time (PT) and activated partial thromboplastin time (APTT)
- Aggressive fluid management
- Close neurologic monitoring
- Continuation of other medication as part of SAH treatment

Posttreatment Clinical Management

Acute Care

The patient is admitted to the NCCU for acute care, serial neurologic assessments, and hemodynamic monitoring to prevent potential complications. Patients are maintained on bed rest with the head of the bed elevated 30 degrees. Patients not restricted to bed rest should have supervised ambulation because nimodipine can precipitate postural hypotension. Routine monitoring of neurologic status and vital signs, including cardiac monitoring, is advised until the patient is stable and free of complications. Normoglycemic control is achieved by close monitoring of blood glucose and insulin therapy as needed with careful titration. Observation for vasospasm is essential. This can be done with daily transcranial Doppler examination of the arterial flow velocity and postoperative angiogram. A preoperative Doppler study assists in comparing the postoperative flow velocities. It is important to maintain hypervolemia and to avoid dehydration with strict monitoring of CVP or pulmonary wedge pressure (or both). Serum electrolytes should be checked every day. Early postoperative mobilization along with physiotherapy helps minimize complications from prolonged immobility. Triple-H therapy is frequently instituted in vasospasm, which is previously described.

Potential posttreatment changes to monitor are shown in Box 18-1.

Nutritional Considerations

Acute nutritional considerations have been discussed. Recovery can present significant issues due to loss of appetite, weight loss, and lack of energy, causing "fatigue syndrome," which can cause difficulties for some patients. Dietary consultation, eating six small meals per day, scheduled periods of rest, and dietary supplements are recommended. Fresh fruits and vegetables, with the addition of natural bran in the diet and fruit juices as natural laxatives, improve bowel regularity.

BOX 18-1	Potential Posttreatment Changes to Monitor

- Change in level of consciousness (LOC): May include confusion or agitation that waxes and wanes.
- Motor deficits: May include pronator drift, weakness, or hemiparesis.
- Cardiac changes: May include hypertension; dysrhythmias; congestive heart failure (CHF) and pulmonary edema from fluid therapy; and "sympathetic storms" from increases in intracranial pressure (ICP).
- Increased ICP: May require ventriculostomy with ICP monitoring for elevated ICP that may respond to drainage of cerebrospinal fluid (CSF) or mannitol administration.
- Edema: May occur with cranial nerve deficits in relationship to the affected artery; may involve visual, motor, and sensory dysfunctions.
- Decreased oxygenation: May require intubation and controlled ventilation.
- Meningeal irritation: May occur as head, neck, or back pain (primary components to assess).
- Ischemic injury: May occur from prolonged temporary arterial occlusion or intraoperative hypotension, injury to surrounding veins, or intraoperative aneurysm rupture.
- Pain and headache: Require pain assessment and interventions.
- Loss of appetite: May signal vasospasm or deterioration in the LOC.
- Infection: Fever may be warning signal that heralds complications.
- CSF drainage: Occurs from a dural leak.
- Electrolyte imbalance (hyponatremia): Occurs in 10% to 34% of patients and can cause confusion and lead to seizures or progress to coma in patients not treated

appropriately. Cerebral salt wasting (CSW) versus syndrome of inappropriate antidiuretic hormome (SIADH) must be determined. If the cause is CSW with failure of the central nervous system to regulate sodium absorption, the treatment is to increase fluid intake. For SIADH the intervention is to restrict fluids, which allows the serum sodium level to rise, or in severe cases volume replacement may be needed (see Chapter 5).
- Fluid imbalance: Crystalloid and colloid solutions are used to counter vasospasm; imbalances can result in diabetes insipidus (DI), SIADH, or CSW (described above).
- Seizures: Occur in approximately 25% of patients because of the disruption in blood flow and irritation of the brain from the blood. Administration of anticonvulsants is recommended.
- Increased ICP: Can occur immediately following the aneurysm rupture and fluctuates as the patient's condition waxes and wanes; results in cerebral ischemia.
- Deep vein thromboses (DVTs) and pulmonary embolism (PE): Risk requires close monitoring and early detection.
- Rebleeding: Occurs if the aneurysmal clip is not totally occlusive or is improperly placed.
- Severe onset of neurologic deficits: May occur if an adjoining cerebral vessel was inadvertently clipped during the placement of the aneurysmal clip. Requires immediate notification of the surgeon and immediate imaging with possible return to the operating room (OR) and reclipping of the aneurysm.
- Vocal cord swelling: May occur from prolonged surgery and intubation.

Constipation and straining during bowel movements are to be avoided. Energy-saving tips and exercise instructions from the rehabilitation team to use large muscles to relieve tension and restlessness are useful in stimulating the appetite.

For the brain to heal, the patient must have a balanced and adequate diet to meet increased nutritional needs. Depending on the patient's age, diagnosis, and ability to tolerate oral nutrition, a complete nutritional assessment and therapeutic diet plan should be initiated by the hospital dietitian. A comprehensive plan includes a goal for ideal weight, daily food and fluid intake, supplemental oral feedings such as Ensure, restriction of any foods that interact with prescription medications, recommendations for the types and amounts of food for rapid recovery, and a diet diary or calorie count. Goals of the diet plan are to achieve the ideal body weight and to maintain a well-balanced diet with no adverse outcomes.

ALERT: Patients with an impaired gag and swallow reflex are at risk for aspiration. Speech and language therapists are consulted in the early period to evaluate the patients and to indicate to the treating team when oral feedings are appropriate.

Psychosocial Considerations

Patients recovering from cranial surgery need psychosocial support for any temporary or permanent deficits, complica-

tions, or body image changes (e.g., hair loss, edema and swelling of the face, or changes in speech and language, motor and sensory functions, and cognition). Sensitivity and support are needed to help the patient cope with fear, anxiety, and depression and with any other effects of the cranial surgery on the patient's recovery and future life. Patients should be encouraged to talk about their feelings and emotions, and their responses should be evaluated. The need for referral and professional psychologic or psychiatric follow-up should be evaluated. (See Chapters 7 and 11 for psychosocial considerations in relation to brain tumors and traumatic brain injury, respectively.)

Postoperatively and before discharge, it is important to defuse the stress and anxiety of the family members. They may be exhausted from worry and their constant vigilance at the bedside, particularly if the patient experienced periods of "waxing and waning." Families are central participants of the caregiver team for psychosocial support to meet the early and continuous needs of the patient. The family's attitude of confidence and satisfaction with the patient's treatment is imparted to the patient and begins the stages of positive psychosocial adaptation. This concept is not well understood by all caregivers. It is important to identify the important needs of family members of critically ill neurosurgical patients and to explore the differences in perception of needs by family members and clinicians.

Important needs of family members may include designating a specific number or person for the family to call at the hospital when unable to visit, visitation at any time (if hospital policy permits), and the ability to see the patient frequently and participate with the patient's physical care. Families are intimidated with the seriousness of the loved one's condition and all the medical equipment at the bedside. They appreciate directions for what to do and what not do at the bedside. The family's anxiety level is decreased with explanations about the environment before going to the bedside. Family conferences with the treating team and frequent updates from the staff are needed, particularly when transfer or discharge plans are being made. When visiting hours do not start on time, the family may fear the worst and should be given assurance that there is no crisis and information concerning any delay (e.g., physician and team rounds were delayed or the respiratory therapist was at the bedside).

Communication and information to the family by clinicians who demonstrate compassion and caring can empower families for improved patient and family outcomes following emergency events, such as an SAH.

Older Adult Considerations

A large group of patients with SAH were classified into three groups to compare outcome: (1) ages 59 or younger, (2) ages 60 to 69, and (3) age 70 and over. The overall outcome at 1 year after SAH was significantly poorer in group 3 than in groups 1 and 2. No differences were found between groups 1 and 2. The overall mortality rate for all patients was 35%. The rate of patients in group 1 surviving in good condition or in a disabled but independent condition at 1 year was 93%.[31] Older adults should therefore not be denied the benefits of surgery solely on the basis of their age.[11] The functional outcome in older patients with SAH is disappointing, even if they are considered suitable for surgical treatment. Even though the operability rate for older patients 70 to 79 years of age has increased, resulting in improvements in both surgical and management outcomes, functional outcomes are still unsatisfactory.[31]

Posttreatment Potential Complications Specific to Subarachnoid Hemorrhage

For complications during the acute posttreatment recovery, the reader is also referred to Chapter 9 for a comprehensive review of potential complications.

Rebleeding. The risk of rebleeding is definitely reduced by surgical clipping or endovascular treatment of the aneurysm. Ruptured aneurysms should be obliterated as soon as possible to prevent this complication.[62]

Hydrocephalus. The incidence of acute ventricular dilatation after SAH is about 20%.[26,34] Ventricular drainage may be required to relieve acute hydrocephalus in patients with depressed sensorium and increased ICP. Clinically significant acute hydrocephalus is more likely to occur with increasing age, poor clinical grade, intraventricular hemorrhage, diffuse SAH, focal thick SAH, posterior circulation aneu-

rysms, use of antifibrinolytic agents, hyponatremia, and preexisting or postoperative systemic hypertension. An external ventricular drain may be perioperatively instituted to achieve brain relaxation at the time of surgery.[49] The drain can be left in place postoperatively to monitor ICP, drain CSF, and instill fibrinolytic agents if indicated.

Chronic hydrocephalus is documented in 10% to 20% of patients who had aneurysmal SAH.[71] Symptomatic patients with hydrocephalus need permanent CSF diversion with a ventriculoperitoneal shunt (see Chapter 13).

Intraventricular Hemorrhage. Major intraventricular hemorrhage with aneurysmal SAH is documented in 13% to 28% of patients.[34,50] Anterior communicating and basilar tip aneurysms are the most common causes of intraventricular hemorrhage. Over 50% of patients with large intraventricular bleeds are admitted in poor grade, and their mortality rate exceeds 64%.[50]

Increased Intracranial Pressure. Increased ICP may occur in the absence of ventricular dilation.[2] The possible causes for raised ICP include acute hydrocephalus, intraventricular or intracerebral hemorrhage, brain swelling, ischemic brain edema, and increased resistance to CSF outflow, probably due to blockade of arachnoid villi by blood (see Chapter 10). The advantages of placing an external ventricular drain in such cases include the ability to measure ICP and reduce ICP by draining CSF, thereby improving CPP. Risks include infection, hematoma, and aneurysmal rebleeding.[33,55]

Treatment of the increased ICP after SAH includes removal of large intracranial hematoma, placing an external ventricular drain, mechanical ventilation, sedation, intravenous mannitol with or without furosemide, and short periods of hyperventilation (see Chapter 10 for increased ICP and monitoring).

Intracerebral Hemorrhage. About 34% of ruptured aneurysms cause intracerebral hematoma.[56] Small deep-penetrating arteries may bleed into the brain parenchyma or the major lobes of the brain, basal ganglia, ventricles, and areas of the brainstem or cerebellum. Patients with a history of uncontrolled hypertension are at risk.

Because of significant morbidity and mortality risks, the decision to evacuate the hematoma depends on the size and location, as well as level of sensorium with features of herniation. Patients may have increased ICP and displacement of structures from compression by the clot and edema with rapid deterioration. Emergency resuscitation measures are performed followed by diagnostic studies that may include CT, MRI, and angiography for accurate diagnosis. Interventions are performed to prevent hypoxia and further deterioration that may include intubation with mechanical ventilation and ventriculostomy for escalating ICP. Careful control of blood pressure and aggressive management to prevent complications are continued in the intensive care setting. Guidelines for the use of factor VIIa in warfarin-anticoagulated patients with a traumatic or nontraumatic spontaneous intracranial hemorrhage can be found in Chapter 11, Box 11-11.

Surgical decisions are made by the neurosurgical team regarding evacuation of the clot. A ruptured aneurysm can be dealt with at the time of clot evacuation. Postoperative management as described previously is continued, and measures are taken to prevent secondary complications and improve outcome (described later).

Seizures. The literature reports an incidence of seizures in about 20% of patients with SAH[25] (see Chapter 23). Risk factors for the development of late epilepsy include younger age, middle cerebral artery aneurysms, intracerebral hematoma, poor clinical grade, postoperative neurologic deficits due to cortical infarction, history of seizures, medial temporal lobe retraction, and shunt-dependent hydrocephalus.[63] Treatment with anticonvulsants, such as phenytoin (Dilantin), carbamazepine (Tegretol), phenobarbital (Solfoton), valproic acid (Depakote), or lamotrigine (Lamictal), is recommended for most SAH patients in the first few days covering the perioperative period. Anticonvulsants can be discontinued in most cases except those with high risk factors (see Chapter 24 for comprehensive management of seizures and epilepsy). Clinicians should be aware of drug-drug interactions (e.g., certain anticoagulants and antiseizure medications) and check for incompatibilities.

Cerebral Vasospasm. Neurologic deterioration subsequent to initial stabilization is frequently attributed to vasospasm. Patients may have depression in sensorium or drowsiness. Surgery is usually deferred in patients in whom there is clinical suspicion or angiographic demonstration of vasospasm. Vasospasm is thought to be caused by the breakdown product of blood that has accumulated in cisterns around vessels of the circle of Willis.

Postoperative vasospasm can be demonstrated by **transcranial Doppler (TCD)** evaluation. A daily bedside evaluation to measure the changes in flow velocities that correlate with the degree of arterial narrowing can be performed. This noninvasive bedside technique provides immediate feedback to the neurosurgical team, allowing them to decide on therapeutic management. Alternatively, vasospasm can be demonstrated by an angiogram.

Clinical evidence of vasospasm occurs between days 4 and 10 following hemorrhage, with maximal narrowing at around day 7. Vasospasm has been observed up to 21 days after the SAH.[70] The amount of blood or large, thick clots in the basal cistern appears to correlate well with the degree of vasospasm or delayed ischemic deficit.[12] Symptoms are initially subtle but tend to progress very rapidly. Symptoms include confusion, agitation, decreased LOC, cranial nerve palsies, seizures, dysphasias, and motor or sensory deficits. Vasospasm is potentially treatable and reversible, if it is detected and treated early. Continuous monitoring is needed for early detection of this condition.

The treatment regimen for vasospasm generally consists of triple-H therapy (hypervolemia, hemodilution, and hypertension). Phenylephrine and dopamine are the most commonly used pressors. The aim of this treatment should be an increase in MAP of approximately 20 to 30 mm Hg above "baseline" systolic pressure. Intravenous fluids and the administration of dobutamine, which selectively improves the cardiac output without much change in MAP, is increasingly used in the management of vasospasm. The hematocrit should be reduced to the low 30s, which usually occurs as a result of hypervolemia. Transluminal angioplasty is indicated when conventional therapy has failed.

Other Potential Medical Complications

Respiratory Complications. Respiratory complications in SAH contribute to about 50% of deaths from medical causes, which are more common with advancing age and poor clinical grade.[66] The most frequently encountered respiratory complications are pulmonary edema, hypostatic pneumonia, atelectasis, aspiration, pneumothorax, and pulmonary emboli. Pulmonary edema may complicate the course of patients with aneurysmal SAH and may be either cardiogenic or noncardiogenic (neurogenic, or secondary to pulmonary insults such as aspiration). The treatment includes endotracheal intubation, adequate oxygenation, mechanical ventilation with positive end-expiratory pressure, furosemide, and measures to reduce ICP, especially if it is neurogenic in origin.

Venous Thromboembolism. Incidence of symptomatic deep vein thrombosis in SAH patients is about 2%, of which half result in pulmonary embolism.[42] Risk factors for venous thromboembolism include advanced age, heart failure, direct trauma to limbs, previous history of thromboembolism, varicose veins, use of oral contraceptive pills, pregnancy and puerperium, obesity, malignancy, infection, duration of surgery over 4 hours, limb weakness, or paralysis.[13] Graduated compression stockings and pneumatic compression devices are regularly used to prevent this complication. If deep vein thrombosis or pulmonary embolism develops, treatment includes anticoagulation or placement of an inferior vena cava filter.

Cardiovascular Complications. Cardiovascular abnormalities are commonly encountered in aneurysmal SAH, including changes in ECG, dysrhythmias, and alteration in blood pressure. These changes are attributed to sympathetic overactivity following SAH. ECG abnormalities include peaked P waves; pathologic Q waves; increased QRS voltages; ST-segment depression or elevation; peaked, flattened, diphasic, or inverted T waves; sinus bradycardia or tachycardia; and large U waves.[45] Various arrhythmias such as sinus tachycardia, multifocal ventricular extrasystoles, supraventricular extrasystoles, and sinus arrhythmias can occur with aneurysmal SAH. These patients should be continuously monitored with electrocardiography and frequently monitored for serum electrolytes, especially potassium.

Fluid and Electrolyte Disturbances. The commonly encountered electrolyte abnormalities after aneurysmal SAH are hyponatremia, hypernatremia, and hypokalemia.[69] SAH produces excessive sodium loss through the urine, leading to negative sodium balance, decreased body weight, and increased blood urea nitrogen. This hyponatremic state could be due to two conditions: syndrome of inappropriate antidiuretic hormone secretion (SIADH) or cerebral salt-wasting syndrome (CSWS) (see Chapter 5). It is important to differentiate these two conditions to treat hyponatremia accurately. The differentiating feature is that the blood volume status is decreased in CSWS, unlike in SIADH. CSWS is treated with adequate water and sodium replacement to maintain normovolemia and normal serum sodium. In the case of SIADH, fluid restriction followed by sodium supplementation is needed.

Diabetes insipidus (DI) can complicate a small number of cases with SAH, and is associated with anterior communicating artery aneurysm (ACoA) rupture. Treatment includes the replacement of fluid with a hypotonic solution such as 5% dextrose or half-normal saline (0.45%). Chronic DI is usually treated with ADH supplementation.

Gastrointestinal Complications. Mucosal ulceration (stress ulceration) in the stomach may occur following aneurysmal SAH. The accepted treatment includes H_2 antagonists. Sucralfate is a promising drug for stress ulcer prophylaxis without affecting gastric pH. Stool softeners are administered to prevent straining. Nimodipine may be associated with gastrointestinal pseudo-obstruction and ileus.[42] A small percentage of patients (4%) may develop significant hepatic dysfunction, which may be related to liver congestion, systemic inflammation, and drugs.[66]

ARTERIOVENOUS MALFORMATION

Intracranial AVMs are relatively uncommon but may cause serious neurologic problems, hemorrhage, or even death. Intracranial AVMs can cause serious neurologic symptoms or morbidity related to hemorrhage or seizure,[48] but advances in diagnostic neuroimaging techniques are increasing the detection of lesions before rupture.[7] An AVM can be described as complex tangles or coils of arteries and veins. AVMs may be connected by fistulas to a vascular conglomerate separated by sclerotic tissue or "nidus." There is no capillary bed that serves to nourish the brain tissue from the arterial system or remove waste by-products by way of the venous system. High-velocity arteriovenous shunting takes place by way of the fistulas, and over time these veins may become severely dilated and at risk for rupture and bleeding. If congenital, the AVM may enlarge over time and begin to show symptoms when the individual is between 15 and 40 years of age, often beginning with a headache. Hemorrhage and seizure may be the first indication that the individual is harboring an AVM.

There have been significant changes in the management of intracranial AVMs over the last decade owing to improvements in microsurgical, endovascular, and radiosurgical techniques.

Epidemiology

The incidence and prevalence of intracranial vascular malformations are not clearly known. The available data suggest that there is an overall incidence of AVMs in about 3% of the population.[22]

Clinical Presentation

Intracranial AVMs are typically diagnosed before the patient has reached 40 years of age. More than 50% of AVMs cause

intracranial hemorrhage, with a mortality rate between 10% and 15%.[9] Intracerebral hemorrhage is more common than subarachnoid and intraventricular hemorrhages and can be a lethal and devastating event. Seizure is the next most common manifestation, occurring in about 20% to 25% of cases.[10] Seizures can be either focal or generalized, which may be an indicator of the location of the lesion. Other manifestations include headaches, focal neurologic deficit, and, rarely, pulsatile tinnitus. Children under 2 years of age may have high-output CHF and large head due to hydrocephalus. Vascular malformation–related steal phenomena that cause focal neurologic deficit by altering perfusion in the brain in the vicinity of the AVM are rare.[43] Intracranial aneurysms can be associated in 7% to 17% of patients.[8] They can occur on the feeding artery to the AVM. These may involute after resection or obliteration of the brain AVM.

Spetzler-Martin Grading System for AVMs

The Spetzler-Martin grading system described in Table 18-5 helps predict the likelihood of satisfactory outcomes if an attempt at surgical resection is made.[67] The Spetzler-Martin grade is determined by adding the three individual scores from the table. High-grade AVMs are more difficult to resect, and therefore neurologic deficits from the surgery are more likely.

Neurodiagnostic and Laboratory Studies

Intracranial AVMs are diagnosed with a variety of diagnostic imaging studies. **Computed tomography (CT) without contrast** has a low sensitivity, but calcification and enhancement following contrast administration may be seen.[36] **Magnetic resonance imaging (MRI)** is highly sensitive, showing an inhomogeneous signal void on T1- and T2-weighted sequences, commonly with hemosiderin, suggesting prior hemorrhage. MRI can also provide information regarding the location and topography of an AVM, which could be useful in planning treatment.[35] MRI is a reliable form of imaging following intervention, especially after radiosurgery. Ideally, an MRI study and a four-vessel angiogram should be obtained to delineate the anatomy of an AVM. **Arteriography** is considered the "gold standard" to define the arterial and venous anatomy.

Treatment Options

Currently four major treatment options are available to patients with an AVM of the brain: conservative observation, microneurosurgery, endovascular treatment, and radiosurgery. The lesion can be conservatively observed with the understanding that the patient could have the risk of hemor-

TABLE 18-5	Spetzler-Martin Grading of Arteriovenous Malformations				
Size of Arteriovenous Malformation		**Eloquence of Adjacent Brain**		**Pattern of Venous Drainage**	
Small (<3 cm)	1	Noneloquent	0	Superficial only	0
Medium (3–6 cm)	2	Eloquent	1	Deep component	1
Large (>6 cm)	3	—		—	

rhage or other neurologic symptoms such as seizures or focal deficits. The goal of intervention should be complete AVM obliteration since suboptimal therapy does not protect the patient from subsequent hemorrhages. Each treatment option has associated potential risks and benefits.

Microsurgical Resection

Anesthetic and Perioperative Considerations for Microsurgical Resection. AVM resection is usually an elective procedure. All preexisting medical conditions should be optimized before AVM resection. An important consideration throughout the operative period is the potential for massive, rapid, and persistent blood loss.

Surgical Procedures. The following steps are needed for patient preparation:

- Placement of arterial and central lines
- Electrophysiologic monitoring, including EEG and somatosensory-evoked potentials (SSEPs)
- Positioning (usually supine with the head placed in a three-point head fixation device)
- Craniotomy procedure, often with interactive image guidance localization

Craniotomy. The patient is transported to the operating room. After routine preparation, the patient is positioned and draped for the procedure, which is performed with the patient under general anesthesia. A craniotomy is performed and the craniotomy flap is reflected. The dura is opened, and careful microdissection of the AVM begins with exposure of the nidus, which is composed of a coiled tangle of abnormal vessels. In the next step, the feeding arteries are identified and controlled. The draining veins should then be dissected and controlled. After confirming that all the feeders are controlled effectively, the nidus is excised completely and the remaining bed is inspected for residual nidus or source of bleeding. Meticulous hemostasis is critical in AVM resection. Hemorrhage, cerebral edema, cerebral ischemia, and parenchymal brain injury are potential intraoperative complications.

Postoperative Care. The recommendations for postoperative care include neurologic intensive care monitoring for at least 24 hours. Blood pressure is monitored with an arterial catheter and urine output with an indwelling catheter. Typically, normotensive and euvolemic conditions are maintained; however, tight blood pressure control with agents that do not act on the central nervous system may be appropriate for selected individuals. Postoperative hyperthermia may be detrimental and may even be exacerbated by mild, intraoperative-induced hypothermia. Therefore careful attention should be paid to the control of patient temperature in the ICU.

Perioperative antibiotics, steroids, and seizure medications are used variably. After the initial postoperative period of monitoring in the ICU, the patient is transferred to a surgical floor with early mobilization. An angiogram may also be performed to document complete resection of the AVM during the immediate postoperative period. A new neurologic deficit after surgery is usually investigated with a CT scan to rule out a hemorrhage or complications attributed to surgical procedure. MRI scanning with diffusion-weighted imaging may be preferred to document infarct.

In summary, AVM surgery is usually elective and frequently preceded by preoperative embolization. Surgical approach allows complete resection of the nidus, with selective ligation of the feeding vessels and the draining veins.[77] Management of associated aneurysms is determined on an individual basis.

Endovascular Treatment

Technical advances in interventional neuroradiology/endovascular neurosurgery have afforded new avenues in the management of cerebral AVMs. Flow-directed and flow-assisted microcatheters have allowed for accuracy and safer delivery of embolic materials. Various embolic materials are used in the endovascular treatment of AVMs, including N-butyl cyanoacrylate (NBCA), which has recently been approved by the FDA for use in brain AVMs.[54] Embolization of cerebral AVMs is just one aspect of a multimodality approach to these lesions.

Current indications include the following:

1. Presurgical embolization in large or giant cortical or subcortical AVMs can be done to reduce the nidus size and to occlude surgically inaccessible or deep arterial feeders, to facilitate surgical excision, and to treat intranidal aneurysms and high-flow fistulas, thereby promoting progressive thrombosis of the nidus of the AVM.[74]
2. Preradiosurgical embolization. There are three potential goals of embolization before radiosurgery: (a) to decrease target size to less than 3 cm in diameter because smaller volumes have a higher cure rate with less morbidity; (b) to eliminate angiographic predictors of hemorrhage, such as intranidal or venous aneurysms or high-flow fistulas; and (c) to attempt to reduce symptoms related to venous hypertension.[41] Most centers recommend the use of more permanent agents, such as polymers of cyanoacrylate, for embolization. However, numerous studies indicate that the use of such agents may also result in a recanalization rate of 14%.[16] There is no evidence that flow reduction alone without reduction of the AVM volume provides any benefit before radiosurgery, and it may make it more difficult to provide a dose plan at the time of radiosurgical planning.[23]
3. Palliative embolization can be used in large AVMs with progressive neurologic deficits secondary to high-flow or venous hypertension that are not suitable for microsurgical or radiosurgical treatment. The aim of treatment is to reduce the flow and halt symptom progression.[54]
4. Aneurysms in relation to AVMs can also be treated with endovascular intervention.

Anesthetic and Perioperative Considerations for Endovascular Therapy. Although many of the risks and responses of microsurgery and endovascular treatment are conceptually the same, there are many important differences in the working environment. The procedure can be done under general endotracheal anesthesia or intravenous sedation. Premedication includes corticosteroids, anticonvulsants, aspirin, calcium channel blockers, and antibiotics.

Direct invasive monitoring of arterial blood pressure is mandatory, due to the manipulation of systemic pressure with vasoactive agents. The femoral artery introducer sheath, as well as the coaxial (guiding) catheter, can be used to monitor arterial pressure. Placement of an additional pulse oximeter on the foot that will receive the femoral introducer catheter provides an early warning of femoral artery obstruction or distal thromboembolism. Indwelling urinary catheters assist in fluid management, as well as patient comfort. Patients who received sedatives should be on supplemental oxygen.

The primary goals of anesthetic choice for intravenous sedation include alleviation of pain or discomfort, alleviation of anxiety, and patient immobility. If neurologic testing is required, there should be a rapid decrease in level of sedation. Patients who are intravenously sedated are prone to develop upper airway obstruction. Placement of nasopharyngeal airways should be done before anticoagulation. Careful management of coagulation is required to prevent thromboembolic complications during and after procedures. Profound deliberate systemic hypotension may be induced while the interventionist prepares the glue for injection.

Radiosurgery

Stereotactic radiosurgery is a highly effective and relatively noninvasive treatment technique for the management of cerebral AVMs. The purpose of radiosurgery is to subject the blood vessels of the AVM to a high dose of radiation, causing progressive luminal obliteration and preventing subsequent hemorrhage. Stereotactic delivery minimizes radiation to surrounding normal parenchyma.

Indications for AVM Radiosurgery. Radiosurgery is most appropriate for patients with small AVMs, especially when they are located in eloquent brain locations. Lesions most effectively treated with radiosurgery have volumes of less than 10 cm^3 or a maximum diameter less than 3 cm.[14,59,68] Candidates for treatment are selected on the basis of AVM volume and location, patient age, and relative risk analysis compared with surgical and endovascular therapies as predicted by the Spetzler-Martin grading scale.

Multimodality Treatment of Cerebral AVM

AVMs are often treated by more than one treatment modality. It is done either as a planned maneuver, with embolization followed by surgical resection or radiosurgery, or if one treatment modality fails and a second treatment modality is necessary to obliterate the AVM.[54]

Continuum of Care

Home Care and Rehabilitation

Patients who survive the crisis of a ruptured aneurysm, its surgical clipping or other interventions, and the subsequent postoperative therapy are still faced with a long recovery. Patients need to be monitored carefully and observed for late-onset vasospasm. Nimodipine is continued for the 21-day regimen, and patients are instructed to continue good hydration and fluid intake. The goal of returning the patient

home and to the highest level of physical, psychologic, and cognitive functioning is challenging.

Consultation with a physiatrist for a rehabilitation plan of care and therapy in the outpatient setting or home may be necessary to improve cognition, ameliorate speech and motor deficits, and strengthen muscles. Memory loss may be temporary or long term and can be frustrating. Strategies to reduce fatigue include avoiding sensory overload, keeping a daily planner to limit activities, and using a tape recorder and writing notes. Fatigue becomes a limiting factor in the patient's activities of daily living (ADLs). Complaints of headache may persist for months and insomnia may interrupt sleep patterns. Migraine headaches secondary to cerebral hemorrhage have been reported by some patients. Headaches may last for months or years and cause much distress if a headache was the first symptom of a subarachnoid hemorrhage. Acetaminophen, with or without codeine, as well as warm packs or a heating pad applied to the back of the neck, may offer some relief for headaches.

Recognition of the signs and symptoms of hydrocephalus should be reinforced, since this complication may develop over time. Hydrocephalus may require a return to the hospital for placement of a shunt (see Chapter 8).

Depression is not unusual for a patient who faces this long and complicated recovery. Psychosocial support for the patient and family should continue until they can successfully cope and deal with these conditions. Physical changes and brain healing may be temporary, and the patient may take months to adjust. Talking to other survivors in a support group encourages sharing of feelings to realize this is "normal" following a major insult to the brain.

Speech and language impairment may persist, causing the patient to perform these skills more slowly. Visual impairment may decrease or limit the ability to read. Neuropsychologic evaluation is recommended for dementia in individuals who may have cognitive deficits even when they do not have obvious neurologic defects. (See Chapter 13 for stroke rehabilitation.) The Brain Aneurysm Foundation (BAF) (see Resources) has information on BAF support groups around the country (contact office@brainfound.org). Many deficits are possible, but most will respond to time and treatment.

Case Management Considerations

There is nothing as frightening to a patient and the family as "brain surgery" for a ruptured aneurysm or AVM. Depending on the patient's age, prognosis, and level of function, case management may be required to coordinate individualized, comprehensive services. The goal is to help the patient return home, recover, or adapt to a life with temporary or permanent functional alterations without complications or the need for rehospitalization. Assessment and planning include the following:

- Interview of the family and caregivers
- Neurologic assessment: for deficits, pain, and complications (e.g., hydrocephalus)
- Rehabilitation: with a plan of care that may include physical, occupational, and speech therapy

- Consultation for medical complications, including return appointments with arrangements for transportation
- Support groups and resources in the community for individuals with disabilities
- Assessment of home living arrangements to determine barriers to ADLs, potential for injury and harm, and equipment needs (e.g., home care, special bed, bath, or toileting needs)

Case management may be needed for only a short period of time, or it may be needed for the lifetime of a patient with severe neurologic problems. Case management helps afford the patient the best possible quality of life and the ability to function at his or her highest level of care.

CONCLUSION

Rapid diagnosis and early treatment of aneurysmal and vascular surgical patients and aggressive management by a skilled team of neuroscience nurse clinicians contribute significantly to decreased morbidity and mortality rates. Prevention and treatment of neurologically detrimental complications (e.g., vasospasm) improves outcomes for a good recovery and early discharge. During hospitalization, recovering patients and their families learn about the risk factors associated with their condition and receive important education on how to improve their health and lifestyle to avoid future embolic risks. Advanced technology, new devices, and improved techniques, combined with sophisticated pharmacologic treatments, hold promise for minimally invasive procedures and improved therapies in the future. The search continues for techniques to repair damaged brain tissue that will reduce disability and save more lives. Our challenge is to implement clinical management based on the latest knowledge and best practices for this population of patients with life-threatening neurologic conditions.

RESOURCES

American Association of Neurological Surgeons (AANS): www.aans.org

American Association of Neuroscience Nurses (AANN): www.aann.org

American Heart Association: www.stroke.org

Brain Aneurysm Information: www.brainaneurysm.com

Brain Aneurysm Foundation: www.bafound.org

Congress of Neurological Surgeons: www.neurosurgeon.org

Society of Neurosurgical Anesthesia and Critical Care: www.snacc.org

REFERENCES

1. Adams HP Jr, Putnam SF, Kassell NF, Torner JC: Prevalence of diabetes mellitus among patients with subarachnoid hemorrhage, *Arch Neurol* 41:1033–1035, 1984.
2. Bailes JE, Spetzler RF, Hadley MN, et al: Management of morbidity and mortality in poor grade aneurysm patients, *J Neurosurg* 72:559–566, 1990.
3. Berenstein A, Graeb DA: Convenient preparations of ready-to-use particles in polyvinyl alcohol foam suspension for embolization, *Radiology* 145:846, 1982.
4. Broderick JP, Brott T, Tomsick T, Huster G, Miller R: The risk of subarachnoid and intracerebral hemorrhages in blacks as compared with whites, *N Engl J Med* 326:733–736, 1992.
5. Broderick JP, Brott T, Tomsick T, Miller R, Huster G: Intracerebral hemorrhage more than twice as common as subarachnoid hemorrhage, *J Neurosurg* 78:188–191, 1993.
6. Bromberg JE, Rinkel GJ, Algra A, et al: Outcome in familial subarachnoid haemorrhage, *Stroke* 26:961–963, 1995.
7. Brown RD, Wiebers DO, Forbes G, et al: The natural history of unruptured intracranial arteriovenous malformations, *J Neurosurg* 68:352–357, 1988.
8. Brown RD, Wiebers DO, Forbes GS: Unruptured intracranial aneurysms and arteriovenous malformations: frequency of intracranial hemorrhage and relationship of lesions, *J Neurosurg* 73:859–863, 1990.
9. Brown RD, Wiebers DO, Torner JC, et al: Frequency of intracranial hemorrhage as a presenting symptom and subtype analysis: a population-based study of intracranial vascular malformations in Olmsted County, Minnesota, *J Neurosurg* 85:29–32, 1996.
10. Brown RD Jr, Flemming KD, Meyer FB, Cloft HJ, Pollock BE, Link ML: Natural history, evaluation, and management of intracranial vascular malformations, *Mayo Clin Proc* 80(2):269–281, 2005.
11. Cheung RB: Neurosurgical intensive care. In Fulmer TT, Walker MK, editors: *Critical care nursing of the elderly,* New York, 1992, Springer.
12. Claassen J, Bernardini GL, Kreiter K, et al: Effect of cisternal and ventricular blood on risk of delayed cerebral ischaemia after subarachnoid haemorrhage: the Fisher scale revisited, *Stroke* 32:2012–2020, 2001.
13. Collins R, Scrimgeour A, Yusuf S, Peto R: Reduction in fatal pulmonary embolism and venous thrombosis by perioperative administration of subcutaneous heparin. Overview of results of randomized trials in general, orthopedic, and urologic surgery, *N Engl J Med* 318(18):1162–1173, 1988.
14. Colombo F, Pozza F, Chierego G, et al: Linear accelerator radiosurgery of cerebral arteriovenous malformations: an update, *Neurosurgery* 34:14–20, discussion 20–21, 1994.
15. Davis PH, Hachinski V: Epidemiology of cerebrovascular diseases. In Anderson DW, Schoenberg DG, editors: *Neuroepidemiology: a tribute to Bruce Schoenberg,* Boston, 1991, CRC Press.
16. Dawson RC III, Tarr RW, Hecht ST, et al: Treatment of arteriovenous malformations of the brain with combined embolization and stereotactic radiosurgery: results after 1 and 2 years, *AJNR Am J Neuroradiol* 11:857–864, 1990.
17. Dehdashti AR, Rufenacht DA, Delavelle J, Reverdin A, De Tribolet N: Therapeutic decision and management of aneurysmal subarachnoid haemorrhage based on computed tomographic angiography, *Br J Neurosurg* 17:46–53, 2003.
18. *Detailed diagnoses and procedures, national hospital discharge survey, 1990,* DHHS pub no PHS 92–1774, series 13, Hyattsville, MD, 1992, US Department of Health and Human Services.
19. Dorsch NWC: Review of cerebral vasospasm in aneurysmal subarachnoid hemorrhage. II. Management, *J Clin Neurosci* 1:78–92, 1994.

20. Drake CG, Hunt WE, Sano K, et al: Report of World Federation of Neurological Surgeons Committee on a Universal Subarachnoid Hemorrhage Grading Scale, *J Neurosurg* 68:985, 1988.

21. Fisher CM, Kistler JP, Davis JM: Relation of cerebral vasospasm to subarachnoid hemorrhage visualized by computerized tomographic scanning, *Neurosurgery* 6:1–9, 1981.

22. Gault J, Sarin H, Awadallah NA, Shenkar R, Awad IA: Pathobiology of human cerebrovascular malformations: basic mechanisms and clinical relevance, *Neurosurgery* 55(1):1–16, 2004.

23. Gobin YP, Laurent A, Merienne L, et al: Treatment of brain arteriovenous malformations by embolization and radiosurgery, *J Neurosurg* 85:19–28, 1996.

24. Guy J, McGrath BJ, Borel CO, Friedman AH, Warner DS: Perioperative management of aneurysmal subarachnoid hemorrhage: part 1. Operative management, *Anesth Analg* 81:1060–1072, 1995.

25. Hart RG, Byer JA, Slaughter JR, et al: Occurrence and implication of seizures in subarachnoid hemorrhage due to ruptured intracranial aneurysms, *Neurosurgery* 8:417–421, 1981.

26. Hasan D, Vermeulen M, Wijdicks EF, et al: Management problems in acute hydrocephalus after subarachnoid hemorrhage, *Stroke* 20:747–753, 1989.

27. Hunt WE, Hess RM: Surgical risk as related to time of intervention in the repair of intracranial aneurysms, *J Neurosurg* 28:14, 1968.

28. Inci S, Spetzler RF: Intracranial aneurysms and arterial hypertension: a review and hypothesis, *Surg Neurol* 53:530–540, 2000.

29. Ingall TJ, Whisnant JP, Wiebers DO, O'Fallon WM: Has there been a decline in subarachnoid hemorrhage mortality? *Stroke* 20:718–724, 1989.

30. Ingall TJ, Wiebers DO: Natural history of subarachnoid hemorrhage. In Whisnant JP, editor: *Stroke: populations, cohorts, and clinical trials,* Boston, 1993, Butterworth-Heinemann.

31. Jarpe MB: Nursing care of patients receiving long-term infusion of neuromuscular blocking agents, *Crit Care Nurse* 12(7):58, 1992.

32. Jayaraman MV, Mayo-Smith WW, Tung GA, et al: Detection of intracranial aneurysms: multi-detector row CT angiography compared with DSA, *Radiology* 230:510–518, 2004.

33. Kasuya H, Shimsu T, Kagawa M: The effect of continuous drainage of cerebrospinal fluid in patients with subarachnoid hemorrhage, retrospective analysis of 108 patients, *Neurosurgery* 28:56–59, 1991.

34. Kassel NF, Torner JC, Haley ECJ, et al: The international cooperative study on the timing of aneurysm surgery. I. Overall management results, *J Neurosurg* 73:37–47, 1990.

35. Kucharczyk W, Lemme-Pleghos L, Uske A, et al: Intracranial vascular malformations: MR and CT imaging, *Radiology* 56:383–389, 1985.

36. Kuman AJ, Fox AJ, Vinuela F, et al: Revisited old and new CT findings in unruptured larger arteriovenous malformations of the brain, *J Comput Assist Tomogr* 8:648–655, 1984.

37. Lanzino G, Guterman L, Hopkins LN: Endovascular treatment of aneurysms. In Winn HR, editor: *Youmans neurological surgery,* ed 5, New York, 2004, WB Saunders.

38. Linn FH, Rinkel GJ, Algra A, van Gijn J: Headache characteristics in subarachnoid haemorrhage and benign thunderclap headache, *J Neurol Neurosurg Psychiatry* 65:791–793, 1998.

39. Linn FH, Rinkel GJ, Algra A, van Gijn J: The notion of "warning leaks" in subarachnoid haemorrhage: are such patients in fact admitted with rebleed? *J Neurol Neurosurg Psychiatry* 68(3):332–336, 2000.

40. Longstreth WT Jr, Nelson LM, Koepsell TD, van Belle G: Cigarette smoking, alcohol use, and subarachnoid hemorrhage, *Stroke* 23:1242–1249, 1992.

41. Lunsford LD, Kondziolka D, Flickinger JC, et al: Stereotactic radiosurgery for arteriovenous malformations of the brain, *J Neurosurg* 75:512–524, 1991.

42. MacDonald RL, Weir B: Perioperative management of subarachnoid hemorrhage. In Youmans JR, editor: *Neurological surgery: a comprehensive reference guide to the diagnosis and management of neurosurgical problems,* ed 5, Philadelphia, 2003, WB Saunders.

43. Mast H, Mohr JP, Osipov A, et al: "Steal" is an unestablished mechanism for the clinical presentation of cerebral arteriovenous malformations, *Stroke* 26:1215–1220, 1995.

44. Mayer PL, Awad IA, Todor R, Harbaugh K, Varnavas G, Lansen TA, et al: Misdiagnosis of symptomatic cerebral aneurysm. Prevalence and correlation with outcome at four institutions, *Stroke* 27(9):1558–1563, 1996.

45. Mayer SA, LiMandri G, Sherman D, Lennihan L, Fink ME, Solomon RA, et al: Electrocardiographic markers of abnormal left ventricular wall motion in acute subarachnoid hemorrhage, *J Neurosurg* 83(5):889–896, 1995.

46. Mayer SA, Lin J, Homma S, Solomon RA, Lennihan L, Sherman D, et al: Myocardial injury and left ventricular performance after subarachnoid hemorrhage, *Stroke* 30(4):780–786, 1999.

47. McGrath BJ, Guy J, Borel CO, Friedman AH, Warner DS: Perioperative management of aneurysmal subarachnoid hemorrhage: part 2. Postoperative management, *Anesth Analg* 81(6):1295–1302, 1995.

48. Michelson WJ: Natural history and pathophysiology of arteriovenous malformations, *Clin Neurosurg* 26:307–313, 1978.

49. Milhorat TH: Acute hydrocephalus after aneurysmal subarachnoid haemorrhage, *Neurosurgery* 20:15–20, 1987.

50. Mohr G, Ferguson G, Khan M, et al: Intraventricular hemorrhage from ruptured aneurysm, retrospective analysis of 91 cases, *J Neurosurg* 58:482–487, 1983.

51. Molyneux AJ, Kerr RS, Yu LM, et al, International Subarachnoid Aneurysm Trial (ISAT) Collaborative Group: International Subarachnoid Aneurysm Trial (ISAT) of neurosurgical clipping versus endovascular coiling in 2143 patients with ruptured intracranial aneurysms: a randomized comparison of effects on survival, dependency, seizures, rebleeding, subgroups, and aneurysm occlusion, *Lancet* 366(9488):809–817, 2005.

52. Mount LA, Brisman R: Treatment of multiple aneurysms—symptomatic and asymptomatic, *Clin Neurosurg* 21:166–170, 1974.

53. Niemi T, Tanskanen P, Taxell C, Juvela S, Randell T, Rosenberg P: Effects of nonsteroidal anti-inflammatory drugs on hemostasis in patients with aneurysmal subarachnoid hemorrhage, *J Neurosurg Anesthesiol* 11:188–194, 1999.

54. Ogilvy CS, Stieg PE, Awad I, et al: Recommendations for the management of intracranial arteriovenous malformations. A statement for healthcare professionals from a special writing group of the Stroke Council, American Stroke Association, *Stroke* 32:1458, 2001.

55. Pare L, Delfino R, Leblanc R: The relationship of ventricular drainage to aneurysmal rebleeding, *J Neurosurg* 76:422–427, 1992.

56. Pasqualin A, Bazzan A, Cavanazzi P, et al: Intracranial hematoma following aneurysmal rupture, experience with 309 cases, *Surg Neurol* 25:6–17, 1986.

57. Peerless SJ: Pre- and postoperative management of cerebral aneurysms, *Clin Neurosurg* 26:209–231, 1979.

58. Pickard JD, Murray GD, Illingworth R, et al: Effect of oral nimodipine on cerebral infarction and outcome after subarachnoid haemorrhage: British aneurysm nimodipine trial, *BMJ* 298:636–642, 1989.

59. Pollock BE, Flickinger JC, Lunsford LD, Maitz A, Kondziolka D: Factors associated with successful arteriovenous malformation radiosurgery, *Neurosurgery* 42(6):1239–1244, discussion 1244–1247, 1998.

60. Rinkel GJE, Feigin VL, Algra A, Vermeulen M, van Gijn J: Calcium antagonists for aneurysmal subarachnoid haemorrhage (Cochrane Review). In *The Cochrane Library,* Issue 2, Oxford, 2003, Update Software.

61. Ronkainen A, Hernesniemi J, Puranen M, Niemitukia L, Vanninen R, Ryynänen M, et al: Familial intracranial aneurysms, *Lancet* 349:380–384, 1997.

62. Rosenorn J, Eskesen V, Schmidt K, Ronde F: The risk of rebleeding from ruptured intracranial aneurysms, *J Neurosurg* 67:329–332, 1987.

63. Sbeih I, Tamas LB, O'laoire SA: Epilepsy after operation for aneurysms, *Neurosurgery* 19:784–788, 1986.

64. Scievnik WI, Schaid DJ, Micheles VV, et al: Familial subarachnoid hemorrhage, a community based study, *J Neurosurg* 83:426–429, 1995.

65. Selman WR, Tarr RW, Ratcheson RA: Intracranial aneurysms and subarachnoid hemorrhage. In Bradley WG et al, editors: *Neurology in clinical practice,* ed 3, Boston, 2000, Butterworth-Heinemann.

66. Solenski NJ, Heley ECJ, Kassel NF, et al: Medical complication of aneurysmal subarachnoid hemorrhage. A report of multicentre, cooperative aneurysm study, *Crit Care Med* 23:1007–1017, 1995.

67. Spetzler RF, Martin NA: A proposed grading system for arteriovenous malformations, *J Neurosurg* 65:476–483, 1986.

68. Steiner L, Lindquist C, Adler JR, et al: Clinical outcome of radiosurgery for cerebral arteriovenous malformations, *J Neurosurg* 77:1–8, 1992.

69. Takaku A, Shindo K, Tanaka S, Mori T, Suzuki J: Fluid and electrolyte disturbances in patients with intracranial aneurysms, *Surg Neurol* 11(5):349–356, 1979.

70. Treggiari-Venzi MM, Suter PM, Romand JA: Review of medical prevention of vasospasm after aneurysmal subarachnoid haemorrhage. A problem of neurointensive care, *Neurosurgery* 48:249–262, 2002.

71. Vale F, Bradley EL, Fisher WS: Relationship of subarachnoid hemorrhage and need for postoperative shunting, *J Neurosurg* 86:462–466, 1997.

72. Vega C, Kwoon JV, Lavine SD: Intracranial aneurysms: current evidence and clinical practice, *Am Fam Physician* 66(4):601–608, 2002.

73. Vermeulen M: Subarachnoid haemorrhage: diagnosis and treatment, *J Neurol* 243(7):496–501, 1996.

74. Vinuela F, Dion J, Duckwiler G, Martin N: Combined endovascular embolisation and surgery in the management of cerebral arteriovenous malformation, experience with 101 cases, *J Neurosurg* 75:856–864, 1991.

75. Wiebers DO, Torner JC, Meissner I: Impact of unruptured intracranial aneurysms on public health in the United States, *Stroke* 23(10):1416–1419, 1992.

76. Wilson SR, Hirsch NP, Appleby I: Management of subarachnoid haemorrhage in a non-neurosurgical centre, *Anaesthesia* 60(5):470–485, 2005.

77. Yasargil MG: AVM of the brain: clinical considerations, general and special operative techniques, surgical results, non-operated cases, cavernous and venous angiomas. In Yasargil MG, editor: *Microneurosurgery,* Stuttgart, 1988, Thieme.

78. Yong-Zhong G, van Alphen HA: Pathogenesis and histopathology of saccular aneurysms: review of the literature, *Neurol Res* 12:249–255, 1990.

CHRISTINA M. WHITNEY,
BRIAN N. MADDUX,
DAVID E. RILEY

CHAPTER 19

Management of Parkinson's Disease and Movement Disorders

The field of movement disorders consists of conditions associated with involuntary movements, as well as some that impair an individual's ability to command the body's movement. There is currently no cure for most movement disorders, but many symptoms can be adequately treated. In some cases the patient and the patient's family must confront the possibility that the disorder may be genetically transmitted. Movement disorders discussed in this chapter include Parkinson's disease, tremor, chorea, dystonia, tardive syndromes, tics, and restless legs syndrome. The effect of movement disorders on the patient's lifestyle is discussed, as well as psychosocial, rehabilitation, nutritional, and case management considerations.

PARKINSON'S DISEASE

Parkinson's disease (PD) is a slowly progressive degenerative disorder of the central nervous system (CNS) affecting brain centers that regulate movement. PD is characterized by tremor at rest, rigidity, and slowness or difficulty in initiating and executing movement (akinesia or bradykinesia). This combination of clinical features is collectively known as **parkinsonism.** Parkinsonism is a syndrome with numerous causes, of which PD is the most common.[1] Although tremor is the most notorious symptom of PD, it is the akinesia interfering with voluntary movement that usually proves more disabling for patients. Practice guidelines dealing with several aspects of PD were published in April of 2006 by the American Academy of Neurology (AAN) and can be accessed through their website at www.aan.com/pd.

Epidemiology

PD occurs worldwide and is present in all races. There is a slight male preponderance,[1-3] with a mean age of onset in the late fifties to mid-sixties.[3] The prevalence of PD increases with age, affecting approximately 1% of persons over age 60.[3] Young-onset PD, starting between 21 and 40 years of age, affects 5% to 10% of PD patients.[3] With proper treatment, individuals live longer lives but may not enjoy the same quality of life as a person not affected by PD.

Etiology

The etiologic classification of parkinsonism is divided into **Parkinson's disease** and secondary parkinsonism. PD is **idiopathic** (i.e., it has no known cause). It is currently believed that the etiology of PD is genetic, environmental, or most likely a combination of the two, with individuals having PD for different reasons.[2] This chapter focuses on PD as the most common form of the syndrome of parkinsonism. Other types of parkinsonism ("secondary parkinsonism") are caused by other disorders (e.g., neoplasm, multiple cerebral infarcts, infection, or trauma). Drug-induced parkinsonism is the most common secondary form and is usually reversible. Causative drugs include the following:

- **Neuroleptics** (e.g., haloperidol, risperidone, olanzapine, aripiprazole)
- **Antiemetics** (e.g., prochlorperazine, metoclopramide)

Other forms of parkinsonism are caused by other degenerative disorders, in which symptoms of parkinsonism are usually combined with other neurologic deficits. Many of the clinical features of these syndromes resemble those of PD, yet patients fail to respond to conventional antiparkinson drug therapy. These disorders include the following:

- **Progressive supranuclear palsy (PSP):** a progressive disorder characterized by parkinsonism, early and frequent falling, eye movement abnormalities (slowness of vertical saccades), eyelid apraxia, dysphagia, and speech problems.[4] This aggressive disease causes disability and death from complications of immobility, often in less than 10 years.
- **Multiple system atrophy (MSA):** a progressive disorder characterized by parkinsonism, early and frequent falling, autonomic dysfunction (orthostatic hypotension, bladder and bowel incontinence, sexual dysfunction, disordered sweating), and cerebellar dysfunction (slurred speech, incoordination, ataxia).[5,6] It also has a poorer prognosis than PD.

- **Alzheimer's disease (AD)** with parkinsonism: Alzheimer's disease is often accompanied by mild signs of parkinsonism.

Pathophysiology

Pathologic findings of PD include the following:

- Principal neurochemical change: depletion of dopamine; dopaminergic underactivity, particularly in the nigrostriatal pathway.
- Characteristic abnormalities: depigmentation and neuronal loss in the substantia nigra and the presence of cytoplasmic inclusion bodies (Lewy bodies) in surviving substantia nigra nerve cells. Lewy bodies stain positively for **alpha-synuclein,** a key protein that accumulates in abnormally large quantities in substantia nigra neurons in PD.
- Site: basal ganglia and several large gray nuclei at the base of the brain.

The components of the basal ganglia are the substantia nigra, the caudate nucleus, the putamen, the globus pallidus, and the subthalamic nucleus. The globus pallidus and the putamen together make up the lenticular nucleus.

Assessment

The diagnosis of PD is based on the individual's history and clinical presentation. Symptoms begin on one side of the body, progress at a variable but generally slow rate, and ultimately involve both sides of the body asymmetrically. The clinician's assessment should focus on the presence or absence of the four cardinal features of PD: resting tremor, rigidity, akinesia, and postural instability.

- **Resting tremor** is the most common reason why individuals seek medical evaluation. A resting tremor occurs when the arms or legs are in repose (rest). The tremor is usually present in the upper and lower limbs, but can occur in the lips, chin, or tongue. A resting tremor will abate or significantly diminish with purposeful movement. As with most involuntary movements, it resolves during sleep and worsens during periods of physical or emotional stress.
- **Rigidity** is an increase in tone when the patient's extremities are moved passively through a range of motion (ROM). "Cogwheeling" is a ratchet-like movement that appears when muscles cannot be extended or flexed smoothly, but can be moved only in staccato fashion. Cogwheeling is a passive phenomenon that can accompany tremors, and it is often confused with rigidity.
- **Akinesia** is taken from a Greek term meaning a lack of movement. There are three major facets to akinesia:
  - **Bradykinesia:** slowness of initiation and execution of movement
  - **Hypokinesia:** a reduced size of movements, resulting in softening of the voice **(hypophonia),** shortening of the stride while walking, or small handwriting **(micrographia)**

- **Oligokinesia:** a diminished quantity of movement, such as a lack of spontaneous blinking or facial expression **(hypomimia),** lack of arm swinging while walking, or lack of adjustment of posture while sitting

Assessment of akinesia includes the following:

- Repetitive movements such as finger and toe taps (assess speed and amplitude)
- Ability to get in and out of a chair; ask about ability to get out of bed and to turn over in bed
- Gait (speed, stride, arm swing, posture); note if there is any start hesitation or freezing—a sudden inability to initiate or complete a step; freezing is most likely to occur when turning, walking through a doorway, or in narrow spaces (e.g., bathroom, elevator)

Postural disturbances consist of two components. These are a tendency to a stooped or **flexed posture,** and disequilibrium or **postural instability.** Postural instability occurs in the more advanced stages of PD and contributes to falling. **Retropulsion** is a common manifestation of postural instability that involves an inability to prevent oneself from going backward; **propulsion** is a similar phenomenon of forward motion.

To assess postural instability, the clinician performs the "pull test" by standing behind the patient and tugging briskly on the shoulders. Normally a person should take no more than two steps to recover balance. The clinician must be ready and able to catch the patient in case the patient is unable to recover his or her balance (Fig. 19-1).

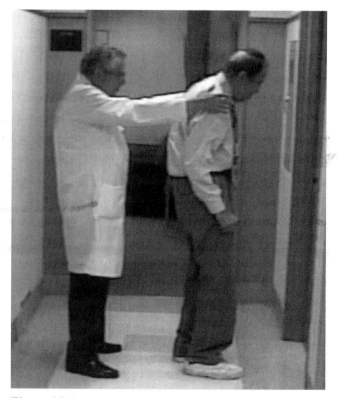

Figure 19-1 Flexed posture and pull test in a patient with Parkinson's disease. The physician is performing a pull test to determine postural stability.

While motor manifestations of PD are the most visible, **nonmotor symptoms** occur frequently and, for some, are more disabling than the motor symptoms.[7] Nonmotor symptoms fall into four general categories: dysautonomia, cognitive and psychiatric disturbances, sleep disturbances, and sensory complaints. The clinician needs to assess each of these areas.

- **Dysautonomia:** drenching sweats, facial flushing, dyspnea, urinary frequency and urgency, gastrointestinal dysfunction (especially constipation), dysphagia, sialorrhea (drooling), orthostatic hypotension, and sexual dysfunction (impotence, decreased libido)
- **Cognitive and psychiatric disturbances:** anxiety, apathy,[8] mental fatigue,[9] irritability, impaired executive function,[10] depression (affects about 40% to 50% of persons with PD),[11] psychosis (hallucinations, delusions),[12] and dementia
- **Sleep disturbances:** fragmented sleep with frequent awakenings; rapid eye movement (REM) sleep-behavior disorder,[13] restless legs syndrome, excessive daytime sleepiness, and sleep attacks[14]
- **Sensory complaints:** pain,[15] restlessness, and akathisia

As PD progresses, many of the motor and nonmotor symptoms of PD are associated with the "off" state. The "off" state is the period when a dose of medication, most commonly carbidopa/levodopa, has lost its effectiveness and the next dose has not kicked in yet. This period can be minutes to hours. It is important for the clinician to ask individuals with PD if their symptoms fluctuate with the timing of their medication. This will guide treatment decisions.

PD is typically classified by the worsening of clinical manifestations. The Modified Hoehn and Yahr Scale is one method used to rate the severity of PD:[16,17]

- **Stage 0:** no evidence of PD
- **Stage 1:** unilateral involvement
- **Stage 1.5:** unilateral and axial involvement
- **Stage 2:** bilateral involvement, balance is intact
- **Stage 2.5:** bilateral involvement, recovery on pull test
- **Stage 3:** mild to moderate impairment with postural instability
- **Stage 4:** severe impairment but still able to stand or walk unassisted
- **Stage 5:** confinement to a wheelchair or bed

Neurodiagnostic and Laboratory Studies

The clinician takes a thorough patient history and performs a complete neurologic examination to make the diagnosis of PD. Clinical evaluation and response to therapy usually confirm the diagnosis. Neurodiagnostic studies such as computed tomography (CT) or magnetic resonance imaging (MRI) of the head are sometimes helpful to rule out secondary causes of parkinsonism.

Conventional criteria for diagnosis include the following:[18]

- Presence of two or more of the cardinal features (akinesia, plus rest tremor, rigidity, or postural instability)
- Absence of clinical or radiologic evidence that would point to an alternate diagnosis (e.g., history of encephalitis, head trauma, neuroleptic use, supranuclear gaze palsy, cerebellar signs, hydrocephalus on CT or MRI)
- Three or more of the following:
  - Unilateral onset
  - Persistent asymmetry (affecting side of onset more)
  - Rest tremor
  - Progressive disorder
  - Clinical course lasting 10 years or more
  - Excellent initial response (70% to 100%) to levodopa
  - Responsiveness to levodopa for 5 years or more
  - Severe levodopa-induced dyskinesias (slow, rhythmic, involuntary movements that can involve the head, face, trunk, and limbs)

Treatment

Medical Management

The treatment of PD is geared toward restoring, promoting, or substituting for missing dopamine in the nigrostriatal tract. This is primarily achieved through the use of medications. Once patients begin "symptomatic" therapy for PD, they usually continue such treatment for the rest of their lives. To date, no form of treatment has been proven to alter the rate of progression of PD.

Not everyone diagnosed with PD requires immediate intervention. Some patients do not find their symptoms troubling enough to warrant embarking on daily, lifelong medication. The decision to initiate treatment rests on a judgment of the relative merits of the benefits and risks of the proposed treatment. The severity of the patient's symptoms will determine the potential benefits. The "risks" comprise the side effects of the medication, plus expenses incurred and the inconvenience of taking medication that usually requires multiple daily doses.

There are six drugs or drug classes currently available to treat PD: anticholinergics, amantadine, dopamine agonists, levodopa, type B–selective monoamine oxidase (MAO) inhibitors, and catechol-O-methyl-transferase (COMT) inhibitors.

Anticholinergic medications are effective for the rest tremor of PD, but little else. Movement disorder specialists usually prefer to use trihexyphenidyl from this group because it has the least amount of sedating antihistamine effect. Benztropine and diphenhydramine are other well-known members of this drug class. Side effects include dry mouth, constipation, urinary retention, blurred near vision, and problems with short-term memory. All antiparkinsonian medications can cause confusion and psychosis, and particularly visual hallucinations, but the anticholinergic class is the most likely to do so. Anticholinergics are notoriously toxic in elderly patients. They are best reserved for young persons with a prominent rest tremor.[11]

Amantadine (Symmetrel) is an antiviral drug that was serendipitously found to benefit patients with PD. Amantadine has relatively modest benefit for PD, but unlike anticholinergics it is typically effective for symptoms related to akinesia, as well as tremor. It is available as a syrup and in tablet form. Amantadine is generally well tolerated, but it can cause edema or a mottling of the skin (livedo reticularis), usually of the lower limbs, that necessitates dose reduction or discontinuation of the drug. Amantadine is now recognized as the most effective adjunctive therapy for the dyskinesias induced by the dopaminergic medications described below.

The two definitive treatments of PD are levodopa and a class of drugs known as **dopamine agonists.** The latter derive their name from their design as synthetic imitators of dopamine that bind with receptors for dopamine and mimic its chemical actions in the brain. The four dopamine agonists available for oral treatment of PD in North America are bromocriptine, pergolide, pramipexole, and ropinirole. Bromocriptine is measurably less effective than the others, and pergolide has been associated with severe fibrosis, particularly of cardiac tissue resulting in valve regurgitation.[19] Thus the current dopamine agonists of choice are pramipexole and ropinirole. These drugs represent a close second in terms of efficacy to levodopa, and have important advantages in terms of a lesser tendency to lead to dose-related motor fluctuations and dyskinesias associated with levodopa. However, they are more prone to causing cognitive side effects, edema, and orthostatic hypotension. Experience with dopamine agonists also indicates that they can cause severe sedation, with some patients reported to fall asleep while driving, and disinhibited behaviors such as pathologic gambling and hypersexuality.[14,20–22] Another dopamine agonist, apomorphine, is available as a rapidly acting subcutaneous injection to "rescue" patients whose oral medication has worn off.[23] Apomorphine use can be complicated by severe nausea and orthostatic hypotension. The cumbersome and costly measures necessary to prevent side effects, to establish the optimum dose, and to prepare each injection have limited its usefulness.

The most effective treatment for PD is **levodopa.** Levodopa is an amino acid from which the brain manufactures dopamine. The brain will not absorb dopamine from the bloodstream, but levodopa is able to cross the blood-brain barrier, and it provides an ingenious way of getting dopamine into the brain. Levodopa is available in regular, extended-release, and orally dissolvable preparations of carbidopa/levodopa, as well as a combined formulation with entacapone. Levodopa is the mainstay of medical treatment of PD, and virtually all patients will end up taking carbidopa/levodopa. Levodopa is also the least likely of all antiparkinson medications to cause cognitive side effects.

Nausea is the only common early side effect of levodopa, so it is formulated with carbidopa to lessen this side effect. Carbidopa, a decarboxylase inhibitor, was added to levodopa to block the conversion of levodopa to dopamine in the periphery, thereby reducing nausea. However, some patients still experience intolerable nausea. Nausea can be managed by taking levodopa after meals or taking extra carbidopa with each dose of carbidopa/levodopa. Definitive therapy for levodopa-induced nausea is provided by domperidone, an antiemetic that must be imported to the United States.

As time goes by and PD progresses, an increasing proportion of patients note that the beneficial effect of levodopa tends to wear off in a dose-related fashion. They experience cycles of improvement lasting a few hours from each dose of medication, followed by wearing off of benefit manifested by a return of parkinsonian symptoms. These cycles of "on" and "off" periods throughout the course of the day are known as fluctuations. Fluctuations are typically managed by manipulating the dosage of levodopa or adding other medications in an attempt to fill in the gaps in treatment.

Dyskinesias are another long-term complication of PD that are strongly related to the current dosage of levodopa. Dyskinesias most commonly occur at times of the peak effects of a dose; however, they may occur at the end of a dose interval or during both time periods. Dyskinesias are addressed by manipulating levodopa dosages (usually downward) or adding amantadine.

The remaining two classes of antiparkinsonian drugs block enzymes that cause premature breakdown of levodopa, and are used primarily to treat motor fluctuations associated with levodopa treatment. The **type B–selective monoamine oxidase (MAO) inhibitors** are selegiline and the more potent rasagiline. **Catechol-O-methyl-transferase (COMT) inhibitors** include tolcapone and entacapone. Tolcapone is the more potent of the two, but has been associated with rare but potentially fatal liver disease that requires periodic monitoring of liver function with blood tests. Entacapone requires no monitoring. It is available as a stand-alone drug, or in a formulation combined with carbidopa/levodopa. COMT inhibitors must be taken in conjunction with carbidopa/levodopa; on their own, they have no antiparkinson effects.

A majority of PD patients will experience motor fluctuations or dyskinesias, and frequently both, within 5 years of initiation of levodopa. These problems tend to increase in severity over time, and fluctuations and dyskinesias represent the most common long-term management problems in PD.

Other common complications include nonmotor manifestations of PD such as dementia, psychosis, depression, and autonomic nervous system problems. All of these issues are largely addressed in the same fashion as they are in people without PD. Dementia is managed with a cognition-enhancing medication such as donepezil, galantamine, rivastigmine, or memantine. Both the dementia of PD and antiparkinsonian medications cause hallucinations, and treatment with antipsychotics may be necessary. Quetiapine and clozapine are the members of this class least likely to aggravate PD, with quetiapine the preferred drug because of the strict monitoring of white blood cell count required with clozapine.[24,25] The use of atypical antipsychotics for behavioral problems in demented elderly patients requires caution because of a reported increase in cerebrovascular events and death in this population.

Autonomic nervous system problems such as orthostatic hypotension, sialorrhea, and constipation are amenable to pharmacologic intervention. Orthostatic hypotension responds to fludrocortisone or midodrine. Midodrine can cause supine systolic hypertension; therefore patients are advised to remain upright after taking midodrine and avoid taking it after 4:00 PM. Most oral medications used to treat sialorrhea have the potential to cause or aggravate confusion and should be avoided in elderly persons with PD. However, sialorrhea can be very effectively treated with botulinum toxin injections into the parotid gland.[26,27] Constipation is controlled with stool softeners along with the traditional nonpharmacologic treatments (e.g., fluid, exercise). Autonomic nervous system dysfunction, when present, significantly impairs quality of life. The clinician must identify and treat nonmotor symptoms.[28]

Treatment of PD with medication is highly individualized. Many patients develop intricate schedules with varying combinations of medications at different doses, which are based on a long experience of trial and error. Guiding principles of medication therapy include the following:

- Dopamine agonists are preferred in patients younger than age 60, because that is the age-group most susceptible to levodopa-related fluctuations and dyskinesias.
- Levodopa is preferred in patients over 70 years of age, because of its lesser tendency to cause cognitive side effects.
- Small doses of multiple drugs tend to cause fewer side effects than large doses of any single drug.
- The lowest dose that produces a satisfactory effect is the preferred dose.

Surgical Management

Over the years, a variety of surgical procedures have been performed for PD, but a consensus has emerged that the best combination of safety and efficacy is achieved with deep brain stimulation (DBS). DBS is the delivery of high-frequency electrical stimulation to a select target in the brain. The target is selected based on the disorder being treated. For PD, targeting the globus pallidus internus (GPi) or the subthalamic nucleus (STN) is effective in reducing "off" time and improving the patient's ability to complete activities of daily living (ADLs).[29] The STN is often the preferred site because it allows for a greater reduction in antiparkinson medication.[29]

DBS is indicated in PD patients who, using available medications, do not achieve consistent control of symptoms. DBS works best in patients who (1) have idiopathic PD; (2) enjoy a robust response to levodopa but experience problematic fluctuations or side effects, particularly dyskinesias; (3) are not demented; (4) are not depressed; (5) are healthy enough to undergo two surgical procedures; and (6) have adequate social support.[30]

All potential candidates for DBS should undergo extensive neuropsychologic evaluation preoperatively and at preset intervals postoperatively.[31] In the past, DBS has been found to not work well in patients who never obtain significant relief from their medication. However, DBS is effective for treating tremor that is not well controlled by medication. Older patients (>75 years of age) may not respond as well to DBS surgery as younger patients.[32]

At most centers, the neurosurgeon performs DBS surgery in two stages. In the first surgery, a lead that consists of four insulated wires with four electrodes at the tip is stereotactically implanted, often with the guidance of microelectrode recording, in the STN or GPi bilaterally (Fig. 19-2). In the second surgery, about 7 to 10 days later, the intracranial leads are connected to an extension wire that is tunneled subcutaneously from the head to the upper chest under general anesthesia. Next, the surgeon creates a pocket in the upper chest wall just below the clavicle for the neurostimulator. The two parts of the system are then connected.

About 3 weeks later the patient returns to the office for initial programming of the neurostimulators. The clinician noninvasively adjusts the neurostimulator using a programmer that communicates with the neurostimulator via radio telemetry.[33] The clinician adjusts stimulator parameters, including selection of active electrodes, electrode polarity, amplitude (intensity of the stimulus), pulse width, and pulse frequency to achieve the best possible symptom control. These programming options lead to an enormous variety of combinations of generator settings. The end result is a great deal of flexibility in applying the treatment, but it often requires multiple clinic visits with multiple trials of different settings along with medication adjustments to find the optimal combination.[33]

Potential side effects of the neurostimulation include dysarthria, paresthesias, visual disturbances, light-headedness,

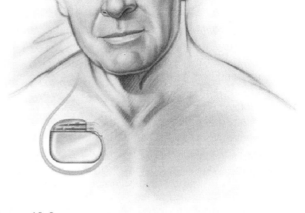

Figure 19-2 Patient with an implanted deep brain stimulator (DBS).
(Courtesy of Medtronic Neurosurgical.)

and involuntary movements. The side effects will abate with a change in stimulation parameters or by turning the system off.

The neurostimulators are susceptible to electromagnetic interference (EMI). For example, EMI from theft detectors, airport security devices, or refrigerator doors could turn the system on or off, or the person may feel a brief increase in stimulation. However, EMI from an MRI scan is more hazardous, particularly if the transmit coil extends over the chest area, resulting in excessive heating of the implanted hardware. This could cause serious injury or death. In select circumstances it is possible to perform MRI safely, but only of the head, and only if strict guidelines are followed. In addition, **diathermy** (e.g., therapeutic ultrasound) used by dentists, physical therapists, chiropractors, sports medicine physicians, and others is likely to cause heating of tissue along the lead, resulting in severe injury or death. Therefore diathermy is an absolute contraindication for anyone with an implanted neurostimulator system. Before performing any procedure, it is wise to check with the movement disorders team.

Successful treatment with DBS usually results in patients being at their best for longer periods of the day than they were with medication alone. Most patients are able to reduce their intake of medication, resulting in a lower prevalence of side effects. In PD, the neurostimulator batteries last approximately 3 to 5 years, depending on the amount of stimulation needed to control the symptoms. The neurostimulators should be replaced before the batteries are completely drained. It appears that the benefits of DBS do not wane over time, but PD continues to progress.[29,34] Long-term follow-up is required, and patients and families need detailed teaching to avoid complications.

Clinical Management
Nonpharmacologic Treatment. In addition to the medical and surgical treatment of persons with PD, nonpharmacologic measures are a useful adjunct in the management of PD symptoms. Some of these measures include the following:

- Mobility training and physical therapy: exercise programs (combined active and passive exercises), fall prevention, and the use of assistive devices for walking (e.g., a cane or walker). Unfortunately, canes and walkers have a mixed track record in minimizing the risk of injury. Patients should be taught how to overcome a **freezing episode.** Most patients can overcome a freezing episode by using visual cues (e.g., stepping over another person's foot, stepping onto a different-color floor tile) or auditory cues (e.g., a marching sequence such as one-two-three and step).
- Speech therapy: the Lee Silverman Voice Treatment (LSVT), an intensive voice and speech program, improves both hypophonia and speech clarity.[35,36] If dysphagia is a problem, speech therapists should be consulted for a swallowing evaluation and treatment if indicated.
- Sleep: establish good sleep hygiene such as going to bed and arising at the same general time, avoiding

naps during the day, exercising regularly but not too close to bedtime, limiting fluid intake after dinner, and voiding before going to bed. If turning over in bed is a problem, consider sleeping on satin or other low-friction sheets. The clinician should consider possible concomitant disorders such as depression, restless legs syndrome, REM sleep behavior disorder, and obstructive sleep apnea.
- Orthostatic hypotension: increase fluid and salt intake, wear thigh-high support stockings, sleep with the head of the bed elevated (place blocks under the headboard), and sit on the edge of the bed for several minutes before standing.
- Constipation: increase fluid intake to 2 L/day and dietary fiber in the form of raw fruits and vegetables; establish a bowel routine, and encourage exercise (particularly walking).
- Eye problems: three common eye problems in PD are eye irritation, trouble reading, and diplopia. Eye irritation can result from a decreased blink rate and from medications that dry the mucous membranes (e.g., anticholinergics). Washing the eyelids twice a day with a "no-tears" baby shampoo and using artificial tears can reduce eye irritation. Trouble reading is often caused by subnormal convergence of the eyes during near vision. This problem is exaggerated when the person with PD wears bifocals, trifocals, or progressive lenses. Single-vision glasses for distance, reading, or working at the computer are the most effective treatment of this problem. Convergence insufficiency can also cause diplopia. In this case, prisms can be added to the glasses to eliminate the diplopia.[37]
- Patient and family education: rationale for medications and their potential side effects; importance of adhering to the medication schedule;[38] need for medication titration as the disease progresses; and, if the patient is experiencing fluctuations, the benefit of keeping a diary noting symptom onset in relationship to timing of medication. Inform patient and family of local support groups and community agencies that can provide needed services.
- Psychosocial/emotional: assess for appropriate coping mechanisms, depression, and family support. Help the person with PD participate in activities that promote a sense of well-being and provide the person with meaning and purpose in life.[39] Referral for counseling may be appropriate.

Nutritional Considerations. There is no known nutritional deficiency that causes parkinsonism, nor is there any food, special nutrient, vitamin, or mineral that is known to have a therapeutic or protective effect. Several nutrients, particularly pyridoxine (vitamin B_6), L-tryptophan (an amino acid), and choline, may interfere with levodopa metabolism when consumed in large doses. A minority of persons with PD notice sensitivity to protein; that is, they report that their medication (carbidopa/levodopa) is less effective after consuming a protein-rich meal. This may occur because levodopa

When selecting any therapy it is important to consider concomitant medical conditions and potential side effects. For example, propranolol (a nonselective beta-adrenergic blocker) would not be the treatment of choice if a person with ET also suffered from chronic obstructive pulmonary disease (COPD), unstable heart failure, or bradycardia.

Surgical Management

Stereotactic neurosurgical intervention for ET is reserved for persons with severe, medically refractory tremor.

Thalamotomy, creating a lesion in the ventrointermedius (VIM) nucleus of the thalamus, is effective in reducing contralateral tremor but carries a significant risk of complications such as cognitive decline, dysarthria, hemiparesis, and gait disturbances. The risk increases, particularly for persistent dysarthria and dysphonia, if bilateral thalamotomy is performed. For this reason, bilateral thalamotomy is no longer recommended for the treatment of ET.[50]

Deep brain stimulation (DBS) is another surgical intervention available for those with medically refractory ET. For tremor, the preferred DBS target is the VIM nucleus of the thalamus. Stimulation of the VIM thalamus is effective in reducing contralateral limb tremor.[50] It is less clear how effective DBS is in reducing head, voice, and trunk tremors.[50]

Unilateral DBS of the VIM thalamus will reduce the risk for complications. The side chosen to implant the first lead is usually determined by severity of tremor or handedness. For example, a right-handed person with severe ET is likely to have the first lead implanted in the left VIM thalamus. Later, the person may choose to have DBS surgery on the other side.

Thalamic DBS is a very effective treatment for medically refractory ET. A significant reduction in tremor leads to more independence with ADLs such as eating, drinking, dressing, and writing, and this leads to an improved quality of life.[51]

DYSTONIA

Dystonia is a disorder of intermittent or sustained contraction of muscles that results in abnormal postures or movements of the affected body part. Dystonic movements are[52,53]

- Repetitive (direction of the contraction is consistent)
- Patterned (involving the same group of muscles)
- Triggered by voluntary movement (action dystonia)
- Of variable speed, but at some point during the movement there is a sustained posture
- Often lessened by using sensory tricks (e.g., touching the chin or back of the head to straighten the neck; talking, singing, or chewing to keep eyes open)

Dystonia can involve any voluntary muscle, including muscles of the face, larynx, neck, trunk, limbs, hands, or feet. As with most movement disorders, dystonia is aggravated when a person is tired or during periods of physical or emotional stress.[52] In most instances, dystonia will abate during deep sleep.

Dystonia is often classified based on what body parts are affected: focal, segmental, multifocal, hemidystonia, and generalized dystonia.[53]

Focal dystonias involve a single body part. There are many types of focal dystonias, including blepharospasm, oromandibular dystonia, spasmodic dysphonia, cervical dystonia, and writer's cramp.

Blepharospasm results in involuntary closure of the eyes. This can range from frequent blinking to forcible closure of the eyes rendering the person temporarily blind. Other symptoms include dry eyes and a sense of grittiness in the eyes. Blepharospasm usually begins after age 50 and is much more common in women.[53] It is often aggravated by driving, walking, reading, and watching television and by eye irritants such as smoke, wind, and bright lights. Because of the increased sensitivity to bright lights, many people with blepharospasm are more comfortable wearing sunglasses, even indoors.

Oromandibular dystonia (OMD) involves the muscles of the lower face, jaw, and mouth. OMD can cause grimacing, twitching around the mouth, tongue protrusion, or spasms of jaw opening or closing. OMD can interfere with speech, swallowing, and chewing.

Spasmodic dysphonia involves either the adductor or, less commonly, the abductor muscles of the larynx. When the adductor muscles are affected, the person's voice sounds very strained and hoarse. If the abductor muscles are affected, the voice will have a breathy, whispered quality.[53]

Cervical dystonia (CD), or spasmodic torticollis ("twisted neck"), the most common focal dystonia, results in abnormal neck and head postures. The head may rotate toward either side (rotational), tilt backward (retrocollis), tilt forward (anterocollis), or tilt toward a shoulder (laterocollis). Some persons with CD have a combination of abnormal head postures, such as a left head turn with a right tilt. For some persons with CD their head is tonically deviated in one direction. Others may experience a combination of intermittent tonic deviation with a jerky, tremor-like movement. The shoulder on the side to which the chin turns is often elevated.[53] Unlike other dystonias, pain is a common feature of CD. The pain is usually localized to one side of the neck or along the shoulder. Persons with CD are at increased risk for degenerative joint disease of the cervical spine.[53]

Writer's cramp involves contraction of the hand and forearm muscles resulting in an abnormal posture when writing. A similar phenomenon may occur in musicians when their fingers take on an abnormal posture while playing an instrument.[54] When the activity ceases, the hand returns to a relaxed and normal posture.

Segmental dystonia involves two or more adjacent regions such as a combination of blepharospasm and oromandibular dystonia. A **multifocal dystonia** involves two areas of the body that are not contiguous, such as combination of cervical dystonia and a leg dystonia. **Hemidystonia** affects one side of the body and is usually the result of a structural lesion in the contralateral cerebral hemisphere. To be classified as a **generalized dystonia,** one or both legs, the trunk, and another body part are involved.[53]

The course of dystonia is variable. Generally, the older the onset, the more likely the dystonia will plateau and remain as a focal dystonia. Dystonia that begins in childhood is more likely to progress over time and involve more than one body part.

Etiology

Dystonia is also classified based on etiology: primary (idiopathic), secondary (symptomatic), dystonia-plus syndromes, and heredodegenerative diseases.[55]

Primary Dystonia

The clinician considers a diagnosis of primary dystonia if dystonia is the only symptom. Primary dystonia is either sporadic or inherited. The majority of people with primary dystonia do not have an affected relative with dystonia. Typically, sporadic primary dystonia begins in adulthood, has a gradual onset, and starts as an action dystonia.

Genetic testing should be considered if the dystonia begins in childhood or if there is a positive family history of early-onset dystonia. Childhood-onset dystonia is more likely inherited in an autosomal dominant pattern. Several gene mutations that cause primary inherited dystonia have been mapped (e.g., DYT1, DYT6, DYT7, DYT13).[53] The DYT1 gene accounts for most of these cases. About one third of those who carry the DYT1 gene will express the gene clinically.[53] The prevalence of DYT1 dystonia is significantly higher in the Ashkenazi Jewish population than in the non-Jewish population.[53,55] DYT1 dystonia typically manifests in mid to late childhood, starts in a limb (e.g., hand, foot), and progresses to generalized dystonia in the ensuing 5 years. These children are intellectually normal. The degree of disability can vary from mild to profound.[55]

Secondary Dystonia

A diagnosis of secondary dystonia requires an identifiable cause. Possible indicators of secondary dystonia include the following:[52,53]

- Abnormal (excluding the dystonia) neurologic examination (e.g., cognitive changes, seizures, spasticity, weakness, cerebellar dysfunction)
- Abnormal laboratory or imaging studies
- Sudden onset, rapid progression, or occurring primarily at rest
- Atypical site of onset (e.g., cranial onset in a child)
- Hemidystonia

Secondary dystonia may result from the following:[53,56]

- Brain insult (e.g., hypoxia, trauma, tumor, vascular injury)
- Spinal cord injury or lesion
- Infectious or inflammatory processes (e.g., encephalitis, lupus, Reye's syndrome)
- Peripheral injury
- Electrical injury
- Drug exposure (particularly to dopamine-receptor blockers)
- Toxin exposure (e.g., carbon monoxide, cyanide, manganese)
- Perinatal trauma

The onset of secondary dystonia may occur months to years after the neurologic insult.

Dystonia-Plus

A diagnosis of dystonia-plus is considered when a person has dystonia plus one other neurologic problem.[55] In most instances, this would be parkinsonism or myoclonus, which is a rapid jerk of a muscle or a group of muscles.

Dystonia in combination with parkinsonism suggests a dopa-responsive dystonia (DRD). DRD is typically inherited in an autosomal dominant pattern, although there are reports of spontaneous mutations.[57] Penetrance is incomplete, with women more likely to manifest symptoms than men.[57] Characteristics of DRD include the following:[52,53,55,57]

- Onset in childhood (usually by 12 years of age, although adolescent- and adult-onset cases have been reported)
- Often begins with a foot dystonia while walking or running
- Worse in the evening, better in the morning after a good night's sleep
- Signs of parkinsonism preceding, concurrent with, or after onset of dystonia
- Significant and sustained response to low-dose levodopa

Myoclonic dystonia is another type of autosomal dominant inherited dystonia with incomplete penetrance. Characteristics of myoclonic dystonia include the following:[52,53,55]

- Onset in the first or second decade of life
- Myoclonus and dystonia may affect the same or different muscles
- Neck and arms more likely to be involved
- Alcohol responsive
- Benign course

Heredodegenerative Dystonia

Heredodegenerative causes of dystonia are inherited neurodegenerative disorders in which dystonia may or may not be the prominent feature.[55] Most will exhibit other neurologic signs and symptoms such as dementia, psychosis, dysarthria, chorea, ataxia, spasticity, or abnormal eye movements. Examples include Lubag (X-linked recessive), Rett's syndrome (X-linked dominant), Huntington's disease (autosomal dominant), and Wilson's disease (autosomal recessive).[55]

Pathophysiology

The pathophysiology of dystonia is not well understood. Dysfunction of the basal ganglia, thalamus, and cortical sensorimotor pathways is believed to play a significant role in the development of dystonia.[58,59] A better understanding of changes in neuronal activity will emerge as advances are made in functional neuroimaging studies and data are gathered through microelectrode recordings performed during DBS surgery.

Assessment of Dystonia

The person's history and clinical presentation will help the clinician determine the type of dystonia and as a result guide the diagnostic evaluation and treatment. The clinician should obtain the following information from the person with dystonia:[60]

- Age at onset and pattern of progression
- Affected body parts
- Situations that aggravate or alleviate symptoms (ask about sensory tricks)
- Family history of dystonia or other movement disorders
- Peripheral or CNS trauma
- Metabolic abnormalities
- Current medications
- Drug exposure (past and present)

In addition to performing a thorough neurologic examination, the clinician should examine the person during actions or activities that enhance dystonia and assess the following:

- Abnormalities on examination that might indicate a diagnosis other than primary dystonia
- Characteristics of the abnormal movements (e.g., direction of pull, speed of movement)
- Severity and social/functional disability

Neurodiagnostic and Laboratory Studies

Age of onset and clinical presentation will guide the diagnostic evaluation. The purpose of diagnostic studies is to identify an underlying cause that is potentially treatable. In most people with adult-onset dystonia and a normal neurological examination (excluding the dystonia), no structural abnormalities will be found on imaging studies.[53] Genetic testing and counseling is considered if the primary dystonia begins before age 26 or if there is a positive family history of early-onset dystonia.[60] In addition, Wilson's disease, an autosomal recessive inherited disorder of copper metabolism, must be ruled out in persons younger than 50 years of age with dystonia plus other systemic, psychiatric, or neurologic signs.[56,60]

Treatment

There is no cure for dystonia; therefore the treatment goals are to alleviate symptoms, avert contractures, improve function, and enhance quality of life.[60] There are three principal approaches to treatment: (1) oral medications, (2) botulinum toxin injections, and (3) surgery. In some cases of secondary dystonia, treating the underlying disorder may bring relief of the dystonia.

Medical Management: Oral Medications

Medications that have been used to treat dystonia include anticholinergics (e.g., trihexyphenidyl), benzodiazepines (e.g., clonazepam, lorazepam, diazepam), skeletal muscle relaxants (e.g., baclofen administered orally or via an intrathecal pump), anticonvulsants (e.g., carbamazepine), dopaminergic agents (e.g., levodopa), and dopamine depletors (e.g., tetrabenazine, not yet available in the United States, or reserpine).[60,61] Unfortunately, oral medications rarely produce sustained benefit and are often limited in use by their side-effect profile.

Medical Management: Botulinum Toxin Injections

To date, chemodenervation with botulinum toxin injections is the most effective treatment for dystonia. Botulinum toxin blocks the release of acetylcholine at the neuromuscular junction, thereby preventing contraction of the muscle.[62] Therefore injections of botulinum toxin into the dystonic muscle will temporarily weaken the muscle, allowing it to assume a more normal posture. Side effects are generally limited to transient weakness of the injected muscles. For example, injections around the eye to treat blepharospasm may result in a droopy eyelid or diplopia. Injections of cervical muscles may cause dysphagia or a sense that one's head is too heavy; for example, it may require more effort to lift one's head off the pillow. The side effects, if they occur, gradually resolve over 2 to 3 weeks, whereas the benefit is sustained for an average of 3 to 4 months. Once symptoms begin to return the person can be reinjected with botulinum toxin. To reduce the likelihood of developing antibodies to the toxin, the interval between injections should be kept to a minimum of 10 to 12 weeks.

Two types of botulinum toxin currently are available in the United States: botulinum toxin type A and botulinum toxin type B. A multicenter, randomized, double-blind study compared the efficacy of botulinum toxin types A and B in the treatment of CD. Both toxins, at 4 weeks after injection, demonstrated comparable benefit in relieving symptoms of CD. Participants receiving type A had a slightly longer duration of improvement. Participants receiving botulinum toxin type B reported more dry mouth and dysphagia.[63]

Unfortunately, a small percentage of people never respond to botulinum toxin or after a period of successful treatment become refractory to the toxin. In the latter case it is believed that the individual has developed antibodies to the toxin. For some of these individuals, surgical therapy is an option.

Surgical Management

Surgical therapy for select dystonias had been limited to destructive or ablative procedures such as thalamotomy, pallidotomy, selective myectomies (removing part of the overactive muscle), or rhizotomies (severing the nerves that innervate the overactive muscle). In 2003 the U.S. Food and Drug Administration (FDA) approved, as part of its humanitarian device exemption (HDE) program, unilateral or bilateral deep brain stimulation (DBS) of the globus pallidus internus (GPi) or subthalamic nucleus (STN) for the treatment of chronic, drug-refractory primary dystonia, including generalized dystonia, cervical dystonia, segmental dystonia, and hemidystonia in persons age 7 or older. GPi has been the preferred target.[64-67] Unlike DBS for PD or ET, the benefit from DBS in persons with dystonia is delayed by several months, with the majority reaching maximum improvement by 12 months after activation of the stimulators.[66,67]

TARDIVE DYSKINESIA

The term *tardive dyskinesia* (TD) comprises a cluster of iatrogenic movement disorders. These result from exposure to the same dopamine receptor blocking agents that cause drug-induced parkinsonism, namely antipsychotics (e.g., haloperidol, risperidone, olanzapine, and aripiprazole) and antiemetics (e.g., prochlorperazine and metoclopramide). There is evidence that the newer atypical antipsychotics have a lower risk of tardive complications than the traditional agents.[68] The name "tardive" comes from the French word for "late," reflecting the fact that classic TD usually does not occur until long after a patient is first exposed to continuous therapy with the offending agent, usually a year or more. However, certain forms of TD may begin after a much briefer exposure. It is estimated that 20% of patients on long-term dopamine blockade therapy will develop TD. Those at highest risk appear to be older adults and women. Other risk factors may include greater total drug exposure, preexisting drug-induced parkinsonism, a history of treatment for depression, alcoholism, and smoking.

The distribution of classic TD is mainly oral and facial, and the movements often represent a combination of licking, smacking, and chewing. Limb, truncal (producing rocking movements), or respiratory (producing erratic, gasping breathing) musculature is variably involved. TD may begin during ongoing treatment with causative medications, or within 3 months of their discontinuation. Because of the pharmacologic peculiarities of TD, an exacerbation of TD may occur shortly after cessation of the offending drug, and resumption of treatment may suppress the movements. However, it is widely believed that continued exposure will ultimately result in a worsening of TD.

TD is a particularly feared complication of use of dopamine receptor blockers because many cases are irreversible. Approximately 60% of patients with TD eventually recover without treatment, but in the other 40% the TD is unrelenting and prolonged. The patient's best chance for a remission lies in stopping the offending drug as soon as possible; thus early recognition is paramount in treatment. However, it is important to remember that many psychiatric patients need their antipsychotics to function well, and that untreated psychiatric illness can be life threatening, whereas TD is not.

A number of "tardive" disorders have different clinical presentations but share the same relationship to dopamine-blocking medications, in terms of both acute dosage and cumulative exposure. The major categories are as follows:

- **Classic TD:** as described above. The movements are patterned and repetitive, and have been called "stereotypies."
- **Tardive dystonia:** sustained postures that resemble idiopathic focal dystonia. The dystonia here usually involves the face and neck, and is often quite severe. Young men are at greatest risk, possibly due to treatment with high doses of medication. The length

of exposure required is shorter than that for classic TD, and may be measured in weeks. Prognosis is poorer; remission is rare.[69]
- **Tardive akathisia:** a sense of inner restlessness, tension, emotional unease, and aversion to remaining still. Patients are often seen to pace about, or engage in rubbing movements. Akathisia commonly occurs as a subacute phenomenon with dopamine blocker treatment, in which case it resolves with dose reduction or discontinuation. In tardive akathisia, symptoms begin after prolonged exposure, typically worsen immediately after drug discontinuation, and are suppressed by increased doses.

Assessment

- Repetitive facial and oral movements, possibly in combination with irregular, gasping respirations, truncal rocking, pelvic thrusting, or rapid writhing movements of the extremities. Oral movements are typically diminished during voluntary movement such as maintaining a protruded tongue.
- Alternatively, cranial or cervical dystonia, or severe restlessness, during ongoing therapy with antipsychotics or antiemetics.
- Patients are usually less aware of the abnormal movements than outside observers are.

Treatment

The first step is to minimize the dose of the causative medication, or stop it if possible. Patients should be warned that their symptoms might promptly worsen, but that this will improve their long-term outcome. Presynaptic dopamine-depleting agents, such as reserpine or tetrabenazine, are the most effective symptomatic treatments. This approach provides relief in most cases of classic TD and akathisia. Patients with tardive dystonia may benefit more from anticholinergics, such as trihexyphenidyl, or botulinum toxin injections. Deep brain stimulation surgery has been used with marked success in a small number of patients with severe tardive dystonia.[70,71]

CHOREA

Chorea, from the Greek word for "dance," is a motor phenomenon that consists of nonrhythmic, rapid, irregular, unpredictable, brief, jerky movements that flow from one part of the body to another in a continuous and random fashion. Variants include athetosis (slow, writhing chorea) and ballism (more proximal chorea, with flinging and rotatory character). The entire body is commonly affected, including all four limbs, as well as trunk, neck, and facial muscles. However, focal chorea may occur.

Chorea may be associated with a wide variety of neurologic disorders, including hereditary degenerative diseases (see subsequent discussion of Huntington's disease). Infrequently, chorea may be the result of a small infarct in the basal ganglia, an autoimmune process, or endocrine disturbances.

Treatment addresses the underlying cause if it is identifiable. Pharmacologic therapy is used to suppress the movements. Pharmacologic treatments may include dopamine antagonists (e.g., neuroleptic antipsychotics), dopamine depletors (e.g., reserpine) and other agents such as amantadine, whose mechanism of action is unclear.

HUNTINGTON'S DISEASE

Huntington's disease (HD) is a devastating, relatively rare hereditary disease that results in a gradual loss of motor coordination and mental function. Although this disorder has been called "Huntington's chorea" in the past, chorea usually represents only a fraction of the total symptom burden. In fact, patients with HD may manifest chorea, dystonia, rigidity, gait instability (ataxia), and speech and swallowing dysfunction, as well as numerous cognitive and emotional impairments with significant personality changes. Motor symptoms may not be as prominent or as early as psychiatric symptoms; many patients are misdiagnosed with primary psychiatric disorders if HD is not recognized. One study found that 90% of patients were demented by a mean age of 48.3 years and that dementia preceded the onset of chorea in about one fourth of the patients.[72]

The onset is insidious, typically around age 35 (range of onset: younger than 5 to older than 75), and the disease is relentlessly progressive. Individuals lose their ability to ambulate, perform basic self-care functions, and communicate (Fig. 19-3). Fall-related complications such as fractures and intracranial hemorrhages may be significant. Patients with advanced HD are susceptible to urinary tract infections, aspiration pneumonia, and decubitus ulcers. Death occurs 10 to 20 years after the onset of symptoms, often related to such complications of chronic debility. There is no known cure.

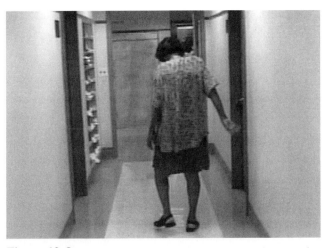

Figure 19-3 Stuttering, uncoordinated gait due to chorea and right arm posturing owing to chorea/dystonia in a patient with Huntington's disease.

Etiology, Prevalence, and Incidence

HD is caused by a totally penetrant autosomal dominant gene. Offspring of an affected parent have a 50% chance of inheriting the gene. Everyone who carries the gene will develop the disease. Recombinant DNA techniques and genetic research led to the discovery of the abnormal gene on the short arm of chromosome 4 in 1993.[73] The gene is called IT-15, and the protein product is called *huntingtin*.

The abnormal gene contains a "triplet repeat" mutation. Near one end of the normal gene, the DNA base sequence "C," "A," "G" is repeated several times. The CAG triplet codes for the amino acid glutamine when the DNA is translated into protein by the cell machinery. The normal protein thus includes a string of glutamine near one end. The functions of the normal *huntingtin* protein and its polyglutamine component are not known. The abnormal gene contains a larger number of CAG repeats, and thus a longer polyglutamine segment. Currently available evidence suggests that the expanded polyglutamine string is somehow toxic to neurons.[74]

The length of the CAG repeat expansion carries significant implications for the health of the affected individual. In general, age of onset and rapidity of progression are inversely related to the length of the expansion.[75] Patients with modestly abnormal mutations (40 to 45 repeats) usually experience their onset of symptoms in midlife, with typically slow progression. Markedly expanded (70 to 100) CAG repeats may result in onset of symptoms in childhood or adolescence with a much more aggressive and rapidly fatal course.

Triplet repeat mutations may expand from one generation to the next. A person who inherits HD from his or her mother will usually have a gene with about the same number of repeats as the mother. Therefore the age of onset can be expected to be similar to that of the mother. However, genes transmitted from the father may contain even longer CAG repeat sequences. Therefore the first symptoms may occur much earlier in the offspring. This phenomenon is known as "genetic anticipation."

The prevalence of HD is estimated at 5 to 10 per 100,000.[76] An estimated 30,000 individuals in the United States are affected, and more than 125,000 are believed to be at risk for inheriting HD. HD is most prevalent in people of western European ancestry,[77] but it affects men and women of all races. In about 10% of patients, HD has a juvenile onset (at 4 to 19 years of age), and the individual may have symptoms of diminishing school performance, rigidity, akinesia, and dystonia (the Westphal variant). Children with HD rarely live to adulthood, with death occurring in 5 to 10 years. The father is consistently the affected parent.[78]

Pathophysiology

The genetic mutation causes loss of neurons in specific regions of the brain. The most affected parts of the brain are the basal ganglia (specifically the striatum) and the frontal lobes of the cerebral cortex. In patients with advancing HD, atrophy of these regions is apparent on imaging studies such as MRI or CT scan, or at autopsy on gross macroscopic examination of the brain. In the most advanced cases of HD, more widespread brain atrophy is apparent, involving the entire cerebral cortex. At autopsy, brain weight may be decreased by 30%. Microscopically, cell loss can be seen in the striatum and in the other regions. Cell loss is mild before the symptoms appear, and is more severe with advancing disease.

In the degenerating regions of brain, neurons are observed to contain abnormal intracellular inclusions. These inclusion bodies have been found to contain aggregates of the abnormal *huntingtin* protein.[74] Current concepts suggest that the normal cellular machinery for clearing and recycling proteins may be unable to degrade the mutated *huntingtin* product. The buildup of a mass of abnormal protein appears to be toxic, though the molecular mechanisms leading to cell death are not yet clear.

Cell loss in the basal ganglia results in the characteristic motor, cognitive, and emotional impairments. The basal ganglia are part of a major circuit in which information from all parts of the cerebral cortex is processed and returned ultimately to the cerebral cortex, apparently to assist in planning and execution of behaviors. Several neurotransmitters are involved, including acetylcholine (Ach), gamma-aminobutyric acid (GABA), and dopamine (DA). Understanding of the functions of each of these transmitters and the balance among them remains incomplete. In a necessarily oversimplified view, chorea and certain psychiatric symptoms may result from overabundance of dopamine. Contrast this with Parkinson's disease, in which symptoms result from insufficient dopamine. Although this scheme cannot explain all of the manifestations of HD, it does allow a rational basis for pharmacologic treatment.

Assessment

Hallmark symptoms include intellectual decline and abnormal movements, together or separately. The patient may report subjective symptoms of forgetfulness and problems with speech, swallowing, clumsiness, coordination, and balance. Falling may be a frequent event. Early diagnosis is therefore based on reported symptoms, observed clinical signs, and a positive family history. Remarkably, even in the early twenty-first century, not all affected individuals are aware of a family history, so the clinical specialist must carry an index of suspicion even in the absence of such. The initial assessment focuses on the following:

- The historical account (by the patient or family members) of cognitive or emotional problems, clumsiness, gait impairment, and involuntary movements.
- A thorough family history and a standard family pedigree.
- Speech and swallowing. Dysarthria and dysphagia are common and should be assessed in every patient.
- Cognitive and emotional state. Document using standard neuropsychologic and psychiatric scales. Identify severe depression and suicide risk.
- Motor examination. Identify and document motor impairment, including chorea, dystonic posture, and gait disturbance.
- Weight. Obtain baseline weight, since weight loss may be progressive as a result of excessive caloric need and poor eating.
- Confirmation of the clinical diagnosis in patients with overt symptoms may be made with the gene test.

Individuals at risk for HD (with a known family history but no overt symptoms) may choose to be evaluated. The initial evaluation of these patients is similar to those in whom HD is already manifested. Sometimes clinical evidence of HD can be gathered in patients unaware of their motor or cognitive decline. A normal clinical evaluation generally does not rule out future development of HD in an at-risk presymptomatic individual. After the clinical evaluation is complete, it may be appropriate to perform the test for the genetic mutation. However, testing of presymptomatic individuals is not to be taken lightly. This should be considered only after neuropsychologic and psychiatric evaluations, as well as genetic counseling. People at risk for depression and suicide can be identified and supported. Confidentiality of test results is always a concern because of the serious and fatal outcome of HD. Before being tested, presymptomatic individuals often consider the benefits and risks of knowing test results for themselves and their families. Some individuals may opt not to be tested for fear of discrimination from employers or insurance companies.[79]

Neurodiagnostic and Laboratory Studies

- **Genetic marker:** The abnormal gene for HD contains 40 or more CAG repeats. The gene mutation can be detected before symptoms occur. The specificity and sensitivity are sufficiently high that this test is all that is needed to confirm the diagnosis.
- CT or MRI may demonstrate evidence of gross wasting of the caudate nucleus and putamen and later atrophy in the frontal or temporal lobes.

Treatment

Medical Management

At this time, no neuroprotective or neurorestorative treatment is available. Several agents have been investigated or are currently being explored. Therefore medical management of HD remains essentially supportive and symptomatic. Medication may help the patient maintain or temporarily regain control of movement and better cope with changes in mood. The following types of medications may be used:

- Dopamine receptor blockers (neuroleptics). Haloperidol, risperidone, and others may be used for suppression of chorea, agitation, and psychotic symptoms. Side effects include sedation, dystonia, weight gain, and (long-term) possible tardive dyskinesia.
- Dopamine-depleting agents. Reserpine may suppress chorea but may worsen depression and cause

hypotension, so it is less commonly used. A related agent, tetrabenazine (TBZ), is less likely to cause side effects but is not FDA approved in the United States.

- Amantadine. The mechanism of this agent is unclear, but it is frequently effective for suppression of chorea and is generally well tolerated. Side effects may include pedal edema and livedo reticularis.
- Antispasmodics. Baclofen may reduce motor tone in juvenile-onset HD.
- Benzodiazepines. Clonazepam (longer half-life) or lorazepam (shorter half-life) may be used for panic or anxiety.
- Antidepressants. Fluoxetine, paroxetine, and other selective serotonin reuptake inhibitors (SSRIs) may stabilize mood and improve anxiety. Tricyclic antidepressants such as imipramine or nortriptyline may also be effective. Some antidepressants are "activating," others are sedating; the specific agent selected will depend on individual need.
- Anticonvulsants. Valproate and other agents may stabilize mood.
- Cholinesterase inhibitors. Donepezil, galantamine, and rivostigmine may improve cognition.

Surgical Management

There is currently no surgical intervention for HD. Transplantation of fetal or stem cells is in the early stages of investigation.

Clinical Management

A multidisciplinary team approach is ideal for the treatment of patients and may include a neurologist, psychiatrist, internist, geneticist, genetic counselor, clinical nurse specialist, neuropsychologist, physical therapist, occupational therapist, speech therapist, dietitian, and social services representative. Each member of the team can anticipate and handle problems that commonly occur in HD.

Education of the patient and family is paramount. Patients and their siblings may have experience with the deterioration of previous family members with HD. However, spouses and children of these patients may not have such background. Education and counseling should be targeted to all levels of experience and make few assumptions about what is already known. A concise description of HD itself should be presented, as well as an explanation of how current symptoms relate to the disease, and an outline of the expected course and future problems to be anticipated. With a realistic understanding of the prognosis, changes in the structure and function of the home environment may be planned (for example, a move to a single-level home or installation of grab bars in the bathtub). Options for eventual long-term care in the home or in an institution can be discussed. Consultation with legal and financial advisors may be arranged as needed. Disability benefits and other social services may be secured. Patients should be encouraged to make their wishes clear regarding issues such as use of a feeding tube or cardiopulmonary resuscitation and artificial ventilation. It should be apparent that this educational mission cannot be accomplished in one visit.

An essential part of education is counseling. At a minimum, patients and families should be led to understand the autosomal dominant nature of the disorder, that each of their offspring has a 50% risk of inheriting the disease. Unfortunately, because symptoms are usually not manifest until after peak reproductive age, it may be too late for the affected pair to decide not to have children. Presymptomatic siblings or children of affected patients may wish to be tested for possible diagnosis of HD. Testing of presymptomatic individuals (and particularly minor children) is not a casual decision. Proper consultation with a psychologist or psychiatrist, genetic counselor, and neurologist is required prior to sending the blood sample for CAG repeat analysis.

The disorder has a devastating effect on the present and future lives of all family members. HD is a family disease, beyond the simple transmission of the gene. Newly diagnosed patients may carry disturbing memories of a relative with HD. Risk of self-harm and suicide is high in individuals with HD,[80] and also in family members who do not carry the gene. At the time of diagnosis, affected individuals may have judgment and behavioral problems that are already affecting the integrity of family function. Psychiatric and psychologic support are essential for the patient, and counseling should be provided for spouses and children to deal with caregiver burden and other losses related to quality of life. Fear of the development of HD in at-risk individuals must be dealt with realistically and supportively (see also discussion of genetic counseling earlier). At more advanced stages, support is necessary to deal with the impending death of a loved one.

Physical, occupational, and speech therapy is recommended to improve the quality of life as appropriate. Swallowing and maintenance of adequate nutrition usually become a major problem and should be actively followed. Regular dental care may improve ability to take nutrition and reduce the risk of infection from tooth decay.

TIC DISORDERS

Tics are abrupt, brief, purposeless, stereotypic, coordinated movements (behaviors) that vary in intensity and are repeated at irregular intervals. The movements are most often brief and jerky (clonic tics). Slower, more prolonged movements (tonic or dystonic tics) may occur. Sounds, such as sniffing, grunting, or words, may be produced.

Individuals usually experience an irresistible urge to execute a behavior, which is temporarily relieved by its performance (Table 19-1). Tics may be suppressible for some period of time, particularly in a socially sensitive situation (at the workplace or school or even in the doctor's office), but may then rebound in a flurry when the active suppression stops. As with other movement disorders, tics may be more frequent or intense during periods of anxiety, fatigue, and stress, and they may decrease during periods of relaxation. Tics may occur in sleep, in contrast to other movement disorders that disappear during sleep.[81]

Tics may exist as single behaviors or as part of an entire repertoire. Specific tic behaviors may come and go with time. Most tic disorders make their first appearance in childhood,

TABLE 19-1	Tics	
Simple Tics	**Complex Tics**
Eye blinking	Finger cracking
Nose flaring	Hitting or biting oneself
Head jerking	Jumping or twirling about
Tongue protrusion	Touching other people or things,
Lip smacking	rubbing, skipping, smelling
Shoulder shrugs	objects
Fist clenching	Obscene gestures or uttering words
Sphincter tightening	or phrases out of context and
Pelvic thrusts	obscene words (**copropraxia,**
Facial grimacing	**coprolalia**)
Throat clearing	Imitating other people's behavior
Sniffing	(**echopraxia**)
Tongue clicking	

though occasionally adults may have new onset of tics. Tics in childhood may be transient, spontaneously resolving in less than a year. Tics may occur in neurodegenerative disorders such as HD or as a result of drug abuse (particularly cocaine).[82]

GILLES DE LA TOURETTE'S SYNDROME

Tics are the cardinal feature of Tourette's syndrome (TS). Multiple tics are present, including at least one sound-producing behavior. Although the general public is aware of socially inappropriate or obscene utterances (coprolalia) in TS, this phenomenon is actually present in only a minority (perhaps 15%) of patients. An affected individual may repeat another person's words (echolalia), mimic another's behaviors (echopraxia), or exhibit suggestibility.

Onset is typically in early childhood, and the peak symptoms occur around early adolescence.[83] Specific tic behaviors are known to come and go, and overall to wax and wane over time. Tics must be present for more than 1 year and negatively affect quality of life, according to the widely accepted definition. Although tic frequency and severity are reported to diminish by age 18, the number of adults with residual symptoms is not insubstantial.[84]

An association with comorbid psychiatric disorders in pediatric patients is well described. These include attention-deficit/hyperactivity disorder (ADHD), obsessive-compulsive disorder (OCD), depression, and anxiety.[85]

Incidence

TS was once thought to be rare, but many studies in the last 20 years have documented prevalence as high as 1% to 2% or even higher.[85] Males usually outnumber females by a factor of 3 to 4. TS occurs worldwide, and symptoms appear to be independent of culture or ethnic background.

Etiology

The etiology is not yet clear. Genetic transmission is well documented.[85,86] In February 2000 the National Institute of Neurological Disorders and Stroke (NINDS) awarded the Tourette Association's International TS Genetic Consortium (a six-nation group) $8.5 million to search for a genetic cause. Individuals with TS commonly report family members with TS, ADHD, or OCD, or some combination, suggesting the possibility of a common genetic link between all three disorders.

Some investigations have reported a possible role of infections and immune response in the development of TS and other "PANDAS" (pediatric autoimmune neuropsychiatric disorders associated with streptococcal infection),[87] but this is not likely to be a major factor in most patients with TS.

Pathophysiology

The dysfunction in the nervous system has long been believed to involve the basal ganglia and related connections with the cerebral cortex and thalamus. Examination of brains at autopsy has not revealed specific findings. Likewise, specialized imaging techniques in living patients have provided variable results. At least some component of the abnormality appears to involve the function of dopamine; by the late 1970s, it was apparent that dopamine blockers could suppress tics. The basal ganglia are a major target of the dopaminergic system projecting from the brainstem. Other neurotransmitters, such as serotonin, GABA, and acetylcholine, may be involved as well.

In current concepts of normal basal ganglia function, the system is optimized to select desired movement programs and suppress competing or unwanted movements.[88,89] In tics and other hyperkinetic movement disorders, malfunction of the system results in inability to suppress undesired behavior. Because the system contains not only motor but also pathways serving cognitive and emotional functions, dysfunction of the basal ganglia commonly results in behavioral and affective disturbances. This may explain the high incidence of obsessive-compulsive symptoms and behaviors in TS.

Assessment

The diagnosis of TS is made on clinical grounds. Careful history and physical examination focus on the following information:

- Careful descriptions of the current "repertoire" of tic behaviors, including sound-producing tics. Historical descriptions of tics that may no longer be performed. Document waxing and waning of tic behaviors and factors that exacerbate or relieve them.
- Report the earliest recollection of behaviors that could be classified as tics, even if they were too mild to result in medical evaluation, or had gone unrecognized as such.
- Gauge the relative impact of tics on social and economic quality of life, compared to the impact of comorbid symptoms (if present) such as obsessive-

compulsive symptoms, attention-deficit symptoms, or depression.

- Medical history should include other neurologic diseases and current and prior medications. Specifically ask about neuroleptics, antidepressants, and stimulants. Do not ignore over-the-counter and alternative therapies. Patients should be asked about smoking and drugs of abuse. Determine the relative timing of onset of tics with respect to the time of the prior medication use or drug abuse.
- Inquiry into the family history should include not only others with TS, but also ADHD, OCD, depression, anxiety, and other psychiatric and neurologic disorders.

The following widely accepted diagnostic criteria are published by the American Psychiatric Association's *Diagnostic and Statistical Manual,* 4th edition (DSM-IV).[90]

- Onset before age 18
- Presence of multiple motor tics
- Presence of at least one sonic tic
- Duration of symptoms for more than 1 year
- Symptoms are bothersome to the patient or family members

Neurodiagnostic and Laboratory Studies

No biochemical, electrophysiologic, radiologic, or genetic marker tests assist in the diagnosis of TS. MRI studies do not reveal useful distinguishing features. Electroencephalogram (EEG) and evoked potential findings are either nonspecific or normal.

Treatment

Treatment is symptomatic. Conservative treatment is tried first, because some patients' symptoms resolve over time with no therapy. Medical treatment initially addresses the symptoms that cause the most difficulties for the individual, particularly those that are functionally disabling. Many individuals with TS report that they lead productive lives and are able to manage their symptoms, sometimes without any medications. Benefits of medications must be weighed against their side effects.

Pharmacologic treatment for TS has focused on typical neuroleptics (haloperidol, pimozide, fluphenazine, and others), atypical neuroleptics (risperidone and others), presynaptic catecholamine depletors (reserpine, tetrabenazine), or central α_2-adrenergic receptor blockade (clonidine, guanfacine).[88,91] Benzodiazepines (such as clonazepam) are also used. An accepted conservative approach is to avoid neuroleptics until other options have been exhausted, due to the side effects of dopamine blockers.

Psychiatric comorbidities are also treated. SSRIs such as fluoxetine and certain tricyclic antidepressants such as clomipramine are helpful for OCD symptoms, as well as depression or anxiety, common in patients with TS. However, these agents are not particularly effective for tic behaviors.[91]

Tics are rarely eradicated entirely; the goal of medication is to achieve maximum control with minimal side effects.

Some patients (children and adults) remain symptomatic with clinically disabling tics despite maximal medical therapy.

Several specific behavioral techniques, as well as alternative treatments, have been investigated. However, these methods are incompletely studied or of limited efficacy.[88] On the other hand, psychotherapy to help patients and family members cope with the social burden of TS may be very helpful. Individuals with TS may face public ostracism, difficulty in school and the workplace, and potential medication side effects. Constructive teaching is needed to help individuals manage TS. Health care providers can provide patient/family support and help the individual find the most appropriate treatment.

Surgical treatment, specifically deep brain stimulation (DBS), is investigational and is not yet recommended. However, results of individual cases and small series of patients with DBS implants in the thalamus globus pallidus have been encouraging.[92,93]

RESTLESS LEGS SYNDROME

Restless legs syndrome (RLS) is a common, though underrecognized, neurologic disorder. Persons with RLS experience an uncomfortable sensation deep inside their legs and sometimes in their arms that is only relieved by movement. (See Chapter 6 for the relationship of RLS and sleep.) Words people have used to describe these sensations include tingling, pulling, itching, burning, creeping, and crawling sensations underneath their skin.[94,95] These sensations occur at rest, when the person sits or lies down, and disappear with movement, particularly walking. When the movement ceases the sensations often return. The symptoms are worse in the evening and at night, significantly interfering with sleep. Once asleep, persons with RLS often experience periodic limb movements of sleep (PLMS) particularly of the legs. PLMS can result in frequent awakenings, adding to a person's already disturbed sleep.[96]

Etiology and Prevalence

The prevalence of RLS in the general population has been reported to be from 6% to 24%, increasing with age until about 60 years, and more common in women.[97-99] The majority of persons with primary (idiopathic) RLS have a positive family history.[100,101] Ondo and colleagues[100] studied 12 identical twin pairs where at least one of the twins reported symptoms of RLS. They found that in 10 of 12 twin pairs both had definite RLS and 11 of 12 pairs had a positive family history. This suggests an autosomal dominant pattern of inheritance with high penetrance.[100] The age of onset for primary RLS is variable. It can begin in childhood or early adulthood. Those with a positive family history tend to have a younger age of onset than those with a negative family history.[101]

Causes of secondary RLS include iron deficiency (ferritin <50 mcg/L), pregnancy, uremia in persons with end-stage renal failure, neuropathies, and radiculopathies.[95,96] Some medications such as antihistamines, tricyclic antidepressants,

SSRIs, lithium, dopamine antagonists, and caffeine may uncover or worsen RLS.[95,101]

Pathophysiology

Although the pathophysiology of primary RLS is not well understood, it is believed to be a disorder of the CNS.[46] One possible mechanism is an abnormal iron metabolism that leads to a reduction in the formation of central dopamine.[101]

Assessment

Rarely are the symptoms of RLS evident on examination. A diagnosis of RLS is dependent on meeting four criteria:[94,99] (1) an urge to move the legs usually associated with an uncomfortable sensation in the legs, (2) symptoms occur at rest, (3) symptoms are relieved with movement (e.g., walking, stretching), and (4) the symptoms are worse in the evening or at night.

The clinician obtains a history that includes the following:[95,101,102]

- Symptom onset, frequency, and intensity
- Body parts involved (legs or arms, unilateral or bilateral)
- Correlation between symptoms and time of day
- Activities that relieve or exacerbate symptoms
- Sleep history
- Sleep pattern (ask bed partner about periodic movement of limbs during sleep)
- Daytime sleepiness or fatigue; difficulty concentrating
- Family history of RLS
- Current medications
- Alcohol, caffeine, and tobacco use
- Medical history
- Impact on quality of life

Neurodiagnostic and Laboratory Studies

There are no diagnostic studies to confirm a diagnosis of RLS. Diagnostic studies are conducted to rule out secondary causes of RLS.[95,101] Serum ferritin levels and iron saturation studies are done to rule out iron deficiency. Polysomnography is not part of the standard evaluation for RLS but is helpful if sleep apnea is suspected or if sleep disturbances persist after successful treatment of RLS.[94]

Treatment

Treatment of RLS involves nonpharmacologic and pharmacologic therapies. Nonpharmacologic interventions include maintaining regular sleep habits; engaging in mild to moderate daily exercise; and avoiding caffeine, alcohol, and tobacco.[101,102] Using relaxation techniques such as massage, biofeedback, and hot baths may also provide temporary relief.[101,102]

When to initiate pharmacologic treatment will depend on the severity and frequency of symptoms. Medications used to treat RLS include dopaminergic agents (e.g., ropinirole, pramipexole, levodopa), antiepileptic agents (e.g.,

gabapentin), opiates (e.g., propoxyphene), and benzodiazepines (e.g., clonazepam).[101,103] Dopaminergic medications are the most effective and, unless contraindicated, should be tried first. The doses of the dopaminergic drugs needed to treat RLS are much less than what is required to treat PD. One disadvantage of the dopaminergic agents is the potential for augmentation or rebound of symptoms.[101] Augmentation is the development of symptoms beginning earlier in the evening and resulting in the need to take medication at an earlier time.[103,104] The rebound phenomenon is when symptoms return with greater intensity than before treatment. Augmentation and rebound are more likely to occur with the shorter-acting dopaminergic agents such as levodopa.[104]

In cases of secondary RLS, treating the underlying disorder often brings relief of the RLS. RLS due to pregnancy often improves within weeks after the birth of the baby. RLS due to end-stage renal failure often improves after successful kidney transplant.[95]

RLS is a lifelong disorder that significantly interferes with a person's quality of life. Poor sleep affects the person's ability to function the following day. People with RLS may avoid activities that require prolonged periods of sitting such as traveling, going to the movies, or eating at restaurants.[94] Early detection and treatment will improve quality of life for persons with RLS.

CONCLUSION

The term *movement disorders* may refer to abnormal movements or to syndromes that cause abnormal movements. They include a variety of conditions that may be described as hypokinetic, hyperkinetic, or movements that are abnormally coordinated. Conditions include parkinsonism, tremors, dystonia, chorea, tic disorders, Tourette's syndrome, restless legs syndrome, and others. It is important for health care providers to be knowledgeable in early identification and current treatment options for each disorder. The advances in treatment offer new hope for strategies to provide symptom control and an improved quality of life for many individuals. Research continues as scientists endeavor to discover the cause and a cure that will someday eradicate these neurologic disorders.

RESOURCES

American Parkinson Disease Association: 135 Parkinson Ave., Staten Island, NY 10305; 800-223-2732; www.apdaparkinson.org

Benign Essential Blepharospasm Research Foundation, Inc.: PO Box 12468, Beaumont, TX 77726-2468; 409-832-0788; www.blepharospasm.org

Dystonia Medical Research Foundation: One E. Wacker Drive, Suite 2430, Chicago, IL 60601-1905; 312-755-0198; www.dystonia-foundation.org

Huntington's Disease Society of America: 505 Eighth Ave., New York, NY 10018; 800-345-4372; www.hdsa.org

International Essential Tremor Foundation: PO Box 14005, Lenexa, KS 66285-4005; 888-387-3667; www.essentialtremor.org

The Lewy Body Dementia Association: PO Box 11393, Tempe, AZ 85284-0024; 800-539-9767; www.lewybodydementia.org

Michael J. Fox Foundation for Parkinson's Research: Grand Central Station, PO Box 4777, New York, NY 10163; 800-708-7644; www.michaeljfox.org

National Parkinson Foundation, Inc.: 1501 NW Ninth Avenue, Bob Hope Road, Miami, FL 33136-1494; 800-327-4545; www.parkinson.org

National Spasmodic Torticollis Association: 9920 Talbert Ave., Fountain Valley, CA 92708; 800-487-8385; www.torticollis.org

Parkinson's Disease Foundation, Inc.: 1359 Broadway, Suite 1509, New York, NY 10018; 800-457-6676; www.pdf.org

Restless Legs Syndrome Foundation: 819 Second Street SW, Rochester, MN 55902-2985; 507-287-6465; www.rls.org

Society for Progressive Supranuclear Palsy: Executive Plaza III, 11350 McCormick Rd, Suite 906, Hunt Valley, MD 21031; 800-457-4777; www.psp.org

Tourette Syndrome Association: 42-40 Bell Boulevard, Bayside, NY 11361; 718-224-2999; www.tsa-usa.org

We Move: 204 West 84th Street, New York, NY; 800-437-6682; www.wemove.org

Wilson's Disease Association International: 1802 Brookside Drive, Wooster, OH 44691; 800-399-0266; www.wilsondisease.org

REFERENCES

1. De Lau LML et al: Incidence of parkinsonism and Parkinson disease in the general population: the Rotterdam study, *Neurology* 63:1240–1244, 2004.
2. Tanner CM, Goldman SM: Epidemiology of Parkinson's disease, *Neurol Clin* 14:317–335, 1996.
3. Samii A, Nutt JG, Ransom BR: Parkinson's disease, *Lancet* 363:1783–1793, 2004.
4. Nath U et al: Clinical features and natural history of progressive supranuclear palsy: a clinical cohort study, *Neurology* 60:910–916, 2003.
5. Tison F et al: Parkinsonism in multiple system atrophy: natural history, severity (UPDRS-III), and disability assessment compared with Parkinson's disease, *Mov Disord* 17:701–709, 2002.
6. Chaudhuri KR: Autonomic dysfunction in movement disorders, *Curr Opin Neurol* 14:505–511, 2001.
7. Witjas T et al: Nonmotor fluctuations in Parkinson's disease frequent and disabling, *Neurology* 59:408–413, 2002.
8. Pluck GS, Brown RG: Apathy in Parkinson's disease, *J Neurol Neurosurg Psychiatry* 73:636–642, 2002.
9. Alves G, Wentzel-Larsen T, Larsen JP: Is fatigue an independent and persistent symptom in patients with Parkinson's disease? *Neurology* 63:1908–1911, 2004.
10. Green J et al: Cognitive impairments in advanced PD without dementia, *Neurology* 59:1320–1324, 2002.
11. The Movement Disorder Society Task Force: Management of Parkinson's disease: an evidenced-based review, *Mov Disord* 17(suppl 4):S1–S166, 2002.
12. Marsh L et al: Psychiatric comorbidities in patients with Parkinson disease and psychosis, *Neurology* 63:293–300, 2004.
13. Gagnon JF et al: REM sleep behavior disorder and REM sleep without atonia in Parkinson's disease, *Neurology* 59:585–589, 2002.
14. Paus S et al: Sleep attacks, daytime sleepiness, and dopamine agonists in Parkinson's disease, *Mov Disord* 18:659–667, 2003.
15. Djaldetti R et al: Quantitative measurement of pain sensation in patients with Parkinson disease, *Neurology* 62:2171–2175, 2004.
16. Hoehn MM, Yahr MD: Parkinsonism: onset, progression, and mortality, *Neurology* 17:427–442, 1967.
17. Paulson HL, Stern MB: Clinical manifestations of Parkinson's disease. In Watts RL, Koller WC, editors: *Movement disorders: neurologic principles and practice,* New York, 1997, McGraw-Hill.
18. Gibb WR, Lees AJ: The relevance of the Lewy body to the pathogenesis of idiopathic Parkinson's disease, *J Neurol Neurosurg Psychiatry* 51:745–752, 1988.
19. Baseman DG et al: Pergolide use in Parkinson disease is associated with cardiac valve regurgitation, *Neurology* 63:301–304, 2004.
20. Gschwandtner U et al: Pathologic gambling in patients with Parkinson's disease, *Clin Neuropharmacol* 24:170–172, 2001.
21. Driver-Dunckley E, Samanta J, Stacy M: Pathological gambling associated with dopamine agonist therapy in Parkinson's disease, *Neurology* 61:422–423, 2003.
22. Klos KJ et al: Pathological hypersexuality predominantly linked to adjuvant dopamine agonist therapy in Parkinson's disease and multiple system atrophy, *Parkinsonism Relat Disord* 11:381–386, 2005.
23. Hagell P, Odin P: Apomorphine in the treatment of Parkinson's disease, *J Neurosci Nurs* 33:21–34, 2001.
24. Fernandez HH et al: Long-term outcome of quetiapine use for psychosis among parkinsonian patients, *Mov Disord* 18:510–514, 2003.
25. Reddy S et al: The effect of quetiapine on psychosis and motor function in parkinsonian patients with and without dementia, *Mov Disord* 17:676–681, 2002.
26. Lipp A et al: A randomized trial of botulinum toxin A for treatment of drooling, *Neurology* 61:1279–1281, 2003.
27. Ondo WG, Hunter C, Moore W: A double-blind placebo-controlled trial of botulinum toxin B for sialorrhea in Parkinson's disease, *Neurology* 62:37–40, 2004.
28. Magerkurth C, Schnitzer R, Braune S: Symptoms of autonomic failure in Parkinson's disease: prevalence and impact on daily life, *Clin Auton Res* 15:76–82, 2005.
29. Rodriguez-Oroz MC et al: Bilateral deep brain stimulation in Parkinson's disease: a multicentre study with 4 years follow-up, *Brain* 128:2240–2249, 2005.
30. Okun MS et al: Development and initial validation of a screening tool for Parkinson disease surgical candidates, *Neurology* 63:161–163, 2004.
31. Langston JW et al: Core assessment program for intracerebral transplantations (CAPIT), *Mov Disord* 7:2–13, 1992.
32. Russmann H et al: Subthalamic nucleus deep brain stimulation in Parkinson disease patients over age 70 years, *Neurology* 63:1952–1954, 2004.
33. Hunka K et al: Nursing time to program and assess deep brain stimulators in movement disorder patients, *J Neurosci Nurs* 37:204–210, 2005.
34. Krack P et al: Five-year follow-up of bilateral stimulation of the subthalamic nucleus in advanced Parkinson's disease, *N Engl J Med* 349:1925–1934, 2003.
35. Ramig LO, Fox C, Shimon S: Parkinson's disease: speech and voice disorders and their treatment with the Lee Silverman Voice Treatment, *Semin Speech Lang* 25:169–180, 2004.

36. Liotti M et al: Hypophonia in Parkinson's disease: neural correlates of voice treatment revealed by PET, *Neurology* 60:432–440, 2003.

37. Flanders M, Sarkis N: Fresnel membrane prisms: clinical experience, *Can J Ophthalmol* 34:335–340, 1999.

38. Grosset KA et al: Measuring therapy adherence in Parkinson's disease: a comparison of methods, *J Neurol Neurosurg Psychiatry* 77:249–251, 2006.

39. Whitney CM: Maintaining the square: how older adults with Parkinson's disease sustain quality in their lives, *J Gerontol Nurs* 30:28–35, 2004.

40. Pincus JH, Barry K: Influence of dietary protein on motor fluctuations in Parkinson's disease, *Arch Neurol* 44:270–272, 1987.

41. Riley D, Lang AE: Practical application of a low-protein diet for Parkinson's disease, *Neurology* 38:1026–1031, 1988.

42. Chen H et al: Weight loss in PD, *Ann Neurol* 53:676–679, 2003.

43. Noyes K et al: Economic burden associated with Parkinson's disease on elderly Medicare beneficiaries, *Mov Disord* 21:362–372, 2006.

44. Deuschl G et al: Consensus statement of the Movement Disorder Society on tremor. Ad Hoc Scientific Committee, *Mov Disord* 13(suppl 3):2–23, 1998.

45. Deuschl G, Volkmann J: Tremors: differential diagnosis, pathophysiology, and therapy. In Jankovic JJ, Tolosa E, editors: *Parkinson's disease and movement disorders,* ed 4, Philadelphia, 2002, Lippincott Williams & Wilkins.

46. O'Sullivan JD, Lees AJ: Nonparkinsonian tremors, *Clin Neuropharmacol* 23:233–238, 2000.

47. Sharott A, Marsden J, Brown P: Primary orthostatic tremor is an exaggeration of a physiological response to instability, *Mov Disord* 18:195–199, 2003.

48. Soland VL et al: Focal task-specific tremors, *Mov Disord* 11:665–670, 1996.

49. Deuschl G et al: The pathophysiology of tremor, *Muscle Nerve* 24:716–735, 2001.

50. Zesiewicz TA et al: Practice parameter: therapies for essential tremor, *Neurology* 64:2008–2020, 2005.

51. Hariz GM, Lindberg M, Bergenheim AT: Impact of thalamic deep brain stimulation on disability and health-related quality of life in patients with essential tremor, *J Neurol Neurosurg Psychiatry* 72:47–52, 2002.

52. Bressman SB: Dystonia update, *Clin Neuropharmacol* 23:239–251, 2000.

53. Jankovic JJ, Fahn S: Dystonic disorders. In Jankovic JJ, Tolosa E, editors: *Parkinson's disease and movement disorders,* ed 4, Philadelphia, 2002, Lippincott Williams & Wilkins.

54. Schuele S et al: Botulinum toxin injections in the treatment of musician's dystonia, *Neurology* 64:341–343, 2005.

55. Németh AH: The genetics of primary dystonia and related disorders, *Brain* 125:695–721, 2002.

56. Langlois M, Richer F, Chouinard S: New perspectives on dystonia, *Can J Neurol Sci* 30(suppl 1):S34–S44, 2003.

57. Furukawa Y, Lang AE, Trugman JM, et al: Gender-related penetrance and de novo GTP-cyclohydrase I gene mutations in dopa-responsive dystonia, *Neurology* 50:1015–1020, 1998.

58. Trot M: Dystonia update, *Curr Opin Neurol* 16:495–500, 2003.

59. Vitek JL: Pathophysiology of dystonia: a neuronal model, *Mov Disord* 17(suppl 3):S49-S62, 2002.

60. Goldman JG, Comella CL: Treatment of dystonia, *Clin Neuropharmacol* 26:102–108, 2003.

61. Horn S, Comella CL: Treatment of dystonia. In Jankovic JJ, Tolosa E, editors: *Parkinson's disease and movement disorders,* ed 4, Philadelphia, 2002, Lippincott Williams & Wilkins.

62. Comella CL, Jankovic J, Brin MF: Use of botulinum toxin type A in the treatment of cervical dystonia, *Neurology* 55(suppl 5):S15–S21, 2000.

63. Comella CL et al: Comparison of botulinum toxin serotypes A and B for the treatment of cervical dystonia, *Neurology* 65:1423–1429, 2005.

64. Yianni J et al: Globus pallidus internus deep brain stimulation for dystonic conditions: a prospective audit, *Mov Disord* 18:436–442, 2003.

65. Krause M et al: Pallidal stimulation for dystonia, *Neurosurgery* 55:1361–1370, 2004.

66. Bittar RG et al: Deep brain stimulation for generalised dystonia and spasmodic torticollis, *J Clin Neurosci* 12:12–16, 2005.

67. Vidailhet M et al: Bilateral deep-brain stimulation of the globus pallidus in primary generalized dystonia, *N Engl J Med* 352:459–467, 2005.

68. Margolese HC et al: Tardive dyskinesia in the era of typical and atypical antipsychotics. Part 2. Incidence and management strategies in patients with schizophrenia, *Can J Psychiatry* 50:703–714, 2005.

69. Skidmore F, Reich SG: Tardive dystonia, *Curr Treat Options Neurol* 7:231–236, 2005.

70. Schrader C et al: Unilateral deep brain stimulation of the internal globus pallidus alleviates tardive dyskinesia, *Mov Disord* 19:583–585, 2003.

71. Trottenbert T et al: Treatment of severe tardive dystonia with pallidal deep brain stimulation, *Neurology* 64:344–346, 2005.

72. Caselli RJ, Boeve BF: The degenerative dementias. In Goetz CG, editor: *Textbook of clinical neurology,* ed 2, Philadephia, 2003, Saunders.

73. Huntington's Disease Collaborative Research Group: A novel gene containing a trinucleotide repeat that is expanded and unstable on Huntington's disease chromosomes, *Cell* 72:971–983, 1993.

74. Biglan KM, Shoulson I: Huntington's disease. In Jankovic JJ, Tolosa E, editors: *Parkinson's disease and movement disorders,* ed 4, Philadelphia, 2002, Lippincott Williams & Wilkins.

75. Andrew SE et al: The relationship between trinucleotide (CAG) repeat length and clinical features of Huntington's disease, *Nat Genet* 4:398–403, 1993.

76. Pritchard C, Cox DR, Myers RM: The end in sight for Huntington's disease? *Am J Hum Genet* 49:1, 1991 (editorial).

77. Paulus-Thomas J, Gross M, Thull DL: Huntington disease: the long and short of it, *Genet Pract* 4:1–2, 1997.

78. Marsden CD: Functional neuroanatomy and chemistry of the basal ganglia. In Fahn S et al, editors: *A comprehensive review of movement disorders for the clinical practitioner,* New York, 1992, Columbia University Press.

79. Williams JK et al: Adults seeking presymptomatic gene testing for Huntington's disease, *J Nurs Schol* 31:109–114, 1999.

80. Schoenfeld M et al: Increased rate of suicide among patients with Huntington's disease, *J Neurol Neurosurg Psychiatry* 47:1283–1287, 1984.

81. Jankovic J: Tics and Tourette's syndrome. In Jankovic JJ, Tolosa E, editors: *Parkinson's disease and movement disor-*

ders, ed 4, Philadelphia, 2002, Lippincott Williams & Wilkins.

82. Jankovic J: Differential diagnosis and etiology of tics, *Adv Neurol* 85:15–29, 2001.

83. Leckman JF et al: Course of tic severity in Tourette syndrome: the first two decades, *Pediatrics* 102:14–19, 1998.

84. Pappert EJ et al: Objective assessments of longitudinal outcome in Gilles de la Tourette syndrome, *Neurology* 61:936–940, 2003.

85. Robertson MM: Tourette syndrome, associated conditions, and the complexities of treatment, *Brain* 123:425–462, 2000.

86. Leckman JF et al: Phenomenology of tics and natural history of tic disorders, *Adv Neurol* 85:1–14, 2001.

87. Swedo SE et al: Pediatric autoimmune neuropsychiatric disorders associated with streptococcal infections: clinical description of the first 50 cases, *Am J Psychiatry* 155:64–71, 1998.

88. Leckman JF: Tourette's syndrome, *Lancet* 360:1577–1586, 2002.

89. Mink JW: Basal ganglia dysfunction in Tourette's syndrome: a new hypothesis, *Pediatr Neurol* 25(3):190–198, 2001.

90. American Psychiatric Association: Tic disorders. In *Diagnostic and statistical manual of mental disorders,* ed 4, Washington, DC, 1994, American Psychiatric Association.

91. Riddle MA, Carlson J: Clinical psychopharmacology for Tourette syndrome and associated disorders, *Adv Neurol* 85:343–354, 2001.

92. Visser-Vandewalle V et al: Chronic bilateral thalamic stimulation: a new therapeutic approach in intractable Tourette syndrome. A report of three cases, *J Neurosurg* 99:1094–1100, 2003.

93. Maddux BN et al: Clinical efficacy and video analysis of deep brain stimulation for medically intractable Tourette syndrome, *Mov Disord* 19:1123, 2004 (abstract).

94. Earley CJ: Restless legs syndrome, *N Engl J Med* 348:2103–2109, 2003.

95. National Center on Sleep Disorders Research, National Heart, Lung, and Blood Institute, National Institutes of Health: *Restless legs syndrome: detection and management in primary care,* NIH pub no 00-3788, 2000.

96. Allen RP, Earley CJ: Restless legs syndrome: a review of clinical and pathophysiologic features, *J Clin Neurophysiol* 18:128–147, 2001.

97. Högl B et al: Restless legs syndrome: a community-based study of prevalence, severity, and risk factors, *Neurology* 64:1920–1924, 2005.

98. Berger K et al: Sex and the risk of restless legs syndrome in the general population, *Arch Intern Med* 164:196–202, 2004.

99. Nichols DA et al: Restless legs syndrome in primary care: a prevalence study, *Arch Intern Med* 163:2323–2329, 2003.

100. Ondo WG, Vuong KD, Wang Q: Restless legs syndrome in monozygotic twins: clinical correlates, *Neurology* 55:1404–1406, 2000.

101. Thorpy MJ: New paradigms in the treatment of restless legs syndrome, *Neurology* 64:28–33, 2005.

102. Cuellar N: Restless legs syndrome: a case study, *J Neurosci Nurs* 35:193–201, 2003.

103. Ondo W et al: Long-term treatment of restless legs syndrome with dopamine agonists, *Arch Neurol* 61:1393–1397, 2004.

104. Comella CL: Restless legs syndrome treatment with dopamine agonists, *Neurology* 58(suppl 1):S87–S92, 2002.

CHAPTER 20

ALIZA BITTON BEN-ZACHARIA,
MAURA L. DEL BENE

Inflammatory Demyelinating Diseases

Immune-mediated inflammatory demyelinating disorders of the central nervous system (CNS) are common. Immune dysregulation in the CNS and the peripheral nervous system (PNS) is not uncommon. Environmental, genetic, and immunologic factors have been postulated to be involved in the development of the variable neurologic disorders. Major immune-mediated neurologic diseases of the CNS include multiple sclerosis and acute disseminated encephalomyelitis. Immune-mediated diseases of the PNS include myasthenia gravis, Guillain-Barré syndrome, chronic inflammatory demyelinating polyneuropathy, idiopathic polymyositis, and dermatomyositis.[7]

Understanding the immune mechanisms of each disease and uncovering potential therapeutic targets are essential for the design of new treatments and new combinations of treatments. The epidemiology, pathogenesis, and therapeutic approaches to the major neuroimmunologic diseases facilitate the understanding of their effects on individuals.[7] The effects of these diseases result in neurologic deficits.[30] These neurologic symptoms vary in the different disorders and may have an unpredictable course that can progress and affect overall quality of life. This chapter reviews multiple sclerosis, acute disseminated encephalomyelitis, optic neuritis, acute nontraumatic transverse myelitis, and other variant forms of multiple sclerosis.

MULTIPLE SCLEROSIS

Multiple sclerosis (MS) is a chronic neurologic disease first described by Carswell in 1838, Cruveilhier in 1841, and Charcot in 1868.[33] It is the most common demyelinating disease of the CNS and is the most common neurologic illness affecting young adults. The two basic clinical forms of MS include relapses and progression (Fig. 20-1). Relapses are considered the clinical manifestation of inflammatory demyelination, and progression of disease is considered representation of chronic demyelination and axonal loss.[31] It causes episodes of neurologic symptoms that may be followed by neurologic deficits.[45] Deficits and disability are incurred due to incomplete recovery from acute exacerbations and by ongoing deterioration. It is also believed that MS exacerbations produce a measurable and sustained effect on disability.[30]

An increase in prevalence over the past 10 years has been attributed to increased longevity, improved epidemiologic reporting, consistent diagnostic criteria, and technologic advances such as magnetic resonance imaging (MRI). The annual cost of MS is estimated at over $34,000 per person, translating into an estimate of national annual cost of $6.8 billion, and a total lifetime cost per case of $2.2 million.[53]

Incidence

The onset of MS ranges from 10 to 50 years of age, with an average age of onset of 30 years. However, new-onset MS cases have been described in children and in the elderly. MS is more common in women. The female-to-male ratio is approximately 2:1 based on epidemiologic studies. Based on a small study, the ratio is higher in children at approximately 3:1.[12] Whites are most commonly affected. The rate of MS in African Americans is approximately half of the rate of white Americans.[27]

Prevalence figures vary by geographic location. The prevalence in North America and northern Europe (50 degrees latitude) is 30 to 80 cases per 100,000 population. In equatorial areas the prevalence drops to 1 case per 100,000 population. Prevalence rates range from fewer than 5 cases per 100,000 in the southern latitudes to 200 cases per 100,000 population in the north. Studies suggest that if migration occurs after age 15, the risk remains that of the area of origin. Estimates for the total number of cases range between 350,000 and 450,000 in the United States and 1.1 million worldwide.[19,37]

Etiology

The precise etiology of MS remains unknown. The triad involved in MS includes genetic susceptibility, environmental exposure, and dysregulation of the immune system. The destruction in the CNS, including demyelination and axonal loss leading to degeneration, involves immune mechanisms. MS is probably triggered by an environmental factor in persons who are genetically susceptible. The roles of genes and the environment are not fully understood in MS. Although the evidence is indirect, it is believed that the environmental agent is a virus or bacterium, and a few

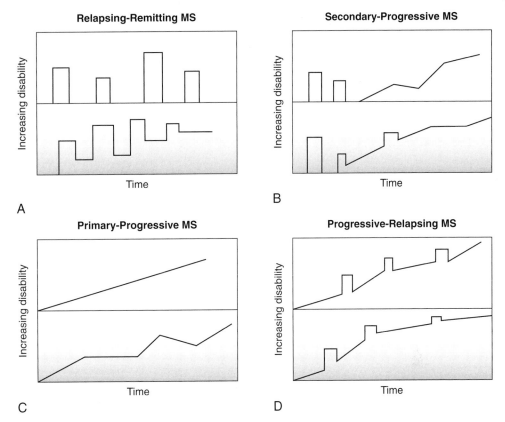

Figure 20-1 **A,** Relapsing-remitting (RR) MS is characterized by acute attacks with full recovery or with partial recovery. **B,** Secondary progressive MS starts with an RR course followed by progressive phase. **C,** Primary progressive (PP) MS is characterized by progression from onset of disease without acute relapses. **D,** Progressive relapsing (PR) MS is characterized by progression from onset of disease with acute relapses.
(Adapted from Lublin F, Reingold S: Defining the clinical course of multiple sclerosis: results of an international survey, Neurology *46:907–911, 1996.)*

researchers believe that a single infectious agent causes the condition. No active or latent virus has consistently been demonstrated in cultures of the cerebrospinal fluid (CSF) of patients with MS. Close contact has not been implicated, because conjugal MS has not been reported. It has also been shown that no single gene causes MS; multiple genes are involved. The multiple epidemiologic studies support a polygenic hereditary predisposition to MS. The genes that were identified in MS do not directly cause the disease, but increase the risk of the development of the disease.[29] One of the definite genes identified in MS is the human leukocyte antigen (HLA) DR2 carriership, which is associated with an increased risk for MS. However, studies show that 60% of MS patients in northern Europe are DR2 haplotype positive compared with 30% in healthy individuals. Therefore the risk caused by the DR2 haplotype is small, and it is neither necessary nor sufficient for development of MS.[11] How these genes operate and interact with the environmental agent is largely unknown. Familial tendency in MS plays a major role in the understanding of genetics and environmental factors in MS.[13,46]

Pathophysiology

MS is a heterogeneous illness characterized by inflammatory demyelination and degeneration in the CNS. Early axonal damage or injury is common in acute cases involving MS plaques, and early atrophy of the brain and the spinal cord can be seen. It is thought that one or more environmental agents in a genetically susceptible individual trigger an autoimmune attack on the myelin sheath. Damage to the myelin

interrupts conduction through the nerves. Over time, remyelination by oligodendrocytes can occur but may not be able to keep up with sustained and repeated damage to the myelin. The loss of oligodendrocytes and persistent demyelination results in axonal loss. Lesions of inflammation and myelin loss (plaques) are seen in affected areas of the CNS.[19,31] Plaques range in size from 1 mm to 4 cm and are found scattered throughout the white matter and, to a lesser degree, in the gray matter. Areas that show a predilection for plaque development include the optic nerves; cortical and juxtacortical regions; the perivenous and periventricular regions of the cerebrum; and the cerebellum, brainstem, and cervical and thoracic spinal cord. Periventricular plaques are found in almost 90% of MS cases.

The disease process of MS may be initiated by an immune response against an environmental agent that cross-reacts with myelin or oligodendrocyte cells, possibly because of molecular mimicry. Both the humoral and cell-mediated immune systems have been implicated in the disease process. Support for a role for the humoral immune system comes from the presence of oligoclonal immunoglobulin G (IgG) and evidence of increased synthesis of immunoglobulins in the CSF in most patients with MS.[33] Although this finding was reported 30 years ago and the test is an element in the diagnostic workup for MS, the antigen to which the antibodies are directed remains unknown. Oligoclonal IgG and increased synthesis of immunoglobulin in the CNS may reflect defective regulation of B cells. Support for a role for the cellular immune response in MS derives in part from studies of experimental autoimmune encephalomyelitis (EAE), an animal model of MS in which symptoms and

Elements of the MS Lesion

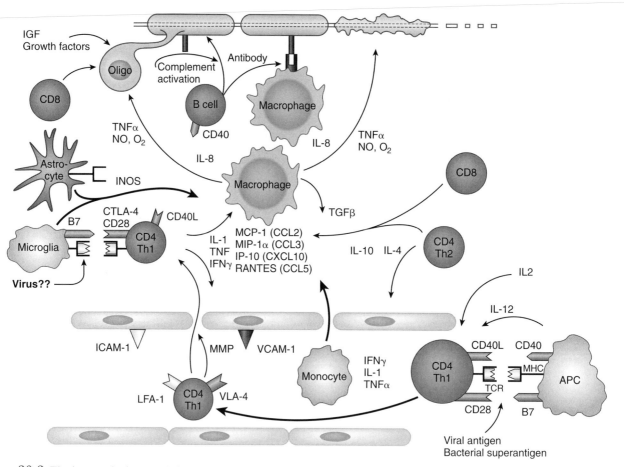

Figure 20-2 The immunologic cascade in multiple sclerosis. *(Courtesy of Dr. H. McFarland.)*

pathologic conditions similar to those found in MS result from a T-cell–mediated response to immunization with CNS tissue. Studies of T-cell function in peripheral blood and CSF show that CD8 lymphocytes are reduced in the progressive form of MS. One current hypothesis is that a defect in suppressor T-cell function lowers the threshold of T-cell activation. Certain immune system signal molecules such as cytokines (i.e., tumor necrosis factor and interleukin-2), interferon, and prostaglandins are thought to play a role in the regulation of cellular and humoral immune responses and have been implicated in MS and other autoimmune disorders.[45,46] In summary, T cells and B cells are present in plaques in MS; therefore they are both involved in MS pathophysiology and the autoimmune response.

The immunopathologic sequences of events that may lead to MS (Figs. 20-2 and 20-3) involve CD4 T cells that are activated by a triprocess. The presence of an antigen, the antigen-presenting cell, and a specific T-cell receptor leads to the activation of T cells. Costimulatory molecules and adhesion molecules are a vital part in assisting the migration of T cells through the blood-brain barrier (BBB) into the CNS. Once in the CNS, the T cells become up-regulated in response to a CNS antigen, probably a macrophage. These up-regulated T cells release proinflammatory cytokines

and chemokines, which cause myelin and oligodendrocyte destruction leading to tissue damage.[33]

One of the challenges in understanding MS is the observation that plaques can be clinically silent. This was suggested by serial MRI studies in which new lesions occurred with a much higher frequency than did clinical exacerbations. Although the use of MRI to measure the outcome of new immunologic treatments is a potentially exciting development, there is no direct relationship between the number of lesions visualized on MRI and the severity of clinical symptoms.[19,51] The clinical course of the four types of MS (relapsing-remitting, secondary progressive, progressive relapsing, and primary progressive MS) are categorized in Fig. 20-1.

The different variants of multiple sclerosis include acute disseminated encephalomyelitis, clinically isolated syndromes, Devic's neuromyelitis optica (NMO), Marburg disease, tumefactive MS, and Balo's disorder (Box 20-1).

ACUTE DISSEMINATED ENCEPHALOMYELITIS

Acute disseminated encephalomyelitis (ADEM) is a monophasic syndrome, which usually follows an infectious process. Therefore it is also called postinfectious encephalitis. Often,

MS Immune Response

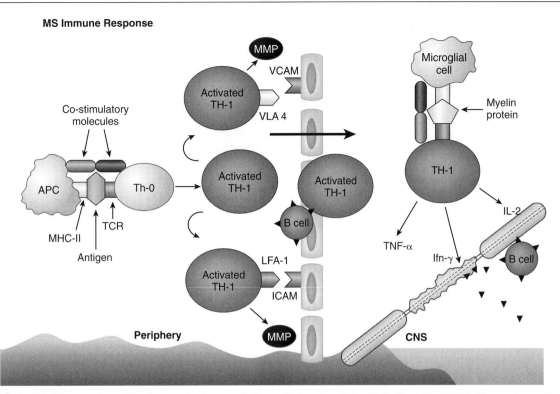

Figure 20-3 A simplified version of the immunologic cascade in multiple sclerosis by Katie Costello (TEVA Neuroscience, Inc.).

BOX 20-1	Variant Forms of Multiple Sclerosis

Monophasic syndromes
• Acute disseminated encephalomyelitis (ADEM)
• Clinically isolated syndromes (CISs)
  • Transverse myelitis
  • Optic neuritis
  • Isolated brainstem/cerebellar syndrome
Devic's NMO
Marburg variant MS
Tumefactive MS
Balo's concentric sclerosis

Adapted from Miller AE, Lublin FD, Coyle PK: *Multiple sclerosis in clinical practice,* London, 2003, Martin Dunitz.

a respiratory infection precedes ADEM. ADEM can also follow different vaccinations, and most of the fatal ADEM cases reported were after measles and smallpox vaccination.[31] ADEM may also follow immunizations of rubella, mumps, and varicella. Most cases are characterized by a self-limited single attack with multiple neurologic deficits and dramatic changes on MRI.

Imaging Studies

MRI of the brain demonstrates diffuse lesions throughout the white matter and multiple gadolinium-enhancing lesions.[8,31,33] It is sometimes difficult to distinguish between ADEM and MS. The lesions in the brain tend to be bilateral and symmetric in ADEM, which distinguishes it from MS. Periventricular lesions are not common, whereas in MS most patients have periventricular lesions. Basal ganglia lesions are common in ADEM.

Lumbar Puncture

Spinal fluid shows pleocytosis in ADEM. Oligoclonal bands and IgG production are uncommon in ADEM as opposed to MS.[33]

Treatment

The most common treatment is intravenous steroids. Plasma exchange is considered when the intravenous steroids have been ineffective. Follow-up for neurologic symptoms and changes on the MRI is critical in determining the diagnosis of MS over time.

CLINICALLY ISOLATED SYNDROMES

Clinically isolated syndromes (CISs) can manifest as a single postinfectious attack or may be the first attack of MS. Early treatment of CIS can minimize the development of definite MS remarkably. The most common CISs are optic neuritis and transverse myelitis.

OPTIC NEURITIS

Optic neuritis (ON) is a common cause of acute visual loss. It is typified by sudden onset of visual impairment or vision loss and pain with eye movements, followed by spontaneous complete recovery or partial recovery of vision over months. Often patients with ON experience visual fields defects, central scotoma, and decreased color vision. Pathologically, ON is an acute demyelinating event affecting the optic nerve. The disease may occur in isolation or may herald MS. ON may result as a consequence of MS, and the most common cause of vision loss in MS is ON.

Other conditions may cause ON, such as meningitis, encephalitis, nutritional deficiencies (tobacco-alcohol amblyopia), poisonings (e.g., lead, carbon monoxide, methanol, and quinine), antitubercular drugs, and ischemia of the nerve from temporal arteritis or atherosclerosis. In addition, differential diagnosis should be done to rule out sarcoidosis, lyme, lupus, or syphilis. Demyelinating ON usually evolves over days to 2 weeks and is associated with pain. Therefore a longer course of vision loss with absence of pain and failure to recover should raise the suspicion of other disorders.

In acute ON, the optic nerve is inflamed and edematous resulting in rapid compromise in vision associated with scotomas, visual field losses, and pain on movement and palpation. The funduscopic examination reveals the optic nerve to be pale and edematous with blurred margins.

Neurodiagnostic and Laboratory Studies

- Visual evoked potential (VEP): VEP is performed to diagnose ON.
- MRI: Brain MRI, orbital MRI, and cervical spine MRI should be done as baseline testing and to rule out MS or other diagnoses.
- Computed tomography (CT)/MRI: These studies may be ordered to rule out the presence of foreign bodies, hemorrhage, fractures, or orbital damage from trauma, or to assist in the diagnosis. Two or more lesions consistent with MS may be found on MRI of the brain. The brain and orbital MRI may show optic nerve inflammation and other demyelinating lesions, which are positive predictors for conversion to clinically definite multiple sclerosis (CDMS). According to the 10-year ON trial, even one demyelinating brain lesion can increase the risk for MS.
- Neuro-ophthalmologic testing: This is done to identify visual defects, including perimetry and tangent visual screening. The funduscopic examination may be normal during the acute phase.
- Lumbar puncture (LP): Spinal fluid may be tested to rule out infectious or inflammatory diseases.
- Chest CT or radiographic testing: This test may be done to rule out sarcoidosis if there is suspicion of systemic involvement.
- NMO antibodies: This is checked if there is major vision loss.

Treatment

Once the diagnosis of ON is confirmed, treatment usually includes corticosteroids, such as methylprednisolone 250 mg intravenously (IV) every 6 hours or methylprednisolone 1000 mg daily for 3 to 5 days followed by prednisone taper. The ON trial compared patients treated with intravenous methylprednisolone, oral prednisone, or placebo. Oral prednisone was associated with increased recurrence of ON. Most patients are expected to recover vision to near baseline or baseline.[2] Patients with CIS have a high risk of developing MS. Therefore, based on the examination and diagnostic tests of each patient, discussion about initiation of a disease-modifying drug should be done before establishing a definite diagnosis of MS. The CIS studies showed a remarkable reduction in conversion to definite MS with early treatment.[3,24]

ACUTE NONTRAUMATIC TRANSVERSE MYELITIS

The clinical characteristics of acute nontraumatic transverse myelitis (ANTM) and MS are fairly well known. Acute transverse myelitis is a focal inflammatory disorder of the spinal cord, resulting in motor, sensory, and autonomic dysfunction. It has been described as an immune-mediated process that causes neural injury to the spinal cord. Acute transverse myelitis is an acute attack of spinal cord inflammation involving both sides of the spinal cord.[31] Because of the acute onset, patients typically are seen in the emergency department (ED). The diagnosis can be made by an emergency physician, although transverse myelitis can be difficult to diagnose because of the variable signs and symptoms.

The pathophysiology is poorly understood. Patients may report a rapid onset of symptoms with paraparesis or tetraparesis. ANTM is usually accompanied by neck or back pain followed by sensory symptoms, motor symptoms, and sphincter issues. Most patients with transverse myelitis have sensory symptoms (e.g., bandlike sensation, paresthesias, and numbness) and bladder and bowel dysfunction.[48] Bladder dysfunction includes urinary urgency, incontinence, or urinary retention characterized by inability to void. Bowel dysfunction usually encompasses bowel constipation.[47] It is important to quickly rule out other causes of the spinal cord symptoms, such as anterior spinal cord syndrome, ischemia of the spinal cord from interruption of the anterior spinal cord artery, spinal tumors or hemorrhage (cauda equina syndrome), Brown-Séquard's syndrome, polyradiculoneuritis, infections of the CNS or spinal cord, and psychologic causes. ANTM may be the first manifestation of MS. Patients with asymmetric clinical findings and predominantly sensory deficits are more likely to develop MS.[48]

Neurodiagnostic and Laboratory Studies

- MRI: Brain and spine MRIs with or without gadolinium help confirm the diagnosis by detecting lesions in the brain and spine. The MRI helps distinguish between MS and ANTM, as lesions in MS involve the peripheral cord and the brain, and ANTM involves the central cord. Patients with small spinal MRI lesions (less than two spinal segments) and abnormal brain MRI are more likely to be diagnosed with MS.[48] Long-segment spine lesions may raise the suspicion of NMO or other disorders (e.g., vision loss, tumor).
- LP and CSF analysis: Presence of oligoclonal bands and elevation of IgG index or synthetic rate can

increase the risk of developing MS in the future.[48] CSF analysis can rule out other causes of spinal symptoms, such as infection or tumor.

- Evoked potentials (EPs): Abnormal EP test consistent with MS can increase the risk for MS in the future.
- NMO antibodies titer.

Treatment

Intravenous corticosteroid is the mainstay treatment of ANTM. Plasma exchange treatment should be considered if patients do not respond to the steroid course. Immunoglobulin infusion may be considered. When the risk for developing MS is high, patients should initiate treatment with one of the disease-modifying agents (DMAs). The possible diagnoses are idiopathic transverse myelitis versus disease-associated transverse myelitis, MS, ADEM, or NMO.[48] Identification of etiologies of transverse myelitis may suggest treatment; however, there is no established treatment for idiopathic transverse myelitis.[48]

NEUROMYELITIS OPTICA (DEVIC'S SYNDROME) OR OPTICOSPINAL MULTIPLE SCLEROSIS

NMO, or Devic's syndrome, usually involves the optic nerves and the spinal cord. NMO was initially described by Eugene Devic. It is characterized by optic neuritis and myelitis. There is a continued controversy about Devic's syndrome being a variant of MS or a completely different disease. The NMO-IgG autoantibody test, which is done at Mayo Clinic, is a biologic marker for Devic's syndrome but not for MS.[31] Distinguishing between the two affects their treatments. It seems, based on experience, that NMO patients do not respond to DMAs, but do respond to pulse steroid courses, azathioprine, and plasmapheresis (plasma exchange). Devic's syndrome is usually associated with a worse outcome mainly related to respiratory failure.[54]

Neurodiagnostic and Imaging Studies

- MRI: Brain and spine (cervical and thoracic) MRIs are done to rule out MS versus Devic's syndrome. Devic's syndrome patients usually do not have any lesions in the brain but have extensive abnormality in the spine and inflammation around the optic nerves. NMO patients might have a few lesions in the brain.
- LP: The spinal fluid is tested for presence of oligoclonal bands and IgG production for MS. It is rare to have oligoclonal bands and increased IgG production in Devic's syndrome. Spinal fluid characterized by pleocytosis greater than 50 white blood cells per cubic millimeter or greater than 5 neutrophils per cubic millimeter and increased protein are more likely to be present in NMO.[33]
- VEP: The VEP test is helpful to distinguish between transverse myelitis and Devic's syndrome when patients are treated initially for myelitis.

Treatment

The reported effective treatments are intravenous steroids and oral azathioprine. Intravenous immunoglobulin and plasma exchange have been used and have showed some effect. Other chemotherapy drugs, such as methotrexate and cyclophosphamide, did not show any positive effect.[33] New data support treatment with rituximad (Rituxan), a monoclonal antibody. Patients with NMO do not respond to the DMAs, such as interferon.

OTHER SYNDROMES

Acute Marburg Disease

Acute Marburg disease is a fulminant disease associated with rapid progression and death.[31] This disorder, identified by Otto Marburg in 1906, is characterized by a severe course with brainstem lesions or mass effect with herniation.[31,33] It may be difficult to distinguish between ADEM and Marburg disease.[33] There can be PNS involvement.[31]

Imaging Studies
MRI imaging demonstrates multiple and confluent lesions throughout the white matter.[32,33] Usually there are lesions in the brainstem. The MRI usually shows a diffuse demyelination throughout the white matter.[31]

Treatment
Intravenous corticsteroids may ameliorate the disease. Death occurs when the brainstem is involved.

Tumefactive Multiple Sclerosis

Tumefactive MS represents a unilateral mass lesion leading to an acute attack characterized by a remarkable edema, mass effect, and enhancing lesion seen on brain MRI. Patients usually have changes in consciousness, aphasia, or seizures.[33]

Diagnosis and Treatment
Though similar to that for MS, it is important to rule out other disorders (e.g., tumor), which requires CT studies and repeat MRI.

Balo's Concentric Sclerosis

Balo's concentric sclerosis is a rare variant of MS. The disorder is progressive and severe. It may end in death related to increased cranial pressure and cerebral herniation.[31,33] This disorder is typified by an acute onset followed by rapid progression to major disability and death within a few months.[31]

Neurodiagnostic Studies
The brain MRI shows diffuse large demyelinating lesions.[31] Cerebrospinal fluid is positive for oligoclonal bands and IgG.

Treatment
Treatment is with steroids, immunosuppressives, and plasma exchange.

Diagnosis of Multiple Sclerosis

The diagnosis of MS is based on dissemination in time and place in the CNS. The evidence of neurologic dysfunction

Expanded Disability Status Scale

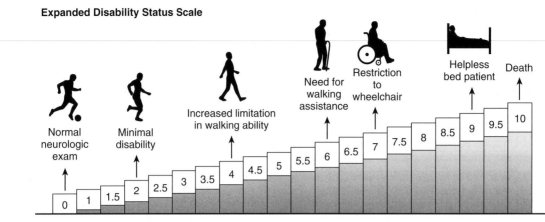

Figure 20-4 The Expanded Disability Status Scale (EDSS).

involves more than two sites in the nervous system (predominantly in the white matter) and is separated by at least 1 month or appears at different times along the disease course. Because no single test confirms the diagnosis, the diagnosis is based on patient history, supplemental documents from referring providers, and a physical examination in which there is no better explanation of symptoms. The assessment includes the following:

- Thorough history: past subjective episodes; health records of visual loss, hand numbness, and other neurologic signs and symptoms
- Complete neurologic assessment and examination: mental status; cranial nerve, motor, sensory, cerebellar, and reflex examinations; common associated clinical manifestations
- Clinical pattern of exacerbations and remissions: a wide variety of manifestations present during an exacerbation and a normal examination during remission versus a chronic progressive pattern from the outset

Several standardized assessment tools are used to follow the course of illness longitudinally, including the Expanded Disability Status Scale (EDSS)[27] (Fig. 20-4) and the Multiple Sclerosis Functional Composite (MSFC) tool. To further explicate a potential problem, other tests are used along the course of the disease (e.g., neuropsychologic testing, urodynamic studies, and neuro-ophthalmologic evaluation).

The initial signs and symptoms of MS (Table 20-1) vary widely and may include a history of various previous events and disorders with motor, sensory, visual, or coordination deficits, such as the following:

- Acute optic neuritis: transient unilateral ON (visual loss); Marcus Gunn pupil (a light shone directly into the eye will cause the pupil to dilate rather than constrict), also known as afferent pupillary defect (APD) (see Chapter 2)
- Internuclear ophthalmoplegia (INO) (impaired eye movement)
- Lhermitte's sign (an electrical sensation occurring throughout the extremities or the back while flexing the neck forward)

TABLE 20-1	Clinical Manifestations of Multiple Sclerosis
Area of Dysfunction	**Symptoms**
Cranial nerve dysfunction	Blurred vision, faded colors, blind spots (optic neuritis)
	Diplopia
	Dysphagia
	Facial weakness, numbness, pain
Motor dysfunction	Weakness
	Paralysis
	Spasticity
	Abnormal gait
Sensory dysfunction	Paresthesias
	Lhermitte's sign (electric shock–like sensation radiating down spine into the extremities)
	Decreased proprioception
	Decreased temperature perception
Cerebellar dysfunction	Dysarthria
	Tremor
	Incoordination
	Ataxia
	Vertigo
Bowel and bladder dysfunction	Fecal urgency, constipation, incontinence
	Urinary frequency, urgency, hesitancy, nocturia, retention, incontinence
Cognitive and emotional dysfunction	Decreased short-term memory
	Difficulty learning new information
	Word-finding trouble
	Short attention span
	Decreased concentration
	Mood alterations (depression, euphoria)
Sexual dysfunction	Women: decreased libido, decreased orgasmic ability, decreased genital sensation
	Men: erectile, orgasmic, and ejaculatory dysfunction
Fatigue	Overwhelming weakness not overcome with increased physical effort

From Beare PG, Myers J: *Principles and practice of adult health nursing*, ed 2, St Louis, 1994, Mosby.

- Acute transverse myelitis (acute inflammation in the spinal cord)
- Fatigue
- Motor dysfunctions: changes in gait
- Coordination issues: dysmetria, clumsiness of hands
- Sensory dysfunction: numbness, "pins and needles," tingling, itch
- Temperature intolerance: especially heat (increased body temperature leads to temporary worsening of MS symptoms)

- Pain: trigeminal neuralgia (paroxysmal facial pain)

The diagnosis of MS is based mainly on the history and the physical examination of the individual. The Poser and McDonald/Polman criteria base the diagnosis of MS on dissemination in time and place. However, the McDonald/Polman criteria heavily base the diagnosis on the neurodiagnostic studies, especially the MRI findings (see Neurodiagnostic/Laboratory Studies paragraph, Boxes 20-2 and 20-3, and Table 20-2).

BOX 20-2	**2005 Revised McDonald Multiple Sclerosis Diagnostic Criteria**

Clinical (Attacks)	Objective Lesions	Additional Requirements to Make Diagnosis
2 or more	2 or more	None
		Clinical evidence alone will suffice; additional evidence desirable but must be consistent with MS
2 or more	1	Dissemination in space by MRI or 2 or more MRI lesions consistent with MS plus positive CSF *OR* await further clinical attack implicating other site
1	2 or more	Dissemination in time by MRI or second clinical attack
1	1	Dissemination in space by MRI or 2 or more MRI lesions consistent with MS plus positive CSF *AND* dissemination in time by MRI or second clinical attack
0 (progression from onset)	1 or more	Disease progression for 1 year (retrospective or prospective) *AND* 2 out of 3 of the following: • Positive brain MRI (9 T2 lesions or 4 or more T2 lesions with positive VEP) • Positive spinal cord MRI (2 or more focal T2 lesions) • Positive CSF

From Polman CH et al: Diagnostic criteria for multiple sclerosis: 2005 revisions to the "McDonald" criteria, *Ann Neurol* 58:840–846, 2005.

TABLE 20-2	**The 2005 Revisions to the McDonald Diagnostic Criteria for Multiple Sclerosis**

Clinical Presentation	Additional Data Needed for MS
Diagnosis	
2 or more attacks; objective clinical evidence of 2 or more lesions	None
2 or more attacks; objective clinical evidence of 1 lesion	Dissemination in space, demonstrated by MRI OR 2 or more MRI-detected lesions consistent with MS plus positive CSF OR Await further clinical attack implicating a different site
1 attack; objective clinical evidence of 2 or more lesions	Dissemination in time, demonstrated by MRI OR Second clinical attack
1 attack; objective clinical evidence of 1 lesion (monosymptomatic presentation clinically isolated syndrome)	Dissemination in space, demonstrated by MRI OR 2 or more MRI-detected lesions consistent with MS plus positive CSF AND Dissemination in time, demonstrated by MRI OR Second clinical attack
Insidious neurologic progression suggestive of MS	1 year of disease progression (retrospectively or prospectively determined) AND 2 out of 3 of the following: • Positive brain MRI (9 T2 lesions or 4 or more T2 lesions with positive visual evoked potentials • Positive spinal cord MRI (two or more focal T2 lesions) • Positive CSF

From Polman CH et al: Diagnostic criteria for multiple sclerosis: 2005 revisions to the "McDonald" criteria, *Ann Neurol* 58:840–846, 2005.

BOX 20-3	Paraclinical Evidence in MS Diagnosis

What Is a Positive MRI?*†

1 Gd-enhancing brain or cord lesion OR 9 T2
    hyperintense brain and/or cord lesions if there is no
    Gd-enhancing lesion
1 or more brain infratentorial or cord lesions
1 or more juxtacortical lesions
3 or more periventricular lesions
    Note: Individual cord lesions can contribute along with
    individual brain lesions to reach the required number of T2
    lesions.

What Provides MRI Evidence of Dissemination in Time?

A Gd-enhancing lesion detected in scan at least 3
    months after onset of initial clinical event at a site
    different from initial event
OR
A new T2 lesion detected in a scan done at any time
    compared to a reference scan done at least 30 days
    after initial clinical event

What Is Positive CSF?

Oligoclonal IgG bands in CSF (and not serum) OR
    elevated IgG index

What Is Positive VEP?

Delayed but well-preserved wave form

Courtesy of the National MS Society, USA. Reprinted by permission of
The National MS Society; McDonald WI et al: Recommended diagnostic
criteria for multiple sclerosis: guidelines from the International Panel on
the Diagnosis of Multiple Sclerosis, *Ann Neurol* 50:121–127, 2001. (See
Table 20-2.)
These diagnostic criteria were developed through the consensus of the
International Panel on the Diagnosis of Multiple Sclerosis. See cited
articles for details.
*Barkhof et al: Comparison of MR imaging criteria at first presentation
to predict conversion to clinically definite MS, *Brain* 120:2059–2069,
1997.
†Tintoré et al: Isolated demyelinating syndromes: comparison of different
imaging criteria to prediction-version to clinically definite MS, *Am J
Radiol* 21:702–706, 2000.

Differential Diagnosis

The differential diagnosis of MS is critical (Box 20-4). Multiple diagnoses can mimic the presentation of MS. Misdiagnosis of MS occurs in approximately 5% to 10% of the cases.[21] A thorough history and neurologic examination should be the basis for making a diagnosis of MS. MRI findings help confirm the diagnosis of MS. However, the diagnosis should not be based only on the MRI films. Clinical clues such as a normal examination, an atypical clinical presentation, or normal MRI studies should raise the possibility of other disorders.

Neurodiagnostic and Laboratory Studies

Magnetic Resonance Imaging: Cerebral and Spinal

In 2002, the International Panel on the Diagnosis of Multiple Sclerosis published revised diagnostic criteria that include the use of new technology. The recommendations preserve the traditional criteria of two attacks of disease separated in space and time, but add specific MRI, CSF, and evoked

BOX 20-4	Differential Diagnosis of Multiple Sclerosis

Genetic Disorders
- Hereditary spastic paraparesis
- Adrenoleukodystrophy (ALD)
- Cerebrovascular malformation syndrome
- Leber optic neuropathy
- Wilson disease

Infectious Diseases
- Viral diseases
  - Herpes virus infection
  - JC virus (progressive multifocal leukoencephalopathy)
  - Human T-cell lymphotropic virus type I (HTLV-1)
  - Human immunodeficiency virus (HIV)
- Bacterial diseases
  - Lyme disease
  - Syphilis
  - Chlamydia pneumonia

Inflammatory Diseases
- Neurosarcoidosis
- Myasthenia gravis
- Bechet disease
- Systemic lupus erythematosus
- Sjögren disease
- Systemic sclerosis

Vascular Disorders
- CADASIL
- Antiphospholipid syndrome
- Vascular headache
- Vasculitis
- Susac syndrome

Neoplastic Disorders
- Lymphoma
- Paraneoplastic syndrome
- Brain tumor
- Metastatic tumor

Structural Conditions
- Arachnoid cyst
- Arnold-Chiari malformation
- Syrinx
- Cervical spondylosis
- Spinal cord disk disease
- Vascular malformation

Psychiatric Disorders
- Anxiety disorder
- Depression

Adapted from Miller AE, Lublin FD, Coyle PK: *Multiple sclerosis in
clinical practice,* London, 2003, Martin Dunitz.
CADASIL, Cerebral autosomal dominant arteriopathy with subcortical
infarcts and leukoencephalopathy.

potential findings as means of identifying the second attack. Results from these modalities are used in conjunction with clinical criteria to diagnose MS, possible MS, or not MS. Dissemination in space based on MRI studies requires that three out of the four criteria be established: nine T2 hyperintense brain and spine lesions or one gadolinium-enhancing lesion, at least one juxtacortical lesion, at least one infratentorial lesion, and at least three periventricular lesions (see Boxes 20-2 and 20-3 for the McDonald criteria). The Poser and the McDonald/Polman criteria both require dissemination in time and space to make a diagnosis of MS.

The MRI data can support the increased suspicion for MS and possible initiation of treatment without dissemination in time characterized by two clinical attacks separated by at least 1 month. The fluid-attenuated inversion recovery (FLAIR) image has a predominant contrast and therefore can show burden of disease better than other views. However, infratentorial lesions are better seen on T2-weighted scan. Brain atrophy may also be evident in early stages of MS. The MRI films may demonstrate the chronic inflammatory process, including demyelination, black holes that correlate with axonal loss, and atrophy, even in the absence of clinical signs and symptoms, and may be partially used for follow-up management.

Evoked Potentials

Slow, absent, or abnormal visual evoked responses are seen in 85% of patients with definite MS and are the most useful. Brainstem auditory evoked responses detect pontine lesions in 67% of patients with MS. Somatosensory evoked responses detect sensory abnormalities in people with normal findings on clinical examination and are positive in 77% of cases.

Lumbar Puncture

CSF analysis is required if other tests are inconclusive. Elevated CSF IgG and the presence of oligoclonal bands (OCBs) distinct from serum are indicative of CNS inflammation. Although common in 90% of cases, OCBs can also be seen in patients with infections or other inflammatory diseases of the CNS, and other causes should be ruled out.[1,19] In summary, a positive spinal fluid increases the suspicion for a demyelinating disease such as MS, and a negative spinal fluid does not rule out MS.

Electroencephalogram

Electroencephalogram (EEG) may reflect plaques and indicate a risk of seizures.

Positron Emission Tomography Scan

When available, positron emission tomography (PET) shows metabolism and the presence of plaques.

Nonconventional Magnetic Resonance Imaging

Nonconventional MRI tests can assist in establishing the diagnosis of MS and the severity of the disease. Magnetic resonance spectroscopy (MRS) has capacity to demonstrate low parameters of N-acetyl aspartate, which is a metabolic marker, and magnetic transfer imaging, which is a structural marker showing the magnitude of axonal loss in MS lesions and in normal-appearing white matter.

Treatment

MS management begins with an early, accurate diagnosis and includes medical management, functional assessment, and rehabilitation. Individuals with MS are managed in settings that include the home and inpatient or outpatient settings. The goals of therapy are to control relapse, delay disability, reverse disability, alleviate or modify symptoms, and enhance quality of life.[4]

There is no available prevention or cure for MS and no medication or therapy that completely prevents MS relapses. Because the management of MS is complex, an interdisciplinary team that offers a multitude of services should provide comprehensive care. In general, patients may be offered treatment with the potential to alter the natural course of MS, reduce the frequency and severity of relapses, and slow the onset and progression of disability. Early diagnosis and aggressive treatment to reduce inflammation are recommended to slow the progression. Management includes simultaneous treatments to enhance recovery from acute exacerbations, disease-modifying interventions, and symptom management.[19,20,39]

Acute and Postacute Care

Acute respiratory failure can result from demyelinating lesions in the cervical spinal cord or medulla or from aspiration, atelectasis, and community-acquired pneumonia. Respiratory failure caused by restrictive lung disease is rare. Respiratory failure is more common in Devic's syndrome. Sepsis, usually from urinary tract infection or pneumonia, is another cause of acute admission. The acute care patient may require short-term ventilatory support until the primary process improves. In addition, fever can increase weakness by impairing the conduction of already compromised nerves. During an acute admission, patients may be at high risk for injury, particularly falls.

Surgical Management

For individuals with severe spasticity who become intolerant of medical therapy or suffer undesirable side effects of oral therapy, the option of a surgically implantable intrathecal baclofen (ITB) pump to receive the medication intrathecally can be an effective alternative (see Chapter 13). There are no systemic side effects of ITB, and precise dosing can be achieved. ITB therapy is usually reserved for individuals in whom all other interventions are unsuccessful. After admission for a test dose of intrathecal baclofen with positive results, as well as the individual being determined to be a candidate for surgical implantation of a pump, the surgical procedure is planned. This is followed by a period of rehabilitation. The pump is refilled on a scheduled basis as an outpatient procedure, and the battery is surgically replaced about every 5 to 8 years. Other surgical approaches to treat spasticity are adductor tenotomy and dorsal rhizotomy. Surgical diversion to treat severe urinary retention, incontinence, and infection, as well as plastic surgery to close decubiti, is used to treat severe complications in end-stage MS. There are no surgical interventions to alter the course of MS.

Management of Acute Exacerbations

The treatment of acute exacerbations of MS has focused on corticosteroids and adrenocorticotropic hormone (ACTH). The standard of care is treating patients with high-dose intravenous corticosteroids for 3 to 5 days; based on patients' recovery or tolerance, this may be followed by an oral steroid taper. A few studies show an advantage of using high-dose corticosteroids compared with placebo measured by EDSS score.[34] In addition, the ON trial demonstrated that high-dose intravenous steroids were more effective than comparable oral steroids measured by recurrent episodes of ON.[2,3] Plasmapheresis (plasma exchange) is considered as a treatment for acute relapses for individuals who completely fail to recover after intravenous steroid treatment.[52]

Medical Management

There is no medical cure for MS. Medical management by a interdisciplinary team offers the individual with MS a multitude of services and therapies that are complex and comprehensive. Disease-modifying drug therapy that modulates the body's immune activity in order to hinder the MS disease process is available.[5] Generally speaking, MS is almost always progressing. Recommendations usually include early and continued use of disease-modifying therapy to reduce the frequency of relapses and to limit disability progression. The pharmacologic treatment of MS symptoms is described next and summarized in Table 20-3.

Interferon β-1a (Avonex).

The antiviral agent Avonex is a glycosylated recombinant product with an amino acid sequence identical to that of natural interferon; it is injected at a dose of 30 μg intramuscularly weekly. The interferon β-1a (Avonex) pivotal trial showed a significant annual relapse rate reduction of 18% for all patients who were on the study the whole time and 32% for patients who completed 2 years. In addition there was a 37% reduction in disability progression.[30] Avonex is approved for clinically isolated syndrome based on the CHAMPS study, and for relapsing-remitting MS.[24] The CHAMPS study showed a reduction of 44% in developing a second attack in the Avonex-treated group.[25,30] The most common side effect was flu-like symptoms.

Interferon β-1a (Rebif).

The antiviral Rebif is a glycosylated recombinant product with an amino acid sequence identical to that of natural interferon; it is injected at a dose of 44 μg subcutaneously (SC) three times weekly. The interferon β-1a (Rebif) trial showed a 27% relapse rate reduction in the group treated with 22 μg three times a week and a 33% reduction in the 44 μg group.[40] The secondary-progressive Rebif trial (SPECTRIMS) did not show a significant difference between the treated group and placebo in progression of disability as measured by the EDSS.[30] The ETOMS trial treating clinically isolated syndromes with Rebif 22 μg once weekly or placebo showed that the Rebif group had a 24% reduction in developing a second attack and establishing a diagnosis of MS.[30] The most common side effects were flu-like symptoms and injection site reactions.

Interferon β-1b (Betaseron).

Betaseron is a nonglycosylated recombinant product with one change in the amino acid sequence from natural interferon beta; it is injected at a dose of 0.25 mg (8 MIU) SC every other day. Interferon β-1b (Betaseron), the first DMA approved in the United States, showed a significant reduction by almost one third in the annual relapse rate compared to placebo.[22,23] Two secondary progressive trials showed conflicting results about the efficacy of Betaseron. The European trial demonstrated that the Betaseron-treated group had a 22% reduction in progression of disability based on the EDSS, whereas the North American trial did not show a positive effect.[14] The BENEFIT

TABLE 20-3	Pharmacology Summary: Multiple Sclerosis
Symptom	**Medication**
Spasticity	Baclofen (Lioresal)
	Diazepam (Valium)
	Dantrolene (Dantrium)
	Tizanidine (Zanaflex)
Tremor	Isoniazid (INH)
	Propranolol (Inderal)
	Clonazepam (Klonopin)
Bladder dysfunction (failure to store)	Oxybutynin (Ditropan)
	Propantheline bromide (Pro-Banthine)
	Tolterodine (Detrol)
	Solifenacin (VESIcare)
	Trospium (Sanctura)
	Vitamin C
Failure to store and empty	Terazosin (Hytrin)
	Doxazosin (Cardura)
	Tamsulosin (Flomax)
Nocturnal urgency or incontinence	Desmopressin (DDAVP) nasal spray
	Desmopressin (DDAVP) tablets
Bowel dysfunction	Senekot
	Colace (stool softener)
	Enemas
	Lactulose and Miralax (osmotic laxatives)
Bowel incontinence	Psyllium (Metamucil) bulk-forming agent
Fatigue	Modafinil (Provigil)
	Amantadine hydrochloride (Symmetrel)
	Selective serotonin reuptake inhibitors
Depressive disorders	Selective serotonin reuptake inhibitors
	Tricyclic antidepressants
	Bupropion hydrochloride (Wellbutrin)
	Duloxetine hydrochloride (Cymbalta)
	Venlafaxine hydrochloride (Effexor)
	Buspirone hydrochloride (BuSpar)
Anxiety disorders	Selective serotonin reuptake inhibitors
	Benzodiazepines
Bipolar disorders	Carbamazepine (Tegretol)
	Valproic acid (Depakote)
	Lithium
Emotional lability	Amitriptyline (Elavil)
	Selective serotonin reuptake inhibitors
Cognitive dysfunction	
Short-term memory loss	Donepezil hydrochloride (Aricept)
Neuropathic pain	Carbamazepine (Tegretol)
	Gabapentin (Neurontin)
	Oxcarbazepine (Trileptal)
	Tricyclic antidepressants (e.g., amitriptyline [Elavil])
	Pregabalin (Lyrica)
Erectile dysfunction	Vardenafil (Levitra)
	Papaverine
	Sildenafil (Viagra)
	Tadalafil (Cialis)

trial treating clinically isolated syndromes with Betaseron 8 MIU every other day showed a reduction of 55% in developing a second attack and establishing a diagnosis of MS. The most common side effects of interferon β-1b include flu-like symptoms and injection site reactions.

Glatiramer Acetate (Copaxone). Copaxone is a synthetic copolymer with immunologic similarities to myelin basic protein injected at a dose of 20 mg SC daily. Glatiramer acetate (Copaxone) has shown a 29% reduction in annual relapse rate compared to placebo.[26] The European-Canadian trial demonstrated a 33% reduction in relapse rate.[9,30] Copaxone is unrelated to the interferons with no evidence of neutralizing antibodies and does not require monitoring of liver function or complete blood count. The primary progressive trial was terminated prematurely because it did not show a significant difference between the treated and the placebo group. However, this trial provided us with data about the characteristics of primary progressive MS, including radiologic features. In addition, the oral Copaxone trial did not show a significant difference between the treated groups and the placebo groups. The probable reasons may include dosing issues, the route of administration and absorption, and the characteristics of the patients enrolled in the groups. The common side effects include injection site reactions and immediate postinjection reaction, which is a brief systemic reaction characterized by shortness of breath, palpitations, dizziness, and gastrointestinal side effects.

Mitoxantrone (Novantrone). Mitoxantrone 12 mg/m^2 is given intravenously once every 3 months and was approved for three forms of MS: secondary progressive, progressive relapsing, and worsening relapsing-remitting MS. The mitoxantrone trial showed a reduction in relapse rate and a decrease in progression of disability. The patients treated with mitoxantrone who had progressed by 1 point on EDSS were 64% better than the placebo group. The mitoxantrone group also showed a 69% relapse rate reduction, but the results should be interpreted with caution because an unblinded physician diagnosed the presence of relapses. Mitoxantrone as induction therapy may have an impact on the inflammatory process and on the evolution of disability. The major toxicity of mitoxantrone is cardiac, which limits the lifetime dosage of the total medication. Other side effects include alopecia, amenorrhea, leukopenia, and secondary leukemia.[50]

Other Treatments

Cyclophosphamide (Cytoxan). Cytoxan is an agent that has cytotoxic and antiinflammatory effects. There are conflicting data about the efficacy of Cytoxan in MS. Major toxicities include hemorrhagic cystitis, sterility, and malignancy.[44]

Azathioprine (Imuran). Imuran is an agent that impairs DNA and RNA synthesis. In a meta-analysis, Imuran was shown to reduce relapse rate.[50,55]

Methotrexate. Methotrexate impairs DNA and RNA synthesis. It was studied in progressive MS and demonstrated a positive effect on upper extremity function but not on ambulation. In addition it showed a reduction in T2-weighted total lesion in the treated group compared to the placebo group.[18]

Cladribine (Leustatin). Cladribine is an immunosuppressant agent. Several studies showed that cladribine had a favorable effect on relapse rate and MRI outcomes in relapsing and progressive MS.[49] Major side effects include bone marrow suppression and gastrointestinal symptoms.[42,43]

Cyclosporine (Sandimmune). Cyclosporine is an agent that suppresses T helper cells. In a large multicenter trial, it had a modest effect on progression of disability with considerable toxicity, mainly renal failure and hypertension.[36]

Pulse Steroids. Routine intermittent steroid treatment (1 g for one day monthly or 1 g for 5 days every 6 months) for patients with relapses and increased disability is considered as a disease treatment. However, benefit has not been demonstrated based on monthly high-dose methylprednisolone over a 2-year period.[17,56]

Natalizumab (Tysabri). The anti-α4β1 integrin monoclonal antibody, natalizumab (Tysabri), is an agent that blocks adhesion molecules. The adhesion molecules promote the interaction between the T cells and the endothelial cells of the cerebral vasculature (BBB), and allow the migration of activated T cells into the CNS, causing inflammation, demyelination, and axonal damage. Therefore antibodies to the adhesion molecules lessen the inflammatory process in the CNS. The randomized double-blind, placebo-controlled trials (natalizumab as monotherapy and in combination with interferon) showed a tremendous reduction in relapse rate (approximately 60%) and a reduction in the number of new, enlarging, or enhancing lesions (approximately 90%) in patients with relapsing-remitting MS. Natalizumab (Tysabri) was suspended due to multiple cases of progressive multifocal leukoencephalopathy (PML) in the natalizumab group in combination with interferon β-1a (Avonex) and has been re-released based on ongoing research.

Intravenous Immunoglobulin. Intravenous immunoglobulin (IVIG) has antiinflammatory and immune-regulatory effects. Several studies have demonstrated conflicting results related to IVIG efficacy in multiple sclerosis. A few studies showed a significant effect on relapse rate reduction and a significant reduction in gadolinium-enhancing lesions.[15,50] However, other studies have not shown effect on disease activity. Additional studies are required to test the efficacy of IVIG in MS.

Bone Marrow/Stem Cell Transplantation. Small studies have been done on the use of bone marrow/stem cell transplantation in MS and they have shown some clinical and radiographic effects. However, no controlled studies have been performed yet. In addition, there was a high mortality rate associated with this procedure in MS.[6,50]

Symptom Management

Fatigue Management

Fatigue is the most common symptom in MS and usually affects quality of life. Overall, 75% to 90% of MS patients report having fatigue and 50% to 60% report it as the worst symptom of their disease.[4,49] Fatigue is a subjective lack of physical or mental energy that is perceived by the patient or caregiver to interfere with usual and desired activities. The pathophysiologic nature of fatigue is unclear, but is probably multifaceted. Patients with MS should be evaluated for other medical conditions such as thyroid disease, anemia, sleep disorder, and depression, and medications such as benzodiazepines and gabapentin. A balance of exercise and rest increases cardiovascular status, reduces stress, decreases body fat, strengthens muscles, and increases energy. The pharmacologic agents that are used commonly to manage fatigue with modest success include amantadine, modafinil, and antidepressants (selective serotonin reuptake inhibitors [SSRIs]). In summary, management strategies for fatigue include education, energy conservation techniques, and medications.[4]

Pain Management

Pain can be a part of the MS patient's symptoms. The pain can range from mild sensory disturbances to severe, unrelenting primary pain. Pain in MS can be acute, subacute, and chronic. Acute pain syndromes of MS occur as a result of ectopic excitation at sites of demyelination and include trigeminal neuralgia, Lhermitte's syndrome, ticlike extremity pain, dysesthetic pain, and painful tonic seizures. Subacute pain can include ocular pain as a result of optic neuritis, and pain associated with bladder spasms and pressure sores. Chronic pain includes dysesthetic extremity pain, back pain, and painful leg spasms. Approximately 40% of patients with MS experience chronic pain characterized by persistent pain.[49] Neuropathic pain or dysesthetic pain can be experienced as burning or electrical. It often does not respond well to traditional opioids and nonopioids. Neuropathic pain can be relieved with either tricyclic antidepressants (nortriptyline, amitriptyline) or anticonvulsants (gabapentin, Trileptal, or carbamazepine). Nonpharmacologic modalities include acupuncture, therapeutic touch, yoga, and other relaxation techniques (see Chapter 23).

Paroxysmal Symptoms

Paroxysmal symptoms are characterized by brief, repetitive attacks that are probably a result of abnormal electrical discharges from partially demyelinated nerve fibers.[38] The symptoms usually last a few seconds or a few minutes and may occur several or multiple times each day. Common paroxysmal symptoms in MS include trigeminal neuralgia, tonic spasms, dysarthria, and ataxia.[45,49] Trigeminal neuralgia is an uncommon but troublesome symptom related to MS. The incidence of trigeminal neuralgia in patients with MS is greater than in the general population (apporoximately 3%), and the paroxysmal episodes can occur more than 100 times per day. Medications such as carbamazepine (Tegretol), gabapentin (Neurontin), lamotrigine (Lamictal), pregabalin (Lyrica), or amitriptyline (Elavil) may be beneficial. However, trigeminal neuralgia can be refractory to conventional treatment, and surgical procedures such as glycerol injections, rhizotomy, and radiofrequency should be considered.

Spasticity Management

Approximately 70% of patients with MS experience spasticity with big muscles affected. The legs are affected more than the arms. Spasticity can have a major effect on individuals with MS and is characterized by increased tone and muscle spasms in the extremities. Spasticity results from pathology in the corticospinal tract and the associated descending motor pathways.[45] Spasticity can be a double-edged sword with some individuals using spasticity and the stiffness of the legs for weight bearing and to give them strength for transfers or ambulation.

Spasticity can result from sensory disturbances, such as restrictive clothing, a kinked urinary catheter, constipation, or an ingrown toenail. Bladder infection, urinary tract infection, or any other infection can cause spasticity to increase, which may serve to alert the individual to the infection. Initiating interferon therapy may increase spasticity, and the use of steroids may decrease spasticity. Spasticity can adversely affect quality of life and daily function.[4] When spasticity is severe enough to interfere with function and cause pain or interrupt sleep, it requires aggressive therapy.

Assessment of the individual can determine the onset of spasticity, the severity, and response to treatments. The modified Ashworth scale is a tool to measure spasticity (see Chapter 13). The caregiver can contribute to the assessment and describe "caregiver burden" related to spasticity. The individual's spasms can be evaluated by observation of the gait or rising from a seated position, and by performing a pain and neurologic assessment with specific evaluation of muscle tone. Interventions can begin with a regimen of gently stretching and a prescribed exercise regimen. If no relief is obtained, the next phase is oral medications.

A commonly used initial medication to relieve spasticity is baclofen (Lioresal) because it has a wide range of dosing and can be increased as tolerated. Lioresal can also decrease muscle tone, but as the dose is increased the side effects may also increase and become unacceptable. Tizanidine (Zanaflex) does not contribute to muscle weakness but can cause fatigue and may be appropriate for nighttime administration. Patients can try both agents and decide which provides the best outcome or try a combination of both drugs at smaller doses. Other oral medications include gabapentin (Neurontin), dantrolene (Dantrium), and benzodiazepines (e.g., clonazepam [Klonopin]). Focal spasticity may be treated without a systemic effect with intramuscular injections of botulinum toxin (Botox) and repeated injections every 3 months.[49] A combination of stretching exercises, a physical therapy program, and medication may provide relief of spasticity (see Table 20-3).

Severe spasticity may lead to complications, such as contractures, impaired ability to ambulate, interrupted sleep, and pain and discomfort. When other interventions fail and the individual has becomes intolerant of oral medications, intrathecal baclofen with surgical placement of a programmable pump can be considered in patients with severe spasticity (see Chapter 13).

Surgical Management of Spasticity and Other Conditions

The option of a surgically implantable intrathecal baclofen (ITB) pump to deliver intrathecal medication can be an effective alternative for selected individuals who are suitable candidates (see Chapter 13). There are no systemic side effects of ITB, and precise dosing can be achieved. ITB therapy is usually reserved for individuals in whom all other interventions are unsuccessful. Patients may experience improved functionality, relief of pain, and an improved quality of life. The pump can be programmed to deliver different doses of ITB throughout the day to match the patient's level of spasticity and the need for relief when performing activities of daily living (ADLs), exercises, and other tasks, as well as when sleeping.

Other surgical approaches to treat spasticity are adductor tenotomy and dorsal rhizotomy. Surgical diversion to treat severe urinary retention, incontinence, and infection, as well as plastic surgery to close decubiti, is used to treat severe complications in end-stage MS. There are no surgical interventions to alter the course of MS.

Bladder Management

Approximately 80% of patients with MS experience bladder dysfunction. Bladder dysfunction in MS is associated with demyelinating plaques in the spinal cord and in the pontine cerebellar micturition control areas, or along the connecting points between the brainstem/cerebellum and spinal cord. Bladder dysfunction can impair social and vocational activities, and can be complicated by urinary tract infection, renal and bladder stones, renal disease, and urosepsis.[45] Neurogenic bladder in MS may be characterized by hyperreflexia (urinary urgency or incontinence) or hyporeflexia (urinary retention). Patients with MS may also experience detrusor sphincter dyssynergia (DSD), which is characterized by incompatible detrusor and sphincter activity.[10] Bladder training and education are the mainstays of bladder management. These include education about the importance of fluid intake, trial void, pelvic floor exercises, and biofeedback. Other procedures include postvoid residual measurement, intermittent catheterization, medications, and surgical procedures. Bladder incontinence may be treated with anticholinergics and bladder training, including education. Bladder retention can be treated by intermittent catheterization, an indwelling Foley catheter, or surgical procedures such as insertion of a suprapubic tube.

Bowel Management

Bowel issues in MS may include constipation or incontinence (or both). Approximately 70% of patients with MS experience bowel dysfunction. The etiology of bowel dysfunction in MS is not well understood, but may be complicated by inadequate fluid intake, poor dietary habits, immobility, and medications such as anticholinergics.[45] A bowel routine, timed bowel evacuation, hydration (adequate fluid intake), high-fiber diet, activity, and medications address bowel management in MS. Constipation can be managed by change to a high-fiber diet, increased hydration, increased activity, and medications.[10,19,20] Bowel incontinence can be managed by a bowel routine with timed evacuation daily or every other day using medications.

Sexuality Dysfunction Management

Sexuality often goes unaddressed in patients with MS. Approximately 70% to 80% of patients with MS experience sexual dysfunction.[49] Involvement of the lower spinal cord may contribute to sexual dysfunction in MS. For young adults, which is the population most affected by MS, sexuality is an important developmental and personal issue. Intimacy, communication, friendship, and socialization are important and should be addressed along with genital sexuality. Other indirect reasons that can lead to sexual problems include physical problems (fatigue, weakness, numbness, spasticity, bowel and bladder issues), psychologic issues (depression, low self-esteem), and social issues (isolation, decreased friendship).[10] Sexual dysfunction is present in approximately 80% of patients with MS. Common symptoms in men include mainly erectile dysfunction and in women include decreased vaginal lubrication, sensation, and orgasm. Decreased libido is common in both genders. Several devices and medications (e.g., sildenafil, vardenafil, tadalafil) are available to increase erection in males, but reduced genital sensation is a typical female complaint and rarely responds to medications or treatments. Topical creams can be used for vaginal lubrication. Vibrators and vacuum devices may enhance orgasm and satisfaction. The Eros device is a vacuum device placed over the clitoris and may increase arousal and orgasm.[49]

Speech and Communication Issues

Approximately 40% of patients with MS experience impaired speech. Dysarthria, dysphonia, and rarely aphasia can be seen in MS. Often, patients with speech difficulties are referred to speech and language pathologists.[4] Therapy includes oral exercises, modifying the speech by controlling rate and number of words. Medications for spasticity or augmentation systems may be considered for speech problems in MS.

Swallowing Dysfunction

Approximately 30% of patients with MS have impaired swallowing. Reduced peristalsis and delayed swallowing reflex are the most common features in MS. Clinical evaluation and assessment of swallowing are used for the analysis of swallowing difficulty and planning an effective rehabilitation program. Dysphagia therapy may prevent complications, such as aspiration pneumonia, dehydration, and malnutrition. Oral motor exercises, including active and passive exercises for the tongue and the lips, are designed to increase strength and range of motion.[4] Modification of diet and liquids is based on the individual assessment.

Emphasis on symptom management, patient education, and clinical support may not alter the disease course but can be beneficial in treating neurologic deficits, emotional problems, and psychosocial problems. Symptom management, education, and support enhance quality of life.

Psychosocial Considerations

Psychosocial is formally defined as the psychologic and social aspects of a person's being and functioning, which encompasses the emotional, social, and intellectual realms. It includes issues of self-esteem, insights into adaptations to illness and its consequences, communication, and relationships. Challenges in the psychosocial arena may affect the ability of the individual to cope with and adapt to the multitude of changes imposed by the variable architecture of MS. These challenges may include depression, anxiety, emotional lability, and changes in interpersonal relationships. Given the average age of onset of 30, the lived experience of MS covers more than three quarters of life's developmental process. Consequences of impaired psychosocial functioning can have serious deleterious effects on social, fiscal, vocational, and spiritual facets of the individual and subsequently society.

Variables in the provision of psychosocial care are the ability and willingness to participate in an educational process, premorbid psychologic functioning and coping, support system, financial and health-related resources, spiritual basis, concurrent stressors, cultural orientation, and the experience of grief as a result of the diagnosis. It is essential that treating clinicians provide validation of the patient's perception of the medical events, options, and tools for preserving an emotional balance and skills to address the unpredictable nature of the disease. Education and support in the area of disease management (disease-modifying treatments), symptom management for intrusive and residual chronic symptoms, and acute treatment for exacerbations are essential to communicate at the time of diagnosis and address accordingly throughout the disease.

MS as a neuropsychiatric disease offers an array of different challenges to the interdisciplinary team. Psychiatric complications are a direct manifestation of demyelination and inflammation along with the necessity to constantly adapt to the unpredictability of disease. Features of anxiety, depression, euphoria, irritability, cognitive impairment, delirium, apathy, emotional lability, and psychosis are becoming more prominent in the list of concerns in the management of MS.[35] In MS, the lifetime prevalences of depression and bipolar illness are 50% and 15%, respectively. The literature supports a multifaceted rationale, including reaction to diagnosis, chronicity of disease, neuropathology of MS, and specifically for treatment of depressive symptoms with beta-interferons.[16] It is important to differentiate between depressive symptoms and major depression, mood swings and bipolar disorders, and emotional lability and moodiness when considering treatment options. Referral to a psychiatric mental health professional for evaluation and treatment is more prevalent in many MS centers given the complicated nature of neuropsychiatric symptoms and the potential risk to self and psychosocial functioning with untreated affective disorders. Treatment of affective disorders in MS encompasses traditional psychopharmacologic interventions, psychotherapy, and group therapy.

Cognitive impairment exists in 45% to 65% of patients with MS, ranging from mild to moderate severity. Approximately 5% to 10% of individuals have severe impairment, such that they are unable to function without supervision and assistance. Similar to depression and other affective changes in MS, disease severity is not indicative of the severity of cognitive impairment.[28] Specific cognitive symptoms include decreased memory recall, poor attention, slow information processing, altered executive functioning, difficulty with calculations, and decreased visuospatial perception. Mini mental status examinations are not sensitive to the neuropsychologic changes experienced in MS. Patients themselves, caregivers, and professional staff often identify mild inconsistencies and alterations in cognitive function, which warrant acknowledgment and subsequent referral for neuropsychologic testing. The potential for social and vocational dysfunction secondary to cognitive change can negatively affect quality of life and have potential implications for mood disorders if left untreated.[41] Treatment normally involves a multimodal approach including neuropsychologic and occupational therapeutic interventions of cognitive therapy, cognitive-behavior training, compensatory techniques, and group and family therapy.

Other Considerations

Complementary and Alternative Medicine

One third of patients with MS may be using complementary and alternative medicine (CAM), such as St. John's wort for depression. Valerian may be used for insomnia but may cause sedation and increase MS fatigue. Ginkgo biloba is popular but has not been shown to be effective for MS attacks. Because of potential drug-CAM interactions, patients are encouraged to discuss the use of any CAM before experimenting.

Nutritional Considerations

Common nutritional alterations in MS are weight loss with malnutrition, obesity, and bowel dysfunction. Weight loss can be attributed mostly to changes in swallowing function. Dysphagia occurs due to demyelination in the brainstem sensorimotor pathways and can often take a relapsing-remitting course along with exacerbations. Patient report of swallowing changes is usually in more advanced disease states (50%) rather than early in the disease course (19%).[10] Contributing factors in the assessment and management of dysphagia are cognition and fatigue. Severe dysphagia that requires a feeding tube is less common with MS yet should be introduced according to risk of aspiration, body mass index, and after thorough patient and family education on the implications for the intervention. Immobility and the influence of corticosteroids on nutritional status are primary culprits leading to excessive weight gain, which is viewed as a far greater problem than malnutrition. Introduction of caloric guidelines and referral to a physical therapist are essential for weight maintenance. Constipation is common due to swallowing or chewing dysfunction, altered mobility, and neurologic changes.

Family Planning

Family planning is a vital concern for many people with MS. MS does not affect fertility, and studies indicate that pregnancy does not worsen MS. In fact, it is believed that pregnancy may have a protective effect, particularly during the last trimester. It is possible that pregnancy has a protective effect because of the immune changes occurring during pregnancy and the presence of high levels of hormones, blocking antibodies, and alpha fetoprotein, which is a pregnancy immunoregulator. Clinical trials have shown that the frequency of relapses decreases during pregnancy, especially in the third trimester. However, the relapse rate increases in the first 3 months postpartum, as compared with the relapse rate during the year before the pregnancy. Exacerbations or disease instability that occurs during pregnancy can be treated with corticosteroids with the mutual consent of the neurologist, patient, and obstetrician.

The effects of DMAs (e.g., Avonex, Copaxone, Rebif, Betaseron) on the fetus are unknown. Therefore the recommendations are to discontinue the DMAs 2 to 3 months before conception, resume the injectable treatments immediately after giving birth, and forgo breastfeeding. Some MS specialists allow women to continue glatiramer acetate (Copaxone) during pregnancy after thorough discussion with women and their partners because Copaxone is considered pregnancy category B, as opposed to interferons, which are considered pregnancy category C.

Special considerations in family planning and counseling include physical and cognitive capabilities before planned conception, available resources and existing support system regarding caring for a child, and the impact of fatigue.

Older Adult Considerations

Aging with MS is an expected experience because most patients have only a slightly reduced life span; one study estimated that the average patient lived only 6 to 7 years less than patients without MS. However, patients with a severe progressive disability often have a life span up to four times less than that of control populations. Healthier lifestyles and an emphasis on wellness related to bone density, diet, and cardiovascular health may further reduce complications and increase longevity in patients with MS. Financial planning should include health care resources (long-term care insurance and disability policy) associated with provision of care for ADLs and choice in living environment, should the need arise, and documentation of who will serve as custodian to the estate and assist with decision making in the presence of cognitive impairment.

Individuals with more significant physical or cognitive impairment may need placement in an assisted-living or skilled nursing facility if older caregivers precede them in death or if they cannot manage at home. MS patients are often the youngest patients in nursing homes. The care needs of patients with MS may be complex. Over time, the pathophysiologic changes and age-associated illnesses may complicate the management of MS patients in older adult facilities. Further chronic illnesses (e.g., osteoporosis, stroke, diabetes) imposed by age can compound the management of these patients.

Rehabilitation

Across the disease course, patients with MS will require either in-home or outpatient assistance to establish and then continue an exercise and rehabilitation program. Programs provided by in-home or certified rehabilitation facilities or the Commission on Accreditation of Rehabilitation Facilities (CARF) may help the patient with chronic progressive MS, particularly if there is an appearance of new functional deficits and cognitive alterations that are not amenable to medication treatment and individualized interventions.

Acute Rehabilitation

Neurologic rehabilitation incorporates traditional rehabilitation principles with cognitive-behavioral interventions for specified disease populations such as MS. The interdisciplinary team includes neurology, physiatry, neuropsychology, psychology, occupational therapy, physical therapy, speech therapy, vocational therapy, and a social worker. Clinicians initiate an integrated and aggressive rehabilitation program during an inpatient stay. Most acute neurologic rehabilitation admissions last at least 7 to 14 days, depending on the severity of the admitting status and insurance coverage. The goal of acute inpatient rehabilitation is to provide a program to improve the functional and cognitive aspects of affected patients. Patients who live long distances from therapeutic services or those who are unable to integrate the concepts from each discipline might benefit from a neurologic rehabilitation admission.

Initial rehabilitation teaching focuses on narrowing the knowledge gap experienced by patients newly diagnosed with MS. Patients may experience symptoms for months or years before they are correctly diagnosed and begin treatment. Some express emotions of anger, grief, or sadness after confirmation of the diagnosis, whereas others express relief that they finally know the cause of their symptoms and can receive treatment. Nearly all patients express a need to know what symptoms to expect and how MS will affect them, as well as a need for their families to understand how their MS-related difficulties will affect them. Patients also need current information regarding MS management, research toward a cure, and new treatments or drug information. They need to have someone to talk with about their disease. Social workers are a pivotal resource for providing counseling and education for psychosocial and mental health services, connecting MS patients with ancillary services and support groups in the community, registering patients at local MS chapters, and arranging for transportation services for follow-up visits with health care providers.

Continuity of rehabilitative care, regardless of the location, with physical and emotional support and physical and occupational therapies is needed to help the patient maintain maximum strength and function. These therapies include the following:

- Each member of the rehabilitation team completes a comprehensive evaluation and a plan individualized to the specific disability of the patient.
- Assistive devices (e.g., foot and ankle orthotics, braces, walkers, and canes) are essential to increase mobility and remain independent.
- Compliance with a daily exercise regimen prevents stiffness and decreases spasticity (see Chapter 13).
- Moderately ambulatory and nonambulatory patients are measured for manual or power wheelchairs.
- Measures of functional ability, such as the Multiple Sclerosis Functional Composite (MSFC) and the

Kurtzke (EDSS) Scale, are favored by most neurologic comprehensive care centers. These scales are MS specific, reliable, and valid and are used commonly throughout the country in clinical research to measure improvement and relapses.

- Environmental control devices and units should be introduced to maintain independence in the home and work environment for those with occupational therapy deficits. Such systems should be investigated and include special telephones, intercoms, security devices, and computer-driven lighting, lifts, and meal preparation devices.
- Fatigue, bladder, and bowel changes need to be addressed both pharmacologically and nonpharmacologically.
- Aquatic or hydrotherapy programs (in a pool heated to approximately 82° F to support "no sweat, no heat" exercise) are highly regarding in MS rehabilitation programming. Water has 12 times the resistance of air. Instead of exercising one muscle at a time, hydrotherapy works to strengthen multiple muscles.
- Yoga and tai chi are excellent forms of exercise.
- Home assessment should be performed by a physical or occupational therapist to assess barriers to independence and durable medical equipment (DME) needs, provide therapy, and provide instructions in ADLs. A home health aide can assist with ADLs and provide light housekeeping until the patient's caregiver can assume care of the patient.

A supportive network and a backup caregiver are mandatory for MS patients to enable them to live alone safely for extended periods. Supportive apartments, group residences, and adult day treatment are relatively new concepts for promoting independence and reducing the rate of nursing home placement of patients with severe MS. The clinician should explore ways to provide support to caregivers, such as respite admission and adult day treatment. Extensive home care services may be costly, and families may have difficulty affording extended, privately paid long-term care. Alternative community resources should be investigated.

Long-Term Rehabilitation
Many individuals with MS may continue to be ambulatory after 20 to 30 years with only a slightly reduced life span. Weakness and fatigue can be managed with an outpatient, home, or long-term rehabilitation plan of care that may include a period of physical or occupational therapy for strengthening, stretching, range of motion, gait training, bracing, ambulation, transfers, and safety measures. The use of assistive devices (e.g., a cane, crutches, or walker) helps prevent falls and injury, increase independent ambulation, and save energy. If the individual uses a wheelchair, proper measurement, including a seating evaluation, may enable the patient to return to work or live independently (see Chapter 13). Home programs require compliance in order to maintain muscle strength and tone.

Case Management
The role of case management is to monitor the progression of the disease over time and offer appropriate services to meet the individual's needs as they change in frequency, duration, and severity. The case manager can investigate and coordinate services for the following:

- Assistive devices as the need changes over time
- Follow-up with health care providers and therapies
- Funding for supplies and medications required for the patient's lifetime
- Equipment for bowel and bladder disorders (urinary tract infection)
- Sleep and pain disorders
- Nutritional needs, especially for individuals with swallowing problems, weight loss or gain, and tube feedings
- Chronic fatigue that can trigger chronic sorrow, depression, and the need for interventions and assistance to help with coping
- Health teaching and education for dealing with symptom management, sexuality, and family needs of children and spouses
- Assistance during pregnancy or child-rearing support
- Community resources for patient and family with local support groups and membership in MS chapters
- Transportation
- Other unmet needs (e.g., obtaining an air conditioner, a scooter, or other equipment)
- A canine partner
- Assisted-living facilities at the end of the patient's life span, hospice/palliative care

CONCLUSION

Living with MS poses unique challenges and rewards. Advances in basic science and new developments promise to improve the lives of individuals with MS. From the time of diagnosis until end-stage MS, nurse clinicians can offer a spectrum of services and health teaching for a quality of life that is meaningful, productive, and satisfying for men and women, and also children and adolescents, who live each day with this progressive neurologic disorder.

RESOURCES

International Multiple Sclerosis Support Foundation: www.msnews.org

Multiple Sclerosis Association of America: 706 Haddonfield Road, Cherry Hill, NJ 08002

Multiple Sclerosis Foundation: 6350 North Andrews Avenue, Fort Lauderdale, FL 33309-2130; www.msfacts.org

National Institute of Neurological Disorders and Stroke: www.ninds.nih.gov

National MS Society: www.nmss.org

REFERENCES

1. Anderson M et al: Cerebrospinal fluid in the diagnosis of MS: a consensus report, *J Neurol Neurosurg Psychiatry* 57:897–902, 1994.

2. Balcer LJ, Galetta SL: Treatment of acute demyelinating optic neuritis, *Semin Ophthalmol* 17:4–10, 2002.

3. Beck RW et al: High- and low-risk profiles for the development of multiple sclerosis within 10 years after optic neuritis: experience of the optic neuritis treatment trial, *Arch Ophthalmol* 121:944–949, 2003.

4. Ben-Zacharia A, Lublin F: Palliative care in patients with multiple sclerosis, *Neurol Clin* 19:801–827, 2001.

5. Ben-Zacharia A, Lublin F: The near future of multiple sclerosis immunotherapies, *Multiple Sclerosis Quarterly Report* 22:9–16, 2003.

6. Burt RK et al: T cell depleted autologous hematopoietic stem cell transplantation for multiple sclerosis: report on the first three patients, *Bone Marrow Transplant* 21:537–541, 1998.

7. Chitnis T, Khoury S: Immunologic neuromuscular disorders, *J Allergy Clin Immunol* 111(2 suppl):S659–S668, 2003.

8. Cohen O et al: Recurrence of acute disseminated encephalomyelitis at the previously affected brain site, *Arch Neurol* 58:797–801, 2001.

9. Comi G et al: European/Canadian multicenter, double blind, randomized placebo controlled study of the effects of glatiramer acetate on MRI—measured disease activity and burden in patients with RRMS. European/Canadian Glatiramer Acetate Study Group, *Ann Neurol* 49:290–297, 2001.

10. Costello K, Halper J, Harris C: *Nursing practice in multiple sclerosis,* New York, 2003, Demos.

11. De Jong BA et al: Evidence for additional genetic risk indicators of relapse onset MS within the HLA region, *Neurology* 59:549–555, 2002.

12. Duquette P et al: Multiple sclerosis in childhood: clinical profile in 125 patients, *J Pediatr* 111:359–363, 1987.

13. Ebers GC et al: A genetic basis for familial aggregation in multiple sclerosis, *Nature* 377:150–151, 1995.

14. European Study Group on Interferon β-1b in Secondary Progressive MS: Placebo controlled multicentre randomized trial of interferon β-1b in treatment of secondary progressive MS, *Lancet* 352:1491–1497, 1998.

15. Fazekas F et al: Randomized placebo controlled trial of monthly intravenous immunoglobulin therapy in RRMS. Austrian Immunoglobulin in Multiple Sclerosis Study Group, *Lancet* 1997:349, 589–593, 1997.

16. Goldman Consensus Group: The Goldman consensus statement on depression in multiple sclerosis, *Multiple Sclerosis* 11:328–337, 2005.

17. Goodkin DE et al: A phase II study of IV methylprednisolone in secondary-progressive multiple sclerosis, *Neurology* 51:239–245, 1998.

18. Goodkin DE et al: Low dose oral methotrexate reduces the rate of progression in chronic progressive multiple sclerosis, *Ann Neurol* 37:31–40, 1995.

19. Halper J, Holland N: Part I: new strategies, new hope: meeting the challenge of multiple sclerosis: treating the person and the disease, *Am J Nurs* 98(10):26, 1998.

20. Halper J, Holland N: Part II: new strategies, new hope: meeting the challenge of multiple sclerosis, *Am J Nurs* 98(11):39, 1998.

21. Herndon RM, Brooks B: Misdiagnosis of multiple sclerosis, *Semin Neurol* 5:94–98, 1985.

22. IFNB Multiple Sclerosis Study Group, University of British Columbia MS/MRI Analysis Group: Interferon β-1b in the treatment of multiple sclerosis: final outcome of the randomized controlled trial, *Neurology* 45:1277–1285, 1995.

23. IFNB Multiple Sclerosis Study Group: Interferon β-1b is effective in relapsing-remitting MS. I. Clinical results of a multi-center, randomized double blind, placebo controlled trial, *Neurology* 43:655–661, 1993.

24. Jacobs LD et al: Intramuscular interferon β-1a therapy initiated during a first demyelinating event in multiple sclerosis. CHAMPS Study Group, *N Engl J Med* 343:898–904, 2000.

25. Jacobs LD et al: Intramuscular interferon β-1a for disease progression in relapsing MS. The Multiple Sclerosis Collaborative Research Group (MSCRG), *Ann Neurol* 39:285–294, 1996.

26. Johnson KP et al: Copolymer 1 reduces relapse rate and improves disability in RRMS: results of a phase III multicenter, double blind placebo controlled trial. The Copolymer 1 Multiple Sclerosis Study Group, *Neurology* 45:1268–1276, 1995.

27. Kurtzke JF, Wallin MT: Epidemiology. In Burks JS, Johnson KP, editors: *Multiple sclerosis: diagnosis, medical management, and rehabilitation,* New York, 2000, Demos.

28. LaRocca NG: Cognitive and emotional disorders. In Burks JS, Johnson KP, editors: *Multiple sclerosis: diagnosis, medical management, and rehabilitation,* New York, 2000, Demos.

29. Li YJ et al: Age at onset in two common neurodegenerative diseases is genetically controlled, *Am J Hum Genet* 70:985–993, 2002.

30. Lublin FD et al: Effect of relapses on development of residual deficit in multiple sclerosis, *Neurology* 61(11):1528–1532, 2003.

31. Lucchinetti CF et al: The pathology of multiple sclerosis, *Neurol Clin* 23:77–105, 2005.

32. Mendez MF, Pogacar S: Malignant monophasic multiple sclerosis or Marburg disease, *Neurology* 38:1153–1155, 1998.

33. Miller AE, Lublin F, Coyle PK: *Multiple sclerosis in clinical practice,* London, 2003, Martin Dunitz.

34. Miller DM et al: A meta-analysis of methylprednisolone in recovery from multiple sclerosis exacerbations, *Multiple Sclerosis* 6:267–273, 2000.

35. Mitchell AJ et al: Quality of life and its assessment in multiple sclerosis integrating physical and psychological components of wellbeing, *Lancet* 4:556–566, 2005.

36. Multiple Sclerosis Study Group: Efficacy and toxicity of cyclosporine in chronic progressive MS: a randomized double blind placebo controlled clinical trial, *Ann Neurol* 27:591–605, 1990.

37. Murray TJ: The history of multiple sclerosis. In Burks JS, Johnson KP, editors: *Multiple sclerosis: diagnosis, medical management, and rehabilitation,* New York, 2000, Demos.

38. Ostermann PO, Westerberg CE: Paroxysmal attacks in multiple sclerosis, *Brain* 98:189–202, 1975.

39. Polman CH, Uitdehaag BM: Drug treatment of multiple sclerosis, *BMJ* 321(7529):490, 2000.

40. PRISMS, Prevention of Relapses and Disability by Interferon β-1a Subcutaneously in MS, Study Group: Randomized double blind placebo controlled study of interferon β-1a in relapsing remitting MS, *Lancet* 353:1498–1504, 1998.

41. Rao SM et al: Cognitive dysfunction in multiple sclerosis. II. Impact on employment and social functioning, *Neurology* 41(5):692–696, 1991.

42. Rice GP et al: Cladribine and progressive MS: clinical and MRI outcomes of a multicenter controlled trial. Cladribine MRI Study Group, *Neurology* 54:1145–1155, 2000.

43. Romine JS et al: A double blind placebo controlled randomized trial of cladribine in RRMS, *Proc Assoc Am Physicians* 111:35–44, 1999.

44. Rudick RA et al: Management of multiple sclerosis, *N Engl J Med* 337(22):1604, 1997.

45. Rudick RA: Contemporary diagnosis and management of multiple sclerosis, *J Neuroophthalmol* 21(4):284–291, 2001.

46. Sadovnick AD, Ebers GC, Dyment D, Risch NJ, Canadian Collaborative Study Group: Evidence for the genetic basis of multiple sclerosis, *Lancet* 347:1728–1730, 1996.

47. Sakakibara R et al: Micturition disturbance in acute transverse myelitis, *Spinal Cord* 34:481–485, 1996.

48. Transverse Myelitis Consortium Working Group, Kerr D, et al: Proposed diagnostic criteria and nosology of acute transverse myelitis, *Neurology* 59:499–505, 2002.

49. Tullman M: Symptomatic therapy in multiple sclerosis, *Continuum: Multiple Sclerosis* 10(6), December 2004.

50. Tullman MJ et al: Immunotherapy of multiple sclerosis—current practice and future directions, *J Rehabil Res Dev* 39:273–285, 2002.

51. Van Walderveen MA et al: Correlating MRI and clinical disease activity in MS: relevance of hypointense lesion on short-TR/short-TE (T1 weighted) spin echo images, *Neurology* 45:1684–1690, 1995.

52. Weinshenker BG et al: A randomized trial of plasma exchange in acute central nervous system inflammatory demyelinating disease, *Ann Neurol* 46:878–886, 1999.

53. Whetten-Goldstein K et al: A comprehensive assessment of the cost of multiple sclerosis in the United States, *Multiple Sclerosis* 4(5):419–425, 1998.

54. Wingerchuck DM et al: The clinical course of neuromyelitis optica (Devic's syndrome), *Neurology* 53:1107–1114, 1999.

55. Yudkin PL et al: Overview of azathioprine treatment in multiple sclerosis, *Lancet* 338:1051–1055, 1991.

56. Zivadinov R et al: Effects of IV methylprednisolone on brain atrophy in relapsing remitting MS, *Neurology* 57:1239–1247, 2001.

JANET S. CELLAR,
JAFFAR KHAN, JAMES J. LAH,
MERAIDA POLAK

CHAPTER 21

Management of Dementia and Motor Neuron Disease

Individuals diagnosed with dementia or the motor neuron disease amyotrophic lateral sclerosis (ALS) are faced with devastating neurologic disorders for which there is no recovery, only symptom management. This chapter reviews the dementias with a focus on Alzheimer's type, the most common cause of the degenerative dementias. Many other conditions can result in dementia, including vascular dementia, dementia with Lewy bodies, and frontotemporal dementia. ALS is the most common adult-onset motor neuron disease. Management of neurologic diseases where there is no hope for a cure or recovery requires knowledge of the pathophysiology, diagnosis, and management of the disease process to help patients and their families cope with these diseases and provide support as the disease progresses through the terminal phases.

DEMENTIA

Dementia is a term used to describe a clinical syndrome marked by decline in cognitive abilities compared to an individual's previous baseline level of functioning. The decline must be of sufficient severity to affect an individual's social or occupational abilities, and the changes must occur in a clear state of consciousness. A diagnosis of dementia is used to describe the overall level of function; it does not specify a cause. In addition to Alzheimer's disease, many other conditions can result in dementia (Box 21-1). Dementias that are potentially reversible are rare (e.g., metabolic disorders related to hypothyroidism, vitamin B_{12} deficiencies with associated neurologic symptoms, infection caused by neurosyphilis, or psychiatric disturbances that result in severe depression). Identification of dementias with a reversible etiology and instituting appropriate treatments may totally reverse the condition, may prevent progression to more significant impairment, and may decrease the likelihood of permanent impairments. Consensus criteria have been developed to provide guidelines for the accurate diagnosis of diseases causing dementia and can provide valuable guidelines for diagnosis in clinical practice as well.

Advanced age and family history have long been recognized as the most significant risk factors for dementia. Studies have associated other risk factors, including lower levels of education, past history of head injury, and depression. Some cases of dementia, including some familial forms of Alzheimer's disease and frontotemporal dementia, are inherited as an autosomal dominant disease that is transmitted as simple mendelian traits. If the disease occurs in an individual, his or her children will each have a 50% chance of suffering from the same disease through transmission of the mutant gene. These relatively pure genetic variants are very rare, but they have revealed a great deal about the basic biology of the more common, sporadic forms.

Neurodegenerative diseases are increasingly being viewed as disorders of protein production and metabolism within the brain. The brain has a special system of proteins that help maintain the ability of neurons to communicate. Although each of the neurodegenerative diseases may have a distinct pattern of symptoms, it is recognized that they have different disorders of protein metabolism. More information is now known about the changes in protein metabolism. The exact cause of the abnormal processing and how to treat it remains unknown. The disordered production or metabolism of all of these proteins ultimately leads to cell injury, loss of neurons, and clinical symptoms of dementia.

In the early stages of dementia, problems are often subtle and easily missed. Some studies suggest that as many as 75% of individuals with moderate to severe dementia go undetected in primary care settings.[8] In 2001 the Quality Standards Subcommittee of the American Academy of Neurology published guidelines recommending the evaluation and monitoring of individuals using screening instruments to detect dementia in individuals at risk, including the elderly and those with complaints of memory impairment.[43]

Obtaining a detailed medical history for suspected dementia is important to define the initial problem, pattern of onset, duration, and course. Determining if there are other symptoms (e.g., change in sleep, change in urinary habits, gait disturbance, change in vision, weakness, difficulty with coordination, or significant fluctuations in functioning with slowly or rapidly progressive continued decline) can assist with the diagnosis. Coexisting medical conditions and medication history should be obtained because they may be causing or contributing to the problem. Although by definition all dementias result in impairment in an individual's cognitive and functional abilities, the onset of symptoms, as

BOX 21-1 Causes of Dementia

Potentially Reversible Causes of Dementia

Infection
Neurosyphillis
Meningitis
Encephalitis
Normal pressure hydrocephalus
Chronic subdural hematoma
Nutritional deficiencies
Vitamin B_{12} (cobalamin) deficiency
Vitamin B_1 (thiamine) deficiency
Pellagra
Chronic drug intoxication
Alcohol
Sedatives
Metabolic disorders
Thyroid abnormalities
Chronic hepatic encephalopathy
Cerebral vasculitis
Sarcoidosis
Some types of tumor
Frontal and temporal lobe
Pseudodementia of depression
Medication side effects
Anticholinergics
Antihypertensives
Antihistamines

Irreversible Causes of Dementia

Neurodegenerative disorders
Alzheimer's disease
Dementia with Lewy bodies
Frontotemporal dementia
Pick's disease
Huntington's disease
Parkinson's disease
Vascular disease
Binswanger's disease
Amyloid angiopathy
Vascular dementia
Multiinfarct
Strategic single infarct
Infection
Creutzfeldt-Jakob disease (CJD)
Postencephalitic dementia
Dementia associated with HIV

HIV, Human immunodeficiency virus.

well as their course, may vary. Deteriorations in functional abilities such as financial and medication management are often closely related to diminished cognition. Behavioral problems are common in dementia, complicate care, and often present the greatest challenges to caregivers. A comprehensive evaluation of cognitive and functional abilities, as well as evaluation of possible psychiatric or behavioral problems, is important to diagnosis, treatment, and quality of life. Dementia can affect a patient's recognition of his or her impairments (anosognosia); therefore information should also be obtained from a reliable informant such as a family member or close friend.

Cognitive assessment for dementias should include testing of performance in a number of cognitive domains, including memory, language, judgment, reasoning, problem solving, and visuospatial skills. Cognitive testing may reveal aphasia, apraxia, agnosia, or impaired executive function. Brief cognitive screening assessments have been developed to test an individual's cognitive abilities, such as the Folstein Mini Mental State Examination (MMSE).[18] The MMSE is the most widely used screening test of cognitive ability (Box 21-2). It is a 30-point measurement assessing orientation (10 points), immediate and delayed recall (6 points), attention and calculation (5 points), and language (9 points). A score of 25 or higher is considered to be within the normal range; scores of 20 to 24 indicate mild impairment, scores of 10 to 20 indicate moderate impairment, and scores below 10 indicate severe dementia. The MMSE and other brief screening

BOX 21-2 Examples of Questions From the Mini Mental State Examination

Orientation to time: "What is the date?"
Registration: "Listen carefully. I am going to say three words. You say them back after I stop. Ready? Here they are: APPLE [pause], PENNY [pause], TABLE [pause]. Now repeat those words back to me." (Repeat up to five times, but score only the first trial.)
   Naming: "What is this?" (Point to a pencil or a pen.)
   Reading: "Please read this and do what it says." (Show examinee the words on the stimulus form.) CLOSE YOUR EYES.

assessments used for routine evaluation are often not sensitive to very mild difficulty. It is not unusual for an individual with a high level of education to score within the normal range on the MMSE but be impaired on more detailed neuropsychologic assessment. Other assessments such as **clock drawing,** a simple bedside test in which an individual is asked to draw a clock with the numbers and hands drawn to indicate a specified time, can be sensitive to early cognitive decline. Obtaining a more detailed cognitive assessment of areas including verbal and visual memory may be warranted if problems are suspected despite a negative screening examination. An individual's **functional performance** or **instrumental activities of daily living (IADLs)** (see Chapter 13) should also be assessed. In mild dementia, activities of daily living (ADLs) may remain intact while higher-level functions (IADLs), such as financial management, driving, or cooking, may be subtly affected. Functional assessment tools such as the Functional Activities Questionnaire (FAQ) can be administered over the course of the disease to address safety issues and caregiver burden of disease.[24,30,44]

Behaviors that can have a negative impact on the individual and family, such as mild depression, anxiety, or agitation, may contribute to a decline in function with dementia. Depression should be assessed and, if indicated, treated, which in some cases may result in improved cognition. Depression screening tools, such as the Geriatric Depression Scale (GDS) or the Beck Depression Inventory (BDI),[3,62] can be helpful in identifying coexisting depression. Assessing for other possible behavioral changes using tools such as the Neuropsychiatric Inventory (NPI)[12] is important for diagnosis, as well as for planning care.

Early in a dementia, the **physical and neurologic examination** may be normal. As the dementia progresses, extrapyramidal symptoms such as **bradykinesia, muscle rigidity,** and **postural instability** may emerge. Assessment should include baseline weight, vital signs, and skin integrity. Hearing and vision are important because they may compound already existing cognitive impairment, resulting in excess disability. Vascular risk factors such as hypertension or diabetes mellitus should be addressed because there is growing evidence that they may contribute to disease progression.

Neurodiagnostic and Laboratory Studies

Practice recommendations for the diagnosis of dementia published by the Quality Standards Subcommittee of the American Academy of Neurology include both laboratory evaluations and imaging of the brain[27] (Box 21-3). None of the imaging tests are of sufficient sensitivity or specificity to diagnose the specific cause of the dementia, and in most cases, they are used to exclude other disorders. For dementias in general, the following diagnostic studies may be ordered:

Laboratory tests: to rule out infection, anemia, vitamin deficiencies, or metabolic causes of dementia.

Computed tomography (CT) or magnetic resonance imaging (MRI): to exclude possible reversible causes and establish patterns of atrophy or shrinkage of the brain (e.g., medial temporal atrophy or enlarged ventricles). Enlarged ventricles, out of proportion to the degree of atrophy, may suggest normal pressure hydrocephalus (NPH) (see Chapter 13). Atrophy in the temporal and parietal areas of the brain with pronounced hippocampal atrophy is typically seen in Alzheimer's disease.

BOX 21-3	**Practice Parameter: Diagnosis of Dementia**[27]

Laboratory Evaluation
- Recommended
  - CBC
  - Serum electrolytes (including calcium)
  - Glucose
  - BUN/creatinine
  - LFTs
  - Thyroid function tests (generally TSH)
  - Vitamin B_{12} levels
- Optional
  - Syphilis serology
  - Erythrocyte sedimentation rate
  - Serum folate
  - HIV (per CDC protocol)

Brain Imaging—Recommended
- Structural imaging:
  - Noncontrast CT scan
  - MRI (especially if vascular component possible)

Brain Imaging—Optional
- Functional imaging (Medicare has recently approved reimbursement for functional imaging when diagnosis uncertain)
- SPECT
- PET

Other Testing
- EEG
- Carotid ultrasound

BUN, Blood urea nitrogen; *CBC,* complete blood count; *CDC,* Centers for Disease Control and Prevention; *EEG,* electroencephalogram; *HIV,* human immunodeficiency virus; *LFTs,* liver function tests; *MRI,* magnetic resonance imaging; *PET,* positron emission tomography; *SPECT,* single-photon emission computed tomography; *TSH,* thyroid-stimulating hormone.

Positron emission tomography (PET) or single-photon emission computed tomography (SPECT) scans: to identify decreased glucose metabolism or hypoperfusion, for example, a pattern of hypoperfusion in the temporal and parietal regions of the brain, which is commonly seen in Alzheimer's disease, or experimental scans that demonstrate beta-amyloid deposits. The Center for Medicare and Medicaid Services has recently approved the use of functional neuroimaging (experimental scan) for diagnosis in cases where there is some diagnostic uncertainty even after a comprehensive evaluation.

Interventions

To date there have been no treatments developed that have been shown to halt or reverse the cognitive and functional decline of dementia. Pharmacologic and nonpharmacologic treatments have been identified that are helpful in treating cognitive symptoms while also having a beneficial effect on function and behavior.

Whereas pharmacologic agents may provide modest relief from symptoms, there can be an equally measurable benefit from nonpharmacologic interventions. The term *excess disability* has been used to describe functional impairments or behavioral problems that appear out of proportion to the degree of cognitive impairment.[6] Once recognized, these problems can be addressed, which can result in improved function and resolution of behavioral problems. The conceptual model of progressively lowered stress threshold has identified five common stressors that can contribute to behavioral problems and functional decline: fatigue, disruptions in normal routine, understimulation or overstimulation, demands that exceed functional abilities, and physical stressors such as pain.[21] Other models have focused on the association of problem behaviors such as repeated vocalizations with boredom, loneliness, or social isolation and have used music and increased social contact to modify the behavior. Behavioral/learning models have focused on the relationship between possible antecedents and reinforcement of behaviors and have been referred to as the antecedent-behavior-consequence (ABC) models of intervention. The growing availability of **adult day programs** designed specifically to meet the needs of individuals with dementia has been a valuable resource for patients and caregivers. These programs provide activities that are designed for individuals experiencing cognitive impairment while providing them with social support.

Pharmacologic treatments are available to help manage associated symptoms and behaviors that can be common in all dementias. Although nonpharmacologic approaches should be the first treatments considered for the management of behavioral disturbances, pharmacologic therapies may be necessary for brief periods of time if nonpharmacologic approaches do not provide adequate symptom relief. When necessary, these medications should be started at low doses and slowly titrated as needed to achieve the desired effect (Table 21-1).

Treatment of psychosis or agitation with newer "atypical" neuroleptics, such as quetiapine or risperidone, or mood stabilizers such as valproic acid may be necessary when behavioral problems are acute or affect the safety of the patient or caregivers. Studies on the use of many of the medications used in the treatment of behavioral problems secondary to dementia in a geriatric population are quite limited, and no medications have been tested and approved by the U.S. Food and Drug Administration (FDA) for this use. After reviewing the results of a number of research studies, in April 2005 the FDA issued a health advisory that atypical neuroleptics have increased associated mortality rates compared to treatment with a placebo. As a result, all atypical neuroleptics received a "black box" warning from the FDA. However, older neuroleptics such as haloperidol are associated with greater Parkinson's-like side effects, which can result in motor disability and gait changes that can increase the risk of falls. Likewise, the use of sedative-hypnotics in elderly dementia patients can worsen cognition and increase the risk of falls. Although the paucity of rigorously controlled clinical trials of "atypical" neuroleptics in the elderly should raise significant concerns about their use in dementia patients, it should be noted that many, if not most, experienced clinicians continue to favor their use when the need for behavioral management becomes acute.

Acute agitation is often seen as a result of a **delirium** secondary to an acute medical illness such as a urinary tract infection, the result of a stressor such as the death of a spouse, or a side effect from a medication used to treat a coexisting medical illness. Attempts should be made to identify and address potential precipitants to these behaviors, thereby allowing doses of medications to be reduced or discontinued.

Depression with dementia is common in the early stages. It can be difficult to differentiate between decreased motiva-

TABLE 21-1	Pharmacologic Management of Behavioral Problems		
Type and Drug	**Initial Daily Dose**	**Suggested Maximum Dose**	**Targeted Symptoms**
Atypical Antipsychotic			
Risperidone (Risperdal)	0.25–0.5 mg	2 mg/day	Agitation and psychosis
Quetiapine (Seroquel)	12.5–25 mg	200 mg/day	
Olanzapine (Zyprexa)	2.5–5 mg	10 mg/day	
Aripiprazole (Abilify)	5 mg	15 mg/day	
Mood Stabilizer			
Divalproex sodium (Depakote)	125 mg bid	750–2000 mg/day	Agitation
Carbamazepine (Tegretol)	50–100 mg	500–800 mg/day	
Antidepressant (SSRI)			
Citalopram (Celexa)	10–20 mg	40 mg/day	Depression, irritability, and compulsive behaviors
Paroxetine (Paxil)	5–10 mg	20 mg/day	
Fluoxetine (Prozac)	5–10 mg	20–40 mg/day	
Sertraline (Zoloft)	25–50 mg	100–150 mg/day	
Duloxetine (Cymbalta)	20 mg	30 mg/day	
Antidepressant (Atypical)			
Venlafaxine (Effexor)	25–50 mg	75 mg/day	Depression and irritability
Mirtazapine (Remeron)	7.5–15 mg	45 mg/day	
Bupropion (Wellbutrin)	75–100 mg	200 mg/day	

tion and loss of initiative common to dementia from decreased interest and energy seen in depression. Depression may manifest itself in the more typical pattern of sadness and loss of interest; however, increased somatic preoccupation, irritability, and generalized anxiety may also be seen. When these symptoms begin to affect a patient's quality of life, a trial of an antidepressant medication may be warranted. Although different antidepressants may be equally effective, there is evidence that the newer selective serotonin reuptake inhibitors (SSRIs) may be better tolerated. Older classes of antidepressants, especially tricyclics, have significant anticholinergic properties, which can worsen confusion and result in a mild delirium. Trazodone, a heterocyclic antidepressant that also inhibits serotonin reuptake, has been shown to be helpful in treating mild anxiety, as well as sleep difficulty.

ALZHEIMER'S DISEASE

Alzheimer's disease (AD), a nonreversible dementia, is the most common cause of the degenerative dementias, accounting for an estimated 50% to 70% of all dementias. The onset of symptoms in patients with AD is typically slow and insidious with gradual worsening over time. There are normal changes in cognition experienced with age. Generally, cognitive changes associated with healthy aging are very mild and do not result in significant limitations. The term **mild cognitive impairment (MCI)** is now being used to describe the earliest clinically identifiable stages of a dementing illness such as AD. MCI criteria have been refined to identify specific subtypes depending on the area of cognitive functioning most affected. The subtype that is most relevant to AD has been termed **amnestic mild cognitive impairment (AMCI),** recognizing that a decline in short-term memory is the most common complaint in individuals who may ultimately progress to a diagnosis of AD. This subtype includes a subjective memory complaint, objective memory impairment detected via clinical examination, normal general cognitive functioning in other areas, and intact IADLs. Prospective studies have determined that approximately 12% to 15% of individuals who meet criteria for AMCI will go on to develop AD each year as compared with 1% to 2% of normal controls.[42]

Risk of developing AD is intimately linked to aging. It has been estimated that the risk of AD doubles for every 5 years between ages 65 and 85. For those over 85, the risk of AD is close to 50%.[16] In light of the aging of millions of baby boomers and increasing life expectancy, unless effective treatments are developed that can prevent or halt disease progression, the incidence of dementia in the general population will continue to grow. Approximately 4.5 million individuals were diagnosed with AD in the U.S. population in 2000. It has been estimated that by 2050 this number will rise to between 11 and 16 million. As the number of individuals in each age-group shifts over time, it is anticipated that by 2050 the number of 75- to 84-year-olds with AD will double to 4.8 million and the number of people older than 85 with AD will reach 8 million. Only the group of people with AD between 65 and 74 years of age is expected to remain stable.[23]

Etiology

Although the exact cause of AD remains a mystery, the chemical and biologic changes associated with the disease are apparent. Epidemiologic studies have helped identify possible risks, as well as protective factors that provide clues aiding in the development of potential treatments. Advanced age represents the most significant risk factor in the development of AD. The incidence of AD is higher in women than men, in individuals with lower educational levels, and in those with a past history of significant head injury.[29] **Genetics** plays a role, with a family history of AD increasing an individual's risk of developing the disease. It has been estimated that the risk of developing AD is approximately 30% in individuals with a family history of AD in comparison to 10% in individuals who have no known family history. Individuals who develop AD before age 60 are considered to have an early-onset form of the disease. Specific genetic defects can cause early-onset familial AD, including mutations in the APP gene on chromosome 21, presenilin-1 gene on chromosome 14, and presenilin-2 gene on chromosome 1. Although the discovery of these genes provided valuable insight into the cause of AD, they account for less than 5% of all Alzheimer's cases.

A specific form or allele of the apolipoprotein E (apo E) gene has been identified as an important genetic risk for developing common late-onset forms of AD. The apo E gene located on chromosome 14 has three different alleles: $\varepsilon 2$, $\varepsilon 3$, and $\varepsilon 4$. Each individual inherits two copies of the apo E gene, a separate allele from each parent. The $\varepsilon 3$ allele is most prevalent; however, the $\varepsilon 4$ gene has been associated with an increased risk of AD. The lifetime risk of developing AD is approximately 20% for an individual without an $\varepsilon 4$ allele in comparison to 47% for an individual with at least one copy and 91% for an individual with two copies of the apo E $\varepsilon 4$ allele.[10] Although having one or two copies of the $\varepsilon 4$ allele increases an individual's risk of developing AD, it does not guarantee that an individual will develop AD; conversely, having no copies of the $\varepsilon 4$ allele is no guarantee of remaining disease free. This genetic test is commercially available, but the interpretation is complex. There is unanimity among professional groups, including the American Academy of Neurology, and advocacy groups, including the Alzheimer's Association, that apo E genotype testing should not be done on asymptomatic individuals. Even among dementia patients, the genetic testing should only be performed when adequate education and genetic counseling can be provided to the patient and family.

Pathophysiology

In 1907, Dr. Alois Alzheimer was the first to identify the amyloid plaques and neurofibrillary tangles that have become recognized as the hallmark neuropathologic changes in the brains of individuals affected by a disease later named for him. The amyloid precursor protein (APP) and tau are key proteins identified in the pathophysiology of AD. The **amyloid hypothesis** of AD suggests that the deposition of amyloid in the brain initiates a cascade of events including inflammation leading to neurotoxicity and cell death. The

amyloid precursor protein (APP) is a transmembranous protein found in high concentrations in synaptic terminals. APP plays a key role in the formation of *extracellular* plaque. Aβ is a normal product of APP metabolism throughout life and is formed by the enzymatic cleavage of APP by a combination of β and γ secretases, resulting in the release of the Aβ peptide. Secreted Aβ can form insoluble protein aggregates in **neuritic or senile plaques. Tau** is an axonal protein crucial for microtubule assembly and stability. In AD, tau aggregates due to hyperphosphorylation forming *intracellular* twisted paired helical filaments recognized as **neurofibrillary tangles.** Some researchers believe that this process is triggered by the aggregation of extracellular Aβ.[22]

The **cholinergic hypothesis** of AD recognizes that loss of neurons in the nucleus basalis of Meynert, where cholinergic neurons involved in memory and cognition originate, has been associated with the depletion of the neurotransmitter acetylcholine. Acetylcholine has been identified as one of the neurotransmitters crucial to memory formation, and the depletion of acetylcholine is correlated with disease severity. The identification of these changes in the neurotransmitter system led to the development of cholinesterase inhibitors, the first drugs approved by the FDA for the treatment of AD.

It is well established that the coexistence of cerebrovascular disease can act in concert with AD to accelerate the progression of dementia.[58] Recent studies suggest that there is a relationship between the presence of vascular risk factors such as hypertension or diabetes mellitus in patients with unremarkable neuroimaging findings and both the risk for AD and the pattern of cognitive impairments.[20,25,26]

Diagnosis

Though a definitive diagnosis of AD may only be made in many cases following examination of brain tissue, newer PET scans have demonstrated beta-amyloid deposits. Clinical criteria have been developed that can assist in diagnosis. Criteria described in the DSM-IV-TR[15] for dementia of the Alzheimer's type include the following: development of multiple cognitive deficits manifested by memory impairment and one or more cognitive disturbances (e.g., aphasia, apraxia, agnosia, or disturbances in executive functioning; these cognitive deficits result in significant impairment in social or occupational functioning and represent a significant decline from previous level of functioning); the course is one of gradual onset and progressive decline, and the cognitive deficits are not the result of another central nervous system (CNS) condition that could result in progressive cognitive decline; a systemic condition that is known to cause dementia; a substance abuse condition; and the deficits do not occur exclusively during the course of a delirium.

As noted in the DSM-IV-TR[15] criteria for AD, the earliest cognitive change is most typically memory loss, with impairments in other areas developing slowly over time. Early changes are often subtle and easily missed by both family and health care providers. A request for evaluation may be triggered by a crisis such as an individual getting lost while driving or an episode of acute confusion as a result of a medical illness.

As in the evaluation of any dementia, assessment should include laboratory evaluations and neurodiagnostic studies to rule out potentially reversible causes of decline or identify coexisting medical conditions (e.g., elevated cholesterol levels or diabetes mellitus) that may not be identified as the cause of a dementia but can potentially contribute to the rate of decline. Imaging of the brain with CT, MRI, or experimental scans is described earlier in this chapter. Detailed assessment of cognitive and functional abilities is important to establish a level of performance while also documenting baseline functioning. The MMSE is useful to track cognitive abilities over time. Detailed neuropsychologic testing can provide a more accurate assessment of an individual's strengths and areas of impairment. On average, AD patients decline 2 to 4 points on the MMSE each year. A diagnosis of AD requires a decline in cognitive abilities that significantly impairs an individual's social and occupational functioning, necessitating a detailed assessment of functional performance. The assessment of functional abilities and behavioral problems described previously is especially important to identify areas of concern that will need to be addressed as part of a person's care.

Course of the Disease

The course of AD is one of slowly progressive decline in both cognitive and functional abilities. Table 21-2 details the progression of cognitive, functional, and behavioral changes commonly seen in AD. The length of time from diagnosis to end-stage disease averages between 7 and 10 years with a range of 2 to 20 years. Progression of disease can be affected by many variables, including a person's age and physical health at the time of diagnosis. Changes in a person's health status have a significant impact on morbidity, with progressive compromise in mobility and nutritional status increasing an individual's risk of infection, which is often the most immediate cause of death.

Treatment

Medical Management

Pharmacologic treatments have been developed that have been shown to treat the cognitive and behavioral symptoms of AD without affecting disease progression (Table 21-3). In 1993, tacrine (Cognex) was the first drug approved by the FDA for the treatment of mild to moderate AD. Tacrine, an acetylcholinesterase inhibitor, works by inhibiting the breakdown of acetylcholine in the synapse, thereby increasing its availability. Although it was a less than perfect treatment, requiring dosing multiple times through the day and with associated side effects including possible hepatotoxicity, it provided hope for the millions of individuals diagnosed with AD. Since then three other cholinesterase inhibitors, donepezil (Aricept), rivastigmine (Exelon), and galantamine (Razadyne, previously called Reminyl), have been approved by the FDA for the treatment of mild to moderate AD. These later drugs are both easier to administer and relatively free

TABLE 21-2 Stages of Alzheimer's Disease

Mild Cognitive Impairment	Early-Stage AD	Middle-Stage AD	Late-Stage AD	End-Stage AD
MMSE 25+	MMSE 21–25 (mild)	MMSE 10–20 (moderate)	MMSE 0–9 (severe)	
Common Cognitive Changes				
Mild memory loss Retains awareness of problems	Short-term memory loss Repeats questions Forgets conversations Geographic disorientation Mild word-finding difficulty May minimize problems	Significant decline in short-term memory Word-finding difficulty May no longer recognize impairments	Short- and long-term memory impaired Impaired expressive and receptive language Loss of recognition of deficits	Little or no meaningful communication May no longer recognize family
Common Changes in Function				
May not require assistance, but tasks take longer to complete	May have difficulty: Driving Managing medications Cooking	May require assistance with: Bathing Dressing No longer able to: Drive Cook Intermittent loss of bladder control	Dependent in personal care May need assistance with eating Bladder incontinence Intermittent bowel incontinence	Unable to assist with any personal care tasks May have difficulty with chewing and swallowing Walking difficult Incontinent of bowel and bladder
Common Changes in Behavior				
Depression Mild anxiety	Depression Suspiciousness Anxiety Apathy Social withdrawal	Apathy Agitation with personal care Anxiety Suspiciousness	Delusions Wandering Aggression Agitation	May become upset with personal care May be fearful of being moved

AD, Alzheimer's disease; *MMSE*, Mini Mental State Examination.

TABLE 21-3 Medications for Alzheimer's Disease

Cholinesterase Inhibitors

Medications	Dosage*	Possible Side Effects
Donepezil (Aricept 5 mg, 10 mg)	5–10 mg/day; increase the dose after 4–6 weeks	GI upset, sleep disruption, vivid dreams, leg cramps
Rivastigmine (Exelon 1.5 mg, 3 mg, 4.5 mg, 6 mg)	1.5 mg bid titrated slowly to 6 mg bid increasing the dose every 4–6 weeks	GI upset
Galantamine (Razadyne 4 mg, 8 mg, 12 mg)	4 mg bid titrated slowly to 12 mg bid increasing the dose every 4–6 weeks	GI upset
(Razadyne ER 8 mg, 16 mg, 24 mg)	8 mg/day titrated slowly to 24 mg/day increasing the dose every 4–6 weeks	GI upset

Other Drug Classes

Medications	Dosage	Possible Side Effects
Memantine (Namenda 5 mg, 10 mg)	5 mg qd titrated to 10 mg bid increasing dose by 5 mg each week	Dizziness, anxiety

*Side effects are minimized if dose is slowly titrated to therapeutic level as tolerated.
GI, Gastrointestinal.

of hepatotoxicity. The effects of these drugs have proven to be modest; however, there is no question that they can play an important role in helping to improve symptoms while providing some stability for short periods of time. There is some indication that the earlier in the disease these drugs are introduced the better the response, suggesting that early identification of problems and intervention may affect disease progression. Whereas early studies focused on the effect these drugs had on cognitive function alone, subsequent studies have documented a beneficial effect on both maintaining functional independence and treating behavioral problems. Although patients and families often focus on improvement in memory, the cholinesterase inhibitors have proven to be more effective in improving apathy, initiation, and attention.

In 2003, memantine (Namenda) was approved by the FDA for the treatment of moderate to severe AD. Memantine is a weak N-methyl-D-aspartate (NMDA) receptor antagonist that may decrease abnormal excitatory neurotransmission in the brain resulting from excess levels of glutamate. Memantine was tested in groups of individuals with moderate to severe AD given as a monotherapy, as well as in combination with the acetylcholinesterase inhibitor donepezil, and was shown to be modestly effective in maintaining higher levels of function in individuals in the later stages of AD.

A number of neuroprotective treatments have been studied; however, high-dose vitamin E (1000 IU twice a day) has been the only treatment to date that has shown an impact on disease progression.[54] Nonsteroidal antiinflammatory drugs and estrogen replacement have been studied, but none of the prospective, placebo-controlled treatment trials completed to date have shown any effect on disease progression.

Psychosocial Considerations

The availability of FDA-approved medications to treat symptoms of AD throughout the course of the disease has provided patients and their caregivers with hope; however, in the absence of a treatment that can halt or reverse the progression of the disease, ongoing education and support remains a crucial part of disease management. Educational needs vary throughout the course of the disease. In the early stages of AD, legal and financial issues (including decisions related to advance directives) are important to address while an individual is able to participate in future care planning. With increased awareness of the significance of early memory loss, support groups are being developed to meet the needs specific to this group. Providing the necessary support and structure can allow an individual to continue functioning independently for as long as possible. Ensuring that patients and caregivers are aware of all available services is important as they plan for care throughout the disease.

Caregiver Stress

The stress of caregiving can become overwhelming for both family and professional caregivers. Educational and support groups can help caregivers manage the unique challenges confronted at each stage of the disease. Studies have established the benefit of comprehensive educational and support programs for both patients and caregivers. The Alzheimer's Association provides educational programs and ongoing support groups in local communities that provide caregivers with valuable information about strategies to manage the many challenges of the disease.

Case Management

Each stage of the disease has potential safety issues that need to be addressed. **Decisions related to driving** safety are important and are often a point of contention between patients and families. Health care providers are often asked to make recommendations regarding a patient's ability to continue driving. Driving assessment programs that can provide both written and on-the-road assessments of an individual's driving safety are available through some rehabilitation facilities. Often health care providers will make recommendations based on the family's observations and the patient's level of cognitive and functional impairment. For some patients the concern is with becoming lost while driving. Enrolling patients in the **Alzheimer's Association's Safe Return program** can help ensure that if a patient does become lost his or her family will be able to be contacted.

Early in the disease, independent **management of household activities,** such as cooking and financial management, is important. **Medication management and compliance** is particularly important given the number of prescription drugs that many patients are taking. The use of a pill dispenser may help with maintaining medication compliance in the early stages of the disease. Family members may need to assume some tasks, or, if living alone, consideration may be given to providing help in the home or alternative living arrangements.

Assisted living facilities, also called **personal care homes** in some areas of the country, can be alternatives providing additional support to patients while allowing them to maintain some degree of independence. Many facilities have dementia-specific units that are designed to meet the special needs of patients in the later stages of the disease while still providing a more homelike environment. Some families may choose to arrange for additional **in-home care** such as homemakers or home health aides who can help provide care at home.

In the later stages of the disease, patients begin to have more difficulty with maintaining their ADLs, and providing assistance can become a challenge. Episodes of agitation or anxiety are often associated with assistance with personal care activities such as bathing or toileting. Incontinence and disrupted sleep are often identified as the leading precipitants to nursing home placement. Establishing regular toileting schedules can be helpful in maintaining continence, and encouraging regular exercise, daytime exposure to light, and avoidance of daytime naps helps maintain regular sleep patterns. Delusions and hallucinations may emerge, further complicating care. Individuals may have difficulty identifying their family members or they may no longer recognize their house as their "home." Attempts to reorient individuals or to correct their misperceptions can contribute to increased agitation. Educating caregivers to redirect or distract instead of confronting helps minimize escalating behavior. *Sun-*

downing is a term commonly used to describe agitation that becomes more prominent late in the day.

In the end stages of AD, hospice services can provide the education, support, and care that are crucial to families and caregivers. Hospice services are available to provide both home care and inpatient services that can help ease the burden of the disease.

Future Research

A number of different strategies, developed as a direct result of the increased understanding of the pathophysiology of AD, are being evaluated for the possible treatment of Alzheimer's disease. The focus of research has shifted to approaches that not only treat the symptoms of AD but may also have an impact on halting or slowing disease progression. Techniques are being developed to improve diagnostic accuracy while also identifying the disease in the earliest possible stages. Improved imaging techniques including the testing of new compounds used in imaging such as PET may prove helpful in allowing accurate measurement of amyloid deposition in the brain. These imaging techniques may provide a mechanism to assess the effects of new treatments on the actual pathology in the brain, which could facilitate the testing of new drugs.

Drugs are being developed that may be effective in altering the accumulation of insoluble amyloid plaques in the brain by inhibiting β and γ secretase, which play a role in the abnormal processing of APP. Immunotherapy techniques are being developed that have the potential to decrease amyloid plaques in the brain. A vaccine was developed and tested in mice that were genetically altered to produce excess levels of amyloid deposition in their brains. Although the vaccine was successful in halting and in some cases reducing the amyloid depositions in the brains of the mice, when the vaccine was tested in humans a number of subjects developed CNS inflammation leading to the early termination of the study. Alternative methods of vaccination are currently under investigation.

3-Hydroxy-3-methylglutaryl coenzyme A reductase inhibitors (statins) are currently being investigated as potential treatments to slow the progression of AD. It has been postulated that this class of drugs may have a positive effect on disease-associated brain inflammation while also affecting the accumulation of insoluble amyloid plaque.

Elevated plasma homocysteine has been identified as an independent risk factor for AD,[57] which may have a direct impact on AD pathology or serve to increase an individual's cardiovascular risk for coexisting vascular changes in the brain. Trials are currently underway investigating strategies to reduce levels of plasma homocysteine and slow the rate of disease progression.

VASCULAR DEMENTIA

Vascular dementia (VaD) is the second leading cause of dementia representing approximately 15% to 20% of diagnosed cases of dementia throughout the world.[49] Increased recognition is being given to the impact that vascular changes in the brain can have on the rate of progression of neurodegenerative diseases such as AD and the relative infrequency of pure vascular pathology as the sole cause of dementia.

Etiology

VaD has been defined as the loss of cognitive function resulting from ischemic, hypoperfusion, or hemorrhagic brain lesions due to cerebrovascular disease or cardiovascular pathology.[50] VaD may occur acutely after stroke associated with large-vessel disease, multiple strokes (referred to as multiinfarct dementia), or a single strategically located stroke. VaD can also occur when small vessels are occluded and thus block the arterial blood supply to small areas of the brain. The resulting death of brain tissue can produce a slowly progressive decline in cognitive function.

Assessment

Assessment for dementia has been described previously with criteria for diagnosis of vascular dementia developed by the NINDS-AIREN international work group in 1993.[51] It requires the presence of cognitive loss, most often affecting subcortical brain functions, vascular brain lesions demonstrated by brain imaging, a temporal link between stroke and dementia, focal signs on the neurologic examination, and the exclusion of other causes of dementia. DSM-IV-TR[15] criteria for VaD do not require the exclusion of other causes of dementia. They do require that changes are not associated with a delirium. In contrast to AD, individuals with VaD typically have impairment in executive function, such as difficulty with judgment and reasoning abilities, whereas memory impairment may be mild or nonexistent. Gait is often affected in VaD typically demonstrated as shuffling with short steps similar to a parkinsonian gait. Problems with urinary frequency or urgency can be seen, as well as changes in mood and personality such as depression or emotional incontinence. Focal findings on a neurologic examination such as hemiparesis or asymmetric deep tendon reflexes may be seen in VaD.

Treatment

Treatment of VaD has focused on preventing further decline while also using medications to help treat symptoms. Aggressive management of underlying risk factors such as atrial fibrillation, hypertension, hyperlipidemia, and diabetes mellitus may help limit the progression of cognitive decline. Antiplatelet medications and the use of anticoagulants such as daily aspirin or the use of warfarin may help prevent recurrent stroke. If patients have significant carotid stenosis, surgical intervention may also reduce the risk of further stroke. Although no drugs have been approved to date by any regulatory agencies for the treatment of VaD, there is some evidence, given the identification of cholinergic deficits in VaD, to support the use of cholinesterase inhibitors currently approved for the treatment of AD. As in the other dementias, the use of neuroleptics or antidepressants may be appropriate to treat psychiatric or behavioral symptoms.

DEMENTIA WITH LEWY BODIES

Dementia with Lewy bodies (DLB) and a group of related diseases known as **frontotemporal dementia** may account for more cases of the neurodegenerative dementias than previously appreciated, but these diseases are still poorly recognized and underdiagnosed.[41,47,59] Although less prevalent, DLB has gained recognition as a leading cause of dementia, with some studies identifying it as the second most common form of dementia seen in the elderly population.[35] DLB is estimated to be responsible for 11% to 20% of all dementing illnesses in the elderly.[2,59] Onset of symptoms is typically seen around age 75, but the range can be between 50 and 80. Males are affected at a slightly greater rate than females, and the course of the disease is shorter than AD with an average duration of 5 to 6 years.[46] Accumulation of α-synuclein aggregates, which form Lewy bodies, is the hallmark feature in the brains of patients with DLB.

Diagnosis

As in other dementias, the core feature required for a diagnosis of DLB is cognitive decline of sufficient severity to impair functional abilities. Decline in cognitive performance is seen most typically on tests of visuospatial abilities and executive function along with fluctuating levels of attention. In addition, the cognitive decline is most often seen in the presence of other distinctive features, including the presence of behavioral disturbances such as visual hallucinations and depression early in the course of the disease. The extrapyramidal system is affected early, manifesting in problems with gait and mobility. Although fluctuations in attention have been recognized as being a core feature of DLB, fluctuations can be difficult to assess. One study identified four features as being reliable in differentiating between DLB and AD: daytime drowsiness and lethargy, daytime sleep of 2 or more hours, staring into space for long periods, and episodes of disorganized speech.[17]

Treatment

Studies examining the use of cholinesterase inhibitors in DLB have documented benefit in treating both behavioral and cognitive symptoms, with improvement in apathy, anxiety, sleep, and hallucinations. Neuroleptics have been effective in treating some of the behavioral problems, including hallucinations; however, they should be used with caution given DLB patients' increased sensitivity to extrapyramidal side effects. Motor symptoms may respond to treatment with levodopa, but the response is typically less robust than in individuals diagnosed with Parkinson's disease.

FRONTOTEMPORAL DEMENTIA

Previously believed to be rare, frontotemporal dementia (FTD) has recently been recognized as a common cause of dementia in younger individuals. One of the first of the FTDs identified was **Pick's disease,** named after Dr. Arnold Pick,

a psychiatrist, who first described symptoms of the disease in 1892. Recent studies suggest that FTD may represent the most common cause of dementia in individuals under age 70.[47] Pathologic changes identified in FTD include gliosis, spongiosis, and neuronal loss. Tau plays an important role in FTDs such as Pick's disease, in which abnormal phosphorylation leads to aggregation of tau in Pick bodies, one of the hallmark neuropathologic features of this disease. Other degenerative diseases associated with dementia and tau pathology include progressive supranuclear palsy and corticobasal ganglionic degeneration. The term *tauopathy* has begun to be used referring to this group of neurodegenerative diseases. Deficits in the neurotransmitter serotonin have been identified and linked to the prominence of some of the behavioral problems such as repetitive compulsive behaviors, as well as depression and irritability.

Recent research has identified frontal dementia syndromes in patients diagnosed with ALS and the corresponding identification of a subgroup of patients with FTD who develop motor neuron syndromes. In one study, 14% of patients with a diagnosis of FTD also met criteria for a diagnosis of ALS with an additional 36% of patients exhibiting early features of ALS.[31] In another study examining the cognitive function of patients diagnosed with ALS, 15% met criteria for a diagnosis of FTD.[48]

Diagnosis

In contrast to many of the other dementias, one of the earliest hallmark symptoms of FTD is significant personality change, most frequently a change in social or personal conduct. Families often describe disinhibited or impulsive behavior. There is a measurable decline in cognitive abilities, with language and executive functions such as reasoning, planning, and judgment being affected early in the course of the disease.

As the name suggests, imaging techniques such as CT or MRI show a prominence of atrophy in the frontal and temporal regions of the brain. PET scans can show a pattern of hypometabolism in the frontal and temporal regions of the brain. Symptoms correlate with the function of the brain region with the greatest amount of atrophy or hypometabolism.

Treatment

Treatment of FTD has focused on managing the often difficult behavioral symptoms. There has been no evidence to date that would suggest that the use of the cholinesterase inhibitors approved for the treatment of symptoms in AD provide any benefit for patients with FTD. The use of SSRIs has been shown to be of some benefit in treating the depression and irritability, as well as the compulsive stereotypic behaviors. Anticonvulsants such as sodium valproate and carbamazepine have been used to treat agitation and aggressive behaviors sometimes associated with the disease. The use of atypical antipsychotics such as risperidone or quetiapine may also be beneficial in treating these symptoms. Caregiver support and education is crucial to minimizing the impact of the behavioral symptoms associated with FTD.

Psychosocial Considerations

Because of the early age of onset and the prominent behavioral changes, FTD presents unique challenges for care. Early changes are subtle, and familial relationships can be seriously affected before symptoms reach a level of severity such that a diagnosis of possible dementia is considered. Often impulsive decisions related to employment or finances have disastrous consequences, affecting patients' and families' available resources. Dealing with prominent behavioral problems can be exhausting, making the need for help in the home or the provision of respite services crucial for both patients and caregivers.

MOTOR NEURON DISEASE

Motor neuron diseases (MNDs) are a category of neuromuscular disorders that are related to degeneration of the anterior horn cell. In MNDs, the cells that control voluntary movement are damaged, leaving the sensory system essentially intact.[39] MNDs include the spinal muscular atrophies, Kennedy's disease (bulbospinal muscular atrophy), postpolio syndrome, and amyotrophic lateral sclerosis.

AMYOTROPHIC LATERAL SCLEROSIS

The most common adult-onset MND is **amyotrophic lateral sclerosis (ALS),** a degenerative disease characterized by the loss of both upper and lower motor neurons. ALS causes weakness and atrophy of the voluntary muscles (muscles of the hands, arms, legs, and trunk, as well as respiratory, bulbar, and facial muscles). The term **amyotrophic** (without muscle nutrition or progressive muscle wasting) refers to the lower motor neuron (LMN) component of the syndrome. **Lateral sclerosis** refers to the demyelination and gliosis that occur in the corticospinal tracts of the lateral column of the spinal cord. These areas harden and degenerate, causing a scar or **sclerosis.** This causes the upper motor neuron (UMN) component of the syndrome. ALS was first described by Charcot in 1869. However, it was not until Lou Gehrig, the famed "Iron Man" of the New York Yankees, was diagnosed with the disease in 1939 and later died that ALS gained more recognition and became known as **Lou Gehrig's disease.** Unfortunately, research conducted over the past century has not found a cause or a cure. Progress is being made, and one drug has been approved for the treatment of ALS; several more are in various phases of clinical development.[40]

The clinical picture of ALS is heterogeneous; some people have a predominantly LMN picture, whereas others show mostly UMN signs (Table 21-4). Rarely, an individual will have pure UMN or LMN syndrome. Usually, these patients will develop the signs that were initially absent. When this occurs, the diagnosis becomes ALS. When it does not occur, the pure UMN syndrome is labeled **primary lateral sclerosis (PLS)** and the pure LMN syndrome is called **progressive muscular atrophy (PMA).** Patients with PMA tend to live longer than ALS patients, and people with PLS have a life

TABLE 21-4	Upper and Lower Motor Neuron Signs	
Upper Motor Neuron Signs	**Lower Motor Neuron Signs**
Spasticity	Weakness
Hyperreflexia	Muscle wasting
Clonus	Fasciculations
Extensor spasms	Cramps

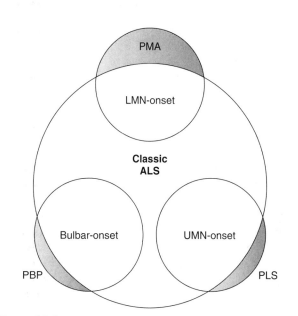

Figure 21-1 ALS manifests with lower motor neuron (LMN) involvement, upper motor neuron (UMN) involvement, or bulbar involvement.

expectancy longer then both. Pure bulbar disease is called **progressive bulbar palsy.** This nearly always becomes bulbar-onset ALS[39] (Fig. 21-1).

Epidemiology

ALS occurs equally around the world with no ethnic, racial, or socioeconomic differences. The most common age of onset is between ages 40 and 70, but the disease can occur at any adult age. It affects 1.6 men for every woman, but the ratio begins to equalize after menopause. In the United States, the incidence is about 2 per 100,000 people, which means that about 5000 new cases are diagnosed annually. A recent study of mortality rates from ALS in the United States shows a greater frequency in states at higher latitudes. Suspicions that the disease is increasing in frequency have neither been proven nor disproven. The average length of time from symptom onset until death in most cases is 2 to 5 years.[55]

The majority of cases of ALS are sporadic, but between 5% and 10% are familial, usually displaying an autosomal dominant pattern of inheritance. In 1993, mutations in the superoxide dismutase-1 gene on chromosome 21 were discovered.[53] This genetic mutation can be detected in 15% to 25% of families with two or more members having ALS.[1,40,52]

Etiology

The cause of ALS is unknown, but the understanding of the cell death process has improved in the last decade.[9,52] Several highly plausible mechanisms of both LMN and UMN degeneration have been suggested. Investigators believe that the neuronal degeneration may result from the final common pathway of programmed cell death, or apoptosis. This includes theories of glutamate excitotoxicity, free radical injury resulting in increased oxidative stress, the accumulation of neurofilaments resulting in axonal strangulation, and mitochondrial dysfunction.[52] These theories form the foundation of current and future basic science and clinical research, which may someday lead to a cure.

Assessment

Initial History

Patients may be typically in the 50- to 60-year-old age range and may first notice limb weakness. Patients will commonly report a gradual onset of asymmetric, progressive, painless weakness. When onset is in the lower extremity, the symptoms may be tripping, falling, decreased endurance, or a change in gait. Upper extremity onset causes reduced dexterity leading to functional loss. Difficulty swallowing or breathing may be reported. Slurred speech indicates bulbar onset and occurs from weakness of the tongue (Fig. 21-2), facial, and oropharyngeal muscles. The patient may give a history of symptoms spreading within a region or from one region to another.

Although there have been a few reports through the decades of cognitive changes in ALS patients, until recently, ALS patients have been told that the disease would not affect their cognition. In 2002, definitive evidence that ALS patients sometimes have FTD and that FTD patients frequently have undiagnosed motor neuron disease was found.[31,32] In obtaining the initial history, the clinician should be alert to indications from family members that there has been a personality change. Individuals with FTD might have deficits in reasoning, planning, attention, and awareness (see the section on FTD earlier in this chapter).

Initial Physical Examination

A neurologic assessment will include inspection of the muscles. Weak areas will reveal muscle atrophy. In the upper extremity, this will commonly be seen in the first dorsal interossious muscles, located on the top of the hand, between the thumb and second finger. In the lower extremity, wasting of the tibialis anterior causes the tibia to become prominent due to loss of the muscular bulge. LMN signs include muscle atrophy and the presence of **fasciculations,** which are involuntary contractions or twitching of muscle fibers that can be seen under the skin or tongue. UMN signs include a Babinski sign and hyperreflexia (see Table 21-4).

When **spasticity** is present, the examiner will note resistance to passive movement of the limb. This increase in muscle tone may result in a spastic gait or spastic dysarthria.

Patients with **bulbar symptoms** usually have a tongue with scalloped edges and a rutted appearance. It will move slowly and be unable to fully extend, making mastication difficult. The finding of fasciculations in the tongue is especially important because it is a specific and sensitive sign for the diagnosis of ALS.[60] When fasciculations are present, the tongue has undulating and quivering movements while at rest. Functional rating scales are available and may be used in some settings, for example, the revised ALS Functional Rating Scale (ALSFRS-R) or the ALS Assessment Questionnaire–40, or measure-of-life scales.

Ongoing Assessment

At each patient contact, the patient's current status is assessed (Box 21-4). The clinician will be alert to the milestones of disease progression and associated interventions (Box 21-5). Many of the symptoms of people with ALS (PALS) are amenable to treatment (Table 21-5).[19]

Diagnostic Testing

A single laboratory test, radiographic image, or neurophysiologic study specific for the diagnosis of ALS does not exist. The diagnosis of ALS is clinical and requires the presence of evidence of upper and lower motor neuron degeneration with progressive spread of symptoms or signs within a region

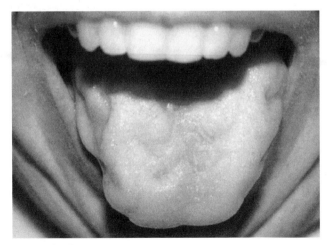

Figure 21-2 Atrophy of the tongue in ALS.

BOX 21-4	Assessment of Persons With Amyotrophic Lateral Sclerosis

- Nutrition: weight, length of time to complete meals, elimination
- Respiratory: seated vital capacity (VC), negative inspiratory force (NIF); supine vital capacity when concerned that seated test has failed to demonstrate suspected weakness
- Mobility: gait abnormalities, range of motion
- Psychosocial: disability status, insurance status, individual and family coping mechanisms, family support, community support, status of advance directives
- Constitutional: quality and quantity of sleep, pain, mood

BOX 21-5 Milestones and Interventions

- Dysphagia with or without weight loss
  - Placement of feeding tube before vital capacity drops below 50%, for optimal safety
- Vital capacity 50% of predicted
  - Eligible for BiPAP based on criteria for restrictive thoracic and neuromuscular disorders
- Negative inspiratory force > –60
  - Eligible for BiPAP based on criteria for restrictive thoracic and neuromuscular disorders
- Vital capacity 30% of predicted
  - Eligible for hospice under Medicare guidelines

BiPAP, Bimanual positive airway pressure.

or to other regions along with the absence of electrophysiologic, pathologic, or radiologic evidence of other disease processes.[7] However, the grave prognosis of ALS usually prompts additional testing in hope of finding an alternative diagnosis. Routine testing normally includes a limited number of studies (Table 21-6).

Typically, the clinical suspicion is confirmed by the opinion of a neurologist who has substantial experience with motor neuron diseases and electrophysiologic testing. Testing includes the following studies:

- **Nerve conduction studies (NCSs)** are performed to assess the integrity of the sensory and motor peripheral nerves and reveal loss of motor axons in multiple limbs with sparing of the sensory axons.
- **Electromyography (EMG)** involves the placement of a needle electrode into muscle to obtain recordings of electrical activity. EMG shows fibrillations, a sign of

TABLE 21-5 Symptom Management

Symptom	Pharmacologic Options	Nonpharmacologic Options
Anxiety	Alprazolam, lorazepam, clonazepam	Referral to mental health professional for counseling
Constipation	Bowel stimulants	Increased water, increased fiber, bowel training, enema
Depression	SSRI, tricyclic, or atypical antidepressants	Referral to mental health professional for counseling
Dry mouth	Guaifenesin	Increased water, room humidifier
Dyspnea	Morphine oral or inhaled, transdermal fentanyl	NIPPV, elevated head of bed
Emotional incontinence	SSRI, tricyclic, or atypical antidepressants	Patient and family education
Fatigue	Pyridostigmine, modafinil, other stimulants	Energy conservation techniques, NIPPV
Insomnia	Zolpidem, temazepam, trazadone, other hypnotics	Referral to mental health professional for counseling
Muscle cramps	Quinine, baclofen, clonazepam	Stretching exercises
Musculoskeletal pain	NSAIDs and narcotic analgesia	Massage, heat, cold, physical therapy
Sialorrhea	Glycopyrrolate, hyoscyamine, atropine, scopolamine	Suction machine
Spasticity	Baclofen, tizanidine, dantrolene	Stretching exercises, massage
Thick phlegm	Guaifenesin	Cough assist device, increased water, room humidifier

NIPPV, Noninvasive positive pressure ventilation; *NSAIDs*, nonsteroidal antiinflammatory drugs; *SSRI*, selective serotonin reuptake inhibitor.

TABLE 21-6 Diagnostic Testing

Laboratory Test	Reason
Erythrocyte sedimentation rate	Inflammation/malignancy: nonspecific
Serum protein electrophoresis with immunofixation	Monoclonal gammopathy
Thyroid function tests	Hyperthyroidism
Vitamin B$_{12}$ level	Subacute combined degeneration of the spinal cord
Serum calcium level/parathyroid hormone	Hyperparathyroidism
Creatine kinase	Myopathy
Heavy metal screen—24-hour urine collection	Lead toxicity

Additional Testing	Reason
Brain/cervical spine MRI	Spondylosis with spinal cord compression, herniated disk, tumor, syringomyelia
Nerve conduction studies	Demyelinating neuropathy: multifocal motor neuropathy with conduction block
Electromyography	Polymyositis

active denervation, and neurogenic motor unit recruitment in multiple muscles of different peripheral nerve territories, nerve root territories (myotomes), and levels of the nervous system (bulbar, cervical, thoracic, lumbosacral).

- **MRI** of the cervical spine that reveals cervical spondylosis may provide an alternative explanation for the patient's clinical picture, especially those without bulbar symptoms and signs.

Through these tests, an examiner can determine the likelihood of motor neuron disease and exclude alternative etiology, of degeneration of the motor neurons. It is not uncommon for the diagnosis to be delayed because of the presence of only limited physical signs and electrophysiologic abnormalities early in the course of the disease. Therefore several clinical examinations and EMG/NCSs may be required over time before a conclusive diagnosis can be made. On occasion, findings from a thorough investigation may lead to a treatable diagnosis such as a demyelinating peripheral neuropathy or an inflammatory myopathy.

Medical Management

The American Academy of Neurology has published a practice parameter for ALS patients, and this should guide the management for all ALS patients.[36] Riluzole is the only drug approved by the FDA for the treatment of ALS. It was introduced into the market after clinical trials showed a modest improvement in survival.[4,28] These initial trials showed a survival benefit of only 2 months; however, data from long-term, uncontrolled studies have shown survival benefits of up to 20 months.[37] Side effects can include fatigue, gastrointestinal upset, and dizziness. Most of the side effects are dose related and many disappear after continued dosing. Because of the limited effect on survival, the high cost, and the terminal nature of the disease, many people choose not to take Riluzole, the only medication proven to alter the natural course of ALS (Box 21-6).

A multidisciplinary team approach is the optimal way to provide care to PALS. The primary goals of medical management are to support nutrition and respiration and manage symptoms, both physical and emotional. Early in the course of the disease, PALS with bulbar dysfunction should be introduced to the idea of a feeding tube to maintain nutrition (see Nutritional Considerations). Placing the tube is a relatively simple and safe procedure when patients have reasonable strength of breathing muscles. As breathing strength deteriorates, the risk of the procedure increases and the recovery time lengthens. To minimize the avoidable risks of the procedure, a goal is to place the tube before the vital capacity (VC) drops below 50% of predicted[36] (Box 21-7; see also Box 21-5). Primary reasons for resistance include the mistaken belief that after the tube is placed, the person will be unable, or not permitted, to eat. When placed early, patients may continue to take their nutrition orally and use the tube only for supplementary water or medications that are unpleasant or difficult to swallow. As dysphagia slowly worsens, they will begin to supplement their oral intake, and

---

> **BOX 21-6   Riluzole**
>
> Riluzole is a tablet that is administered twice daily on an empty stomach. Before the first dose, liver function tests (LFTs), specifically alanine aminotransferase (ALT) and aspartate aminotransferase (AST), should be obtained as a baseline and checked at 1, 2, 3, 6, and 12 months. Some people tolerate it best when started at half dose (one tablet once daily) for the first week.

> **BOX 21-7   Feeding Tube Options***
>
> **Percutaneous Endoscopic Gastrostomy (PEG)**
> Placed by gastroenterologist or general surgeon with expertise in endoscopic procedures. Performed with mild sedation or monitored anesthesia care (MAC). Tube is threaded down the esophagus and pulled out through an opening in the skin.
> **Radiographically Inserted Gastrostomy (RIG)**
> Placed by interventional radiologist. Performed with mild sedation or MAC. Tube is placed from the outside to the inside through the small surgical opening.

*Both methods are safe and effective, and both are most safely done while vital capacity exceeds 50% of predicted. Choice of procedure is based on availability of specialist, availability of follow-up care, and center preference.

---

gradually shift to using the feeding tube for the bulk of calories.

Respiratory management is guided by the results of easily measured parameters (see Box 21-5). VC and negative inspiratory force (NIF) should be measured at regular intervals. Intervention with **noninvasive positive pressure ventilation (NIPPV)** is started as indicated by these measurements. Sometimes PALS with abnormal respiratory measurements do not experience, or deny experiencing, respiratory symptoms, and this may contribute to resistance to using NIPPV. In this situation, it is helpful to remind them that NIPPV has been proven to prolong survival.[5] In addition, this intervention will reduce the patient's work of breathing and improve fatigue. Aggressive management of sialorrhea and anxiety will improve tolerance of NIPPV.

Also useful in the management of respiratory issues is the cough assist device. Patients with ALS will develop a weak cough and an inability to clear their airway. The cough assist allows someone with a weak or even absent cough to generate an involuntary cough and clear the airway of obstruction.[61] Insurance, including Medicare, pays for the device. Suction machines provide additional help by allowing the removal of secretions from the mouth.

The disease will progress relentlessly, and there will come a time when NIPPV is inadequate to manage respiratory symptoms. Optimally, the patient will have made and communicated his or her decision related to end-of-life care. If the choice is to have life prolonged with advanced technology, this will be the time to proceed to tracheotomy and invasive ventilation. It may be difficult for social services to arrange for discharge to a nursing facility or home care managed by family members or home health services around the clock. Management is complex and requires training of caretakers before discharge to successfully manage an individual who is totally dependent and will require close follow-up by a team that may include respiratory services, nursing, therapists, hospice, and a case manager.

If invasive ventilation is declined and symptomatic management is preferred, referral to hospice is indicated. Opiates can alleviate air hunger and often do so without excessive sedation.

Surgical Management

There is no surgical treatment of ALS but there are procedures useful in easing some of the symptoms, including dysphagia/malnutrition and spasticity. Percutaneous endoscopic gastrostomy (PEG) feeding tube or other feeding routes are usually performed using one of two techniques: radiographic insertion or endoscopic placement[14] (see Box 21-7). For patients who have elected to receive long-term invasive positive-pressure ventilation, a tracheostomy may be performed during the hospitalization. There are a few reports of ALS patients with severe spasticity or patients with primary lateral sclerosis who may benefit from the placement of a baclofen pump[33,34] (see Chapter 13).

Research

Since the discovery that a mutation of the **superoxide dismutase 1 (SOD1)** gene causes familial ALS, over 100 different mutations have been reported. However, these mutations account for only 20% to 25% of the familial ALS cases.[1] Finding mutations that explain the remaining 75% continues to be a focus of research.

Between 1990 and 2005 several novel agents, currently approved drugs and nutritional supplements that showed promising results in animal models of ALS, were studied in clinical trials with ALS patients. Unfortunately, none showed efficacy in altering the natural history of the disease. These clinical trials included testing of creatine, coenzyme Q_{10}, Celebrex, topiramate, Neurontin, minocycline, and several growth factors.[11,38,56] We are awaiting results on coenzyme Q_{10} and minocycline.

Recently, a consortium of scientists has screened thousands of currently approved drugs and compounds. Several of these agents look promising, and it is likely that some will reach the clinical trial phase. Current clinical trials can be found at www.clinicaltrials.gov.

Dr. James Thompson at the University of Wisconsin developed a technique to use human embryonic stem cells for research in 1998. The possibility of a renewable source of replacement cells is the first hint of a therapy that could possibly reverse the loss of function in ALS. Though promising, this area of study is complex and has been associated with political and ethical ramifications. For now, safe and effective treatment is still far away.

Gene therapy is another research direction providing hope to patients. This approach attempts to treat diseases at the molecular level by correcting what is wrong with defective genes. The idea is to prevent the gene product, a protein, from causing disease by restoring the normal function, providing new function, or enhancing the existing functions of the proteins.

Health Teaching

Patients usually learn of their diagnosis in stages. Initially a physician may inform them of the suspicion of ALS or provide the less specific label of motor neuron disease or anterior horn cell disease. When the diagnosis is confirmed, it is rarely a surprise and for a few reasons this is an ideal time to begin teaching. Patients usually are accompanied by individuals who are their primary support system. Addressing the group will increase the likelihood that information about the diagnosis will be retained after the visit. Access to the Internet allows patients to obtain information about their disease. It is important that patients and their families check with the health care providers or the ALS organizations to verify information. It is important for patients to receive information about community resources (the Muscular Dystrophy Association (MDA) and the ALS Association [ALSA]) and other sources of information (American Neurologic Association, World Federation of Neurology, and the National Institutes of Health [NIH]) that are listed at the end of the chapter. Patients should be advised that they may choose to receive care from their physician or from a clinic with a multidisciplinary team, including physicians, nurses, therapists, dietitians, social workers, and others who are knowledgeable about their condition and available to them throughout the course of their illness. ALS clinics can be located by contacting either MDA or ALSA.

Patients may be overwhelmed with the diagnosis of a terminal illness. They may react with grief, depression, or anger and with mixed emotions. Some may discuss their condition freely, ask specific questions about what to expect as the disease progresses, and make plans to put their affairs in order. Others may use denial as a method of coping. It is important for clinicians to be perceptive in providing information when the patient is ready and to determine the best time to discuss sensitive issues. Clinicians may use open-ended statements such as the following: "Many ALS patients wonder about the later stages of ALS. If you would like to discuss these issues or have questions, members of the ALS team can help you."

Questions may arise concerning the legitimacy of complementary and alternative medicine (CAM), massage, tai chi, or acupuncture. It is important to encourage open, honest, and compassionate discussions and encourage participation in ALS support groups.

ALS patients of childbearing potential need to know that their fertility is not affected. Birth control is needed to avoid an unwanted pregnancy. All patients benefit from discussions regarding sexual activity. Their previous patterns of sexual expression may change as their mobility changes, and they can be instructed on how to continue sexual or intimate relationships. Patients can be taught about **emotional incontinence** or **emotional lability** with episodes of uncontrollable crying or laughter that is not congruent with their current emotional state. This is a neurochemical response seen in patients with UMN signs and is often seen with dysarthria and dysphagia. It is not a sign of psychiatric dysfunction but rather part of the illness. Although emotional incontinence is different from depression, it usually responds to treatment with antidepressant medications.

ALS patients and their families can experience feelings of loss of control. Although it is not possible to change the diagnosis or the rate of progression, it is possible for PALS to remain in charge of many aspects of their lives. Providing patients with information and options regarding their care can empower them with a sense of control.

Nutritional Considerations

A dietitian can conduct a nutrition assessment to ascertain the ALS patient's eating capabilities, nutrition-related complications, and nutritional status. Based on these determinations, the dietitian can assess the patient's nutritional needs and educate the patient and caregivers on how to most comfortably and easily meet these needs.

Patients are most often referred to the dietitian because of weight loss. The causes of weight loss in ALS patients are often multifactorial, with the most problematic one being a decreased ability to swallow. This often manifests along with slurred speech and coughing while drinking water. As dysphagia progresses, the ALS patient becomes more wary of eating and drinking, slows down, feels full earlier, and may become too fatigued to finish the meal. Other patients experience a dramatic increase in metabolic rate due to the increased effort it takes to breathe.

Once the primary causes of weight loss are determined, the dietitian can work with the patient and caregivers to improve the patient's intake. Foods can be made calorie-laden and power-packed by adding extra fats, sugars, and protein. "Double strength" milk (powdered milk added to milk) can be used in preparing hot cereal, soups, and sauces. If the speech-language pathologist has recommended modifications of food or fluid consistencies, the dietitian will review appropriate foods to be included, or the use of thickening agents. Sometimes the challenge is identifying appropriate meal and snack foods that the patient can open and self-feed. The patient and caregivers frequently need new ideas on what they can readily prepare and easily consume. Liquid meal substitutes are often recommended to augment the patient's intake.

In addition to solutions for combating weight loss, the dietitian manages nutrition via feeding tube (see Medical Management). The patient's needs are determined and the enteral formula and regimen are recommended. Bolus feedings are most frequently used; however, patients occasionally follow nighttime or continuous feeding regimens.

Inadequate fluid intake, diminished mobility, and decreased intake of fiber-rich food all contribute to constipation. Patients frequently limit their fluid intake to decrease the number of times they will need to urinate, particularly if they have limited mobility or spend numerous hours alone. The dietitian can work with the patient and caregivers to improve liquid and fiber intake, as well as recommend natural and pharmaceutical laxatives that may be beneficial.

Some ALS patients take herbal supplements and an assortment of vitamin-mineral compounds. The dietitian evaluates what the patient takes and explains the costs, benefits, and risks of the specific supplements. A standard multivitamin mineral complex is recommended.

Psychosocial Considerations

The psychologic impact of ALS permeates all dimensions of life. Depression, anxiety, emotional lability, and changes in interpersonal relationships can occur. Depression and anxiety are assumed to be highly prevalent in any disease with a progressive course and no known cure, but this is not necessarily true in ALS. A recent study indicated that depression is rare in advanced ALS. Intermittent symptoms of depression may, however, occur throughout the course of the illness.[45] Pervasive mood symptoms that do occur can be treated aggressively with psychopharmacologic agents.

ALS affects every member of the family. Although healthy relationships are often made stronger during this challenging time, unhealthy relationships are often made worse. An option is referral for family-based psychotherapy to assist family members and help them maintain a sense of normalcy and develop mutual support.

Discussion of advance directives may include the physician, nurse clinician, or social worker (see Chapter 25). The clinician must present unbiased facts that the patient can incorporate into his or her personal, cultural, and religious beliefs. The *living will* and the *durable power of attorney for health care* forms can be provided by the social worker. Common misconceptions about these forms are that they need to be notarized, that a lawyer is necessary, or that they are the same as a do not resuscitate (DNR) order (see Chapter 25). The social worker will be knowledgeable about forms and will encourage everyone in the family to have them in place.

The decision to go on disability is difficult for many people, and conversations are best initiated by the PALS. Options are short- or long-term disability policies that are associated with one's employment and Social Security disability. One does not necessarily preclude the other. The patient needs to speak with human resources in his or her workplace to maximize the work-related benefits. A social worker can play an important part in helping initiate the Social Security application by making sure that the PALS and the case worker in the Social Security office are knowledgeable of the special exceptions made for PALS. In July 2001, the 24-month waiting period for Medicare was waved for ALS patients (www.ssa.gov/legislation/legis_bulletin_012201.html).

Another difficult but universal topic is care in the home. Even the most supportive families will find that the day-to-day responsibility of providing care can become overwhelming. This need is best met with long-term care insurance, which few people have. The social worker will seek out the resources that are available in the area. Encourage PALS to speak with their insurance company to find out what services are covered. People are often confused about the term *home health* and are surprised to learn that Medicare does not pay for help with activities of daily living (ADLs). Some states have programs associated with Medicaid that can help.

Most people neither qualify for Medicaid nor own long-term care insurance and must consider private pay. Obtaining and keeping adequate caregivers may be one of the biggest challenges facing the family with ALS. The social worker can help people explore options by suggesting ways to find help. Agencies that provide caregiver services are always an option, but the cost is greater than hiring privately. Information can be obtained from www.respitematch.com, a Web site run by an ALS patient that can be helpful in finding caregivers. It is important for the health care team to be attuned to those family members who are providing the care. Talking openly about the stress of this role and the importance of regular relief is crucial.

When one member of the family is severely disabled, his or her partner has to choose between staying home to be the caregiver and going to work to support the family and pay for other caregivers. This causes severe financial strain on families. A social worker may know of resources to help out in specific areas, such as pharmaceutical assistance programs and charitable agencies that provide services or help in other ways, such as building ramps.

Rehabilitation

Speech-Language Therapy

The speech-language pathologist's (SLP's) role in the treatment of ALS patients focuses on identifying compensatory techniques for deficits in swallowing and speech intelligibility. Diagnosis of dysphagia and dysarthria is critical in maintaining a patient's least restrictive diet and maximizing his or her expressive communication.

Deficits in swallowing due to ALS may affect respiratory function, hydration, and nutrition. The SLP will perform a clinical swallowing evaluation at the bedside or tableside to examine the oral mechanism and assess for deficits in the oral phase (mastication and posterior transfer of bolus) and pharyngeal phase (trigger of swallow response, any clinical signs of aspiration) of the swallow. Varied consistencies of solids and liquids are used. Further evaluation via modified barium swallow (MBS) or flexible endoscopic evaluation of swallowing (FEES) may be used for further objective assessment of the swallowing mechanism.

An MBS study is performed by the SLP in conjunction with a radiologist. Under videofluoroscopy, while in an upright position, the patient consumes varied quantities and consistencies of solids and liquid barium. The MBS provides an objective assessment of the structure and function of the swallowing mechanism, as well as details regarding adequacy of airway protection.

A FEES may be conducted instead of an MBS. Using a flexible, fiberoptic endoscope directly inserted into and through the patient's nasal cavity into the hypopharynx, the SLP assesses the structure and function of the swallowing mechanism while the patient actively manages saliva and consumes solids and liquids.

When swallowing becomes impaired, the SLP recommends compensatory strategies (i.e., chin tuck, multiple swallows, alternate solids/liquids, small bites/sips), if it remains safe for the patient to continue oral intake. Nonoral nutrition may be recommended if the patient is at high risk for aspiration or not meeting nutritional needs.

As ALS progresses, a patient may experience a reduction in speech intelligibility. The SLP's role in dysarthria management includes intervention that focuses on maintenance of expressive communication rather than reduction of dysarthria. The SLP assesses the structure and function of the oral mechanism, the current communication method, vocal quality, vocal intensity, resonance, and the percentage of speech that is intelligible in conversation and in oral reading.[13] Immediate needs may include implementation of strategies to conserve energy for communication, increase breath support, overarticulate, use direct eye contact, and decrease environmental distractions during communication acts. The use of oral motor exercises is discouraged because they may fatigue muscles to the point at which functional communication may be compromised.

Future needs may include maintaining functional communication via alternative and augmentative communication (AAC). The SLP assesses a patient's potential for use of augmentative communication techniques to maintain functional communication. AAC methods include no-tech (i.e., gestures, head nods/shakes), low-tech (i.e., communication boards, writing), and high-tech (i.e., speech-generating devices) methods. The patient must be able to physically access the device or communication board, as well as cognitively manage the input and output methods. Trials are conducted to determine the most effective method of augmentative communication. A high-tech speech-generating device is recommended if the patient demonstrates cognitive and motor ability to access the device.

Occupational Therapy

The occupational therapist's (OT's) role in the treatment of ALS patients begins with a full assessment of the individual's current level of independence with ADLs. This includes the ability to feed, groom, dress, bathe, toilet, and transfer oneself. If the individual has difficulty with a particular ADL, compensatory techniques and adaptive equipment are recommended to increase the individual's level of independence and to conserve energy as much as possible.

Regarding transfers, caregivers are educated on the best way to help transfer an individual if the PALS is no longer able to do it on his or her own. Proper body mechanics, including bent knees, a straight back, and keeping the patient close, are recommended.

The OT also assesses upper extremity muscle strength and range of motion. PALS can develop stiff and painful shoulders with limited range of motion. This "frozen shoulder" or adhesive capsulitis is most likely due to inactivity from muscle weakness. Treatment includes moist heat to relax the muscles and manual therapy. Passive range of motion exercises are essential to maintain the current range of motion.

Exercises should only be performed in a pain-free range of shoulder flexion, abduction, internal rotation, and external rotation. Often a physiatrist or orthopedist is consulted for intraarticular steroid injection to help manage the pain. As the pain subsides, active-assistive range of motion may be initiated (in supine position).

Splinting is another part of an OT's job with PALS. For patients who have increased muscle spasticity and whose hands tend to curl up, a resting hand splint to prevent joint contracture is recommended. Resting hand splints could also be helpful for patients with low tone or muscle atrophy to help with proper positioning to avoid nerve compression, tingling, and pain. If the patient is in the early stages of ALS and continues to have finger flexion without extension, a dynamic finger extension splint is sometimes helpful.

Edema management also is addressed. Limb weakness causes dependent edema that can be severe. Elevation, icing, retrograde massage, and "exercise" are encouraged by the caregiver. Compression garments may be helpful as well.

Physical Therapy

The physical therapist's (PT's) role in the treatment of ALS patients is best started soon after diagnosis. Early intervention prepares the patient and family for what the PT can offer them throughout the course of the disease, including exercise, guidelines for physical activity, and equipment prescription. The therapist should design a home exercise program and be prepared to modify the program as the disease progresses.

Initially, physical therapy involves teaching home exercise to prevent development of contractures and poor posture as the disease progresses. Stretching exercises are particularly important for preventing frozen shoulders, discouraging kyphotic posture, and preventing pain and discomfort associated with spastic or tight musculature. As the disease progresses, patients need increasingly more assistance to stretch muscle groups that they can no longer stretch on their own.

Patients often request a program to increase the strength of weak muscles. A common concern is that one could speed up denervation and worsen atrophy by the overuse of weakened muscles. However, the effect of exercise on ALS patients is not well documented and the available literature is inconclusive. Patients should be encouraged to continue their regular exercise program; however, high-resistance and high-repetition activity for any weak muscle group should be discouraged because it will likely result in increased fasciculations and fatigue. It is important to encourage patients to vary their normal workouts to involve numerous muscle groups, as well as to match repetitions and resistance training to their current abilities. For patients who do not routinely exercise, it is best to teach stretching exercises and encourage them to stay as active as they can in their daily routine. A reasonable aerobic exercise program is appropriate to optimize muscle strength and endurance. Gentle, low-impact aerobic exercise such as walking, swimming, and stationary bicycling can strengthen unaffected muscles, improve cardiovascular health, and improve fatigue and depression. When spasticity is present, isotonic exercise is useful but low repetition is advised. Isometric and resistive exercises are not recommended because spastic muscles fatigue quickly and cramping is common.

As with the modification of the exercise program as the disease progresses, the PT will consider the natural history of ALS when recommending and prescribing assistive equipment. Needs should be anticipated, and appropriate equipment should adapt to the evolving requirements of the patient. A careful, periodic evaluation of the ALS patient's functional mobility and safety can result in optimizing resources in a timely and sequential manner. Additionally, keeping up to date on third-party payer guidelines is a challenge but may prevent unnecessary delay in obtaining needed equipment.

Ankle-foot orthoses (AFOs) are the most common and useful aids to safe walking when footdrop occurs. The type of AFO is critical to the success of its use. In the absence of spasticity, it is safest to prescribe a solid or semisolid AFO. Quadriceps weakness can be controlled by increasing the rigidity of the ankle with a solid AFO. If the patient feels overly restricted or the brace impairs balance, the AFO can be easily changed to a semisolid type. When patients need bilateral AFOs, the semisolid brace provides ankle flexibility and improved balance control. Initially a single AFO is recommended, allowing the patient to become accustomed to its presence before the other is made. An orthotic clinic is available in most rehabilitation centers where a trial brace can be used to evaluate the patient's gait pattern and compliance before a final decision is made.

Transfer aids such as sliding boards or hydraulic lifts are almost always necessary at some point during the disease course. Sliding boards can be helpful for car transfers but are temporary as PALS will lose sitting balance in time. Hydraulic lifts work well for many families. A "U"-type or "wrap-around sling" is recommended so patients can easily be placed in the sling while seated. The sling must have head support.

Once ambulation becomes less functional, a qualified therapist should be involved in prescribing an appropriate wheelchair to meet the patient's evolving needs. Wheelchair prescription, seating, and positioning has become a subspecialty for PTs, OTs, and equipment providers. Understanding ALS and the progressive course is vital in determining an appropriate wheelchair for independent mobility, comfort, postural control, and pressure relief (Boxes 21-8 and 21-9).

Special considerations are needed when the patient enters the very late stages of the disease. The patient's end-of-life decisions must be known because the wheelchair will need to accommodate a tray if mechanical ventilation is desired. A "vent tray" placed on the chair allows continued mobility while using assistive breathing devices. When the patient is seen for the first time late in the disease course, or if the patient is unable to drive a power chair, a manual, adjustable, solid-backed chair with pressure relief cushion is considered.

Today's technology provides options that PALS have never had before. Education in the evaluation process is very important to the success of the outcome. Some patients will choose to avoid having to deal with a world that is not inherently accessible or amenable to wheelchairs and high-tech equipment. Overall it is up to the patients to choose how they

BOX 21-8	Considerations When Planning for a Power Wheelchair

- Programmable electronics to accommodate disease progression
- Midwheel drive option for maneuverability and access
- Tilt or recline allows postural control, head control, rest, and pressure relief
- Elevating leg rests, for discomfort associated with dependent edema
- Supportive and soft cushions for seat and back
- Wide-profile arm rests or troughs
- Contoured head rest with potential for anterior head strap or use with a cervical collar

BOX 21-9	Choosing an Equipment Supplier for Power Wheelchairs

- There are no consistent rules regarding who can provide this equipment.
- The National Registry of Rehabilitation Technology Suppliers (NRRTS) has identified suppliers who are qualified to provide high-quality rehabilitation technology and related services to people with disabilities through their registry (www.nrrts.org).
- NRRTS membership confirms that a supplier has demonstrated work experience, received recommendations from professional associates, adheres to a "Code of Ethics," and commits to ongoing continuing education.
- A Certified Rehabilitation Technology Supplier (CRTS) is an NRRTS member in good standing who has successfully completed the Rehabilitation Suppliers of North America (RESNA) credentialing examination. Passing the examination alone qualifies the individual as an Assistive Technology Supplier (ATS).
- Ideally, the patient will work with an experienced therapist in the area of assistive technology or seating and positioning. There is a certification process for therapists in this area, the Assistive Technology Practitioner (ATP).

want to live, and it is the job of the therapist to provide options allowing them to make an informed decision.

Case Management Considerations

The following are tips for the case manager working with patients with ALS:

- Obtain an accurate assessment of insurance coverage.
- Refer the patient to an ALS center to maximize efficiency and minimize the cost of care.
- Review the standard of care for ALS patients published by the American Academy of Neurology and use it as a minimum standard.
- Refer patients to the MDA and ALSA for additional support, clinical trial information, and educational materials.

- Facilitate and attempt to eliminate delays in obtaining the usual durable medical equipment that any homebound person would need.
- Verify that a qualified seating specialist has prescribed the wheelchair.
- Assist the patient in planning for private home care.
- Encourage the patient to complete advance directives. Patients who choose a natural death (with or without NIPPV) have the right to continuous, comprehensive management of symptoms associated with the dying process.
- Depending on their insurance coverage, patients with mechanical ventilation may be able to access skilled nursing care in the home; ultimately, however, long-term planning is necessary.
- Feeding tubes and NIPPV do not prohibit entry into hospice.

Home Care

ALS is a fatal neuromuscular disease that leads to progressive paralysis of the muscles. The goal of care is to individualize each patient's services to enhance or to maintain the patient's quality of life until death.

Most ALS patients are cared for in the home. Those without families or without families able or willing to provide care will seek long-term care facilities. Funding this option is even more challenging than funding care in the home (see Psychosocial Considerations). Most patients will have to pay out of pocket until their resources are exhausted. At that point they will switch to public support.

PALS who choose long-term invasive ventilation face enormous challenges because only a tiny percentage of long-term care facilities will accept ventilator patients without weaning potential. Most PALS on vents are cared for at home by family members. These patients eventually become quadriplegic and mute, so communication systems must be obtained in advance to prevent them from being locked in (see Speech-Language Therapy).

The majority of PALS do not choose tracheostomy and ventilation but choose to receive symptomatic treatment and end-of-life care at home. Hospice provides highly effective palliative care to ALS patients and their families. The hospice philosophy is life affirming and supports PALS in maintaining their dignity and comfort through this last phase of the disease.

CONCLUSION

The most important role of the ALS team is to talk to patients and their families about how the disease is affecting their lives. This is not always easy, and a level of trust is necessary for it to be of value. Listening is primary. People want answers, but more important, they want to be heard. Having the strength and the willingness to sit still for a moment and listen as these brave people slowly and courageously face their future is probably worth more than anything else that a health care provider can do.

Acknowledgments

The following contributors are acknowledged for the content they submitted for this chapter. Nutritional considerations: Elizabeth Kustin, dietitian; psychosocial considerations: Martha Giardina, social worker; rehabilitation considerations: Diane Beckwith, physical therapist; Kathleen Herrelko, speech-language pathologist; Melissa Tober, occupational therapist, Emory University Hospital, Atlanta, GA.

RESOURCES

ALS Association: 818-880-9007; www.alsa.org

Alzheimer's Association: 800-272-3900; www.alz.org

Alzheimer's Disease Education and Referral Center (ADEAR): 800-438-4380; www.alzheimers.org

Association for Frontotemporal Dementia: 866-507-7222; www.FTD-Picks.org

Family Caregiver Alliance/National Center on Caregiving: 800-445-8106; www.caregiver.org

Lewy Body Dementia Association: 800-539-9767; www.lewybodydementia.org

Muscular Dystrophy Association: 800-572-1717; www.mda.org

National Institute of Mental Health (NIMH): 866-615-6464; www.nimh.nih.gov

National Institute on Aging (NIA), National Institutes of Health, Department of Health and Human Services: 800-222-2225; www.nia.nih.org

Robert Packard Center for ALS Research: www.alscenter.org

World Federation of Neurology Research Group on ALS: www.wfnals.org

www.clinicaltrials.gov: provides regularly updated information about federally and privately supported clinical research in human volunteers

www.quackwatch.com: nonprofit corporation whose purpose is to combat health-related frauds, myths, fads, and fallacies

REFERENCES

1. Anderson PM et al: Sixteen novel mutations in the Cu/Zn superoxide dismutase gene in amyotrophic lateral sclerosis: a decade of discoveries, defects and disputes, *Amyotroph Lateral Scler Other Motor Neuron Disord* 4:62–72, 2003.
2. Barker WW et al: Relative frequencies of Alzheimer's disease, Lewy body, vascular and frontotemporal dementia and hippocampal sclerosis in the state of Florida brain bank, *Alzheimer Dis Assoc Disord* 16:203–212, 2002.
3. Beck AT et al: An inventory for measuring depression, *Arch Gen Psychiatry* 4:561–571, 1961.
4. Bensimon G, Lacomblez L, Meininger V, et al: A controlled trial of riluzole in amyotrophic lateral sclerosis, *N Engl J Med* 330(9):585–591, 1994.
5. Bourke SC, Tomlinson M, Williams TI: Effects of non-invasive ventilation on survival and quality of life in patients with amyotrophic lateral sclerosis: a randomized controlled trial, *Lancet Neurology* 5:140–147, 2006.
6. Brody EM et al: A longitudinal look at excess disabilities in the mentally impaired aged, *J Gerontol* 29:79–84, 1974.
7. Brooks BR et al: El escorial revisited: revised criteria for the diagnosis of amyotrophic lateral sclerosis, *Amyotroph Lateral Scler Other Motor Neuron Disord* 1:293–299, 2000.
8. Callahan CM, Hendrie HC, Tierney M: Documentation and evaluation of cognitive impairment in elderly primary care patients, *Ann Intern Med* 122:422–429, 1995.
9. Cleveland DW, Rothstein JD: From Charcot to Lou Gehrig: deciphering selective motor neuron death in ALS, *Nature Reviews Neuroscience* 2(11):806–819, 2001.
10. Corder EH et al: Gene dose of apolipoprotein E type 4 allele and the risk of Alzheimer's disease in late onset families, *Science* 261:921–923, 1993.
11. Cudkowicz ME et al: A randomized, placebo-controlled trial of topiramate in amyotrophic lateral sclerosis, *Neurology* 61(4):456–464, 2003.
12. Cummings JL et al: The Neuropsychiatric Inventory: assessing psychopathology in dementia patients, *Neurology* 44:2308–2314, 1994.
13. Darley FL, Aronson AE, Brown JR: *Motor speech disorders,* Philadelphia, 1975, Saunders.
14. Desport JC et al: Complications and survival following radiologically and endoscopically-guided gastrostomy in patients with amyotrophic lateral sclerosis, *Amyotroph Lateral Scler Other Motor Neuron Disord* 6(2):88–93, 2005.
15. *Diagnostic and statistical manual of mental disorders DSM-IV-TR,* Arlington, VA, 2004, American Psychiatric Association, pp 157–158.
16. Evans DA et al: Prevalence of Alzheimer's disease in a community population of older persons, *JAMA* 262:2551–2556, 1989.
17. Ferman TJ et al: DLB fluctuations: specific features that reliably differentiate DLB from AD and normal aging, *Neurology* 62:181–187, 2004.
18. Folstein MF, Folstein SF, McHugh PR: Mini-mental state: a practical method for grading the cognitive state of patients for the clinician, *J Psychiatr Res* 12:189–198, 1975.
19. Forshew DA, Bromberg MB: A survey of clinicians' practice in the symptomatic treatment of ALS, *Amyotroph Lateral Scler Other Motor Neuron Disord* 4:258–263, 2003.
20. Goldstein FC et al: Hypertension and cognitive functioning in African-Americans with probable Alzheimer's disease, *Neurology* 64:899–901, 2005.
21. Hall G: Caring for people with Alzheimer's disease using the conceptual model of progressively lowered stress threshold in the clinical setting, *Nurs Clin North Am* 30:129–141, 1994.
22. Hardy J, Selkoe DJ: The amyloid hypothesis of Alzheimer's disease: progress and problems on the road to therapeutics, *Science* 297:353–356, 2002.
23. Hebert LE et al: Alzheimer's disease in the US population: prevalence estimates using the 2000 census, *Arch Neurol* 60:1119–1122, 2003.
24. Katz S et al: Studies of illness in the aged, *JAMA* 185:914–919, 1963.
25. Kivipelto M et al: Midlife vascular risk factors and Alzheimer's disease in later life: longitudinal, population based study, *BMJ* 322:1447–1451, 2001.
26. Kivipelto M et al: Apolipoprotein E c4 allele, elevated midlife total cholesterol level, and high midlife systolic blood pressure are independent risk factors for late-life Alzheimer disease, *Ann Intern Med* 137:149–155, 2002.
27. Knopman DS et al: Practice parameter: diagnosis of dementia (an evidence-based review). Report of the Quality Standards Subcommittee of the American Academy of Neurology, *Neurology* 56:1143–1153, 2001.
28. Lacomblez L et al: Dose-ranging study of riluzole in amyotrophic lateral sclerosis, *Lancet* 347(9013):1425–1431, 1996.

29. Launer LJ et al: Rates and risk factors for dementia and Alzheimer's disease: results from EURODEM pooled analyses, *Neurology* 52:78–84, 1999.

30. Lawton MP, Brody EM: Assessment of older people: self maintaining and instrumental activities of daily living, *Gerontologist* 9:179–186. 1969.

31. Lomen-Hoerth C, Anderson T, Miller B: The overlap of amyotrophic lateral sclerosis and frontotemporal dementia, *Neurology* 59:1077–1079, 2002.

32. Lomen-Hoerth C et al: Are amyotrophic lateral sclerosis patients cognitively normal? *Neurology* 60:1094–1097, 2003.

33. Marquardt G, Lorenz R: Intrathecal baclofen for intractable spasticity in amyotrophic lateral sclerosis, *J Neurol* 246(7):619–620, 1999.

34. Marquardt G, Seifert V: Use of intrathecal baclofen for treatment of spasticity in amyotrophic lateral sclerosis, *J Neurol Neurosurg Psychiatry* 72(2):275–276, 2002.

35. McKeith IG et al: Consensus guidelines for the clinical and pathologic diagnosis of dementia with Lewy bodies (DLB): report of the consortium on DLB international workshop, *Neurology* 47:1113–1124, 1996.

36. Miller RG et al: Practice parameter: the care of the patient with amyotrophic lateral sclerosis (an evidence-based review): report of the Quality Standards Subcommittee of the American Academy of Neurology, *Neurology* 52:1311, 1999.

37. Miller RG et al: Riluzole for amyotrophic lateral sclerosis (ALS)/motor neuron disease (MND), *Cochrane Database of Systematic Reviews* 2:CD001447, 2002.

38. Miller RG: Phase III randomized trial of gabapentin in patients with amyotrophic lateral sclerosis, *Neurology* 56(7):843–848, 2001.

39. Mitsumoto H, Chad DA, Pioro EP: *Amyotrophic lateral sclerosis. Contemporary neurology series,* New York, 1998, Oxford Press.

40. Murry B, Mitsumoto H: Disorders of upper and lower motor neurons. In Bradley WG et al, editors: *Neurology in clinical practice,* Philadelphia, 2004, Butterworth Heinemann.

41. Papka M, Rubio A, Schiffer RB: A review of Lewy body disease: an emerging concept of cortical dementia, *Neuropsychiatry Clin Neurosci* 10:267–279, 1998.

42. Peterson RC et al: Mild cognitive impairment: clinical characterization and outcome, *Arch Neurol* 56:303–308, 1999.

43. Peterson RC et al: Practice parameter: early detection of dementia: mild cognitive impairment (an evidence based review). Report of the Quality Standards Subcommittee of the American Academy of Neurology, *Neurology* 56:1133–1142, 2001.

44. Pfeffer RI, Kurosaki TT, Harrah CH: Measurement of functional activities in older adults in the community, *J Gerontol* 37:323–329, 1982.

45. Rabkin JG et al: Prevalence of depressive disorders and change over time in late-stage ALS, *Neurology* 65(1):62–67, 2005.

46. Ransmayr G: Dementia with Lewy bodies: prevalence, clinical spectrum and natural history, *J Neural Transm Suppl* 60:303–314, 2000.

47. Ratnavalli E et al: The prevalence of frontotemporal dementia, *Neurology* 58:1615–1621, 2002.

48. Ringholz GM et al: Prevalence and patterns of cognitive impairment in sporadic ALS, *Neurology* 65:586–590, 2005.

49. Roman GC: Stroke, cognitive decline and vascular dementia: the silent epidemic of the 21st century, *Neuroepidemiology* 22:161–164, 2003.

50. Roman GC: Vascular dementia: distinguishing characteristics, treatment, and prevention, *J Am Geriatr Soc* 51:S296–S304, 2003.

51. Roman GC et al: Vascular dementia: diagnostic criteria for research studies. Report of the NINDS-AIREN International Workshop, *Neurology* 43:250–260, 1993.

52. Rowland LP, Shneider NA: Amyotrophic lateral sclerosis, *N Engl J Med* 344(22):249, 2001.

53. Rosen DR, Siddique T, Patterson D, et al: Mutations in Cu/Zn superoxide dismutase gene are associated with familial amyotrophic lateral sclerosis, *Nature* 362:59–63, 1993.

54. Sano M et al: A controlled trial of selegeline, alpha-tocopherol, or both as treatment for Alzheimer's disease, *N Engl J Med* 336:1216–1222, 1997.

55. Sejvar JJ: Amyotrophic lateral sclerosis mortality in the United States, 1979–2001, *Neuroepidemiology* 25:144–152, 2005.

56. Shefner JM et al: A clinical trial of creatine in ALS, *Neurology* 63(9):1656–1661, 2004.

57. Seshadri S et al: Plasma homocysteine as a risk factor for dementia and Alzheimer's disease, *N Engl J Med* 346:476–483, 2002.

58. Snowdon DA, Greiner L: Brain infarction and the clinical expression of Alzheimer's disease. The Nun study, *JAMA* 277:813–817, 1997.

59. Stevens T et al: Islington study of dementia subtypes in the community, *Br J Psychiatry* 180:270–276, 2002.

60. Swash M: An algorithm for ALS diagnosis and management, *Neurology* 53(8 suppl 5):S58–S62, 1999.

61. Unterborn PC et al: Pulmonary complications of chronic neuromuscular diseases and their management, *Muscle Nerve* 29(1):5–27, 2004.

62. Yesavage JA et al: Development and validation of a geriatric depression screening scale: a preliminary report, *J Psychiatr Res* 17:37–49, 1983.

CHAPTER 22

MARCIA S. LORIMER,
BERNADETTE TUCKER-LIPSCOMB,
DONALD B. SANDERS

Neuromuscular Junction and Muscle Disease

Chronic muscle weakness, fatigue, and restlessness are common symptoms with many possible causes. Diseases that affect the neuromuscular junction and muscle fibers may produce weakness and other complex symptoms. The primary focus of this chapter is myasthenia gravis (MG) and related disorders of the neuromuscular junction. Information about myopathies and restless legs syndrome (RLS) is also presented.

There have been many advances in the diagnosis and treatment of these disorders in recent years; however, the choice of treatment for individual patients requires clinical acumen and experience. Additional research is needed to identify more targeted and efficacious treatments that have minimal adverse effects.

NEUROMUSCULAR JUNCTION DISORDER

Myasthenia Gravis

Myasthenia gravis (MG) is the most common primary disorder of neuromuscular transmission. It is a chronic autoimmune disorder that results from a defect in the transmission of nerve impulses at the postsynaptic membrane of the neuromuscular junction. This leads to the hallmark symptoms of variable and fatigable weakness of voluntary muscle groups. Related disorders include **Lambert-Eaton myasthenic syndrome (LEMS)** and **congenital myasthenia gravis (CMG) syndromes.** LEMS is also autoimmune and results from a defect at the presynaptic terminal of the neuromuscular junction. Patients with LEMS typically have proximal muscle weakness, especially in the lower limbs, and frequently have associated carcinomas. CMG syndromes are rare inherited forms of myasthenia. Symptoms of weakness are generally milder and present at birth or in early life. The information in this chapter focuses on autoimmune or acquired MG with brief descriptions of related disorders. A cure remains elusive, despite extraordinary advances in the understanding and treatment of MG. Without recognition and treatment, MG may be life threatening when the muscles supporting respiration are involved.

Etiology and Prevalence

The etiology of MG is an acquired autoimmune process. The immunologic basis for MG was established in the 1970s when antibodies directed against the acetylcholine receptor (AChR) on the motor end-plate were identified.[12] This breakthrough led to the development of an experimental animal model. MG is perhaps the best understood autoimmune disease, although understanding of what triggers the immunologic process responsible for the disorder is incomplete. There is considerable variation in muscle group involvement leading to differences in the course of illness among individual patients. MG symptoms are usually more variable and fulminating in the first few years after onset. Multiple therapeutic interventions have been tried but few are supported by scientific evidence from carefully designed studies. The Medical/Scientific Advisory Board of the Myasthenia Gravis Foundation of America formed a task force to address the need for a universally accepted clinical classification system that could be used to study various therapeutic interventions. The classification system helps to identify subgroups of individuals with MG who have similar clinical attributes. The Task Force also developed a system to define responses to treatment and recommended methods to measure disease severity that can be used in clinical treatment trials.[17]

Population-based studies have demonstrated MG to be an uncommon disorder, affecting approximately 20 per 100,000 or approximately 60,000 people in the United States.[13] The reported prevalence rates have increased over the past several decades, most likely because of better recognition of MG, earlier diagnosis, and more specific treatments resulting in decreasing mortality. Although MG occurs in all ethnic groups and in both men and women, the most common age of onset is the second and third decades in females and the seventh and eighth decades in males. Early studies showed that women were more often affected than men. Because the general population is aging and living longer, the average age at onset has increased and males are now more affected than females.[19] These demographic changes suggest that health professionals can expect to encounter greater numbers of MG patients in the future.

LEMS is a rare disorder that results from an antibody attack against voltage-gated calcium channels (VGCCs) on the presynaptic motor nerve terminal. VGCCs control the release of the neurotransmitter acetylcholine (ACh) at the neuromuscular junction. LEMS has a deduced prevalence of 1 per 100,000 or approximately 2800 people in the United

States. Fifty-three percent of patients with LEMS are male, and the usual onset is in middle to late life. Forty percent of patients with LEMS have a carcinoma; the most common is small-cell lung cancer.[14]

CMG syndromes are rare genetic disorders of the neuromuscular junction. There are many types of CMG syndromes, which are classified by location of the defect in the neuromuscular junction. Defects can be presynaptic, synaptic, or postsynaptic.

Pathophysiology

The weakness of MG results from the destructive and inflammatory action of circulating antibodies that disrupt neuromuscular transmission. The neuromuscular junction is a synapse that transmits nerve impulses from the nerve terminal to the motor end-plate on the muscle. This is accomplished by the release of the neurotransmitter ACh, which is synthesized and stored in synaptic vesicles in the motor nerve terminal. Each vesicle contains a quantum of ACh molecules. For muscle contraction to occur the many quanta must cross the synaptic cleft and bind to AChRs on the motor end-plate of the postsynaptic muscle membrane, causing an action potential.

In autoimmune MG, the concentration of AChRs is reduced, the postsynaptic muscle membrane becomes distorted and simplified, and AChR antibodies become attached to the membrane. ACh is released normally, but its effect on the postsynaptic membrane is reduced and muscle weakness ensues (Fig. 22-1). Most patients with MG have measurable circulating AChR antibodies in their blood, although these antibodies may not be detectable in the initial months of symptoms. In approximately 15% of MG patients, AChR antibodies cannot be detected using the usual assay techniques. These patients are referred to as having seronegative MG.

Some patients who are seronegative for AChR antibodies have detectable antibodies to muscle-specific receptor tyrosine kinase (MuSK), which is a polypeptide found on the muscle side of the neuromuscular junction. MuSK has been identified as being necessary for the formation of AChR clusters.[4] Patients who test positive for MuSK antibodies frequently have a different clinical presentation than those who are AChR antibody positive. They are frequently young adult females with bulbar, neck, or respiratory muscle weakness. By studying the clinical phenotypes of patients with AChR and MuSK antibodies and learning more about the mechanism of anti-MuSK antibody actions, researchers hope to identify more targeted treatments for patients.[15,20] It is suspected that other, not yet identified antibodies, may be responsible for neuromuscular dysfunction in patients who do not have anti-MuSK or anti-AChR antibodies.

The role of the thymus in the pathophysiology of MG is unclear but thymic abnormalities are common and may be responsible for causing the immune attack on the AChR in MG. Hyperplasia and tumors of the thymus are frequently found in MG patients. Thymectomy, the removal of the thymus, seems to improve the clinical course in most patients. Thymoma is a rare thymic tumor that occurs in about 10% to 15% of patients with MG. Most of these patients have antibodies to striated muscle.

Assessment

MG is characterized by fluctuating skeletal muscle weakness and fatigue that is exacerbated by exercise. A high index of suspicion is important in diagnosing the disorder. When providing subjective data, the MG patient typically reports

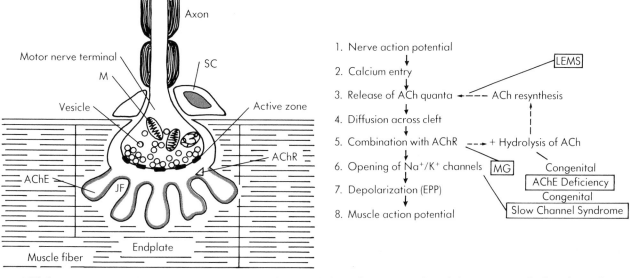

Figure 22-1 Pathophysiology of neuromuscular junction disorders. Schematic representation of the neuromuscular junction and summary of presynaptic and postsynaptic processes in neuromuscular transmission. The locations of the acquired lesions in MG and other myasthenic syndromes are indicated. *ACh,* Acetylcholine; *AChE,* acetylcholinesterase; *AChR,* acetylcholine receptor; *LEMS,* Lambert-Eaton myasthenic syndrome; *EPP,* end-plate potential; *JF,* junctional fold; *M,* mitochondria; *MG,* myasthenia gravis; *SC,* Schwann cell. *(Modified from Kim YI: Neuromuscular transmission in myasthenia gravis,* Semin Neurol 2[3]:199, 1982.)

fluctuating fatigable weakness that increases as the day progresses and improves with rest. Patterns of weakness are individual and may fluctuate from muscle group to muscle group in some patients. In addition, stressors such as emotional upset, infection, immunizations, menses, pregnancy, increased body temperature, hypothyroidism or hyperthyroidism, and drugs affecting neurotransmission may exacerbate weakness.

A variety of clinical presentations may occur but the earliest symptoms most commonly involve the ocular muscles, with patients reporting diplopia and/or ptosis. Diplopia may manifest itself as blurred or double vision. Ptosis may be reported as unilateral or bilateral but is typically asymmetric. Nasal speech quality, nasal regurgitation, and difficulty chewing and swallowing are initially reported in a smaller number of patients. Still fewer patients report limb weakness as the initial symptom. The symptoms typically progress over time from limited ocular symptoms to more generalized weakness including difficulty holding the head erect, dyspnea, and girdle and limb weakness. In approximately 15% of patients, symptoms remain limited to ocular muscles alone (ocular myasthenia).

The technique used in the objective assessment should detect fluctuating and fatigable weakness in specific muscle groups. Examination of the cranial nerves in patients with MG usually reveals asymmetric weakness of the extraocular muscles, lid ptosis, and weakness of eyelid closure. Patients may also have facial weakness and lack of facial expression, inability to fully raise the eyebrows, inability to frown or smile (attempts to smile may resemble a sneer), inability to tightly close the eyelids, and inability to puff out the cheeks. Pharyngeal and palatal weakness is exhibited as nasal speech, difficulty swallowing, and regurgitation of liquids through the nares. Other cranial nerve findings may include trapezii weakness on shoulder shrug against resistance, sternomastoid weakness against resistance, and tongue weakness with accompanying inarticulate speech.

MG patients with generalized weakness may have difficulty walking or rising from sitting because of proximal weakness. Coordination will be intact and tandem walking will not demonstrate ataxia. Grip and arm muscles may be weak. In the motor assessment, the MG patient may display an abnormal body position because of weakness. For example, the patient with severe neck muscle weakness may sit supporting his chin on his hand. Involuntary movements are not present. Muscle bulk should be normal, although atrophy may occur if chronic weakness has been untreated. Tone may be diminished because of weakness.

Muscle strength should be assessed after repeated use and after rest (see Chapter 2). The Quantitative MG Score for Disease Severity and manual muscle testing may be used to objectively assess muscle strength.[16] The speed of rapid alternating movements may be affected by weakness but the rhythm and smoothness will be unaffected. Point-to-point movements are accurate and smooth. Pain, temperature, position sense, vibration, light touch, and discrimination are all intact in the sensory assessment. Stretch reflexes are normal to slightly diminished.

The results of a mental status assessment may be influenced by MG weakness particularly when there is respiratory insufficiency. Appearance and behavior may be affected. The patient may appear depressed if facial muscles are weak. If there is air hunger, the patient may be anxious and confused. The quality, rate, volume, and fluency of speech and language may be affected by weakness but there will be no aphasia. Mood may be affected by weakness and reaction to illness. Thoughts and perceptions are not affected. Memory and attention may be affected by respiratory insufficiency but orientation to time, place, and person are intact. Finally, cognition may be affected when there is insufficient air exchange.

MG patients should have an assessment of respiratory effort. They should be observed for positions that suggest dyspnea or orthopnea. Patients with respiratory compromise may yawn frequently or sigh deeply. Evaluate any cough for aspiration of saliva, liquids, or solid foods. The use of pulmonary function tests (e.g., spirometry) can help quantify respiratory effort, and the use of pulse oximetry will quantify oxygen saturation.

Neurodiagnostic and Laboratory Studies

In addition to a careful history and physical examination, neurodiagnostic studies help to confirm the diagnosis of MG. Electrophysiologic, pharmacologic, and serologic testing are commonly used in diagnosis.

- **Repetitive nerve stimulation (RNS)** is the most common electrophysiological test used to evaluate neuromuscular transmission. RNS measures muscle action potentials after rapidly repeated nerve stimulation. In MG, there is a decremental muscle response.
- **Single fiber electromyography (SFEMG)** is an electrophysiologic test that is considered to be the most sensitive clinical test of neurotransmission. If appropriate muscles are tested, almost all patients with MG will have increased "jitter."[9]
- **Edrophonium chloride (Tensilon)** is an intravenous (IV) pharmacologic agent that has rapid onset and short duration. It increases neurotransmission by inhibiting cholinesterase in the neuromuscular junction (Box 22-1).
- **AChR antibody titers** are serologic tests that are generally regarded as being the most specific for autoimmune MG. Approximately 85% of patients with generalized MG have circulating AChR antibodies.[21]
- **Anti-MuSK antibody test** is a serologic assay that identifies antibodies to MuSK. A positive test confirms MG in AChR antibody seronegative patients.
- **VGCC antibody test** is a serologic assay that identifies antibodies directed against the VGCC on the presynaptic nerve terminal. It is positive in most LEMS patients.
- **Ice pack test** is a simple and quick method sometimes used to determine whether lid ptosis is caused by MG. An ice pack is applied to the eye for 2 minutes. Improvement in ptosis is considered a positive response.
- **Muscle biopsy** may be performed in MG patients who are seronegative for antibodies and have normal or indeterminate electrodiagnostic findings. Muscle biopsy is used in the diagnosis of CMG.

BOX 22-1	Edrophonium Chloride (Tensilon) Test

The most important task in preparing for an informative edrophonium test is to select a focal area of weakness to test. The experienced clinician can objectively evaluate ocular or pharyngeal weakness by observing the degree of ptosis or diplopia, or by assessing the patient's ability to count to 100 (noting the number at which dysarthria or dysphonia becomes evident). Other muscle groups, which require a more subjective evaluation of improved weakness, are less reliable.

The edrophonium dose that produces improvement in weakness varies among patients. IV administration of edrophonium typically begins with the preparation of 1 ml of edrophonium (10 mg) in a 1-ml syringe. The experienced provider should administer 0.2 ml (2 mg) IV push as a test dose. If there are no adverse events, additional edrophonium (between 3 and 5 mg) is administered via a very slow IV push. An abrupt and observable improvement in symptoms lasting for a few minutes is a positive response.

ALERT: The edrophonium test is not without risk. Patients with bronchospasm or cardiac dysrhythmias are generally excluded from edrophonium testing. Atropine (0.6 mg for intramuscular or intravenous injection) must be at the bedside to counter any adverse effects.[9] The patient's pulse must be monitored, and special attention must be given to older patients, patients with a cardiac history, and patients taking beta blockers or digoxin.

- **Computed tomography (CT) scan** of the mediastinum is performed to detect thymoma or hyperplasia of the thymus.
- **Thyroid function tests** are frequently performed to evaluate for any coexisting autoimmune thyroid disease.

Treatment

Medical Management. Anticholinesterases are the first line of treatment for MG. **Pyridostigmine bromide (Mestinon)** is the principal agent prescribed. It prolongs the effect of ACh in the neuromuscular junction by reducing the action of cholinesterase. Anticholinesterases temporarily improve muscle strength through this action but they do not treat the underlying autoimmune MG defect. There is no standard dose schedule. Doses are individually adjusted, and the patient and provider must work together closely to determine the most effective regimen, which is aimed at reducing weakness in the muscles that cause the greatest disability with minimal adverse effects. Patients with MuSK antibodies frequently do not respond to anticholinesterases.

ALERT: It is important to give pyridostigmine on time and exactly as ordered. A delay in administration may find the patient too weak to swallow the pills. Administration at intervals shorter or longer than ordered should be avoided, even if the time deviations are within those generally acceptable for hospital procedure.

Overdose of anticholinesterase agents may result in cholinergic weakness that may be difficult to distinguish from myasthenic weakness. Patients taking pyridostigmine should be monitored for adverse effects, which may be indicative of overdose. These result from ACh accumulation at the muscarinic receptors on smooth muscle and autonomic glands and at the nicotinic receptors of skeletal muscle. The most common adverse effects are gastrointestinal (GI) discomfort, loose stools, diarrhea, nausea, and vomiting. Other adverse effects include increased bronchial and oral secretions and may further compromise patients with swallowing or respiratory symptoms. Muscle fasciculations and cramps are common adverse effects also. All adverse reactions must be reported to the MG-treating provider.

Not all pyridostigmine preparations are equal. Regular-release pyridostigmine is available in tablet and syrup formulations. A slow-release pyridostigmine tablet (Mestinon Timespan) is also available as a bedtime dose for patients who are too weak to swallow a pill upon awakening. Overdosage and underdosage are more likely to occur with Mestinon Timespan because its absorption and effect are sometimes erratic. Some providers prefer to schedule nighttime doses of regular-release pyridostigmine rather than use the slow-release preparation. Milligram for milligram, regular- and slow-release formulations are not equal. Pyridostigmine is available also in a parenteral solution (Regonol Solution for Injection) for the patient who cannot take anything by mouth. The provider will generally order one thirtieth of the usual oral regular-release pyridostigmine dose by intramuscular (IM) injection or very slow IV administration.

Plasmapheresis or **plasma exchange (PEX)** is another short-term treatment for autoimmune MG. This procedure involves the removal of plasma, which contains the disease-producing circulating antibodies. Patients with AChR and MuSK antibodies, as well as those without detectable autoantibodies, usually have improved MG weakness after PEX. PEX is used to induce improvement when there has been a rapid increase in muscle weakness especially if it involves oropharyngeal or respiratory compromise. A course of PEX is often performed just before surgery to reduce moderate to severe weakness. Finally, PEX may be added if current treatments are insufficient to control debilitating weakness. The procedure takes from 1 to 3 hours and is generally performed in a series of alternate-day exchanges over a 10-day period. PEX works quickly and most patients begin to have improved strength within a few days of treatment. Benefit is sustained typically for 3 to 6 weeks. Limiting factors include the expense and possible adverse effects. Placement of a central line catheter may be required for venous access and the patient must be monitored for infection, bleeding, clotting problems, hypotension, and toxic reactions.[7]

Intravenous immunoglobulin (IVIg) treatment involves the administration of pooled human gamma globulin, which usually produces a relatively quick and short-term relief of MG weakness. IVIg is thought to have a suppressive effect on the patient's immune system. Indications for IVIg are similar to those for PEX. It is administered by slow IV infusion and patients must be monitored closely for headache and aseptic meningitis. If used in selected patients on a long-term adjunctive basis, one to three treatments per month are commonly required.

Immunosuppressant Agents

Prednisone is a corticosteroid that is an effective and inexpensive treatment for autoimmune MG. It produces rapid and significant improvement in most patients by suppressing the immune system. Significant adverse effects (Table 22-1) may occur and are related to the dose and length of time that it is used. The initial prednisone dose may be as much as 60 to 80 mg per day and may cause worsening of MG symptoms. For this reason, patients may be hospitalized for close monitoring. This regimen will be continued until sustained improvement occurs, usually 2 to 4 weeks. An alternate-day schedule will then be ordered to minimize adverse effects. Using this approach, the dose of prednisone will be kept constant until maximum improvement is achieved. Then the dose is gradually tapered over a period of several months to the minimum maintenance dose required to sustain improvement. An alternative approach is to begin with smaller doses of prednisone daily (typically 5 to 10 mg), increase gradually until maximum improvement occurs, then switch to alternate-day administration. When a maintenance dose of prednisone (5 to 10 mg per day) does not sufficiently sustain clinical improvement, additional immunosuppressive agents may be ordered with the goal of eventually eliminating the need for prednisone and minimizing the use of pyridostigmine.

Azathioprine is a nonsteroidal immunosuppressant that is typically added when patients relapse, do not respond, or have unacceptable side effects while on prednisone. It may be used also as the initial immunosuppressant, with or without prednisone. Azathioprine is available in tablet formulation; initial dosing is 50 mg per day, which is increased weekly to the typical maintenance dose of 150 to 200 mg per day. After obtaining baseline values, complete blood count (CBC) and liver function tests must be monitored weekly for 1 month and then every month for 6 months after initiating therapy. Response to therapy may not be evident for 3 to 12 months. A hypersensitivity reaction may occur in as many as 20% of patients taking azathioprine, usually about 2 weeks after initiation. The reaction may include flu-like symptoms, fever, rash, or malaise. The patient should stop taking azathioprine and immediately contact the provider if this occurs.

Cyclosporine is an immunosuppressant agent that is prescribed to help patients lower the dose of prednisone required to maintain improvement. It is available in capsule or liquid form and is typically taken at 12-hour intervals after a meal. Clinical improvement usually begins within 1 to 2 months after initiating treatment. The dose of cyclosporine is adjusted based on trough plasma cyclosporine levels drawn 12 hours after the last dose. Blood pressure checks and creatinine levels to assess for renal toxicity are performed at monthly intervals for the first 6 months, and less frequently thereafter. Other adverse effects include hirsutism, hypertension, gum hyperplasia, nausea, and tremor.

Mycophenolate mofetil (CellCept) is a relatively new immunosuppressant being studied for safety and efficacy in MG patients. Like cyclosporine, improvement typically begins in the first months after initiating treatment. By using mycophenolate, clinicians hope to lower or eliminate prednisone required to sustain improvement in weakness. An early retrospective study indicates that mycophenolate is safe, well tolerated, and produces clinical improvement in 75% of treated patients. Few adverse effects were reported, with diarrhea most common.[8] Baseline and monthly CBC monitoring is performed.

Cyclophosphamide (Cytoxan) and **methotrexate** are potent immunosuppressive agents used rarely for MG patients who are unresponsive to other therapies.

Other medications may exacerbate MG weakness. A variety of medications have been reported to increase MG or LEMS weakness by impairing neuromuscular transmission (Box 22-2). Much of this information is anecdotal but should

---

TABLE 22-1   Adverse Effects of Prednisone Treatment

Adverse effects are usually related to dose and length of time prednisone is used. Patients should take prednisone exactly as prescribed. Stopping prednisone abruptly may result in adrenal insufficiency. Alternate-day dosing may reduce adverse effects.

Reaction	Monitoring/Intervention
Insomnia and mood changes such as depression or euphoria	Prednisone should be taken as a single dose in the morning to reduce insomnia.
Increased appetite and weight gain	Monitoring caloric intake and maintaining an exercise plan will minimize weight gain.
Hyperglycemia	Monitor for steroid-induced diabetes. Reduce dietary intake of simple carbohydrates.
Dyspepsia or peptic ulcer	Take prednisone with food, milk, or antacids.
Fluid retention secondary to sodium retention and potassium depletion	A sodium-restricted diet and increased dietary potassium intake may help to reduce fluid retention.
Osteoporosis (long-term use)	Monitor through bone density studies. Increase dietary and supplemental calcium and vitamin D. Drugs to prevent osteoporosis may be prescribed.
Cushingoid features, acne, skin atrophy (long-term use)	Alternate-day dosing may reduce adverse effects.
Cataracts and glaucoma (long-term use)	Yearly screening ophthalmologic exams are recommended.

BOX 22-2	Myasthenia Gravis Drug Alert

1. D-penicillamine and interferon alpha should never be used in myasthenic patients.
2. The following drugs produce worsening of weakness in most MG patients who receive them. Use with caution and monitor patient for exacerbation of myasthenic symptoms:
   Succinylcholine, d-tubocurarine, vecuronium or other neuromuscular blocking agents
   Quinine, quinidine, or procainamide
   Certain antibiotics, particularly tobramycin, gentamicin, kanamycin, neomycin, streptomycin, colistin, erythromycin, telithromycin, and fluoroquinolones (ciprofloxacin, norfloxacin, ofloxacin, pefloxacin)
   Beta-blockers: propranolol, timolol maleate eye drops
   Calcium channel blockers
   Iodinated contrast agents
   Magnesium, including Milk of Magnesia, Maalox, and Epsom salt
3. Many other drugs are reported to exacerbate the weakness in some MG patients. All MG patients should be observed for increased weakness when a new medication is started.

not be dismissed because of lack of evidence. The patient and provider should be alert to the possibility of symptom exacerbation whenever a new medication is prescribed. A reference for health professionals is available online at http://www.myasthenia.org/drugs/reference.htm.

Surgical Management. Thymectomy is one of the most frequently used interventions for MG but its efficacy remains controversial because of lack of evidence-based studies. An international multicenter study supported by the National Institutes of Health (NIH) is underway to determine the benefits of thymectomy in the treatment of MG. Although it is known that patients who undergo thymectomy are more likely to experience a drug-free remission and to have improvement in their MG weakness, it is not known which patients are most likely to benefit, when thymectomy should be performed, and what type of surgical procedure is best for thymus removal. Even though most patients do improve, they do not respond immediately. Positively attributing benefit to thymectomy is complicated by the natural fluctuating course of MG.

A number of techniques are used to remove the thymus, and there is debate over which technique will produce the most desirable results. The thymus is located primarily in the anterior mediastinum but extends into the neck. The thymus consists of multiple lobes; varying amounts of thymic tissue may be found in the fat surrounding these lobes. It is involved in the development of the immune system and has been implicated in the pathogenesis of MG. Approximately 70% of MG patients have hyperplasia of the thymus; 10% have thymoma, a tumor of the thymus, which is rarely malignant. Thymectomy should almost always be performed when thymoma is present. For patients without thymoma, thymectomy is generally offered to relatively healthy patients who have impairing MG weakness. Some clinicians suggest that thymectomy should be performed early in the course of the disorder for maximum benefit.

Three types of surgical approaches are currently used for thymus removal: transsternal, transcervical, and videoscopic. These approaches remove varying amounts of thymus tissue. Proponents of the extended form of the transsternal approach claim that this technique is superior in removing the most thymus tissue because there is more complete visualization of the chest and neck. Advocates of the transcervical and videoscopic procedures prefer these approaches because they are less invasive. Without head-to-head comparison studies, it is not possible to say which of these approaches is best.

Clinical Management
Acute Care
Because of improved treatments, MG patients need much less acute care than in years past. The patient undergoing thymectomy requires expert hospital management by experienced clinicians. This team includes neuromuscular specialists, surgeons, respiratory care specialists, anesthesiologists, and intensive care physicians and nurses. Patients should choose a hospital center that manages large numbers of thymectomy cases. Preoperative care typically includes a course of PEX or IVIg to maximize the patient's strength and to minimize oropharyngeal or respiratory weakness. Patients undergoing chronic steroid therapy may require extra "stress" doses during the perioperative period. Most MG centers discontinue the use of anticholinesterase agents during the day of surgery and in the immediate postoperative period to reduce possible excess pulmonary secretions.

Patients should expect to be in an intensive care unit (ICU) and be maintained on a ventilator in the immediate postoperative period. The length of time that ventilatory support is required is variable and is influenced by the patient's preoperative status and the use of muscle relaxants during anesthesia. Patients are taught deep breathing and coughing techniques before surgery so that after extubation they can clear pulmonary secretions. Chest splinting with a pillow during coughing or repositioning helps to reduce pain and discomfort. Chest percussion and suctioning will help to prevent pooling of secretions. Chest tubes may be in place postoperatively. Pain medications are offered for discomfort and the patient is monitored closely for any resultant respiratory depression. Depending on the surgical technique used and the degree of MG debilitation, the patient can expect to remain in the hospital from several days to a few weeks.

The term *crisis* denotes a medical emergency involving rapidly increasing weakness affecting the oropharyngeal and respiratory muscles. **Myasthenic crisis** is attributed to factors that exacerbate MG weakness, such as infection. **Cholinergic crisis** results from excess pyridostigmine or other anticholinesterases. Myasthenic crisis is most likely to occur early in the illness, before effective treatment has begun. A major goal of treatment is to improve strength and to recognize potentially exacerbating factors before crisis occurs.

Emergency Assessment
Important principles in managing medical emergencies of this nature include early recognition, keeping the airway open, supporting respiration for adequate air exchange, and

removing excess respiratory secretions. Patients experiencing severe respiratory difficulty will have shortness of breath at rest, air hunger, inability to lie flat, restlessness, anxiety, and fatigue. Patients with severe oropharyngeal weakness will have gagging, choking, inability to swallow medications or food, restlessness, and anxiety. Physical assessment includes the evaluation of airway patency, breathing effort, and circulation. The patient should be placed in an ICU for close monitoring. PEX or IVIg is typically ordered to induce quick improvement. During the period when the patient is profoundly weak, the following may be required: total assistance in personal care, nutritional support via nasogastric tube, special skin care, frequent repositioning to avoid complications of immobility, chest percussion, and suctioning to avoid pneumonia.

Psychosocial Considerations

Assess the patient's and family's understanding of the disorder, coping methods, and their reaction to the present situation. Because early fluctuating symptoms of MG may be attributed to a psychogenic cause by the uninformed clinician, the patient may have been treated inappropriately for psychiatric illness. Recognize that the patient may experience a grief reaction from the loss of body function. Encourage the patient to discuss fears and uncertainties and provide realistic reassurance. Refer for mental health services if the patient has significant anxiety or depression.

Nutritional Considerations

Encourage good nutritional practices. If the patient is taking pyridostigmine, offer meals 45 minutes to an hour after dosing for peak strength. Assess for difficulty with chewing, swallowing, and potential for aspiration. Offer soft foods and frequent meals that are less fatiguing. Patients taking prednisone may have increased appetite, and weight gain may be a problem. Excess caloric intake, foods high in sugar, and salty foods should be avoided. These patients should have adequate calcium intake to prevent loss of bone density. Supplemental calcium, vitamin D, and prescription medicines preventing osteoporosis may be ordered.

Older Adult Considerations

Preexisting medical conditions related to aging complicate MG treatment decisions. The use of prednisone is a particular concern in the older patient who is more prone to osteoporosis, cardiac disease, diabetes, and cataracts.

Health Teaching

Education begins with a comprehensive health teaching plan that includes clear verbal and written explanations of the disease process, medications and other therapeutic interventions, tests, procedures, and patient management strategies. Stress the importance of taking medicines on time and at the correct dose. Patient education materials can be obtained online from the Myasthenia Gravis Foundation of America (MGFA) and other resources.

Continuum of Care

Home Care and Case Management Considerations. After discharge, the MG patient needs ongoing management. Stress the importance of keeping regular appointments and close communication with the MG specialist. Ensure that the patient knows how to reach the MG medical specialist during office and evening hours in case urgent advice is needed. Primary care providers and family members should be educated about MG, particularly about how to avoid and manage factors that may exacerbate weakness. If the patient has significant weakness at the time of discharge, community resources will be required. These may include referral to occupational therapy for help with activities of daily living (ADLs), home health care nursing for home-based treatments, patient support groups, and resources for financial assistance if needed. Patients with MG should obtain a medical identification alert tag or bracelet from MedicAlert or a similar group. A wallet medication information card can be obtained from MGFA with a list of drugs to be avoided or used with caution in MG.

All MG patients who continue to experience weakness should be taught energy conservation strategies to manage ADLs. Those patients who have well-controlled symptoms may fully engage in regular activities and even in carefully designed exercise programs.

When MG affects women of childbearing age, they should be offered preconception counseling and high-risk obstetric services. The potential adverse effects of certain MG therapies on the fetus should be discussed when making pregnancy and treatment choices. Successful pregnancy and delivery is maximized by the close collaboration of the obstetrician, neurologist, neonatologist, and well-informed patient. Like other stressors, pregnancy can unpredictably alter the course of MG. Delivery should take place at a hospital center that has expertise with the management of MG patients and their neonates. Approximately 10% to 20% of mothers with autoimmune MG deliver neonates who have transient neonatal MG, which can last for a few weeks. Because it is not possible to predict which infants will be affected, all neonates born to mothers with MG must be monitored carefully for signs of weakness, respiratory problems, and feeding difficulties in the first few days. This is best accomplished in a neonatal intensive care unit (NICU). Maternal antibodies may cross the placenta and produce weakness in the fetus, which when severe, can cause arthrogryposis. To detect this, fetal movements should be monitored regularly and appropriate treatment instituted if necessary. The decision to breastfeed should always be discussed with the managing providers but is generally not contraindicated unless the mother is debilitated or taking certain immunosuppressive agents.[5]

MG is an uncommon and serious disorder. With expert management, current treatments provide significant improvement in most patients. These treatments will not cure MG, but in some cases, the disorder will go into remission for a time. Continued research is essential to further understand the various clinical presentations of MG and to develop targeted therapeutic choices that are more specific.

Myopathy

Myopathy is a general classification term used to describe a broad range of disorders of primarily skeletal muscle tissue; these disorders have common presentation patterns. Myopathies can be acquired or inherited. Intermittent or persistent muscle weakness is the primary symptom, but cramping, stiffness, and spasm are common. The many different types of myopathies have varying etiologies. **Inflammatory myopathies** are a heterogeneous group of idiopathic, immune-mediated disorders. The three most common are dermatomyositis (DM), polymyositis (PM), and inclusion body myositis. In addition to inflammatory myopathies, there are inherited myopathies and myopathies related to other systemic conditions. Inherited myopathies will not be reviewed; however, the major characteristics of the muscular dystrophies are outlined in Table 22-2.[10]

Dermatomyositis (DM) is a chronic multisystem autoimmune disorder that affects both adults and children. In adults, the incidence is 0.5 to 1 per 100,000. Females are affected twice as often as males; blacks are affected more frequently than whites. The average age at diagnosis is 40 years. The etiology is thought to be an immune-mediated vasculopathy that results in injury to the epithelial lining of small vessels, causing swelling and necrosis. Initial manifestations are cutaneous changes including a photosensitive, confluent, reddish-purple rash over the eyelids, cheeks, nose, back, upper chest, elbows, knees, and knuckles (Gottron's sign). The rash may be pruritic. Proximal and axial muscle weakness progresses over days, weeks, or months. Patients should be screened for systemic manifestations, which may be life threatening. Some older patients with DM have associated malignancies.[6]

Polymyositis (PM) literally means "inflammation of many muscles." It is currently considered the least common of the inflammatory myopathies based on new understandings of histologic findings.[18] PM occurs chiefly in individuals older than age 20 and mostly affects those in their 40s and 50s. PM presents with insidious symmetric proximal weakness of the upper and lower extremities that develops over weeks to months. Weakness of the neck flexors is common. Oropharyngeal and esophageal involvement occurs in about a third of patients, causing dysphagia. Patients with PM usually have elevated levels of the muscle enzymes serum creatine kinase and aldolase. PM has been associated with connective tissue and viral disorders but its etiology remains unknown.

Inclusion body myositis (IBM) is the most common inflammatory myopathy affecting individuals older than age 40. It is often diagnosed when a patient is found unresponsive to therapy prescribed for the diagnosis of PM. Patients with IBM have slowly progressive asymmetric distal weakness that frequently begins in the quadriceps, wrist and finger flexors, or pharyngeal muscles.[3] IBM is generally painless and males are three times more affected than females. Intracellular amyloid deposits, similar to the plaques found in Alzheimer's disease, have been found in the vacuolated muscle fibers of IBM patients.[1]

Assessment

The subjective assessment of a patient suspected to have a myopathy includes a detailed history of the onset, duration, pattern, and progression of the symptoms. Gather history about weakness, pain, tenderness, difficulty swallowing, ability to rise from a chair, walk, or perform daily tasks such as dressing or bathing. Ask if the symptoms are variable or constant. Gather information about any skin rashes and lesions. Question the patient about any coexisting disorders.

TABLE 22-2	Major Characteristics of Muscular Dystrophies			
Type	**Age of Onset**	**Inheritance/Gender Affected**	**Muscles First Affected**	**Progression**
Myotonic muscular dystrophy	Early childhood to adulthood; newborn period for congenital form	Autosomal dominant/ males and females	Face, feet, hands, front of neck	Slow
Duchenne muscular dystrophy	2 to 6 years	X-linked/males	Pelvis, upper arms, upper legs	Slow, sometimes with rapid spurts
Becker muscular dystrophy	2 to 16 years	X-linked/males	Pelvis, upper arms, upper legs	Slow
Limb-girdle muscular dystrophy	Teens or early adulthood	Autosomal recessive and dominant forms/males and females	Hips, shoulders	Usually slow
Facioscapulohumeral muscular dystrophy	Teens or early adulthood	Autosomal dominant/ males and females	Face, shoulders	Slow, sometimes with rapid spurts
Congenital muscular dystrophy	At birth	Autosomal recessive/ males and females	Generalized	Slow
Oculopharyngeal muscular dystrophy	40s, 50s, 60s	Autosomal dominant/ males and females	Eyelids, throat	Slow
Distal muscular dystrophy	Adulthood	Autosomal recessive and dominant forms/males and females	Hands or lower legs	Variable
Emery-Dreifuss muscular dystrophy	Childhood to early teens	X-linked recessive/males	Upper arms, lower legs	Slow

BOX 22-3   Neuromuscular Examination Tips

Proximal Muscle Weakness
- Ask patient to rise from a chair with arms folded across chest.
- Ask patient to rise from a squat.
- Ask patient to lift arms over head for 60 seconds, then straight forward for 60 seconds.

Distal Muscle Weakness
- Ask patient to walk on toes and then heels.
- Ask patient to spread fingers against resistance.

Atrophy
- Proximal: Observed in upper arm (deltoid) and top of thighs (quadriceps).
- Distal: Observed in pad under thumb (thenar eminence) and shin (tibialis anterior).

Increased Tone in Extremities
- Passively move all extremities in a relaxed patient.

Ask about family and social history. A complete physical examination with a careful neurologic assessment is important. Some physical examination tips specific for the neuromuscular patient are listed in Box 22-3.

Neurodiagnostic and Laboratory Studies

Diagnostic tests may include the following:
- **Serum creatine kinase (CK).** Levels of CK are typically elevated.
- **Electromyography (EMG).** This test may demonstrate myogenic changes with short duration–low amplitude action potentials.
- **Muscle biopsy.** Histologic changes observed are confirmatory and differentiate the diagnosis.
- **Myositis-specific or associated antibodies.** Laboratory analysis of a series of specific or associated antibodies is performed. Identifying certain antibodies can help to differentiate the diagnosis.
- **Erythrocyte sedimentation rate (ESR).** These levels are typically elevated.

Treatment

Medical Management. Current treatments are ineffective for IBM. Treatment of DM and PM involve the following:
- Corticosteroids: Prednisone is typically the first therapy prescribed
- Immunosuppressants: azathioprine, methotrexate, cyclosporine, tacrolimus, and mycophenolate mofetil
- IVIg
- Topical preparations: hydrocortisone or tacrolimus for the cutaneous manifestations of DM

Clinical Management

Acute and Nonacute Care and Rehabilitation

Most patients do not require hospitalization except for complications of compromised mobility or for respiratory failure, which is rare. Physical therapy is directed at providing symptom relief.

Health Teaching

Patients benefit from a comprehensive care plan including explanations of the disease process, medications, tests, procedures, and patient coping strategies. Those with difficulty walking should receive a home safety evaluation and information about mobility aids. Information about community resources and peer support groups is included in the plan.

Psychosocial Considerations

Monitor response to chronic disease and bodily changes. Assess for anxiety and depression and refer to a mental health provider if significant.

Older Adult Considerations

Older adults with myopathies require increased monitoring for injury from falls. Conditions such as osteoarthritis and osteoporosis impede recovery from a fall. Chronic age-related conditions may reduce the number of treatment options. The use of prednisone is a particular concern in the older adult.

Continuum of Care

Rehabilitation and Home Care. A rehabilitation plan is useful to teach patients new ways of coping with weakness. Physical therapy and exercise programs help to maintain strength and prevent contractures. A healthy lifestyle and routine primary care visits enhance wellness. The use of adaptive equipment may maximize functional independence.

Case Management Considerations. Complex patients require case management and coordination of care. Patients with DM tend to require more health services than those with PM. Patients with IBM tend to have a slowly progressing course and poor response to treatment. The patient with an inflammatory myopathy may require mobility aids in the home including cane, walker, wheelchair, or scooter. These aids must be properly fitted for the individual patient. Assistive devices such as lifts for bathing and other ADLs (reacher, button holer, zipper puller) may increase independence.

Restless Legs Syndrome

RLS is thought to be a primary dopaminergic movement disorder that causes sufferers to have uncomfortable or painful sensations (paresthesias), accompanied by an irresistible urge to move the legs (see Chapter 6). This condition may have life-altering consequences. RLS is more prominent during times of inactivity, especially at night. Movement of the legs gives a brief period of relief. It is a common and treatable condition that often interferes with sleep and can lead to disturbed sleep and daytime somnolence. Women may be affected more than men. Carefully designed studies have not yet established the prevalence of RLS. The syndrome should be evaluated and treated when the quality of life is affected as demonstrated by nighttime sleep deprivation and excessive daytime sleepiness.

The pathophysiology of RLS is unclear. Familial cases suggest a genetic origin for primary RLS. Secondary causes of RLS may include iron deficiency, neurologic lesions, pregnancy, uremia, drug side effects, and caffeine. RLS may be associated also with neuropathies.

A high index of suspicion facilitates early recognition and treatment of this underdiagnosed syndrome. Suggested criteria for RLS diagnosis include (1) an urge to move the legs, usually accompanied by unpleasant sensations; (2) unpleasant "quivering and crawling" sensations that begin or worsen during rest or inactivity; (3) movement partially or completely ameliorates unpleasant sensation; and (4) unpleasant sensations are worse in the evening. Suggested supportive criteria include positive family history, positive treatment response to dopaminergics, and the presence of periodic limb movements.[2]

Assessment includes gathering a complete history, including family history of RLS, and evaluation for any of the conditions that may produce or exacerbate this syndrome. The clinician should obtain a careful sleep and quality of life history or ask the individual to keep a sleep log. Secondary causes of RLS should be assessed and treated. Management entails nonpharmacologic and pharmacologic approaches. Suggested nonpharmacologic approaches are relaxation and stress-reduction techniques and elimination of caffeine, tobacco, and alcohol. In patients with significant dysfunction, pharmacologic treatment may be initiated with ropinirole (Requip), a dopamine precursor (e.g., levodopa). Dopamine agonists, opioids, benzodiazepines, and anticonvulants are also prescribed. Clonidine, propranolol, and amantadine may be effective also.[2,11]

CONCLUSION

Individuals with muscle weakness, fatigue, and restlessness may not have a life-threatening disorder but do have a disorder that disrupts the quality of their life that may affect their occupation, quality of life, and ability to function at their highest level. Diseases affecting the neuromuscular junction and muscle fibers produce weakness that must be accurately diagnosed and treated appropriately.

New advances in the diagnosis and treatment of these disorders require a dedicated team of knowledgeable clinicians. As additional research targets new and efficacious treatments with minimal adverse effects, patients will be able to manage their symptoms and reduce the sequelae of these neurologic conditions.

RESOURCES

Muscular Dystrophy Association: 3300 E. Sunrise Drive, Tucson, AZ 85718; www.mdausa.org

Myasthenia Gravis Foundation of America: 1821 University Avenue West, Suite S256, St. Paul, MN 55104; www.myasthenia.org

The Myositis Association: 1233 20th St NW, Suite 402, Washington, DC 20036; www.myositis.org

Restless Legs Syndrome Foundation: 819 Second Street SW, Rochester, MN 55902; www.rls.org

REFERENCES

1. Askanas V, Engel WK: Molecular pathology and pathogenesis of inclusion-body myositis, *Microsc Res Tech* 67(3–4):114–120, 2005.

2. Avecillas JE, Golish JA, Giannini C, Yataco JC: Restless legs syndrome: keys to recognition and treatment, *Cleve Clin J Med* 72(9):769–786, 2005.

3. Badrising UA, Maat-Schieman ML, van Houwelingen JC, van Doorn PA, van Duinen SG, van Engelen BG, Faber CG, Hoogendijk JE, de Jager AE, Koehler PJ, de Visser M, Verschuuren JJ, Wintzen AR: Inclusion body myositis: clinical features and clinical course of the disease in 64 patients, *J Neurol* 252(12):1448–1454, 2005.

4. Cartaud A, Strochlic L, Guerra M, Blanchard B, Lambergeon M, Krejci E, Cartaud J, Legay C: MuSK is required for anchoring acetylcholinesterase at the neuromuscular junction, *J Cell Biol* 165(4):505–515, 2004.

5. Ciafaloni E, Massey JM: The management of myasthenia gravis in pregnancy, *Neurol Clin* 22(4):771–782, 2004.

6. Katsambas A, Stefanaki C: Life-threatening dermatoses due to connective tissue disorders, *Clin Dermatol* 23(3):238–248, 2005.

7. Keesey J: Clinical evaluation and management of myasthenia gravis, *Muscle Nerve* 29(4):484–505, 2004.

8. Meriggioli MN, Ciafaloni E, Al-Hayk KA, Rowin J, Tucker-Lipscomb B, Massey JM, Sanders DB: Mycophenolate mofetil for myasthenia gravis: an analysis of efficacy, safety, and tolerability, *Neurology* 61(10):1438–1440, 2003.

9. Meriggioli MN, Sanders DB: Myasthenia gravis: diagnosis, *Semin Neurol* 24(1):31–39, 2004.

10. Muscular Dystrophy Association: *Facts about muscular dystrophy (MD),* http://www.mdausa.org/publications/fa-md-9.html.

11. NHLBI Working Group on Restless Legs Syndrome: *Restless legs syndrome: detection and management in primary care,* 2000, NIH; http://www.nhlbi.nih.gov/health/prof/sleep/rls_gde.pdf.

12. Patrick J, Lindstrom J: Autoimmune response to acetylcholine receptor, *Science* 180(88):871–872, 1973.

13. Phillips LH: The epidemiology of myasthenia gravis. Myasthenia gravis and related disorders, *Ann N Y Acad Sci* 998:407–412, 2003.

14. Sanders DB: Lambert-Eaton myasthenic syndrome: diagnosis and treatment, *Ann N Y Acad Sci* 998:500–508, 2003.

15. Sanders DB, El Salem K, Massey JM, McConville J, Vincent A: Clinical aspects of MuSK antibody positive seronegative MG, *Neurology* 60:1978–1980, 2003.

16. Sanders DB, Tucker-Lipscomb B, Massey JM: A simple manual muscle test for myasthenia gravis: validation and comparison with the QMG score, *Ann N Y Acad Sci* 998:440–444, 2003.

17. Task Force of the Medical Scientific Advisory Board of the Myasthenia Gravis Foundation of America: Myasthenia gravis. Recommendations for clinical research standards, *Neurology* 55(1):16–23, 2000.

18. van der Meulen MFG, Bronner IM, Hoogendijk JE, Burger H, van Venrooij WJ, Voskuyl AE, Dinant HJ, Linssen WHJP, Wokke JHJ, de Visser M: Polymyositis: an overdiagnosed entity, *Neurology* 61(3):316–321, 2003.

19. Vincent A, Clover L, Buckley C, Grimley Evans J, Rothwell PM: Evidence of underdiagnosis of myasthenia gravis in older people, *J Neurol Neurosurg Psychiatry* 74:1105–1108, 2003.

20. Vincent A, Leite MI: Neuromuscular junction autoimmune disease: muscle specific kinase antibodies and treatments for myasthenia gravis, *Curr Opin Neurol* 18(5):519–525, 2005.

21. Vincent A, McConville J, Farrugia ME, Bowen J, Plested P, Tang T, Evoli A, Matthews I, Sims G, Dalton P, Jacobson L, Polizzi A, Blaes F, Lang B, Beeson D, Willcox N, Newsom-Davis J, Hoch W: Antibodies in myasthenia gravis and related disorders, *Ann N Y Acad Sci* 998:324–335, 2003.

PART THREE

Neurologic Conditions

653

ELLEN BARKER,
JOYCE S. WILLENS

CHAPTER 23

Management of the Neuroscience Patient With Pain

Pain is a common condition for neuroscience patients and can originate from many different sites of the nervous system. Pain may be acute, chronic, and disabling. In some instances, pain becomes more debilitating than the disease itself. It is recognized that chronic pain disables more people than cancer or heart disease. Head and spine trauma, central nervous system (CNS) tumors and infections, spinal dysfunction and disease, cranial and peripheral nerve injury, vascular diseases, and inflammatory conditions may result in acute pain that is only temporary or chronic pain that can literally take control of a person's life. Numerous studies have indicated that pain is widely undertreated in the United States. The medical community is often criticized for not treating an individual's pain with an effective pain management plan of care or acknowledging its emotional, physical, and financial impact. With adequate education and in-depth knowledge of the pathophysiology of pain and the new advancements in pain treatments, pain management can be provided to neuroscience patients to restore a quality of life that is free of pain or allow patients to effectively take control of their pain. Clinicians can tell neuroscience patients that they don't have to live with pain.

Pain has been called a silent epidemic in this country, with an estimated 50 million Americans partially or totally disabled because of pain. Pain management is a high priority for neuroscience nurses. Pain is costly, not only in terms of human suffering, but also in terms of financial hardship. Americans spend upwards of $100 billion on medications for chronic pain each year, with the majority of the U.S. population experiencing some type of painful condition. Misconceptions of pain (e.g., in poorly understood painful conditions such as neuropathic pain), even within the nursing community, may prevent clinicians from providing adequate pain relief to their patients. Fear of overdosing or patient addiction must be replaced by recognition that underlying psychosocial factors may coexist. These conditions should be assessed early and treated aggressively along with the pain interventions. This chapter will review the neuroanatomy and neurophysiology of pain, clinical manifestations of acute and chronic pain in the neuroscience patient population, comprehensive pain assessment, and treatment options with a multidisciplinary approach that highlights the important roles of nurse clinicians.

DEFINITION OF PAIN

Having an accurate definition of pain is important in effectively managing pain. The International Association for the Study of Pain (IASP) defines pain as "an unpleasant sensory and emotional experience associated with actual or potential damage or described in terms of such damage."[38] Pain is a subjective experience that patients sometimes have difficulty communicating. A classic and often cited definition is, "pain is what the experiencing person says it is, existing whenever he says it does."[36] This definition underscores the subjective experience of pain. The best expert about patient pain is the patient.

EPIDEMIOLOGY

It is estimated that one third of Americans suffer from a chronic painful condition, with 50% to 60% of these individuals partially or totally disabled by pain, either transiently or permanently. An estimated $79 billion is spent annually on health care, Workers' Compensation, and litigation, amd 40 million visits to health care practitioners are for chronic painful conditions.[6] Low back pain, for example, is the most common musculoskeletal pain syndrome. It is estimated that between 58% and 84% of the population will report an episode of low back pain at some point, with an excess prevalence in women.[15] The epidemiology of pain may have psychologic and psychosocial factors when accompanied by high levels of depression, anxiety, or adverse life events. Social disadvantage may place an individual at increased risk for general pain. Genetic influences may play a role, and mechanical factors related to workplace activities that require lifting heavy weights, kneeling, squatting, pulling, or pushing are associated with low back pain. Women report more severe pain and more frequent and persistent pain. Increased age reflects degenerative changes with an increase in joint pain. Risk factors vary at different ages and are influenced by psychologic, cultural, and social factors.[34]

PATHOPHYSIOLOGY

The portions of the nervous system responsible for the sensation and perception of pain may be divided into three areas:

(1) the afferent pathways, (2) the CNS, and (3) the efferent pathways. The afferent portion of the system is composed of **nociceptors** (pain receptors) in the tissues. Afferent nerves carry signals to the spinal cord network, which transmits the signals to the brain. The portions of the CNS involved in the interpretation of pain signals are the limbic system, reticular formation, thalamus, hypothalamus, medulla, and cortex. The efferent pathway is responsible for modulation or inhibition of afferent pain signals.[31] **Nociception** (pertaining to a neural receptor or painful stimuli) results from an injury with stimulation of receptors known as "nociceptors" and begins in the periphery on the skin, subcutaneous tissue, or visceral or somatic structures (Fig. 23-1). It can be perceived as well localized and constant. Transmission begins when a painful substance comes in contact with a pain receptor.[10] Nociceptors respond to chemical, thermal, or mechanical noxious stimuli. Inflammation results after tissue damage that causes the release of a barrage of noxious stimuli (bradykinin, substance P, prostaglandins).

Two types of fibers transmit the pain impulse. **Unmyelinated C fibers** transmit nociception from the periphery to the spinal cord. They are small in diameter and slow to conduct the impulse; therefore they transmit pain that is poorly localized. The **AO or A-delta fibers** are thinly myelinated, large-diameter, fast-conducting fibers that transmit well-localized pain.[44] Both fibers transmit nociception from the periphery to the dorsal horn and ascend to the brainstem and thalamus. The thalamus relays the information to the cortex where the pain can be processed.

As the pain signal enters the brain, the descending pathway begins to work to inhibit pain. The neuronal pathways start at the brainstem and descend to the dorsal horn of the spinal cord. The descending pathways release endogenous opioids, serotonin (5-hydroxytryptamine [5-HT]), and norepinephrine. Combined they act to provide analgesia. The perception of pain is the outcome of the neural transmission of the peripheral nervous system and the descending pathways. The perception of pain can be influenced by behavioral, emotional, and other factors.

CLINICAL MANIFESTATIONS OF PAIN

Types of Pain

Pain is often classified temporally, by location, by pathophysiology, and/or by cause. The IASP defines **acute pain** as sudden or slow onset of any intensity from mild to severe pain with an anticipated or predictable end. The duration is less than 6 months. Acute pain is a "symptom" usually in response to tissue trauma and is usually nociceptive. It can be classified as **somatic pain** (coming from the skin or close to the surface of the body), **visceral pain** (in internal organs, the abdomen, or the skeleton), or **referred pain** (present in an area removed or distant from its point of origin).[31]

Acute pain is a warning of actual or impending tissue injury.[31] Characteristic behaviors of acute pain may include protective behaviors (e.g., guarding; gestures, facial mask); sleep disturbances evidenced by eyes that are lackluster; impaired thought; reduced interaction with people; and restlessness, pacing, moaning, or crying. Physiologic responses include increased heart and respiratory rate, elevated blood pressure, pallor, or flushing. In addition, blood glucose may be elevated, gastric acid secretion and motility decrease, and blood flow to the viscera and skin decrease. Nausea occasionally occurs.[31]

The IASP defines **chronic pain** as sudden or slow onset of any pain intensity from mild to severe, constant or recurring without an anticipated or predictable end, and duration of greater than 6 months. It can be nociceptive, neuropathic, or both. Chronic pain is long-lived, debilitating, not protective, serves no useful purpose, and occurs longer than expected despite no apparent tissue injury. Low back pain is an example of chronic pain that is prolonged and may be persistent. Other examples include central pain caused by a lesion or dysfunction in the CNS such as a traumatic injury,

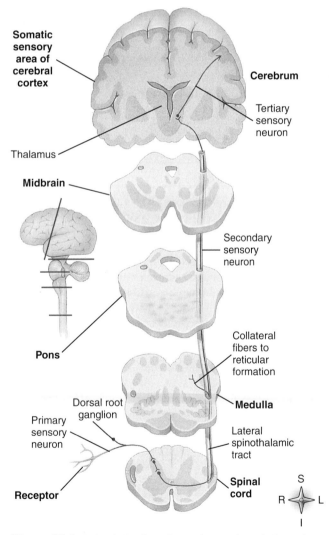

Figure 23-1 Spinothalamic pathway that conducts information about pain and temperature.
(From Thibodeau GA, Patton KT: Anatomy and physiology, *St Louis, 2003, Mosby.)*

or thalamic pain from a lesion in the thalamus.[31] Characteristics of chronic pain may include weight loss/gain, muscle atrophy, depression, fatigue, fear of reinjury, lack of sexual activity, decreased socialization, and preoccupation with the pain. Avoidance of any stimuli that will provoke pain may affect quality of life. The individual's physiologic response may depend on whether the pain is persistent or intermittent. Persistent pain for prolonged periods allows the sufferer to adapt with little or no changes in vital signs even though the pain is not relieved. This type of pain is the most difficult to treat, is expensive to manage, and may require rehabilitation. Intermittent chronic pain produces a response similar to acute pain.

Patients may experience both acute and chronic pain simultaneously. For example, a postoperative patient operated on for failed back syndrome may have acute pain from the surgical manipulations and incision and continue to experience the chronic pain from long-standing nerve compression during the postoperative recovery phase.

Multidisciplinary Pain Team and Clinics

Team Approach
A multidisciplinary team approach is effective in comprehensive pain management that can offer a wide range of treatment techniques and develop successful practice parameters and pathways. Nurse clinicians may practice in various roles (e.g., clinical nurse pain specialists) and serve as integral members of the pain team or specialty practice. Pain teams or clinics may provide a modality-oriented, disease-oriented, or multidisciplinary service.

A pain clinic may focus on interruption of the pain behavior reinforcement cycle, rewards for healthy behavior, appropriate goals, measurement of improvement of pain by pain level, and psychosocial adjustment. Pain management programs are focused on improved management of the pain and designed to reduce but not necessarily eliminate pain. The goal is to increase the patient's functional capabilities. Exercise is emphasized but is focused on what the patient can perform, with progressive increases. Patients receive help in changing their beliefs that their pain is insurmountable. They are instructed to monitor thoughts and behaviors and to concentrate on positive thoughts while minimizing the negative. This may help patients feel more in control of their pain versus the pain controlling them. Patients are taught how to channel their pain complaints and behaviors by using therapeutic strategies rather than continuing to focus on the pain.[60] The following disciplines may comprise a pain team to offer specialized pain programs or clinics to evaluate and treat chronic pain:
- Pain physician who specializes in the diagnosis and treatment of pain
- Nurse clinician pain specialist
- Anesthesiologist
- Psychiatrist/psychologist
- Pain counselor
- Neurosurgeon
- Physiatrist and rehabilitation team
- Case manager
- Vocational counselor
- Social worker
- Pharmacist
- Dietitian

ASSESSMENT

Individuals who suffer pain from head and spine trauma, CNS tumors and infections, spinal dysfunction and disease, cranial and peripheral nerve injury, vascular diseases, and inflammatory conditions may have severe acute or chronic pain. The most important factor for successful pain management is accurate assessment of the patient's pain.[52] Without a thorough assessment, good pain management is impossible. Pain that is not recognized cannot be treated, whereas treatment initiated without adequate assessment is potentially dangerous.[23] Patient assessments should include more than just the sensory features of pain. The clinician should also evaluate the patient to determine if the pain has become overwhelming and demands immediate attention or is disrupting ongoing behavior and thought.[37] Evaluation of diagnostic studies is correlated with the clinical presentation, with the recognition of study limitations in some cases.

The measurement of pain is important to[37]:
- Determine pain intensity, quality, and duration
- Aid in diagnosis
- Help decide on the choice of therapy
- Evaluate the relative effectiveness of different therapies

Areas that should be questioned to define the pain include the following[52]:
- Temporal relationship to the onset of pain and changes in the character of the pain over time.
- Severity of the pain, including the impact on quality of life, sleep, and the psychologic state of the patient.
- Quality of the pain. What descriptor does the patient use? These descriptors are often useful in establishing the pain as neuropathic or nociceptive in origin.
- Intensity of pain, which is usually measured using various pain scales. The consistent recording of pain levels is helpful when reevaluating a patient to track the patient's response to therapy. A patient with mild pain and minimal loss of function usually reports a pain level of 1 to 3. Pain that is reported as moderate (on a scale of 4 to 6) causes significant reduction in function. Patients with severe pain (on a severity scale of 7 to 10) often cannot function at all.
- Location and distribution of pain. A patient often easily localizes superficial pain. Deeper sources of pain are more difficult to localize and can be referred over a wide area. The patient can be asked to mark the location of pain on a diagram of the body.
- Identification of exacerbating and relieving factors. This information is used to further define the potential mechanisms sustaining the pain, as well as to formulate treatment strategies.
- PQRST: **P**ain location, **Q**uality, **R**elieving factors, **S**everity, and **T**iming.

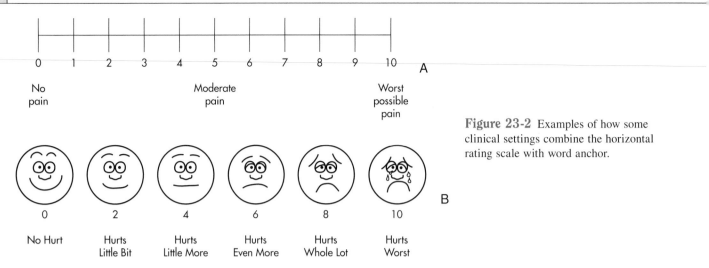

Figure 23-2 Examples of how some clinical settings combine the horizontal rating scale with word anchor.

- The effect of the pain on the individual's quality of life, sleep and rest, interpersonal relationships, and appetite with weight loss or gain.
- History of substance abuse and treatments.

Nursing assessment of pain as the "fifth vital sign" is an effective means of validating the importance of the patient's pain, recognizing the severity, locating the source of pain, and evaluating response to therapy in the overall management of neurologic disease. In some cases, members of the family may contribute by reporting pain intensity based on firsthand knowledge of the individual's expressions or behavior with past pain experiences.[59] Every attempt must be made to prevent any clinician bias because research has repeatedly shown that health care providers frequently rate patients' pain intensity lower than what patients report.[9,48,61]

The **numeric pain scale (NPS)** illustrated in Fig. 23-2, *A,* is now most commonly used in clinical settings to assess pain intensity. The NPS is appropriate for use in cognitively intact patients. The **Faces Pain Scale Revised (FPS-R)** is a revised scale designed to determine how a child feels (Fig. 23-2, *B*) and is appropriate for adults as well. Evidence of reliability and validity has been established.[29] Many neuroscience patients are scheduled for rehabilitation. Knowledge of the relationship between pain intensity and activity can be managed with appropriate pain interventions that will allow the patient to comfortably engage in prescribed therapeutic modalities (see Fig. 23-2). Pain assessment is followed by a neuroassessment to further define and clarify how the neurologic disease process and pathologic lesions are causing pain and need to be treated. Gentle inspection and palpation of the painful site can be correlated with the patient's emotional and behavioral response to the neurologic illness. A comprehensive pain management plan can be integrated with the medical plan of care to prevent pain from interfering with function and activities of daily living (ADLs) during recovery and rehabilitation.

The McGill Pain Questionnaire is a valid and reliable tool that is useful to measure an individual's acute or chronic pain experience. It can be read to the individual or filled out by the patient (Fig. 23-3). The Questionnaire includes a list of descriptors in subclasses 1 to 20, with the explicit instruction that patients choose only those words that describe their feelings and sensations at that moment.

Pain Assessment With an Altered Level of Consciousness

The assessment of pain in the patient with an altered level of consciousness (LOC) requires increased diligence. When a self-report of pain cannot be obtained from the patient, then other assessment criteria must be used. Assume that gross sensation is intact if the comatose patient has responded to painful stimuli. If there is a pathologic condition likely to cause pain, it should be assumed that pain is present, and it should be treated preemptively. The next most reliable indicators of pain are the patient's own behaviors followed by reports of pain by proxy from the patient's significant other(s).[59] The least reliable indicator of pain is an increase in the patient's vital signs. The clinician can use observed behaviors (e.g., grimacing, moaning, withdrawing, restlessness, guarding) to assess pain in patients unable to communicate.

Factors Affecting Perception of Pain

How a person perceives pain may be influenced by gender, culture, experience, the meaning of pain, and age. Emotional distress is an intrinsic and the most undesirable feature of painful experiences. Past experiences, as well as social and cultural differences, generate individual perception of pain. In addition to the inevitable discomfort, fear and anxiety often accompany pain, although other aversive emotional qualities are often observed, including depression, anger, and disgust. Anticipatory fear and avoidance of pain-related thought patterns, or "catastrophizing," can predispose and exacerbate pain severity and disability, serve as a source or consequence of pain, or require investigation as concurrent psychologic disorders.[11] Gender differences, for example, in analgesic responses to kappa-like opioids (pentazocine, nalbuphine, and butorphanol) provided greater analgesia in females compared with males.[39] It is interesting that the pain threshold has been found to be influenced by women's

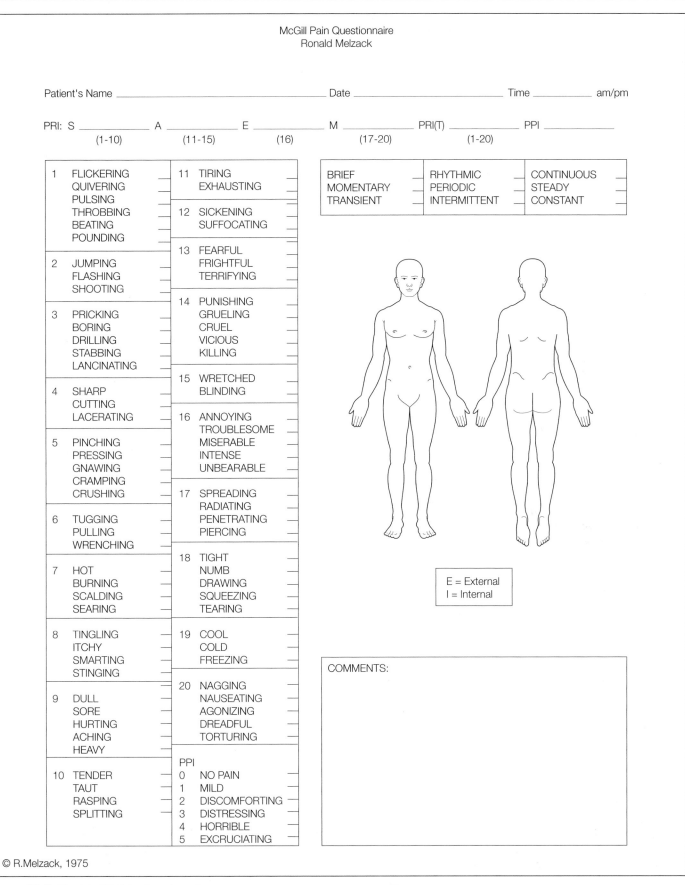

Figure 23-3 The McGill Pain Questionnaire.

menstrual cycles. Pain threshold was highest in the follicular phase and lowest in the luteal phase.[1] The brainstem may induce powerful analgesia in response to noxious stimuli. In addition, cognitive processes also produce a dramatic effect in the perception of pain. If a person believes that the return of pain signals a recurrence of cancer, that person may report greater pain. If the noxious stimulus is perceived during the end course of Guillain-Barré syndrome, the patient may be excited about the return of sensation and report less pain.

Older Adult Considerations

Pain is common in older adults, especially those with painful neurologic disorders and those who have become immobile to reduce their pain. There has been a steady increase of research into pain and aging over the past decade because of the growing number of older adults in society and the increasing demand this group will create for better pain management. Older adults are at high risk for inadequate pain management.[23] As people age there are functional, structural, and biochemical changes in the peripheral nerves. The density of myelinated and unmyelinated fibers decreases by age 60.[25] Age-related changes in pain mechanisms are more apparent when decreased functional reserves are exceeded. When stimuli are brief and at peripheral or visceral sites it is more likely that the threshold for pain will be increased.[25] Another issue is the cognitively impaired older adult who may be unable to verbally communicate his or her pain. Intense pain that interferes with cognitive or physical functioning in the older adult is not a normal part of aging and should never be accepted as such. Observations of behaviors and emotions of pain are substituted for verbal reporting before and after pain therapies to measure pain relief and psychologic interventions.[23]

Chronic Pain Assessment

Distressed and dysfunctional patients who seek treatment for chronic pain require a more complete patient and pain history and a comprehensive neurologic assessment (see Chapter 2). Data obtained from the patient or significant others often indicate the need for a psychologic evaluation and intense psychologic therapy.

The assessment is essential to the correct diagnosis of the pain origin and should focus on key indicators that usually correlate with the pain history, such as increased or decreased pinprick or touch sensation (i.e., hyperesthesia, hypoesthesia, or anesthesia). A **Neuropathic Pain Scale** has been developed as an assessment tool for clinicians to assist in the diagnosis and treatment of neuropathic pain.[24] A list of neuropathic pain syndromes in included in Box 23-1. A **pain diary** or tape recorder is useful to reflect the temporal and spatial aspects of the pain, record exacerbating or relieving pain, and highlight the particular physiologic or psychologic events that increase or decrease the pain perception. Patients should be encouraged to keep their pain diaries with them every day and write down a word, sentence, or comment about their pain beginning when they wake up in the morning. An entry should be made if the pain changes intensity with ADLs,

BOX 23-1	Neuropathic Pain Syndromes

Peripheral Neuropathic Pain Syndromes
- Chemotherapy-induced neuropathy
- Complex regional pain syndrome
- HIV sensory neuropathy
- Painful diabetic neuropathy
- Postherpetic neuralgia
- Postmastectomy pain
- Trigeminal neuralgia
- Alcohol polyneuropathy
- Entrapment neuropathies (carpal tunnel)

Central Neuropathic Pain Syndromes
- Central poststroke pain
- Multiple sclerosis pain
- Parkinson disease pain
- Spinal cord injury pain
- Nerve compression
- Phantom limb pain
- Tic douloureux (trigeminal neuralgia)
- Syringomyelia
- Radiculopathy (cervical, thoracic, lumbosacral)

From Dworkin RH: An overview of neuropathic pain: syndromes, symptoms, signs and several mechanisms, *Clin J Pain* 18(6):343–349, 2002.
HIV, Human immunodeficiency virus.

before or after medications, and after home or outpatient therapies. It often serves as a catharsis and becomes therapeutic to keep a journal and write down how pain affects a patient's mood and emotions. Some individuals may draw sketches. Pain diaries are especially helpful in gauging the effectiveness of both pharmacologic and nonpharmacologic pain interventions. Patients reporting to an office, clinic, or hospital setting can bring a copy of their pain diary to be placed in their medical records.

Types of Pain and Pain Syndromes

Postoperative incisional pain is generally short-lived and is readily treated with nonopioid and opioid analgesics.

Procedural pain can be managed several ways. Communication about what to expect is important. Depending on how invasive and painful the procedure, providing sedation while also providing analgesia is important.[12] Clinicians can use eutectic mixture of local anesthetics (EMLA) to decrease pain during intravenous (IV) cannulation.[56] EMLA takes as long as 60 minutes to take effect and this may not always be feasible. A newer topical anesthetic liposomal lidocaine 4% cream has an onset of action in 30 minutes and is effective for IV insertion.[24] For more painful procedures physicians can use procedural sedation and analgesia. Propofol and a fast-acting opioid such as fentanyl are used.[24] Hydromorphone and morphine are also acceptable but the onset of action is slower.

Common cancer pain syndromes include bone metastases, epidural metastases, spinal cord compression, and brain tumors. Management of these syndromes is beyond the scope of this text. The reader should consult a cancer resource.

BOX 23-2 | **Characteristics of Complex Regional Pain Syndrome Types I and II**

Type I

- Presence of an initiating noxious event, or a cause of immobilization
- Continuing pain, allodynia, or hyperalgesia that is disproportionate to any inciting event
- Evidence at some time of edema, changes in skin color or temperature (difference from homologous body part), or abnormal sudomotor activity in the region of pain
- This diagnosis is excluded by the existence of conditions that would otherwise account for the degree of pain and dysfunction

Type II

- Presence of continuing pain, allodynia, or hyperalgesia after a nerve injury, not necessarily limited to the distribution of the injured nerve
- Evidence at some time of edema, changes in skin color or temperature, or abnormal sudomotor activity in the region of pain
- This diagnosis is excluded by the existence of conditions that would otherwise account for the degree of pain and dysfunction

Data from Galer BS, Schwartz L, Allen RJ: Complex regional pain syndromes—type I: reflex sympathetic dystrophy, and type II: causalgia. In Loeser JD, editor: *Bonica's management of pain,* ed 3, Philadelphia, 2001, Lippincott Williams & Wilkins.

Complex regional pain syndrome (CRPS) is a poorly defined pain disorder clinically characterized by pain; abnormal regulation of blood flow and sweating; edema of skin and subcutaneous tissues; active and passive movement disorders; and trophic changes of skin, appendages of skin, and subcutaneous tissue. It is classified into **Type I CRPS,** formerly known as **reflex sympathetic dystrophy,** or **Type II CRPS,** previously known as **causalgia.**[4] Type I CRPS is not considered a neuropathic pain syndrome.

Minor injuries or fracture of a limb may precede Type I and usually no obvious nerve lesion is present. Soft tissue injury is thought to be the cause. A well-defined nerve injury is thought to cause Type II because the syndrome usually develops after injury to a peripheral nerve.[4] It is not always possible to determine whether a person's CRPS followed injury to a nerve, soft tissue, or both. Box 23-2 shows differences between Type I and Type II CRPS. The cause is unknown and many theories have been proposed.[24] These include but are not limited to dysfunctional sympathetic nervous system, CNS abnormality, and psychogenic factors. A multidisciplinary treatment plan should be implemented immediately and focus on restoration of full return of function.

In addition to a detailed history and physical assessment, diagnostic tests may be needed. The following studies are used to validate the clinical diagnosis: nerve conduction studies, electromyography (EMG); computed tomography (CT), magnetic resonance imaging (MRI), or functional MRI (fMRI); positron emission tomography (PET) or single photon emission computed tomography (SPECT); myelogram; nerve blocks to identify specific nerves involved; a three-phase bone scintigraphy; plain radiographs and x-ray bone densitometry; quantitative sensory testing (QST); autonomic testing with quantitative sudomotor axon reflex test (QSART); and skin temperature measurements to detect thermoregulatory changes of sympathetic activity.[4] Psychosocial evaluation (e.g., the Brief Battery for Health Improvement [BBHI], which is a self-report battery of psychomedical questions regarding depression, functionality, level of pain, emotional distress, and defensiveness) is recommended.

Treatment may include nonsteroidal antiinflammatory drugs (NSAIDs) for mild to moderate pain. Opioids could and should be used as part of a comprehensive pain treatment program (Table 23-1). Other treatments may include a stepwise program beginning with transcutaneous electrical nerve stimulation (TENS), physical therapy, and occupational therapy. Pharmacologic therapy is added and in severe cases evaluation may include the option for a thoracoscopic or surgical sympathectomy.[4] Treatment will vary according to symptoms and the person's response to therapy. Medications are prescribed for pain, anxiety, and depression. In addition, nonpharmacologic interventions (e.g., psychotherapy, cognitive behavioral psychotherapy) may be added. Neurologic interventions may include epidural clonidine, calcium channel blockers, calcitonin, intrathecal opioids, and implantable devices (see Table 23-1).

Neuropathic pain is defined by the IASP as pain initiated or caused by a primary lesion or dysfunction in the nervous system. There are two types of neuropathic pain: peripheral and central. A distinction also needs to be made between acute and chronic neuropathic pain. Pain that persists beyond the expected healing time is considered chronic neuropathic pain. The **dysesthetic** or abnormal quality of neuropathic pain is often described by patients as burning, shooting, or like an electric sensation. The types of neuropathic pain syndromes are listed in Box 23-1.

When a telephone cable is cut, the signals at both ends fall silent; damaged neurons behave differently. Nerve injury and disease trigger a range of metabolic and functional responses in the sensory cell soma and beyond that are ultimately responsible for positive sensory symptoms including chronic neuropathic pain. Electrical hyperexcitability and abnormal impulse generation (ectopic electrogenesis) develop in the injured primary sensory neurons that can cause spontaneous paresthesias, dysesthesia, frank pain, pain evoked by weight-bearing movement, and deep palpation and tenderness to stimuli in the partially denervated body part (allodynia, hyperalgesia).[4]

The types of nerve damage that cause chronic, often intractable neuropathic pain syndromes are many, including infections, trauma or disease affecting peripheral nerves, metabolic abnormalities, chemotherapy, surgery, radiation, neurotoxins, nerve compression, inflammation, and tumor infiltration.[17] When considering the symptoms of neuropathic pain it is important to distinguish between stimulus-evoked pain and spontaneous pain, which is not caused by stimulation. Spontaneous pain, not produced by stimulation, can be either continuous or intermittent. Most patients describe

TABLE 23-1	Overview of Medications Useful for Pain		
Medication Class	**Examples**	**Mechanism of Action**	**Uses for Pain Management**
Opioids	Multiple different compounds, such as morphine, fentanyl, dilaudid, hydrocodone, oxycodone	Primary analgesic action is on the mu receptor	Primary role in acute and cancer pain Adjuvant role in neuropathic pain
Nonopioids	Acetaminophen	Possible COX-3 receptor effect	As primary analgesic or in combination with opioids
Nonsteroidals	Both mixed NSAIDs and selective CDX-2	Both peripheral and central effect, to varying degrees	Nociceptive pain, possible use in neurophatic pain
Psychotropics	Psychostimulants, antipsychotics, benzodiazepines	Different mechanisms	Adjuvant role as antiemetic, helpful for sedation, delirium
Anticonvulsants	Most useful first-generation agents include carbamezepine; second-generation agents include gabapentin, lamotrigine, topiramate, oxcerbazepine, and others	Increased inhibitory transmitters, sodium channel blockade and others	Neuropathic pain; possible role as adjuvant in acute pain
Membrane stabilizing agents	Local anesthetics, mexiletine	Sodium channel blockade	Neuropathic pain
Topical medications	Various over-the-counter medications, Lidoderm patch (lidocaine), Doxipan, capsaicin, TCAs, compounded drugs	Topical anesthetics, substance P depletion	Localized hyperalgesia
NMDA antagonists	Ketamine, dextropmethorphan, memantine	NMDA receptor	Potantial opioid analgesia, neuropathic pain, modulate opioid tolerance
Muscle relaxants	Baclofen, diazepam and other benzodiazepines, cerisoprodol, chlorzoxazone, metaxalone, methocerbamol, orphenadrine, clonidine, tizanidine, cyclobenzaprine	Various mechanisms. Usually attributed to a central effect	Acute myofascial pain syndromes
Alpha agonists	Clonidine, tizanidine	Enhance opioid analgesia, helpful for withdrawal symptoms	Headache, neuropathic pain
Antidepressants	Tricyclics, SSRIs	Blockade of norepinephrine reuptake; SSRIs controversial if they are analgesic	Generalized analgesic, specific helpful with neuropathic pain

COS, Cyclo-oxygenase; *NMDA*, N-methyl-D-aspartate glutamate; *NSAIO*, nonsteroidal antiinflammatory drug; *TCA*, tricyclic antidepressant.

many qualities of their pain, such as burning, throbbing, and shooting. Spontaneous intermittent pain is usually short in duration.

The stimuli in stimulus-evoked pain vary and are a response to a normally nonpainful stimulus (allodynia). Stimuli that have been used to evaluate stimulus-evoked pain include thermal, vibration, dynamic (punctate), and static (blunt). Diagnosis is usually based on a comprehensive history and assessment and comprehensive neurologic examination. Drugs used to treat neuropathic pain have effects in the CNS on the levels of calcium, 5-HT, and norepinephrine[44] (Table 23-2). These chemicals may be important in the central processing of nociceptive input.

When conventional oral medications fail and/or the patient becomes intolerant of the side effects, an intrathecal drug delivery system (IDDS) with infusion directly into the cerebrospinal fluid (CSF) can be started after a successful screening process and surgical implantation of the pump (see Chapter 13). The intrathecal route has several advantages that include selective perfusion of CNS regions, avoidance of the blood-brain barrier (BBB), and constant programmed drug delivery so that levels of analgesia can be maintained.[45] Intrathecal morphine and other drugs have been used routinely. For patients who do not respond to conventional therapies and are unable to obtain relief, ziconotide is a new therapy that has been approved for individuals with chronic

TABLE 23-2   Medications Effective for Neuropathic Pain

Drug Class	Representative Medications	Comments
Antidepressants	Desipramine Nortriptyline	Secondary amines
	Amitriptyline Imipremine Doxepin	Tertiary amines
	Venlafaxine Duloxetine	Has a combination effect from a selective serotonin reuptake inhibitor and a tricyclic antidepressant
Anticonvulsants	Carbamazepine Valproate Phenytoin	First-generation anticonvulsants, require monitoring of liver function and blood counts
	Clonazepam	A benzodiazepine
	Gabapentin Topiramate Pregabalin Lamotrigine	Second-generation, generally fewer side-effects
Opioids	Oxycodone Morphine Fentanyl Methadone	Usual in a adjuvant role, with sustained-release preparations. Methadone may have unique properties for neuropathic pain.
Topical agents	Lidocaine patch Topical creams	Most useful with limited areas of pain
Oral local anesthetics	Mexiletine	Should be used after failure of antidepressants and anticonvulsants
α_2-Agonists	Clonidine Tizanadine	Sedation can be a problematic side effect

pain. Ziconotide (Prialt) is the newest Food and Drug Administration (FDA)-approved drug delivered intrathecally from a surgically implanted pump.[3] Advantages of ziconotide should be noted. Ziconotide does not lead to tolerance, can be discontinued abruptly if needed, and does not bind to opioid receptors or cause respiratory depression. It works by blocking N-type calcium channels on nerves that normally transmit pain signals.[3] Side effects may include dizziness, nausea, confusion, headache, sleepiness, nystagmus, and weakness. Ziconotide must be titrated very slowly, should be used cautiously in older adults, and is contraindicated for individuals with a history of psychiatric symptoms.[3]

Anticonvulsants suppress epileptic seizure activity and are specialized analgesics for neuropathic pain. The mechanism is not well understood but may act by decreasing the excitability of nerves and reducing the number and strength of the pain signals that are sent to the brain, as membrane-stabilizing drugs or in reducing the pain transmission. Gabapentin (Neurontin) is used more frequently than any other anticonvulsant largely because of its ease of administration, lack of need for monitoring, and a relatively low incidence of serious adverse events. Gabapentin may be prescribed as first-line therapy for neuropathic pain and occasional patients may tolerate and benefit from escalated dosages above 3600 mg/daily, which is the therapeutic range listed in the literature.[2] The side effect of somnolence is the most common limiting factor for gabapentin. Pregabalin (Lyrica) has more recently been FDA approved at 300 mg/day with up to 600 mg/day. Other anticonvulsants include carbamazepine (Tegretol), oxcarbazepine (Trileptal), and levetiracetam

(Keppra). The anticonvulsant lamotrigine (Lamictal) has been shown to be effective for neuropathic pain (e.g., trigeminal neuralgia [TN]). The side effects of carbamazepine, including sedation, dizziness, nausea, unsteadiness, and the potential to produce bone marrow suppression (leukopenia), may limits its use[42] (Table 23-3). Trial and error is needed for the best pain adjuvant analgesia. Antidepressants have been prescribed for analgesia and may work by increasing the neurotransmitters serotonin and norepinephrine in the CNS that help to suppress pain signals that travel up the spinal cord to the brain. Antidepressants may include amitriptyline (Elavil), imipramine (Tofranil), duloxetine (Cymbalta), venlafaxine (Effexor), and others. Combination therapies may be effective in targeting multiple pain pathways or providing potentially synergistic analgesic effect.

Neurosurgical management of neuropathic pain, in particular entrapment neuropathies, is best handled with neurolysis, transposition, or decompression.[14] In patients with focal neuropathies therapy begins with the least invasive and continues an aggressive course up to invasive treatment until the patient finds relief. Effective therapies for neuropathic pain relief are few and the number of patients suffering from unrelieved chronic neuropathic pain remains large.[2]

NEURODIAGNOSTIC AND LABORATORY STUDIES

For some neuroscience patients with chronic pain the first step is to find the neurologic lesion and to establish an initial

TABLE 23-3   Anticonvulsants Used to Treat Neuropathic Pain

Drug	Dose (mg)	Frequency	How Supplied	Comments
First-Generation Anticonvulsants				
Carbamazepine (Tegretol)	100–1000	bid to qid	100, 200, 20 mg/mL suspension, also 200 and 300 mg CR tablets	Requires monitoring for liver toxicity and anemia.
Phenytoin (Dilantin)	100–300	qd	50, 100 mg, also 100 mg CR capsule, 25 mg/mL suspension	Not very helpful for neuropathic pain, significant side effects
Valproic Acid (Depakote)	150–1000	tid	125, 250, 500 mg coated tablets	Not very helpful for neuropathic pain; indicated for third-line migraine prophylaxis.
Clonazepam (Klonopin)	0.25–2.0 mg/day	tid	0.5, 1.0 and 2.0 mg tablets	Limited evidence for efficacy as an analgesic, must be weaned off slowly because of potential of seizures.
Second-Generation Anticonvulsants				
Pregabalin (Lyrical)	75–300 mg/day		75, 100 and 150 mg capsules	Not yet available; similar to Gabapentin in mechanism of action; linear pharmakinetics with easier dose titration.
Gabapentin (Neurontin)	900–3600	tid	100, 300, 400 mg capsules, 600 and 800 mg tablets	Indicated for postherpatic neuralgia. Doses should be titrated upward to 3600 mg at least before determined to be ineffective.
Lamotrigine (Lamictal)	150–500	bid	25, 100, 150, 200 mg tablets and 5, 25 mg dispersion tablet	Slow titration at 25 mg/week to avoid Stevens-Johnson syndrome. Also associated with nausea, vomiting, and visual disturbances.
Topiramate (Topamex)	25–200	bid	15, 25 mg capsules, 25, 100, 200 mg tablets	No consistent evidence for neuropathic pain, FDA for migraine prophylaxis. Associated with weight loss.
Oxcarbazepine (Trileptal)	150–300	bid to qid	150, 300, 600 mg tablets	Monitor sodium levels.
Levetiracetam (Keppra)	1000–4000	bid to qid	250, 500 mg tablets	Well tolerated, little evidence for efficacy.
Zonisamide (Zonagrem)	100–400	qd	100, 200, 300, 400 mg tablets	Titrate slowly, to avoid sedation; little evidence for efficacy.
Tiagabine (Gabitril)	2–32	bid to qid	2, 4, 12, 16 mg tablets	Small trials show some efficacy.

diagnosis of the underlying nervous system disorder. After the neurologic diagnosis has been determined, the source and location of chronic pain can be investigated. The following studies may be performed[42]:

- **Conventional x-ray films, CT, MRI:** The neuroradiologic tests that are most commonly used to evaluate the structural integrity of the nervous system to locate the source of pain.
- **Myelogram:** Occasionally needed when other studies are inconclusive because hemorrhage, hematomas, tumors, infections, and degenerative processes must be ruled out as causative factors for pain.
- **Nerve blocks:** Injection of an anesthetic agent into the peripheral nerve or plexus or the spinal epidural or subarachnoid space. This is often done before more

definitive treatment options are used to facilitate the identification of the specific nerves that are involved in the pain transmission problem and can predict the outcome of surgical or chemical interventions. The preganglionic autonomic fibers are most susceptible to these agents, followed by C fibers and then A-delta fibers.

- **Sweat test, pilomotor and/or vasomotor response, histamine flare, skin temperature:** Specialized tests of autonomic function studies that help to identify peripheral nerve pathologic conditions (e.g., CRPS) and guide interventions.
- **Ultrasound scans, endoscopic or laparoscopic procedures:** May be required when pain originates in the viscera.

- **EMG; nerve conduction studies; brainstem auditory evoked response (BAER), visual evoked response (VER), and somatosensory evoked response (SSER) potentials:** Used diagnostically to assess alterations in electrophysiologic function and intraoperatively to guide surgical interventions. If there is a need for a surgical approach to pain control, the surgeon can use the appropriate evoked potentials to monitor nerve function in areas adjacent to the operative target. This minimizes patient risk for damage to motor and other sensory functions.
- **PET, SPECT, regional blood flow studies, fMRI:** The application of these diagnostic imaging technologies to pain studies is an exciting new trend in testing to assist in diagnosing pain etiologies and revealing new information about the physiology of pain transmission.[10] The use of these studies in clinical practice, however, is still quite limited.
- **Psychologic evaluation:** A psychologic evaluation or neuropsychologic battery of tests may be useful to determine the emotional, cognitive, behavioral, social, or vocational factors involved in the pain perception.

TREATMENT

Medical Management

Efficacy is the ability of a drug to produce a specific result, regardless of dosage. Opioids have a nearly identical efficacy but require various dosages to obtain the effect. Drug **potency** is the amount of a drug it takes to achieve a target effect. Thus, because it takes smaller dosages of fentanyl than morphine to achieve the same degree of analgesia, morphine is less potent than fentanyl. However, both fentanyl and morphine have equal efficacy. That is, titrated properly, they both achieve the same degree of analgesia. The **half-life** of a drug is the time required to reduce a drug level to half of its initial value. Drugs commonly have four to five half-lives to achieve a **steady state.** If, for example, fentanyl has a half-life of approximately 4 hours, and it is given every 4 hours for 24 hours, it will reach a steady state in approximately 1 day (4 hours × 5 half-lives = 20 hours) and can be titrated on a daily basis.[27] The clinician often evaluates a patient's need for and response to the simultaneous administration of short-acting analgesics given for **breakthrough pain** while the patient is also receiving long-acting analgesics for chronic pain, as in the case of a transdermal patch with a half-life of 17 hours.

Issues about the **placebo effect** surround the concept of whether an inactive substance (e.g., saline, sterile water, glucose) or a less-than-effective dose of a harmless substance should ever be prescribed as if it were an effective dose of a needed pain medication. Placebos are frequently used in clinical trials to compare the effects of an inactive substance with those of the experimental drug. Trial participants given the placebo may report beneficial changes reflecting their expectations for a positive outcome. Recent research reported in the media described how Fabrizio Benedetti, M.D., from the University of Torino Medical School in Italy demon-

strated that the power of expectations has physical and not just psychologic effects. When individuals he studied knew that the nurse was giving opioid injections through a computerized system, the drug was up to 50% more effective. His work with individuals diagnosed with Alzheimer's disease, and unable to expect a pain medication to be effective, found that pain medication did not work nearly as well. Media coverage on new research by neurologist Tor Wager, M.D., from Columbia University in New York, found that an individual's expectations can have profound effects on the brain. Dr. Benedetti believes that there is probably not a single placebo effect but many placebo effects that differ by illness. New research is underway to show direct evidence that the placebo effect can actually trigger neurologic pathways to release endorphins that block transmission of pain signals comparable to prescription medications.

In the postoperative setting, patients undergoing craniotomy procedures may be undermedicated for pain because of concerns about increased sedation, inability to accurately assess the LOC, respiratory suppression, and the overall effects on cerebral blood flow (CBF) and intracranial pressure (ICP). Research has demonstrated that the undertreated pain can itself have negative effects on intracranial physiologic mechanisms.[29] Patients who have undergone craniotomy procedures report varying degrees of pain (see Chapter 8). Those who have had frontal craniotomies tend to report the greatest amount of postoperative pain.[16]

Pharmacologic Options for Pain Management

Options for competent and compassionate acute and chronic pain management include the use of NSAIDs, opioids, anticonvulsants, antidepressants, antispasmodics/muscle relaxants, corticosteroids, and other agents[47] (Tables 23-4, 23-5, and 23-6). Drug therapy must be highly individualized. The three-step analgesic ladder proposed by the World Health Organization (WHO)[62] is described in Fig. 23-4. The pharmacokinetics of each drug must be the basis of the dosing strategy. Blood flow, cardiac output, and protein binding influence drug clearance and the volume of distribution. Blood concentrations are also influenced by hepatic metabolism and clearance. The route of administration (i.e., intravascular or extravascular) regulates the magnitude and time course of plasma drug concentrations. For constant or chronic pain, drug concentrations require a consistent therapeutic blood level for pain to be well controlled.

Analgesic drugs are the cornerstone of acute and chronic pain management. Nonopioid analgesics are recommended for the relief of mild to moderate pain. For the relief of moderate to severe pain—whether acute, chronic nonmalignant, or cancer in origin—opioid analgesics are usually recommended. Depending on the etiology and/or characteristics of the pain, treatment with adjuvant drugs may also be indicated (Figs. 23-5 and 23-6).

Nonsteroidal antiinflammatory drugs (NSAIDs) are available over the counter (OTC) and often recommended as first-line analgesics. Examples include ibuprofen (Motrin), naproxen (Naprosyn), and aspirin. Indomethacin (Indocin) requires a prescription. NSAIDs act at the peripheral nervous system level (Table 23-7). They inhibit the release of

TABLE 23-4   Medications Used for Acute Pain

Medication	Site of Action	Why It Is Useful	Potential Routes of Administration
Opiates	CNS primarily. Peripheral effects potentially clinically important with further development.	Mainstay of treatment for acute pain. Binds to opiate receptors found in selected areas within the CNS.	Epidural, intrathecal for severe pain IV for most acute inpatient situations, usually PCA devices PO routes desirable, use timed-release formulations for tolerant patients
Nonsteroidal anti-inflammatory medications	Well-documented peripheral effects. Potentially useful CNS COX-2 inhibition reducing chance of wind-up.	Potent analgesics. Consider using selective COX-2 for perioperative and acute injuries where bleeding is a concern.	IV for katorolac and parecoxib, rest are PO only, consider long acting forms for preemptive effects
Local anesthetics	Peripheral and central nervous system	Can be used for regional blockade and as a adjuvant for epidural analgesia.	Injection and epidural infusion, also can be used through topical approaches
Anxiolytics, such as benzodiazepines	CNS	Anxiety increases the perception of pain.	Generally PO
NMOA antagonists, such as ketamine	CNS	Can reduce opiate requirements and improve neuropathic pain states.	Commonly IV, compounding pharmacies can make oral forms
Anticonvulsants	CNS	Improves neuropathic pain states.	Primarily PO
Muscle relaxants	CNS Usually only for short-term use.	Relieves acute muscle sprains and strains.	Primarily PO, orphenadrine and mathocarbamol are available in injectable form

CNS, central nervous system; *COX-2*, cycle-oxygenase-2.

TABLE 23-5   Chronic Pain Treatment Approaches

Treatment Modality	Description
Medication	Different types of medication can target different types of pain and associated symptoms. See Table 5 for more specific management discussion.
Relaxation training	Anxiety and unmanageable stress enhance a patient's pain perception. Learning relaxation techniques can combat anxiety and stress.
Biofeedback	These approaches can provide patient-initiated nonpharmacological treatment and helps give patients a sense of control
Nerve blocks and trigger point injections	Interventional treatments that can be helpful even when patients have not responded to noninvasive therapies.
Transcutaneous electrical nerve stimulation	Noninvasive device that can be helpful for select patients. Electrical energy is applied to the skin through electrodes.
Acupuncture and other alternative medicine approaches	Alternative medicine therapies have been very helpful for relaxation and analgesia in wall-selected patients as part of the treatment plan.
Nutrition counseling	Many patients with chronic pain are obese and require weight loss as part of a treatment plan.
Occupational and physical therapies	A must for almost all chronic pain patients to restore function.
Support and education, group and individual	Using groups and individual approaches, learning about what chronic pain is and how a patient can restore self-control can be very helpful.
Psychotherapy	Depression and other comorbid psychological conditions can stand in the way of meaningful progress in chronic pain management. Psychotherapy helps alleviate psychological conditions.
Vocational counseling	Very helpful for treatment plans that call for return to work. Should be obtained early in the treatment course to facilitate goal-directed treatment.
Surgery and implantable devices	In certain well-selected patients, implantable devices such as spinal cord stimulators and intrathecal pumps can be very helpful as part of a comprehensive treatment plan.

TABLE 23-6	Medication Classes Useful for Chronic Pain
Drug Class	**Pain Treated/Comments**
Opiates	Nociceptive pain. Helpful with appropriate adjuvants for neuropathic pain.
Nonsteroidal antiinflammatory drugs	Mainly useful for nociceptive pain. The variety of clinical settings in which the cyclo-oxygenase 2 agents can be used has increased.
Tricyclic antidepressants	Neuropathic pain, can improve sleep. Used also as a nonspecific analgesic for many types of pain.
Selective serotonin reuptake inhibitors	Might be helpful in neuropathic pain syndromes. Very helpful for depression, which is common in patients with chronic pain.
Anticonvulsants	Primarily used for neuropathic pain syndromes. Can be useful as adjuvant for opiates and for improving quality of sleep.
NMDA receptor antagonists such as ketamine, and dextromethorphan	Useful as opiate adjuvants, might help to improve responsiveness of neuropathic pain to opiates. Might be helpful to manage opiate tolerance.
Muscle relaxants	Nonspecific analgesics for muscle and myofascial pain syndromes.
Baclofen	Helpful for headaches and myofascial pain syndromes.
α_2-Agonist drugs such as tizanadine or clonidine	Useful for opiate withdrawal, can be helpful for neuropathic pain.
Topical medications such as lidocaine patch, desipramine cream, and other compounded formulations	Localized neuropathic pain or dyesthesias.

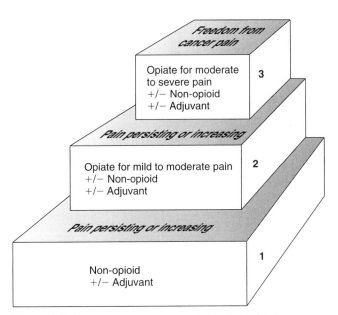

Figure 23-4 World Health Organization's (WHO's) three-step Pain Relief Ladder.

bradykinin and prostaglandins, both of which augment pain messages.[40] Acetaminophen is not an NSAID and has little antiinflammatory action but does have analgesic properties. Although these drugs are effective in the relief of mild pain, there is a recommended dosage ceiling for each. Increasing the dosage beyond the ceiling may not increase pain control yet may potentiate significant side effects. For example, the administration of acetaminophen beyond 4 g per day is associated with liver damage and is not recommended.[55] Yet, many individuals exceed this amount daily through the use of both prescription medications (e.g., acetaminophen/hydrocodone [Vicodin]) and OTC preparations for pain, colds, sleep disturbances, or other symptoms. The maximum dose for ibuprofen is 3.2 g/day and is found in many OTC remedies. Long-term administration of the salicylates produces gastric irritation and inhibition of platelet aggregation.

In selecting an appropriate NSAID for the treatment of pain, it is important to remember that choice is influenced by several factors. Patient response to each of these medications is not equal. Although optimal pain relief is a treatment goal, the presence of side effects must also be considered. In the older patient, compromised hepatic or renal function makes drug selection and dosage titration more difficult.[55] When patient compliance is an issue, those preparations available in once- or twice-a-day dosing may be a better choice. Side effects should also be a concern. For patients who may experience gastrointestinal (GI) bleeding, an NSAID may not be the first choice. Patients for whom renal functioning is a concern may not be candidates because NSAID can cause renal toxicity. Finally, cost is an additional factor to be considered. In general, preparations that are time-released for convenience are usually more expensive.

Acetylsalicylic acid (aspirin) is a nonselective cyclooxygenase (COX) inhibitor and a nonsteroidal salicylate that inhibits prostaglandin synthesis (see Table 23-6). It acts on the hypothalamus heat-regulating center and blocks prostaglandin synthetase action. Aspirin is recommended for mild to moderate pain and reduces the amount of nociceptive signals generated. Aspirin reduces inflammatory response and intensity of pain stimulus reaching sensory nerve endings. The drug is rapidly absorbed from the GI tract with a half-life of 15 to 20 minutes. High doses of aspirin may produce GI bleeding and toxicity.[40]

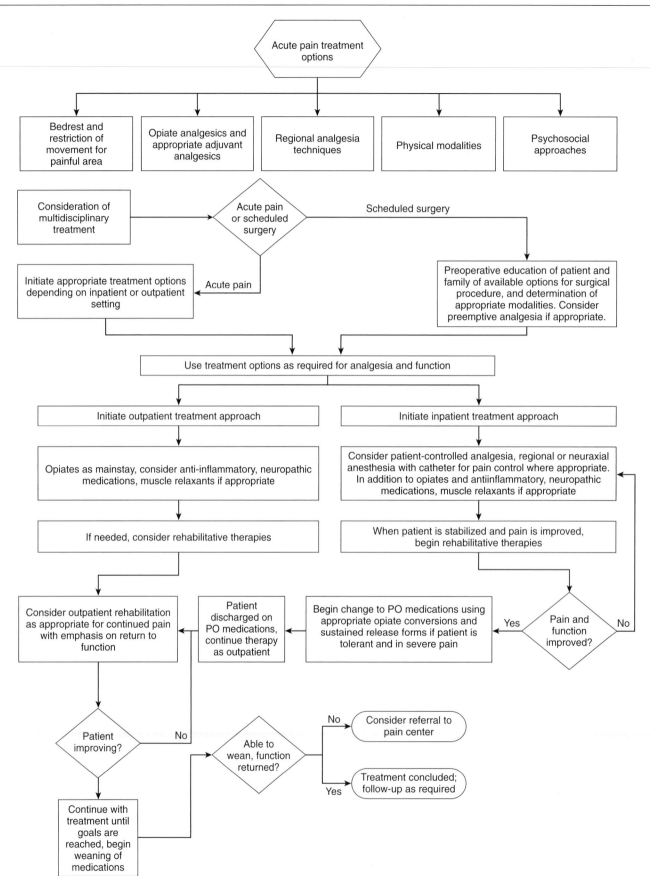

Figure 23-5 Acute pain treatment overview.

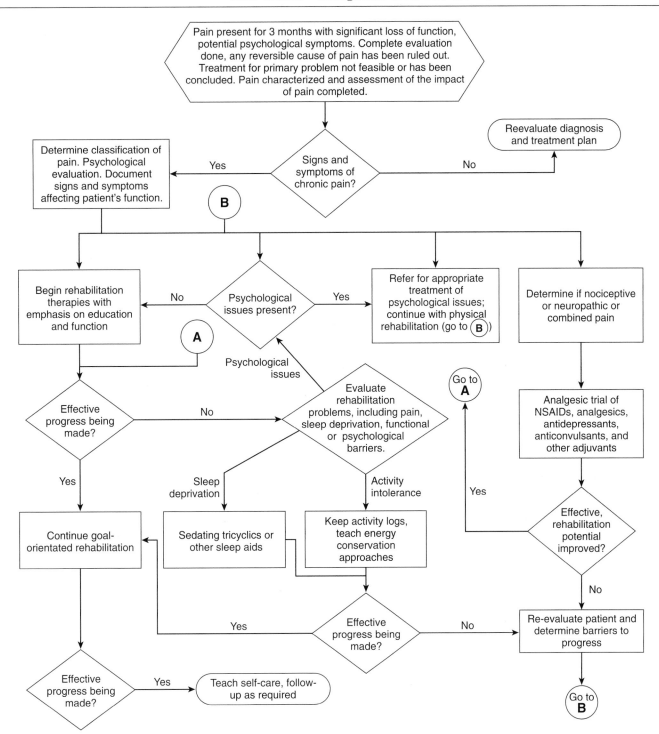

Figure 23-6 Treatment approach for chronic pain.

Nonselective COX inhibitors are recommended for mild to moderate pain. The group includes OTC drugs (e.g., ibuprofen [Advil, Nuprin, and Motrin], naproxen [Naprosyn]) (see Table 23-6). These drugs share characteristics similar to aspirin; therefore, patients should not combine these drugs. It has been estimated that more than 100,000 hospitalizations and 16,500 deaths from GI side effects occur annually, particularly in the older adult population.[27]

Acetaminophen (Tylenol) is an OTC central analgesic for mild to moderate pain (see Table 23-6). Its exact mechanism is unknown but the drug appears to inhibit prostaglandin synthesis in the CNS and, to a lesser extent, block pain impulses through peripheral action for an analgesic effect.[40] Tylenol does not promote bleeding and is considered safe following perioperative neurosurgical procedures. Acetaminophen is rapidly, completely absorbed from the GI tract and metabolized in the liver with a half-life of 1 to 4 hours. Because of liver metabolism, this drug is contraindicated in active alcoholism, liver disease, or viral hepatitis, which can increase the risk of hepatotoxicity. The dose should not

TABLE 23-7	Dosing and Characteristics of Common Nonopioid Analgesics				
Drug	Dose (mg)	Peak Effect (hour)	Duration of Action/ Half-Life (hour)	Precautions/ Contraindications	Comments
Acetaminophen	325–1000 mg q4–6 hr	2	4–6/0.25	Avoid combining with alcohol	Found as a combination with many drugs, especially opioids
Aspirin	325–1000 mg q4–6 hr	2	4–6/0.25	Irreversible platelet effects	Used in combination with some opioids
Diflunisal	200–500 q12 hr	1–2	>12/8–20	Platelet effects	
Choline salicylate with magnesium salicylate	870–1740 q3–4 hr	0.5–1.0	>12/8–20	Tinnitus in high doses	
Indomethacin	25–75 mg	2	6–8/2–3	Headache and psychosis	Easily penetrates the CNS
Sulindac	150–200 mg	1–2	12		Prodrug
Etodolec	200–400 q6–8 hr	2	4–6/6		
Ketorolec tromethamine	IM 60 mg IV 30 mg <120 mg/day 10 mg q4–6 hr	05–1.0	6/5		
Diclofenec sodium	50 mg q8 hr	1	8/1–2		
Naproxen	250–500 q8–12 hr	2	8–12/12–15		Over-the-counter formulation
Ketoprofen	50–100 q6–8 hr	1–2	6/1–35		Easily penetrates the CNS
Ibuprofen	200–800 q8–12 hr	1–2	4–6/2		Used in combination with some hydrocodones
Oxaprozin	1200 qd	3–6	24/59		
Piroxicam	20 q12–24	2–4	>24/45	Low acting NSAIDs increase gastrointestinal risk	
Meloxicam	7.5–15 mg	1–3	4–6/16–20	Low dose range is generally subtherapeutic	Some selectivity to COX-2 in low doses only
Nabumetone	1000–2000 qd	9–12	24/24	Increased incidence of liver toxicity	
Calecoxib	200–600 qd	3	6–8/11.2		Small risk of allergy in patients with history of sulfa allergies Cardiovascular concerns have been raised
Valdecoxib	10–40 qd	3	24/18		Cardiovascular concerns have been raised

CNS, central nervous system; *NSAIDs,* nonsteroidal antiinflammatory drugs.

exceed 4000 mg per day. The antidote for toxicity is acetylcysteine.[40]

Opioids are the oldest class of analgesic medicine and still the most effective, primarily used to relieve intense pain and anxiety that accompanies it.[27] They bind to opioid receptors in the CNS to block pain impulses in the brain. Opioids (e.g., morphine sulfate [short acting], codeine) are naturally occurring substances isolated from the sap of the opium poppy (Table 23-8). All opioids cause side effects, with respiratory depression the most serious side effect.

ALERT: Prescribing or administering two long-acting agents (e.g., methadone and opioids) is questionable, is a duplication of pain therapy, and may place the individual at risk for respiratory depression and medi-

cation toxicity. Generally, it is not recommended to prescribe or administer two analgesics from the same class unless one is sustained release used on a round-the-clock basis and the other is for instant release of breakthrough pain.

Constipation is experienced by most patients (Table 23-9). This requires initiating a bowel program that emphasizes adequate hydration, stimulant laxatives, and stool softeners as adjunct therapy.[27]

Fentanyl (Duragesic) is a strong agonist that has 80 to 100 times the analgesic potency of morphine. It has a rapid onset and short duration with an IV half-life of 2 to 4 hours. It is also available as a transdermal patch. Meperidine (Demerol) is prescribed for acute pain and produces less of an increase

TABLE 23-8	**Equianalgesic Opiate Doses**

Drug	Equianalgesic Doses (mg)		Available Doses	Comments
	IM/IV	Oral		
Morphine	10	30 (chronic)	Liquid 10 and 20 mg/5 mL, 20 mg/mL	Kadian 20, 30, 50, 60, 100 mg and Avinza 30, 60, 90, 120 mg both labeled for 24-hour release
		60 (acute)	SR or CR 15, 30, 60, 100, 200 mg	
			IR dose 15, 30 mg and injectable forms	
Hydromorphone	1.5	7.5	Supp 3 liquid 5 mg/5 mL	Palladone doses of 12, 16, 24, and 32 mg, to be used only in opioid tolerant patients
			Tablets 2, 4, 8 mg	No active metabolite accumulation with renal failure.
			Injectable forms	
Oxycodone	N/A	20	CR tablet 10, 20, 40, 80 mg	Parcodan and Percocet combination medications with acetaminophen
			IR dose 5 mg	
			Liquid 5 mg/mL or 20 mg/mL	
Codeine	130	200	Elixir 15 mg/mL	Very weak opiate
			Solution 15 mg/mL	
			Tablets 15, 30, 60 mg	
Fentanyl	0.1 or 100 µg	N/A	Transdermal 25, 50, 75, 100 µg/hr	25 µg patch equivalent to 50 mg of morphine per day. For orelat dosing, see below.
			Oralet 200, 400, 600, 800, 1200, 1600 µg	
			Injectable	
Oxymorphone	1	10 (rectal)	Supp 5 mg and injectable	Oral formulation in clinical trials
Merperidine	75	300	Tablets 50, 100 mg	Avoid chronic dosing, metabolite nomar-pyridine can cause central nervous system excitation
			Syrup 50 mg/5 mL	
Proproxyphene	N/A	130–200	Suspension 50 mg/ 5 mL	Short-acting analgesic with metabolite accumulation. Infrequent clinical use
			Tablet Darvocot N-100	
Levorphanol	1 (chronic)	1 (chronic)	Tablet 2 mg	Long half-life
	2 (acute)	4 (acute)	Injectable	Accumulates on day 2–3
Methadone	10 (acute)	20 (acute)	Liquid: 1 and 10 mg/mL	Shorter acting analgesic than metabolic half-life
	2–4 (chronic)	2–4 (chronic)	Tablet 5, 10, and 40 mg wafer	
			Injectable	
Hydrocodone	N/A	10 mg	2.5, 5, 7.5, and 10 mg with acetaminophen doses including 325, 500 and 750 mg	Available only as combinations with acetaminophen
Tramadol	N/A	N/A	50 mg single dose or 37.5 mg with acetaminophen 325 mg	Slight opioid activity

Balow is a list of partial agonist and antagonist medications. These are not commonly used for chronic pain. They will cause withdrawal symptoms in opioid-tolerant patients.

Drug	Doses		Comments
	SL	IM	
Buprenorphine	0.4–0.8	0.3–0.6	Very lipid soluble, could be used sublingually, also long acting
Butorphanol	N/A	2	Hallucinations and other cognitive disturbances
Nalbuphina	N/A	10–20	Hallucinations and other cognitive disturbances but less than pentazocine
Pentazocine	50–200	40–60	Hallucinations and other cognitive disturbances

CR, Controlled release; *IR*, immediate release; *SR*, sustained release; *Supp*, suppository.

TABLE 23-9	Opioid Side Effect Management	
Side Effect	Treatment Approach	Comments
Nausea	Antiemetics or pro-peristaltic agents	Ensure the patient is not constipated.
Sedation	Psychostimulants such as methylphenidate or modafinil	Use low doses and administer in AM to avoid sleep difficulties. Consider depression with this side effect.
Euphoria	Trial of methadone	This can be a troubling side affect for many patients.
Constipation	Bowel program	Use prophylatic measures to avoid this routine side effect.
Loss of libido	Hormonal replacement therapy	High-dose opiates cause suppression of the hypothalamic pituitary axis.
Loss of appetite	Anabolic steroids or dronabinol (Marinol)	Also a symptom of depression.
Dizziness	Consider scopolamine patch	Opioids can have an effect on the inner ear balance mechanism.
Urinary retention	Trial of bladder muscle stimulant such as bethanechol	If using a tricyclic or other anticholinergic, consider stopping or changing medication.
Respiratory depression	Usually not needed; tolerance builds rapidly	If respiratory depression is noted, look for new developing pathologic condition.
Myoclonus	GABA agonists such as baclofen, benzodiazepines	Rare with oral routes, consider reducing opioid doses if able, opioid rotation or alternate routes such as epidural or intrathecal route.

in urinary retention than morphine.[40] Methadone is 10 times more potent than morphine sulfate and a strong agonist and synthetic oral opioid with a half-life of 15 to 25 hours. This drug is inexpensive and used in the controlled withdrawal of addicts from heroin and morphine.

Oxycodone (OxyContin) is a semisynthetic strong opioid and one and a half to two times more potent than morphine sulfate. The short-acting agent is OxyFAST; OxyContin is the extended release form that can be administered every 12 hours.

ALERT: Patients taking OxyContin should avoid alcohol, which may cause the release of all the medication at once.

Hydromorphone (Dilaudid) is also a semisynthetic strong opioid. When opioids are used in combination with nonopioid analgesics, there is a dual peripheral and CNS action. The net effect of this synergism is reduction of the opioid dosage needed to achieve pain control. Although most μ opioid agonists have no clinical ceiling, unacceptable side effects can include nausea, vomiting, pruritus, constipation, sedation, and respiratory depression. Management of side effects may require the concomitant use of antiemetics, antihistamines, and laxatives/stool softeners. Patients must be treated prophylactically for the prevention of constipation, especially those who must avoid Valsalva maneuvers (e.g., subarachnoid hemorrhage [SAH], increased ICP [IICP]). In the patient with an altered LOC, medications to treat side effects should be chosen judiciously. Antihistamines (e.g., diphenhydramine [Benadryl], hydroxyzine [Vistaril]), as well as some antiemetics (e.g., phenothiazines) can result in a significant increase in sedation and constipation. Stimulants such as methylphenidate (Ritalin) can be useful for counteracting the sedative effects of opioids and potentiate the analgesia.[51,63] Tolerance and physical dependence are seen after sustained opioid administration. Therapeutic analgesic effects are maintained by increases in dosage as needed.

Tolerance to the drug does not necessarily mean addiction. When treatment is no longer needed, dosages should be slowly tapered to prevent signs and symptoms of opioid withdrawal.

Tramadol (Ultram) is an atypical opioid that binds to μ opioid receptors and inhibits reuptake of norepinephrine. It can produce less sedation and respiratory depression than a pure opioid agonist. This makes it a viable option for the neurologically compromised patient in whom sedation is an issue. It is contraindicated, however, in the patient with a seizure history or a high potential for seizure activity, and it can accumulate in patients with renal dysfunction.

Codeine is often overused in the neurosurgical patient population. Although it can be effective in the treatment of mild to moderate pain, it is not an effective choice for moderate to severe pain and can cause significant constipation for some patients. Preferred opioid choices include morphine, hydromorphone, and fentanyl for this patient population.

Opioids are appropriate to use for selected patients with chronic nonmalignant pain when there is no relief from other methods.[46] With many neuropathic pain states, opioids are not the primary pharmacologic choice, yet they can still provide some degree of pain control. When opioids are used to treat the patient with chronic nonmalignant pain, the use of an opioid contract can assist the clinician in providing clear boundaries and in establishing defined patient expectations.[20]

Anticonvulsants have been used for many years for the treatment of pain, particularly neuropathic pain (described earlier). These drugs have not been found to be as useful in the treatment of somatic or visceral pain (see Table 23-3). Anticonvulsants, such as carbamazepine (Tegretol) and phenytoin (Dilantin), are thought to stabilize the neuronal membranes and suppress spontaneous firing (e.g., sharp, shooting, lancinating pain) of TN and other pain problems. The exact mechanism by which gabapentin (Neurontin) facilitates pain relief is still not understood, but it is now used more prevalently in the treatment of neuropathic pain syndromes than it is in the treatment of seizure disorders. Additional anticonvulsants (e.g., lamotrigine) are being used in various clinical settings and trials for the treatment of specific pain conditions.[18] Cymbalta is a new drug approved for treatment of fibromyalgia and painful diabetic neuropathy.

It is presumed that pain transmission can be blocked with these agents by the suppression of paroxysmal neuronal discharges in which anticonvulsants block seizure activity. Dosages of anticonvulsants used for the treatment of pain should be individualized and titrated judiciously to effect. Common side effects of anticonvulsants include sedation, dizziness, and nausea. Rapid-dose titration can lead to more patient reports of side effects and perceived drug intolerance.

Antidepressants are widely acknowledged for their efficacy in treating depression but have a role in the treatment of pain, particularly neuropathic pain, with and without concurrent depression, anxiety, insomnia, or depression. Pain transmission results in the physiologic depletion of serotonin and norepinephrine within the CNS. Antidepressants play a significant role in the treatment of pain by blocking the reuptake of these neurotransmitters and enhancing pain modulation. Tricyclic antidepressants (TCAs), such as amitriptyline (Elavil), nortriptyline (Pamelor), and desipramine (Norpramin), remain highly effective as a treatment of specific neuropathic pain conditions (e.g., diabetic neuropathy, postherpetic neuralgia). The analgesic effects of these medications may occur at doses lower than those given to treat primary depression, but the anticholinergic (e.g., decreased salivation) and adrenergic (e.g., orthostatic hypotension) side effects of these medications persist. Selective serotonin reuptake inhibitors (SSRIs) such as paroxetine (Paxil) and fluoxetine (Prozac) have given clinicians additional options for treating pain, especially in patients who cannot tolerate TCAs. Although clinicians continue to use SSRIs for the treatment of pain, results of studies demonstrating efficacy are mixed. Dosages of all antidepressants used to treat pain must be individualized and cautiously titrated to effect, especially in older patients. When appropriate, single-dose administration before bedtime is the preferred method. This minimizes daytime drowsiness and facilitates more restful sleep for the individual experiencing pain.

The choice of antidepressants must be individualized. The older medicines in this class (e.g., amitriptyline [Elavil]) have a broader spectrum of side effects, such as dizziness and drowsiness. For example, they might not be the best choice for an elderly man with trigeminal pain, because of the risk of urinary problems related to benign prostatic hypertrophy. Elavil has a half-life of 10 to 26 hours. Side effects may include rapid eye movement sleep rebound, characterized by vivid dreaming near awaking.[27] Oral dosage for pain management for adults ranges from 25 to 100 mg one hour before bedtime.[40] A newer medication option, recently approved by the FDA for treating neuropathic pain, is the serotonin norepinephrine reuptake inhibitor (SNRI) duloxetine (Cymbalta).

Skeletal **muscle relaxants** are used to treat acute musculoskeletal pain. The primary mechanism of action is through the CNS. A common mistake made with these medications is assuming that all the drugs in a given class have the same effects (Table 23-10). Muscle relaxants and antispasmodics, such as baclofen (Lioresal), metaxalone (Skelaxin), and tizanidine (Zanaflex), relieve the pain of muscle spasms.

Baclofen has been found to inhibit monosynaptic and polysynaptic pain transmissions within the spinal cord and possibly even at the supraspinal level. Baclofen, which is chemically similar to the inhibitory neurotransmitter GABA, is often used intrathecally to treat severe spasticity associated with conditions such as multiple sclerosis (MS) or cerebral palsy (CP).[22]

When there is soft tissue swelling and edema, **corticosteroids** are effective in reducing the edema and as a consequence may improve pain (Table 23-11). For example, dexamethasone (Decadron) 4 mg every 4 hours may be prescribed for reduction of cerebral edema in the case of IICP from cerebral metastasis. In the case of neuropathic pain from compressive tumors in the head, cortisteroids may have a role.[30] Awareness of the serious side effects requires tapering the dosage to the lowest effective dose for the shortest period of time. Weight gain, peripheral edema, and cushingoid features can appear rapidly.[40]

Topical Medications. Newer insights into the physiologic changes that occur with pain reveal that sensitization changes do not just occur within the CNS (Table 23-12). Peripheral sensitization is also very important in the initial response to acute injury and seems to play a role in the perpetuation of some chronic pain states as well. When the patient applies topical applications there is no concern for undesirable side effects. Usually only small areas can be treated. Patients may have to seek out compounding pharmacies to obtain these topical medications. Lidocaine 5% dermal patches are used to treat herpetic neuralgia. Capsaicin topical cream in Lidocaine may be prescribed or administered to relieve neuralgia pain (e.g., diabetic neuropathy, postherpetic neuralgia) and is thought to deplete and prevent reaccumulation of substance P in peripheral sensory neurons. OTC topical analgesics with lidocaine or capsaicin may not be as effective because they have weaker strengths than the prescription drug, but they could be tried to check the response.[52]

Medication and Routes of Delivery

Dosing Tables/Scales. Opioid equianalgesic dosing tables and charts are now readily available in most pain textbooks and clinical resource manuals (see Table 23-8 for equianalgesic dosing).[19] Dosage recommendations must be individualized to the patient and titrated to the desired analgesic effect. Caution should be exercised in initiating treatment in the opioid-naive patient who has had minimal previous exposure to opioids. Patients with traumatic brain injury or who have undergone neurosurgery should be carefully monitored, ideally within an intensive care environment, because opioids are administered and titrated slowly to achieve analgesia. Frequent evaluation of sedation and respiratory status should occur at least hourly for the first 24 to 48 hours of treatment. The clinician should use a sedation scale ranging from awake to severely sedated for monitoring the LOC. The goal for opioid therapy is to achieve maximum analgesia with minimal side effects of treatment.

TABLE 23-10 Muscle Relaxants: Dosing, Effects, and Pharmacological Profile

Agent	Dose	Onset of Action	Duration of Action/ Half-Life	Precautions/Contraindications	Special Effects
Baclofen	5–10 mg tid up to 80 mg/day	3–4 d	3–4 d/2.5–4 hr	Renal impairment, can cause depression, rebound effects common	Can be used for chronic pain conditions
Carisoprodol	350 mg tid/qid	30 min	4–6 hr/8 hr	Dependency liability of metabolite meprobamate	Additive effects with alcohol end central nervous system depressants
Chlorzoxazone	250–750 mg tid/qid	1 hr	3–4 hr/1–2 hr	Rare hepatocellular toxicity	No known pharmacokinetic interactions
Cyclobenzaprine	5–10 mg tid	1 hr	12–24 hr/24–72 hr	Several drug interactions, especially monoamine oxidase inhibitors	Tricyclic effects, indicated for short-term treatment only
Diazepam	2–10 mg tid/qid	30 min	Variable duration/ 20–50 hr	Abstinence syndrome with abrupt discontinuation	Caution in addiction-prone patents
Metaxalone	800 mg tid/qid	1 hr	4–6 hr/1–2 hr	Avoid in patients with renal or hepatic dysfunction	No significant drug interactions; avoid in patients with history of drug-induced anemia
Methocarbamol	750–1500 mg qid	30–60 min	4–6 hr/1–2 hr	Avoid IV form in patients with seizure disorders or renal failure	IV form available
Orphenadrine	100 mg bid	1 hr	12 hr/14–72 hr	Potential anticholinergic effects	Few drug interactions
Tizanidine	4–8 mg tid/qid, max 36 mg/day	2 wk	8 wk/2.5 hr	Potential for liver injury, avoid in patients using oral contraceptives and with renal impairment because of decreased clearance	Can be used for spasticity and myofascial pain syndromes

Routes for Medication Administration. The routes available for opioid administration are extensive. Minimally invasive routes (e.g., transdermal, oral, buccal, rectal) should be used as much as possible. The medications available for these routes are generally effective when titrated correctly. Fentanyl is currently available in a transdermal preparation, which is a useful option for patients unable to take medication by mouth. This route is convenient but can be more costly for the patient. Intramuscular (IM) injections should be avoided because of unpredictable medication absorption, associated pain at the injection site, and the potential for tissue damage. Systemic intravascular administration of opioids is commonly used in the acute care setting.

Patient-Controlled Analgesia. **PCA** is an alternative method of pain relief for the cognitively intact patient to self-administer opioids. With IV PCA the patient injects the drug intravenously within prescribed parameters using a computer-controlled infusion device. The patient must be able to understand how to use the device to control the pain. Pharmacologic advantages of PCA include greater stability of opioid blood levels, minimal delay between pain and relief, greater dose flexibility, and titration capability. In addition, improved analgesia can be associated with psychologic benefits, including enhanced patient control, participation in care, and patient satisfaction. The patient must be closely monitored (e.g., the IV site should be observed for signs and symptoms of infiltration and phlebitis, with close attention paid to the alarms and proper working condition of the equipment). In addition, the clinician should assess patient response to treatment on a regular basis and verify that the pain treatment goals are being met.

In the acute care setting, IV PCA is most commonly used for pain control after surgery. It can also be used for other patients who have uncontrolled pain, especially when they are unable to tolerate medications by the oral route. Some acute care settings use oral PCA for appropriate patients. In this case patients self-medicate as needed for pain per physician order instead of ordering the administration of as-needed analgesics. IV PCA can also be found in home care, hospice, and long-term care settings. Alternatively, subcutaneous PCA may be used when IV access or maintenance becomes problematic for the patient. Fentanyl transdermal patch 25 mcg/hr is also available and has been found to be equivalent to PCA IV use.

Other Routes. There are other routes for the administration of analgesics (e.g., the epidural or intrathecal space). Neuraxial opioid administration into the epidural or intrathecal space produces analgesia with less sedation. The pain relief is mediated by direct action on the spinal cord opiate receptors. These receptors bind in the dorsal horn receptors and

TABLE 23-11   Steroids for Chronic Pain

Drug	Dose	How Supplied	Indications	Comments
Oral Steroids				
Dexamethasone (Decadron)	1–4 mg qid	0.5, 0.75, and 4 mg for oral use, 24 mg/mL for injection	Cancer pain emergencies. Helpful as an antiemetic and treatment of cachexia.	Should be used short-term if possible, reduce dose as able, as other medications are titrated up and become effective
Prednisone (Deltasone, Cortan, and others)	No specific dose recommendations for pain conditions	1, 2.5, 5, 10, 20, 50 mg tablets	Inflammatory indications	Short-term use
Methylprednisolone (Medrol)	No specific dose recommendations for pain conditions	2, 4, 8, 16, 24, 32 mg tablets	Acute headache management and other acute pain crises	Dose packs for short-term bolus therapies
Depot Steroids for Injection				
Methylpredisolone (Depo-Medrol)	1–3 mL depending on use	40 and 80 mg/mL	Used with nerve blocks, epidurals, joint injections, and other procedures	Epidural use requires preservative-free formulation
Triamcinolone (Aristocort)	Same as above	25 mg/mL	Same as above	Same use, small particle size
Anabolic Steroids				
Magestrol	160–800 mg/day	20 and 40 mg tablets	Both anabolic and antiemetic effects	Progestational steroid, avoid use in patients with estrogen-dependent cancers
Oxymetholone (Anadrol)	150–200 mg/day	50 mg tablet	Both anabolic and antiemetic effects. Delayed effect, up to 3 months	Androgenic drug, avoid use in patients with testosterone-dependent cancers

produce pain relief at the level of injection. Rostral caudal spread of the medication is affected by the injected fluid volume and by the pharmacologic properties of the medications. The opioids most commonly used for intrathecal administration are morphine, fentanyl, and hydromorphone. When administered via the epidural route, fentanyl, with lipophilic characteristics, diffuses rapidly through the dura into the CSF and is then taken up quickly by the vessels and fat within the epidural space. There is rapid onset of action and little rostral-caudal spread from the level of injection or infusion. Morphine and hydromorphone, which are both hydrophilic, have difficulty moving through the lipid-rich dura. After they transverse the dura, they dissolve quickly in an aqueous solution such as CSF and can circulate rostrally within the CSF.[49] Preparations are generally preservative free, and other agents such as local anesthetics (e.g., bupivacaine) or alpha-2 agonists (e.g., clonidine) may be added to potentiate desired therapeutic effects. The addition of local anesthetics allows a reduction in the amount of opioid and does not exert sensory effects when kept to a low percentage.

In the acute care setting epidural and intrathecal opioid administration are being used with increasing frequency for postoperative and posttraumatic pain. These methods result in excellent pain relief with lower medication doses and generally with fewer side effects. Administration of spinal opioids can be either single-bolus medication injection (e.g., morphine [Duramorph] every 24 hours) or continuous infusion through a temporary catheter and using a computer-controlled device to regulate the infusion. Epidural PCA is also an available option for patients. In this instance patients are able to administer epidural bolus doses within prescribed parameters set into the infusion device. All patients should be monitored closely for increased sedation, depressed respirations, sensorimotor deficits, urinary retention, and orthostatic hypotension. For patients with temporary epidural catheters, additional responsibilities include (1) ensuring that the catheter does not become disconnected, dislodged, or kinked; (2) keeping the insertion site free of contamination; and (3) inspecting the site for leakage, bleeding, or signs and symptoms of infection.[54] It is imperative when removing the catheter to inspect the entire catheter to make certain the tip was not left inside the body.

Epidural pain management also plays a role in providing pain relief for patients in home, hospice, and extended care settings. Permanent catheters, tunneled from posterior to anterior via the subcutaneous space, are used for providing

TABLE 23-12	Topical Medications for Pain Management			
Drug Class	**Examples**	**Mechanism of Action**	**Pain Conditions**	**Comments**
Local anesthetics	EMLA Lidoderm (lidocaine impregnated patch)	Blockade of sodium channels important in neuropathic pain and a local anesthetic effect	Postherpetic neuralgia, localized hyperalgesia, myofascial pain	Because of irritation from the adhesive, lidoderm patch is used intermittently, 12 hours on and 12 hours off
Capsaicin	Multiple brand names (e.g., Zostrix)	Substance P depletion	Hyperalgesia, takes 2–4 weeks for benefit	Difficult to tolerate, leads to substantial noncompliance
Topical tricyclic antidepressants	Doxapin (Zonulon), emitryptaline, nortripraline, desipramine	Sodium channel blockade, block reuptake of norepinephrine, serotonin, indirect action on the opiate receptor and NMDA receptor blockade	Use in areas of hyperalgesia and intractable itch, such as chronic pain from burns, eczema, postherpetic neuralgia	Avoid large areas of treatment because of systemic toxicity
Anticonvulsants	Gabapentin, trileptal	GABA or sodium channel blockade	Neuromas, local neuropathic pain	Small uncontrolled studies support use
Opiates	Morphine, dilaudid	Peripheral opiate receptors	Decubitus ulcers, burns	Peripheral opiate receptors seen only in acute inflammatory states
NSAIDs	Aspirin, ketoprofen, nebumetone (Relafen), diclofenec (Cataflam), piroxicam (Feldene)	Reduces production of peripheral prostaglandins	Acute muscloskeletal injuries and myofascial pain. Less effect on chronic rheumatic conditions.	Can have significant systemic absorption, with same side effects as oral use; also local rash and pruritus
Nitrates	Nitroglycerin	Smooth muscle relaxation	Tendon and musculoskeletal disorders, thrombophlebitis	Common side effect is headache
α-Agonists	Clonidine (Catepress)	Alpha receptor is involved in analgesia	RSD, causalgia, diabetic neuropathy	Use as a patch or topical cream
NMDA receptor antagonists	Ketamine, dextromorphan	NMDA receptor blockade	RSD, causalgia, other local neuropathic pain disorders	Ketamine has more data for efficacy

EMLA, Enteric mixture of local anesthetic; *NSAID*, nonsteroidal antiinflammatory drug; *RSD*, reflex sympathetic dystrophy.

long-term epidural pain control to these patients. Although catheter migration is less of a problem, monitoring for medication side effects and signs of infection should continue.

A surgically implanted **intrathecal pump** for an IDDS is an option for patients with chronic, intractable pain who are intolerant of oral opioids with pain refractory to high-dose opioids and concerned about dependency.[58] Aggressive pain control can be achieved because the IDDS provides direct drug distribution to target specific receptors in the nervous system that are generating the discomfort for improved pain relief. Patients receiving IDDS therapy drugs have easier drug titration, reduced dosages, and enhanced pain control with minimal side effects. Factors for considering IDDS as an option include appropriate patient selection, a screening

trial, surgically cleared for pump implantation, and compliance for long-term follow-up and monitoring.

Patients with failed back syndrome, arachnoiditis, or severe neuropathies that are opioid responsive may be candidates for an implanted device (see Chapter 13). After the device is implanted and the dosage is programmed to deliver maximum analgesia, patients can enjoy being free of external equipment from the intrathecal administration of the medication.[33]

Fentanyl (Duragesic) is available as a transdermal patch in 25 mcg/hr, 50 mcg/hr, 75 mcg /hr or 100 mcg/hr. Instruct the patient on how to apply and remove the patch and the importance of maintaining an exact schedule to avoid an overdose. The skin should be cleansed thoroughly with only water and dried and the patch applied to nonhairy areas where the skin is intact on the upper torso. Press the patch firmly against the skin evenly for 10 to 20 seconds to ensure adhesion is in full contact with the skin and the edges are completely sealed. Rotate the sites and fold the used patch over so that the edges adhere to themselves. Instructions may indicate to discard the used patch in the toilet.[40]

Various Treatment Approaches for Successful Pain Management

Comprehensive pain management may employ various modalities and medications (Table 23-13). Interventions for acute pain begin with the least invasive and continue until the pain management plan is successful. For patients who have pain present for 3 months or longer with significant loss of function and psychologic symptoms, a different approach is needed.

Adjuvant drugs are commonly used for pain control, especially when there is a neuropathic pain component present. These drugs either have analgesic properties of their own or work synergistically to increase the effects of other analgesics. New uses in pain management are being found for many medications traditionally associated with the treatment of other conditions. Clonidine (Catapres), a blood pressure medication, affects pain receptors at the central and peripheral levels. This alpha-2 adrenergic agonist can provide pain relief either when administered alone in a transdermal patch or in a spinal infusion, where it is usually used in conjunction with an opioid, whose effects it potentiates.

A more recent example is dextromethorphan, an N-methyl-D-aspartate (NMDA) receptor antagonist that suppresses coughing and is found in many OTC preparations. It also has been found at higher doses to provide analgesia and is used concurrently with morphine to enhance the clinical effectiveness of the opioid without increasing side effects. Its clinical mechanism of action is to inhibit central sensitization of spinal NMDA receptors; thus it is termed an NMDA receptor antagonist.[26] Dextromethorphan-morphine (MorphiDex) is undergoing final U.S. FDA studies before commercial release.

There are seven distinct serotypes of botulinum toxin with two serotypes A and B approved by the FDA in the United States. When injected into a muscle, botulinum toxin blocks the release of acetylcholine, as substance necessary for muscular contraction, at the neuromuscular junction. Several areas of a muscle may be injected for maximum benefit. The effects of Botox may last as long as 2 to 3 months and injections must be separated by at least 3-month intervals. Botox can produce neutralizing antibodies and become ineffective. In selected patients with postherpetic neuralgia, Botox has demonstrated positive outcomes. Injections into the region of the zygomatic arch have become effective in treating refractory TN. Botox is now used in the treatment of pain from severe spasticity or dystonia. A physician injects the medication intramuscularly into the painful region. Often a series of injections must be given to obtain optimal results.[53] A gradual increase in the dose may be required or over time the effectiveness may decrease. In general, therapy with Botox is appropriate for a targeted area and considered a safe procedure with only transient side effects that are mostly local and reversible. Few systemic side effects occur because little toxin reaches the systemic circulation. Botox may work best when combined with other treatments (e.g., physical therapy).

TABLE 23-13 Acute Pain Treatments

Approach	Examples	Goal
Restriction of movement	Bedrest, splinting of involved area	Initial restriction of movement is helpful for analgesia. Should be used for only a short period of time.
Analgesics	Numerous types of medications (e.g., opioids, NSAIDs, anxiolytics) and delivery systems (e.g., topical, oral, transcutaneous, and intravenous)	Provide analgesia compatible with treatment, venue of care, PD status, with goal to facilitate rehabilitation and avoid noncompliance because of pain.
Regional anesthetic approaches and neuraxial analgesia	Various regional anesthetic techniques (e.g., epidural blocks), neuraxial approaches	Specialized approaches usually used for inpatient pain relief. Appropriate when other treatment approaches are not helpful. Can be continued on outpatient basis in well-selected patients.
Physical modalities	Heat, cold, electroanalgesia such as transcutaneous electrical nerve stimulation, accupuncture, other physical modalities	Physical modalities are helpful for analgesia early on. Should not replace active approaches later in the course of treatment. Can be used to facilitate rehabilitation when needed.
Psychosocial approaches	Relaxation, distraction, imagery	When used for appropriate patients and situations, can reduce anxiety, improve analgesia, and reduce need for medication.
Rehabilitation	Physical therapy, occupational therapy	Physical activity and restoration of function. Begin as soon as possible after the acute pain period is over.

Immune-Modulating Medications

The effectiveness of tumor necrosis factor (TNF)-α blockade among herniated disk patients was studied by Karppinen et al. in a recent study reporting 1-year results. Their results demonstrated that a single infusion of infliximab was highly effective in reducing sciatic pain by a mean of 49% within 1 hour of the infusion. This benefit was maintained even 6 months after infusion, with the result that none of the subjects underwent surgery and all returned to work within 1 month of the infusion.[32a]

Because anxiety is associated with both acute and chronic pain states, anxiolytics have come to be associated with pharmacologic pain management interventions.[31] However, benzodiazepines, such as alprazolam (Xanax) and lorazepam (Ativan), do not appear to have any primary analgesic properties. Because benzodiazepines tend to increase sedation, clinicians may limit the use of effective analgesics to treat the pain. In a patient with severe anxiety and pain, benzodiazepines treat the anxiety, not the pain. Although decreased anxiety and muscle tension can help with pain management efforts, patients with pain should be treated with appropriate doses of analgesics to control their pain.[55]

Local anesthetics are used in the treatment of pain, especially neuropathic pain. Most commonly the local anesthetics are administered into the epidural or intrathecal space. However, oral administration of mexiletine or transdermal administration of lidocaine (Lidoderm) directly on the affected area can be used to block sodium channels within pathways involved in pain transmission.[43]

Rehabilitation

Comprehensive physical rehabilitation has been prescribed for neuroscience patients with acute and especially chronic pain to prevent disuse, deconditioning, depression, and disability. The goal is to maximize the individual's ability to function physically and emotionally despite pain, reduce pain intensity, minimize pain, and prevent the individual from falling back into a cycle of depression, drug dependency, and other emotional states that can worsen the pain experience.

Physical therapists and occupational therapists are becoming more involved in pain management for neuroscience patients as members of the multidisciplinary team. Rehabilitation therapists offer therapeutic modalities for recovery of the neurologic illness using a cognitive-behavioral approach that helps patients cope with their pain and improve function. Therapy may begin with heat and gentle stretching and progress to a manual therapy, massage, or programmed exercise regimen program that can be continued at home. Remaining in bed or lack of movement and exercise can result in up to 20% loss of muscle strength, muscle atrophy, cardiopulmonary deconditioning, bone mineral loss, and increased risk for deep vein thrombosis (DVT) and pulmonary embolus.

Patients who have experienced neurotrauma, stroke, or other neurologic illnesses may receive a variety of rehabilitation interventions for the management of pain states. The physiatrist may prescribe physical therapy, occupational therapy, manipulation, heat, cold, ultrasound, and/or massage for acute and chronic pain problems. Range-of-motion (ROM), slow stretching, and other exercises help to reestablish strength and function but are primarily prescribed for pain relief.

Invasive Pain Relief Strategies

Invasive procedures for pain management include nerve blocks, neuroaugmentive or stimulation procedures, decompressive procedures, and ablative procedures.

The usefulness of **epidural steroid injections** in management of chronic pain is controversial.[21] Epidural steroid injection may have a role in reducing pain related to inflamed tissue and is one of the invasive procedures performed for pain caused by peripheral nerve compression, usually from a herniated intervertebral disk, spinal stenosis, or other structural spine problem. The steroid is injected via a spinal needle into the epidural space at the spinal level(s) causing pain. The steroid assists in reducing swelling and inflammation of involved nerve roots, such as in the presentation of sciatic nerve pain. Often the patient may require 2 to 3 injections done 1 to 2 weeks apart to achieve optimal results. Pain relief can range from complete and permanent to minimal and temporary.

Nerve blocks interrupt the sensory, including nociceptive, pathways through the injection of local anesthetics or neurolytic agents. Xylocaine 1% is an example of an amide anesthetic that inhibits conduction of nerve impulses. It causes temporary loss of feeling and sensation. Nerve blocks may be used diagnostically to locate the site and specific pathway, to predict the effect of the prolonged interruption produced by destructive (ablative) neurosurgical procedures, and therapeutically to continuously relieve pain. Nerve blocks for acute or chronic pain may include occipital, peripheral, median, ulnar, sural, tibial, peroneal, and saphenous nerves, as well as intravertebral and sympathetic blocks.

Intervertebral facet nerve blocks are common procedures done when the pain originates from degenerative changes in the vertebral facet joints. For sympathetically mediated pain involving the arms, hands, or face, a stellate ganglion block may be appropriate. Celiac plexus blocks are effective for visceral abdominal pain. Nerve blocks are usually less effective in the long-term management of chronic pain because of the complexity of transmission mechanisms and neuroplasticity. Extensive chemical destruction of major afferent nerves from repeated injections can be beneficial. Neurolytic agents, usually alcohol or phenol, are used for more permanent blocks of pain transmission.[35]

Acupuncture is an invasive technique referred to as an alternative treatment that involves insertion of fine needles into strategic points on the skin. These points tend to be located where nerves enter muscles. The needles have low resistance and high conductivity electrically. The needles are often stimulated using a pulse generator to produce low frequencies. With these lower frequencies it may take longer to achieve pain relief, but the effects last longer. The sensations induced at the site are variously described as tingling, soreness, numbness, or heaviness. The mechanisms of action of acupuncture are thought to be (1) large-fiber input inhibiting small-fiber input, (2) endorphins and related substances being released, and (3) the autonomic nervous system being influenced. Acupuncture can also be used in conjunction with other pain management strategies.

Surgical Management

Patients with complex and complicated pain problems who fail to respond to traditional pain relief measures can be evaluated for invasive surgical interventions.

Neuroaugmentive procedures are based on endorphin-mediated pain suppressor mechanisms. Local release of beta-endorphins is increased, and activation of the descending serotonergic inhibitor system blocks pain transmission. Electrodes are implanted along the dorsal column to electrically stimulate neural structures, thereby inhibiting pain sensations. The electrode assembly is connected to a radiofrequency receiver buried under the skin. The patient is given an external radiofrequency transmitter that enables the patient to control the intensity and frequency of stimulation as the pain is experienced. The patient with chronic pain from a syndrome of back pain that has failed to respond to intervention or with deafferentation pain of a phantom limb can benefit from dorsal column stimulation. If this intervention is successful, the patient's medication needs are usually decreased. The risks of stimulation procedures include infection, breakage or migration of the electrode or wires, and inadvertent neural damage.

Peripheral nerve stimulators (PNSs) are an additional option for more localized pain. Pain confined to the distribution of a single peripheral nerve (e.g., posttraumatic neural-

gia) may be amenable to electrode placement proximal to the injury. First, temporary percutaneous electrical nerve stimulation is used to test the efficacy of pain relief. If this proves useful in pain reduction, a permanent peripheral nerve stimulator is surgically implanted with an electrode inserted around the nerve (Fig. 23-7). There appears to be a high correlation between significant temporary pain relief with a peripheral nerve block and long-term PNS success. The internal receiver is surgically implanted on the chest wall at the waist level, which allows the patient to activate the system for maximum pain control. PNS has proven to be a good long-term treatment for patients with pain in the distribution of one major peripheral nerve.[28]

Spinal cord stimulation (SCS) is an implantable device typically used for severely disabled patients (e.g., failed back and neck surgeries, CRPS, chronic painful benign or malignant conditions). SCS can be a very effective therapy for carefully selected patients. The process includes a screening test to determine if SCS will provide adequate relief.

Patients must understand the limits and risks of therapy and demonstrate a willingness to work with the treatment team, as well as be willing and able to use the therapy. A temporary electrode is placed percutaneously within the selected level (e.g., the cervical epidural space). During the screening trials, the electrode is connected to an external battery-operated stimulator. A home-testing period takes place. If the pain is reduced by 50% or is "much improved" using scoring pain, the pain is returned to the operating room (OR). The temporary lead is removed and a permanent epidural electrode is tunneled subcutaneously and surgically

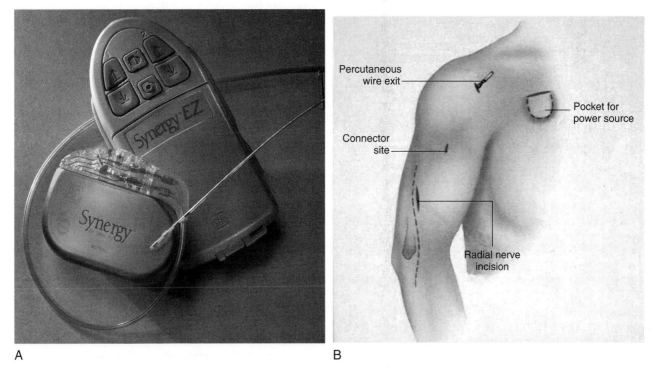

A   B

Figure 23-7 A, Example of electrodes and implantable pulse generator showing the Medtronic Synergy neurostimulation system as an aid in the management of chronic intractable peripheral nerve pain. **B,** During a trial of peripheral nerve stimulation, a temporary percutaneous trialing wire is connected to the electrode lead, tunneled subcutaneously, and brought out through a stab incision, proximal to the location of the stimulation electrode implant site. The location of the power source in the infraclavicular fossa is shown.

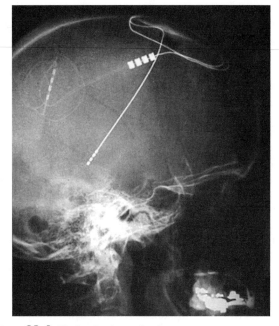

Figure 23-8 Thalamic electrode placement.

connected to a subcutaneous pulse generator that contains a battery so that the power source is implanted in the abdominal site and connected to the electrode by a tunneled extension lead. After the skin is closed, the pulse generator can be activated using a programmer. The parameters are set by the physician via an external programmer that "talks to" the implanted pulse generator (IPG) through the skin via telemetry. The patient also has a hand-held programmer that turns the IPG on and off and can adjust certain settings (Fig. 23-8). After careful monitoring for the required period of time to assess for any changes, the patient is discharged. Follow-up with physical therapy with graded exercises for strength, mobility, and function of the affected site for as long as 6 months may be beneficial for return of function. Complications are minor and may include headache, infection, defective lead, or unsatisfactory positioning of the electrode.

Selection of patients for analgesic **deep brain stimulation (DBS)** depends on two factors: the location of the patient's pain and the etiology of the pain. Thus, DBS is used primarily for pain involving the head, neck, and cranial nerves, or pain generated within the CNS secondary to damage to the brain or spinal cord that is not accessible for stimulation of peripheral nerves or the spinal cord. The most common indications arising from the CNS are **central pain states** (e.g., posttraumatic brain injury, poststroke pain, thalamic syndrome, pseudothalamic syndromes) and postoperative central pain states involving the face and neck but also including the arm, trunk, and leg.[50] Box 23-3 lists general selection criteria for DBS in the chronic pain patient.

As part of the presurgical workup for DBS, the treating team may completely withdraw patients from all opioids and all benzodiazepines for detoxification as long as 2 weeks before surgery. Patients may be required to undergo psychologic testing and/or psychiatric evaluation to diagnose and treat any emotional disorders before surgery. A stereotaxic

frame is applied and after stereotactic CT/MRI anatomic target location, the patient is transferred to the OR where the procedure is done under local anesthesia. A burr hole is made anterior to the coronal suture. After the dura is opened and coagulated, the pia is entered and the target area is explored. Physiologic confirmation of the target location is done with microelectrode recording and stimulation or microstimulation. The patient can be questioned before stimulation and during placement testing. The patient may experience pain reduction, including a feeling of warmth or coolness of the face or cheek. This indicates that the electrode is in the proper location.[50] If good pain relief is obtained in the OR, the electrode is locked in place for later internalization and the patient is discharged (see Fig. 23-8). With reports of adequate pain relief 3 to 5 days postoperatively, the patient is readmitted for internalization of the system using the Medtronic Soletra pulse generator and extension. The connector is placed between the extension and electrode in a burred grove behind the mastoid air cells to prevent migration of the connector[50] (see Fig. 23-8). Approximately 1 week after electrode implantation, the patient is seen for testing and can be started on stimulation of the target nucleus. An example of stimulation voltage parameters by the treating team is stimulation for 10 to 30 minutes two to four times a day. Patients are not allowed to self-adjust their voltage or parameters. During this period, patients may be prescribed amitriptyline 25 to 50 mg/day to enhance activation of the periventricular gray matter.[50] Stimulation of the sensory nucleus or internal capsule is titrated much like that for patients with SCS, with the patient allowed to adjust the stimulation to his or her needs using an external voltage control device.

The complications of DBS include intracranial hemorrhage, infection with the possibility of secondary abscess formation, seizures, and pneumocephalus; the rates are below 5%.[49] Transient postoperative weakness and numbness are not uncommon and long-term effectiveness has been successful in up to 82% in some centers.

Destructive (ablative) procedures continue to play an important role in the management of patients with peripheral nerve injury and chronic intractable pain (Fig. 23-9). There are both advantages and disadvantages to destructive pain

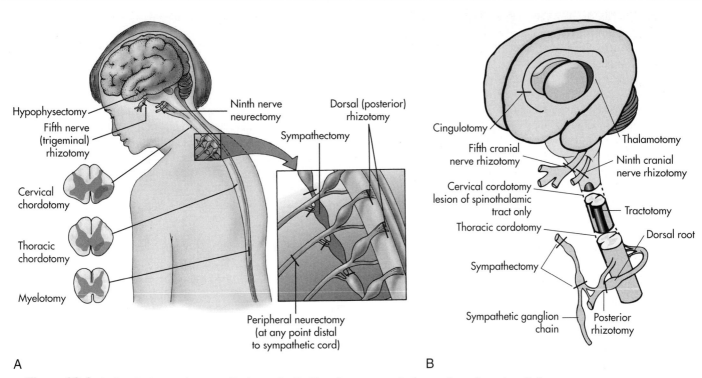

Figure 23-9 A, Surgical procedures to alleviate pain. **B,** Sites for neurosurgical procedures for pain relief.

procedures. Disadvantages are (1) destructive procedures are irreversible, (2) they carry the risk of neurologic morbidity, and (3) the analgesic efficacy of most destructive procedures cannot be tested with the degree of certainty that is present with augmentative procedures (e.g., electrical stimulation, IDDSs).[41] Advantages include (1) the procedure can be performed as a single-stage procedure, (2) the patient experiences immediate analgesia, (3) an effective ablative procedure allows the patient more freedom because it eliminates follow-up visits for refilling an implanted reservoir or reprogramming an implanted device, and (4) the cost may be lower.[41]

Dorsal rhizotomy may have limited application, especially in the treatment of cancer pain and in patients with nonmalignant pain.[57] Rhizotomy has no role in the treatment of spontaneous steady pain and in fact leads to further deafferentation. However, rhizotomy may have a role in relieving hyperpathia limited to a radicular distribution, particularly if the pain is relieved by a local anesthesia block. Rhizotomy has been used for pain in the occipital and upper cervical regions with variable degrees of success. Rhizotomy has been used for traumatic arm pain, nerve roots trapped in thoracic fractures, and in highly selected cases of pain generated from lumbar regions. Percutaneous rhizotomy procedures can be performed as radiofrequency electrocoagulation (hyperthermia) that completely destroys the nerve, cryoanalgesia (hypothermia) that partially destroys the nerve, or chemical neurolysis using phenol preparations. Compared with other techniques, radiofrequency rhizotomy (RFR) completely destroys the nerve.

Interventions that destroy the sensory division of a peripheral or spinal nerve are classified as neurectomies, rhizotomies, ganglionectomies, and sympathectomies (see Fig.

23-7). A dorsal rhizotomy is the surgical destruction of the sensory nerve root via a percutaneous radiofrequency (thermal) lesion, cryotherapy lesion, or open surgery. Ablative procedures are usually done only after the patient has had good pain relief from at least one temporary or diagnostic nerve block. There are overlapping fibers that transmit nociceptive information to the dorsal horns; therefore rhizotomies must cover several unilateral spinal levels to be effective.

Depending on patient symptoms, bilateral radiofrequency lesions may be needed. Most commonly, radiofrequency lesioning is done for pain originating in the lumbosacral vertebral facet joints. This procedure may also be appropriate for postherpetic pain of the trunk or abdomen. Percutaneous trigeminal rhizotomy is the procedure of choice in the older patient with TN who is a poor surgical risk for other, more extensive neurosurgical procedures. Although pain is relieved, the procedure also produces ipsilateral facial analgesia. Patients with deafferentation pain do not respond to rhizotomy. Even after technically satisfactory ablative lesions are used and there is initial pain relief, over time the pain tends to return. With radiofrequency lesioning the patient can expect good pain relief for an average of 6 months or more.[7]

A **ganglionectomy** may be indicated for pain of peripheral origin involving the neck, trunk, or abdomen; conditions (e.g., intractable occipital neuralgia) that have not responded to electrical stimulation; or high cervical or peripheral neurectomy. It differs from a rhizotomy in that the dorsal root ganglia are removed.[57] Based on the large number of failures with dorsal rhizotomy, dorsal root ganglionectomy is now generally the preferred technique that may provide the best outcomes.[41] The surgical procedure obviates a laminectomy and an intradural exposure and therefore reduces the anesthetic time, reduces the risk of a CSF leak, and makes localization somewhat easier.[41]

Sympathectomy is a procedure with the most common indication today for symptomatic hyperhidrosis. As far as pain is concerned, the major indication for sympathectomy is for the treatment of patients with CRPS who display sympathetically maintained pain (SMP), especially in the upper extremity. After several successful sympathetic blocks from which the patient obtains either complete or nearly complete pain relief, a surgical sympathectomy may be considered. The procedure can be accomplished through local anesthetic injection of the stellate ganglion of the head/neck and upper extremity, lumbar sympathetic chain of the lower extremity, or celiac plexus of the abdomen.

Intradiscal electrothermoplasty (IDET) is a relatively new technique that is being used for limited decompression procedures. A wire is inserted percutaneously into the herniated disk and then heated to a fixed temperature. The heating causes changes in the protein matrix of the disk that result in a decrease in disk volume over time. Although the patient may start to feel improvement in 3 weeks or more, complete results may take as long as 6 months as the disk protein slowly consolidates. This procedure is particularly useful for patients who are poor surgical candidates for laminectomy procedures.

Cordotomy involves interruption of pain fibers in the spinothalamic tract. In patients being considered for cordotomy, several factors are critical: (1) All noninvasive methods of pain control should have been attempted without success, (2) the patient should have no medical contraindications to surgery, and (3) the pathophysiology and somatic localization of the patient's pain should be carefully considered. Patients with neuropathic pain after a spinal injury may be considered candidates for cordotomy.[5] Generally, cordotomy is limited to individuals with limited life expectancy with severe unilateral pain, such as patients with cancer, to improve their quality of life and survival. The cordotomy procedure can be performed as a percutaneous or open procedure with good reduction in pain for carefully selected patients.

Dorsal root entry zone (DREZ) may be achieved with a percutaneous needle electrode and radiofrequency current. The DREZ may be an option for patients with localized neuropathic pain. Destruction of Lissauer's tract, substantia gelatinosa, and a superficial portion of the dorsal horn results in a profound ipsilateral sensory deficit over the affected dermatomes. The DREZ lesions are effective in intractable pain from brachial plexus avulsion injuries and the central pain of spinal cord injury.

Implantable pumps, devices that are designed to dispense medications into the intrathecal space, are used for the control of pain, as well as spasticity. The medication is dispensed within fixed, programmable parameters set using an external telemetry unit. Morphine is typically used to treat the pain, although other opioids such as hydromorphone and fentanyl have been used. Local anesthetics such as bupivacaine may be used in combination with the opioid or, less often, alone. Clonidine can also be used in combination with the opioid.

For treatment of spasticity, baclofen[13] is used (see Chapter 13). Initially the use of implantable pumps was limited to patients with cancer pain. However, this modality is now used in the treatment of carefully screened patients with chronic, intractable nonmalignant pain. With intrathecal medication administration, patients can significantly decrease their pain while experiencing fewer medication side effects than with other systemic routes. Complications include infection; bleeding; CSF leak; and catheter obstruction, kinking, or disconnection. The most common side effects are constipation, urinary retention, impotence in men, nausea, and vomiting.[33]

Research

Researchers and scientists from the University of California at Los Angeles (UCLA) and the University of Cambridge, United Kingdom, reported the first clinically suitable method using nerves as a means of delivery of high doses of pain killers at the Society for Neuroscience conference in November 2001. Neurosurgeons used "axonal transport" to deliver pain medication to the spinal ganglia and spinal cord, where it was transported to the axon nerve endings and ultimately to the core tissues of the nervous system involved in pain sensation. For example, one administration of the pain medication intraoperatively travels only to the nerves involved during surgery and could eliminate the pain sensations for as long as 4 days. Clinical trials of axonal transport to treat neuropathic pain, as well as other exciting trials, are in progress for improved pain management.

Classically, pain modulatory circuits have been conceptualized as being composed solely of neurons. However, current research has provided evidence on the role of activated spinal cord microglia and astrocytes of the spinal cord and peripheral nerves. These cells release a variety of substances upon activation, such as nitric oxide, superoxide, and other free radicals; chemokines and proinflammatory cytokines, prostaglandins, leukotrienes, and arachidonic acid; and glutamate and other excitatory amino acids and nerve growth factors. This is an exciting discovery in pain research because microglia and astrocytes outnumber neurons about 10:1, so activation of these cells could be expected to significantly affect the function of neurons in the area. Glial cells are activated by neurotransmitters, such as substance P and glutamate aspartate. Glial cells are also activated by immune challenges (e.g., trauma, viruses, bacteria).[14a,60a,60b,60c]

Clinical Management

The effective management of pain for the neuroscience patient can be challenging and complicated. The patient's right to effective pain control is a priority and should be included as part of all other treatment decisions. Good pain relief with the application of one or more of the modalities described in this chapter is an attainable goal in the overwhelming majority of neuroscience patients. In considering the concept of **neuroplasticity** that may have the ability to remodel the nervous system in response to repeated pain, it is important to prevent the affected nerves from becoming "hypersensitive" to pain or become resistant to the antinociceptive system. Chronic pain signals may become imbedded into the CNS cells and allow the pain signals to continue after the injury has resolved, forming a pain "memory."

The initial assessment is followed by an individualized plan of pain management for neuroscience patients. Patients are continuously monitored for their neurologic and pain status and should receive pain relief based on their level of pain and previous response. Activities such as dressing changes, invasive procedures, and treatments may exacerbate the patient's pain. Clinicians should provide pain relief before painful procedures and patients should be instructed to request medication as needed. Evaluation of the neurologic condition as the underlying cause of pain, together with the pain assessment, will determine the need for adjustments in medications and therapy.

Outpatient or clinic patients are encouraged to keep a pain diary for monitoring. The diary is reviewed at follow-up visits to analyze the pain relief obtained, side effects, and patient compliance. Hospitalized patients or those who return for follow-up after discharge and who have been unable to obtain pain relief require a more aggressive approach. These individuals require referral to a specialized pain team, specialists, or clinics if the pain continues to interrupt their functional abilities, ability to sleep, and ability to achieve a satisfactory quality of life. The multidisciplinary pain team offers comprehensive evaluation and care with additional alternatives, including invasive therapies or surgical options described earlier.

Nonpharmacologic Interventions

The treatment of pain also focuses on pain elimination, or reduction, to increase the patient's ability to cope with the pain experience. The interventions are designed to increase a patient's sense of control, promote relaxation, and modify cognitive activity. Modalities include the use of superficial or deep heat and/or cold, massage, exercise, mobilization, traction, and electrical stimulation (e.g., physical therapy, described earlier) as adjuncts to pharmacologic management.

Dermal cutaneous stimulation involves techniques to stimulate the skin, thereby relieving pain. These techniques include superficial and deep massage, vibration, application of heat and cold/ice, mentholated substances, and TENS. Although cutaneous stimulation methods are not curative, they are palliative in the relief of pain. Pain intensity is reduced during or after stimulation. The most effective stimulation site varies and may be adjacent to or distant from the site of the pain. **Massage therapy** tends to soothe and relax muscle tension. **Acupressure** developed more than 5000 years ago is referred to as Jin Shin Do, or "the way of companionate spirit simultaneously," during which pressure is applied, usually with the hands, at acupoints in order to release muscular tension. Acupressure allows chi to flow through the medians and relieve pain by releasing endorphins or sensory gating. Acupressure can lower blood pressure, particularly in those taking antihypertensive medications. Japanese practitioners developed a form of acupres-

sure known as **shiatsu.** The practitioner applies pressure using the thumb, elbow, or knee perpendicularly to the skin at acupoints, combined with passive stretching and rotation of the joints for pain relief. **Vibratory massage** is a type of therapy in which a mechanical device delivers a light, rhythmic quivering effect that can cause numbness or anesthesia of the stimulated areas.

Applications of heat and cold can relieve pain, either used alone or in alternating combinations, especially when pain is of musculoskeletal origin. The advantage of heat/cold therapy is that patients can apply many of these therapies in the home setting with proper education and guidelines. **Heat therapy** may include hot packs, deep heat with ultrasound diathermy, fluidotherapy with a machine that allows the patient to dip the affected part into heated finely ground corn or particles, hot water bottles, moist compresses, heating pads, paraffin wax, chemical and gel packs, hydrotherapy, and whirlpools.[60] Heating the painful area can be direct by way of conduction heat, or by convection with a current. Heat modalities increase the temperature at the painful site, relax muscles, and dilate blood vessels for increased blood flow and oxygen supply. Heat is usually applied for 20 to 30 minutes and removed. It is never used continuously because it can cause a burn or cause the blood vessels to become engorged and painful.

Cold therapy has a counterirritant effect. Cold applications are frequently used in acute injuries (e.g., painful sports injury). Cold contact activates relief by a different mechanism than heat with the use of ice or cold packs, vaporized coolants, or dipping the body part in cold water. Freezing a cup of water in a Styrofoam cup and then peeling off the lower half when frozen makes cold pack that can be used for a manual ice massage by holding the top half and gently rubbing the painful area. Warn the patient that the initial contact with the skin will produce a cold sensation for a minute or so, then a burning sensation for a few minutes, and lastly a numbing sensation with pain relief. Cold therapy restricts blood supply, reduces nerve conduction velocity, including the pain nerves, and reduces painful spasms.[60] Cold packs are applied for approximately 15 minutes and should always be wrapped (i.e., using a terry cloth material) to prevent direct contact with the skin that could cause a "cold burn." Cold therapy may provide longer pain relief than heat.[60] The application of a substance containing menthol also serves as a counterirritant as it acts in a cooling manner much like ice.

Transcutaneous electrical nerve stimulation (TENS) is used in the management of both acute and chronic pain. The patient can achieve maximum and prolonged pain relief by using a device to induce neuronal transmission. Stimulation of large myelinated fibers (A-alpha fibers) inhibits pain transmission at the level of the spinal cord. In addition, endogenous opiates (endorphins) are produced in response to the electrical stimulation. TENS units are programmed to send a mild, controlled electrical current along the skin that blocks pain sensations (Fig. 23-10).

Cognitive-behavioral therapies (CBTs) (e.g., distraction, imagery, relaxation, hypnosis, biofeedback) are among the psychologic approaches to the management of pain.

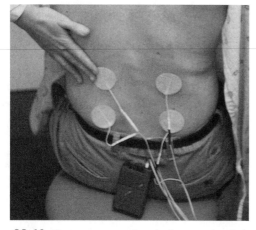

Figure 23-10 Transcutaneous electrical nerve stimulation (TENS).

Clinicians often use cognitive techniques for managing patient pain, because these techniques are easily adaptable to a variety of clinical settings.[8] Cognitive techniques increase coping ability by focusing attention on stimuli other than pain sensation. The choice of hearing, vision, touch, or movement depends on individual preference and energy levels. Concentrating on other sensory input decreases the attention being placed on pain. Pain tolerance is increased, and intensity is decreased. The pain is more acceptable or bearable, but it does not go away. When pain remains on the periphery of awareness, the sense of control is increased.

CBT is an alternative psychologic approach to the management of chronic pain. Patients are assisted in understanding their pain triggers and how to minimize them. Their individual pain modifiers are also identified, and they are taught how to use them more effectively. The emphasis of the therapy is to facilitate increased functional capacity, decrease reliance on pharmacologic interventions, and diminish pain behaviors. Chronic pain patients are taught effective coping mechanisms to better deal with ongoing pain that might not be completely relieved.[51]

Relaxation techniques (e.g., meditation, hypnosis, visualization, progressive muscle relaxation) seek to achieve a self-induced state that is incompatible with pain. The decrease in muscle tension results in decreased pain and anxiety. Relaxation techniques use mental, physical, and environmental modifications. A passive attitude, comfortable position and clothing, and a quiet environment combined with deep breathing and peaceful images reduce muscle tension and increase pain tolerance.

Guided imagery is the use of the imagination or mental images to reduce pain by distracting, relaxing, or producing an image of pain relief. Patients with prolonged pain can benefit from guided imagery. They are taught to systematically create or recreate situations and to proceed through them in an altered sensory state. These sensory images (e.g., numbness, coolness) are more pleasant and acceptable or provide a nonpainful substitute for pain, which therefore reduces pain intensity.

The use of **hypnosis** is one of the oldest and most documented psychologic interventions for the reduction of pain and suffering. Scientists may differ on the theories that explain hypnosis but many individuals who use hypnosis report less pain and a reduced need for pain medications. The patient can be taught how to enter and exit a relaxed, hypnotic state. During the relaxed state the patient is in an altered state of awareness evidenced by increased alertness and intense concentration. The concentration is so highly focused that peripheral awareness, including pain, is diminished. Hypnosis should not be used with patients who fear loss of control or being controlled, or with those who hope for a magical cure.

Biofeedback is based on the assumption that there is a physiologic pain component that the patient can learn to control. Instruments are used to amplify a physiologic response (e.g., muscle tension, heart rate, respirations) and convert it to visual or auditory signals that give immediate needle, tone, or digital feedback. Biofeedback for pain patients can use EMG to reduce muscle tension, skin temperature measurement to alter the sympathetic nervous system (dermal blood flow and temperature), cephalic blood volume pulse measurement to control temporal artery pulsation, and electroencephalography (EEG) to increase alpha brain wave activity. Biofeedback may be incorporated into a comprehensive pain management program with relaxation therapy and other interventions.

Psychologic Interventions

Operant conditioning (OP) is a behavior modification approach used when environmental factors are a major part of the pain behavior. The goals of OP are to reduce positive reinforcement of pain behavior, increase positive reinforcement of well behavior, and teach significant others to continue this approach. Baseline data are obtained concerning the use of medications, exercise and activity tolerance, and attention from others. The treatment team manipulates the schedule of medications, activity, and exercise until drug usage has decreased with a concomitant increase in activity and exercise. Significant others and friends must understand that they can no longer provide positive reinforcement for pain behavior. Rest and attention should not be used to reinforce pain behavior. OP is effective for patients who have minimal organic disease and a good psychosocial support system, with everyone willing to participate in the process.

COMPREHENSIVE PATIENT MANAGEMENT

Health Education

Individuals who have pain need health education in relation to the cause, prevention, and relief measures that will allow them to take control of their pain problem. After the cause of the pain is recognized, effective teaching will focus on instructing the patient, family, and caregivers about medications as a significant part of pain management. Timing, dosage, side effects, and complications of medications (e.g., NSAIDs, acetaminophen overusage, self-medicating with

OTC preparations) are just a few of the important issues. Patients often are unaware of the potential drug interactions between vitamin and nutritional supplements they self-prescribe and the medications prescribed by the professional. When adjuvant drugs are prescribed for the treatment of pain, it is important for the patient to understand the indications for which the medication has been prescribed. Many of the adjuvant drugs do not list "pain" as a clinical indication. Patients can get confused, panic, or simply not take the medication if they do not clearly understand that the anticonvulsant or antidepressant was correctly prescribed as treatment for their pain.

Fear of opioid addiction should be discussed and teaching should focus on the differences between tolerance, addiction, and physical dependence. The many myths and misconceptions of pain and its management provide numerous opportunities to provide patient education. As always, for health teaching to be effective, it is important to assess not only patients' understanding of their pain but also their readiness and willingness to learn.

The use of positioning, assistive devices, and other comfort measures will give patients confidence to take charge. Medical alert identification is stressed, including the use of a wallet card that lists all medications. Instructions include how to recognize and report untoward reactions and when to call for medical assistance or 911 for emergencies.

CONTINUUM OF CARE

Standards of practice for pain management should be defined for all clinical settings, especially when the patient is discharged and has fewer contacts with health care providers. The Joint Commission on Accreditation of Healthcare Organizations (JCAHO) pain standards require that pain be evaluated and treated appropriately wherever patients seek medical care from licensed professionals (e.g., emergency departments [EDs], mental health centers, hospitals, long-term facilities, ambulatory centers, the home).[32] Some basic rules for achieving effective pain management are summarized in Table 23-13 and are applied as guiding principles.

Case Management Considerations

Case managers are in a unique position as an advocate to assist the patient who has persistent pain, and their family, to receive appropriate services for pain management. The case manager facilitates continuity of care after surgery, hospitalization, or diagnosis of a neurologic disorder and persistent pain. Patient and family education is essential along with the ability to perform a neurologic assessment and pain assessment in coordinating care. The case manager should have knowledge of current pain treatment options and pain specialists who can provide comprehensive pain management care that is cost-effective.

Chronic pain lasting longer than 6 months may require referral to a rehabilitation or pain clinic setting. After review of all records and completion of the initial patient neurologic and pain assessment (see Chapter 2), the case manager will develop a holistic plan of care that includes functional assessment, vocational evaluation, and therapeutic modalities with realistic goals. It is important to evaluate the patient's quality of life and the effect of lost work and earnings, interpersonal relationships with family and caregivers, coping strategies, barriers to health care providers, transportation needs, and the costs of care. For patients with an implanted pump, the schedule for pump refills must be adhered to or the patient can develop drug withdrawal symptoms and suffer unnecessarily. The plan of care should include pharmacologic and nonpharmacologic interventions and identify available local community resources. It is important to also have knowledge of advance directives, as well as cultural preferences that may be different from the case manager's.

The case manager assesses the home environment for safety, energy conservation, comfort (hospital bed, bedside commode, patient lift), and required services (home health aide, physical therapy, occupational therapy, infusion therapy, aquatic therapy) and coordinates all components of the home management plan of care. Case managers also monitor the individual's response to each component and evaluate their effectiveness and long-term use. They intervene as needed to promote pain relief, improve psychologic well-being, and improve the individual's overall functional status and quality of life.

With each visit, documentation of the patient's response to the plan of care, caregiver burden, any adverse effects, or aberrant behaviors that signal abuse or noncompliance should be part of the follow-up. Urine testing may be requested in some cases. Drug tolerance and unpleasant side effects of long-term opioid use, for example, should be carefully assessed with follow-up for appropriate interventions. Good pain control will reduce ED visits and unnecessary visits to health care providers and costs of pain treatment.

Home Rehabilitation

The patient's plan of care from an inpatient or outpatient setting may be continued after discharge. Home rehabilitation may include biofeedback, aquatics, home or health club exercise programs, and behavior modification to address both pain management and lifestyle adaptation. Education about the etiology and pathology of the pain, as well as information about nonpharmacologic alternatives to pain control, gives the patient new strategies to manage his or her pain and minimize its consequences. Rehabilitation may be through an acute rehabilitation hospital, freestanding Commission on Accreditation of Rehabilitation Facilities (CARF)-accredited program, or a combination of a therapy center and a physician/pain clinic. Support groups and educational meetings often prove particularly beneficial for patients with chronic pain who are undergoing rehabilitation.

Home Care Management

Patients may be discharged to their home with acute pain that requires competent home health providers with expertise in acute pain management. For the patient with a progressive, debilitating neurologic disease process, palliative home care may be an option. This growing area of health care can be both effective in the symptomatic treatment of pain and cost-efficient. As the patient's pain increases, pain control measures can easily be adapted in the home care environment, offering a wide range of treatment choices. Figure 23-5 is an example of a critical pathway developed for the treatment of pain in the home setting. When the treatment of pain is incorporated into the overall plan of care through the use of critical pathways or other similar systematic methods, the potential for achieving positive patient outcomes is much greater.[12] The patient may benefit from sleep restoration strategies to improve sleep, education on the use of the "relaxation response," modifying behaviors to exercise and be more active, or advice to patients who "overdo" and need to pace their activities.

CONCLUSION

With the expanded knowledge of pain management and the growing number of new and improved options for acute and chronic pain, neuroscience patients can expect significant relief or reduction of their pain. Holistic management with realistic evaluation of the pain experience as a biopsychosocial disorder is needed. Nurse clinicians who are involved in the care of neuroscience patients in every setting recognize the high prevalence of pain in this patient population and the adverse consequences of inadequate pain management. They are challenged to the difficult task of listening and responding to each patient with assurance that their suffering will not be ignored or undertreated but managed with the understanding that truly epitomizes today's competent, caring neuroscience nurse.

GLOSSARY OF TERMS

The following terms are provided to broaden the reader's pain vocabulary and terminology:

Addiction: A behavioral pattern of substance use characterized by a compulsion to take the drug primarily to experience its psychic effects.

Agonist: A substance that when combined with the receptor produces the drug effect or desired effect. Endorphins and morphine are agonists on the opioid receptors.

Algogenic: Causing pain.

Allodynia: Pain from a non-noxious stimulus. Also called stroking hyperalgesia.

Antagonist: A substance that blocks or reverses the effects of the agonist by occupying the receptor site without producing the drug effect. Naloxone (Narcan) is an opioid antagonist.

Balanced analgesia: Using more than one form of analgesia concurrently to obtain more pain relief with fewer side effects.

Breakthrough pain: A sudden and temporary increase in pain occurring in a patient being managed with opioid analgesia.

Dependence: Occurs when a patient who has been taking opioids experiences a withdrawal syndrome when the opioids are discontinued; often occurs with opioid tolerance and does not indicate an addiction.

Endorphins and **enkephalins:** Morphine-like substances produced by the body. Primarily found in the CNS, they have the potential to reduce pain.

Hyperalgesia: There is an increased response to a pain stimulus; an excess response to pain.

Nociception: Activation of sensory transduction in nerves by thermal, mechanical, or chemical energy impinging on specialized nerve endings. The nerves involved convey information about tissue damage to the CNS.

Nociceptor: A receptor preferentially sensitive to a noxious stimulus.

Non-nociceptor: Nerve fiber that usually does not transmit pain.

Opioid: A morphine-like compound that produces bodily effects including pain relief, sedation, constipation, and respiratory depression. This term is preferred over **narcotic.**

Pain threshold: The point at which a stimulus is perceived as painful.

Pain tolerance: The maximum intensity or duration of pain that a person is willing to endure.

Patient-controlled analgesia (PCA): Self-administration of analgesic agents by a patient instructed about the procedure.

Placebo effect: Analgesia that results from the expectation that a substance will work, not from the actual substance itself.

Prostaglandins: Chemical substances that increase the sensitivity of pain receptors by enhancing the pain-provoking effect of bradykinin.

Referred pain: Pain perceived as coming from an area different from that in which the pathology is occurring. An example would be the perception of left arm or jaw pain in a person having a myocardial infarction.

Sensitization: A heightened response seen after exposure to a noxious stimulus. Response to the same stimulus is to feel more pain.

Tolerance: Occurs when a person who has been taking opioids becomes less sensitive to their analgesic properties (and usually side effects). Tolerance is characterized by the need for increasing doses to maintain the same level of pain relief.

RESOURCES

Agency for Healthcare Research and Quality: www.ahrq.gov
American Academy of Pain Management: www.aapainmanage.org
American Chronic Pain Association: www.theacpa.org
American Pain Foundation: www.painfoundation.org
American Pain Society: www.ampainsoc.org
American Society for Pain Management Nursing: www.aspmn.org

International Association for the Study of Pain: www.iasp-pain.org

The Mayday Pain Project: www.painandhealth.org

National Chronic Pain Outreach Association: www.chronicpain.org

National Foundation for the Treatment of Pain: www.paincare.org

Partners Against Pain: www.partnersagainstpain.com

Trigeminal Neuralgia Association: www.tna-support.org

REFERENCES

1. Aloisi AM: Sensory effects of gonadal hormones. In Fillingim RJ, editor: *Progress in pain research and management,* Seattle, 2000, IASP Press.

2. Backonja M, Rowbotham MC: Pharmacological therapy for neuropathic pain. In McMahon SB, Koltzenburg M, editors: *Wall and Melzack's textbook of pain,* ed 5, Philadelphia, 2006, Churchill Livingstone.

3. Barker E: A new approach to chronic pain, *RN* 68(5):32–33, 2005.

4. Baron R: Complex regional pain syndromes. In McMahon SB, Koltzenburg M, editors: *Wall and Melzack's textbook of pain,* ed 5, Philadelphia, 2006, Churchill Livingstone.

5. Binder DK, Barbaro NM: Cordotomy. In Follett KA, editor: *Neurosurgical pain management,* Philadelphia, 2004, Saunders.

6. Bloodworth D, Calvillo O, Smith K, Grabois M: Chronic pain syndromes: evaluation and treatment. In Braddom RL, editor: *Physical medicine and rehabilitation,* ed 2, Philadelphia, 2000, WB Saunders.

7. Buijs EJ, van Wijk RM, Weesman RR, Stolker RJ, Groen GG: Radiofrequency lumbar facet denervation: a comparative study of the reproducibility of lesion size after 2 current radiofrequency techniques, *Reg Anesth Pain Med* 29(5):400–407, 2004.

8. Butler AC, Chapman JE, Forman EM, Beck AT: The empirical status of cognitive-behavioral therapy: a review of meta-analyses, *Clin Psychol Rev* 26:17–31, 2006.

9. Clark L, Jones K, Pennington K: Pain assessment practices with nursing home residents, *West J Nurs Res* 26(7):733–750, 2004.

10. Costigan M, Woolf CJ: Pain: molecular mechanisms, *J Pain* 1(3 suppl 1):35–44, 2000.

11. Crain KD: Emotions and psychobiology. In McMahon SB, Koltzenburg M, editors: *Wall and Melzack's textbook of pain,* ed 5, Philadelphia, 2006, Churchill Livingstone.

12. Darcy Y: Managing procedural pain, *Nursing 2004* 34(12):76, 2004.

13. Dario A, Scamoni C, Picano M, Casagrande F, Tomei G: Pharmacological complications of the chronic baclofen infusion in the severe spinal spasticity. Personal experience and review of the literature, *J Neurosci Nurs* 48(4):177–181, 2004.

14. Dawson D: *Entrapment neuropathies,* Boston, 1983, Little, Brown and Company.

14a. DeLeo JA, Colburn RW: Proinflammatory cytokines and glial cells: their role in neuropathic pain. In Watkins L, editor: *Cytokines and pain,* New York, 1999, Birdhouse.

15. Dionne CE: Low back pain. In Crombie IK, Croft PR, Linton SJ, Le Resche L, Von Korff M, editors: *Epidemiology of pain. A report of the Task Force on Epidemiology of the International Association of Pain,* Seattle, 1999, IASP Press.

16. Dunbar PJ, Visco E, Lam AM: Craniotomy procedures are associated with less analgesic requirements than other surgical procedures, *Anesth Analg* 88(2):335–340, 1999.

17. Dworkin RH: An overview of neuropathic pain: syndromes, symptoms, signs and several mechanisms, *Clinical J Pain* 18(6):343–349, 2002.

18. Eisenberg E, Shifrin A, Krivoy N: Lamotrigine for neuropathic pain, *Expert Rev Neurother* 5(6):729–735, 2005.

19. Fine PG, Portenoy RK: *A clinical guide to opioid analgesia,* New York, 2004, McGraw-Hill.

20. Fishman SM, Kreis PG: The opioid contract, *Clin J Pain* 18(4S):70–75, 2002.

21. Follett KA: Failed back syndrome. In Follett KA, editor: *Neurosurgical pain management,* Philadelphia, 2004, Saunders.

22. Franciso GE, Hu MM, Boake C, Ivanhoe CB: Efficacy of early use of intrathecal baclofen therapy for treating spastic hypertonia due to acquired brain injury, *Brain Inj* 19(5):359–364, 2005.

23. Gagliese L, Melzack R: Pain in the elderly. In McMahon SB, Koltzenburg M, editors: *Wall and Melzack's textbook of pain,* ed 5, Philadelphia, 2006, Churchill Livingstone.

24. Galer BS, Jensen MP: Development and preliminary validation of a pain measure specific to neuropathic pain: the neuropathic pain scale, *Neurology* 48:332–338, 1997.

25. Gibson SJ, Farrell M: A review of age differences in the neurophysiology of nociception and the perceptual experience of pain, *Clin J Pain* 20(4):227–239, 2004.

26. Glen VL, St. Marie B: Overview of pharmacology. In St. Marie B, editor: *Core curriculum for pain management nursing,* Philadelphia, 2002, Saunders.

27. Haddox JD: Pharmacologic therapies for pain. In Follett KA, editor: *Neurosurgical pain management,* Philadelphia, 2004, Saunders.

28. Hassenbusch SJ: Peripheral nerve stimulation. In Follett KA, editor: *Neurosurgical pain management,* Philadelphia, 2004, Saunders.

29. Hicks CL, von Baeyer CL, Spafford PA, van Korlaar I, Goodenough B: The Faces Pain Scale—revised: toward a common metric in pediatric pain measurement, *Pain* 93:173–183, 2001.

30. Hoskin PJ: Cancer pain: treatment overview. In McMahon SB, Koltzenburg M, editors: *Wall and Melzack's textbook of pain,* ed 5, Philadelphia, 2006, Churchill Livingstone.

31. Huether SE, Leo J: Pain, temperature regulation, sleep, and sensory function. In McCance KL, Huether SE, editors: *Pathophysiology: the biologic basis for disease in adults and children,* ed 4, St Louis, 2002, Mosby.

32. Joint Commission on Accreditation of Healthcare Organizations, http://www.jcaho.org; accessed October 1, 2005.

32a. Karppinen J, Korhonen T, Malmivaara A, Paimela L, Kyllönen E, Lindgren KA, Rantanen P, Tervonen O, Niinimäki J, Seitsalo S, Hurri H: Tumor necrosis factor-α monoclonal antibody, Infliximab, used to manage severe sciatica, *Spine* 28:750–754, 2003.

33. Lind G, Meyerson BA, Winter J, Lindroth B: Intrathecal baclofen as adjuvant therapy to enhance the effect of spinal cord stimulation in neuropathic pain: a pilot study, *Eur J Pain* 8(4):377–383, 2004.

34. Macfarlane GJ, Jones GT, McBeth J: Epidemiology of pain. In McMahon SB, Koltzenburg M, editors: *Wall and Melzack's textbook of pain,* ed 5, Philadelphia, 2006, Churchill Livingstone.

35. Mailis A, Furlan A: Sympathectomy for neuropathic pain, *Cochrane Database Syst Rev* (2):CD002918, 2003.

36. McCaffery M: *Nursing practice theories related to cognition, bodily pain, and man—environmental interactions,* Los Angeles, 1968, University of California at Los Angeles Student's Store.

37. Melzak R, Katz J: Pain assessment in adult patients. In McMahon SB, Koltzenburg M, editors: *Wall and Melzack's textbook of pain,* ed 5, Philadelphia, 2006, Churchill Livingstone.

38. Merskey H, Bogduk N: *Classification of chronic pain: descriptions of chronic pain syndromes and definitions of pain terms,* Seattle, 1994, IASP Press.

39. Miaskowski C, Levine JD: Does opioid analgesia show a gender preference for females? *Pain Manag Nurs* 8(1):34–44, 1999.

40. *Mosby's 2005 drug consult for nurses,* St Louis, 2005, Mosby.

41. Osenbach RK: Peripheral ablative techniques. In Follett KA, editor: *Neurosurgical pain management,* Philadelphia, 2004, Saunders.

42. Pagana KD, Pagana TJ: *Mosby's diagnostic and laboratory test reference,* ed 7, St Louis, 2005, Mosby.

43. Pasero C: Lidocaine patch 5%, *Am J Nurs* 103(9):75–78, 2003.

44. Pasero C: Pathophysiology of neuropathic pain, *Pain Manag Nurs* 5(4)(suppl 1):3–8, 2004.

45. Penn RD: Neuraxial analgesic administration. In Follett KA, editor: *Neurosurgical pain management,* Philadelphia, 2004, Saunders.

46. Portenoy RK: Current pharmacotherapy of chronic pain, *J Pain Symptom Manage* 19(suppl 1):16–20, 2000.

47. Portenoy RK: Opioid therapy for chronic nonmalignant pain: a review of the critical issues, *J Pain Symptom Manage* 11(4):203–217, 1996.

48. Puntillo K, Neighbor M, O'Neil N, Nixon R: Accuracy of emergency nurses in assessment of patients' pain, *Pain Manag Nurs* 4(4):171–175, 2003.

49. Rezai AR, Lozano AM: Deep brain stimulation for chronic pain. In Burchiel KJ, editor: *Surgical management of pain,* New York, 2002, Thieme.

50. Richardson DE: Intracranial stimulation therapies: deep-brain stimulation. In Follett KA, editor: *Neurosurgical pain management,* Philadelphia, 2004, Saunders.

51. Ririe DG, Ririe KL, Sethna NF, Fox L: Unexpected interaction of methylphenidate (Ritalin) with anesthetic agents, *Pediatr Anesth* 7(1):69–73, 1997.

52. Ross EL: *Hot topics in pain management,* Philadelphia, 2004, Hanley & Belfus.

53. Slawek J, Bogucki A, Reclawowicz D: Botulinum toxin type A for upper limb spasticity following stroke: an open-label study with individualized, flexible injection regimens, *Neurol Sci* 26(1):32–39, 2005.

54. Steffen P, Seeling W, Essig A, Stiepan F, Rockemann MG: Bacterial contamination of epidural catheters: microbiological examination of 502 epidural catheters used for postoperative analgesia, *J Clin Anesth* 16(2):92–97, 2004.

55. St. Marie B, Loeb JL: Gerontologic pain management. In St. Marie B, editor: *Core curriculum for pain management nursing,* Philadelphia, 2002, Saunders.

56. Taddio A, Soin HK, Schuh S, Koren G, Scolnik D: Liposomal lidocaine to improve success rates and reduce procedural pain in children: a randomized controlled trial, *CMAJ* 172(13): 1691–1695, 2005.

57. Taha JM: Dorsal root ganglionectomy and dorsal rhizotomy. In Burchiel KJ, editor: *Surgical management of pain,* New York, 2002, Thieme.

58. Valentino L, Pillay KV, Walker J: Managing chronic nonmalignant pain with continuous intrathecal morphine, *J Neurosci Nurs* 30(4):233–239, 243–244, 1998.

59. Voepel-Lewis T, Malviya S, Tait AR: Validity of parent ratings as proxy measures of pain in children with cognitive impairment, *Pain Manag Nurs* 6(3):239–248, 2005.

60. Wasserman MY, Vasudevan SV: Physical medicine and rehabilitation in pain management. In Follett KA, editor: *Neurosurgical pain management,* Philadelphia, 2004, Saunders.

60a. Watkins LR, Maier SF: Illness-induced hyperalgesia: mediators, mechanisms and implications. In Watkins LR, Maier SF: *Cytokines and pain,* Boston, 1999, Birkhäuser Verlag.

60b. Watkins LR, Maier SF: The pain of being sick: implications of immune-to-brain communication for understanding pain, *Annu Rev Psychol* 51:29–57, 2000.

60c. Watkins LR, Milligan ED, Maier SF: Glial activation: a driving force for pathological pain, *Trends Neurosci* 24(8):450–455, 2001.

61. Weiner D, Peterson B, Ladd K, McConnell E, Keefe F: Pain in nursing home residents: an exploration of prevalence, staff perspectives, and practical aspects of measurement, *Clin J Pain* 15(2):92–101, 1999.

62. World Health Organization's Pain Relief Ladder, http://www. who.int/cancer/palliative/painladder/en; accessed October 1, 2005.

63. Yee JD, Berde CG: Dextroamphetamine or methylphenidate as adjuvants to opioid analgesia for adolescents with cancer, *J Pain Symptom Manage* 9(2):112–125, 1994.

DIANA ABSON KRAEMER,
ELLEN BARKER

CHAPTER 24

Management of Seizures and Epilepsy

Epilepsy has been recognized as a unique disorder for thousands of years, and references to its symptoms have been made as far back as the Mesopotamian writings from the fifth millennium BCE.[1] Epilepsy and seizures are a major health problem that affects 2.3 million Americans of all ages, their families, and society. Almost 200,000 Americans develop seizures and epilepsy every year. The estimated annual cost of epilepsy is $12.5 billion in direct and indirect costs, approximately the same as lung cancer. Because they live so many years with this condition, the young bear an inordinate burden.[2]

Many new medications have been introduced for the treatment of epilepsy. Refinements in electroencephalogram (EEG) monitoring technology and in functional and structural neuroimaging have increased the number of patients undergoing epilepsy surgery. Yet, with all the advances, no cure has been found. Societal attitudes have improved, but myths and misconceptions about epilepsy remain. Health care professionals recognize that despite new medications, technologic advances, and public education, a stigma still exists for many Americans with epilepsy that fuels discrimination and personal hardships. The intent of this chapter is to focus on the classification of seizures, diagnosis, medical and surgical treatment, status epilepticus, psychosocial issues, and case management.

DEFINITIONS

Seizures are abnormal paroxysmal electrical discharges in the cerebral cortex. Epilepsy comes from the Greek word *epilambanein,* meaning "to seize" or "to attack." Another author has defined epilepsy as a sudden, intermittent alteration in consciousness or function, resulting from excessive discharges of cerebral neurons.[3] Clinically, a seizure manifests as an alteration in sensation, behavior, movement, perception, or consciousness. The clinical presentation of seizures reflects the region of the brain in which the discharge arises or spreads. The discharge may remain localized to a small area or, like a ripple in a pond, spread to involve the entire brain. During a seizure, oxygen consumption increases by 60% and cerebral blood flow (CBF) by 250%.[4] A seizure is generally not fatal but creates the poten-

tial for injury from falling, as well as the potential for other serious injuries.

Seizures are classified as being provoked (an acute insult leads to a seizure) or unprovoked, meaning they occur for no apparent reason. Provoked seizures can occur in isolation as a result of some acute disorder of the central nervous system (CNS). After the cause of the disorder is corrected, these seizures often do not recur or may decrease. Examples of isolated provoked seizures are childhood febrile convulsions; drug or alcohol withdrawal seizures; seizures related to metabolic disturbances (e.g., hypoglycemia); or acute seizures resulting from head injury. (See Chapter 11 for more details on seizures and head injury.) **Epilepsy** is defined as the occurrence of two unprovoked seizures.[5]

The phases of a seizure are **preictal** (the period before the seizure), **ictal** (the period during the seizure), **postictal** (the period immediately after the seizure), and **interictal** (the period between seizures). The duration of each phase is specific to each seizure type and to the individual. For example, some seizures have no postictal period whereas a generalized, tonic-clonic seizure may have a postictal period for many hours. Likewise, some patients with partial seizures have a very short postictal phase and can talk or function immediately, whereas others have a prolonged postictal disturbance lasting up to several hours.

All people with epilepsy have seizures; however, not everyone who has a seizure has epilepsy. Epilepsy has no single cause but can be caused by any number of conditions that injure or affect the brain. Epilepsy can affect anyone, at any age, at any time (Box 24-1).

EPIDEMIOLOGY

Incidence refers to the number of new cases of a disease in a population over a period of time. It has been estimated that the cumulative incidence of epilepsy to age 80 is between 1.3% and 3.1%.[6,7] The risk of having an isolated seizure in one's lifetime is about 6%. People under age 20 have the highest incidence rate. The incidence of epilepsy then declines until age 60, when it increases again, and may be related to the strokes, brain tumors, and Alzheimer's disease seen in older adults or may be due to aging of the brain. **Prevalence**

- Perinatal problems (e.g., toxemia, low birth weight, hypoxia, neonatal seizures)
- Head trauma
- Central nervous system (CNS) infections
- Brain tumors
- Brain attack/stroke, cerebrovascular disease, aneurysm, arteriovenous malformation (AVM)
- Complex febrile convulsions
- Alcohol or drug abuse
- Family history of epilepsy and febrile convulsions
- Toxic and metabolic disturbances
- Anoxia
- Degenerative diseases: Alzheimer's disease and multiple sclerosis
- Cerebral palsy (CP)
- Mental retardation
- Congenital malformations of the CNS
- Genetic predisposition

Modified from Hauser WA, Hesdorffer DC: *Epilepsy frequency, causes and consequences,* New York, 1990, Demos Publications.

refers to the number of cases present at a specified time. The estimated prevalence of active epilepsy is 6.42 per 1000.[7]

ETIOLOGY

Epilepsy can be caused by any process that disrupts the stability of the cellular environment (see Box 24-1). Some people have a lower threshold for seizures as a result of either genetic factors or an acquired condition such as a structural injury. All individuals have the capacity to have seizures given the right circumstances and provocations.[1]

CLASSIFICATION

Epilepsy has been classified according to the age of onset, cause, area of origin, EEG abnormalities, and clinical seizure type. To manage epilepsy effectively and to study and evaluate the effectiveness of treatment options, it is useful to have a uniform way of classifying seizures.

In 1964, the **International League Against Epilepsy (ILAE)** appointed a commission on classification and terminology to create a uniform system of seizure classification. In 1969, the **International Classification of Epileptic Seizures** was published. In response to improved technology and monitoring capabilities, a revision was adopted in 1989. The 1989 International Classification of Epileptic Seizures is based on clinical seizure types and interictal and ictal EEG patterns. Further attempts to reclassify the epilepsies occurred in 2001 and 2005, but have not been formally adopted.[5,8] The current classification, based on the 1989 document, is divided into partial (focal), generalized, and unclassified seizures.[9] Table 24-1, Box 24-2, and Fig. 24-1 can be used as references when considering the seizure types discussed here.

TABLE 24-1   ILAE Classification of the Epilepsies and Epileptic Syndromes

1. Localization-related (focal, local, partial) epilepsies and syndromes
   - 1.1 Idiopathic (with age-related onset)
     - Benign childhood epilepsy with centrotemporal spikes
     - Childhood epilepsy with occipital paroxysms
   - 1.2 Symptomatic
     - Chronic progressive epilepsia partialis continua of childhood
     - Syndromes characterized by seizures with specific modes of precipitation
     - Temporal lobe epilepsies
     - Frontal lobe epilepsies
     - Parietal lobe epilepsies
     - Occipital lobe epilepsies
   - 1.3 Cryptogenic
2. Generalized epilepsies and syndromes
   - 2.1 Idiopathic (with age-related onset)
     - Benign neonatal familial convulsions
     - Benign neonatal convulsions
     - Benign myoclonic epilepsy in infancy
     - Childhood absence epilepsy
     - Juvenile absence epilepsy
     - Juvenile myoclonic epilepsy
     - Epilepsy with grand mal seizures on awakening
     - Other generalized idiopathic epilepsies not defined above
     - Epilepsies with seizures precipitated by specific modes of activation
   - 2.2 Cryptogenic or symptomatic
     - West syndrome (infantile spasms)
     - Lennox-Gastaut syndrome
     - Epilepsy with myoclonic-astatic seizures
     - Epilepsy with myoclonic absences
   - 2.3 Symptomatic
   - 2.3.1 Nonspecific etiology
     - Early myoclonic encephalopathy
     - Early infantile epileptic encephalopathy with burst suppression
     - Other symptomatic generalized epilepsies not defined above
   - 2.3.2 Specific syndromes
3. Epilepsies and syndromes undetermined, whether focal or generalized
   - 3.1 With both generalized and focal features
     - Neonatal seizures
     - Severe myoclonic epilepsy in infancy
     - Epilepsy with continuous spike waves during slow wave sleep
     - Acquired epileptic aphasia (Landau-Kleffner syndrome)
     - Other undetermined epilepsies not defined above
   - 3.2 Without unequivocal generalized or focal features
4. Special situations
     - Febrile convulsions
     - Isolated seizures or isolated status epilepticus
     - Seizures occurring only when there is an acute toxic or metabolic event

BOX 24-2	Seizure Types and Symptoms		
Type	**Subtype**	**Symptoms**	**Comments**
Partial			
Simple (no loss of consciousness)	Motor	"Jacksonian" march Movement of eye, head, and body to one side Stopping of movement or speech	Spreads topographically Limited to one body part
	Sensory or somatosensory	Tingling, numbness of body part Visual, auditory, olfactory, or taste sensations Dizzy spells	
	Autonomic forms	Pallor, sweating, flushing, piloerection, pupillary dilation Dysphagia	
	Psychic forms	Déjà vu ("already seen") Dysmnesic phenomena Distortion of time sense Fear illusions Micropsia—objects appearing small Macropsia—objects appearing large Teleopsia—objects appearing far away	
Complex (alteration of consciousness)		Automatisms (simple, lip smacking, or picking with hands) Automatisms (complex, verbal automatisms, bicycling movements of feet, washing dishes, wandering) Antisocial or aggressive behavior if restrained	Partial seizures can generalize if discharge spreads to other sites Amnesia for the ictal event
Generalized			
Absence	Simple Atypical	Staring spell lasting 2–15 seconds Staring spell, possibly with myoclonic, tonic, or atonic seizures	
Myoclonic	—	Brief jerk of one or more muscle groups	
Clonic	—	Repetitive jerking of muscle groups	
Tonic	—	Stiffening of muscle groups	
Tonic-clonic	—	Starts with the stiffening or tonic phase, followed by the jerking or clonic phase Unconsciousness Tongue biting Bowel and bladder incontinence	
Atonic	—	Drop attack or abrupt loss of muscle tone	

Modified from Petit JM: *Primary neurologic care,* St Louis, 2001, Mosby.

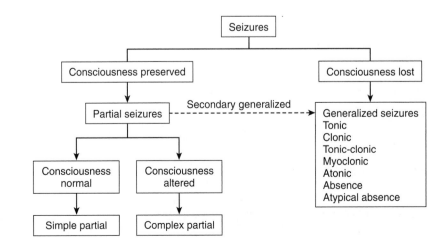

Figure 24-1 ILAE classification of seizures.

Partial (Focal) Seizures

Partial seizures arise from focal area of the brain (see Box 24-2). Partial seizures may be simple or complex. Partial seizures may progress to generalized tonic-clonic seizures if the seizure discharge spreads beyond its focal origin to affect the whole brain. In describing partial seizures, one must be aware of the degree to which consciousness is impaired. Impairment of consciousness is not defined as a total loss of consciousness but instead is an alteration of consciousness that affects the ability of the person to make contact with the outside world.

Simple Partial Seizures

Simple partial seizures are epileptic seizures characterized by motor, sensory, autonomic, or psychic symptomatology during which consciousness is preserved. There is no alteration or loss of consciousness. Simple partial seizures involve a small, focal area of the brain, and symptoms depend on where in the brain the electrical discharge occurs.[10] For example, a simple partial seizure that begins in motor cortex will be manifest by motor movements without loss of consciousness. Seizures that begin in the limbic system may lead to viscero-sensory perceptions such as an epigastric sensation, a smell, or a sound. These sensory perceptions are often referred to as **auras** (Greek for "breeze"). The term *aura* is reserved for subjective symptoms of epileptic origin reported by the patient in the absence of objective signs. An aura has been defined as that portion of the seizure that occurs before consciousness is lost and for which memory is retained afterward.[11]

Simple partial seizures begin in a focal area of the brain. Approximately 50% of simple partial seizures will spread to a regional area (lobe) of the brain and evolve into a complex partial seizure. If a simple partial seizure spreads to involve both hemispheres, a secondarily generalized tonic-clonic seizure will occur. Because simple partial seizures often involve relatively small areas of brain, scalp EEG recordings may be normal.

Complex Partial Seizures

Complex partial seizures are also referred to as **psychomotor seizures.** Complex partial seizures are associated with an **alteration in consciousness, but not with complete loss of consciousness.** The seizure may begin with a motionless stare or arrest of activity followed by oral-alimentary or hand motions, eye movements, speech disturbances, or automatic behavior. **Automatisms** are a frequent manifestation of complex partial seizures, and refer to a simple action performed during a seizure, such as lip smacking, chewing, or picking at clothes. These automatic behaviors are performed even though consciousness is impaired. Automatism tends to be stereotypic, occurring in the same way over time. However, different patients have different automatisms: one person might have lip smacking, another patient might have repetitive speech or hand movements.

Approximately half of partial seizures begin as complex partial seizures with aura (simple partial seizures), and half begin without aura.[6,7,12] The neurologist may report that the EEG demonstrates focal or lateralized sharp waves, spikes, or spike and slow wave complexes; however, nearly one third

of the routine outpatient EEGs performed in people with epilepsy will be normal.[1]

Partial seizures may be **idiopathic** or **symptomatic,** but the majority are symptomatic partial epilepsies, meaning that an underlying cause can be identified (trauma, hippocampal sclerosis, brain tumor, etc.). Partial epilepsies are the most common seizure type in adults, but occur frequently in children as well. In children, the most common causes of symptomatic partial epilepsy are developmental malformations, such as cortical dysplasia or tuberous sclerosis, or perinatal insult, such as intraventricular hemorrhage. Between ages 16 and 45, the most common causes of partial seizures are mass lesions, such as tumors, or head trauma with contusion or hemorrhage. Cardiovascular disease is the most common cause of new-onset partial epilepsy in adults over age 60.[13]

Children may also have **idiopathic partial epilepsies.** Childhood epilepsy with occipital paroxysms (CEOP) and autosomal dominant nocturnal frontal lobe epilepsy (ADNFLE) are examples of genetic epilepsies that manifest with partial seizures. Idiopathic partial seizures are less common than symptomatic partial seizures. The type of seizure seen in the patient will depend on where the seizure begins and how it spreads, more than on whether the partial seizure is idiopathic or symptomatic.

Partial Seizures With Secondary Generalization

A partial seizure can occur in isolation, or it can progress to become a secondarily generalized seizure. The patient may or may not have premonitory symptoms, including headache, mood change, anxiety, irritability, lethargy, change in appetite, dizziness, and light-headedness. This preictal phase is different from an aura and is difficult to describe; however, many patients report that they "feel a seizure coming on" for hours or days before the event. Seizures may begin with or without a recognizable partial seizure (especially if the patient always progresses to a generalized seizure, in which case the partial seizure may not be recognized or remembered). Initially, patients usually enter into a tonic phase, when all muscles become rigid. This rigidity may involve muscles of respiration, resulting in a cry or moan. Then follows the clonic, rhythmic jerking phase (any combination of tonic and clonic activity, i.e., tonic-clonic, clonic-tonic, or tonic-clonic-tonic can occur). During the seizure, the patient may become cyanotic, but breathing resumes when the seizure ends. Tongue biting and urinary or fecal incontinence may occur. Patients may be confused, complain of a headache, or sleep afterward.

Some patients may have a **Todd's paralysis** after a generalized seizure, usually lasting 30 minutes or less, characterized by focal weakness of an extremity. This focal weakness indicates that the partial seizure originated from the contralateral hemisphere. Occasionally, a clinician may confuse this postictal state with a stroke, particularly in new-onset seizures or when a patient is unknown to the evaluating facility.

Generalized Seizures

Primary generalized seizures involve both cerebral hemispheres from the onset (see Box 24-2). There are more seizure types in the generalized epilepsies than in the partial epilepsies. The most common are absence, myoclonic, atonic, tonic, clonic, and tonic-clonic seizures, described in the following sections. In general, the primary generalized epilepsies are most commonly seen in childhood and less often begin in adulthood.

Most primary generalized epilepsies are either idiopathic or symptomatic. Many of the **idiopathic generalized epilepsies** are thought to have genetic defects that alter neuronal firing. Childhood absence epilepsy and juvenile myoclonic epilepsy are examples of idiopathic epilepsies that are genetic. The **symptomatic generalized epilepsies** can occur for many different reasons, such as tumor, severe birth anoxia, or cortical developmental malformation.

Absence Seizures

Absence seizures are classified as typical or atypical. A typical **absence seizure**, formerly called *petit mal seizures*, is an electrographic seizure lasting from 1 to 15 seconds. Electrographic activity that lasts more than 2 or 3 seconds may be associated with a loss of contact, such as staring. Typical absence seizures are characterized by sudden behavioral arrest, staring, and unresponsiveness, after which the child returns to normal activity without a postictal period. Absence seizures may occasionally be accompanied by eyelid or facial clonus; automatisms; and autonomic, tonic, or atonic features. Brief absence seizures of 1 to 2 seconds might not be recognized by the child or an observer; prolonged absences rarely exceed 15 seconds.[1] Absence seizures are seen on EEG as a highly characteristic pattern with 3-second spike and wave activity. Childhood absence epilepsy is one of the most common types of childhood epilepsy. Approximately 40% of patients with childhood absence epilepsy develop generalized tonic-clonic seizures, often 5 to 10 years after the onset of the absences.[14] In childhood absence epilepsy, seizures become less frequent through adolescence and about 80% remit by adulthood.[15] When one hears of childhood epilepsy that responds to medicine and in which the family has been told that "the child will outgrow the seizures," one is often referring to childhood absence epilepsy.

Atypical absence seizures are characterized by a specific EEG pattern and generally exceed 10 seconds in duration. Atypical absence seizures often occur along with tonic, atonic, or myoclonic seizures.[16] Clinically, the seizures may have associated mild clonic components (eye fluttering) or atonic components (seizures with falls) or automatisms. The EEG shows an atypical, slow spike and wave pattern, which is characteristic of the disorder. Atypical absence seizures do not regress after childhood and are associated with a more ominous clinical outcome.

Myoclonic Seizures

Myoclonic seizures can involve either a single muscle group or multiple muscle groups, sometimes causing the patient to fall. Myoclonic seizures are single or repetitive rapid muscular contractions. Because the EEG shows bilaterally symmetric epileptiform discharges, these seizures are classified as generalized seizures; however, there is no loss of consciousness. When myoclonic seizures are severe, the patient may fall forward or backward. Myoclonic seizures often occur early in the morning, and a person with myoclonic seizures may also have generalized tonic-clonic seizures as well. Juvenile myoclonic epilepsy is the most frequent type of myoclonic seizure type, making up about 6% to 11% of all childhood epilepsies. Persons with juvenile myoclonic epilepsy will often have generalized tonic-clonic seizures as well. The disorder does not regress after childhood but persists into adulthood.[15]

Atonic Seizures

Atonic seizures manifest as a loss of muscle tone. They may be mild, resulting in a brief head nod. This "head nod" may be the only manifestation of an atonic seizure. Atonic seizures that last longer (1 to 2 seconds) or involve more muscle groups may manifest with more significant loss of tone. Clinically, these may be seen, for example, as a fall forward at the waist or a loss all tone and a fall. These seizures are often referred to as **"drop attacks."** Consciousness is impaired only momentarily, and patients usually get up immediately. Many patients experiencing atonic seizures wear helmets to prevent injury from falls. These seizures are often refractory to pharmacologic therapy.

Tonic Seizures

Tonic seizures are characterized by sustained muscle contractions involving flexion of the upper extremities and flexion or extension of the lower extremities. Impairment of consciousness and autonomic alterations occur. The seizures usually last less than 10 seconds but may last up to 1 minute. Tonic seizures are abrupt in onset, and may precipitate a fall. Tonic seizures are followed by a rapid return to baseline. They commonly occur in clusters during drowsiness or sleep, frequently occurring dozens of times per day.

Clonic Seizures

Generalized **clonic seizures** are relatively uncommon; they consist of regular, short contractions of various muscle groups. Clonic seizures may be confused with tonic-clonic seizures, the difference being that tonic-clonic seizures begin with an initial period of stiffening, followed by muscle jerking (common), whereas clonic seizures occur without initial stiffness (rare). Clonic seizures seldom manifest as a specific seizure type but are more likely to be recognized during video-EEG monitoring.

Tonic-Clonic Seizures

Tonic-clonic seizures have been previously described under the partial epilepsies, but can also occur in the primary generalized epilepsies. The difference is that tonic-clonic seizures in primary generalized epilepsy are not thought to begin in a particular part of the brain and then spread, as in partial seizures with secondary generalization, but to begin within the deep brain regions and involve the entire brain simultaneously. Therefore these two types of tonic-clonic seizures most likely have different mechanisms of onset. The final common pathway, the "grand-mal seizure," can look quite similar, and it can be difficult to tell whether a single generalized seizure is the result of a partial epilepsy or of a primary generalized epilepsy unless one is familiar with the patient and knows the underlying epilepsy syndrome with which that patient is affected.

Unclassified Seizures

Some seizures cannot be identified as either partial or generalized seizures, and are therefore described as **unclassified epileptic seizures.** These seizures often have EEG or clinical characteristics that make it difficult to assign them to either the partial or generalized categories or have characteristics of both. Examples of these include some neonatal seizures and occasionally adult patients as well.

The definitions in this section are provided to help the nurse clinician develop a vocabulary to define seizure types. However, it is often more useful to simply describe what one sees during a seizure than to attempt to classify the seizure. When observing a seizure, it is particularly useful to monitor and observe for level of consciousness (LOC), presence of automatisms, motor movements, and degree of postictal impairment. Documentation helps to record information used to classify the seizure type at a later time.

EPILEPSY SYNDROMES

Once the seizure type is identified, it is useful to relate the seizure type to a clinical history or specific pattern on EEG to classify a person's epilepsy into a specific syndrome. Clinicians use the epilepsy syndrome to determine prognosis, choice of antiepileptic medications, appropriateness for surgical treatment, need for genetic counseling, and other medical treatment options. The International League of Epilepsy has established a classification system that is widely used among epileptologists (see Table 24-1).[9] There are currently over 45 different syndromes, which are constantly undergoing revision. The epilepsy syndromes are classified as **idiopathic, cryptogenic,** or **symptomatic.** Idiopathic epilepsy has no underlying brain lesion or neurologic signs and symptoms. The idiopathic epilepsies are presumed to be genetic and are usually age dependent. In symptomatic epilepsy, seizures are the result of one or more identifiable structural lesions of the brain (e.g., stroke, tumor, brain malformation). Cryptogenic epilepsies are those syndromes that are believed to be symptomatic, but no etiology has been identified. Some authors have suggested that the term *cryptogenic* be replaced with the term *probably symptomatic.*[8] As research into epilepsy continues, it is likely that many of the cryptogenic epilepsies will be reclassified as either idiopathic or symptomatic as genetic sequencing and improved neuroimaging provide further detail. Approximately two thirds of cases of epilepsy are idiopathic and one third are symptomatic.

Two syndromes have already been introduced in this chapter when discussing the generalized epilepsies: childhood absence epilepsy and juvenile myoclonic epilepsy. Both are primary generalized epilepsy syndromes that frequently have absence and generalized tonic-clonic seizures; however, the prognosis for long-term outcome is quite different

between the two. Likewise, absence seizures are commonly seen in Lennox-Gastaut syndrome, a catastrophic childhood epilepsy characterized by multiple seizure types, characteristic EEG findings, and developmental delay. Whereas one would never consider doing surgery for childhood absence epilepsy, absence epilepsy associated with Lennox-Gastaut syndrome can be treated with corpus callosotomy or vagus nerve stimulation therapy. Therefore not only seizure type but also the epilepsy syndromes are important to understanding the pathophysiology, medical and surgical treatment options, and prognosis of the epilepsies. When possible, treatment is based on epilepsy syndrome because particular syndromes are likely to respond to the same antiepileptic drugs (AEDs).

SPECIAL CONCERNS

Medically Refractory Epilepsy

Epilepsy is defined as the occurrence of two or more unprovoked seizures. Medically refractory epilepsy describes persistent seizures despite adequate trials of appropriate AEDs. Although response rates vary greatly in relation to seizure type and syndrome, 50% to 70% of patients with newly diagnosed epilepsy will have their seizures fully controlled with medication.[17] Approximately 30% of patients will have seizures that are resistant to medical therapy, despite trials of multiple medications. All different seizure types can be medically refractory, including absence, partial, and generalized seizures.[17,18]

Patients with medically refractory epilepsy represent a minority of people with epilepsy, but are responsible for most of the cost and burden of disease associated with epilepsy. The financial cost of medication(s) is high, but is only the tip of the iceberg. Refractory patients are more likely to utilize emergency services (for seizures or injury) even if compliant with medications. People with medically intractable epilepsy may have more trouble finding or maintaining employment. They usually cannot operate a motor vehicle. Social and financial burdens associated with medically refractory epilepsy are significant.

If seizures are not well controlled, an extensive workup within a specialized epilepsy center is appropriate. Evaluation may include admission for continuous video and EEG monitoring, advanced neuroimaging, and neuropsychiatric studies. Patients may be admitted for differential diagnosis to characterize their clinical events (i.e., epileptic versus nonepileptic seizures), to determine the exact seizure type by EEG (partial versus primary generalized), or to determine the location within the brain in which seizures originate. After the data are collected, the seizure type and syndrome can be appropriately identified and a treatment plan specifically targeted to the individual can be created.

Posttraumatic Seizures

Postictal seizures may appear early (within 7 days after injury) or late (any time after the first 7 days). Acute treatment with anticonvulsants will reduce the possibility of seizures during the hospital stay but does not reduce the long-term risk of acquiring seizures (Box 24-3).[19,20] Refer to Chapter 11 for guidelines for the management and prognosis of severe traumatic brain injury.

Childhood Febrile Seizures

Febrile seizures can occur in up to 5% of the general population. Most are benign, and remit after age 5. They are not a risk factor for long-term epilepsy. Children with a family history of febrile seizures are more likely to have these seizures themselves. A small proportion of children with febrile seizures will have an underlying structural or genetic abnormality as a cause of their seizures, which may make them more susceptible to febrile seizures. In this small subset of patients, seizures may not remit after age 5, and the patients may eventually be diagnosed with epilepsy. Because febrile seizures are provoked events, two or three febrile seizures do not mean that a patient has epilepsy.

A complicated febrile seizure is described as a febrile seizure lasting more than 15 minutes, two febrile seizures within 24 hours, or a seizure with ictal or postictal lateralizing neurologic signs. Complicated febrile seizures can be associated with later epilepsy. Complicated febrile seizures are a risk factor for mesial temporal lobe epilepsy, one of the most common forms of adult partial epilepsies.[21]

Febrile seizures do not require immediate treatment with AEDs. This is largely based on prior practice, where parents and physicians recognized the negative cognitive and behavioral side effects of AEDs in young patients (particularly with phenobarbital). Consequently, most physicians will use expectant care rather than prophylactic AEDs for these seizures, advocating early treatment with acetaminophen or ibuprofen, and tepid baths to decrease fever in the child. Management may also utilize the new AED, Diastat (rectal diazepam), which can be used to decrease the risk of progression to a complicated febrile seizure.[22]

Sudden Unexplained Death in Epilepsy

Sudden unexplained death in epilepsy (SUDEP) is not well understood but is thought to be caused by central respiratory apnea or cardiac arrhythmia. Risk factors include the following:[23]

- Recent generalized tonic-clonic seizures
- Adolescents and young adults
- Subtherapeutic levels of AEDs
- Symptomatic complex partial epilepsy
- Excessive alcohol intake
- Medically refractory epilepsy
- Unwitnessed nocturnal seizures

The possibility of SUDEP emphasizes the need to stay with the individual for several minutes after a seizure, until the seizure is over and vital signs have returned towards baseline and to know seizure first aid (see Case Management Considerations later in this chapter). Sudden death in epilepsy can occur in patients with only occasional seizures and in those who are compliant with medications. Mortality risk in epilepsy emphasizes the need for caution and prevention of seizure activity for individuals with epilepsy who swim, drive a motor vehicle, have depression, and fail to comply with their AED regimen, because there is an increased mortality rate among patients with epilepsy from accidents that are not SUDEP events.[24,25]

Women and Epilepsy

A recent survey by the Epilepsy Foundation found a low level of knowledge and a high degree of uncertainty among health care professionals about best practices in caring for women with epilepsy. Women with epilepsy face epilepsy-related problems throughout their reproductive lives, including difficulties with hormonally sensitive seizures, sexuality, contraceptive failure, and infertility.[26] Contraceptive failure may occur as a result of increased contraceptive metabolism with the use of AEDs; therefore higher-dose contraceptives are required for some AEDs. Polycystic ovary disease is more common in patients taking valproic acid, and in general, fertility among women (and men) with epilepsy is reduced. The American Epilepsy Society and Epilepsy Foundation of America have added special seminars and teaching sessions to its educational activities for doctors and patients to enhance the well-being of women with epilepsy.

Catamenial epilepsy (CE) is the pattern of predominant seizure occurrence or exacerbation of seizure frequency in relationship to the menstrual cycle and appears to occur in one third of women.[27] Many women experience an exacerbation of seizures during ovulation or menstruation that is attributed to changes in estrogen and progesterone levels.[26] Women should be encouraged to keep a seizure diary and dates of menses in order to look for a catamenial pattern.[28] Hormone treatment for catamenial epilepsy has not been as effective as many have hoped. The effects of cyclic hormonal alterations on AED levels, metabolism, and seizures are under renewed research and may lead to new treatments.

Pregnancy and epilepsy is an area in health care that has been receiving attention since the launching of the Women and Epilepsy Initiative as part of the effort by the Epilepsy Foundation to combat the unique problems of women with epilepsy. Well-managed pregnancies can have excellent outcomes. Most women who continue to take their prescribed AED during a planned pregnancy will have a seizure-free pregnancy. The pregnancy category of their medications should be checked for safety. Pregnancy category C indicates risk from animal studies with no studies in women. Category B indicates that either animal studies or those on pregnant women do not indicate a risk to the fetus. Therefore, with a planned pregnancy, the woman can plan early to take an AED that is classified as a category B before and during pregnancy. Women of childbearing age have major questions, for example, whether a woman with epilepsy can become pregnant, the safety of pregnancy for the infant and the mother, the need to adjust AEDs during pregnancy, what vitamins may be recommended by the obstetrician, breastfeeding, and whether the child will inherit epilepsy.

The more common malformations associated with the use of AEDs during pregnancy are cleft lip and palate, heart defects, and mild developmental delays. **Neural tube defects** have been associated with the use of sodium valproate and, to a lesser extent, carbamazepine.

ALERT: Counseling and consideration of a change in medication is appropriate *before* pregnancy.[29-31]

Considerations for the pregnant patient with epilepsy include the following[32] (Box 24-4):

- Approximately 19,000 births occur each year to women with epilepsy.
- AEDs can increase the metabolism of oral contraceptives, so a higher-dose contraceptive may be necessary to avoid pregnancy.
- Planned pregnancy allows the patient's physicians to work together before pregnancy to optimize a positive outcome.
- Women of childbearing age on AEDs should take high-dose folate daily when sexually active and before planned pregnancy to prevent birth defects.
- AED levels can change during pregnancy and require close monitoring.
- Some individuals report their first seizure during pregnancy.

BOX 24-4	**Guidelines for the Management of Epilepsy During Pregnancy**

- Baseline antiepileptic drug (AED) levels (total/free) and folate (serum/red blood cell)
- Folate supplementation 0.5 to 4.0 mg/day
- Maternal alpha fetoprotein at week 15 to 16
- AED levels and fetal ultrasound at 18 to 19 weeks
- Repeat fetal ultrasound at 22 to 24 weeks
- AED levels at 34 to 36 weeks; make adjustments to ensure therapeutic drug levels at term
- Vitamin K 20 mg/day during eighth month or 10 mg IV 4 hours before birth *and* 1 mg IM to newborn at birth
- Monthly AED levels postpartum for 12 weeks

From Goetz CG: *Textbook of clinical neurology,* ed 2, Philadelphia, 2003, Saunders.
IM, Intramuscularly; *IV,* intravenously.

- AED medications can affect sperm count and motility; therefore men with epilepsy should consider an evaluation if infertility is a concern.[33]
- If a woman has been seizure free for 2 years and has a normal EEG, the physician may consider discontinuing AEDs.
- Polytherapy may be reduced to monotherapy if AEDs cannot be discontinued before pregnancy.
- Sleep deprivation that occurs during pregnancy may trigger seizures.
- The risks to mother and fetus from seizures need to be weighed against the risks of AEDs (e.g., a decrease in the woman's heart rate, lactic acidosis, injury from a fall).[34,35]
- Magnetic resonance imaging (MRI) studies can be performed if necessary for the mother's health after the fetus is 1 month old.
- AEDs are secreted in breast milk; breastfeeding is encouraged but may need to be modified if the infant appears sedated or feeds poorly.
- Decisions regarding pregnancy require preplanning and precise medication evaluation and management. The Prospective Pregnancy Registry can be reached by calling 888-233-2344 for more information.

With good perinatal care, more than 95% of women with epilepsy will deliver normal, healthy infants (see Box 24-4).

Pseudoseizures

Psychogenic nonepileptic seizures (PNESs) mimic seizures but may have an underlying psychologic etiology. Up to 20% of individuals diagnosed with epilepsy may not have epilepsy, and they may undergo unnecessary therapy. Patients are frequently admitted to determine whether events are epileptic or nonepileptic. Many events can masquerade as epilepsy:

- Syncope
- Narcolepsy
- Sleep disturbances
- Restless legs syndrome (RLS)

These are examples of physiologic, nonepileptic events. Treatment is then directed toward the underlying medical cause. Alternatively, some patients suffer from PNESs, known in the vernacular as "pseudoseizures." The diagnosis of pseudoseizures is based on the collection of data consistent with the syndrome. Patients often have one of several characteristic "seizure" types consistent with PNESs.[36,37] A normal EEG during these events is inconsistent with seizures; for example, a person having a seizure that involves all four extremities cannot have a normal EEG unless it is a psychogenic event, because a generalized seizure with such behavior would be quite abnormal. The history of psychogenic patients often contains a history of physical or sexual abuse, or one of chronic pain. Neuropsychologic evaluation can be helpful, because certain profiles on the Minnesota Multiple Personality Inventory (MMPI) are more consistent with psychogenic events. The patient is advised of the diagnosis, and a treatment strategy that involves counseling is usually recommended.

EVALUATION OF THE PATIENT WITH SEIZURES

Assessment

When an individual with a new-onset seizure is treated at an emergency department or a clinic, initial concern is over the safety of the patient. Acute toxic or metabolic events are considered first, followed by the consideration of an intracranial process that might precipitate a seizure. Therefore screening diagnostic and laboratory tests are performed. A computed tomography (CT) scan is performed to rule out intracranial hemorrhage. A comprehensive neurologic assessment is directed toward the LOC and to determine the presence of focal neurologic deficits. The initial screening examination for new-onset seizures is summarized in Box 24-5. The exception to this general rule is the occurrence of childhood febrile seizures.

Once a thorough evaluation of seizure activity is completed, a decision is made on whether or not to begin **antiepileptic drug (AED) therapy.** If a toxic or metabolic insult is discovered, the need for AEDs diminishes. If the seizure is unclear, the decision to begin AEDs will rest with the physician and patient. Referral for close follow-up with a primary care physician, neurologist, or health care provider is advisable in such cases. If an individual has two or more unprovoked seizures, the diagnosis of **epilepsy** becomes more likely and treatment with an AED becomes advisable.

Once the diagnosis of epilepsy is raised, the history is crucial to determine seizure type and syndrome. The choice of medication depends on the type of epilepsy. Collection of the following data helps with diagnosis (Box 24-6):

- Precise description: Individuals may be unable to give specifics about their seizures, either because they cannot describe feelings or because they have no memory of the event. Friends and family members who have witnessed the seizures are often better historians. Begin with the very first alterations the patient experiences or those others observe. Individuals are sometimes reluctant to discuss the seizure because the feeling they have is difficult to describe or seems so bizarre that they fear being labeled "crazy." The clinician should give assurance that no one will judge their experiences as a sign of psychiatric illness and that many individuals with epilepsy have similar experiences.
- Seizure progression: A description of any auras, automatisms, falling, jerking, tongue biting, or incontinence, as well as a description of the postictal phase (confusion, sleepiness, headache, behavioral changes), helps determine seizure progression.
- Duration and frequency: The duration of the seizure and postictal period and the frequency at which the seizures occur should be ascertained. Precipitating factors, such as lack of sleep, alcohol, hyperventilation, stress, and menstruation, should be identified. Some patients are unable to identify the situations that precipitate their seizures. Some individuals with seizures will describe that they only occur during sleep, in clusters, or at certain times of the month.

The individual's past medical history is obtained, including the following:
- Birth and development
- Early risk factors (incidents before age 5: meningitis, febrile seizures)[38]
- Previous head injuries (with loss of consciousness)
- Family history of febrile convulsions, seizures, or epilepsy
- Age of onset of first seizure
- Systemic illnesses
- Focal neurologic symptoms
- CNS infections: encephalitis, meningitis, human immunodeficiency virus (HIV) infection
- Tumor or previous brain surgery
- Stroke
- History of migraine headache
- Occupational and social history: exposure to toxins, substance abuse
- Sleep history: Nocturnal events or signs of seizures during sleep
- Physical and neurologic examination: in most individuals with epilepsy the examination is normal; however, abnormalities may provide clues to the underlying cause; findings may be very subtle, such as a mild hemiatrophy (partial wasting) of the face or

---

| **BOX 24-5** | **Initial Evaluation of New-Onset Seizures** |

Determine whether other seizures (partial or generalized) have occurred or gone unrecognized

Review possible provoking causes (e.g., drugs, alcohol, high fever)

Neurologic Examination

Assess focal findings or other neurologic abnormalities

Laboratory

Assess possible metabolic, infectious, or toxic causes

Neuroimaging

Indicated in most patients except those with identified provoking cause or benign syndrome (e.g., febrile seizure)

Magnetic resonance imaging much preferred to computed tomography

Electroencephalogram

May be referred to neurologist to perform at later date

Indicated in unprovoked seizures

Assess for focal and generalized abnormalities (e.g., slowing, spikes)

Evaluate for possible epileptic syndromic classification

Decision Making

Assess chance of seizure recurrence

Assess risk to patient if seizures recur

Decide whether to recommend antiepileptic drug therapy

Modified from Johnson RT, Griffin JW, McArthur JC: *Current therapy in neurologic disease,* ed 6, St Louis, 2002, Mosby.

BOX 24-6   Seizure Assessment

Subjective Data

Important Health Information

Past health history: Previous seizures; birth defects or injuries; anoxic episodes; CNS trauma, tumors, or infections; hypertension, cerebrovascular disease; metabolic disorders, alcoholism; exposure to metals and carbon monoxide; hepatic or renal failure; fever; pregnancy; systemic lupus erythematosus

Medications: Compliance with antiseizure medications; barbiturate or alcohol withdrawal; use and overdose of cocaine, amphetamines, lidocaine, theophylline, penicillin, lithium, phenothiazines, tricyclic antidepressants, benzodiazepines

Functional Health Patterns

Health perception–health management: Positive family history

Cognitive-perceptual: Headaches, aura, mood or behavioral changes before seizure; mentation changes; abdominal pain, muscle pain (postictal)

Self-perception–self-concept: Anxiety, depression; loss of self-esteem, social isolation

Sexuality-reproductive: Decreased sex drive, erectile dysfunction; increased sex drive (postictal)

Objective Data

General

Precipitating factors, including severe metabolic acidosis or alkalosis, hyperkalemia, hypoglycemia, dehydration, or water intoxication

Integumentary

Bitten tongue, soft-tissue damage, cyanosis, diaphoresis (postictal)

Respiratory

Abnormal respiratory rate, rhythm, or depth; apnea (ictal); absent or abnormal breath sounds, possible airway occlusion

Cardiovascular

Hypertension, tachycardia, or bradycardia (ictal)

Gastrointestinal

Bowel incontinence; excessive salivation

Urinary

Incontinence

Neurologic

Generalized

Tonic-clonic: Loss of consciousness, muscle tightening then jerking, dilated pupils, hyperventilation, then apnea; postictal somnolence

Absence: Altered consciousness (5 to 30 seconds), minor facial motor activity

Partial

Simple: Aura, consciousness, focal sensory, motor, cognitive, or emotional phenomena (focal motor); unilateral "marching" motor seizure (jacksonian)

Complex: Altered consciousness with inappropriate behaviors, automatisms, amnesia of event

Musculoskeletal

Weakness, paralysis, ataxia (postictal)

Possible Findings

Positive toxicology screen or alcohol level; altered serum electrolytes, acidosis or alkalosis, very low blood glucose level, elevated blood urea nitrogen or serum creatinine, liver function tests, ammonia; abnormal CT scan or MRI of head, lumbar puncture; epileptiform discharges on EEG

From Lewis SM, Heitkemper MM, Dirksen SR: *Medical-surgical nursing: assessment and management of clinical problems,* ed 5, 2000, St Louis, Mosby.

CNS, Central nervous system; *CT,* computed tomography; *EEG,* electroencephalogram; *MRI,* magnetic resonance imaging.

posturing of the hand or stressed gait, indicating motor dysfunction; or bruising, as well as tongue injuries

Seizure observation and documentation skills are integral components of seizure and epilepsy management. This can be accomplished with a **"seizure diary,"** which is essential to the recognition and ongoing treatment of individuals with seizures.[39] Individuals with epilepsy (or those who have seizures not related to epilepsy) and their families often require education by the team of health professionals to learn how to accurately describe and record seizures.

Neurodiagnostic and Laboratory Studies

For new-onset epilepsy, initial evaluation includes an EEG to differentiate between generalized and partial epilepsy. If a patient has one of the common primary generalized epilepsies, neuroimaging is not an indication. However, if the EEG is normal or suggests partial epilepsy, MRI to screen for structural lesions is appropriate. Typical diagnostic/laboratory studies for new-onset epilepsy include the following:

Laboratory studies: performed to identify metabolic disturbances that might cause seizures. Glucose, electrolytes, blood urea nitrogen (BUN), thyroid panel, and a toxicology screen help determine metabolic or toxic causes.

EEG: the noninvasive recording of the electrical activity of the brain to evaluate the brain's function.

Neuroimaging: to identify brain lesions that could trigger seizures. It is essential to rule out a structural abnormality that may be causing seizures.

CT: used in the emergency department to screen for acute processes (hemorrhage, infection, and tumor). CT is the better study for identifying certain calcified and bony abnormalities. However, CT is inadequate for evaluating epilepsy, other than in the acute setting, because many lesions that cause seizures will not be seen on CT.

MRI: considered superior to CT for the subtle abnormalities often seen in patients with epilepsy (cortical malformations, low-grade tumors). MRI coronal images of the temporal lobes are necessary in any MRI done for epilepsy, because subtle lesions of the temporal lobes frequently cause epilepsy. MRI may be impractical in the emergency setting, but if more than one seizure has occurred, referral for MRI is appropriate. MRI cannot be done if there is metal with magnetic properties in the brain.

For medically refractory epilepsy, a more extensive evaluation using advanced neuroimaging and neuropsychologic evaluation can be performed using some of the following tests:

Single-photon emission computed tomography (SPECT): measures CBF and is used in patients with partial epilepsy who are being evaluated for surgery. Usually, CBF is elevated in the region where a seizure initiates during the seizure, and is decreased in the seizure onset zone between seizures. Ictal SPECT (injection of the radioactive isotope during a seizure) can be performed during inpatient video-EEG monitoring. Since ictal SPECT can be difficult to interpret, a baseline, interictal SPECT is often obtained while the patient is not seizing to compare with ictal SPECT. The two are coregistered and subtracted from one another, leaving only the areas with the most change. Subtraction ictal SPECT is more accurate in defining an epileptic zone than either ictal or interictal SPECT used alone.[40-42]

Positron emission tomography (PET): measures glucose metabolism, oxygen metabolism, and CBF. The most commonly used tracer is F-fluorodeoxyglucose (FDG). PET is frequently used in the presurgical evaluation of epilepsy. Like SPECT, regions where seizures begin may use less glucose than normal brain between seizures. PET is usually performed only in the interictal state because it is impractical to obtain ictal PET.[43,44]

Magnetoencephalography (MEG): a new technique that attempts to localize a magnetic dipole created by interictal spikes. It has the advantage over EEG that the scalp and skin do not interfere with measuring magnetic dipoles. This emerging technology is available in only a few epilepsy centers, but is increasing.[45,46]

Neuropsychologic evaluation: an extensive battery of tests that can screen for intelligence quotient (IQ), as well as for strengths and weaknesses in certain cognitive areas that suggest localization to particular lobes. For example, verbal memory impairment is a sign that dominant mesial temporal lobe function is compromised and is common in patients with mesial temporal lobe epilepsy with hippocampal atrophy, a syndrome that responds well to surgery.[47] Other tests (e.g., the MMPI) can detect certain characteristics that are more prominent with a person's psychologic makeup. Though not diagnostic, certain profiles are more often associated with particular syndromes and can be useful, especially when performing an evaluation for nonepileptic seizures.[48]

Psychologic or psychosocial evaluation: helpful in assessing the patient's emotional function in association with the diagnosis of seizures and epilepsy, possible comorbid mood disorder, integration into society, compliance, mitigating circumstances affecting treatment, and safety issues.[49-56]

Electroencephalogram Assessment and Monitoring

Electroencephalogram

The EEG records the electrical potentials of the brain from electrodes placed on the scalp. These potentials are recorded as the difference in voltage between two electrodes. The activity being recorded is generated by outer layers of the cerebral cortex (see Chapter 3). EEG is performed in the laboratory over a 2- to 4-hour period, with an attempt to capture awake and sleep recordings. In some cases, extended monitoring using ambulatory monitoring with a device similar to a **24-hour Holter monitor** can be used. The EEG is essential in diagnosing and classifying epilepsy. It can be used to help differentiate epilepsy from other disorders, to localize partial seizures, and to differentiate seizure types.

The **international 10/20 system** is a method used for electrode placement when recording the EEG (Fig. 24-2). It is a means for recording in a uniform and symmetric way that is standard in all EEG laboratories. All electrodes are anatomically positioned on the scalp with a fixed distance between electrodes that is replicable. The electrodes are identified anatomically and by number. Odd numbers represent the left side of the head, and even numbers represent the right. A montage is the sequence of electrodes that is compared during the recording of the EEG. At least three montages are used when an EEG is performed: (1) a reference (monopolar) sequence; (2) a parasagittal-temporal chain sequence; and (3) a transverse sequence. The montages are used to help localize abnormalities.

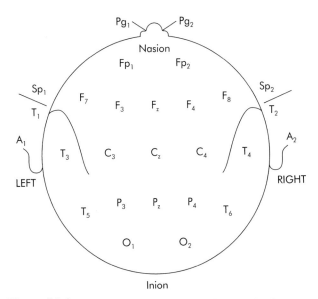

Figure 24-2 International 10/20 system of electrode placement for EEG recording.
(*From Spehlmann R:* EEG printer, *Amsterdam, 1981, Elsevier Biomedical Press.*)

It is not uncommon for patients with epilepsy to have normal EEGs. Physiologic activation procedures are often performed with EEGs in an attempt to enhance or produce abnormalities. Hyperventilation, sleep, and photic stimulation are commonly used. Hyperventilation is performed for a period of 3 to 5 minutes. This may provoke absence seizures or accentuate abnormalities in patients with partial seizures. Sleep can also bring out or enhance epileptiform abnormalities. Natural sleep is preferred, but sleep induced by medication such as chloral hydrate is acceptable. Photic stimulation (rapidly flashing light) may produce a paroxysmal epileptiform response in some patients with primary generalized epilepsy.

Surface scalp electrodes are not always capable of picking up epileptiform abnormalities from structures deep within the brain. Additional electrodes may be used in more comprehensive evaluations to record the medial temporal region (nasopharyngeal, sphenoidal, minisphenoidal, and anterior temporal), including the hippocampus and amygdala. Nasopharyngeal electrodes can be inserted through the nose to the nasopharynx. Discharges are recorded from the deep medial temporal structures. The patient experiences minor discomfort.

Sphenoidal electrodes are inserted through a 1-inch spinal needle anterior to the tragus immediately under the zygomatic arch. This allows recording from the mesiobasal structures, which include deep regions of the frontal and temporal lobes. They are often used in long-term EEG monitoring because they record spikes during ictal events slightly earlier than scalp electrodes. The risks associated with sphenoidal electrodes include infection, bleeding, and focal paresthesias. The patient may experience initial discomfort in opening the mouth wide or chewing. This usually lasts 1 day. Minisphenoidal electrodes are needle electrodes inserted under the zygoma and are easier to place than spenoidal electrodes. They record electrical activity from regions similar to those of sphenoidal electrodes.

Temporal electrodes are placed on the cheek at T1 and T2 on the skin to record medial temporal activity; they compare favorably with nasopharyngeal electrodes. Temporal electrodes can be applied without discomfort. Some centers prefer temporal electrodes to sphenoidal electrodes to avoid discomfort.

If the patient is treated with medication and has a normal EEG recording but continues to have seizures, an alternative type of EEG may help confirm the diagnosis. Options include ambulatory EEG monitoring and long-term continuous video and EEG.

Ambulatory Electroencephalogram Monitoring

Ambulatory EEG monitoring can be used to clarify suspected seizures that are occurring frequently. Typically, four to eight channels of EEG activity are recorded for 24 hours. Signals are transmitted to a tape recorder that the patient carries in a pouch (similar to a Holter monitor). The patient has complete freedom of movement and is able to go to school or work. The patient keeps a log of all activities, including seizures, during the 24-hour period. A disadvantage of this system is that the small number of channels presents a limited sampling of the brain's electrical activity. There is also no video monitoring capability to record clinical behavior during events or to correlate behavior with electrical abnormalities. The EEG record may be difficult to read at times because of artifact related to movement and muscle.

Continuous Video and Electroencephalogram Monitoring

Patients with medically refractory epilepsy may require continuous video and EEG (VEEG) monitoring. Patients are admitted to the hospital for continuous, 24-hour (around the clock), multiday observation. VEEG monitoring can be performed to characterize clinical event (differential diagnosis, i.e., epileptic versus nonepileptic seizures), to determine the exact seizure type (partial versus primary generalized), to determine the location within the brain where the seizures are originating for presurgical localization, or to gain information about the frequency of seizures (particularly in the generalized epilepsies). Treatment recommendations are made based on the results of the inpatient admission.

Continuous video and EEG monitoring can be very useful in the diagnosis of epilepsy. VEEG has the capability of recording 16 to 128 channels of EEG activity, depending on the system. Simultaneous EEG and video recording is performed, enabling correlation between clinical behavior and EEG abnormalities. A routine EEG montage, with or without temporal or sphenoidal electrodes, is placed on the patient's head and attached to recording equipment with a long cable. The goal of VEEG recording is to record the patient's "typical" seizures. Seizures can be identified in one of four ways. First, a push button is available for the patient or family member to mark a seizure. Second, software programs within the monitoring unit are programmed to recognize changes in EEG frequency and amplitude, which are flagged for review by a clinician. Third, nurses can record a seizure or postictal behavior that suggests a seizure has occurred. Finally, either a technician or physician can review the entire file visually to look for seizure activity. Family members or friends are encouraged to stay with the patient throughout the hospitalization, and a sleeping cot is placed in the patient's room for this purpose. Family members are crucial to determine whether a recorded event is typical of the patient's usual seizures. Attempts are made to capture several typical seizures. To do so, AEDs are frequently reduced or stopped altogether to increase the probability of capturing multiple events. Family members are then crucial to watching for escalation of seizures and alerting nursing personnel. VEEG is considered the "gold standard" of diagnosis and has been considered by some to revolutionize seizure diagnosis.

VEEG can be used for a number of purposes. It can be used to determine whether or not a person has epilepsy, and if so, which type. For example, a young female observed with "staring spells" and brief episodes of quiet behavior may be thought to have partial seizures based on a history of severe birth anoxia. If the individual is placed on an AED without cessation of these events, follow-up with several EEGs is nondiagnostic, and an MRI is normal, it would be important to admit the individual for VEEG monitoring. With 24-hour

VEEG monitoring an accurate diagnosis can be established for primary generalized, childhood absence epilepsy. Without a comprehensive evaluation, the correct diagnosis may have been missed, particularly if the family history was negative. The medication can be changed to an AED suited for her seizures with a good outcome expected.

VEEG is crucial for the evaluation of patients for epilepsy surgery. Seizure type and syndrome are categorized so that the epilepsy team can determine what type of surgery, if any, might be beneficial. Partial epilepsies are localized to a specific region of the brain (frontal, temporal, etc.) and correlated with other diagnostic tests to determine the next course of action. Multiple seizures might need to be recorded to ensure that all seizures are similar and arise from one part of the brain (unifocal) and exclude patients with multifocal epilepsy who would not benefit from surgery.

Assessment in the Monitoring Unit

Assessment in the VEEG monitoring unit incorporates neurologic, respiratory, and cardiovascular patient monitoring. Observation and documentation are recorded preictally and ictally, with descriptions of the characteristics of seizure activity, time of onset, duration, automatisms, and the individual's status. Behavior is recorded postictally. Respiratory assessment is needed to evaluate pulmonary status and to detect impaired oxygenation. Elevating the head of the bed and side-lying positioning help prevent aspiration that can cause pneumonia. Supplemental oxygen and suctioning equipment should always be available. Intravenous (IV) access for medications should be maintained for rapid administration of medications during an emergency. Seizure protocols are initiated on admission and may include having side rails up at all times except during patient care and the use of special padding that can be attached with the bed maintained in the low position. The seizure assessment guidelines proposed by the American Association of Neuroscience Nurses (AANN) can be used in any setting, including the monitoring unit.[11,57]

Ictal Phase

- Is the patient fully conscious and able to respond appropriately to the environment, and is the patient aware of self?
  - If the patient is fully conscious, ask about an aura and obtain a description.
  - Observe motor features.
  - Observe autonomic signs.
  - Ask about somatosensory, psychic, special sensory, or autonomic symptoms.
- Does the patient's level of consciousness return to baseline?
  - If yes, note the time when the episode ends. If no, reassess the LOC.
  - If the patient is unconscious, reassess airway, breathing, and circulation (the ABCs) and follow the algorithm.
  - If the patient has altered consciousness (eyes open, not responding appropriately to environment), reassess and follow the algorithm.
- Have features ceased?

Postictal Phase

- Assess the postictal condition, as well as injury and incontinence.
  - Postictal examination: The patient should be examined for level of consciousness and neurologic findings.
  - Document the episode (use a seizure flow chart if available).

Events Before the Ictal Phase. When the episode has ceased, interview the patient when consciousness returns and ask the patient or witnesses about events before and during the ictal phase:

- What were the preictal conditions?
- Precipitating factors?
- Behavioral changes?

Documentation: Use a chronologic sequence of events with time and interventions.

After it is safe to leave the individual, assessment of the need for more seizures during the monitoring period is discussed with the epilepsy team and decisions are made regarding AED therapy. The events are explained to the patient and family, and provisions are made so that the individual will be observed and monitored carefully for more seizures. Someone should remain with the patient until he or she is fully responsive and able to call or signal for help.

Potential Complications. Complications may include hypotension, aspiration, metabolic changes, injury (tongue biting, dental injury, shoulder dislocation, fracture from a fall), anoxia, renal problems, and rhabdomyolysis. The patient's urine is monitored for a red or cola color, which may signal **rhabdomyolysis** or **myoglobinuria** from muscle damage.

HEALTH TEACHING

After the diagnosis of epilepsy is established, the patient needs accurate information about epilepsy, its manifestations, etiology, and treatment. This information can be disseminated in several ways. The clinician can begin with a session with the patient and family to explain epilepsy and how it may affect their lives. Printed educational materials, tapes, and videos on epilepsy give the patient an opportunity to review the information at a convenient time and may stimulate further questions (see Resources at the end of this chapter).

All community resources should be identified, not only for diagnosis and treatment but also for support groups, educational conferences, employment information, and school alert and other programs. After the patient has had been discharged and has made contacts with community resources, follow-up appointments should be made to discuss the plan of care, further concerns, or questions. The individual with seizures and the individual's family must gain the knowledge, skills, and preparation to assume day-to-day management and treatment. Continued consultation with and support from health care providers with whom the individual with seizures and the individual's family have developed a positive relationship and good rapport is necessary. Explanations and education should be tailored to the individual's and family's educational level, age, attitudes, religious and cultural beliefs, and health beliefs.

Education is essential to review how the medication works, the half-life, side effects, and any drug-drug interactions with other medications the patient may be taking and should be emphasized with every patient interaction. Comprehensive education increases medication effectiveness and improves compliance. It is important to discuss the cost of medications, if the individual has adequate medication health care coverage, or if the individual needs assistance in applying for free medications if eligible. Poor compliance results in breakthrough seizures and can be related to inadequate teaching, lack of understanding about AED administration, poor relationships with treating health care providers, inability to pay, poor family support, and health care beliefs incompatible with medication use.

Goals include good seizure control, minimal medication side effects, good medication compliance, a healthy lifestyle, and self-management of common concerns (e.g., school, work, driving, interpersonal relationships, and sexuality, as well as menstruation and pregnancy for women). During this period of adjustment, psychosocial support and close monitoring from an informed nurse clinician and health care professionals is essential. Each individual patient and family member will have different coping skills. The clinician needs to identify individual needs when presenting education and counseling to help the patient and family adjust to the long-term treatment regimen.

TREATMENT

Medical Treatment

The goal of medication management in epilepsy is to control seizures with the minimum number of medication side effects. Knowledge of the seizure type and epilepsy syndrome is particularly useful in optimizing antiepileptic drug treatment, because specific seizures and syndromes respond differently to the different antiepileptic drugs.

AEDs changed little until the early 1990s. The widely studied and well-known agents are commonly known as the conventional AEDs (Table 24-2). Beginning in 1993, a number of AEDs (referred to in this text as "new AEDs") have been introduced into the North American markets that have greatly expanded the treatment options available to the practitioner. A number of medications that were not developed as AEDs are occasionally used as antiepileptic medications (unconventional AEDs). In Table 24-2, mention is made of the experimental drugs, not because they are currently important in the treatment of epilepsy, but because some of them will eventually receive U.S. Food and Drug Administration (FDA) approval. For example, pregabalin recently received FDA approval and is no longer investigational.[58]

Some medications are relatively specific in their action; for example, ethosuximide is very successful in treating absence epilepsy but is ineffective in treating the partial epilepsies. Other medications are proving to be "broad spectrum" agents, and treat both generalized and partial epilepsies; valproic acid and lamotrigine are good examples. Each medication has unique mechanisms of action, metabolic profiles, pharmacodynamics, specific risks, and side effects that affect each patient uniquely. The need to interact with the patient while titrating AEDs makes the practice of treating epilepsy a mixture of both art and science. Approximately 70% of patients with epilepsy are well controlled with AEDs, which are currently the cornerstone of epilepsy treatment. About 30% of patients with epilepsy are not well controlled and have medically refractory epilepsy despite adequate trials of AEDs.

Drugs of Choice by Seizure Type and Epilepsy Syndrome

AEDs should be selected based on the epilepsy syndrome or seizure type if the syndrome is not known (Table 24-3). All

---

TABLE 24-2 Conventional, New, Unconventional, and Experimental Antiepileptic Drugs

Conventional	New	Unconventional	Experimental
Carbamazepine (CBZ) (Tegretol)	Felbamate (FBM) (Felbatol)	Adrenocorticotropic hormone (ACTH)*	Clobazam (Frisium)[†‡]
Ethosuximide (ESM) (Zarontin)	Gabapentin (GBP) (Neurontin)		Eterobarb[‡]
Phenobarbital (PB)	Lamotrigine (LMT) (Lamictal)	Acetazolamide (Diamox)	Ganaxolone[‡]
Phenytoin (PHT) (Dilantin)	Levetiracetam (LEV) (Keppra)	Amantadine (Symmetrel)*	Losigamone[‡]
Primidone (PRM) (Mysoline)	Oxcarbazepine (OXC) (Trileptal)	Bromides*[§]	Nitrazepam (Mogadon)[†‡]
Valproic acid (VPA) (Depakene)	Tiagabine (TGB) (Gabitril)	Clomiphene (Clomid)*	Piracetam (Nootropil)[‡]
	Topiramate (TPM) (Topamax)	Ethotoin (Peganone)	Progabide[‡]
	Zonisamide (ZNS) (Zonegran)	Mephenytoin (Mesantoin)	Remacemide[‡]
		Mephobarbital (Mebaral)	Rotigotine[‡]
		Methsuximide (Celontin)	Retinamide[‡]
		Trimethadione (Tridione)	SPM927 (Harkoseride)[‡]
	Pregabalin (Lyrica)		Stiripentol[‡]
			Vigabatrin (Sabril)[†‡]

Modified from Rakel RE, Bope ET, editors: *Conn's current therapy 2005,* ed 57, Philadelphia, 2005, WB Saunders.
*Not FDA approved for this indication.
[†]Approved in other countries.
[‡]Investigational drug in the United States.
[§]May be compounded by pharmacists.

TABLE 24-3	Drugs of Choice by Seizure Type and Epilepsy Syndrome	
Seizure or Syndrome	Effective Drugs	Ineffective Drugs
Partial seizures	Carbamazepine, felbamate, gabapentin, lamotrigine, levitiracetam, oxcarbazepine, phenobarbital, phenytoin, primidone, tiagabine, topiramate, valproic acid, zonisamide, pregabalin	Ethosuximide
Generalized seizures		
Absence seizures	Ethosuximide, lamotrigine, valproic acid	Carbamazepine, gabapentin, tiagabine
Myoclonic seizures	Lamotrigine, valproic acid, benzodiazepines	
Tonic, clonic, and tonic-clonic seizures	Carbamazepine, phenobarbital, phenytoin, primidone, valproic acid, felbamate, lamotrigine topiramate, zonisamide	
Epilepsy syndromes:		
Juvenile myoclonic epilepsy	Lamotrigine	
Lennox-Gastaut	Felbamate, lamotrigine, topiramate, valproic acid	

Modified from Rakel RE, Bope ET, editors: *Conn's current therapy 2005*, ed 57, Philadelphia, 2005, WB Saunders.

types of **partial seizures** respond to the same medications, so they can be considered together. The available data suggest that all conventional and new AEDs, except for ethosuximide (Zarontin), are equally effective. Therefore, to select among them, consideration must be given to the relative importance of the side effect profile, dosing interval, pharmacokinetics, and cost for each patient. In general, the new AEDs have less frequent side effects, daily or twice-daily dosing, and simple pharmacokinetics, which suggest that they are more desirable than conventional AEDs. On the other hand, conventional AEDs are familiar, have a proven track record, can often be administered intravenously, and are inexpensive. It is common practice to start therapy with a conventional AED, but move quickly to a new AED if necessary. New AEDs are gradually starting to replace conventional AEDs for the initial treatment of partial seizures.[59]

The types of *generalized seizure* must be considered individually. Generalized tonic-clonic (GTC) seizures, tonic seizures, and clonic seizures seem to respond to the same AEDs as partial-onset seizures, but this may be because historically there was little distinction between primary generalized seizures and partial seizures with secondary generalization (all being classified as "generalized" without further distinction) during drug development. All conventional AEDs, except ethosuximide, seem to be effective. There have been few published studies of the efficacy of new AEDs, but lamotrigine (Lamictal), felbamate (Felbatol), topiramate (Topamax), and zonisamide (Zonegran) seem to be effective against generalized seizures; the others are unknown. *Absence seizures* respond to valproate (Depakote), ethosuximide (Zarontin), and lamotrigine, but not to carbamazepine (Tegretol), gabapentin (Neurontin), or tiagabine (Gabitril). The efficacy of other new AEDs has yet to be demonstrated. *Myoclonic seizures* respond to valproate and lamotrigine, and occasionally to benzodiazepines.[59] Guidelines for the use of conventional and new AEDs to treat particular seizure types are summarized in Table 24-3.

A few **epilepsy syndromes** in adults and adolescents respond particularly well to specific AEDs. Myoclonic and GTC seizures occurring in juvenile myoclonic epilepsy respond well to valproate or lamotrigine. Atonic, tonic, and atypical absence seizures occurring as part of the Lennox-Gastaut syndrome respond very well to valproate, lamotrigine, and topiramate. Approximately 30% of patients with childhood absence epilepsy have seizures that persist into adulthood, and valproate or lamotrigine is usually a better alternative than ethosuximide when they have GTC seizures in addition to absence seizures.[59]

Once thought has been given to the type of epilepsy syndrome and seizure type, the pharmacokinetics of the medication must be considered (Table 24-4). The biologic **half-life** of the drug determines how often the drug should be given. The half-life is the time required for the serum level to fall by 50%. Drugs with short half-lives require more frequent dosing, and drugs with longer half-lives do not need to be given as often. In general, a dosing interval should not exceed a half-life. The **steady state** is the amount of time required for a medication to reach a relatively constant level in the blood. A steady state is usually reached when a drug has been taken for about five half-lives. A half-life is the amount of time required for half of the drug to be metabolized. If a drug has a half-life of 24 hours, a period of 5 days is required to reach a steady level after any increase. The half-life of a drug may vary among individuals, particularly when multiple AEDs are being used and drug-drug interactions affect half-life. Determining the half-life on an individual basis may improve seizure control and the maintenance of therapeutic levels throughout the day in some patients with refractory epilepsy (see Table 24-4).

Frequently, AEDs must be used at the higher end of tolerability to achieve seizure control. **Toxicity** may be encountered shortly after taking a dose of medication as it enters the bloodstream. This phenomenon is referred to as peak-dose toxicity. One solution is to prescribe smaller doses of the drug more frequently (e.g., the patient may experience side effects when taking the drug twice daily but not when taking smaller doses three times a day). In such cases the total daily dose is constant but individual doses are smaller, so that the peak dose falls below the level that causes acute side effects. Table 24-5 lists the common side effects associated with the AEDs, for both peak-dose and chronic side effects.

TABLE 24-4   Pharmacokinetics of Conventional and New Antiepileptic Drugs

Drug	Metabolized by Inducible Enzymes (Mechanism)	Induces Hepatic Enzymes	Half-Life (hour)	Protein Bound (%)
Carbamazepine (Tegretol)	Yes (oxidized)	Yes	12–17	76
Ethosuximide (Zarontin)	Yes (oxidized)	No	30–60 (30 in child)	0
Felbamate (Felbatol)	Yes (multiple mechanisms)	No	20–23	25
Gabapentin (Neurontin)	No	No	5–7	<3
Lamotrigine (Lamictal)	Yes (glucuronidated)	No	25 alone 60 with valproate 12 with EI	55
Levetiracetam (Keppra)	No	No	6–8	<10
Oxcarbazepine (Trileptal)	Yes (converted to MHD → glucuronidated)	Mixed	9–11 (for MHD)	67
Phenobarbital	Yes (hydroxylated, glucuronidated)	Yes	80–100	45
Phenytoin (Dilantin)	Yes (hydroxylated, glucuronidated)	Yes	22	90
Pregabalin (Lyrica)	No	No	6	0
Primidone (Mysoline)	Yes (similar to phenobarbital)	Yes	8–15 (shorter with EI)	20
Tiagabine (Gabitril)	Yes (glucuronidation, oxidation)	No	7–9 (alone) 4–7 (with EI)	96
Topiramate (Topamax)	Yes (hydroxylated, hydrolyzed, glucuronidated)	No	20–24	13–17
Valproic acid (Depakene)	Yes (glucuronidated, oxidized)	No	9–16 (shorter with EI)	70–90 (varies with level)
Zonisamide (Zonegran)	Yes (acetylated, reduced)	No	63	40

Modified from Rakel RE, Bope ET, editors: *Conn's current therapy 2005*, ed 57, Philadelphia, 2005, WB Saunders.
EI, Enzyme inducer; *MHD*, monohydroxy derivative.

Therapeutic blood levels are established for all AEDs. The lower limit represents the level below which the majority of patients continue to have seizures. The higher limit is the level above which the majority of patients experience side effects. These ranges are only guides and should not dictate the patient's treatment; some patients require high levels of medication to attain seizure control, whereas others have toxic reactions at subtherapeutic levels. Blood levels are best measured as trough levels. Trough levels are usually drawn in the morning before taking medication. This is done to ensure adequate levels throughout the rest of the day. Falsely high levels (peaks) may be seen if the sample is drawn soon after a drug is taken. Patients should be instructed not to switch from trade name AEDs to the generic formulations without consulting their physician, because **bioavailability** can alter between brand name and generic drugs. Patients who are taking generic AEDs should not switch from one generic drug to a different manufacturer, because bioavailability often changes between manufacturers. Bioavailability is the amount of an administered drug that becomes available after absorption into the bloodstream; this can change between different formulations of the same drug, whether generic or brand name, causing either breakthrough seizures or toxicity. Bioavailability is also affected by protein binding in the bloodstream, because drugs that are highly protein bound will be less available.

BOX 24-7   Blood Antiepileptic Drug Monitoring
- After starting drug at steady state
- When adding or subtracting an interacting drug
- When side effects are occurring
- When seizures are uncontrolled or break through
- When needed to assess compliance

The primary AED chosen for treatment should be initiated at a low to moderate dose to avoid side effects and then increased as tolerated (Table 24-6 shows guidelines). Several drugs induce their own metabolism by inducing production of hepatic microsomal enzymes (CYP 450 enzymes), a process known as **autoinduction.** Carbamazepine is the classic example of autoinduction: Initially, a patient will have therapeutic drug levels of medication, but approximately 1 month after beginning therapy the drug level falls due to autoinduction. Most clinicians anticipate this phenomenon and adjust the level as needed to avoid breakthrough seizures. Box 24-7 lists guidelines on when blood levels may be helpful.

If a therapeutic level of an AED is needed immediately, a loading dose may be given. Loading doses are given according to the milligrams-per-kilogram formula and are usually given over a 24-hour period. Phenytoin and phenobarbital

TABLE 24-5   Side Effects of Antiepileptic Drugs

Drug	Dose Dependent	Often Idiosyncratic
Phenobarbital	Lethargy, dizziness, ataxia Cognitive disturbance Hyperactivity, emotional disturbance Sleep disturbance, headache	Rash Megaloblastic anemia Liver toxicity
Phenytoin (Dilantin)	Lethargy, dizziness, ataxia, nystagmus Coarse facies, hirsutism, gingival hyperplasia Osteomalacia	Rash Blood dyscrasias, variable Liver toxicity Lymphadenopathy
Primidone (Mysoline)	Lethargy, dizziness, ataxia Behavioral changes	Rash Megaloblastic anemia, leukopenia
Ethosuximide (Zarontin)	Lethargy, dizziness, ataxia, headache Behavioral changes Nausea, vomiting, stomach pain, hiccups	Rash Blood dyscrasias, variable (rare) Systemic lupus–like syndrome
Carbamazepine (Carbatrol, Tegretol)	Lethargy, dizziness, ataxia, nystagmus, diplopia Nausea, vomiting, abdominal pain Liver toxicity Hyponatremia	Rash Blood dyscrasias, aplastic anemia
Valproate (Depakene, Depakote)	Lethargy, dizziness, ataxia, headache Thrombocytopenia Nausea, vomiting, weight gain Alopecia, tremor	Rash Liver toxicity Pancreatitis
Felbamate (Felbatol)	Ataxia, headache, insomnia Anorexia, abdominal pain	Liver toxicity Aplastic anemia
Gabapentin (Neurontin)	Lethargy, dizziness, ataxia Nausea, vomiting, weight gain	Rash
Lamotrigine (Lamictal)	Lethargy, dizziness, ataxia, diplopia Headache	Rash
Topiramate (Topamax)	Lethargy, dizziness, ataxia, nystagmus Cognitive slowing, language impairment Weight loss Kidney stones	Acute-angle glaucoma
Levetiracetam (Keppra)	Behavioral changes, psychosis Lethargy, dizziness, ataxia	Rash
Oxcarbazepine (Trileptal)	Lethargy, dizziness, ataxia, headache Nausea Hyponatremia	Rash (30% cross-react with carbamazepine)
Zonisamide (Zonegran)	Lethargy, dizziness, ataxia Psychomotor slowing, difficulty concentrating Nausea, anorexia Kidney stones	Rash Oligohidrosis/hyperthermia
Pregabaline (Lyrica)	Dizziness, somnolence, ataxia, asthenia, blurred vision	

Modified from Rakel RE, Bope ET, editors: *Conn's current therapy 2005,* ed 57, Philadelphia, 2005, WB Saunders.

can be given in loading doses in urgent situations. Because of side effects and the lack of IV formulations, other medications are usually not given this way.

Medication is increased until one of two endpoints is met: seizures are controlled or the patient develops intolerable side effects (toxicity) from the drug. If toxicity occurs and seizures persist, an alternative medication is introduced and increased to therapeutic levels while the first drug is slowly tapered. For some patients whose seizures are not controlled with monotherapy, polypharmacy with two or more drugs may be necessary. The initial steps in choosing an AED are discussed in Box 24-8.

Monotherapy Versus Polytherapy

Monotherapy, the use of a single AED, is the ideal mode of therapy for epilepsy.[60] The current recommended practice is to attempt monotherapy with at least two first-line AEDs targeted to the seizure type or epilepsy syndrome before considering combination therapy (Box 24-9 shows guidelines). Once patients are refractory to two first-line AEDs in high therapeutic doses, the chance of achieving seizure control is significantly reduced. Polytherapy is appropriate for such medically refractory patients, although even with combination therapy (two or even three drugs), control of seizures may be no higher than 20% to 30%.[17,18]

TABLE 24-6 Titration Guidelines for Conventional and New Antiepileptic Drugs

Generic Name	Common Brand Name	Dosing Schedule	Adult			Child	
			Initial Dose	Increment (mg)	Maintenance (mg/d)	Initial Dose (mg/kg/d)	Maintenance (mg/kg/d)
Carbamazepine	Tegretol Tegretol XR, Carbatrol	tid-qid bid	200 bid	200 qwk	600–1800	10	10–35 (for age <6 yr)
Ethosuximide	Zarontin	qd-bid	250 qd	250 q3-7d	750	15	15–40
Felbamate	Felbatol	tid	600–1200 qd	600–1200 q1–2wk	2400–3600	15	15–45
Gabapentin	Neurontin	tid	300 qd	300 q3–7d	1200–3600	10	25–50
Lamotrigine	Lamictal	bid	25 qd	25 q2wk	100 with VPA 400 alone 600 with EI	0.15–0.5	0.5–5 with VPA 5 alone 5–15 with EI
Levetiracetam	Keppra	bid	500 bid	500 qwk	2000–4000	20	40–100
Oxcarbazepine	Trileptal (Generic)	bid	300 qd	300 qwk	900–2400	8–10	30–46
Phenobarbital		qd-bid	30–60 qd	30 q1–2wk	60–120	3	3–6
Phenytoin	Dilantin Kapseals liquid, Infatab	qd bid-tid	200 qd	100 q5–7d	200–300	4	4–8
Primidone	Mysoline	tid	125–250 qd	250 q1–2wk	500–750	10	10–25
Tiagabine	Gabitril	bid-qid	4 qd	4–8 qwk	16–32	0.1	0.4 without EI 0.7 with EI
Topiramate	Topamax	bid	25 qd	25 q1–2wk	100–400	3	3–9
Valproic acid	Depakene, Depakote, Depakote ER	tid-qid bid	250 qd	250 q3–7d	750–3000	15	15–45
Zonisamide	Zonegran	bid	100 qd	100 q2wk	200–400	4	4–12
Pregabalin	Lyrica	bid	75 bid		150–600		

Modified from Rakel RE, Bope ET, editors: *Conn's current therapy 2005*, ed 57, Philadelphia, 2005, WB Saunders.
bid, Twice a day; *EI*, enzyme inducer; *qd*, every day; *qid*, four times a day; *qwk*, every week; *tid*, three times a day; *VPA*, valproic acid.

BOX 24-8 General Guidelines for Beginning Antiepileptic Drug Therapy

- Select an antiepileptic drug (AED) by seizure type and epilepsy syndrome
- Increase dose to maximum tolerated dose (toxicity) before changing
- Substitute one drug at a time in attempt to achieve monotherapy
- All new drugs are equally efficacious for partial seizures
- Select by side effects, dosing, pharmacokinetics, cost
- Refer to an epilepsy center for evaluation of surgery if seizures are refractory to two AEDs

From Perucca E, Levy RH: Combination therapy and drug interactions. In Levy RH, Mattson RH, Meldrum BS, Perucca E, editors: *Antiepileptic drugs*, ed 5, Philadelphia, 2002, Lippincott Williams & Wilkins.

BOX 24-9 Advantages of Monotherapy

- Effective seizure control in most patients
- Minimization of side effects
- Easier clinical management
- Minimization of adverse drug interactions
- Simpler treatment schedule (better compliance)
- Lower treatment cost

Polytherapy is more complicated than monotherapy for many reasons. Side effects are less common when dealing with a single medication than when combining medications. When two medications are given in combination, many different drug-drug interactions can lead to various problems. Examples include alterations in protein binding, competing effects on hepatic microsomal enzymes (autoinduction versus inhibition), and enhanced toxicity. Polytherapy may lower the toxic threshold of one of two medications given together; this interaction can be seen when lamotrigine is added to carbamazepine therapy (the patient becomes toxic on a carbamazepine dose he or she could previously tolerate). Patients need to be advised to watch for such symptoms so that medications can be adjusted as necessary.

Most AEDs are inactivated and eliminated from the body as a result of **biotransformation** (the chemical changes a substance undergoes in hepatic microsomal enzymes) in which AEDs are oxidized into metabolites that are then excreted by the kidneys. Hepatic enzyme induction or inhibition may result in side effects or breakthrough seizures if drug-drug interactions are not anticipated; common examples are the inhibition of lamotrigine metabolism by valproic acid and the induction of lamotrigine metabolism with phenytoin or carbamazepine.[18] Table 24-7 summarizes the most common drug interactions among the AEDs. Frequent monitoring of blood levels may be more necessary with

TABLE 24-7   Antiepileptic Drug Interactions Influencing Serum Concentrations*

Drug Added	Serum Level Influenced												
	CBZ	ESM	FBM	GBP	LMT	LEV	OXC	PB	PHT	TGB	TPM	VPA	ZNS
CBZ	↓	↓	↓	—	↓↓	—	↓	—	↑↓	↓↓	↓↓	↓	↓
ESM	?—	—	?—	?—	—	?—	?—	?—	?↑	?—	?—	?—	?—
FBM	↓ epox ↑	?—	—	?—	—	?—	?—	↑	↑↑	?—	?—	↑↑	?—
GBP	—	?—	?—	—	?—	—	?—	—	—	?—	?—	—	?—
LMT	—	—	—	?—	—	—	?—	—	—	?—	?—	↓	?—
LEV	—	?—	?—	—	—	—	?—	—	—	?—	?—	—	?—
OXC	—	?	?—	?—	↓	?—	—	—	—	?	?—	—	?—
PB	↓	↓	↓	—	↓↓	—	↓	—	—	↓↓	↓	↓	↓
PHT	↓	↓	↓	—	↓↓	—	↓	—	—	↓↓	↓↓	↓	↓
TGB	—	?—	?—	?—	?—	?—	?—	?—	—	—	?—	↓	?—
TPM	—	?—	?—	?—	?—	?—	?—	—	↑	?—	—	↓	?—
VPA	↓ epox. ↑	↑↓	—	—	↑↑	?↑	—	↑↑	—	—	↓	—	—
ZNS	—	—	?—	?—	?—	?—	?—	—	—	?—	?—	—	—
PRE	—				—	—	—	—	—	—	—	—	—

Modified from Rakel RE, Bope ET, editors: *Conn's current therapy 2005,* ed 57, Philadelphia, 2005, WB Saunders.
*Effect of adding the drug listed in the first column on the blood concentration of the drugs listed in the other columns. Clinically significant effects are double arrows; other effects (single arrows) are not usually clinically relevant. Question marks indicate unknown interactions.
CBZ, Carbamazepine; *ESM,* ethosuximide; *FBM,* felbamate; *GBP,* gabapentin; *LEV,* levetiracetam; *LMT,* lamotrigine; *OXC,* oxcarbazepine; *PB,* phenobarbital; *PHT,* phenytoin; *PRE,* pregabaline; *TGB,* tiagabine; *TPM,* topiramate; *VPA,* valproic acid; *ZNS,* zonisamide.

polypharmacy, depending on the combinations of medications employed.

Drug interactions are common with polypharmacy. These can occur between AEDs or with other systemic medications. The induction of phenytoin metabolism by cimetidine is a classic interaction. Clinicians need to be aware of common drug interactions and anticipate management concerns. Almost all AEDs lead to some cognitive or physical side effects, which are compounded with the use of more than one drug, frequently leading to a decreased quality of life for refractory patients. Often, the clinician and patient must weigh the side effects against the benefits of marginally enhanced seizure control, and some patients say they prefer having seizures to "feeling drugged." The balance of medication treatment to side effects varies between the different syndromes, and must be assessed individually.[18]

Noncompliance With Medications

Medication is effective only when it is taken properly. Compliance studies indicate that 15% to 50% of patients are noncompliant. Multiple factors affect compliance (Box 24-10).[61,62] One major factor in compliance is dosing interval: Compliance improves when the dosing schedule is less frequent (once or twice daily). Compliance falls off markedly with dosing three or four times a day.[63] The time of day for taking medication is also effective (e.g., midday doses are more frequently missed because of work or school schedules than doses taken in the morning or evening). Because epilepsy is visible only during seizure activity, patients with epilepsy sometimes think medication can be taken sporadi-

BOX 24-10   Reasons for Noncompliance

- Frequency of dosing of medications (twice vs. four times daily)
- Financial difficulties
- Misunderstanding of instructions
- Lack of information
- Inconvenience of time of medication dosing
- Undesirable side effects
- Prescription expires/delay in getting a refill
- Doing well/denial that they are dependent on medications
- Forgetfulness or memory problems
- Poor family support
- Dependency
- Feelings of powerlessness over epilepsy versus control
- Embarrassment to be seen taking medications in public (e.g., at school or the workplace)
- Lack of knowledge: Not knowing what to do if a dose is missed
- Poor patient-doctor relationship
- Patient's health belief system

cally, either withholding medication until seizures occur or taking "extra" doses with seizure activity. The clinician must focus on the reasons for the noncompliance (see Box 24-10) to understand why a patient may not be adhering to the prescribed therapy.

Patient education can greatly improve compliance. The health care team and the patient work together to find the reason for noncompliance and to develop a solution; it is important not to be accusatory, because this may limit the patient's willingness to be truthful. Setting realistic goals with the patient prevents frustration. Medication doses can be scheduled at a time that is convenient for the patient and is easy to remember, or avoids social concerns such as taking drugs at school or work. Engaging the patient in active participation, for example, by keeping a seizure diary, and identifying barriers to compliance, may help alleviate problems.

Each patient has specific needs that should be addressed individually. Detailed instructions are tailored to the individual's learning ability on how to take medications, what to do if a dose is forgotten, how to refill medication, how often laboratory tests need to be done, how to contact the physician or clinician, and the dangers of abruptly stopping medications. Appropriate *written* instructions must be given to the patient, no matter how minor the change, because many patients have cognitive deficits that make verbal instruction inadequate.

Explanations should be simple to understand and are given in nonscientific language. Emphasizing that epilepsy can be controlled in most cases may help the patient understand the importance of taking medication at the specified time and dose. A brief understanding of steady-state levels and the half-life of the medication may help the patient better understand how medications work, why they must be given at certain times throughout the day, and why they must be taken regularly (Fig. 24-3).

Medication side effects should always be addressed, as well as specific instructions as to how they should be handled. Depending on the side effects, specific suggestions may alleviate the problem. For example, complaints of stomach upset may be remedied by taking medication after meals or with milk. A large portion of the nurse clinician's role is to improve compliance through education.[64-66]

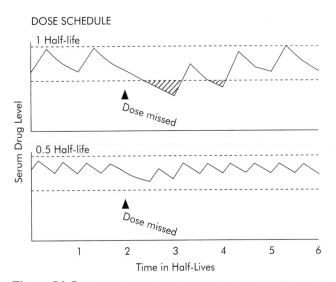

Figure 24-3 Comparison of steady-state levels and half-lives of medications.
(From Engel J: Seizures and epilepsy, *Philadelphia, 1989, FA Davis.)*

Administration of Antiepilepsy Drugs via a Gastrostomy Tube

Administration of AEDs via a gastrostomy tube can pose problems in delivering the correct dose and achieving the desired serum drug level. In a study comparing two groups of head-injured patients receiving phenytoin, the tube feeding was clamped for 1 hour after each phenytoin dose in the first group and in the second group the tube feeding was not interrupted after administering the drug. The investigators found that clamping the gastrostomy tube for only 1 hour after each phenytoin dose improved drug absorption.[67] The formulation of a drug affects its ability to be given via gastrostomy; several of the newer AEDs are packaged as tiny beads within gelatin capsules that can be opened and then made into a slurry for gastrostomy use. Other formulations cannot be opened without altering the pharmacodynamics of the preparation. Special consideration of the patient with a gastrostomy tube must occur so that the medication regimen is optimized.

Discontinuance of Antiepileptic Drug Therapy

Individuals who have been prescribed AED therapy frequently question the need to continue therapy after they have been seizure free for some period of time (e.g., 2 years without seizures while on medications) and are not considered to be at high risk for seizure activity. AEDs are therapeutic but are associated with risks, such as toxicity, teratogenicity, the need for periodic therapeutic monitoring, adverse effects, and other considerations, including high cost. The option to discontinue AEDs requires careful evaluation with expert clinicians of the reasons patients may wish to discontinue medications. Consideration of the type of epilepsy syndrome can be helpful when considering medication discontinuation. Some syndromes, such as juvenile myoclonic epilepsy, respond well to medication but frequently recur when AEDs are stopped; these patients should be counseled to remain on medication. Better candidates for discontinuation include those with partial epilepsy who have been seizure free for 2 years and have a normal EEG. Even among the best candidates, approximately 30% may have a recurrent seizure within 5 years. Discussion between the patient, family, and caregiver must occur to identify motivations for discontinuing medications and to determine whether there are acceptable alternatives to stopping medications (such as reducing medications to decrease side effects or simplifying a drug regimen). Patients must be advised of the risk of seizure recurrence and resulting consequences if medications are to be discontinued. Usually, medications are tapered slowly with a 25% dose reduction every 2 to 4 weeks during which the patient is closely monitored, especially in the early months of tapering. If seizures recur, therapy is reinitiated.

Surgical Treatment

Surgery for epilepsy has been performed since the 1800s. The past 20 years have seen a growth in the number of surgeries performed, yet many patients who could benefit from surgery are not being helped. This is partially because many people consider surgery for epilepsy an option of last resort, whereas others are not aware that surgical intervention is possible. The National Institutes of Health (NIH) has proposed that 2000 to 5000 patients could benefit from epilepsy surgery annually. Currently, far fewer surgeries are being done.[68] The goal of surgery is to remove epileptogenic brain tissue to improve seizure control while avoiding cognitive or neurologic deficits.

Surgery for epilepsy can be divided into **curative** and **palliative procedures** (Fig 24-4). Curative surgery can be performed when a focal epileptogenic region is identified that can be removed safely. Examples of these procedures include lesionectomy, focal cortical resection, lobectomy (frontal, temporal, occipital), or larger resections such as hemispherectomy. Palliative surgery does not remove the epileptogenic region but attempts to make the seizures more tolerable by restricting seizure spread and eliminating seizures that cause physical harm. Corpus callosotomy, multiple subpial transaction, and vagus nerve stimulation are examples of palliative surgery. (See Chapter 1 for anatomy and physiology of the corpus callosum.)

The criteria determining which patients may be eligible for surgery vary among institutions, but several common tenets apply to all centers. Patients should have medically refractory epilepsy or severe side effects from medications. Patients should suffer some level of disability from their seizures so there is appreciable benefit to performing surgery. Some patients are unable to work or go to school because of the frequency and severity of the seizures. Others are unable to work in their own profession because of the inability to maintain a driver's license. Evaluation of the risks versus benefits of surgical intervention should show that the potential benefits of surgery outweigh the risks. Appropriate understanding of these risks and benefits of surgery must be understood by the patient or guardian, and be acceptable. Goals of surgery must be clearly defined (seizure freedom versus seizure reduction). Examples of appropriate candidates are (1) a patient whose seizures can be controlled to one or two seizures per year on three high-dose AEDs with toxic side effects that impair school or work performance, who cannot drive, and who has a vascular malformation that is easily resectable; (2) a patient with hippocampal atrophy with appropriate cognitive memory loss who has weekly seizures who has tried several AEDs in monotherapy or combination therapy; or (3) a patient with Lennox-Gastaut syndrome whose family consents to palliative surgery.

Most patients believe that their lives would change dramatically if they no longer had seizures, and the literature regarding quality of life (QOL) suggests that this is the case.[69,70] Patients who are seizure free after epilepsy surgery will have the greatest improvement in QOL. Patients with persistent seizures, even if these events are rare, will have a significantly reduced QOL compared with patients who are seizure free. Patients must be advised that the goal of surgery is to stop or reduce seizures, and not to discontinue all AEDs, although medications can often be reduced or simplified after surgery. The ultimate goal of epilepsy surgery is seizure freedom, and research is being directed toward this difficult goal.

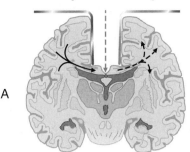

Corpus callosotomy

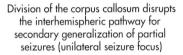

Division of the corpus callosum disrupts the interhemispheric pathway for secondary generalization of partial seizures (unilateral seizure focus)

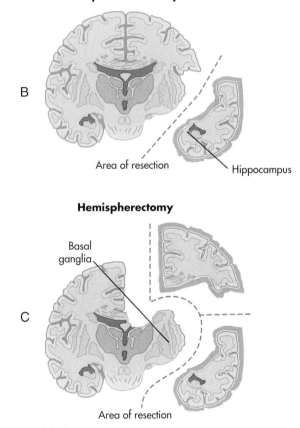

Temporal lobectomy

Area of resection   Hippocampus

Hemispherectomy

Basal ganglia

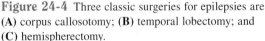

Area of resection

Figure 24-4 Three classic surgeries for epilepsies are (**A**) corpus callosotomy; (**B**) temporal lobectomy; and (**C**) hemispherectomy.
(From Devinsky O: Seizure disorders, Clin Symp 46(1):1–54, 1994. Adapted from an original illustration in Clinical Symposia, illustrated by John Craig, MD, copyright by Ciba-Geigy Corporation.)

There are several contraindications to surgery. Patients who are psychotic are not good candidates for surgery because the risks in these patients usually outweigh the benefits. It is helpful if a patient can cooperate with the evaluation process, although pediatric patients and developmentally delayed patients frequently cannot, and the epilepsy team must identify ways to obtain the information necessary within the limitations set by the patient. A low IQ does not preclude a patient from focal resective surgery; however, a very low IQ does require consideration of widespread disease involving multiple areas of the brain. Ultimately, the presurgical evaluation is tailored to the needs of each patient and his or her family. This is often a fluid process that requires skill and patience from the epilepsy team.

Presurgical Evaluation

Patients with epilepsy who may be candidates for surgery require an extensive evaluation by the epilepsy team known as the presurgical evaluation. Patients are admitted for VEEG because of the need to taper medications and capture multiple seizures. Ictal recordings (i.e., seizure recordings) are considered far more reliable than interictal recordings. Therefore most epilepsy surgery programs rely on ictal recordings to perform surgery and rarely act on the basis of interictal recordings only. Presurgical evaluation frequently includes the following:

- Clinical history and baseline neurologic examination.
- VEEG monitoring is performed to determine seizure type and syndrome, and to provide localizing information for the partial epilepsies.
- Neuropsychologic tests: An extensive neuropsychologic battery of tests is employed to ascertain strengths and weaknesses in verbal and visual-spatial cognitive functions, and in verbal and visual memory, which can help localize regions of dysfunction.[71] Neuropsychologic testing is extremely important to the presurgical evaluation, both for diagnostic purposes and to point out potential injury that could occur if surgery is performed.[72]
- MRI is the procedure of choice for epilepsy evaluation. Special epilepsy protocols have been developed that are designed to screen for lesions that occur in epilepsy. These include T_1- and T_2-weighted sequences, fluid attenuated inversion recovery (FLAIR) sequence, and coronal images. T_1-weighted images are best for looking at anatomy and help identify cortical dysplasias or lesions that might cause epilepsy (Fig. 24-5). T_2-weighted and FLAIR images are more useful for demonstrating signal change in the brain, commonly associated with tumors and hippocampal sclerosis. Special coronal images through the temporal lobes are performed to look for abnormalities in the hippocampus, a common site for epileptogenesis (Fig. 24-6). Hippocampal sclerosis is common in temporal lobe epilepsy and is a positive predictor of surgical outcome.[73-75] It is unclear whether this is the result of previous injury, such as febrile convulsions, and thus the cause of seizures, or whether the sclerosis results from the seizure activity.[76-78] The presurgical evaluation is heavily influenced by the MRI, because the surgical plan for lesional epilepsy is often much different than when the MRI is normal. Functional neuroimaging using MRI-BOLD (brain oxygen level determination) technology allows mapping of motor and sensory function, which can be helpful when

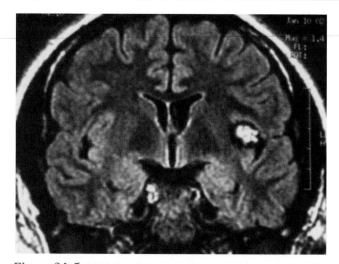

Figure 24-5 MRI showing a vascular malformation in the left insula. This patient's seizures manifest as simple partial seizures of the mouth with secondarily generalized tonic-clonic seizures. The ILAE *seizure* classification is simple partial seizures evolving to generalized seizures. The ILAE syndromic classification is localization-related, symptomatic frontal lobe epilepsy. This patient was seizure free after removal of the vascular malformation.

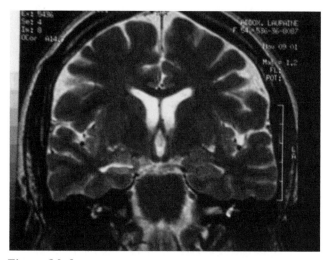

Figure 24-6 Coronal MRI showing right hippocampal atrophy. This patient had complex partial seizures with lip smacking automatisms, without generalization. The formal ILAE classification of this patient's *seizures* would be complex partial seizures with impairment of consciousness at onset without secondarily generalized seizures. The ILAE *syndrome* would be localization-related, symptomatic temporal lobe epilepsy. Commonly, epileptologists refer to this syndrome with the more common term *mesial temporal lobe epilepsy with hippocampal atrophy* (MTLE + HA). Temporal lobectomy for MTLE + HA is the most commonly performed surgical procedure, and has a high success rate.

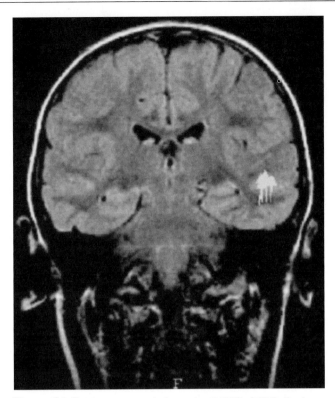

Figure 24-7 Magnetoencephalography (MEG). MEG dipoles are superimposed on an MRI in a patient with acquired epileptic aphasia (Landau-Kleffner syndrome). Such localization can be helpful in localizing the site for surgery, in this case, multiple subpial transection (MST).

planning resection of a tumor adjacent to motor cortex.

- SPECT measures CBF by using gamma-ray tracers labeled with single photon–emitting isotopes to produce images. SPECT detects interictal regions of hypoperfusion in about 50% of patients with complex partial seizures. SPECT scans may demonstrate hyperperfusion in the epileptogenic region during a seizure in several studies. As mentioned previously, subtraction ictal SPECT is more accurate than either interictal or ictal SPECT used alone.

- PET: Several studies have shown that up to 70% of patients with complex partial seizures will have interictal hypometabolism.[79–82] Although difficult to obtain, ictal PET scans may show hypermetabolism in the epileptic focus.

- MEG: In some cases MEG may be helpful. It is particularly useful in a syndrome of acquired aphasia due to epilepsy, called Landau-Kleffner syndrome (Fig. 24-7). MEG is not available in all centers and patients must sometimes travel significant distances for the study. Research suggests that it is a useful adjunctive test in the presurgical evaluation, and its use is increasing.

Intracarotid Amytal Test. The intracarotid Amytal test was developed by Dr. Juhn Wada and is frequently referred to as the Wada test.[83] Since the Wada test is an invasive test, it is usually done after the initial presurgical evaluation dis-

cussed previously is completed and it has been determined that the patient is likely to undergo surgery. The Wada test is performed to determine hemispheric lateralization for language and also tests verbal and nonverbal memory function. It is done in conjunction with a bilateral carotid arteriogram to detect any vascular or flow abnormalities. After the arteriogram is complete, amobarbital (Amytal) is injected into one carotid artery; amobarbital is a short-acting barbiturate that inactivates the hemisphere injected. Language and memory testing is performed sequentially as first one hemisphere is injected, followed after an interval of recovery by the other hemisphere. The results of testing on each hemisphere are compared to the other. Language lateralization is determined by the patterns of aphasia induced by hemispheric injection. If a patient is a candidate for temporal lobectomy, the Wada test simulates the effects of a temporal lobectomy when the side being considered for surgery is inactivated. Memory testing is performed to ensure that the remaining hemisphere has adequate function to support verbal memory, thus the test acts as a safety measure in terms of memory. As technology advances, the value of the Wada test is being questioned, particularly when compared to functional MRI.[84,85] Some epilepsy centers do not perform Wada tests on all patients if other localizing signs and symptoms, such as ictal speech, functional MRI, or neuropsychologic testing, suggest that the nondominant temporal lobe is to be resected.

Barbiturate Activation Study. The barbiturate activation study is an older procedure that is still performed in a few epilepsy centers. Pentothal, a short-acting barbiturate, is used because normal brain cells develop fast beta activity when thiopental is injected. In areas of the brain where there is scarring, gliosis, or tumor, beta activity may not develop.[10] Other activation studies include the methohexital (Brevital) test, which looks for an increase in interictal epileptiform activity. Other agents, such as ketamine, have been used intraoperatively to attempt to localize a seizure focus. The anesthesia department is involved in administering all of these agents because of the potential for respiratory arrest, and most procedures are performed under anesthesia or conscious sedation protocols. All of the activation studies are limited by a number of concerns. First, the data are interictal data, which are usually less specific than ictal data. Second, activations studies may activate a region larger than the epileptic focus, or can lead to false localization. These tests are less frequently used as advanced neurodiagnostic imaging and intracranial electrode studies become more common.

Once some combination of the aforementioned procedures is performed, according to the needs of the individual patient, an assessment of the information obtained is performed by the epilepsy team. If all of the information points to the same region of involvement, the evaluation is considered **concordant.** If the information does not agree, the presurgical evaluation is **discordant.** Patients with concordant data are usually better candidates for epilepsy surgery than patients with discordant data. When data are discordant, further evaluation is often necessary. This frequently involves the use of intracranial electrodes to attempt to resolve conflicting information.

Surgical Options

Surgical procedures can be divided into those that are diagnostic and those that are therapeutic. Placement of intracranial electrodes for intracranial-VEEG monitoring is a diagnostic procedure. Cortical resection, lobectomy, and corpus callosotomy are examples of therapeutic procedures (see Fig. 24-5). Often, the data obtained from the presurgical evaluation are sufficient to proceed to a therapeutic procedure. If the presurgical evaluation is inadequate, an invasive, diagnostic intracranial monitoring session may be necessary to further define the epileptic zone before any surgical resection.

Intracranial Electrode Evaluation. Subdural strip electrodes are thin strips of plastic imbedded with a single string of electrode contacts (Fig. 24-8). Subdural electrodes are larger arrays consisting of multiple rows of electrode contacts designed to cover large areas of the brain. Subdural strips and grids are designed to lie on top of the brain, in direct contact with it. Intracranial depth electrodes are thin tubes of electrodes about the size of a pencil lead that can be safely implanted using stereotactic guidance directly into the brain, particularly into the deep mesial structures of the temporal lobe (hippocampus and amygdala). Less frequently, epidural peg electrodes will be placed through the skull to rest outside the dura mater. Usually, combinations of strips, grids, and depth electrodes are placed so that 64 and 128 contacts are in place on or in the brain. The number and location of intracranial electrodes depends on the surgical plan developed by the epilepsy team after analysis of the presurgical evaluation. Reasons to implant intracranial electrodes are discussed in Box 24-11.

Subdural strips and intracranial depth electrodes are usually placed via burr holes and can be removed percutaneously without a craniotomy. They are often used when large areas of the brain need to be surveyed (i.e., to determine if seizures are frontal or temporal) or when both sides of the brain need to be studied (i.e., to determine which temporal lobe is producing seizures). Subdural grid electrodes are

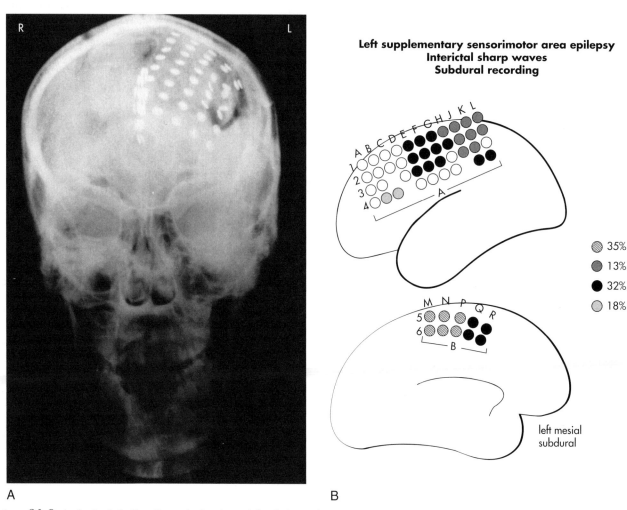

A

B

Figure 24-8 A, Sagittal skull radiograph showing subdural electrodes over the left frontal and parietal convexity and left interhemispheric fissure. **B,** Diagram of the interictal epileptiform discharges recorded from subdural electrodes placed over the mesial and lateral frontoparietal cortex. Most spikes (35%) occurred at electrodes M5 to M6, N5 to N6, and P5 to P6. *(From Lüders HO, Noachtar S:* Atlas of epileptic seizures and syndromes, *Philadelphia, 2001, WB Saunders.)*

BOX 24-11	Indications for Intracranial Electrode Placement

- Seizures are lateralized but not localized (e.g., left frontal lobe vs. left temporal lobe onset).
- Seizures are localized but not lateralized (e.g., both temporal lobes appear to be involved).
- Seizures are neither localized nor lateralized (e.g., complex partial seizures with nondiagnostic scalp VEEG monitoring).
- The presurgical evaluation is discordant.
- The proximity of seizure onset to the motor or language cortex must be determined.
- The relationship of seizure onset to a lesion (or lesions) must be determined (e.g., multiple intracranial lesions).

VEEG, Video and electroencephalogram.

used when the lobe of ictal onset has been identified, but the region within that lobe is in question (i.e., to determine if temporal lobe seizures are medial or lateral). Subdural grids can be used to perform cortical mapping, where either language or motor mapping is performed by stimulating various electrodes on the grid. In such a way, the relationship between seizure onset and critical motor and language cortex can be determined and the risks and benefits of different surgical plans can be discussed with the family before resective surgery. For example, if seizures are found to arise in hand or face motor cortex, the patient and family may decide that seizures are severe enough to sacrifice motor function (as long as language is preserved). On the other hand, if the patient is unwilling to accept a motor deficit in this theoretic example, a lesser resection sparing motor cortex can be performed as a palliative procedure. Figure 24-8 shows a skull x-ray film with subdural electrodes placed over the left frontal and parietal convexity and in the left interhemispheric fissure. A craniotomy must be performed to implant the subdural grid. After a craniotomy, the patient may be monitored in a critical care unit for a brief period of time, after which transfer to the epilepsy monitor unit for VEEG occurs. The patient is monitored until adequate information is obtained, after which the patient is returned to the operating room for grid removal and resective surgery, if indicated.

Presurgical education by the nurse and social worker on the epilepsy team are important to the success of intracranial monitoring. Patients and families are educated as to what to expect when admitted to the monitoring unit. Family members are informed that their presence during monitoring will be required to identify seizures, that medications will most likely be decreased during monitoring, and what the expectations are for the monitoring session. Discussion of financial circumstances may be necessary to accommodate travel or lodging concerns. While hospitalized, astute neurologic nursing care is essential to the success of the monitoring session. The neurologic nurse is the first line of defense in evaluating the patient for altered mental status or neurologic changes that could indicate intracranial hemorrhage, frequent seizures or status epilepticus, or, less commonly, infection, all of which place the patient at risk. The value of

the experienced neuroscience nurse on the epilepsy team cannot be stressed enough.[86] The reader is referred to several additional texts for further discussion of the risks of intracranial monitoring.

Focal Cortical Resection. Focal cortical resection is performed for partial epilepsy. The goal of focal cortical resection is usually to make the patient seizure free. Lesionectomy, cortical excision, lobectomy, and multilobar excisions are all examples of focal cortical resections. When lesionectomy is performed for vascular malformation, tumor, or focal cortical dysplasia, the chances of being seizure free are 60% to 70%.[87,88] Temporal lobectomy for mesial temporal lobe epilepsy with hippocampal atrophy is effective in two thirds of patients.[89] Lobar resections done in patients with no lesion on MRI (nonlesional epilepsy) are less effective, with seizure-free rates of approximately 50%. Multilobar resections have variable outcomes, depending on the syndrome being treated.

The syndrome of mesial temporal lobe epilepsy with hippocampal atrophy (MTLE + HA) deserves special mention because it is the most common cause of partial epilepsy in adults and is the most commonly performed surgical procedure (see Fig. 24-7). The syndrome of MTLE + HA has certain clinical characteristics that are identifiable during the presurgical evaluation, as follows:

- Frequently medically refractory
- Complex partial seizures with automatism, with or without aura
- History of early risk factor present in 40% to 50%
- Typical seizures begin in childhood or adolescence (before age 18)
- Unilateral hippocampal atrophy seen on MRI
- EEG with unilateral or bilateral frontotemporal epileptiform discharges
- Ictal VEEG localized to the side of hippocampal atrophy
- Neuropsychologic tests show memory deficit lateralized to the side of hippocampal atrophy
- Interictal PET and SPECT scans show temporal lobe hypometabolism/hypoperfusion

The syndrome of MTLE + HA is highly amenable to temporal lobectomy and should be considered for surgical resection once several first-line AEDs have not controlled seizures. Unfortunately, the patient with the syndrome of MTLE + HA will, on average, wait 10 to 15 years with refractory epilepsy before being referred for appropriate presurgical evaluation. Attempts are being made to change referral patterns so that patients with lesions (vascular malformations, hippocampal atrophy), which are frequently amenable to surgery, receive earlier referral.

Hemispherectomy. Hemispherectomy is actually the most extensive form of focal cortical resection. There are different degrees of hemispheric resection. The more moderate procedure is referred to as a parieto-occipito-temporal lobectomy, in which the frontal lobe and motor strip are left intact. This procedure is performed in patients who have residual functional motor activity that is to be preserved. More complete procedures remove or disconnect one entire hemisphere. Hemispherectomy is most commonly performed in children with severe (catastrophic) epilepsy. These children typically have extremely frequent partial seizures that impair not only the side on which seizures begin, but impair cognitive function in the contralateral (good) hemisphere as well. Frequently the damaged hemisphere is not removed, but is disconnected (known as functional hemispherectomy).[90,91] Common indications for hemispherectomy include diffuse unilateral cortical dysplasia, prenatal intrauterine stroke, tuberous sclerosis, Rasmussen's encephalitis, and hemimegalencephaly. Surgery is performed in children with medically intractable seizures who have a hemiplegia who are not candidates for a lesser resection. Usually, functional outcome after hemispherectomy is good, particularly when extensive damage to the motor cortex was present preoperatively. The child loses fine motor function of the contralateral hand, but is able to use the hand as an assist device. The child has a mild hemiplegia, but is able to walk and usually ambulates quite well. Although homonymous hemianopsia is usually present, the child adapts to it by increasing head turning; since depth perception remains intact, the child can usually navigate well in space. Cognition frequently improves after surgery. Seizures are controlled in approximately 60% and significantly improved in up to 90% of these patients.[92]

Callosotomy. Patients with symptomatic generalized epilepsy may be candidates for corpus callosotomy. Callosal section is most frequently performed for Lennox-Gastaut syndrome, characterized by multiple seizure types and developmental delay. Patients often have drop attacks from tonic or atonic seizures that lead to injury. Frequent seizures affect cognition and overall function. Corpus callosotomy, known in the lay press as the "split brain operation," can be effective in stopping drop attacks and also treats generalized seizures to a variable extent. Seizures are improved, but not completely controlled, in 40% to 80% of cases.[93] Function and QOL can improve after surgery, but function is often limited by the severe developmental delay present preoperatively.[94,95] Patients and families are told that this procedure is palliative and that the patient will continue to take medication after surgery. Vagus nerve stimulation is also effective in treating drop attacks (but not generalized seizures in Lennox-Gastaut) and is less invasive; therefore it is an alternative therapy to corpus callosotomy.

Vagus Nerve Stimulation. Vagus nerve stimulation (VNS) is FDA approved for the treatment of medically intractable simple or complex partial seizures with or without secondary generalization. VNS reduces seizures by 50% in approximately 40% of those in whom it is implanted. Reports indicate that those who benefit notice a reduction in the number, intensity, and duration of their seizures. Those who benefit with a reduction in seizures may be able to reduce the amount of their AEDs. Improved QOL scores have been reported in VNS therapy.[96] VNS therapy does not usually lead to seizure control, so patients will continue to have occasional seizures and are unable to operate a motor vehicle.

Criteria for patient selection for VNS include the following:

- Patients who have had a previous trial of at least three of the major AEDs without success.

- Patients who are not suitable candidates for surgery. Since lesional epilepsy can be treated effectively with resective surgery with a high chance of seizure freedom, patients being considered for VNS should have a screening MRI to ensure that they are guided toward a curative procedure (resection of an identified lesion) rather than a palliative one (VNS).

The mechanism for decreasing seizures is not completely understood. Original research testing the vagus nerve during stomach surgery showed that stimulation led to desynchronization of the EEG. When the vagus nerve is stimulated, projections to the brainstem may lead to desynchronization of an epileptiform patter and interrupt a seizure.[96]

The vagus nerve stimulator has two components: (1) an implantable pulse generator that contains a battery and computer chip, about the size of a cardiac pacemaker, and (2) electrode wires that are tunneled under the skin during the surgical procedure and attached to the left vagus nerve (cranial nerve X). With the patient under general anesthesia, the surgeon places the generator in a pocket in the chest wall below the clavicle. Stimulator electrodes are wound around the vagus nerve in the neck and then tunneled subcutaneously to the generator in the chest wall. The patient returns 2 weeks after surgery to activate the system. Programming is performed using a laptop computer and a special wand. The VNS applies a current to the vagus nerve at an amplitude and time period determined by the physician; standard settings are to stimulate the nerve for 30 seconds every 5 minutes. This stimulation occurs continuously, whether a person is having seizures or not. In addition, the patient or caregiver can be taught to deliver an additional stimulation epoch when the individual experiences a warning, or an aura, that a seizure is about to begin. Not all patients have auras, and not all auras respond to VNS therapy, but for those that do, having a mechanism that they can control can be very beneficial. Because the vagus nerve innervates the pharynx, heart, lungs, bronchi, and gastrointestinal tract, VNS can cause adverse side effects (e.g., hoarseness, coughing, tingling, shortness of breath, nausea, dysphagia).[97] The patient may or may not accommodate to these symptoms over time. After 3 months of stimulation, about 40% of patients have reported at least a 50% reduction in the frequency of their seizures.[98] In unblinded studies performed 12 months after implant, seizure control improved slightly.[99,100] VNS is not a cure, and it is uncommon for a patient to be seizure free. If the device does not work, the generator can be removed, but removing the electrodes from around the vagus nerve can be more difficult and they are often left in place.

Multiple Subpial Transection. Multiple subpial transection (MST) is a surgical procedure designed to make small cuts in the cortex to stop the spread of seizures as an alternative to removing brain tissue.[101] It is thought that enough tissue remains between cuts to allow preservation of function, but that the cuts interrupt horizontal spread in the cortex via interneurons.[102] It was introduced in the 1980s as an alternative to removing the speech or language cortex.[103,104] MST has been used most frequently in the treatment of Landau-Kleffner syndrome, a syndrome characterized by regression of speech in the presence of seizures or epileptiform discharges, with good results.[103] MST may also be used in the primary motor cortex when the surgeon is unwilling to create a motor deficit. When used for seizure control, MST is more likely to be palliative, reducing seizures rather than stopping them completely.[105]

Deep Brain Stimulation for Epilepsy. Deep brain stimulation for epilepsy is a field undergoing active research.[106,107] Investigators are using several different devices and different target sites within the brain. Some are focusing on the thalamic or subthalamic nuclei to control partial or generalized epilepsy. Others are stimulating the cortex or hippocampus to try to interrupt partial seizures. Reports on small series of patients have shown some improvement in seizures, suggesting that further research into this area is warranted.

Health Teaching in Epilepsy Surgery

Patients admitted for surgery travel to specialized centers for treatment and may be far from home and their loved ones. During hospitalization, the epilepsy team needs to observe the seizures they have been trying to prevent. The patient is hooked up to EEG monitoring equipment, often including an electrocardiogram (ECG), and attached to cables making it impossible for the patient to take a walk or even leave the room. Privacy is impossible because the patient is on camera 24 hours per day. This can be frustrating and confusing to the patient. Adequate patient preparation can help reduce anxiety and fear.

Extensive preparation is needed for surgical candidates and may include education through pamphlets, articles, books, and videotapes. Patients are often concerned about pain, immobility, cutting of the hair, risk of stroke or neurologic deficit, loss of autonomy, and risk of death. Multiple discussions with the patient will often be necessary to identify fears or misconceptions about surgery, whether diagnostic or treatment related. Monitoring while in the ospital includes the risks of seizures and injury associated with video-EEG monitoring, and in addition, the risks of intracranial surgery. In addition, close monitoring of laboratory values for therapeutic levels of anticonvulsants reduces the potential for breakthrough seizures or postsurgical toxicity. Special seizure flow sheets may be part of the patient record. (See Chapter 10 for information about neurosurgery.)

Nutritional Treatment

The **ketogenic diet (KD)** was developed at the Johns Hopkins Medical Institutions in 1940 as a high-fat, low-carbohydrate, low-protein diet that results in ketosis.[108] It appears to be effective for multiple types of seizures for patients not controlled by AEDs or who have intolerable side effects from AEDs. It is thought to be most effective for myoclonic seizures. The KD induces acidosis in the brain partly by burning fat instead of carbohydrates. The change in pH and lack of glucose affect neuronal firing rates and may decrease seizures, although the mechanisms of action are not clear.[109] The diet is difficult and requires an extremely motivated patient and family to not only understand the diet but also comply with it 100%. Everything has to be weighed unless it is administered via tube feedings using a commercially prepared KD. Every product used by the individual must be screened (e.g., toothpaste, over-the-counter drugs, diet drinks, food coloring). It has been estimated that one third of those who try the diet are not helped. The KD does not seem to cause any serious complications, but there have been reports of poor linear growth in children, hypercholesterolemia, poor weight gain, and kidney stones. After about 2 years on the diet, some people have been weaned off during the third year without an increase in seizure activity. The KD has become an accepted alternative for children but has not commonly been used in adults because of the impression that the KD is less effective after childhood. A recent case study was published to show evidence that a young man with intractable epilepsy since childhood was treated with great success by a medium-chain triglyceride KD. The KD not only controlled the seizures but also improved the patient's QOL. The study questions whether the diet should be more widely used.[108]

A hospital admission is usually required to initiate the diet and teach the components of living exclusively on the KD. The initial response for the patient may be drowsiness, lethargy, nausea, and vomiting as the body adapts to the change in metabolism from using glucose to using fats as the primary source of energy. A slower gastric emptying can be expected. If the diet is successful, AEDs may be reduced to monotherapy. Individuals respond differently to the KD and need close monitoring and supervision.[110,111]

General nutrition guidelines apply to individuals with epilepsy, with the nutritionist and clinicians working with the individual and the family to focus on a good nutritional diet, adequate fluids, adequate rest, relaxation to reduce stress, and avoidance of skipping meals.

STATUS EPILEPTICUS AND ACUTE REPETITIVE OR SERIAL SEIZURES

Status epilepticus (SE) is a potentially life-threatening medical emergency that can result in transient or permanent brain damage.[112,113] The frequency in the United States is about 100,000 to 150,000 per year.[114] In 1993 the Epilepsy Foundation of America's Working Group on Status Epilepticus defined the condition as more than 30 minutes of continuous seizure activity, or two or more sequential seizures without full recovery of consciousness between seizures. Any type of epileptic seizure can develop into SE (both primary generalized and partial seizure types can develop into SE). SE can be either **convulsive** (with generalized tonic-clonic seizures) or **nonconvulsive.** Classification for SE is usually generalized status with convulsive or nonconvulsive seizures, or partial (focal) status epilepticus with convulsive or nonconvulsive types. The seizure type most commonly seen in SE is tonic-clonic seizures. An EEG helps distinguish between the types when a diagnosis is unclear. The causes of SE include the following:[1]

- CNS insults (e.g., anoxia or hypoxia related to a brain attack/stroke)
- CNS infection
- Cerebral neoplasms
- Craniocerebral trauma (e.g., head injury)
- Cerebrovascular disease
- Toxic conditions
- Metabolic disorders: respiratory and metabolic acidosis, hyperazotemia, hypokalemia, hyponatremia, hyperglycemia followed by hypoglycemia
- Medication adjustment, noncompliance or withdrawal of AEDs
- Undetermined: approximately one third of cases

Generalized Convulsive Status Epilepticus

Generalized convulsive status epilepticus (GCSE) is the most common and life-threatening form, and is characterized by tonic-clonic seizures without return to full consciousness or the baseline state. GCSE may occur with a single seizure that fails to end, or, more commonly, with multiple seizures in a row without return to full consciousness. GCSE is considered a life-threatening medical emergency because of the hypoxia and neuronal metabolic exhaustion that can occur. Neuronal death in SE may result from prolonged continuous electrical discharges. Immediate treatment should be initiated after two to three seizures, or after 5 minutes of continuous tonic-clonic activity (Boxes 24-12 and 24-13).[115,116]

BOX 24-12   Initial Interventions for Convulsive Status Epilepticus

Emergency protocols should be followed for a tonic-clonic seizure lasting longer than 3 minutes.

Roll patient onto side to minimize risk of aspiration. Remove constricting clothing or items that might cause injury from around patient.

Give lorazepam (Ativan) 0.1 mg/kg intravenous push (IVP) bolus given slowly at 1 to 2 mg/min. May repeat in 5 minutes if seizures persist. Alternatively, diazepam (Valium) 2 mg IVP can be used. If no IV access is established, consider use of rectal diazepam.

Alert

Monitor for respiratory depression.

Flush with 2.5 ml of normal saline immediately. Ask a colleague to place a second IV.

Provide appropriate respiratory support, suction, and oxygenation.

Call the physician immediately for further orders.

If seizures stop, check vital signs every 15 minutes until the patient is back to normal baseline. Order bed rest for 2 hours following administration of lorazepam.

Order phenytoin or fosphenytoin to the unit for use if seizures continue.

Consult with the physician for additional laboratory and medication orders.

If status epilepticus persists, proceed with interventions in Box 24-13.

Modified from Gilbert K: *J Neurosci Nurs* 31(1):27–36, 1999.

Nonconvulsive SE (NCSE) is the presence of repetitive seizures such as myoclonic or absence seizures, without tonic-clonic activity, and may be seen more commonly in young children or adults older than age 60. Multiple seizures may be witnessed, or the patient may appear to be in a trance-like state associated with acute or chronic conditions. NCSE may be precipitated by low levels of AEDs; may be precipitated by changing AEDs; or may occur with a brain tumor, CNS infection, high fever, traumatic brain injury (TBI), stroke, or metabolic disorders, or during alcohol/drug withdrawal. The initial signs and symptoms may include a change in the LOC, pupillary changes, automatisms, or other abnormal behaviors, such as wandering. Individuals with NCSE should have a rapid diagnostic workup, have an EEG, and be aggressively treated as a medical emergency to minimize the risk of neuronal injury.[114,117] The initial management follows

---

BOX 24-13   Management of Status Epilepticus

Step 1

Assess Airway, Breathing, and Circulation

1. Administer O_2, monitor cardiac rhythm, oxygen saturation, and vital signs
2. Establish intravenous line with normal saline
3. Bedside glucose test
4. Draw blood for AED levels, CBC, electrolytes, calcium and magnesium, glucose, and toxicology screen
5. Administer thiamine 100 mg and dextrose 50% 50 ml IV (D_{25} 2 ml/kg in children)
6. Obtain history and perform examination

Step 2

1. Administer intravenous lorazepam 0.1 mg/kg in adults, 0.05 to 0.5 mg/kg in children (up to 2 mg/min) or diazepam 0.25 mg/kg in adults, 0.1 to 1.0 mg/kg in children (up to 5 mg/min); repeat after 10 minutes if seizures persist
2. Administer fosphenytoin 20 PE/kg load (up to 150 PE/min)
3. If seizures persist, give additional fosphenytoin 5 to 10 PE/kg to a total dose of 30 PE mg/kg or serum concentration of 30 µg/ml

Step 3

1. Intubate, place arterial line, and draw arterial blood gas and phenytoin level
2. Consider intravenous phenobarbital 20 mg/kg (100 mg/min or 3 mg/kg/min in children)

Step 4

1. Consider pharmacologic coma with pentobarbital 5 to 8 mg/kg load, followed by continuous infusion of 2 to 4 mg/kg/hr titrated to burst suppression for 6 to 48 hours

OR

2. Midazolam 0.2 mg/kg load followed by continuous infusion beginning at 1 µg/kg/min increasing by 1 µg/kg/min every 15 to 30 minutes as needed to a maximum rate of 10 µg/kg/min

From Goetz CG: *Textbook of clinical neurology*, ed 2, Philadelphia, 2003, Saunders.

AED, Antiepileptic drug; *CBC*, complete blood count; *PE*, phenytoin equivalents.

the emergency protocol of airway, breathing, and circulation (the ABCs), and the underlying cause is investigated and treated, if possible. Establishing an IV line for administration of appropriate antiseizure agents with close monitoring and observation is needed until the individual has no EEG evidence of seizure activity.

Partial Status Epilepticus

Simple partial SE is the second most common form of SE and may last for hours or days. **Partial SE is also known as focal motor status or epilepsia partialis continua.** Repetitive clonic motor activity occurs in one area of the body, usually the face or hand. Consciousness usually remains intact. Partial SE is not life threatening unless the seizure progresses to multiple complex partial or secondarily generalized seizures. Focal seizures can last for hours or days, and can be highly refractory to medical management. Intracranial grid recordings taken during epilepsia partialis continua show epileptiform activity arising in the primary sensorimotor cortex. Focal cortical resection and MST are surgical options available for refractory epilepsia partialis continua.

Complex partial SE manifests as a prolonged confusional state resulting from continuing or recurring seizures. Automatisms and speech difficulty may be present, after which the person's typical complex partial seizure may or may not be seen. The person may be able to make simple statements and may attempt to cooperate with the examiner, but is not fully conscious. If the seizure activity ceases, the patient may enter a postictal confusional state or become sleepy. If another seizure occurs again before the person recovers entirely, the person is in complex partial SE and requires urgent medical therapy.

Acute Repetitive Seizures

Acute repetitive seizures are also known as seizure clusters or serial seizures. Acute repetitive seizures are defined as multiple seizures occurring within a 24-hour period in adults or within a 12-hour period in children.[66] The individual with acute repetitive seizures is likely to be seen multiple times in the emergency department and is at risk for SE even with high levels of multiple AEDs. Rectal diazepam gel (Diastat) may be given at home at the beginning of a seizure cluster to break the cluster and can sometimes prevent a trip to the emergency department.[22,118] The patient with acute repetitive seizures is at risk for psychosocial stigma because of serial seizure activity and is at risk for death related to SE. Closely monitoring and working with the patient to maintain high compliance leads to less risk for acute repetitive seizures and medical emergencies.

Assessment for Status Epilepticus

- ABCs: Airway to ensure adequate air exchange, breathing, and the need for suctioning, and circulation.
- History: From the family (if available), determine if the SE event was the first seizure; a complete past

history should include specific questions regarding epilepsy, prior seizures, drug or alcohol abuse, recent head injury, infection, or headaches. If the patient is taking antiepilepsy medications, obtain the name, dosage, time last taken, and any recent changes in the dosage. Identification of all other medications taken by the patient is essential.
- Medications: Prescriptions, herbal supplements, homeopathic treatments, over-the-counter (OTC) medications, and illicit drug use.
- Neurologic assessment: May reveal a focal deficit indicating the underlying cause.
- Cardiorespiratory assessment.
- Pulse oximetry.
- Transfer to the intensive care unit (ICU).

Neurodiagnostic and Laboratory Studies

Identify the cause, if possible, for appropriate treatment:
Laboratory studies: routine studies; electrolytes to rule out metabolic causes; glucose to rule out hypoglycemia or hyperglycemia; calcium; magnesium; BUN; creatinine; complete blood count (CBC) with differential; liver profile, toxicology screen to rule out alcohol or drug abuse; AED drug levels; arterial blood gas (ABG) studies to rule out hypoxia and acidosis
MRI/CT: obtained as soon as possible to rule out a cerebral lesion in new cases of SE

Treatment

Medical/Clinical Management
Patients with SE are treated as a medical emergency, with full resuscitation measures available to protect the airway, breathing, and circulation. Treatment protocols should be followed, and an anesthetist consulted if the seizures cannot be controlled with treatment or medications within 60 minutes.

The goals of treatment are to stop the firing of the cerebral neurons, to correct the underlying cause, and to limit complications from SE. Guidelines may include the following:[64,114]
- Provide supplemental oxygen to maintain oxygenation; suction to prevent aspiration; intubate as needed.
- Draw blood for the laboratory studies listed above.
- Administer 100 mg of thiamine intravenously before administering 50 ml of 50% glucose if alcoholism or hypoglycemia is suspected.
- Closely monitor vital signs with frequent recordings every 5 minutes or as needed; do temperature checks.
- Monitor the patient's cardiac status.
- Use an indwelling urinary catheter to measure intake and output (I&O).

Prompt treatment is vital in treating tonic-clonic SE to prevent medical complications (Box 24-14). Mortality rates for tonic-clonic SE are 10% to 12%.[119] See Box 24-12 for an example of a protocol for initial interventions and Box 24-13

BOX 24-14	Complications Accompanying Tonic-Clonic Status Epilepticus

- Cardiac dysrhythmias
- Hyperthermia
- Aspiration
- Hypertension
- Hypotension
- Anoxia
- Hyperglycemia or hypoglycemia
- Dehydration
- Lactic acidosis
- Myoglobinuria
- Oral and musculoskeletal injuries
- Death

for management if convulsive seizures persist. If SE persists after the treatments described in Box 24-13, the patient, who has probably been transferred to the ICU, may need to be placed into a medication-induced coma. Sodium thiopental is historically the most common medication used for induced coma, but other anesthetic medications are increasingly being used. The care delivered is the same as that for other patients in a coma.

Nonacute/Home Care.　After discharge from the acute setting, caregivers and family should be taught how to respond when a person with a history of SE experiences a seizure. An immediate assessment of the seizure is needed, with a plan designed to recognize progression to SE and strategies to abort it in place. This can include early use of first aid measures, use of sublingual or rectal benzodiazepines, education as to appropriate use of emergency aid, and a monitoring plan until the individual has recovered. All individuals with epilepsy should carry some type of medical identification.

COMPREHENSIVE PATIENT MANAGEMENT: SEIZURES AND EPILEPSY

Psychosocial Aspects of Epilepsy

The psychosocial aspects of epilepsy may be quite debilitating. As with any chronic illness, every patient goes through a period of adjustment. Because of the unpredictability of seizures, people with epilepsy experience unique problems. They may experience problems at home, work, or play, or with interpersonal relationships. Parents, family, friends, and employers are instrumental in helping an individual adjust to the seizures and the consequences. The age of onset and seizure frequency may affect the patient's ability to cope.

Significant others tend to overprotect the person with epilepsy or to hold back information. This fosters real and imagined dependency. Open and honest communication is necessary among family members, as well as with health professionals. Significant others must balance their own expectations with the expectations and desire of the person with epilepsy to lead a normal life. Special precautions should be taken for individuals with frequent and severe seizures.

Work and household activities must be evaluated carefully for their potential harm. Some activities that are potentially harmful include showers, baths, cooking, and ironing. When seizures occur during one of these activities, any number of injuries may result, such as burns or falls. Drowning has been reported when individuals had seizures with loss of consciousness while bathing or swimming. For example, if an individual has most of his or her seizures in the morning, he or she should shower in the evening. For patients with frequent seizures resulting in falls or injury, the level of precaution may be high. Extreme precautions may involve "bird baths" rather than showering, filling the tub with the least amount of water needed, and bathing with supervision.

Many people with controlled epilepsy are able to work and function normally in society; however, the work environment has many potential hazards for individuals with uncontrolled seizures. Individuals who operate heavy equipment (e.g., truck drivers, forklift operators, printers) or who work under potentially dangerous circumstances (e.g., construction that uses scaffolding) should consider changing to a job that is less likely to involve injury should a seizure occur. Patients with refractory epilepsy frequently lose jobs after having seizures at work, and find it more difficult to obtain new employment. The inability to drive limits employment opportunities. Fear of discrimination often obscures good work judgment. Educational programs are available through some affiliates of the Epilepsy Foundation to make employees more aware of potential problems and better able to handle these should they arise. For those individuals who have lost their jobs or who are having difficulty finding work, referral to a vocational rehabilitation agency may be helpful.[120]

Caution also must be exercised with recreational activities. Individuals with controlled seizures can participate in almost all recreational activities. However, individuals with uncontrolled seizures should take special precautions regarding particular sports. Swimming or aquatic sports should be supervised. It is recommended that helmets always be used when there is a risk for head injury (as in contact sports). Activities that should be avoided include sports that involve physical injury (e.g., boxing) and sports where a loss of consciousness could potentially be fatal (e.g., parachuting, scuba diving, and mountain climbing). Exercise in general should pose no problems for individuals with uncontrolled seizures and should be encouraged to improve health and mitigate depression.

Driving restrictions are especially difficult for individuals with uncontrolled seizures.[121,122] Driving is an important symbol of independence in our society: it is a privilege and skill that most people want to obtain. Driving regulations vary from state to state. Whereas some regulations are restrictive and stipulate that the individual must be seizure free for up to 1 year, others are liberal and state that the decision is left to the physician's discretion. Both health care professionals and people with epilepsy should be aware of their own state's regulations. Individuals with uncontrolled seizures should be told to comply with their state's driving regulations. If individuals do not comply, it may be the responsibility of the physician to inform the licensing bureau. In some states the law may mandate physician reporting. A list of state laws can be found on the Epilepsy Foundation Web site (see Resources at the end of this chapter).

Older Adult Considerations

The incidence of epilepsy increases in older adults and is greater than that seen in children. Acute symptomatic seizures occur most commonly as complex partial seizures. As with the general adult population, the risk factors for seizures include brain attack/stroke, brain tumors, head injury, CNS infections, and substance abuse. Recognition of seizure activity by the patient's physician is often difficult because the patient may not accurately report the event or may live alone and have no witnesses.[86]

Management for older adults is the same as for other adults, with prompt diagnostic testing and treatment. Monotherapy is an important consideration particularly as medication side effects can be more serious in older adults. Drugs to minimize adverse effects on cognition, mobility, and bone health should be considered. It often takes longer for older people to metabolize medications and to eliminate them from the body, leading to toxic levels of AEDs if dosing is not carefully regulated; lower AED dosages may be adequate. People over age 65 may be taking a multitude of medications, some of which can interact with AEDs, resulting in drug-drug interactions and negative side effects. Older patients may be more sensitive to the depressive aspects of AEDs. Osteoporosis is a problem with older adults and may be a larger problem for those with epilepsy because of interference by some AEDs with the metabolism of vitamin D. Special consideration of memory difficulties that might reduce compliance should be addressed. Some solutions include using special pill containers to be refilled weekly by a visiting health care provider or family member, or an electronic device that sounds an alarm when the next dose is due. All individuals with epilepsy, especially older adults, should carry wallet cards containing important medical information and a current list of medications. Newer AEDs (e.g., gabapentin and lamotrigine) may be better tolerated by older adults and have more favorable side effect profiles.[123-125] The absence of research studies on AEDs and pharmacokinetics for older adults increases the possibility of therapeutic failure and adverse reactions in this vulnerable population.

Alternative Care

A topic of importance to patients may be alternative/complementary practices (A/CPs), which are being used by people with epilepsy today. The health care team should carefully review these A/CPs. Some are better than others. Examples of A/CPs include acupuncture, aromatherapy, mind-body approaches, hypnosis, guided imagery, relaxation therapy, therapeutic touch, and biofeedback.[65] Educating patients and their families in choosing A/CPs is an individual choice for clinicians and should be done in concert with the patient and the health care team.[65]

The diagnosis and treatment of the seizures will affect the QOL of the individual and family. Five major variables have been defined: health; family life; personal development; economics; and social, community, and civic activities. Comprehensive health education and management includes more than education about seizures; it also requires management of human responses to the treatment and changes that the seizures impose on the individual's life. A newly developed self-administered QOL questionnaire has been found to represent a useful measure for individuals with epilepsy.[126]

Education is an ongoing process. After the needs of the patient have been assessed, the process of education begins.[127] Pertinent and accurate information is given to enable patients to make ongoing decisions and to be active participants in their care. Knowledge can dispel not only the patient's misconceptions but also those of family members, friends, and employers. Throughout this process, positive behaviors should be reinforced. Patient education materials and information about support groups are available through the Epilepsy Foundation and local and state affiliates. The introduction of a clinical nurse specialist in epilepsy is associated with a significant increase in patient reports that enough advice has been provided. Clinician intervention appears to help those with the least knowledge of epilepsy improve their knowledge scores.[128]

Rehabilitation

Rehabilitation issues need to be assessed in all patients to ensure a smooth transition to home, school, work, and the community. Employment and educational concerns must be addressed as well. Vocational training and placement programs are available through the state office of rehabilitation.

Patients and families must be familiar with seizure first aid so that they can direct the education of others, including friends, employers, colleagues, teachers, and classmates. Information from local Epilepsy Foundation chapters is particularly helpful because it may be reviewed repeatedly and passed on to others.

Alternative modes of transportation may need to be explored if the patient is prohibited from driving. The state department of motor vehicles can provide information on driving regulations and requirements.

Adjusting to a chronic condition can be very difficult, not only for the patient but also for the family and significant others. Individual or family counseling may be warranted. Support groups are often helpful in putting patients and families in contact with others who share their problems and concerns. Information on support groups can be obtained through local social services.

The Epilepsy Foundation or a local affiliate or a comprehensive epilepsy center in the area can help with vocational and educational referrals, driving regulations, and support groups.

Case Management Considerations

In the event that a patient with complicated seizures requires case management, the first step is to discuss with the health care team the type of seizure, characteristics, and potential complications. After a comprehensive review of medications and special needs, the case manager will develop a plan of care with the goal of reducing the incidence of seizures and keeping the patient safe and compliant with the prescribed regimen. Careful documentation is a very important responsibility of the case manager. The records and seizure log and outcomes from the case manager's plan of care will be used by the health care team to measure the patient's progress. Considerations for case management include the following:

- Continuing education and medical updates. Provide verbal and written health teaching for the individual, the family, and all care providers.
- Living and coping with a seizure condition. Identify resources to support individuals who may have a medical disability or other losses.
- Compliance. Stress the importance of taking medications at the right time and the right dose, and of immediately reporting serious adverse events to a 24-hour phone number provided by the case manager (or, in a life-threatening situation, calling 911).
- Seizure first aid. Check to see whether all family members and caregivers know seizure first aid and basic cardiopulmonary resuscitation (CPR).
- Home safety. Have an appropriate professional conduct a home safety check for a safe environment, particularly the kitchen, bath, and bedroom.
- Support. Locate local support groups and encourage the individual and family to participate in them, as well as in Epilepsy Foundation programs.
- Substance abuse. Educate the individual on the need to avoid alcohol and drugs that may interact with or inactivate the AEDs.
- Personal safety. Review the need to never bathe or shower alone, or swim in a pool unsupervised.

CONCLUSION

It is expected that there will be new and improved treatments for epilepsy, as well as methods to prevent it. This expectation has been reinforced by Curing Epilepsy: Focus on the Future, the White House–initiated conference in 2000. Conference objectives included a future that holds promise for a true cure for epilepsy with nothing less than a complete, permanent cessation of seizures with no untoward effects of therapies. Today patients with epilepsy still face many challenges in their lives, both medically and psychosocially. The aim of all epilepsy treatment is to control seizures and minimize complications of treatment: "no seizures, no side effects." This will enable the patient to lead as normal a life as his or her condition permits. Through education, support, and counseling, clinicians influence how the patient and family adjust to living with a chronic disorder. Community education aimed at schools, businesses, and community services may help improve society's understanding of epilepsy.

RESOURCES

American Academy of Neurology: www.aan.com
American Association of Neuroscience Nurses: www.aann.org

American Epilepsy Society: 342 N. Main Street, West Hartford, CT 06117-2507; 860-586-7505; www.aesnet.org
Anita Kaufmann Foundation: www.theanitakaufmannfoundation. org
Antiepileptic Drug Pregnancy Registry: 888-233-2334; www. aedpregnancyregistry.org
Epilepsy Foundation: 4351 Garden City Drive, Landover, MD 20785; 800-332-1000; www.efa.org
National Epilepsy Library Resource Center: 800-332-4686
Partners with Seizures and Epilepsy Education (S.E.E.): Akfoundation@bellsouth.net

REFERENCES

1. Foldvary N, Wyllie E: Epilepsy. In *Textbook of clinical neurology,* Philadelphia, 1999, WB Saunders.
2. *Epilepsy: a report to the nation,* Landover, MD, 2000, Epilepsy Foundation.
3. Lipe H: Common neurological health problems: phenomena of relevance to neuroscience medicine. In Stewart-Amide C, Kunckel JA, editors: *AANN's neuroscience nursing: human responses to neurologic dysfunction,* ed 2, Philadelphia, 2001, WB Saunders.
4. Swearingen PL, Ross DG: *Manual of medical-surgical nursing: interventions and collaborative management,* ed 4, St Louis, 1999, Mosby.
5. Fisher RS, van Emde BW, Blume W, et al: Epileptic seizures and epilepsy: definitions proposed by the International League Against Epilepsy (ILAE) and the International Bureau for Epilepsy (IBE), *Epilepsia* 46(4):470–472, 2005.
6. Hauser WA, Annegers JF, Kurland LT: Prevalence of epilepsy in Rochester, Minnesota: 1940–1980, *Epilepsia* 32:429–445, 1991.
7. Hauser WA, Hesdorffer DC: *Epilepsy frequency, causes and consequences,* New York, 1990, Demos.
8. Engel J Jr: A proposed diagnostic scheme for people with epileptic seizures and with epilepsy: report of the ILAE Task Force on Classification and Terminology, *Epilepsia* 42:796–803, 2001.
9. Commission on Classification and Terminology of the International League Against Epilepsy: Proposal for revised classification of epilepsies and epileptic syndromes, *Epilepsia* 30(4):389–399, 1989.
10. Estes R: A closer look at seizures, *Outlook* 1(2):19–22, 2000.
11. *Seizure assessment. Clinical guideline series,* Chicago, 1997, American Association of Neuroscience Nurses.
12. Escueta AV, Bacsal FE, Treiman DM: Complex partial seizures on closed-circuit television and EEG: a study of 691 attacks in 79 patients, *Ann Neurol* 11:292–300, 1982.
13. Foldvary-Schaeffer N, Wyllie E: Epilepsy. In Goetz CG, editor: *Textbook of clinical neurology,* ed 2, Philadelphia, 2003, WB Saunders.
14. Gastaut H, Broughton R: *Epileptic seizures: clinical and electroencephalographic feature, diagnosis and treatment,* 1972, Thomas.
15. Duncan JS: Idiopathic generalized epilepsy of childhood and adolescence. In Hopkins A, Shorvon SD, Cascino GD, editors: *Epilepsy,* ed 2, New York, 1995, Chapman & Hall.
16. Foldvary N, Lee N, Thwaites G, et al: Clinical and electrographic manifestations of lesional neocortical temporal lobe epilepsy, *Neurology* 49:757–763, 1997.
17. Kwan P, Brodie MJ: Early identification of refractory epilepsy, *N Engl J Med* 342(5):314–319, 2000.

18. Perucca E, Levy RH: Combination therapy and drug interactions. In Levy RH, Mattson RH, Meldrum BS, Perucca E, editors: *Antiepileptic drugs,* ed 5, Philadelphia, 2002, Lippincott Williams & Wilkins.

19. Agrawal A, Timothy J, Pandit L, Manju M: Post-traumatic epilepsy: an overview, *Clin Neurol Neurosurg* 108(5):433–439, 2006.

20. Gottesman RF, Komotar R, Hillis AE: Neurologic aspects of traumatic brain injury, *Int Rev Psychiatry* 15(4):302–309, 2003.

21. Abou Khalil BW, Andermann E, Andermann F, Olivier A, Quesney LF: Temporal lobe epilepsy after prolonged febrile convulsions: excellent outcome after surgical treatment, *Epilepsia* 34:878–883, 1993.

22. O'Dell C, Shinnar S, Ballaban-Gil KR, et al: Rectal diazepam gel in the home management of seizures in children, *Pediatr Neurol* 33(3):166–172, 2005.

23. Langan Y, Nashef L, Sander JW: Case-control study of SUDEP, *Neurology* 64:1131–1133, 2005.

24. Day SM, Wu YW, Strauss DJ, Shavelle RM, Reynolds RJ: Causes of death in remote symptomatic epilepsy, *Neurology* 65(2):216–222, 2005.

25. Strauss DJ, Day SM, Shavelle RM, Wu YW: Remote symptomatic epilepsy: does seizure severity increase mortality? *Neurology* 60(3):395–399, 2003.

26. Herzog AG, Fowler KM: Sexual hormones and epilepsy: threat and opportunities, *Curr Opin Neurol* 18(2):167–172, 2005.

27. Herzog AG, Harden CL, Liporace J, et al: Frequency of catamenial seizure exacerbation in women with localization-related epilepsy, *Ann Neurol* 56(3):431–434, 2004.

28. Weatherford KJ: Catamenial epilepsy: in search of a clinical entity and its prevalence, *J Neurosci Nurs* 31(6):328–331, 2000.

29. Artama M, Auvinen A, Raudaskoski T, Isojarvl I, Isojarvl J: Antiepileptic drug use of women with epilepsy and congenital malformations in offspring, *Neurology* 64(11):1874–1878, 2005.

30. Perucca E: Birth defects after prenatal exposure to antiepileptic drugs, *Lancet Neurol* 4(11):781–786, 2005.

31. Meador KJ, Zupanc ML: Neurodevelopmental outcomes of children born to mothers with epilepsy, *Cleve Clin J Med* 71(suppl 2):S38–S41, 2004.

32. Jeha LE, Morris HH: Optimizing outcomes in pregnant women with epilepsy, *Cleve Clin J Med* 72(10):938–945, 2005.

33. Herzog AG, Drislane FW, Schomer DL, et al: Differential effects of antiepileptic drugs on sexual function and hormones in men with epilepsy, *Neurology* 65(7):1016–1020, 2005.

34. Sahoo S, Klein P: Maternal complex partial seizure associated with fetal distress, *Arch Neurol* 62(8):1304–1305, 2005.

35. Knight AH, Rhind EG: Epilepsy and pregnancy: a study of 153 pregnancies in 59 patients, *Epilepsia* 16(1):99–110, 1975.

36. Vossler DG: Nonepileptic seizures of physiologic origin, *J Epilepsy* 8:1–10, 1995.

37. Wilkus RJ, Dodrill CB: Factors affecting the outcome of MMPI and neuropsychological assessments of psychogenic and epileptic seizure patients, *Epilepsia* 30:339–347, 1989.

38. O'Connor WM, Masukawa L, Freese A, Sperling MR, French JA, O'Connor MJ: Hippocampal cell distributions in temporal lobe epilepsy: a comparison between patients with and without an early risk factor, *Epilepsia* 37(5):440–449, 1996.

39. Wolf JA: Evaluation of seizure observation and documentation, *J Neurosci Nurs* 32(1):27–36, 2000.

40. O'Brien TJ, So EL, Mullan BP, et al: Subtraction SPECT co-registered to MRI improves postictal SPECT localization of seizure foci, *Neurology* 52:137–146, 1999.

41. So EL: Integration of EEG, MRI and SPECT in localizing the seizure focus for epilepsy surgery, *Epilepsia* 41(suppl 3): S48–S54, 2000.

42. Zaveri HP, Duckrow RB, de Lanerolle NC, Spencer SS: Distinguishing subtypes of temporal lobe epilepsy with background hippocampal activity, *Epilepsia* 42(6):725–730, 2001.

43. Chen FA, Farias S, Lima A, Boggan JE, Zusman E, Alsaadi TM: Relevance of 18-fluorodeoxyglucose positron emission tomography in presurgical evaluation of patients with refractory epilepsy, *Epilepsia* 44(suppl 9):79–80, 2003.

44. Henry TR, Van Heertum RL: Positron emission tomography and single photon emission computed tomography in epilepsy care, *Semin Nucl Med* 33(2):88–104, 2003.

45. Knake S, Grant PE, Stufflebeam SM, et al: Aids to telemetry in the presurgical evaluation of epilepsy patients: MRI, MEG and other non-invasive imaging techniques. *Suppl Clin Neurophysiol* 57:494–502, 2004.

46. Wolff M, Weiskopf N, Serra E, Preissl H, Birbaumer N, Kraegeloh-Mann I: Benign partial epilepsy in childhood: selective cognitive deficits are related to the location of focal spikes determined by combined EEG/MEG, *Epilepsia* 46(10):1661–1667, 2005.

47. Hermann BP, Seidenberg M, Schoenfeld J, Davies K: Neuropsychological characteristics of the syndrome of mesial temporal lobe epilepsy. *Arch Neurol* 54:369–376, 1997.

48. Dodrill CB, Wilkus RJ, Batzell LW: The MMPI as a diagnostic tool in non-epileptic seizures. In Rowan AJ, Gates JR, editors: *Non-epileptic seizures,* Boston, 1993, Butterworth-Heinemann.

49. Noeker M, Haverkamp-Krois A, Haverkamp F: Development of mental health dysfunction in childhood epilepsy, *Brain Dev* 27(1):5–16, 2005.

50. Smy J: Improving the lives of epilepsy patients, *Nurs Times* 101(27):44–45, 2005.

51. Meldolesi GN, Picardi A, Quarato PP, et al: Factors associated with generic and disease-specific quality of life in temporal lobe epilepsy, *Epilepsy Res,* March 1, 2006.

52. Powell KW: Seizures in the workplace, *AAOHN J* 53(12):511–513, 2005.

53. Yeager KA, Diiorio C, Shafer PO, et al: The complexity of treatments for persons with epilepsy, *Epilepsy Behav* 7(4):679–686, 2005.

54. Helde G, Bovim G, Brathen G, Brodtkorb E: A structured, nurse-led intervention program improves quality of life in patients with epilepsy: a randomized, controlled trial, *Epilepsy Behav* 7(3):451–457, 2005.

55. Clinical nursing in adult epilepsy, *Axone* 26(3):31–34, 2005.

56. Grabowska-Grzyb A, Jedrzejczak J, Naganska E, Fiszer U: Risk factors for depression in patients with epilepsy, *Epilepsy Behav* 8(2):411–417, 2006.

57. Bader MK, Littlejohns LR: *AANN core curriculum for neuroscience nursing,* ed 4, St Louis, 2004, WB Saunders.

58. French JA, Kugler AR, Robbins MS, Knapp LE, Garafalo EA: Dose-response trial of pregabalin adjunctive therapy in patients with partial seizures, *Neurology* 60(10):1631–1637, 2006.

59. Ranta A, Fountain NB: Seizures and epilepsy in adolescents and adults. In Rakel RE, Bope ET, editors: *Conn's current therapy 2005,* ed 57, Philadelphia, 2005, WB Saunders.

60. Mattson RH: Antiepileptic drug monotherapy in adults: selection and use in new-onset epilepsy. In Levy RH, Mattson RH, Meldrum BS, Perucca E, editors: *Antiepileptic drugs,* ed 5, Philadelphia, 2002, Lippincott Williams & Wilkins.

61. Dodrill CB, Batzel LW, Wilensky AJ, Yerby MS: The role of psychosocial and financial factors in medication noncompliance in epilepsy, *Int J Psychiatry Med* 17:143–154, 1987.

62. Sander JW: The use of antiepileptic drugs—principles and practice, *Epilepsia* 45(suppl 6):28–34, 2004.

63. Cramer JA, Glassman M, Rienzi V: The relationship between poor medication compliance and seizures, *Epilepsy Behav* 3(4):338–342, 2002.

64. Cross C: Seizures. Regaining control, *RN* 67(12):44–50, 2004.

65. Shafer PO, Sierzant TL, Dean P: Alternative and complementary therapies: focus on epilepsy, *Clin Nurs Pract Epilepsy* 4(2):4–8, 1997.

66. Shafer PO: New therapies in the management of acute or cluster seizures and seizure emergencies, *J Neurosci Nurs* 31(4):224–230, 1999.

67. Faraji B, Yu PP: Serum phenytoin levels of patients on gastrostomy tube feeding, *J Neurosci Nurs* 30(1):55–59, 1998.

68. Engel J Jr, Wiebe S, French J, et al: Practice parameter: temporal lobe and localized neocortical resections for epilepsy: report of the Quality Standards Subcommittee of the American Academy of Neurology, in association with the American Epilepsy Society and the American Association of Neurological Surgeons, *Neurology* 60(4):538–547, 2003.

69. Malmgren K, Sullivan M, Ekstedt G, Kullberg G, Kumlien E: Health-related quality of life after epilepsy surgery: a Swedish multicenter study, *Epilepsia* 38:830–838, 1997.

70. Vickery BG, Hays RD, Engel J Jr, et al: Outcome assessment for epilepsy surgery: the impact of measuring health-related quality of life, *Ann Neurol* 37:158–166, 1995.

71. Oyegbile TO, Dow C, Jones J, et al: The nature and course of neuropsychological morbidity in chronic temporal lobe epilepsy, *Neurology* 62:1736–1742, 2004.

72. Wieser HG, ILAE Commission on Neurosurgery of Epilepsy: Mesial temporal lobe epilepsy with hippocampal sclerosis, *Epilepsia* 45(6):695–714, 2004.

73. Berkovic S, Andermann F, Olivier A, et al: Hippocampal sclerosis in temporal lobe epilepsy demonstrated by magnetic resonance imaging, *Ann Neurol* 29:175–182, 1991.

74. Berg AT, Vickery BG, Langfitt JT, et al: The multicenter study of epilepsy surgery: recruitment and selection for surgery, *Epilepsia* 44(11):1425–1433, 2003.

75. Berkovic SF, McIntosh AM, Kalnins RM, et al: Preoperative MRI predicts outcome of temporal lobectomy: an actuarial analysis, *Neurology* 45:1358–1363, 1995.

76. Bernasconi N, Natsume J, Bernasconi A: Progression in temporal lobe epilepsy: differential atrophy in mesial temporal structures, *Neurology* 65(2):223–228, 2005.

77. Cendes F, Andermann F, Gloor P, et al: Atrophy of mesial structures in patients with temporal lobe epilepsy: cause or consequence of repeated seizures? *Ann Neurol* 34:795–801, 1993.

78. Theodore WH, Bhatia S, Hatta J et al: Hippocampal atrophy, epilepsy duration, and febrile seizures in patients with partial seizures, *Neurology* 52:132–136, 1999.

79. Abou Khalil BW, Siegel GJ, Sackellares JC, Gilman S, Hichwa R, Marshall R: Positron emission tomography studies of cerebral glucose metabolism in chronic partial epilepsy, *Ann Neurol* 22:480–486, 1987.

80. Engel J Jr, Kuhl DE, Phelps ME, Rausch R, Nuwer M: Local cerebral metabolism during partial seizures, *Neurology* 33(4):400–413, 1983.

81. Engel J Jr, Kuhl DE, Phelps ME, Mazziotta JC: Interictal cerebral glucose metabolism in partial epilepsy and its relation to EEG changes, *Ann Neurol* 12:510–517, 1982.

82. Theodore WH, Sato S, Kufta CV, Gaillard WD, Kelley K: FDG–positron emission tomography and invasive EEG: seizure focus detection and surgical outcome, *Epilepsia* 38:81–86, 1997.

83. Wada JA: A new method for the determination of the side of cerebral speech dominance: a preliminary report on the intracarotid injection of sodium amytal in man, *Med Biol* 14:221–222, 1949.

84. Cohen-Gadol AA, Westerveld M, varez-Carilles J, Spencer DD: Intracarotid Amytal memory test and hippocampal magnetic resonance imaging volumetry: validity of the Wada test as an indicator of hippocampal integrity among candidates for epilepsy surgery, *J Neurosurg* 101(6):926–931, 2004.

85. Detre JA: fMRI: applications in epilepsy, *Epilepsia* 45(suppl 4):26–31, 2004.

86. Boss B: Nursing management of adults with common neurologic problems. In Beare PG, Myers JL, editors: *Adult health nursing,* ed 3, St Louis, 1998, Mosby.

87. Kraemer DL, Griebel ML, Lee N, Friedman AH, Radtke RA: Surgical outcome in patients with epilepsy with occult vascular malformations treated with lesionectomy, *Epilepsia* 39(6):600–607, 1998.

88. Spencer SS, Berg AT, Vickrey BG, et al: Predicting long-term seizure outcome after resective epilepsy surgery: the multicenter study, *Neurology* 65(6):912–918, 2005.

89. Wiebe S, Blume WT, Girvin JP, Eliasziw M: A randomized, controlled trial of surgery for temporal-lobe epilepsy, *N Engl J Med* 345(5):311–318, 2001.

90. Villemure JG, Mascott CR: Peri-insular hemispherotomy: surgical principles and anatomy, *Neurosurgery* 37:975–981, 1995.

91. Schramm J, Behrens E, Entzian W: Hemispherical deafferentation: an alternative to functional hemispherectomy, *Neurosurgery* 36:509–516, 1995.

92. Jonas R, Nguyen S, Hu B, et al: Cerebral hemispherectomy: hospital course, seizure, developmental, language, and motor outcomes, *Neurology* 62(10):1712–1721, 2004.

93. Roberts DW, Rayport M, Maxwell RE, Olivier A, Marino R Jr: Corpus callosotomy. In Engel J Jr, editor: *Surgical treatment of the epilepsies,* ed 2, New York, 1993, Raven Press.

94. Andersen B, Arogvi-Hansen B, Kruse-Larsen C, Dam M: Corpus callosotomy: seizure and psychosocial outcome. A 39 month follow-up of 20 patients, *Epilepsy Res* 23:77–85, 1996.

95. Yang TT, Wong TT, Kwan SY, Chang KP, Lee YC, Hsu TC: Quality of life and life satisfaction in families after a child has undergone corpus callosotomy, *Epilepsia* 37(1):76–80, 1996.

96. Snively C, Counsell C, Lilly D: Vagus nerve stimulator as a treatment for intractable epilepsy, *J Neurosci Nurs* 30(5):286–289, 1998.

97. Schallert G, Foster J, Lindquist N, Murphy JV: Chronic stimulation of the left vagal nerve in children: effect on swallowing, *Epilepsia* 39(10):1113–1114, 1998.

98. Handforth A, DiGiorgio CM, Schachter SC, et al: Vagus nerve stimulation therapy for partial-onset seizures: a randomized active-control trial, *Neurology* 51:48–55, 1999.

99. Ben-Menachem E, Hellstrom K, Waldton C, Augustinsson LE: Evaluation of refractory epilepsy treated with vagus nerve stimulation for up to 5 years, *Neurology* 52:1265–1267, 1999.

100. Labar D, Murphy J, Tecoma E, E04 VNS Study Group: Vagus nerve stimulation for medication-resistant generalized epilepsy, *Neurology* 52:1510–1512, 1999.

101. Devinsky O, Perrine K, Pacia S, Vazquez B, Buchwald J, Luciano DJ: Multiple subpial transections in language cortex: effects on language functions, *J Epilepsy* 10:247–253, 1997.

102. Telfeian AE, Connors BW: Layer-specific pathways for the horizontal propagation of epileptiform discharges in neocortex, *Epilepsia* 39:700–708, 1998.

103. Morrell F, Whisler WW, Smith MC, et al: Landau-Kleffner syndrome: treatment with subpial intracortical transection, *Brain* 118:1529–1546, 1996.

104. Morrell F, Whisler WW, Bleck TP: Multiple subpial transection: a new approach to the surgical treatment of focal epilepsy, *J Neurosurg* 70:231–239, 1989.

105. Pacia SV, Devinsky O, Perrine K, et al: Multiple subpial transection for intractable partial seizures: seizure outcome, *J Epilepsy* 10(2):86–91, 1997.

106. Oommen J, Morrell M, Fisher RS: Experimental electrical stimulation therapy for epilepsy, *Curr Treat Options Neurol* 7(4):261–271, 2005.

107. Theodore WH, Fisher RS: Brain stimulation for epilepsy, *Lancet Neurol* 3(2):111–118, 2004.

108. Schiff Y, Lerman-Sagie T: Ketogenic diet—an alternative therapy for epilepsy in adults, *Harefuah* 134:529–531, 1998.

109. Dahlin M, Elfving A, Ungerstedt U, Amark P: The ketogenic diet influences the levels of excitatory and inhibitory amino acids in the CSF in children with refractory epilepsy, *Epilepsy Res* 64:115–126, 2005.

110. Hosain SA, La Vega-Talbott M, Solomon GE: Ketogenic diet in pediatric epilepsy patients with gastrostomy feeding, *Pediatr Neurol* 32(2):81–83, 2005.

111. Vining EP: The ketogenic diet, *Adv Exp Med Biol* 497:225–231, 2002.

112. Duncan JS: Seizure-induced neuronal injury: human data, *Neurology* 59:S15–S19, 2002.

113. Fujikawa DG, Itabashi HH, Wu A, Shinmei SS: Status epilepticus–induced neuronal loss in humans without systemic complications or epilepsy, *Epilepsia* 41:981–991, 2000.

114. Gilbert K: An algorithm for diagnosis and treatment of status epilepticus in adults, *J Neurosci Nurs* 31(1):27–36, 1999.

115. Sirven JI, Waterhouse E: Management of status epilepticus, *Am Fam Physician* 68(3):469–476, 2003.

116. Starreveld E, Starreveld AA: Status epilepticus. Current concepts and management, *Can Fam Physician* 46:1817–1823, 2000.

117. Wheless JW: Acute management of seizures in the syndromes of idiopathic generalized epilepsies, *Epilepsia* 44(suppl 2):22–26, 2003.

118. Pellock JM: Safety of Diastat, a rectal gel formulation of diazepam for acute seizure treatment, *Drug Saf* 27(6):383–392, 2004.

119. Delgado-Escueta AV, Wasterlain C, Treiman DM, Porter RJ: Current concepts in neurology: management of status epilepticus, *N Engl J Med* 306:1337–1340, 1982.

120. Fraser RT, Clemmons DC, Dodrill CB, Trejo WR, Freelove C: The difficult-to-employ in epilepsy rehabilitation: predictions of response to an intensive intervention, *Epilepsia* 27:220–224, 1986.

121. DeToledo JC, Lowe MR: Driving restrictions and people with epilepsy, *Neurology* 58(12):1864–1865, 2002.

122. Krauss G: Individual state driving restrictions for people with epilepsy in the US, *Neurology* 58(12):1865, 2002.

123. Meador KJ, Loring DW, Vahle VP, et al: Cognitive and behavioral effects of lamotrigine and topiramate in healthy volunteers, *Neurology* 64:2108–2114, 2005.

124. French JA, Chadwick DW: Antiepileptic drugs for the elderly: using the old to focus on the new, *Neurology* 64(11):1834–1835, 2005.

125. Rowan AJ, Ramsay RE, Collins JF, et al: New onset geriatric epilepsy: a randomized study of gabapentin, lamotrigine, and carbamazepine, *Neurology* 64(11):1868–1873, 2005.

126. McNulty P, Baker JA: Patient-based assessments of quality of life in newly diagnosed epilepsy patients: validation of the NEWQOL, *Epilepsia* 41(9):1119–1128, 2000.

127. Galletti F, Sturniolo MG: Counseling children and parents about epilepsy, *Patient Educ Couns* 55(3):422–425, 2004.

128. Risdale L, Kwan I, Cryer C: Newly diagnosed epilepsy: can nurse specialists help? A randomized control trial, Epilepsy Care Evaluation Group, *Epilepsia* 41(8):1014–1019, 2000.

Legal Considerations

JEAN M. JONES,
ELLEN BARKER

CHAPTER 25

Legal Issues and Life Care Planning for the Neuroscience Patient

The nurse clinician who provides care for the neuroscience patient must be knowledgeable in neuroanatomy and physiology, neurologic assessment, neuropathology, pharmacology, neurodiagnostic studies, and disease management, as well as have the appropriate skills to deliver patient care. In addition, the clinician must understand the legal and ethical parameters that affect health care decisions today. It is important for clinicians to have knowledge of today's health laws in order to understand their legal rights and those of their patients and their patients' families. The material in this chapter is designed to clarify the legal background of neuroscience patient care and management.

In general, applicable laws discussed are state laws, not federal laws. There are some exceptions, including medical device reporting (MDR), the Patient Self-Determination Act, and the Americans with Disabilities Act. State laws are governed by the state legislative intent. It is therefore important that health care providers be familiar with the relevant statutory and case law in the state in which they practice and seek appropriate legal counsel as needed.

This chapter also provides some of the necessary legal background for decision making; clinical illustrations are used as appropriate. The final portion of the chapter is devoted to some common professional liability concerns. This format should not suggest that the threat of professional liability is less important; instead, it is meant to suggest that competent, attentive, and well-documented care is the best protection against a possible professional liability action.

The information that is provided in this chapter should not be construed as legal advice; when appropriate, staff should refer to hospital policy or consult with appropriate hospital personnel. Issues of consent for and refusal of treatment, professional liability concerns, medical device reporting, and life care planning are included.

CLINICAL CARE DECISION MAKING

Decisions about the care of a patient must be made whether or not the patient is competent to make them. If the patient is incapacitated or incompetent, states provide for various types of decision making by others.

The Competent Patient

It has long been a principle of law in the United States and in many Western countries that competent adult patients 18 years of age and older may agree to or refuse treatment. This is true even if the decision made by the patient is deemed medically inappropriate by the health care provider or detrimental to the patient. Courts have confirmed this right. A well-known case involved Abe Perlmutter, a 73-year-old man who suffered from amyotrophic lateral sclerosis (ALS), or Lou Gehrig's disease. Mr. Perlmutter was conscious and competent but ventilator dependent. He had disconnected his ventilator himself on at least one occasion, but it was reconnected when an alarm alerted the nursing staff. Although Mr. Perlmutter found speaking to be difficult and painful, he was able to express how he was suffering and his wish to die. When the hospital refused to discontinue the ventilator, Mr. Perlmutter retained an attorney and petitioned the Broward County (Florida) Circuit Court. After a hearing, the court authorized removal of the respirator.

The state attorney general promptly appealed, arguing that anyone who assisted in removal of the ventilator was guilty of assisting suicide, a criminal offense in Florida. The district court of appeals affirmed the lower court decision and found that Mr. Perlmutter "should be allowed to make his choice to die with dignity." The day after this decision, Mr. Perlmutter summoned his family to his bedside, and his ventilator was disconnected. He died about 40 hours later. The Florida Supreme Court later upheld the court's decision.[32]

When a competent patient refuses treatment or refuses to cooperate with medical recommendations, the health care provider must document the situation objectively and carefully. In addition to stating that the patient refused treatment, the note must also state that the treatment and alternatives were explained, that recommendations were made, and that the patient refused treatment and was informed of the foreseeable or likely consequences of the decision. If the consequence is clear (e.g., death), it should be mentioned in the note. The views of the patient's family may be noted, if known, but the competent adult patient may make a decision of which even family members, including a spouse, disapprove. In these difficult situations, a family meeting, including the patient if the patient so desires, may prove useful in making it clear to the family that it is the patient who is making the decision rather than the health care providers. The risk manager or a representative of the facility's legal department should be notified and should participate in the case.

The Incompetent Patient: Guardians and Conservators

The law contains a presumption that persons are **competent** unless and until a court has declared them incompetent. All states have in place mechanisms by which a person or hospital may petition a court, most often the probate court, to have a disabled person declared incompetent. The state statutes contain definitions of incompetence that the court must follow. For example, in Connecticut one must be incapable of caring for one's self. That means

> a mental, emotional or physical condition resulting from mental illness, mental deficiency, physical illness or disability, advanced age, chronic use of drugs or alcohol, or confinement which results in the person's inability to provide medical care for physical and mental health needs, nutritious meals, clothing, safe and adequately heated and ventilated shelter, personal hygiene and protection from physical abuse or harm and which results in endangerment to such person's health.[12]

A **guardian** is defined as a person or organization judicially appointed to make decisions for the person; this may be a "personal" guardian (making decisions concerning the care, support, comfort, health education, and maintenance of the ward) or an "estate" guardian (making financial decisions concerning the ward and the ward's assets). The word **conservator** means guardian or protector—a person appointed by a court to manage the estate of one who is unable to manage property and business affairs effectively.[5] The procedure for having a guardian or conservator appointed varies from state to state. In general, the procedure commences with an application filed in court. The disabled patient is then served with a notice of the proceeding, and a hearing date is set. Often a lawyer is appointed by the court to represent the patient. Most states require one or more physician evaluations, provided either in writing or in person at the hearing. Other testimony may be taken.

Once the standards are met, a guardian or conservator (the terms are equivalent in this context) is appointed by the judge to act for the disabled person. A guardian may be appointed to protect assets (i.e., a **guardian of the estate/ property**) or to make decisions about health care and other personal matters (i.e., a **guardian of the person**), or both. The persons accepting guardianship appointment may, but need not be, part of the family. Although some states permit appointment of guardians with limited powers, most guardians have the power to make all necessary decisions for patients, regardless of what the patient's family requests.

Appointment of a guardian may take a month or more because the statutes provide for a hearing before the appointment. Where an emergency exists, states have a mechanism for the appointment of a temporary guardian. Since this appointment often occurs without a hearing, the standard for a temporary, emergency appointment is quite high. The health care provider (and often there must be more than one) must allege that the potential harm to the patient is imminent and the consequences dire if a guardian is not appointed to make decisions immediately.

Advance Directives

Today, patients have the right to make their own health care decisions. The patient's physician or another health care provider may advise the patient and make recommendations. The patient, however, has the right to be told about his or her choices of treatment in a way that he or she can understand. Patients have the right to accept or refuse any treatment that is offered and, regardless of their decision, continue to receive the care necessary to keep them comfortable. As a practical matter, guardians are appointed for very few hospitalized patients regardless of their mental capacity. If hospitals and nursing homes were to insist on a guardian for every incapacitated patient, the courts would be overwhelmed. Furthermore, the length of stay in the hospital would be greatly extended while the staff awaited the appointment of the guardian before treatment or placement decisions were made. Finally, there are usually reasonable alternatives to formal court-appointed guardianship.

There are several ways that persons, at a time when they are mentally competent, may inform others as to what their decisions would be regarding medical treatment in the event that they became incapacitated. These include use of a living will, appointment of a health care proxy, and use of a durable power of attorney for health care.

Living Will

Most states have statutes authorizing the use of a living will. A **living will** generally states the kind of medical care patients desire or do not desire if they become unable to make their own decisions. This document is called a living will because it takes effect while a person is still living. Most states have their own living will forms, which can vary from state to state.[46] Living wills may also be advance medical directives in some states. A living will is a document executed by a competent adult; formalities of execution vary among the states, but usually two people must witness the person's signature on the document. Witnesses to a living will must be prepared to testify that the person signing was competent at the time the living will was signed. States may disqualify certain persons as witnesses. For example, some states would invalidate a living will if it were witnessed by a health care provider with the power to directly order health care interventions for the individual. Therefore witnesses to a living will should no have responsibilities involving ongoing care of the patient. Many states also disqualify family members or others who may benefit under a patient's will.

A living will becomes applicable only when the patient is in a terminal condition (or, in some states, is permanently comatose) *and* is incapacitated. A **terminal condition** is usually defined as a condition that is incurable or irreversible and will result in death within a relatively short period of time if life support systems are not provided. **Incapacity** occurs when a patient is unable to understand and appreciate the nature and consequences of health care decisions and to reach and communicate an informed decision regarding the treatment.

Thus when a patient is terminal but still able to reason and communicate, the living will is not applicable. However, when the patient is terminal and loses the ability to formulate and state his or her wishes, the living will goes into effect.

The form used to express wishes may vary. Some state statutes contain recommended forms; patients may use standard or individualized forms in most states. Oral advance directives are also valid in some states under specified sets of circumstances. Whatever the form, it never seems to be detailed enough to cover every possible situation. It is therefore desirable for health care providers to discuss foreseeable decisions with the patient before his or her incapacity. These discussions should be well documented in the medical record. Most states provide that advance directives may be revoked orally, in writing, or by destruction.

States provide for procedures to be followed if a health care provider does not in good faith believe that the advance directive should be followed, and provide immunity for health care providers who in good faith follow an advance directive.

Health Care Proxy/Agent

As early as 1992, 16 states had statutes in place that permit a competent adult to appoint a decision maker, either in addition to a living will or in lieu of that document. The authority to appoint an agent or proxy is usually found within the state's living will statute. Execution formalities are generally the same as those for a living will.

The powers of a health care agent or proxy are usually limited to making decisions about implementation or withdrawal of life-sustaining treatment when a patient is in a terminal condition and is incapacitated. They also may grant the agent the power to make decisions in the patient's best interests if the terms of the living will are unclear or open to interpretation. In effect, these documents appoint a person with whom the health care team may discuss decisions that may seem appropriate under a living will.

Durable Power of Attorney

A **durable power of attorney for health care** is a written document that authorizes an individual, as an agent, to perform certain acts on behalf of and according to the written directives of another, the person executing the document, from whom the agent obtains authority.[39] The durable power of attorney for health care takes effect only on incapacity of the principal and becomes ineffective when and if the principal regains competency. Some patients have executed a general power of attorney. In many states these documents can be used to grant financial, banking, and other powers to manage a person's estate when that person can no longer do so. They can also designate a person to make health care decisions, but that power must be specifically enumerated in the power of attorney document. Some states limit the authority of the holder of the power where health care decisions are concerned, whereas others make the power unlimited if the document so states.

Patient Self-Determination Act

On December 1, 1991, the Patient Self-Determination Act went into effect. This federal statute is applicable to all federally funded facilities that receive Medicare or Medicaid reimbursement for patient care. The law requires that hospitals, nursing facilities, home health care services, hospice programs, and certain health maintenance organizations provide information to adults about their rights concerning decision making in that state. For hospitals this information must be provided to every adult patient on admission, regardless of the diagnosis. This material must include written information about the types of advance directives that are legal in that state. The institution must also describe its own policies regarding the exercise of these. Documentation that the patient has received the information must be placed in the patient's medical record. Proposed regulations (called an interim final rule) state that if the patient is incapacitated on admission, the information may be provided to a family member. This action, however, does not relieve the hospital of its duty to provide information to the patient once he or she is no longer incapacitated.[41]

Surrogate/Proxy Decision Maker (Other Than a Guardian)

Most patients do not have guardians, and many do not have advance directives to guide clinical decision making. When patients can no longer make decisions for themselves and no other guidance is available, hospitals and health care providers consult family members, or, if there are none, close friends, about what the patient would have wanted under the circumstances. Many states and the District of Columbia now have statutes addressing this long-standing practice. These statutes usually establish a list of persons, in order of priority, who may make decisions for an incompetent patient who has not left a living will or other instructions.[14]

Where family members and health care providers agree on the proposed course of medical treatment and it is clinically appropriate, it may proceed. Unfortunately, this is often not the case. The health care team may disagree with the family, or the family members may disagree with each other. Where the health care team disagrees with requests being made by the family, the team may decline to carry out the requests. For example, the family of a patient may request termination of ventilator support when the patient has suffered a brain attack/stroke just 12 hours before. If the prognosis is unclear, the health care team may, and possibly should, decline the request to remove the ventilator at that time. It should be made clear to the family, however, that within a reasonable time the prognosis should become clearer and the question of termination of treatment may be raised again. A member of the ethics committee of a large medical center wrote the following to a newspaper:[36]

We need to face our fear of death and dying. Too often discussions are left until late in the course of illness, when patients are unable to participate in decisions. With the medical technology that is available today, family members often demand that "everything be done" to keep loved ones alive, even against the patient's wishes and best interest. According to the American Medical Association's ethics code, physicians should not give medical care when a cure is no longer possible or the patient is not expected to recover. When there is no chance for recovery, why won't the family let go and permit the patient to be unfettered by feeding tubes, catheters, and ventilators; to be pain-free; and to die with dignity. Is that too much to ask?

There are also situations where family members disagree among themselves as to the proper treatment of a patient. In general, the decisions of the next of kin will prevail when there are conflicts. For example, a spouse has the decision-making authority regardless of the wishes of the adult children. When there is no spouse and there are several children who cannot agree among themselves, most would advise a family meeting to attempt to get a consensus. If the family cannot agree and one member is demanding one course of treatment and another is demanding a different course, the health care providers should refer the case to the committee established in their institution to deal with such situations or to the facility's legal department. In such a situation, the institution may petition a court for appointment of an independent guardian, usually called a guardian *ad litem,* to resolve the situation in accordance with the patient's wishes, insofar as they are known, or the patient's best interests.

SELECTED CLINICAL DECISIONS

Surgical Consent

The **consent for surgery** form should be properly witnessed, dated, and signed by the patient; in some hospitals it may also need to be signed by the physician or health care provider who is performing the procedure. It should also delineate the expected usual, unusual, and rare adverse consequences of the operation or procedure and the risks of nonperformance of the procedure, including the need for, risks associated with, and alternatives to the use of blood products.[23] In addition, alternative treatment options, which are available to the patient in the event of nonperformance of the procedure, should be listed.[23] Some hospitals may use a general consent form and require the physician to document specific risks, alternatives, and other information in the patient's medical record.

Case law confirms that the patient's consent must be obtained for medical and surgical treatment except in special circumstances. Whereas hospital personnel may presume consent when a patient acquiesces to procedures such as venipuncture, invasive radiologic and surgical procedures are handled more formally. In these cases the law requires that the patient be informed of the reasonable alternatives, if any, and the potential risks and benefits of the proposed procedure. It is the responsibility of the health care provider carrying out the procedure to be sure that the patient has been given enough information and has made an informed decision.[45]

In some institutions, consent forms are used to confirm that the patient has given consent; in others a note in the history and progress section of the medical record is considered acceptable. The form or note is more useful legally if the responsible physician has noted at least a few of the serious risks that have been discussed with the patient. Many facilities have eliminated the requirement that the patient's signature on a consent form be witnessed. In other places a clinician may be asked to witness the execution of the form. Unless there is a state statute stating otherwise, a witness to a consent form is simply able to testify that the signature was not a forgery. That witness need not be present during the discussion that precedes the signing of the form and generally is not required to state that the patient had received enough information to give informed consent. If the clinician who witnesses the signature, however, was present during the discussion, that clinician may testify about the content of the discussion.

Two common situations arise when the patient is incapacitated and unable to give consent. First, the patient may be incapacitated and the condition to be treated is a life-threatening emergency. With the assumption being made that the patient has not previously refused the procedure when competent and that it is clinically appropriate, consent is implied. When no informed consent is obtained, the reason why it was omitted should be noted in the medical record. If the decision is made that no expressed informed consent will be required or obtained, there should be no effort made after the completion of the procedure to obtain retrospective consent. Attempting to obtain written consent for a completed procedure after the fact implies that the consent was needed before initiating the procedure.

Second, the patient may be incapacitated and the procedure is indicated but not an emergency. Discussion with the family should occur, and their consent should be obtained.

Some patients do not have family or friends. If the patient is unable to make a treatment decision and consent is necessary, the health care team may do one of two things: (1) it may seek the appointment of a guardian to consent, or (2) it may get a documented second opinion that the procedure is necessary and is likely to benefit the patient (which can include providing pain relief or comfort) and then proceed.

Termination-of-Treatment Orders

Patients and families today are offered the opportunity to make decisions about withholding and termination of treatment that are much more complex than in the past. Do-not-resuscitate (DNR) orders now seem relatively routine as compared with other orders involving discontinuation of life support measures, including ventilator support and fluid and nutrition.

Do-Not-Resuscitate Orders

It has been reported that attempts at cardiopulmonary resuscitation (CPR) had taken place for 30% of patients who died at a major Boston hospital.[2] However, CPR may not be appropriate for all patients who experience a cardiac arrest because it is highly invasive and may constitute a "positive violation of an individual's right to die with dignity."[26] The rates of survival to hospital discharge after cardiopulmonary arrest and resuscitation in and outside the hospital have been shown to be similar and to range from 10% to 20%.[13]

Many states and accrediting organizations require that hospitals have a policy on the "withholding of resuscitative services from patients."[22] These policies should describe how the decisions are made, how conflicts are resolved, and the roles of the various health care providers. Most statutes regulating the use of DNR orders specifically apply to medical emergencies, which occur either (1) in a health care facility (e.g., a hospital or nursing home) or (2) outside the facility (e.g., in a patient's home). Many states authorize the use of a DNR identification device, which the patient wears so that the emergency medical technicians (EMTs) will be aware of and honor the DNR order. Statutes typically provide immunity for health care professionals acting in good faith in accordance with a DNR order.[18]

If a cardiopulmonary arrest occurs without an order in place, resuscitation should take place. A "slow code," where the clinician takes excessive time to call the code or the team takes excessive time to respond, should never be permitted—either resuscitation is indicated or it is not.

Whether to resuscitate a particular patient is a decision that must be made by the attending physician, the patient, and the family. Nurses and other personnel may have input into the decision. The consent of a competent patient should be obtained when a DNR decision is made. When the patient is incompetent and has left no indication of what his or her wishes would have been, the physician and the family make the decision. Where there is disagreement between the physician and the family, hospital policy should address the resolution of conflict.

Once a DNR decision has been made, the order should be written, signed, and dated by the responsible physician. The order should be reviewed periodically. Many hospitals have begun to address questions that arise when a patient with a DNR order goes to the operating room (OR). One article recommends that the DNR order not be suspended. Instead, it recommends that the anesthesiologist refrain from resuscitation only when the cardiac arrest is due to the patient's underlying condition.[8] Others have discussed whether a DNR order should be overridden when the complication is iatrogenic (caused by the therapeutic effort itself). One conclusion is that DNR orders should be honored no matter what the cause of the need for resuscitation, except in rare cases consistent with a person's known intentions.[6a] A new "limited aggressive therapy" order has also been advocated, which would allow patients to authorize CPR for "higher success" situations such as cardiac arrest in the operating room.[7a]

In 1987, New York became the first state to enact a statute addressing the withholding of CPR.[27] The statute states that every patient who has not consented to a DNR order is presumed to consent to resuscitation. It establishes the circumstances under which a family member or surrogate may consent to such an order if the patient is incapacitated; DNR orders are to be renewed every 3 days.[35]

Many other states have now adopted their own statutes concerning DNR orders. They generally address resuscita-

tion responsibilities for providers in the field and in the hospital. As with other forms of directives to withhold treatment, DNR orders may be revoked orally if the patient is capable of doing so.

Termination of Life Support, Fluid, and Hydration

Neuroscience patients in various settings (e.g., the emergency department, OR, intensive care unit [ICU], and other inpatient settings, as well as the home) may require decisions about **end-of-life care.** Ambiguity continues concerning the inability to predict a patient's life expectancy and decisions on effective versus futile treatment, when to limit treatment, comfort and pain management, and whether to perform CPR. The continuation of aggressive therapy is weighed against the potential to prolong death, pain, or suffering. There may not be consensus between the wishes of the patient, family members, and health care providers. Many states have statutes providing that ethically inappropriate and/or medically ineffective treatment is not required, subject to the provisions of the living will, health care agent, and surrogate health care decision maker laws.[48] Courts have been considering questions involving the definition of, use of, and termination of life support since 1976, the year in which the *Quinlan* case was decided in New Jersey. These cases have involved competent and incompetent patients, minors and adults, all afflicted with a condition that would eventually be terminal.

In most states, cases involving ventilator support have been brought to court before those involving other types of life support. The Perlmutter case, discussed previously, is atypical only because Mr. Perlmutter was competent. The majority of cases have involved patients who were incompetent by the time the request to discontinue ventilator support was made. In those cases the courts have generally permitted the use of substitute judgment by others.

Many states have now addressed the issue of withholding and withdrawal of artificially supplied fluid and nutrition. A Connecticut case involved Mrs. McConnell, a 57-year-old woman who had been in a persistent vegetative state for 3 years following an automobile accident. Before the accident, the patient had expressed her views about the maintenance of life when useful recovery is hopeless. The patient was being fed through a gastrostomy tube. After considerable discussion, the family asked that the tube be removed and the patient allowed to die. The nursing home refused to comply without court authorization.

The family commenced a court proceeding. After considerable evidence was presented about what Mrs. McConnell had said about her wishes, the lower court ruled in favor of the family. The case was appealed to the Connecticut Supreme Court. In January of 1989, that court affirmed the lower court's decision. Mrs. McConnell's feeding tube was disconnected. She died on February 28, 1989.

One of the most famous of recent cases concerned Nancy Cruzan, a young woman who suffered anoxic brain damage in an automobile accident. She remained in a persistent vegetative state in Missouri and was fed through a gastrostomy tube. After rehabilitation was unsuccessful, Ms. Cruzan's parents as co-guardians requested the withdrawal of the feeding tube. When employees of the rehabilitation center where she was a patient declined, the Cruzans sought judicial review of their request. After testimony, the trial court approved the parents' request.

On appeal, the Missouri Supreme Court reversed the lower court. It held that Missouri law would not permit surrogate decision making in issues of this importance. Thus, for a patient to exercise these rights, that person must have previously expressed wishes, either orally or in writing. Evidence of those wishes had to meet a high evidentiary standard, a standard the court held was not met in the lower court proceeding.

This case was appealed to the U.S. Supreme Court, and in 1990 it was affirmed on constitutional grounds.[11] After that opinion was issued, the Cruzans returned to the Missouri lower court and presented further evidence concerning what their daughter had expressed while competent. The lower court found that the Cruzans had presented clear and convincing evidence of what Nancy Cruzan would have wished. It then affirmed the right of the co-guardians to authorize withdrawal of the feeding tube. After withdrawal of the tube, Nancy Cruzan died on December 26, 1990.

Some health care providers oppose the withholding or withdrawal of life support (fluid and nutrition in particular) on ethical grounds despite the fact that it may be legal and considered by others as appropriate. Others fear that they will be accused of homicide or assisted suicide. Staff support of one another during these situations becomes critical. Given relevant state law, the hospital or nursing home may have an affirmative duty to comply with reasonable patient or family wishes, but most staffs will have a mechanism in place whereby nurses who are seriously troubled by a particular case may be assigned to other patients during that time.

The preceding discussion has presumed that the patient and family have requested the withdrawal of life support. In recent years, however, as health care providers have become more comfortable with these recommendations, they have met with resistance from families who wish to pursue all possible treatment. Just as some health care providers find it ethically difficult to terminate treatment under some circumstances, others find it improper to continue treatment that is considered inhumane. No law or legal principle requires that extraordinary, but clearly futile, treatment be provided. It is also probably true, however, that health care providers have no legal recourse against families who refuse to withdraw life support unless the patient has left written indication of his or her wishes before incompetency.

There has been one case that has addressed this complicated problem. The case involved Helga Wanglie of Minnesota, who in December 1989, at age 86, broke her hip. After a complicated course, Mrs. Wanglie, who was ventilator dependent and competent, suffered cardiopulmonary arrest. She remained in a persistent vegetative state. Pursuant to the wishes of her family, she was nourished by tube feeding and treated aggressively with antibiotics for recurrent pneumonia.

Hospital staff disagreed with the family's decision in this case and believed that Mrs. Wanglie would not benefit from aggressive treatment. The staff therefore believed that it was not obliged to provide aggressive treatment. The family remained firm in its view that aggressive treatment was what Mrs. Wanglie would have wanted. The hospital ethics committee became involved and advised the hospital staff to follow family wishes as it attempted to resolve the conflicts.

When disagreement remained, the hospital filed an application for the appointment of a nonfamily guardian to decide for the patient. The Minnesota court instead confirmed the husband as guardian, finding that he was in the best position to know the wishes of his wife. The court found that the hospital had requested the appointment of a nonfamily member not because Mr. Wanglie was incompetent to be guardian but because he disagreed with hospital staff.[10] Mrs. Wanglie died 4 days after the court order, still connected to the ventilator.

There has yet to be a case in which hospital staff directly requests a court to discontinue treatment over the objections of the family. Most authorities believe that a hospital would not prevail in making these arguments, at least in cases where the family is available and interested in the patient.

A recent, well-publicized case, *In re Schiavo*,[49] highlighted end-of-life issues when there is family disagreement as to termination of treatment. The case sparked heated public debate about withholding nutrition and hydration, what constitutes a "persistent vegetative state," and the conflicts of interest that may develop among family members concerning who should be surrogate decision makers. A positive result of the publicity surrounding the case is increased public awareness of the need to take all steps necessary before serious illness or incapacity to ensure that end-of-life wishes are followed.

The *Schiavo* matter had a long and convoluted procedural history, involving various court decisions, legislative enactments, and executive orders, at both the state and federal levels. The events began in 1990 when Terry Schaivo suffered cardiac arrest and subsequent anoxic brain injury. The care rendered was the subject of a medical malpractice settlement. Terry's husband, Michael, petitioned the court to be appointed guardian, which was granted. Terry's parents opposed the appointment and petitioned to overturn it. In 1998, Michael was granted permission to discontinue care, including hydration and nutrition, which was provided via a gastrostomy tube. Over the ensuing years, numerous appeals, including to the U.S. Supreme Court, special legislation, and state executive involvement captured national headlines. Eventually, Michael's decisions for Terry were carried out, Terry's feeding tube was removed, hydration was withheld, and she died. Resolution of the case in many ways raised more questions than it answered. Among them are the following: What constitutes a conflict of interest under surrogate decision-making and guardianship statutes? What is the meaning of "persistent vegetative state," and how is it medically defined and determined? What standard of proof is required to determine the preinjury wishes of the patient? What constitutes medical futility? How should the courts balance the patient's or family's right to refuse care versus the state's interest in preserving life? The case compelled many people to engage in personal end-of-life planning, to make their wishes known to close family and friends, and to take all available steps to ensure that courts will not be involved when or if they become incapacitated.

In most instances, problems of terminating treatment need not be resolved in court. Decisions regarding treatment and nontreatment that meet accepted medical and hospital standards and with which the patient concurs are made every day without legal risk. When the patient is incapacitated, family members generally make decisions for the patient. Finally, a distinction should be made between termination of treatment and termination of care. Even patients who are not being treated for their terminal condition require sensitive and competent nursing and medical care so that their final days can be as comfortable as possible. The families of these patients may also require information and support during this difficult period.

Brain Death

In 1968, Harvard criteria established standards for determining brain death.[20] It was recommended that brain, or cerebral, death be adopted as the basis for pronouncing death.[17] The criteria are so reliable that no case has "yet been found that met these criteria and regained any brain functions despite continuation of respirator support."[29] Some states have adopted the Harvard criteria by statute, whereas others have chosen to define brain death in broader, less restrictive terms.

Brain death occurs when all vital functions of the brain, brainstem, and spinal reflexes are irreversibly nonexistent as determined by accepted medical standards.[5] A patient who is brain dead is legally dead, and there is no duty to continue to treat. It is not necessary to obtain court or family approval to remove a ventilator or other life support system from a patient who is brain dead. Most authorities, however, consider it useful to obtain family agreement, if only so that the family will not believe that the patient will miraculously regain consciousness.

Examples of prerequisites that a hospital may use in the declaration of brain death include the following:
- Radiological imaging showing an acute central nervous system (CNS) catastrophe compatible with a clinical diagnosis of brain death
- The exclusion of complicating medical conditions that may confound the clinical assessment (e.g., severe facial trauma that interferes with the assessment of brainstem reflexes, sleep apnea, or severe pulmonary disease that results in chronic retention of CO_2)
- The exclusion of a drug overdose or poisoning (toxic levels of any sedative drugs, aminoglycosides, tricyclic depressants, anticholinergics, antiepileptic drugs, or neuromuscular agents)
- A body temperature of 35° C (95° F) or above
  Criteria for the diagnosis of brain death may include the following:
- Coma and cerebral unresponsiveness with no motor response to pain in all four extremities
- Absence of spontaneous movement, including abnormal flexion, abnormal extension, and seizures (with the exception of spinal reflexes)

- Absence of brainstem reflexes
- Apnea test that follows hospital protocol
  Tests to confirm brain death for a clinical diagnosis may include the following:
- Electroencephalography with electrical silence during at least 30 minutes of recording and when repeated at least 6 hours later
- Cerebral circulation at a standstill as witnessed by the following:
  - Conventional angiography
  - Radioisotope brain scan with no uptake of isotope in the brain parenchyma
  - Transcranial Doppler (TCD)
  - Cerebral blood flow studies

When the established protocols have been met, and the determination of brain death has been made by a physician, documentation is made in the patient's medical records. The mechanical support can then be discontinued by the physician.

If the ventilator is to be discontinued on a patient who is brain dead, care should be taken first to determine that organs are not to be donated. If organ donation is to take place, the institutional protocol for continuing life support should continue. If the original injury leading to the patient's brain death was of a criminal nature, when the patient dies, the charges against the perpetrator may be increased to homicide. If the police are involved, it may be useful to contact them to inform them that life support is to be discontinued and to inquire about necessary documentation of the brain death status. This will assist the prosecutor in avoiding allegations from the accused that the death was caused by the termination of life support and not by the original injury.

Organ Donation

Every state in the United States has a law based on the Uniform Anatomical Gift Act. These statutes establish the legality of organ donation by individuals and their families and establish procedures for making and accepting gifts of organs. In general, the patient, before incompetence, may execute a document indicating his or her desire to donate an organ or organs; despite the fact that the patient may have done this, most facilities will still obtain the consent of the next of kin at the time of death. If the patient has not indicated his or her wishes about donation, most statutes will list those family members, in order of priority, who may give consent for donation. In some states individuals can declare on their driver's license that they wish to be an organ donor.

Many states now also have in place "required request" statutes that require health care providers to ask adult patients about their organ donation status. Where required, the response must be noted in the medical record.

Hospitals should have in place policies to guide the staff in determining which patients may be suitable for organ donation, procedures for inquiring about the possibility of donation, and procedures to be followed if the patient or family agrees that donation is desirable.

Autopsy

Autopsies are the most frequent cause of litigation involving dead bodies and health care providers. Autopsies are performed primarily to determine the cause of death.[39] The laws concerning autopsy are, for the most part, statutory; there has been little change in the laws in the past 20 years.[19] The statutes set forth two types of authority to authorize the conduct of a postmortem examination: autopsies are to be done only with patient or family consent unless a statute confers authority on a third party, such as a coroner or medical examiner.[33] Most states have statutes that require notification of the coroner or medical examiner when a death may be due to violence or suicide, or is unexplained. Some statutes also require notification when the death occurs outside a hospital or nursing home or when it occurs within 24 hours of arrival at a hospital.

Once the medical examiner, who is a physician but who may not be a pathologist, has been notified of the death, he or she is empowered by statute to conduct an investigation. The scope of that investigation may, but need not, include an autopsy. If an autopsy is to be done by the medical examiner, no family consent is needed. Several cases have challenged the medical examiner's authority to conduct an autopsy even over the protests of the next of kin; in most cases this authority has been upheld as long as the case fits within the statutory authority.

In cases where the medical examiner declines to do an autopsy, or when the circumstances of the death do not require medical examiner involvement, the statutes usually list those family members, in order of preference, who may give consent. If the statute does not provide a list, it may simply state that the next of kin, who takes responsibility for burial of the body, may consent. Some statutes explicitly authorize the patient to give predeath permission for his or her own autopsy.

When a patient or family member consents to an autopsy, the autopsy may be limited to a particular body part or system, such as the heart. Any restrictions on the scope of the examination should be noted on the autopsy consent form. Information obtained by the autopsy will be used to complete the death certificate and may be used in civil or criminal proceedings involving the patient's death.[24] Although information on death certificates is public, autopsy records are to be kept confidential like all other medical information, except in those states that make medical examiner findings public. A patient retains the right to confidentiality even after death.

PROFESSIONAL LIABILITY CONCERNS

Professional liability cases involving the care of the neuroscience patient involve the same principles as all other malpractice cases. When a patient or his or her estate sues for injuries alleged to have been caused by professional negligence, or malpractice, monetary damages are sought. **Negligence** is conduct that falls below an accepted standard of care. Although each state defines standard of care in its own way, it is the doing or failure to do what is required of a reasonably competent professional in similar circumstances. Negligence as a "cause of action" has four key elements. In order to sustain a case for medical or nursing malpractice, each of the key elements must be present and proved.[30]

Elements of a Malpractice Case

To win a professional liability or **malpractice** case, the plaintiff must allege and prove the key elements of malpractice—the four *D*'s:

1. **Duty:** What should have been done by the nurse. (The nurse [defendant] had a "duty" to the patient.)
2. **Dereliction of duty** (negligence): Failure to meet the standard of care.
3. **Direct results** (causation): Injury being the direct and legal cause of the deviation from what should have been done by the nurse.
4. **Damages:** Actual loss or medical damages suffered by the patient (plaintiff).

A nurse who cares for a patient assumes a "duty" to that patient to use reasonable care. Although the law does not require the health care provider to always be correct in the judgments made, it does require the **standard of care (SOC)** to have been met. The SOC is set by what the reasonably prudent nurse would have done, or not done, under the same or similar circumstances. It is a prospective standard, not retrospective, and is set at the time of the incident, not at the time the suit is brought or at the time it is tried. The attorney for both the patient plaintiff and defendant clinician will investigate to determine if the clinician, assigned to the patient and therefore responsible for the patient's care for that period of time, either through omission or commission, failed to perform certain functions or performed those functions below the SOC.

The **statute of limitation (SOL)** establishes the time period within which a claim may be filed or within which certain rights can be enforced, which in many states is 2 years. In the case of minors, the statute is usually longer. However, the trend is toward shortening extensions of the SOL afforded to minors as the individual states address "tort reform" issues. By setting a limit, the SOL prevents individuals from waiting years to file, by which time memories have faded and information is more difficult to discover.

All elements of a medical or nursing malpractice case, including establishment of the standard of care, must ordinarily be proven by expert testimony. The type of expert testimony needed will vary depending on the circumstances of the case; it might be provided by a generalist if the issue is assessment of protection of a patient at risk for falling but might be very technical if the issue involves the care of a patient undergoing surgery for epilepsy. Expert testimony will be based on information such as hospital records and policies; nursing literature available at the time of the incident; and statements, standards, and guidelines from various accreditation, nursing, and professional organizations that could be seen as relevant.

The purpose of an **expert witness** is to explain to the jury matters that are outside the realm of knowledge ordinarily possessed by a layperson. This may includes matters that require special skill, knowledge, experience, and/or training, such as the nursing standard of care and causation. The trial judge is vested with the discretion to determine who may testify as an expert witness and on what matters. However, it is still the duty of the jury to consider what weight to give the testimony of an expert witness (along with all other evidence) when deciding upon a verdict.

In many cases, the SOC itself is vigorously disputed, whereas in others the defense does not dispute it. For example, where the allegation involves an intramuscular injection, which is alleged to have damaged the sciatic nerve, the plaintiff and defense should agree on the standard for the proper placement of a gluteal injection.

Once the SOC is established, the plaintiff, who is the party bringing the lawsuit, must prove that the defendant nurse or staff breached it. This means that the plaintiff must show that what the nurse did or failed to do did not comport with the standard required at the time. In most states, a physician may testify to the nursing standard of care and that a nurse breached the standard of care. Conversely, it would be unusual for a court to permit a nurse to testify as to the standard of care for a physician or that the physician's actions fell below it. See, for example, *Broehm v. Mayo Clinic*, 690 N.W 2d 721 (2005), where a geriatric nurse practitioner was found unqualified to render affidavit opinions concerning standard of care for a thoracic surgeon. In disallowing the testimony, the court found that the nurse had neither the practical experience nor the education and training to so testify.

Some states have taken action to prevent physicians from establishing the standard of care for nurses. The Illinois Supreme Court recently held that only a nurse expert witness can establish the standard of care for a defendant nurse.[53] At the time the case went to the Illinois Supreme Court on appeal, the American Association of Nurse Attorneys was in the process of developing a position paper advocating that only nurses should be allowed to testify as to nursing standards of care. They filed an *amicus* brief on the issue. Other states by statute or case law have limited or eliminated the role of the physician in establishing the standard of care for nurses.

Then, the plaintiff must prove that the breach of the standard caused the injuries alleged. This may also be an area of dispute in the lawsuit. Causation must be reasonably proximate and not too remote and unlikely. States differ on the issue of what constitutes proximate causation. Some say that the negligent conduct must be "the proximate cause" of the injury; some say that the conduct must be "a proximate cause"; some hold that the conduct must only be "a substantial factor" in bringing about the injury, and the element of foreseeabilility of the injury may be expressed or implied. A medication error, for example, is almost always a violation of the SOC. However, it may be unrelated to a poor outcome, be part of the cause, or be the direct cause of the outcome, depending on the facts. Medical causation is almost always addressed by a physician expert witness. Only in rare circumstances is an expert nurse permitted to testify that a breach in the standard of care caused a particular injury. For instance, in *Sherman v. Bristol Hospital, et al*, 79 Conn. App. 78, 828 A 2d 1260 (2003), an advanced practice nurse (APN) was called on to testify that postoperative monitoring was negligently performed by a nurse who was caring for an obese patient with heart disease who was receiving morphine. The court allowed that testimony, but would not let the nurse go a step further to testify that the failure to monitor the effects of morphine caused the patient to develop a heart attack and congestive heart failure. While recognizing that a nurse might qualify to testify concerning causation in the appropriate case, this particular witness did not possess such qualifications. When nurses attempt to testify in the area of causation, their qualifications to do so will almost always be challenged by the opposing party.

Finally, the plaintiff must prove damages. Damages are generally divided into two categories: special and general. Special damages are pecuniary losses associated with identifiable, absolute dollar figures. Examples are medical expenses, cost of future care, and lost income. General damages are physical and emotional damages. In most jurisdictions there must be at least some physical injury before damages for "pain and suffering" can be collected. Even a minor injury is compensable; the nature of the injury simply affects the amount of money the case is worth. Many states permit at least some types of cases involving emotional distress only. Special damages such as cost of past and future medical care, past and future lost wages, and future expenses for rehabilitation, housing, vocational training, equipment, and other items that are caused by the defendant's negligence are also available if they can be proven.

Over the last 20 or so years, many states have enacted caps on damages as part of a proposed solution to the "insurance crisis." These caps vary from state to state and can consist of no caps at all, caps on noneconomic damages (pain and suffering), and caps on the total amount of damages, regardless of type. Generally, the jury is not informed of the cap, is permitted to award the amount of damages it deems appropriate, and the award is then reduced by the judge to conform to the applicable cap. There are frequent challenges to the constitutionality of these caps, often on the grounds of equal protection in that they unfairly prejudice the severely injured patients who have experienced great pain and suffering. Caps on damages are a hotly contested and constantly evolving societal and political issue that affects both the injured party and the health care providers involved.

Unfortunately, not all patients experience an expected or optimal clinical outcome. A poor outcome alone does not constitute negligence. The plaintiff must prove with reasonable probability (greater than 50% chance) that the poor clinical outcome was caused by a breach of the standard of care by one or more health care professionals.

Common areas in which nurses and health care agencies are at risk for legal action may include the following:

- Medication errors: the "five rights"—failure to give the right medication, the right dose, the right route, at the right time, to the right patient; injection injury
- Prevention of injury related to the patient's falls, burns, or other injuries
- Failure to carry out and follow physicians' orders

- Failure to detect and to report in a timely manner a significant change in the patient's condition
- Failure to properly assess (e.g., neurologic assessment skills fell below the SOC)
- Failure to observe and promptly report defective equipment
- Failure to communicate correctly a telephone or verbal order from a physician
- Failure to document the patient's condition in the medical record accurately, in a timely and comprehensive manner
- Failure to provide appropriate nursing measures
- Failure to follow established nursing SOC procedures
- Failure to properly supervise ancillary staff or student nurses
- Failure to provide safe and adequate staffing, such as specialty nurses in specialized nursing units (e.g., ICUs)
- Failure to document patient/family teaching, discharge information, medication, or treatment
- Infliction of or failure to relieve pain and suffering
- Inadequate knowledge and skill by the health care professional
- Patient abandonment: abandoning care of a patient without arranging for assumption of that responsibility by another health care provider
- Failure to implement special precautions (e.g., implementing seizure, spinal, and aspiration precautions; keeping the head elevated; having alarms on at all times; leaving side rails up and the bed in the low position; releasing the patient from restraints; turning and repositioning the patient every 2 hours)
- Failure to recognize self-harm or harm to others, suicide potential, wandering, and elopement
- Performing treatments or care outside the scope of practice or the state practice act (or both)
- Destruction or alteration of medical records
- Breach of confidentiality
- Premature or unsafe discharge
- Failure to "go up the chain of command" when physician action or inaction is threatening patient safety

NEUROSCIENCE NEGLIGENCE AND CASE LAW

Prevention of negligence is the best way to avoid legal difficulties. On July 1, 2001, new patient safety standards went into effect; these standards require hospitals to initiate specific efforts to prevent medical errors and to tell patients when they have been harmed during treatment and while hospitalized. The Joint Commission on Accreditation of Healthcare Organizations (JCAHO) evaluates more than 5000 hospitals and is urging hospitals to reevaluate policies and procedures to make sure patient safety is a priority. The commission's goal is to create health care environments in which caregivers feel comfortable not only reporting errors but also participating in system changes that could keep these errors from happening. In addition to actual completion of appropriate care for patients, proper documentation of that care, observation pursuant to providing that care, and the responses to care should all be entered in a timely way in the patient's record.[30] The neuroscience cases presented in this section are intended to illustrate the legal and professional principles that apply in malpractice cases. Not all of these cases occurred in neuroscience units; however, all of them could have.

Patient Falls

A fall may be defined as an untoward event in which the patient comes to rest unintentionally on the floor. This includes patients slipping, patients found lying on the floor, and patients falling during assistance by the nurse.[4] Patient falls are extremely common problems and the reason for numerous lawsuits. Neuroscience and older patients are potential fall victims and may be at high risk for injury from falls for the following reasons:

- Cognitive impairment: Poor judgment, impulsiveness, and failure to use assistive devices or call for assistance may lead to falls.
- Confusion/disorientation: Older patients may have "sundowning" or get confused at night and get out of bed to use the bathroom, or to go home.
- Movement disorders, mobility, dystonia, and problems with balance or gait.
- Medical conditions: Dehydration, dizziness, hypoglycemia, delirium, and cardiac dysrhythmias may predispose patients to falls.
- Sensory impairment: May include deceased vision, glaucoma, cataracts, macular degeneration, and decreased hearing, which contribute to a higher risk for falls.[15]
- Dementia: Alzheimer's and other types of dementia.
- Medicated: Patients may be under the influence of a sedative, harsh laxative or bowel preparation, or mental status–altering drugs; diuretics may cause a patient to climb over the side rail to get out of bed to use the bathroom.
- Seizures: Patients with epilepsy or seizures may fall during the event.
- Braces/walkers/assistive devices: Patients who use assistive devices to ambulate are at higher risk for falls.
- Brain attack/stroke: Cerebrovascular disease may cause a "drop attack" or loss of consciousness in which the patient suddenly loses consciousness and falls.
- Orthostatic hypotension: A drop in blood pressure may cause a patient to suddenly fall.
- Advanced age: Patients older than age 60 are at greater risk.
- Previous history: A patient who has fallen previously is at higher risk.
- Substance abuse: Drug and alcohol abuse increase the patient's risk.
- Ill-fitting footwear: Shoes or slippers that do not fit well or that have slippery soles create a hazard for ambulation.

Many neuroscience patients who fall are older adults. Although 90% of these falls do not result in injury, at least 5% of older adults who do fall sustain fractures.[38] It has been estimated that more than 250,000 people, mostly older adults, break their hips every year in the United States. Only about 25% of patients with a hip fracture make a full recovery, and 20% die within 1 year by some estimates. Older adults are hospitalized for fall-related injuries five times more often than they are for injuries from other causes. Of those who fall, 20% to 30% suffer moderate to severe injuries that reduce mobility and independence and increase the risk of premature death.[7] Patient falls that result in injuries are the primary basis for numerous lawsuits against hospitals and nursing staffs. Although courts will not impose liability under all circumstances, it is clear that the nursing staff must assess patients for risk of falling and institute reasonably appropriate precautions. Factors to be considered include the patient's age, disease state, neurologic and musculoskeletal function, amount of sedation, and mental status.[6]

Neurologic illness often impairs a patient's mental status, sensory-perceptual function, and motor function, creating significant disability.[4] Facilities that have protocols, a performance improvement (PI) process, and aggressive fall prevention programs are able to reduce the incidence of patient falls without the use of restraints by offering the following:

- Educational in-service program with validation of proficiency to create a heightened awareness among staff regarding fall prevention
- Safer environment with the bed in the low position, use of appropriate side rails and a call system, elimination of environmental hazards
- Grab bars and elevated toilet seats in bathrooms
- Every-2-hour toileting assistance for patients taking diuretics or who are dependent
- Bowel and bladder training programs
- Physical therapy for balance and gait training
- Motion detectors and alarm systems, pressure-sensitive alarms under the mattress or wheelchair cushion, closed-circuit television monitoring
- Padding of side rails for seizure patients
- Enlistment of sitters or family members to stay with patients who wander or pose a danger to themselves
- Beds that contain the patient without restraints
- Specially designed reclining chairs that have a high back and cushioning
- Placement of the mattress on the floor until another alternative (e.g., the Safe Keeper bed) becomes available

Courts will consider the same factors, as the following case demonstrates:[37]

Ms. Thompson was admitted to the hospital for treatment of a severe migraine headache. She was considered an ambulatory patient who was permitted out of bed (OOB) ad lib. During the night she fell from her bed onto a stool and then to the floor; no side rails were in place at the time. There was a dispute about the level of patient sedation, with the patient stating that she was heavily sedated and the staff disagreeing. The patient claimed lower spinal injuries as a result of the alleged fall (which had not been documented in the medical record).

The malpractice case was tried. At the conclusion of the plaintiff's case, the judge found for the defendants. The plaintiff appealed. The appeals court held that in order to prevail in the case, the patient must show that the physician had ordered side rails or that the patient's condition was such that hospital employees should have known that side rails were required.

Restraints

Restraints are regulated by the U.S. Food and Drug Administration (FDA) as medical devices. The use of restraints has changed over the years and is now considered a "last resort." Restraints are referred to as **protective devices.** In 1996, new JCAHO restraint and seclusion standards became effective. These 25 standards define how hospitals, physicians, and other caregivers provide care for patients who are being restrained and define the facility's responsibilities concerning restraints and seclusion. The facility, organization, staff education, and resources must support the use of restraints and alternatives. The new standards were developed with the intent of reducing the use of restraints and seclusion through alternatives for the patient.[34] Similar standards have been established by the Centers for Medicare and Medicaid Services (CMS) for facilities that receive Medicare and Medicaid funding as part of its delineation of patient rights.[50] The primary areas of focus concerning restraint usage are as follows:[34]

- Restraints are to be used only when other safe and effective alternatives have been considered or do not protect the patient, caregivers, or family.
- Each order must not exceed 24 hours of restraint for medical patients.
- The physician assesses and documents the continued need for restraints if the original order expires and there remains the need for restraints.
- If a restraint is removed before the ordered time limit and needs to be reapplied for the same behavior, a new order is not necessary.
- If a restraint is part of a medical, surgical, or diagnostic procedure or device, an order is not needed.
- If the restraint is part of a protocol, an order is not needed when qualified staff apply the protocol.

Adherence to the guidelines provides protection to the patient and also to the staff in the reduction of patient falls. It is the responsibility of the nurse to keep the patient safe. The role of the caregivers includes following the agency's policy to identify patients at high risk using a fall assessment; communicating and documenting the implementation of a fall prevention program; and, if a patient should fall, protecting him or her from further injury. Also, after a witnessed or unwitnessed patient fall, the following guidelines should be followed:

- Examine the patient, and determine whether to move the patient or to call for help.
- Use an appropriate patient mover placed under the patient and with an appropriate number of assistants to return the patient to bed; keep the patient immobilized and protected from further injury.

- Stay with the patient, and notify the house officer or physician on call, attending physician, supervisor/nurse manager, and family.
- Complete an initial assessment, compare it with the patient's baseline, and document findings; be alert to patients who are on a regimen of anticoagulants and the increased risk for cerebral hemorrhage.
- After the patient has been examined by the responding physician, implement and record new orders.
- Continue to closely observe, monitor, and frequently reassess the patient, and record the neurologic assessment and vital signs until the patient is stable or until the vital signs return to baseline.
- If the patient is to undergo emergency x-ray studies, computed tomography (CT), magnetic resonance imaging (MRI), or other diagnostic studies, notify the radiology department and plan to transport the patient as ordered.
- If the patient has sustained an injury, prepare for treatment or surgery.
- Document all of the facts and prepare to turn the patient's chart over to the next caregiver (e.g., OR staff).
- Follow policy for completing an adverse or incident report.

Clinical Deterioration: Assessment and Intervention

Another expanding area of professional liability risk for the nursing staff concerns the recognition of and response to clinical deterioration of the patient. As a corollary to the nurse's independent duty of care to a patient, the nurse must also be observant, use appropriate standards for patient assessment, and call for further assistance if necessary. The failure to do this may result in permanent damage to the patient and corresponding liability—if the failure to recognize the patient's condition violated the standard of care.

The following case illustrates this point:[3]

A patient was admitted with a diagnosis of possible pulmonary embolism (PE); she was heparinized on admission with a bolus of 7500 units. Thereafter she received 2000 units/hour intravenously. The patient was in the ICU. At 5:00 AM a medical technician performed a venipuncture at the right antecubital vein to take blood; he was unaware that she was heparinized and had to stick the patient five times before he obtained the needed blood. Beginning at about 7:30 AM, the patient complained of pain at and around the elbow site. An uninflated blood pressure cuff was left on the patient's right arm throughout the night; it remained there after the venipuncture and was used throughout the morning hours. The nurse testified that she examined the right arm and never saw a hematoma. She called the physician, who arrived at about 11:50 AM. He found that the patient had a large hematoma, which he treated. He also decreased the heparin dose. However, the patient suffered permanent neurologic injury to the arm. In the malpractice case that followed, the medical technician and nurse were found liable—the former for not taking proper precautions while drawing blood from an anticoagulated patient and the nurse for failing to recognize and respond to the patient's complaints. The

jury awarded the plaintiff $55,000 in damages plus $2,376 in medical expenses. The verdict was appealed. The court found that the expert testimony of the nurse was convincing and that neither the nurse nor the medical technician had treated the anticoagulated patient with an understanding of the risks of hemorrhage; the original verdict was affirmed.

Documentation

Documentation in the patient's permanent record is primarily a communication tool for the health care team to follow the patient's progress for continuity of care. The patient's record is also used for payers, research, and legal proceedings. Proper and adequate nursing documentation of care probably prevents lawsuits, but the statistics are not known. What is known is that perfectly adequate, but poorly documented, care may be impossible to defend. **Accurate and contemporaneous documentation** is considered the most reliable record of the events of a case. Charting should be done chronologically. To avoid misinterpretation or mistakes, writing should be legible. All entries must be in ink, dated, timed, and signed. Some institutions now require that entries be in blue ink to distinguish between originals and copies. Of course, many institutions now use electronic charting formats.

There are numerous cases in the legal literature in which documentation of the patient's record has affected the outcome of the case. An example is *Collins v. Westlake Community Hospital:*[9]

A 6-year-old boy was admitted with a left leg fracture following an accident. The leg was reduced and placed in a cast. The attending physician instructed the nursing staff to "watch the condition of the toes." That night the nurse on duty noted the condition of the toes and circulation several times in the child's record. The next day the boy did well; his physician saw him at 11:00 PM, and there was adequate circulation. The night nurse on the second night did not chart findings concerning the toes or circulation until 6:00 AM, when she noted that the left foot was cold and dusky. Surgery was performed immediately to remove a clot in the femoral artery; ultimately, the leg was amputated.

In the subsequent malpractice case the nursing staff testified that it was not customary to chart negative findings. However, when the appeals court addressed the question of the directed verdict for the hospital, it noted that "the failure by the nurse who was on duty during the crucial period to make any entry of observations that she made concerning the circulation in [the child's] foot, all could very well have led the jury to draw the inference that no such observations were made between 11:00 PM and 6:00 AM." This case was revised, and a new trial was ordered against the hospital as employer of the nurse.

This case is often cited for the commonly heard proposition that "if it is not documented, it is not done." This truism may not be accurate for routine care, such as checking normal skin for decubiti. However, when there is already a problem requiring nursing attention, when pain medications are administered, when the patient is noncompliant, or when observations are critical to the patient's diagnosis, documentation of even negative findings is required. For example, when neurologic signs are to be checked every hour, the fact that those signs are checked is to be noted even if there is no change from the prior charting. The same is true of vital signs—they are always charted despite the fact that they are often within normal limits (WNL). The use of abbreviations in charting should be limited to hospital-approved abbreviations; use of unusual or ad hoc abbreviations may lead to confusion and errors in patient care.

Record Tampering

No portion of the record is to be obliterated, erased, altered, or destroyed. Because the record is a legal document, any changes made may constitute tampering. Hospital policy usually states that corrections to the record must be made by drawing a single line through the error, with the correction dated and initialed. Nurses should never allow anyone to persuade them to tamper with a patient's medical record by doing the following:

- Deleting information or significant facts previously charted
- Altering a patient's medical record by removing and rewriting previously charted information, especially if the patient had a bad outcome or an adverse event
- Making late changes that are fabrications (e.g., checkmarks or entries on flow sheets to make it appear, for example, that care was provided, including vital sign assessment, treatments, or medications)
- Trying to squeeze information between lines or in blank spaces left in the chart
- Altering or adding information to another nurse's documentation
- Removing, destroying, or hiding any portion of the medical record
- Charting information that the clinician knows is not factual

Alterations in medical records often make defensible cases indefensible. If a jury thinks that a nurse has changed medical records after the fact, the nurse's credibility will be damaged and the case may be lost. Alterations in medical records may also void insurance coverage for the incident. In addition, alteration or destruction of medical records is a criminal offense in some jurisdictions. Any change in the medical record that the nurse deems necessary should be made according to institutional policy. Most facilities have a procedure for making "late notes," which should be followed if changes or additions to the records are made.

Selected Nursing Issues

There are now a number of issues that affect nursing practice but that have not been traditionally thought of as patient care issues. Many of these concerns have developed because of changes in federal legal requirements; others have evolved secondary to changes in the nursing profession.

The **Healthcare Integrity and Protection Data Bank (HIPDB)** was established in 1996 by federal law and began operating in 1999. It was created by the Health Insurance Portability and Accountability Act of 1996 to protect the public against fraud and abuse in the areas of health insurance and health care delivery. The HIPDB contains reports of more than 40,000 cases in which nurses and nurses' aides have been disciplined or in which adverse actions were taken. The Health Resources and Services Administration describes HIPDB as a federal data bank of nurses. Only government agencies are allowed to access the information; this includes all state licensing agencies and state boards of nursing. However, individual nurses may access their personal information.

The **National Practitioner Data Bank (NPDB)** was designed to identify problem health care practitioners and to prevent them from moving from state to state when professional competence or other issues arise. Revocation of clinical privileges and malpractice payments, whether by verdict or settlement, are the type of actions that must be reported. The data in this repository are not available to the public. If a report is made to the bank, the practitioner may respond; that response is made part of the record.

Some states, such as Massachusetts, have enacted their own consumer protection regulations with a **"duty to report"** standard that requires nurses to report nurses who violate state standards. Reportable examples include a nurse who is impaired (e.g., chemical substance or alcohol), patient abuse by a nurse, or diversion of controlled substances. In general, nurses should report a nurse, or any practitioner, who harms a patient or who places a patient's health, safety, or welfare at risk. In addition, most states, as part of their Nurse Practice Act, require peer reporting to the state licensing agency concerning nurses who are violating the act in any manner.

The Patient Safety and Quality Improvement Act of 2005

The Patient Safety and Quality Improvement Act of 2005 (S.544; PL 109-41) was signed into law by President Bush on July 29, 2005. It amends the Public Health Service Act by establishing a confidential reporting system to enable health care professionals to voluntarily report information on errors to Patient Safety Organizations (PSOs). The PSOs are responsible for analyzing the data and formulating safety improvement strategies.

The patient safety information is confidential and cannot be used in any civil, administrative, or criminal proceeding. The goal is to improve patient safety without negative repercussions to the reporting or reported person or entity.

The Health Insurance Portability and Accountability Act of 1996

The Health Insurance Portability and Accountability Act of 1996 (HIPAA) was enacted primarily to ensure that workers could retain their health insurance when they changed jobs. A portion of the statute that was little-recognized at the time of enactment referred to confidentiality of a patient's protected medical information. HIPAA privacy requirements take precedence over all state laws that are less restrictive. It has affected the release of medical records, billing information, and other protected information. Within the context of litigation, records that were routinely produced as part of routine pretrial discovery now must be obtained by an HIPAA-compliant subpoena or an HIPAA-compliant authorization. It has affected the way every health-related office, place of employment, or health care facility handles patient privacy issues. Nurses must be very careful not to discuss a patient's health-related information with anyone but the patient or his or her authorized representative.

Standing Orders and Protocols

Because nurses have sought to bill for their services and the need for documentation to comply with federal and state requirements has increased, nurses have begun developing standing orders and protocols. These documents can be quite useful for nursing orientation, peer review of nursing practice, reimbursement, evaluation of employee performance, and other quality assurance activities. However, these documents also have considerable legal significance and should be drafted and reviewed with care.

A facility's own standing orders and protocols will form part of the basis for the standard of care (SOC) to which the nursing staff will be held in defending any professional liability action. Documentation of nursing standards within the facility is also used by representatives of state health departments and Medicare authorities when they seek to evaluate facility performance in light of a patient's complaint about care.

As a result of these competing uses, the content of nursing standing orders, protocols, and policies should be examined carefully. The requirements set forth in these statements should reflect current practice, not aspirations for the future. They should be drafted with sufficient flexibility that acceptable variations in care can occur without violating the standard. Unless they represent truly minimal care that all patients, regardless of condition, are receiving, they should be called guidelines and used that way. An introduction to the material, stating the uses and variations permitted, can be useful.

Written documents of this type should be reviewed by a number of persons to determine if they are too rigid. Once in place, they should be reviewed at least annually; the fact of that review should be noted on the signature page(s). Copies of outdated protocols and other documents should be retained in the nursing office. These are quite relevant in setting the SOC in a malpractice case. It is important to be able to produce the document that was in effect at the time of the incident, since the relevant standard is not what is being done at the time of the lawsuit. Finally, it is critically important to orient and reorient the staff to the presence and content of written material distributed by the nursing administration. It is no defense to any type of action that the nurse in question did not know of the existence of the written nursing requirements.

Less Than Optimal Staffing

Hospitals in America are experiencing a crisis in staffing. Increased patient acuity, increased patient loads, mandatory overtime, and staffing pressures to care for patients are overwhelming nurses. Although the shortage of nurses has seemed more acute in recent years, staffs have always had to cope with shifts or days where there seemed to be insufficient staff to care for patients. The quality of care is challenged today by serious business considerations facing hospitals daily, such as the need for downsizing and financial cutbacks. The hospital remains liable as a corporate institution if it fails to provide adequate staff for its patients.[16]

Hospital nurses complain that inadequate numbers of nurses, the increase in patient loads, verbal abuse, and a decline in the quality of patient care contribute to "burnout." Frustration, burnout, working extra shifts, and emotional or physical exhaustion can contribute to medication and treatment errors. The Institute of Medicine (IOM) has estimated that medication errors cause approximately 7000 hospital deaths a year nationwide.

If the nurse manager believes that staffing is insufficient, the manager must notify the nursing administration. This must be done even if the manager knows that no one is available to the floor. Once this is done, however, the nursing staff is not relieved of its responsibilities with regard to the care of the patients. The nurse manager or charge nurse must design the patient assignments with the qualifications in mind of those staff that are present. Then each nurse must set priorities for those patients (i.e., which care or treatment is critical and which seems less so and will be omitted). The following case illustrates this point:[21]

> Mr. Horton was admitted to a private room with a window that opened onto a balcony with a railing 3 feet high. The patient had a fever of unknown origin. He was later diagnosed as having pneumonitis. On admission, he was confused at times. At 3:30 PM, Mr. Horton was observed standing on the balcony and calling to construction workers nearby for a ladder. The workers notified the nursing staff, who returned the patient to his room and placed him in restraints. The charge nurse called the attending physician, who instructed the nurses to "keep an eye on the patient." The charge nurse then called the patient's wife at work and asked her to come and sit with her husband, since no hospital personnel were free to do so. Mrs. Horton responded by saying that she would send her mother, who lived a short distance away from the hospital. Mrs. Horton asked the charge nurse to have a nurse stay with her husband until her mother got there but was told that the staff could not "possibly do that." Mrs. Horton called her mother, who left for the hospital immediately. She arrived to find that Mr. Horton had already fallen from the second story to the ground. Mr. Horton survived the fall.
>
> In the lawsuit that followed, evidence showed that the patient unit was at capacity. There were no emergencies; all of the staff were engaged in routine duties that could have been postponed. Furthermore, an aide assigned to the unit was sent to supper at the time the charge nurse indicated that there was not enough staff to sit with Mr. Horton for 15 minutes until a family member arrived. The staff did not place Mr. Horton in additional restraints although they had the authority to do so. The trial court found in favor of the plaintiff in this case; an appeals court affirmed the lower court judgment.

Staff Interactions: Independent Duty of Care to Patients

It has long been held by courts that nurses have an independent duty of care to the patient that is separate from that of the physician. This independent duty carries with it certain responsibilities.

The nursing staff has an obligation to clarify physician orders that seem unclear or that may be inappropriate for the patient. For example, the nurse must inquire about a medication order that omits a route of administration or in which the dose seems excessive. In April 2001, a 9-month-old girl died in a Washington, D.C., hospital after a misplaced decimal point caused a nurse to administer two 5 mg doses of morphine for postoperative pain instead of two 0.5 mg doses only 2 hours apart. The infant went into cardiac arrest and died 4 hours after receiving the second dose of morphine.

In making the inquiry, the nurse should state the objection to the order; this approach should result in clarification, a change in the order, or an explanation as to the medical necessity for an unusual order. If the nurse is not satisfied, hospital policy should define the next steps. Normally, these would include involving the unit nurse manager or a representative of the nursing administration. Ultimately the question may be taken to the chief of staff or other medical officer charged with resolving these problems. If such approaches are unsuccessful, the nurse may refuse to carry out the order. A nurse who takes this action should have a clear safety concern.

It is never acceptable for a nurse to ignore an improper order; follow-up with the physician must occur in order to ensure adequate patient care. The same procedures should apply when a nurse calls a physician and considers the response inadequate, either because the physician did not respond to the call or because the treatment ordered seemed improper. If the patient continues to require physician attention, the nurse must persist in efforts to provide it through the chain-of-command steps established by hospital policy. Documentation of physician response should be factual; documentation should include times, dates, and a description of the information provided to the physician and his or her response. Follow-up efforts should also be documented in the patient record. Documentation in these cases should not include any evidence of nurse anger or frustration.

Equipment Malfunction

There is a duty to refrain from using equipment that is known to be defective or malfunctioning. If the equipment is not adequately maintained, has been making unusual noises, or is erratic in function and has not been repaired, the facility may be liable for damage caused by it. Nursing staff members may also be liable if they knew of problems and used the equipment anyway. The following case illustrates the potential liability:[31]

An infant was being treated with hypothermia after surgery during which she suffered a cardiac arrest. Although the nurse knew that the continuous readout thermometer often malfunctioned, she did not check the infant's temperature with a thermometer. When the infant's temperature began to rise and was accompanied by seizures every 15 minutes, the nurse did not use other methods to lower the temperature, nor did she notify the physician. Some hours later it was determined that

the mechanical thermometer was recording a temperature that was 4.6° lower than the infant's actual temperature. During the night the infant required mechanical ventilation. Although the nurse noticed poor air exchange, she did not correct a kink in the ventilator tubing. Furthermore, despite a physician's order, the nursing staff did not check and record neurologic signs on this infant. The infant suffered permanent neurologic damage and became cortically blind. In the malpractice case that followed, the court found that the injury was proximately caused by the negligence of the hospital's employees and by the defective equipment; the jury awarded $294,777.

Medical devices, defined as virtually anything used in patient care that is not a drug, include obvious devices such as pacemakers and defibrillators, as well as less obvious ones such as bedpans, suture materials, patient restraints, and tampons. Medical devices are regulated by the FDA. Before November 1991, hospitals, their employees, and their staffs were permitted, but not required, to report device malfunctions to the device manufacturer or to the FDA. Medical device reporting (MDR) is the FDA's mechanism to detect and correct serious problems that manufacturers, importers, and user facilities encounter.

On November 28, 1991, the Safe Medical Devices Act of 1990 (SMDA) became effective,[28] just after proposed regulations, called the Tentative Final Rule, were published for comment.[40] Certain amendments concerning reporting standards were signed into law in 1992 as the Medical Devices Amendments of 1992. In 1998, the Food and Drug Administration Modernization Act (FDMA) again modified reporting requirements, which were incorporated into MDR in 2000. This act, as amended, requires "user" facilities, which includes hospitals and ambulatory surgery facilities but not physicians' offices, to report to the manufacturer medical device malfunctions that result in "serious illness or injury" to a patient and to report to the FDA those that result in a patient's death. A **serious illness** or **injury** includes not only a life-threatening injury or illness but also an injury that requires "immediate medical or surgical intervention to preclude permanent impairment of a body function or permanent damage to a body structure."[43]

MedWatch, the FDA's Medical Products Reporting System, uses the Center for Devices and Radiologic Health (CDRH) to handle the reports and follow-up. The CDRH enters the information into a database, evaluates the event, and then determines whether follow-up investigation is warranted. Measures may include a recall, a press release, and public notification. As a result of this legislation, nursing staff will be participating in reporting device malfunctions, even those associated with user error, to a designated hospital department. Personnel in that area are generally responsible for determining which malfunctions engender an obligation to report and to whom.

DEVELOPING HEALTH CARE LAW

Probably one of the main issues that has concerned health care providers in the past few years is infection control. It has been estimated that hospital infections kill as many as

88,000 patients each year. Universal precautions to protect health care providers and patients are needed to prevent the transmission of pathogens.[42]

Legal and ethical issues in this area are complex, and the law is changing rapidly. Since those who have been infected with the human immunodeficiency virus (HIV), whether a health care provider or not, are covered by federal, and some state, antidiscrimination laws, there are complex employment[25,31,47] and labor issues, as well as potential risk to a facility that chooses to retain an HIV-infected health care provider and permits unrestricted practice. The Centers for Disease Control and Prevention (CDC) has stated that mandatory testing of health care providers is not indicated but that limitations on practice for those who are infected may be warranted after individual assessment of the provider's type of practice.

The Americans with Disabilities Act (ADA) prohibits "public accommodation," which includes hospitals and clinics, from discriminating against individuals with infectious diseases in their access to service. The ADA also prohibits job discrimination on the basis of a disability in places of public accommodation. The law applies specifically to any physical or mental impairment that substantially limits an individual (e.g., HIV infection). Patients with acquired immunodeficiency syndrome (AIDS) and those infected with HIV are considered handicapped under the ADA. The Rehabilitation Act has also imposed the same duty on health care facilities that receive Medicare and other federal funds.

AIDS and the HIV status of health care providers in the workplace are a controversial and complex issue. The American Nurses Association (ANA) has been on record in support of voluntary anonymous or confidential testing for HIV and the voluntary disclosure of HIV-positive status, when necessary, by infected health care providers.[5] In a case that involved a hospital's decision to discharge a nurse because he refused to divulge the results of his HIV test, a federal trial court held that because he did not meet the definition of handicapped under Section 504, the hospital had not discriminated against the nurse. The trial court ruled that the hospital fired the nurse because he refused to comply with an infection control policy and not because it perceived him as being HIV positive.[39]

In *Leckelt v. Board of Commissioners of Hospital District No. 1*, a Louisiana court held that a nurse was properly terminated for failing to reveal the results of his HIV test, because the interest of the hospital in learning the test results outweighed the privacy interests of the nurse. The hospital contended that it needed to know the information because the nurse engaged in invasive procedures (starting intravenous [IV] lines) and therefore could present a risk to patients.[39] Some state laws may require clinicians to submit to HIV testing if there has been patient exposure to the blood or body fluid of the clinician.

Health care providers have long been concerned about the risks to their own health that arise from confidentiality provisions meant to protect HIV-positive patients. There has been lobbying in many states by health care practitioners to legislate mandatory HIV testing on patients when a health care practitioner has suffered potential exposure to blood or body fluids and the patient's HIV status is unknown. Many states prevent such testing absent patient consent. Some states have allowed for involuntary patient testing under stringent guidelines with attendant confidentiality. For example, Montana allows for testing absent patient consent on previously collected blood in cases of exposure in a manner that may transit the virus where consent has been sought but denied. However, the facility is not required to perform the testing.[51] On September 30, 2005, the U.S. Public Health Service issued updated guidelines for management of occupational exposure to HIV, including recommendations for postexposure prophylaxis.[52]

Electronic means of practicing health care (telemedicine and e-medicine) raise new and unresolved issues for the health care practitioner. For instance, is giving advice by video linkup, computer, or telephone across state lines practicing without a license in the receiving state? How can patient confidentiality be maintained under these circumstances? With regard to medical records and other health records, what sort of retention policy is required? What are the consequences if medical or other records cannot be produced when requested or subpoenaed due to technical failures? These are issues that will need to be addressed by the courts and legislature as the electronic storage and transmission of important data becomes more prevalent.

Whether a nurse should maintain individual malpractice insurance when she or he is covered by her employer's policy is a frequent source of confusion. There is concern by nurses that if they carry their own policy, they will be personally named as a defendant in lawsuits to get at the extra money source. There is also concern that institutions will decline to support nurses who have their own insurance. Generally, the benefits of an individual policy outweigh the risk. If the insurance company covering the hospital is in bankruptcy or a predecessor to it, the nurse has an additional source of coverage. If the hospital's insurance carrier for any reason declines to cover the nurse's actions, the nurse will have her or his own insurance carrier to pay for defense and verdict or settlement costs. If there is a verdict against the hospital and nurse that is over the limits of the hospital's policy, the nurse will have an additional layer of protection. While an individual insurance policy may trigger the plaintiff's lawyers to name the nurse as a defendant, and the hospital's insurance carrier may want to split costs of defense with the nurse's carrier, the extra protection afforded the nurse from her or his own policy is most likely worth those risks.

LEGAL NURSE CONSULTING

Legal nurse consultants (LNCs) are nurses who serve as a liaison between the legal profession and the health care profession. An LNC's practice may include the plaintiff, the defendant, or both. Many LNCs work part-time as an LNC while working full-time in a hospital or health care facility, or work full-time in a law firm, independent practice, government agency, or insurance company, or in the risk management department of a hospital. The LNC may perform medical research, educate attorneys about a case, testify at trial, or work closely with risk managers to prepare a medical malpractice, personal injury, or other type of case. For more information about LNCs, see Resources at the end of this chapter.

LIFE CARE PLANNING

Life care planning is a subspecialty of many health care professionals. It is an important, dynamic document as a legal tool with implications for individuals with complex medical needs who have suffered catastrophic neurologic diseases and disabilities. Life care planning has emerged as a new trend associated with catastrophic case management.[1] A life care plan (LCP) can be defined as a dynamic document based on published standards of practice, comprehensive assessment, data analysis, and research that provides an organized, concise plan for current and future needs with associated costs, for individuals who have experienced catastrophic injury or have chronic health care needs.[44] Because the LCP is a unique document that outlines present and future lifetime needs, the services of a life care planner may be requested in the following situations: family member with a disabled child, spouse, or parent; money put into a reserve fund for insurance companies; workers' compensation claims; civil litigation; or mediation. Individuals who have suffered catastrophic neurologic injury or illness, such as spinal cord injury (SCI), a severe head injury, anoxic encephalopathy, extreme or chronic disabling pain, birth or congenital injury, or a stroke, may require an LCP for their long-term management to maintain a consistent high level of individualized care that includes provisions for funding and resources over the expected lifetime.

The Neuroscience Nurse as a Life Care Planner

Neuroscience nurses are uniquely qualified to become **life care planners** as a subspecialty area of practice because of their extensive background in and knowledge of neuroanatomy, neurophysiology, neurodiagnostic studies, neurologic assessment skills, neurologic procedures, neurosurgery, neurologic disease management, neuropharmacology, and expanded skills in the complex management of neuroscience patients. Neuroscience nurses have expertise in direct patient care, crisis interventions, case management of patients and families with catastrophic and chronic neurologic illnesses, and neurorehabilitation skills. Neuroscience nurse clinicians are especially qualified life care planners because of their familiarity with sophisticated medical equipment; their experience working with specialists from all disciplines and interacting with members of the medical, behavioral, and therapeutic disciplines (e.g., nutrition, hospice care, geriatrics, and pharmacology); and their knowledge of neuroscience terminology and documentation.

The Life Care Plan Process

The life care planner follows standard steps in the preparation process beginning with the referral. After discussing the case with the attorney or patient, written legal **permission for access to the patient's records** is needed. Complete copies of all medical records, log books, and pertinent documents are needed from the date of injury to the present date. Next, employment and salary (tax return) records are needed for the past 5 years, including performance evaluations, disciplines, awards, and bonuses. These documents demonstrate the preinjury required education and skills necessary for the individual's job performance. For school-age clients, academic and school-related records and test scores should be requested and any after-school or summer employment files. If the individual patient has an attorney, depositions and court-related materials should be requested.

Patient Interview and Assessment

After a thorough review of the medical records, a patient interview is scheduled for a home visit, the patient's current residence, school, or other settings. This visit includes interviews with the patient, family, and caregivers; a comprehensive neurologic evaluation; a list of all medications, supplies, and durable medical equipment (DME); inspection of the residence for special considerations, handicapped accessibility, and safety; and the need for wheelchair ramps, home health nursing, and therapy needs and other equipment. If the home visit and these steps are bypassed for only a **record review** in preparation of an LCP, essential elements may be missed that could seriously jeopardize the ability of the patient to safely and comfortably live at home in the community. Americans with disabilities should have the right to remain in a home setting with essential services provided versus a group home or other institutions.

Patient assessment and observation of the patient's activities of daily living (ADLs) in the home setting verus an office visit with a health care provider encourages family and caregiver input and is a critical guide for recommendations of future therapies, equipment, caregiver burden and home health care, necessary resources, future housing needs, and transportation for the patient and family.

Interdisciplinary Team Consultation

Consultation with members of the treatment team provides recommendations and information to project continuing long-term medical and surgical care and follow-up, future diagnostic studies, therapies, and other health care needs. Copies of past visits from treating team members and an organized file system with a **data collection tool** helps organize the vast volume of patient information. Research time is needed to review appropriate literature and to locate resources for supplies and vendors for medications, equipment, and other services.

LCPs are highly individualized and vary both in structure and content. When all of the data have been analyzed, the LCP is prepared with a brief introduction and narrative summary of the patient's case. The LCP describes the purpose of an LCP, reviews the patient's initial injury or illness, and provides information about the patient's past educational and employment status, past medical history, and current medical condition.[1]

Modules of Care Categories

A series of modules or tables are prepared by separating the patient's present and projected future needs into categories for ease of planning and defining associated costs. The tables may be divided into the following categories to include in the LCP based on the individual needs of the patient:[1]

- **Future evaluations** by members of the present or future health care team (e.g., neurologist, neurosurgeon, orthopedic surgeons, psychiatrist, or physiatrist)
- **Future therapeutic modalities** (e.g., physical therapy, occupational therapy, speech therapy, respiratory therapy, recreational therapy, cognitive therapy, coma arousal therapy, audiology, or visual therapy)
- **Future diagnostic studies**, including X-ray studies, CT, MRI, magnetic resonance angiography (MRA), ultrasound, arteriogram, x-rays, bone scans, and laboratory studies
- **Educational/vocational assessment** for evaluations to return to work or school and educational/vocational needs (e.g., special education to age 21, tutoring, public or private schools for students with special needs and disabilities, coaching for life skills training)
- **Orthopedic/prosthetic equipment** (e.g., braces/splints to control or correct deformities)
- **Nursing and facility needs** for care at home or a health care facility with nurses and health providers
- **Adapted home furnishings and accessories,** including special beds and equipment; fire, smoke, and carbon monoxide detectors for safety; and other items to allow the individual to live safely in a therapeutic home environment
- **Prescription medications** with monthly or annual costs
- **Over-the-counter (OTC) medication/supplies** (e.g., protective pads or undergarments, nonprescription drugs, syringes, skin and personal hygiene items)
- **Future medical/surgical needs** (e.g., botulinum toxin injections, heel-lengthening procedure, shunting for hydrocephalus, intrathecal baclofen or drug pump for medications or percutaneous endoscopic gastrostomy [PEG] tube placement)
- **Wheelchair needs,** ranging from a manual or power wheelchair to a sports all-terrain wheelchair, scooter, and wheelchair accessories
- **Special adaptive footwear and clothing** with easy Velcro fasteners to encourage independent dressing
- **Transportation needs** (e.g., an adapted van with a wheelchair lift and a lock-down wheelchair device, or allowance for local handicapped transit)
- **Home architectural modifications** for accessibility in compliance with ADA guidelines, including bathroom with roll in shower, modified kitchen or bedroom, and other home modifications (e.g., front and rear entrance ramps; an elevator; and enlarged door frames and hallways)
- **Health and strengthening needs** for leisure and recreational activities (e.g., summer or wilderness camps for individuals with disabilities, membership in local community reactional facilities)
- **Aids to independent living** to assist individuals with eating, grooming, and ADLs, and other assistive devices and equipment
- **Independent case management** services to coordinate care, implement the LCP, and improve the quality of care to prevent complications and hospitalizations

Completion of the Life Care Plan

The completed LCP organizes extensive data and condenses multiple reports into a concise plan of care. Physician experts may refer to life expectancy tables and provide input regarding the individual's injury and disability to project an individual's **life expectancy.** This number is used for projections of the associated costs of every item in the LCP. An **economist** is a professional who is frequently called on to compute the **present value** of the future medical needs and the **cost analysis** to calculate the total cost of the LCP.[44] The required services and most costly patient needs in the comprehensive LCP may include the fees for physicians, hospitalizations, nursing care, personal attendants, transportation (adapted van), and modified housing to accommodate wheelchairs and hospital beds and equipment. The total lifetime values of the LCP submitted by the economist may be used in court, to negotiate a legal settlement or to establish a trust fund for the individual.

After the life care planner has completed the LCP, he or she may be requested as a medical expert for the daunting task of testifying in a deposition, legal hearing, or civil court proceeding. This opportunity provides a valuable opportunity for the nurse life care planner to demonstrate competence in charting the course for a patient with neurologic deficits to attain the highest potential for a productive, healthy, and independent future quality of life.

Implementation and Benefits of a Life Care Plan

Once the LCP is approved and funded, a special needs trust fund, guardianship, or structured settlement may be established (see the previous discussion). An independent **case manager** can implement the completed LCP to guide the patient's management for overall care with the assurance that the funds and resources have been preplanned and are available. The LCP is a dynamic document that can be modified and changed to meet the changing needs of the individual (Table 25-1 and Box 25-1). Benefits of a well-designed LCP include the following:

- Improved quality of life
- Potential prevention or a reduction of complications
- Reduced future hospitalizations
- Enhanced opportunity to live as near normal a life as possible
- Available funds and resources to ensure quality care and improved outcomes
- Ensure the availability of appropriate services, supplies, and resources

TABLE 25-1 Life Care Plan: Table of Future Evaluations

Evaluations by Specialists	Age to Initiate	Age/Year to Discontinue	Frequency of Evaluations	Cost	Expected Outcomes	Economic Growth Trends
Physiatrist or Rehabilitation Physician	Age 24/2007	Life expectancy	4 times a year for 4 years, then once a year thereafter	$269 per evaluation	Evaluate progress and prescribe therapies	$14,767
Primary internist	Age 24/2007	Life expectancy	Evaluate 1–2 × beyond routine care	$50 to $150 per evaluation	Monitor to prevent complications and early detection of illness for prompt treatment	$3,360
Neurologist	Age 24/2007	Life expectancy	Once a year	$250 per evaluation	Monitor to detect breakthrough seizures; early detection of CNS changes	$18,298
Orthopedic surgeon	Age 24/2007	Life expectancy	Two times per year	$260 per evaluation	Facilitate mobility and ambulation	$485
Neuropsychologist	Age 24/2007	Life expectancy	Two evaluations over life expectancy	$212 per hour evaluation	Evaluate for cognitive impairments	$395
Family counselor	Age 24/2007	Life expectancy	Once every 10 years for evaluation	$212 per hour evaluation	Monitor family's coping responses	$783
Gastrointestinal multidisciplinary team	Age 24/2007	Life expectancy	Twice a year	$350 to $600 per evaluation	Monitor nutritional status, weight loss or gain	$34,766

CNS, Central nervous system.

BOX 25-1 Sample Life Care Plan

The patient is a 24-year-old woman who was traveling to work on a major highway when she was involved in a motor vehicle crash (MVC). She was immediately treated at the scene by the paramedics and transported by helicopter to the regional trauma center, where she was resuscitated and admitted for severe traumatic brain injury (TBI) and orthopedic injuries.

Before the MVC the patient was in her usual state of good health, lived an independent and active lifestyle, and worked full-time as a computer trainer for a large corporation. Today she suffers severe physical and cognitive impairments. She spends most of her day confined to a power wheelchair and continues to require daily rehabilitation and cognitive retraining. A team of caregivers, under the supervision of a case manager, provides for her daily needs. A modified van, outfitted with a wheelchair power lift to accommodate her power chair, is necessary for her transportation. A life care plan (LCP), designed by a neuroscience nurse life care planner, outlines the services and equipment for the patient's present and future needs. Her life expectancy (LE) is estimated to be approximately 79 years. Categories of care are divided into modules with tables based on today's dollars (see Table 25-1).

Follow-up by the life care planner/case manager is continued and scheduled annually or more frequently if needed, throughout the individual's lifetime. It is important to ascertain that all components of the LCP are being implemented and that the plan is satisfactory and beneficial to the individual. Necessary alterations of the LCP and shifting of funds can be made following an evaluation and communications with the family, health care providers, and treatment team.

CONCLUSION

Practice in the neuroscience area demands a tremendous amount of knowledge, information, and sophisticated skills. Neuroscience is the final frontier in health care and one of the most rewarding of nursing specialties. Many of the same legal issues need to be addressed in this specialty as in others, such as professional liability and occupational protection for health care providers. It is important to remain educated in current practice both technically (to ensure the best possible care of the patient) and legally (to minimize legal risks both to the nurse and to the facility).

RESOURCES

American Association of Legal Nurse Consultants: www.aalnc. org

American Association of Nurse Life Care Planners: www. aanlcp.org

Commission on Health Care Certification for Certified Life Care Planners: www.chcc.com

Healthcare Integrity and Protection Data Bank: www. npdb-hipdb.com

Joint Commission on Accreditation of Healthcare Organizations: www.jcaho.org

MedWatch: 800-FDA-1088; www.fda.gov/medwatch; www.fda. gov/cdrh/safety.html

National Council of State Boards of Nursing, Inc.: www.ncsbn. org

University of Florida/MediPro Seminars: www.mediproseminars. com

REFERENCES

1. Barker E: Evolution/revolution: the life care plan, *RN* 62(3):58–61, 1999.
2. Bedell S et al: Survival after cardiopulmonary resuscitation in the hospital, *N Engl J Med* 309:569–576, 1983.
3. *Belmon v. St. Frances Cabrini Hospital,* 427 So2d 541 (La 1983).
4. Benson C, Lusardi P: Neurologic antecedents to patient falls, *J Neurosci Nurs* 27(6):331–337, 1995.
5. Brent NJ: *Nurses and the law: a guide to principles and applications,* Philadelphia, 1997, WB Saunders.
6. Byers V, Arrington M, Finstuen K: Predictive risk factors associated with stroke patient falls in acute care settings, *J Neurosci Nurs* 22:147–154, 1990.
6a. Casarett DD et al: Overriding a patient's refusal of treatment after an iatrogenic complication, *N Engl J Med* 336:1908–1910, 2006.
7. Centers for Disease Control and Prevention: Assessing your knowledge of fall injuries among older adults, *Int J Trauma Nurs* 6(3):103, 2000.
7a. Choudry NK et al: CPR for patient's labelled DNR: the role of the limited aggressive therapy order, *Ann Intern Med* 138:65–68, 2003.
8. Cohen CB, Cohen PJ: Do-not-resuscitate orders in the operating room, *N Engl J Med* 325:1879, 1991.
9. *Collins v. Westlake Community Hospital,* 312 NE2d 614 (Ill 1974).
10. *In re the conservatorship of Wanglie,* No PX-91–283 (Minn Dist Ct Probate Ct Div, July 1991).
11. *Cruzan v. Director, Missouri Department of Health et al,* 497 US, 261, 111 L Ed2d 224, 110 SCt 2841 (1990).
12. Ct Gen Stat Ann Section 45a-644(c) (1991, amended 1993).
13. Desforges JF: Current concepts: cardiopulmonary resuscitation, *N Engl J Med* 327:1075–1080, 1992.
14. DC Stat Section 21-2210. See also Silfen N: Introduction. In *Refusal of treatment legislation,* New York, 1991, Society for the Right to Die.
15. Elesha-Adams M: Preventing falls in older adults, *Adv Nurses* 2(11):7, 28, 2000.
16. Fiesta J: The nursing shortage: whose liability problem? Part I, *Nurs Manage* 21(1):24–25, 1990; part II, *Nurs Manage* 21(2):22–23, 1990.
17. Fisher CM: Brain death—a review of the concept, *J Neurosci Nurs* 23:330–333, 1991.
18. Fried GN, Rangel JL, Storm GA: Treatment decisions. In Bogart JB, editor: *Legal nurse consulting: principles and practice,* Boca Raton, FL, 1998, CRC Press.
19. Friederici H: Reflections on the postmortem audit, *JAMA* 260:3461–3469, 1988.
20. Harvard Medical School, Ad Hoc Committee Report: The definition of irreversible coma, *JAMA* 205:337–340, 1968.
21. *Horton v. Niagra Falls Memorial Medical Center,* 380 NYS2d 116 (NY App Div 1976).
22. Joint Commission on Accreditation of Healthcare Organizations: *Accreditation manual for hospitals,* Chicago, 1991, The Commission.
23. Joint Commission on Accreditation of Healthcare Organizations: *1996 accreditation manual for hospitals: standards,* Oakbrook Terrace, IL, 1996, The Commission.
24. Landefeld CS, Goldman L: The autopsy in quality assurance: history, current status, and future directions, *Quality Research Bulletin* 15:42–48, 1989.
25. Margolis TE: Health care workers and AIDS: HIV transmission in the health care environment, *J Leg Med* 13:357–396, 1992.
26. *Matter of Dinnerstein,* 380 NE2d 134 (Mass, 1978).
27. McClung JA, Kamer RS: Legislating ethics: implications of New York's do-not-resuscitate law, *N Engl J Med* 323:270–272, 1990.
28. PL 101-629.
29. President's Commission for the Study of Ethical Problems in Medicine and Biomedical and Behavioral Research: *Defining death,* Rockville, MD, 1981, US Government Printing Office.
30. Rini AG: Nursing negligence issues. In Meiner SE, editor: *Nursing documentation: legal focus across practice settings,* Thousand Oaks, CA, 1999, Sage Publications.
31. *Rose v. Hakim,* 335 F Supp 1221 (DDC 1971), affirmed in part, reversed in part, 501 F 2d 806 (DC Cir 1974).
32. *Satz v. Perlmutter,* 362 So2d 160 (Fla Ct App 1978) aff'd 379 So2d 359 (Fla 1980). See also Gaul A, Wilson S: Should a ventilator be removed at a patient's request? An ethical analysis, *J Neurosci Nurs* 22:326–329, 1990.
33. Schmidt S: Consent for autopsies, *JAMA* 250:1161–1164, 1983.
34. Shafer A: Implementing the 1996 restraint standards in acute nonpsychiatric facilities, *Update Rev Curr Trends Nurs* 7(2):1–3, 1996.
35. *State of New York Public Health Law,* Article 29-B, Statute 413A.
36. Tarrant SM: Families must prepare early to allow death with dignity, *News Journal,* Wilmington, Del, Feb 1, 2001.
37. *Thompson v. General Hospital Authority of Upton County,* 151 SE2d 183 (Ga 1966).
38. Tinetti M, Speechley M: Prevention of falls among the elderly, *N Engl J Med* 320:1055–1059, 1989.
39. Trandel-Korenchuk DM, Trandel-Korenchuk KM: *Nursing and the law,* ed 5, Gaithersburg, MD, 1997, Aspen.
40. US Department of Health and Human Services, Food and Drug Administration: Medical devices: medical device, user facility, distributor, and manufacturer reporting, certification, and registration, *Fed Reg* 56:60024, 1991.
41. US Department of Health and Human Services, Health Care Financing Administration: Medicare and Medicaid programs, advance directives, *Fed Reg* 57:8194–8204, 1992; 42 CFR 482.13 (e). Health Care Financing Administration is now known as Centers for Medicare and Medicaid Services (CMS).

42. US Department of Labor, Occupational Safety and Health Administration: Occupational exposure to bloodborne pathogens; final rule, *Fed Reg* 56:64004–64182, 1991.

43. USC 360i(b) (5) (B).

44. Weed RO, editor: *Case management and life care planning handbook,* Boca Raton, FL, 2004, CRC Press.

45. Yorker B: Informed consent, *J Neurosci Nurs* 21:130–132, 1989.

46. Youngberg BL: *Nursing and malpractice risk: understanding the law,* ed 3, Brockton, MA, 1996, Western Schools Press.

47. Zellner K: Employers' dilemma: the AIDS crisis, *For the Defense,* pp 2–10, May 1988.

48. Md Health Code Ann Section 5–611.

49. *In re Schiavo,* 780So2d176 (2001).

50. 42 CFR 482.13.

51. MCA 50-16-1007.

52. *MMWR* 54(RR09), September 30, 2005.

53. *Sullivan v. Edward Hosp.,* no. 95409, 2004 Westlaw 228956 (Ill. February 5, 2004).

JFK Coma Recovery Scale—Revised

The JFK Coma Recovery Scale–Revised (2004) was developed by Joseph T. Giacino, PhD, and Kathleen Kalmar, PhD, at the Center for Head Injuries in Edison, New Jersey, for the JFK Johnson Rehabilitation Institute (affiliated with JFK Medical Centers and SOLARIS Health System). The scale was developed to help characterize and monitor patients functioning at Rancho Level I–IV and has been used widely in both the United States and Europe.

The CRS-R is a specialized assessment instrument designed for use in patients with disorders of consciousness. It was first introduced in rehabilitation settings in the early 1990s. The indicators include diagnostic assessment, outcome prediction, projection of disposition needs, interdisciplinary treatment planning, and monitoring of treatment effectiveness. Administration and Scoring Guidelines can be ordered from the authors by e-mail at jgiacino@solarshs.org or by writing to them at the JFK Johnson Rehabilitation Institute, Center for Head Injuries, 2048, Oak Tree Road, Edison, NJ 08820.

SUGGESTED READINGS

Giacino JT: Rehabilitation of patients with disorders of consciousness. In High W, Sandes A, Struchen M, Hart K, editors: *Rehabilitation for traumatic brain injury,* New York, 2005, Oxford Press.

Giacino JT, Kalmar K, Whyte J: The JFK coma recovery scale—revised: measurement characteristics and diagnostic utility, *Arch Phys Med Rehabil* 85(12):2020–2029, 2004.

Giacino JT, Trott C: Rehabilitative management of patients with disorders of consciousness: grand rounds, *J Head Trauma Rehabil* 19(3):262–273, 2004.

JFK COMA RECOVERY SCALE—REVISED
Record Form

Patient:	**Date:**								
AUDITORY FUNCTION SCALE									
4—Consistent Movement to Command*									
3—Reproducible Movement to Command*									
2—Localization to Sound									
1—Auditory Startle									
0—None									
VISUAL FUNCTION SCALE									
5—Object Recognition*									
4—Object Localization: Reaching*									
3—Pursuit Eye Movements*									
2—Fixation*									
1—Visual Startle									
0—None									
MOTOR FUNCTION SCALE									
6—Functional Object Use†									
5—Automatic Motor Response*									
4—Object Manipulation*									
3—Localization to Noxious Stimulation*									
2—Flexion Withdrawal									
1—Abnormal Posturing									
0—None/Flaccid									
OROMOTOR/VERBAL FUNCTION SCALE									
3—Intelligible Verbalization*									
2—Vocalization/Oral Movement									
1—Oral Reflexive Movement									
0—None									
COMMUNICATION SCALE									
2—Functional: Accurate†									
1—Non-Functional: Intentional*									
0—None									
AROUSAL SCALE									
3—Attention*									
2—Eye Opening w/o Stimulation									
1—Eye Opening with Stimulation									
0—Unarousable									
TOTAL SCORE									

Denotes emergence from MCS†

Denotes MCS*

BRAIN STEM REFLEX GRID ©2004

Record Form

Patient:	Date:						

Pupillary Light	Reactive							
	Equal							
	Constricted							
	Dilated							
	Pinpoint							
	Accommodation							
Corneal Reflex	Absent							
	Present Unilateral							
	Present Bilateral							
Spontaneous Eye Movements	None							
	Skew Deviation							
	Conjugate Gaze Deviation							
	Roving							
	Dysconjugate							
Oculocephalic Reflex	None							
	Abnormal							
	Full							
	Normal							
Postural Responses (Indicate Limb)	Abnormal Extension							
	Abnormal Flexion							

NOTES

CRS-R TOTAL SCORE PROGRESS TRACKING CHART ©2004

Record Form

Patient: **Diagnosis:** **Etiology:**

Date of Onset: **Date of Admission:**

Date																
Week	Adm	2	3	4	5	6	7	8	9	10	11	12	13	14	15	16
23																
22																
21																
20																
19																
18																
17																
16																
15																
14																
13																
12																
11																
10																
9																
8																
7																
6																
5																
4																
3																
2																
1																
0																
CRS-R Total Score																

BASELINE OBSERVATION AND
COMMAND FOLLOWING PROTOCOL ©2004

Commands	Baseline	Trial 1	Trial 2	Trial 3	Trial 4
	1 minute frequency count				
I Object Related Commands					
A. Eye Movement Commands					
Look at the *(object #1)*					
Look at the *(object #2)*					
B. Limb Movement Commands					
Take the *(name object #1)*					
Take the *(name object #2)*					
Kick the *(name object #1)*					
Kick the *(name object #2)*					
II Non-Object Related Commands					
A. Eye Movement Commands					
Look away from me					
Look up *(at ceiling)*					
Look down *(at floor)*					
B. Limb Movement Commands					
Touch my hand					
Touch your nose					
Move your *(object/body part)*					
C. Oral Movement/ Vocalization Commands					
Stick out your tongue					
Open your mouth					
Close your mouth					
Say "ah"					
Spontaneous Eye Opening		Yes:		No:	
Spontaneous Visual Tracking		Yes:		No:	

Resting Posture

RUE:	
RLE:	
LUE:	
LLE:	

APPENDIX B

Family Education

From Coma Emergence Program, University Specialty Hospital, University of Maryland Medical Center.

UNIVERSITY SPECIALTY HOSPITAL
COMA EMERGENCE PROGRAM
FAMILY EDUCATION

SENSORY STIMULATION GUIDELINES FOR CAREGIVERS

The purpose of the sensory stimulation activities is to elicit responses and assist with recovery. The consistency and organization of the stimuli in the environment may help the individual increase his/her level of alertness. After you have received initial training from a member of the Coma Emergence Team, you may participate in providing stimulation.

The following are general guidelines recommended by the Coma Emergence Team for providing sensory stimulation.

1. Introduce yourself to the patient, orient him/her to the date, place as well as what you are going to do.

2. Provide an optimal environment. For example:
   — Turn off the radio or TV.
   — Remove any visually distracting items out of view.
   — Turn on the lights.
   — Limit the amount of people (one to one sessions are optimal).
   — Pull the curtain for privacy if another patient is in the room.

3. Sessions should be limited to 15–20 minutes or as tolerated.

4. Start by presenting one stimulation item such as a picture or a familiar object. Ask the patient to look at it and always give the patient time to respond before presenting the stimulus again or presenting a new one.

5. Each stimulus should be presented in a consistent manner approximately 3–5 times.

UNIVERSITY SPECIALTY HOSPITAL
COMA EMERGENCE PROGRAM
FAMILY EDUCATION

EARLY STAGES OF RECOVERY

How to talk to the patient:

1. Assume that the patient comprehends what you are saying, even if they don't seem to respond.

2. Gently touch the patient and use his/her first name to gain attention.

3. Speak softly, calmly, and slowly to allow the patient time to process what you are saying.

4. Use short, simple age appropriate sentences. Pause between each sentence.

5. Use demonstration and physical prompts as needed (i.e., pictures, familiar items).

6. Talk to the patient. Do not converse with other staff members as though the patient is not present.

7. Do not ask questions unless the patient is capable of responding (in some way) and you are willing to honor the response.

8. Talk primarily about the here and now.

9. Simply state what you are going to do with the patient and what you have just done.

10. Give frequent repetition of orientation information:
    - People: "Hi, I'm Paddy from Occupational Therapy."
    - Place: "You're at University Specialty Hospital in Baltimore, MD now."
    - Date: "Today is (day of the week, month, date and year)."
    - Routine: "I am here to work on _____ with you."

UNIVERSITY SPECIALTY HOSPITAL
COMA EMERGENCE PROGRAM
FAMILY EDUCATION

Be aware that by providing too much stimulation (i.e., too long in duration, too high in frequency, too many at one time), a person can become **OVERLOADED**.

How do you know when overload is occurring?
1. The person stops responding
2. Agitation
3. Hyperactivity

What should you do when overload occurs?
1. Discontinue the activity immediately
2. Give the patient a quiet rest break until the above behaviors decrease
3. Discontinue further stimulation for the day

When overload occurs, one of the two conditions may be present:
1. The person is getting used to it and is no longer able to distinguish
2. The person is over-stimulated and can no longer respond to the incoming stimuli

How can stimulus overload be avoided?
➢ Limit the distractions in the environment.
➢ Allow for frequent rest periods between stimulus presentation and between sessions.
➢ Plan for short sessions.
➢ Check with nursing for updates on patient's overall medical condition to make sure stimulation is appropriate.

If you have any questions, contact any of the Coma Emergence Team members.

UNIVERSITY SPECIALTY HOSPITAL
COMA EMERGENCE PROGRAM
FAMILY EDUCATION

Examples of Stimuli Presentation

1. **Visual (sight):** Try to get the patient to follow an object with his/her eyes.

2. **Auditory (hearing):** Present a noise to the left and right ear individually; wait for the patient to turn their head or look in the direction of the noise.

3. **Tactile (touch):** Wipe/touch face or arms with an object; wait and observe for the patient to respond.

4. **Range of motion:** After demonstration by the occupational or physical therapist, caregivers may provide range of motion to a patient's upper and lower extremities 1–3 times a day.

■ Document responses in the communication notebook located in the patient's room. Remember to include the date and time and sign after each entry.

You may get responses that indicate that stimulation was not well tolerated.

■ Stiffening of limbs and/or increased muscle activity
■ Increased heart rate
■ Increased respiration
■ Redness in the face, sweating
■ Decrease in oxygen saturation

If these responses occur, immediately discontinue presentation of the stimuli and notify nursing if the responses continue.

Pittsburgh Sleep Quality Index

Scoring Instructions for the Pittsburgh Sleep Quality Index

The Pittsburgh Sleep Quality Index (PSQI) contains 19 self-rated questions and 5 questions rated by the bed partner or roommate (if one is available). Only self-rated questions are included in the scoring. The 19 self-rated items are combined to form seven "component" scores, each of which has a range of 0–3 points. In all cases, a score of "0" indicates no difficulty, while a score of "3" indicates severe difficulty. The seven component scores are then added to yield one "global" score, with a range of 0–21 points, "0" indicating no difficulty and "21" indicating severe difficulties in all areas.
Scoring proceeds as follows:

Component 1: Subjective sleep quality
1. Examine question #6, and assign scores as follows:

Response	Component 1 score
"Very good"	0
"Fairly good"	1
"Fairly bad"	2
"Very bad"	3

Component 1 score: _____

Component 2: Sleep latency
1. Examine question #2, and assign scores as follows:

Response	Score
≤15 mintues	0
16–30 minutes	1
31–60 minutes	2
>60 minutes	3

Question #2 score: _____

2. Examine question #5a, and assign scores as follows:

Response	Score
Not during the past month	0
Less than once a week	1
Once or twice a week	2
Three or more times a week	3

Question #5a score: _____

3. Add #2 score and #5a score:

Sum of #2 and #5a: _____

4. Assign component 2 score as follows:

Sum of #2 and #5a	Component 2 score
0	0
1–2	1
3–4	2
5–6	3

Component 2 score: _____

Continued

Component 3: Sleep duration

Examine question #4, and assign scores as follows:

Response	Component 3 score
>7 hours	0
6–7 hours	1
5–6 hours	2
<5 hours	3

Component 3 score: _____

Component 4: Habitual sleep efficiency

1. Write the number of hours slept (question #4) here: _____
2. Calculate the number of hours spent in bed:

   Getting up time (question #3): _____

   – Bedtime (question #1): _____ _____

   Number of hours spent in bed: _____
3. Calculate habitual sleep efficiency as follows:

   (Number of hours slept/Number of hours spent in bed) × 100 = Habitual sleep efficiency (%)

   (_____/_____) × 100 = _____ %
4. Assign component 4 score as follows:

Habitual sleep efficiency %	Component 4 score
>85%	0
75–84%	1
65–74%	2
<65%	3

Component 4 score: _____

Component 5: Sleep disturbances

1. Examine questions #5b–5j, and assign scores for *each* question as follows:

Response	Score
Not during the past month	0
Less than once a week	1
Once or twice a week	2
Three or more times a week	3

#5b score _____

c score _____

d score _____

e score _____

f score _____

g score _____

h score _____

i score _____

j score _____

2. Add the scores for questions #5b–5j:

Sum of #5b–5j: _____

3. Assign component 5 score as follows:

Sum of #5b–5j	Component 5 score
0	0
1–9	1
10–18	2
19–27	3

Component 5 score: _____

Component 6: Use of sleeping medication

1. Examine question #7 and assign scores as follows:

Response	Component 6 score
Not during the past month	0
Less than once a week	1
Once or twice a week	2
Three or more times a week	3

Component 6 score: _____

Continued

Component 7: Daytime dysfunction

1. Examine question #8, and assign scores as follows:

Response	Score
Never	0
Once or twice	1
Once or twice each week	2
Three or more times each week	3

Question #8 score: _____

2. Examine question #9, and assign scores as follows:

Response	Score
No problem at all	0
Only a very slight problem	1
Somewhat of a problem	2
A very big problem	3

Question #9 score: _____

3. Add the scores for question #8 and #9:

Sum of #8 and #9: _____

4. Assign component 7 score as follows:

Sum of #8 and #9	Component 7 score
0	0
1–2	1
3–4	2
5–6	3

Component 7 score: _____

Global PSQI Score

1. Add the seven component scores together:

Global PSQI Score: _____

Questionnaire for Spasticity

Demographics

Patient name: _____ (last) _____ (first) _____ (middle initial)

Address: _____ (city) _____ (state) _____ (zip code)

Phone: _____ (home) _____ (work) _____ (cell phone)

Occupation: _____ (retired) _____

Date of birth: _____/_____/_____ Gender: ____ male ____ female

Marital status: ___ married ___ single ___ divorced _____ widowed ____ significant other

Children: ____ no ____ yes   How many? _____

Name of contact person: _____ Relationship: __ spouse __ family member __ other

Phone number of primary contact person: (area code) _____

Social History: _____ use tobacco: how many packs per day: _____

_____ use alcohol: how may drinks per day _____ per week _____

_____ use street drugs: _____

Significant Family Medical History: _____

Past Medical History

Name of treating primary care physician or health care provider: _____

Phone: _____

Address: _____

Allergies: drugs, over-the-counter, latex, tape, or other: _____

Activities of Daily Living (ADL): With whom do you live? _____

Do you live in a: __ nursing home __ assisted living __ private residence __ apartment

Do you drive: __ no __ yes   Do you use assistive devices: __ cane __ walker ___ wheelchair

Do you need assistance with any of the following (check all that apply)? ___ dressing __ bathing

__ using the bathroom __ walking __ cooking __ eating __ getting in and out of bed/chair

Past Surgical History (list type of surgery, names of surgeons, and dates of surgery):

_____

_____

_____

Current Medications (list prescription drugs, dosage, frequency, and prescribing health care professional):

Name of drug: _____ dosage _____ frequency _____ prescriber _____

Name of drug: _____ dosage _____ frequency _____ prescriber _____

Name of drug: _____ dosage _____ frequency _____ prescriber _____

Name of drug: _____ dosage _____ frequency _____ prescriber _____

Name of drug: _____ dosage _____ frequency _____ prescriber _____

Name of drug: _____ dosage _____ frequency _____ prescriber _____

Evaluation by Health Care Provider

1. Has the individual ever been diagnosed or recovering from one or more of the following brain or spine conditions (check all that apply)?

    ___ cerebral palsy (CP)

    ___ traumatic brain injury (TBI)

    ___ spinal cord injury (SCI)

    ___ multiple sclerosis (MS)

    ___ other (describe) _____

2. Has **spasticity** caused or contributed to any of the following signs or symptoms (check all that apply)?

    ___ tight, stiff muscles involving the flexors of the arms and/or the extensors of the legs

    ___ increased weakness

    ___ increased fatigue

    ___ increased pain and discomfort

    ___ interference with positioning

    ___ interference with movement and function

    ___ interruption of normal sleep patterns

    ___ tripping, falling, or extremity fractures

    ___ difficulty with transfers to and from bed or chair

    ___ changes in bladder control with incontinence

    ___ problems with catheterization (self or caregiver) due to close approximation of thighs

    ___ increased burden, time or difficulty for patient or caregiver in ADL

    ___ confinement to bed related to spasticity

    ___ development of contractures: __ upper extremities __ lower extremities

    ___ Babinski reflex with "upgoing toes"

3. Have assessments of the patient/client with spasticity also identified significant problems with any of the following conditions (check all that apply)?

    ___ pain

    ___ depression

    ___ infections (e.g., urinary tract infection, upper respiratory infections or pneumonia, skin breakdown, pressure ulcer infections) (circle all that apply)

    ___ other (describe) _____

4. Is the patient/client currently receiving any of the following interventions related to spasticity (check all that apply)?

___ medication(s) for pain (list) _____

___ therapeutic stretching exercises

___ orthotics

___ casting (e.g., "serial casting")

___ life skills training

___ continence management for bladder or bowel

___ positioning on a documented 24-hour routine

5. Is the patient/client currently receiving any of the following oral medications for spasticity and list physician or prescribing health care provider (check all that apply)?

___ Lioresal (Baclofen); list current dosage _____

___ Diazepam (Valium); list current dosage _____

___ Clonidine (Catapres); list current dosage _____

___ Dantrolene (Dantrium); list current dosage _____

___ Gabapentin (Neurontin); list current dosage _____

___ Tizadine (Zanaflex); list current dosage _____

6. Has the patient/client received injection therapy (e.g., botulinum toxin [Botox]) targeting specific muscles?

___ yes ___ no

Beginning date and frequency of injections with date and site(s) of last injection: _____

7. Last recorded (if known) score on the Modified Ashworth scale:

___ 0   No increase in muscle tone

___ 1   Slight increase in tone, minimal resistance end of range

___ 1+ Slight increase in tone with minimal resistance throughout less than half the remainder range

___ 2   More marked increase in muscle through most of the range; affected part easily moved

___ 3   Considerable increase in tone, passive movement difficult

___ 4   Part fixed

8. Grading of reflexes:

___ 0   absent

___ 1+ present but diminished

___ 2+ within normal limits

___ 3+ increased but pathological

___ 4+ hyperactive

9. What level of spasticity has the treating team identified for the patient/client?

___ mild

___ moderate

___ severe

10. Is the patient/client receiving any of the following rehabilitation modalities for spasticity (check all that apply)?

___ Physical therapy (PT) ___ inpatient ___ outpatient

___ Occupational therapy (OT) ___ inpatient ___ outpatient

___ Aquatic or hydrotherapy ___ inpatient ___ outpatient

___ Other: described _____ inpatient ___ outpatient

11. Has the patient/client undergone any surgical procedure for the treatment of spasticity? ___ no ___ yes

Describe, with date: _____

Treating surgeon: _____

12. Described patient/client's activity level: ____ ambulatory ___ uses assistive device ___cane ___ walker

____ wheelchair ____ other (describe) _____

13. Has the patient/client been identified as a potential candidate for intrathecal baclofen (ITB) therapy?

_____ no _____ yes

Does the patient/client currently receive ITB therapy? ___ no ___ yes

14. What is the patient's schedule for intrathecal baclofen refills? _____

15. What is the patient's schedule for pump replacement? _____

Summary of Assessment: _____

_____

_____

_____

Review of Diagnostic and Laboratory Tests:

_____

Impressions: _____

Recommended Plan of Care: _____

Prescriptions: _____

Diagnostic/Lab Studies: _____

Referrals: _____

Patient/Family Teaching: _____

Additional Comments: _____

Return Visit: _____

Name of Health Care Provider: _____

Page numbers followed by *f, t,* and *b* indicate figures, tables, and boxes, respectively.